Burket's
ORAL MEDICINE

Edited by MALCOLM A. LYNCH, D.D.S., M.D.

Professor of Oral Medicine and Associate Dean
for Hospital and Extramural Affairs
University of Pennsylvania School of Dental Medicine
Philadelphia, Pennsylvania

Associate
Editors Vernon J. Brightman, D.M.D., M.D.Sc., Ph.D.
Professor of Oral Medicine
University of Pennsylvania School of Dental Medicine and School of Medicine
Attending in Oral Medicine, Department of Dental Medicine
Hospital of the University of Pennsylvania
Dental Consultant, The Children's Hospital of Philadelphia
Philadelphia, Pennsylvania

Martin S. Greenberg, D.D.S.
Professor of Oral Medicine
University of Pennsylvania School of Dental Medicine
Chairman, Department of Dental Medicine
Hospital of the University of Pennsylvania
Philadelphia, Pennsylvania

Nine contributors

Burket's
ORAL MEDICINE

DIAGNOSIS AND TREATMENT

EIGHTH EDITION

J. B. LIPPINCOTT COMPANY
Philadelphia · London · Mexico City · New York
St. Louis · São Paulo · Sydney

The author and publisher have exerted every effort to ensure that drug selection and dosage set forth in this text are in accord with current recommendations and practice at the time of publication. However, in view of ongoing research, changes in government regulations, and the constant flow of information relating to drug therapy and drug reactions, the reader is urged to check the package insert for each drug for any change in indications and dosage and for added warnings and precautions. This is particularly important when the recommended agent is a new or infrequently employed drug.

Acquistions Editor: Lisa A. Biello
Sponsoring Editor: Richard Winters
Manuscript Editor: Kristen B. Frasch
Indexer: Deborah Ziwot, D.M.D.
Art Director: Maria S. Karkucinski
Designer: Patricia Pennington
Production Supervisor: J. Corey Gray
Production Assistant: Barney A. Fernandes
Compositor: Ruttle, Shaw & Wetherill, Inc.
Printer/Binder: The Murray Printing Company

Eighth Edition

6 5 4 3 2 1

Library of Congress Cataloging in Publication Data
Burket, Lester W. (Lester William), 1907-
  Burket's Oral medicine.
  Bibliography: p.
  Includes index.
  1. Mouth—Diseases. 2. Oral manifestations of general diseases. 3. Teeth—Diseases. I. Lynch, Malcolm A.
II. Brightman, Vernon J. (Vernon John), 1930-
II. Greenberg, Martin S. IV. Title. V. Title: Oral medicine. [DNLM: 1. Oral medicine, Diagnosis and treatment. 2. Mouth diseases. WU 140 B9590]
RC815.B83   1984   617'.522   83-9814
ISBN 0-397-52106-5

*To Charles Malcolm Lynch and
Alleyne Alexander Lynch*

Preface

Since the seventh edition of *Burket's Oral Medicine*, greater progress in our understanding of the pathogenesis, diagnosis, and treatment of disease has occurred than perhaps in any other similar interval of time since *Burket's Oral Medicine* was first published in 1946. Reflecting this, all chapters have been brought up to the current state of medical knowledge and virtually all chapters have been completely rewritten or have undergone extensive revision.

There are eight new contributors to this eighth edition. These contributors were especially chosen for their broad-based knowledge and clinical experience in their respective subjects. These authors and their chapters include Dr. Gary Cohen, Renal Disease; Dr. Philip Springer, Disorders of the Temporomandibular Joint and Myofascial Pain Dysfunction Syndrome, Dr. Samuel Wycoff and Dr. Sidney Epstein, Geriatric Dentistry; Dr. Kenneth Kent and Dr. Alan Samit, Oral Cancer; Dr. Ronald Johnson, Odontologic Diseases; and Dr. Mark Snyder, Endocrine Disease and Dysfunction.

Dr. Vernon Brightman continues his scholarly presentations with an extensively rewritten chapter on Laboratory Procedures, which has been changed to reflect the rapid advancements in this field, such as automa-

tion techniques in blood chemistry and hematology and immunofluorescent diagnostic procedures. This updating will acquaint the dental practitioner with the latest in laboratory diagnostic methods. In keeping with the format of the book and organizational consistency, this chapter has been relocated to the first section of the text along with other methods of diagnosis. The chapter on Red and White Lesions, representing a logical pathogenetic combination of subjects that were covered in separate chapters in previous editions has, by necessity, been completely rewritten owing to the many developments in diagnosis and treatment of these lesions. The newly recognized and precancerous importance of red lesions is emphasized for the first time in this chapter. Owing to recognition of the increasing importance of sexually transmitted diseases and the hazards these diseases represent to the dental practitioner because of exposure to blood and saliva, an entirely new chapter has been written to cover this important subject.

Dr. Greenberg has brought his extensive clinical experience in the diagnosis and treatment of oral mucosal disease to fruition in a complete rewriting of the chapter on Ulcerative, Vesicular, and Bullous Lesions, which incorporates the latest in diagnostic and therapeutic modalities. His hallmark research identifying the oral cavity as a primary source of often-fatal septicemia in immunocompromised leukemia patients has contributed to the knowledgeable discussion of these diseases in the chapter on Hematologic Diseases and Related Problems. Rapid changes in immunology since the last edition have necessitated substantial changes in that chapter from the previous edition.

The extensively illustrated chapter on Oral Cancer, although written by two specialists most likely to be involved in diagnosis and treatment of these patients, is oriented towards the needs of the generalist. Dr. Kent brings his expertise as a maxillofacial prosthodontist and Dr. Samit brings his as an oral and maxillofacial surgeon. In the chapter on Ionizing Radiation, Dr. Beideman has addressed the oral mucosal and osseous changes associated with radiation and the dental treatment of the post-therapeutic radiation patient.

A new chapter on a subject not heretofore covered, renal disease, has been contributed by Dr. Gary Cohen. Among other things, this reflects the growing interest in the subject because of the need for dental care of an increasing number of patients whose lives have been prolonged by renal dialysis.

Dr. Ron Johnson's vast experience both as a clinician and as an academic pediatric dentist has made his chapter on Odontologic Diseases a more readable, thorough, and well illustrated coverage of the subject than has ever appeared in any previous edition. Drs. Wycoff and Epstein have presented their new chapter, Geriatric Dentistry, from a thought-provoking and informative point of view.

The many changes in the diagnosis and treatment of cardiovascular disease has necessitated extensive revision of that chapter, including discussion of newer drugs to prevent angina in the dental patient. The chapters on respiratory and gastrointestinal disease have been updated and enhanced by the addition of illustrations of the radiologic changes that are so important in the diagnosis of many of these diseases. A new classification of diabetes by the World Health Organization and rapid advancements in our understanding of pathogenesis and treatment of this disease have made this chapter virtually unrecognizable from previous editions. Dr. Mark Snyder's new chapter on Endocrine Disease incorporates the latest in diagnostic laboratory studies in a rapidly changing field.

Special acknowledgment goes to Dr. Irving Shapiro of the Department of Biochemistry, University of Pennsylvania School of Dental Medicine, for his advice and contribution to the chapter dealing with lead metabolism and plumbism. Special acknowledgment also goes to the enormous amount of effort provided by Mrs. Hazel Dean, without whose constant attention toward keeping all contributors and editors on schedule this edition surely would not have come out on the projected date.

Contributors

Robert W. Beideman, D.M.D.
Associate Professor and Director of Radiology
Department of Radiology
University of Pennsylvania
School of Dental Medicine
Philadelphia, Pennsylvania

Vernon J. Brightman, D.M.D., M.D.Sc., Ph.D.
Professor of Oral Medicine
University of Pennsylvania
School of Dental Medicine and School of
    Medicine
Attending in Oral Medicine
Department of Dental Medicine
Hospital of the University of Pennsylvania
Philadelphia, Pennsylvania

S. Gary Cohen, D.M.D.
Director, General Practice Residency
Hospital of the University of Pennsylvania
Clinical Assistant Professor of Oral Medicine
School of Dental Medicine
University of Pennsylvania
Dental Consultant
The Children's Hospital of Philadelphia
Philadelphia, Pennsylvania

Sidney Epstein, D.D.S.
Clinical Professor, Geriatric Dentistry
Department of Dental Public Health and Hy-
    giene
School of Dentistry
University of California
San Francisco, California
Clinical Professor
School of Medicine
Stanford University
Stanford, California

Martin S. Greenberg, D.D.S.
Professor of Oral Medicine
School of Dental Medicine
University of Pennsylvania
Chairman, Department of Dental Medicine
Hospital of the University of Pennsylvania
Philadelphia, Pennsylvania

Ronald Johnson, D.D.S.
Professor and Chairman
Department of Pediatric Dentistry
University of Southern California
Los Angeles, California

Kenneth Kent, D.M.D.
Chief, Maxillofacial Prosthetics
Veterans Administration Medical Center
Assistant Clinical Professor of Restorative Dentistry
University of Pennsylvania
School of Dental Medicine
Philadelphia, Pennsylvania

Malcolm A. Lynch, D.D.S., M.D.
Professor and Chairman
Department of Oral Medicine
School of Dental Medicine
University of Pennsylvania
Associate Dean for the Hospital and Extramural Affairs
Hospital of the University of Pennsylvania
Philadelphia, Pennsylvania

James C. Pettigrew, Jr., D.M.D.
Assistant Professor of Radiology
Department of Radiology
School of Dental Medicine
University of Pennsylvania
Philadelphia, Pennsylvania

Alan Samit, D.D.S.
Chief, Oral and Maxillofacial Surgery
Director, General Practice Residency Program
Veterans Administration Medical Center
Clinical Associate Professor of Oral and Maxillofacial Surgery
School of Dental Medicine
University of Pennsylvania
Diplomate, American Board Oral and Maxillofacial Surgery
Philadelphia, Pennsylvania

Mark B. Snyder, D.M.D.
Director, Oral Diagnostic Clinic
Assistant Professor of Oral Medicine and Periodontics
School of Dental Medicine
University of Pennsylvania
Philadelphia, Pennsylvania

Philip S. Springer, D.M.D.
Clinical Assistant Professor of Oral Medicine
School of Dental Medicine
University of Pennsylvania
Attending in Oral Medicine
Hospital of the University of Pennsylvania
Philadelphia, Pennsylvania

Samuel J. Wycoff, D.M.D., M.P.H.
Professor
Department of Dental Public Health and Hygiene
University of California
San Francisco, California

Contents

4
ORAL MEDICINE IN THE HOSPITAL   156
Martin S. Greenberg

PART II / ORAL DISEASE

5
ULCERATIVE, VESICULAR, AND BULLOUS LESIONS   163
Martin S. Greenberg

6
RED AND WHITE LESIONS OF THE ORAL MUCOSA   209
Vernon J. Brightman

7
PIGMENTATION OF THE ORAL TISSUES   293
Lester W. Burket

15
GERIATRIC DENTISTRY   560
Samuel J. Wycoff and Sidney Epstein

16
CHRONIC ORAL SENSORY DISORDERS—PAIN AND DYSGEUSIA   576
Vernon J. Brightman

17
ORAL SYMPTOMS WITHOUT APPARENT PHYSICAL ABNORMALITY   616
Vernon J. Brightman

PART III / SYSTEMIC DISEASE

Part I

PRINCIPLES OF DIAGNOSIS

1

Dentistry and Oral Medicine

MALCOLM A. LYNCH

Quoted from their constitution, the objectives of the American Academy of Oral Medicine are

> to promote the study and dissemination of knowledge of the cause, prevention, and control of diseases of the teeth, their supporting structures, and adnexa and related subjects; and to foster a better scientific understanding between the fields of dentistry and medicine.

Oral medicine in its broadest sense might be defined as that area of dentistry that concentrates on diagnosis and treatment of oral mucosal disease (stomatology), diagnosis and treatment of other oral complaints that may reflect either local oral disease or oral manifestations of systemic problems, and those phases of dental practice that are especially concerned with dental treatment of physiologically compromised patients. Physiologically compromised patients require thorough evaluation and consideration of their health status in order that dental treatment may be planned and provided in the patient's best interest as part of comprehensive health care.

Philosophically and in practice, dentistry is similar to one of the varied specialties of medicine, and consequently it is imperative that the dentist understand the medical background of his patients before beginning dental therapy, which might (at the least) fail because of the patient's compromised medical status or (at the worst) result in morbidity or death of the patient. It is no longer sufficient merely to obtain "clearance" from a physician before initiating dental treatment. In these days of increasing malpractice litigation, it has become quite clear that each practitioner is responsible for those things he should know by virtue of his education and experience before initiating treatment. For example, the dentist may not be held responsible for listening to a patient's chest and detecting a heart murmur, but he is responsible for ascertaining from the patient's physician whether a heart murmur is present and for using his judgment whether to premedicate the patient with antibiotics before dental treatment. By stating that a patient with rheumatic heart disease needs to be premedicated to prevent endocarditis "only if teeth are to be extracted," a physician does not exonerate the dentist who produces endocarditis in the patient by performing periodontal surgery. A dentist is likewise responsible for knowing whether his patient has hypertension, and the only sure way to know this is to measure the pressure in the office. Numerous other examples of such professional responsibility and liability are delineated in the text.

The dentist trained in oral medicine should be philosophically atuned to the patient and have knowledge of medically important disease as well as of dental problems. The dentist should be well versed in the use of rational approaches to diagnosis, medical risk assessment, and treatment.

It is apparent today that greater interaction is necessary between *all* health professionals in planning dental care as part of comprehensive health care for the patient, and the dentist must function as a member of a team. No one is better qualified than the dentist who is well trained in oral medicine to diagnose oral lesions or to consult and interact on a professional basis with appropriate medical practitioners in their respective areas of expertise in planning and carrying out dental treatment for the medically compromised patient.

2

Rational Procedures for Diagnosis and Medical Risk Assessment

VERNON J. BRIGHTMAN

Diagnostic procedure can be divided into the following four parts for purposes of description and implementation:

1. Taking and recording the patient's history
2. Examination of the patient (physical examination and laboratory studies)
3. Evaluation of the history and results of the physical examination and laboratory studies, leading to formulation of a diagnosis
4. Medical risk assessment for dental patients

The first part of the diagnostic procedure represents mainly the contribution of the patient and provides a record of the patient's *symptoms*. This information is always subjective (*i.e.*, a report of the patient's own sensory experiences) and may even be second hand, as in the cases of young children, comatose patients, or others unable to communicate for themselves. By contrast, the physical and laboratory examinations allow the clinician to record direct objective information (*signs*) about the patient, and to determine whether important elements in the patient's story are confirmed by appropriate physically demonstrable abnormalities.

A definite routine for performing and recording the history and examination should be established and conscientiously followed. This procedure not only minimizes the chance of overlooking important data but frequently results in obtaining information pertinent to making the diagnosis that the patient did not consider to be related to the present illness (*e.g.*, symptoms or signs in more distant parts of the body) or that may be evidence of other problems of even more significance to the patient's well-being than is the particular problem he or she brings to the dentist or physician.

The time devoted to a comprehensive history and examination is not only useful in making the diagnosis and in planning treatment but is an important means of establishing good dentist–patient relations. It is also of the utmost importance for the dentist to be aware of any systemic disease that may be present, as well as the exact nature of the medications a patient may be taking so that appropriate dental treatment can be planned. A comprehensive history and examination are essential for the diagnosis of the less common diseases of the hard and the soft oral tissues. A carefully taken and evaluated history is not only helpful in determining the cause of the lesion but also gives valuable information on how the patient is reacting to the disease and permits a more intelligent and efficient examination. Together, the history and examination furnish valuable records for the treatment of the patient, for research, and in the event that they are needed, for medicolegal purposes.

Patients seeking routine dental services react most favorably to the taking of a comprehensive evaluation once its importance and necessity have been adequately explained; they appreciate the thoroughness of this approach to their problems.

TAKING AND RECORDING THE HISTORY

A history can be considered to be a planned professional conversation that enables the patient to communicate his symptoms, feelings, and fears to the clinician so that the nature of the patient's real or suspected illness and mental attitudes may be determined.

General Suggestions

Attitudes

The completeness and hence the ultimate value of the patient's history in determining the diagnosis depend to a considerable degree on a constructive dentist–patient relationship. The interest, warmth, and compassion exhibited by the dentist are important factors in establishing patient rapport and in obtaining a meaningful history. One of the best rules to follow is to put oneself in the patient's place and to act accordingly. A kindly and considerate approach is most important in securing and gaining the confidence of the patient. A hurried, impatient, and unsympathetic approach or an attitude of weariness is not likely to produce a complete and significant history.

Indicate to the patient that you are a friend who is keenly interested in him or her as a person. Share the total problems of the patient, and above all be a good active listener. Patients seek treatment not necessarily for what they have but for what they think they have, and this self-diagnosis can often be detected during history-taking. Fortunately, in many instances the worst fears of the patient never are realized, and listening attentively and sympathetically to a patient and making a thorough examination may have greater value than does specific therapy.

An exhaustive list of signs and symptoms does not in itself constitute a complete history (see discussion under Medical Questionnaires that follows). The assignment of the responsibility of history-taking to auxiliary personnel no matter how well trained, is generally undesirable. It suggests to the patient that the importance of this diagnostic procedure is not sufficiently great to warrant your time and attention. If auxiliary personnel are assigned to secure and record both demographic information and that more specifically related to the patient's health problem, this information must be reviewed and commented on in the written history by the responsible clinician. In other words, some aspects of the history can be handled by auxiliary personnel, but the responsibility for accuracy of the data and their interpretation cannot be delegated.

Atmosphere

Ideally, the patient's history should be taken in a consultation room or a private office in which the decor and the furnishings are quite different from those of the dental operatory. This more friendly atmosphere is an important factor in helping the patient to talk freely about his problems. The use of an area different from the operatory permits auxiliary personnel to prepare treatment facilities for the physical examination to follow or for other patients. Another advantage in using a consultation area is that the history can be taken with both the patient and the doctor seated. It is poor technique and poor psychology to seat the patient in the dental chair and then attempt to obtain a useful history.

Building Confidence

Much can be accomplished in winning the patient's confidence during this phase of the diagnostic procedure. As the patient's confidence in you deepens, he will have an increased respect for you as a person as well as a professional in the health field. Make the patient feel that he is a person with an important dental or medical problem. By your manner convey the impression that you have an interest in the patient and have time to listen to his health problems whether they appear to be real or imaginary. Give evidence of sympathy and understanding while retaining a firm control of the interview.

Form and Scope

A better history usually can be achieved if it is volunteered by the patient. Within reasonable limits, give the patient the opportunity to tell his "story" completely. Thus, most patients will enumerate the series of events associated with the chief complaint (see below) in proper chronological order. Do not interrupt the patient repeatedly to ask other questions unless it is absolutely necessary.

Do not confine attention solely to the biological problems, but consider the emotional and psychological problems of the patient and the extent to which you are able to deal with them. Try to determine what the suspected or real chief complaint means to the patient both physiologically and psychologically. These considerations are at times important for the diagnosis and may have major significance when developing the therapeutic regimen for the patient.

Encourage the patient to give the reason for the consultation. It is likewise important to try to determine why he thinks he is ill, and if possible, to establish the chronological relationship of events other than those pertaining to the chief complaint. If possible, use the language used by the patient in asking additional questions or commenting on statements already made by him. This device is helpful in gaining his confidence. On the other hand, do not accept generalized, vague, or indefinite statements or replies. Skillful, repeated questioning usually will elicit a more definite reply. When questions are defined more critically, the resultant information is more significant. If it is necessary to question the patient about personal matters, assure him that all such material is considered confidential.

Components of a Patient's History

The order or sequence of the various parts of the history is largely a matter of personal choice. The sequence of the various components of the history given in this section is commonly employed, however.

Routine Data

The history includes a certain amount of routine information, which can be obtained readily by the secretary, assistant, or hygienist. Include the patient's name, address, telephone number, age, sex, race, and marital status. Always obtain the name of the patient and the name of the physician or the dentist who referred the patient for services, so that an expression of appreciation and, when appropriate, a report of the consultation findings may be made.

It is very important that the name, address, and telephone number of the patient's physician be obtained and recorded prominently on the chart as part of this general routine information in the event that it is necessary to consult the physician at short notice. If the name and the address of the patient's physician are requested only after the history is taken, and the examination is made, the patient may worry unnecessarily.

A printed record form is of assistance in assuring that the necessary routine information is secured.

The complete medical (or dental) history consists of the chief complaint, history of the present illness, past dental history, past medical history, family history, and social and occupational history.

Chief Complaint and History of the Present Illness

A good practical approach is to ask the patient to express his chief complaint or trouble in his own words. Usually, this is recorded in nontechnical language, such as "a painful sore on the tongue." Then ask the patient to tell in narrative or "story" form when (date) the lesion first was observed, the mode of development, the symptoms, and any previous treatment. These complete details explaining the chief complaint constitute the history of the present illness.

Do not interrupt the patient if possible. Avoid all leading questions. Allow the patient to express his emotional feelings and his reactions to his surroundings, but do not allow him to wander too far from the theme of the present illness. It is also unwise to point out any errors in the patient's use of technical terms or misinterpretation of symptoms during any part of the history. If the patient halts in relating the story of his present illness, repeat the last few sentences to give him the stimulus needed to continue.

The reason for seeking dental treatment and the details thereof might appear to be easy to obtain and might seem to be the type of information that should be relegated to auxiliary personnel. In the majority of cases this may be an efficient method of obtaining the information, but in a given patient insight into the real problem is gained not from what he says but rather from the manner in which he states it. For example, the patient may complain of a "lump under the jaw," as did a young college student. His statement of this rather mundane complaint seemed to be accompanied by an unusual degree of anxiety. Further questioning and examination indicated that he had apparently noted the anterior margin of the groove for the facial artery in the lower border of the mandible—a normal landmark—on examination of his jaw the week before. Why had he decided to examine his jaw? His roommate had recently been discovered to have Hodgkin's disease, which first presented as a lump under the jaw.

Another patient, a 35-year-old woman, was concerned about "lumps in her lower lip," stating that they had only come up recently. (They were normal mucous glands.) The patient further elaborated, saying that she was "sure" they were cancer. In stating this she smiled in a rather peculiar fashion as if amused or as if it were someone else's lip she was discussing. Further perusal of her complaints indicated inappropriate affect and depersonalization of her symptoms with definite paranoid ideas about the dentists she had previously consulted. She was referred for appropriate psychiatric diagnosis and treatment, was found to be a paranoid schizophrenic, and was treated for her psychiatric disorder.

A third patient came into the School of Dental Medicine to have dentures made. The chief complaint was delivered in such a hostile manner that it immediately made the attending dentists pursue the subject further. The patient had had three different sets of dentures made in the past 18 months, and "none of them were any good." Apparently she expected a great deal more from artificial dentures than was realistically possible. She was satisfied by an explanation that her present dentures were quite satisfactory, considering that she had almost no lower alveolar ridge. Embarking on making new dentures—which also would have been "no good" when they were completed—would have been an exercise in futility for both the doctor and the patient. The correct diagnosis may be missed if the dentist does not personally take the time to talk with the patient and evaluate his emotional response to questions and the manner of describing his illness.

Past Dental History

In addition to the chief complaint and history of the present illness, it is necessary to elicit a past dental history from the patient. As already discussed, it is often more worthwhile to observe closely the patient's description of the details of previous dental treatment and his reaction to his dentist than it is to have these data recorded by a secretary, assistant, or hygienist. By personally discussing previous dental treatment with the patient and noting nuances of meaning and facial expression, one may get a very accurate idea of the importance he places on good dental treatment and how conscientious he has been (and will be) in pursuing the goal of oral health. Even more important, one should be able to gauge the patient's feelings about his previous dentists. Are they all charlatans out only for the money? Are they father-figures? Was the relationship between doctor and patient a mutually satisfactory one? Is the patient reluctant to talk about previous dentists or previous dental treatment? Perhaps a telephone call to previous dentists might be rewarding—the patient may have an outstanding bill, may be very difficult to please, or may be engaged in litigation with the dentist.

Significant components of the past dental history include previous restorative, periodontic, endodontic, or oral surgical treatment; reasons for loss of teeth; untoward complications of dental treatment; attitudes toward previous dental treatment; experience with orthodontic appliances and dental prostheses; and radiation or other treatment for past oral or facial lesions.

Past Medical History

The past medical history of the patient may not seem as important in dental diagnosis as it is in medical diagnosis; however, it is significant in many oral diseases, such as lichen planus, erythema multiforme, and atrophic glossitis. Even though the past medical history may not contribute to the actual diagnosis of the chief complaint, it furnishes information about the physical makeup of the patient, his susceptibility and reaction to infection, and his emotional reaction to disease, all factors that may influence treatment planning and prognosis.

The past medical history contains information about any significant or serious illnesses a patient may have had (past illnesses continuing symptomatically until the present may be described both in the past medical history and in the review of systems) and is composed of the following subdivisions.

Serious or Significant Illnesses. Because *serious illness* is a rather open-ended term, it is preferable to ask patients to enumerate diseases they have had that required the attention of a physician or have necessitated their being confined to bed for 3 days or more. In addition to inquiring about serious illness in general, specifically ask the patient whether he knows of any history of heart disease, rheumatic fever, "growing pains," heart murmur, or other symptoms suggestive of rheumatic fever or rheumatic heart disease. Unfortunately, because rheumatic fever occurs most commonly between the ages of 6 and 10 years, many patients do not remember this vital information. The relationship between rheumatic heart disease and the endocarditis that can result in patients with rheumatic heart disease as a result of dental procedures is well known, but may need to be explained to a patient.

Hospitalizations. Ask the patient to enumerate all previous hospitalizations and indicate the purposes. It may have been for diagnostic studies or for proven serious illness.

Blood Transfusions. Another subdivision of the past medical history should include the record of any blood transfusions. If there were any, they may have been necessary because of serious illness, and this information serves as a double check on the patient who may have forgotten to mention the illness when questioned about hospitalizations or serious illnesses. Also keep in mind that a patient who recently received a blood transfusion may harbor the hepatitis virus non-A, non-B or cytomegalovirus—a potential danger to anyone exposed to the patient's blood or aerosolized oral secretions.

Allergies. Record known allergic propensities in the past medical history. These include diseases such as asthma, eczema, and hay fever. Differentiate true allergies as manifested by findings such as urticaria, angioedema, skin rash, or respiratory symptoms, and the symptoms of serum sickness from simple psychological aversions of the patient. A history of multiple food "allergies" may turn out on further investigation to be nothing more than increased eructation or flatulence that the patient associates with the disliked food. One patient stated she was allergic to aspirin. In the process of writing her a prescription for another, more expensive analgesic that comes in relatively large capsules, it occurred to the dentist to question her further about the allergy to aspirin. She was happy to provide the information, stating that she could not take aspirin because she could not swallow those "big pills," and had no true allergic symptoms at all.

Because patients tend to forget about allergies, it is wise to ask specifically about allergy to any medication including local anesthetic agents and antibiotics that you intend to administer, and as an obvious reminder and for medicolegal reasons, to record the information about the allergy on the chart.

Medications. Carefully question the patient about any medications he is currently taking or has recently taken (within the past 6 weeks). If he is uncertain about the exact nature of the medication, a letter or phone call to the prescribing physician or pharmacy is advisable. Those "heart pills" may be an anticoagulant rather than digitalis. Sometimes a patient who takes medications regularly will forget to include them in the list of medications taken. A patient with rheumatic heart disease might forget that he takes a daily penicillin tablet, or a woman taking birth control pills might forget to mention them. A patient who regularly takes mineral oil as a laxative may not consider this a "medicine" and could hardly be expected to know that the oil seriously interferes with vitamin K absorption and might lead during dental procedures to hemorrhagic diathesis caused by a lowered prothrombin level.

One patient seen at the Philadelphia General Hospital with acute erythema multiforme of the oral cavity forgot that she was taking a laxative. The laxative contained phenolphthalein (a known allergic sensitizer) and was probably the cause of the erythema multiforme.

Patients must be reminded that "medicine" may include anything taken into the body that is not food.

Review of Systems. This list of symptoms referable to the organ systems of the body (*e.g.*, cardiovascular, gastrointestinal, genitourinary, etc.) is obtained by methodically asking the patient about symptoms that might indicate the presence of disease in the organ system. The review of systems is necessary because the patient may not relate his symptoms to any disease or abnormality and therefore would not think of describing them to the dentist or physician unless specifically questioned. If a patient is asked, for example, "Is there anything wrong with your heart?" he might reply in the negative. A more comprehensive review of the cardiac status of the patient can be obtained by asking the patient if he gets short of breath easily, has exertional pain in the precordial area or down the left arm, ankle edema, cyanosis, dyspnea on exertion, orthopnea, and so forth. In this manner the presence of *symptoms* of cardiovascular disease may be elicited. How many patients would be aware of a relationship between their *heart* and their *ankle* swelling? A detailed description of each of the questions to ask in a thorough systems review may be found in any textbook of physical diagnosis, and those symptoms most likely to indicate systemic disease of interest to the dentist are often included in a health questionnaire (Fig. 2-1).

Family History

The family history is designed to gather information about those diseases that are communicable or tend to occur in families. This includes diseases such as tuberculosis, rheumatic fever, migraine, psychiatric or neurotic disorders, certain types of cancer, allergic disease, and arterial hypertension. Hereditary diseases are common in the nervous system (*e.g.*, Huntington's chorea), and the hereditary nature of the hemophilias and diabetes is well known. The age and state of health of parents, siblings, and children should be recorded, and the cause of death of those not living should be determined.

Social and Occupational History

The social and occupational history will in some cases suggest the diagnosis of the patient's ailment. The strange dark stippling of the marginal gingiva may not seem so strange when it is discovered that the patient works with lead, bismuth, or cadmium. Undue erosion of the teeth is easily explained in a sandblaster, who should be promptly referred to his physician for pulmonary evaluation for evidence of silicosis. The alcoholic patient is a known risk for general anesthetic because he may sustain a prolonged and profound hypotensive episode. Alcoholics also frequently exhibit neutropenia with markedly decreased resistance to infection and may, if hospitalized away from sources of the beverage, go into acute delirium tremens from which death may result.

The likelihood of a patient's having recently traveled overseas can also often be deduced from the social and occupational history. A patient recently traveling out of the country may have contracted an infectious disease that is rare in the United States. Malaria in travelers returning from malaria-endemic areas is an example. Hepatitis B infection is endemic in many countries (see Chaps. 20 and 28), and migrants to the United States from those countries as well as US nationals who have lived "off base" in those areas for many months are customarily screened for hepatitis B_s antigenemia, even in the absence of a history of acute hepatitis.

Medical Questionnaires in History-Taking

Many types of medical questionnaires may be purchased and given to the patient to fill out in order to elicit details of present or past illness. Most of the comprehensive questionnaires include all pertinent questions ordinarily asked in the review of systems or past medical history. There is no doubt that the use of these questionnaires can be timesaving, but they are not a substitute for the time the clinician must personally spend with the patient, checking the thoroughness with which the patient answers the questions, the reliability of his answers, and his personal reaction to such a questionnaire. A "No" answer may mean that the patient never had the symptom or disease. On the other hand, it may mean that he does not feel that the questions are important, especially since all he wants is to have his upper second molar filled; and he may consequently answer the questions in a rather cursory and inattentive manner. These problems may be anticipated and perhaps avoided by discussing the questionnaire with the patient.

The Cornell Medical Index* is often cited as the prototype of screening medical questionnaires. It consists of a series of 195 printed questions that provide a comprehensive review of the patient's past medical history and symptoms referable to the major organ systems. This questionnaire is usually completed by the patient and reviewed by the physician before the patient is examined, and can serve to orient the physician to the patient's history and general symptomatology. The Cornell Medical Index may at times furnish more comprehensive information than the clinical history obtained by the physician. For research purposes, the responses of patients to the Cornell Medical Index can be computerized and scored in terms of individual organ system abnormalities. This

* Cornell University Medical College, 1300 York Ave., New York NY 10021.

MEDICAL HISTORY

Name .... Sex ..... Date of Birth ....
Address...
Telephone .... Height .... Weight ....
Date .... Occupation .... Marital Status ....

DIRECTIONS

If the answer is YES to the question, put a circle around YES.
If the answer is NO to the question, put a circle around NO.
Answer all questions by circling either YES or NO and fill in all blank space when indicated.
Answers to the following questions are for our records only and will be considered confidential.

1. Are you in good health?.. YES   NO
   a. Has there been any change in your general health within the past year? .... YES   NO
2. My last physical examination was on
3. Are you now under the care of a physician?.. YES   NO
   a. If so, what is the condition being treated?
4. The name and address of my physician is
5. Have you had any serious illness or operation?..................................... YES   NO
   a. If so, what was the illness or operation?
6. Have you been hospitalized or had a serious illness within the past five (5) years?......... YES   NO
   a. If so, what was the problem?
7. Do you have or have you had any of the following diseases or problems:
   a. Rheumatoid fever or rheumatic heart disease .... YES   NO
   b. Congenital heart lesions .... YES   NO
   c. Cardiovascular disease (heart trouble, heart attack, coronary insufficiency,
      coronary occlusion, high blood pressure, arteriosclerosis, stroke) .... YES   NO
      1) Do you have pain in chest upon exertion?.. YES   NO
      2) Are you ever short of breath after mild exercise? .... YES   NO
      3) Do your ankles swell?.. YES   NO
      4) Do you get short of breath when you lie down, or do you require extra
         pillows when you sleep? .... YES   NO
   d. Allergy.. YES   NO
   e. Asthma or hay fever .... YES   NO
   f. Hives or a skin rash.. YES   NO
   g. Fainting spells or seizures .... YES   NO
   h. Diabetes .... YES   NO
      1) Do you have to urinate (pass water) more than six times a day? .... YES   NO
      2) Are you thirsty much of the time?.. YES   NO
      3) Does your mouth frequently become dry?.. YES   NO
   i. Hepatitis, jaundice or liver disease.. YES   NO
   j. Arthritis.. YES   NO
   k. Inflammatory rheumatism (painful, swollen joints) .... YES   NO
   l. Stomach ulcers.. YES   NO
   m. Kidney trouble.. YES   NO
   n. Tuberculosis .... YES   NO
   o. Do you have a persistent cough or cough up blood? .... YES   NO
   p. Low blood pressure .... YES   NO
   q. Venereal disease .... YES   NO
   r. Other

Fig. 2-1A.
Example of a screening medical questionnaire for use in dental offices and clinics. (American Dental Association: Accepted Dental Therapeutics, 38th ed. Chicago, American Dental Association, 1979)

8. Have you had abnormal bleeding associated with previous extractions, surgery, or trauma YES   NO
   a. Do you bruise easily? .... YES   NO
   b. Have you ever required a blood transfusion? .... YES   NO
      If so, explain the circumstances.
9. Do you have any blood disorder such as anemia? .... YES   NO
10. Have you had surgery or x-ray treatment for a tumor, growth, or other condition
    of your head or neck? .... YES   NO
11. Are you taking any drug or medicine? .... YES   NO
    If so, what
12. Are you taking any of the following:
   a. Antibiotics or sulfa drugs.. YES   NO
   b. Anticoagulants (blood thinners).. YES   NO
   c. Medicine for high blood pressure .... YES   NO
   d. Cortisone (steroids) .... YES   NO
   e. Tranquilizers... YES   NO
   f. Aspirin .... YES   NO
   g. Insulin, tolbutamide (Orinase) or similar drug.................................. YES   NO
   h. Digitalis or drugs for heart trouble .... YES   NO
   i. Nitroglycerin..
   j. Antihistamine... YES   NO
   k. Oral contraceptive or other hormonal therapy .... YES   NO
   l. Other
13. Are you allergic or have you reacted adversely to:
   a. Local anesthetics .... YES   NO
   b. Penicillin or other antibiotics .... YES   NO
   c. Sulfa drugs... YES   NO
   d. Barbiturates, sedatives, or sleeping pills...................................... YES   NO
   e. Aspirin .... YES   NO
   f. Iodine.. YES   NO
   g. Codeine or other narcotics .... YES   NO
   h. Other
14. Have you had any serious trouble associated with any previous dental treatment?........ YES   NO
    If so, explain
15. Do you have any disease, condition, or problem not listed above that you think
    I should know about?... YES   NO
    If so, please explain
16. Are you employed in any situation which exposes you regularly to x-rays or other
    ionizing radiation?... YES   NO
17. Are you wearing contact lenses? .... YES   NO

WOMEN

18. Are you pregnant?... YES   NO
19. Do you have any problem associated with your menstrual period?..................... YES   NO
Chief Dental Complaint:

                    Signature of Patient

                    Signature of Dentist

MEDICAL HISTORY

Date....................

Name .... Address ....
         Last   First   Middle   Number & Street

....
            City   State.   Zip Code   Home & Business Phone

Date of Birth .... Sex .... Height .... Weight .... Occupation ....

Married .... Spouse .... Single ....

Closest Relative .... Phone ....

If you are completing this form for another person, what is your relationship to that person?

PLEASE ANSWER EACH QUESTION

Check One
Yes   No

1. Have you been a patient in a hospital during the past 2 years? .... □   □
2. Have you been under the care of a physician during the past 2 years? .... □   □
3. Have you taken any kind of medicine or drugs during the past year? .... □   □
4. Has anyone in your family been advised of difficulties during anesthesia? .... □   □
5. Are you allergic to penicillin, codeine or any other drugs or medicine? .... □   □
6. Have you ever had any excessive bleeding requiring special treatment? .... □   □
7. Circle any of the following which you have had:

   heart trouble   asthma   arthritis

   congenital heart lesions   cough   stroke

   heart murmur   diabetes   epilepsy

   high blood pressure   tuberculosis   psychiatric treatment

   anemia   hepatitis   sinus trouble

   rheumatic fever   jaundice

8. (Women) Are you pregnant now? .... □   □
9. Have you had any other serious illnesses? .... □   □

   TO BE ANSWERED ONLY BY PATIENTS RECEIVING
   SEDATION OR GENERAL ANESTHESIA
10. Have you had anything to eat or drink within the last 4 hours? .... □   □
11. Are you wearing a removable dental appliance? .... □   □
12. Are you wearing contact lenses? .... □   □
13. Who is to drive you home today?
    a. Name

Chief Dental Complaint

Reviewed by   Signature

Fig. 2-1B.
Example of an abbreviated screening medical questionnaire designed for use by the patient
before outpatient general anesthetic and minor oral surgery. (American Dental Association:
Accepted Dental Therapeutics, 38th ed. Chicago, American Dental Association, 1979)

method of evaluating the past medical history and the present health status of a patient has been incorporated into numerous other screening medical questionnaires designed for particular patient groups, different categories of disease, or special research projects. A number of questionnaires have been specifically designed for dental use and include questions regarding the past dental history and current dental problems, as well as a sampling of questions relating to the more common medical problems of importance in dental care.

After any questionnaire has been completed, the "Yes" replies can be reviewed in a few minutes and any additional questions asked that may be indicated. At times patients will reply "Yes" when the question is not clearly understood. In general, "Yes" answers justify additional questioning and more extensive evaluation. This health questionnaire is not a substitute for a carefully taken history, but it has been found to be an effective method for evaluating the general health status of the patient and an excellent case-finding tool.

For the past 25 years, a health questionnaire of this type[†] (Fig. 2-1, and earlier versions in previous editions of this text) has been used in the Oral Diagnosis Clinic of the School of Dental Medicine, University of Pennsylvania, and at many other universities and larger clinics with excellent results with respect to the information obtained, the time required, and the patient reaction. The majority of private practitioners now use questionnaires in their offices to obtain necessary medical information and to provide written records and details of previous dental treatment.

Possible errors or fallacies in history-taking may be mentioned. The timid or extremely apprehensive patient will require reassurance and encouragement before a diagnostically significant history can be obtained. Patients who have language problems or hearing defects are handicapped in cooperating with the clinician. Forgetful, untruthful, or mentally disturbed patients contribute little to a diagnostically significant history.

After the patient's history has been reviewed, one or more diagnostic possibilities are usually suggested. It is helpful at this time, before the oral examination is made, to form one or more tentative diagnoses. This also furnishes a basis for additional necessary questioning prior to the clinical examination. With these tentative diagnoses in mind, the examination of the patient can be carried out more intelligently, more effectively, and more efficiently.

EXAMINATION OF THE PATIENT

The examination of the patient represents the second stage of the diagnostic procedure, and it is the clinician's contribution to the diagnostic procedure. An established routine is most important because it minimizes the possibility of overlooking previously undiscovered or unknown lesions. If possible, it is helpful and timesaving to have an assistant record the findings. The examination is most conveniently carried out in a dental operatory, with the patient seated and his head supported in a dental chair. Before seating the patient, the clinician should observe the patient's general appearance and manner of walking into the operatory. Does he walk with ease and without apparent pain, or does he appear to be under stress? Is it painful or exhausting for the patient to get into the room and into the dental chair? Does the patient have any physical deformities or handicaps?

Details of examination procedures are described as follows:

- Vital signs (temperature, pulse, respiratory rate, and blood pressure)
- Blood pressure determination
- Examination of the head, neck, and oral cavity
- Examination of the neck and lymph nodes
- Examination of cranial nerve function
- Special examination of other organ systems
- Laboratory studies (see also Chap. 3)

The routine oral examination (*i.e.*, thorough inspection and palpation of the exposed

[†] The questionnaire now used at the University of Pennsylvania School of Dental Medicine differs little from the longer form prepared by the American Dental Association, as illustrated in Figure 2-1A.

surface structures of the head, neck, and face; detailed examination of the oral cavity, dentition, oropharynx, and adnexal structures as customarily carried out by the dentist) should be carried out at least once annually or at each recall visit. Additional special examination of other organ systems and laboratory studies are required for evaluation of patients with orofacial pain or signs and symptoms suggestive of otorhinologic, salivary gland, or other adnexal tissue disorders. A less comprehensive but equally thorough inspection of the face and oral and oropharyngeal mucosas should also be carried out at each dental visit. The tendency for the dentist to focus only on the tooth or jaw quadrant in question should be strongly resisted and each visit commenced by deliberate inspection of the face and oral cavity, starting at the quadrant farthest from the tooth to be treated and displaying the entire oral mucosa and dentition before returning to the scheduled procedure. The importance of this approach in the early detection of head and neck cancer and in developing the image of the dentist as the responsible clinician of the oral cavity cannot be overemphasized.

Examinations carried out in the dental office are traditionally restricted to inspection and palpation of the superficial tissues of the oral cavity, head, and neck and exposed parts of the extremities. On occasion, evaluation of an oral lesion logically leads to an inquiry about similar lesions on other skin or mucosal surfaces or about enlargement of other regional groups of lymph nodes. While these inquiries can usually be satisfied by directly questioning the patient, the dentist may also quite appropriately request permission from the patient to examine axillary nodes or other skin surfaces provided the examination is carried out competently, with adequate privacy for the patient, and with a female assistant present in the case of a female patient. Similar precautions should be followed when it is necessary for a female patient to remove tight clothing for accurate measurement of blood pressure. Facilities for a complete physical examination, however, are not traditionally available in dental offices and clinics, and a complete physical examination should not be attempted when facilities are lacking or when custom excludes it.

In the case of hospitalized inpatients, dental staff and attending oral surgeons are delegated to carry out preoperative complete physical examinations on the patients they have admitted for operating room procedures and general anesthetic. Instruction in the procedures for carrying out and recording the complete physical examination (i.e., examination of heart, lungs, abdomen, extremities, central and peripheral nervous system, special sensory functions, and musculoskeletal system) is therefore part of the postdoctoral training of oral surgeons. Full details of this examination are not within the scope of this text; readers are referred to the many available texts dealing with physical diagnosis.

The degree of responsibility accorded to the dentist in carrying out a complete physical examination varies from hospital to hospital and from state to state. The dentist's involvement may range from permission to examine extraoral structures for educational purposes only, through permission to carry out certain parts of the complete physical examination under the supervision of a physician who reviews and certifies the findings, to full privileges and responsibility for conducting necessary physical examinations before and after general anesthetic or surgical procedures.

Vital Signs

It is usual for some or all of the vital signs (temperature, pulse, respiration, and blood pressure) to be recorded as part of the patient examination. In addition to being useful indicators of systemic disease, vital signs are valuable as a record of the patient's normal signs for reference should syncope or other untoward medical complication in the dental office significantly affect these values.

It is not always necessary or desirable to take the dental patient's temperature, but when systemic illness is suspected or the patient must be evaluated for the presence of systemic involvement secondary to dental infection (e.g., bacteremia), it is necessary to evaluate his temperature response. The normal oral temperature is 37°C (98.6°F), but oral temperatures under 37.8°C (100°F) are not usually considered significant. Remember that recent drinking of hot or cold liquids or mouth breathing of very warm or cold air may alter the oral temperature. Also, unfortunately, severe oral infection has been shown to alter the *local* temperature in the mouth without causing systemic hyperpyrexia, thereby causing oral temperatures to be an inaccurate measure of systemic response. In such cases, when it is important to determine the patient's actual temperature, it is necessary to take a rectal temperature. Rectal temperatures are about 0.5°C (1°F) higher than are oral temperatures and require a special thermometer more easily inserted into the anal canal. Lubrication of the thermometer with petroleum jelly and requesting the patient to bear down as though passing a stool will make insertion of the rectal thermometer more comfortable.

Always determine the patient's *pulse rate and rhythm.* The normal resting pulse rate is about 72/min. A patient with a pulse rate greater than 130, even with the stress of a dental office visit, should be allowed to rest quietly away from the operatory to allow the pulse to return to normal before beginning dental treatment. If after resting, the patient's pulse rate remains persistently high, medical evaluation of the tachycardia is appropriate because severe coronary artery disease or myocardial disease may be present. Note that the pulse rate normally rises about 5 to 10/min with each degree of fever.

It is just as important to determine the regularity (rhythm) of the pulse as it is to determine the rate. Although the normal person, especially under stress, may have occasional irregularities or premature beats, a grossly irregular pulse can indicate that severe myocardial disease may be present, justifying further cardiac evaluation before dental treatment is instituted. In those patients with known cardiac disease and grossly irregular pulses, it is wise to check with the patient's physician to ascertain whether any special precautions should be taken before or during dental treatment.

It is not usually necessary to measure the patient's respiratory rate in the dental office, unless cardiopulmonary disease is suspected or a general anesthetic or relative analgesia is planned; however, observe whether the patient is breathing very rapidly, is short of breath, or is dyspneic. These symptoms alone may indicate the presence of pulmonary or cardiac disease or anemia.

Blood Pressure Determination

It is important to be aware of a patient's blood pressure because many dental procedures are stressful to the patient and may cause an elevation of his usual pressure. Also, the accidental intravascular injection or rapid absorption (*e.g.,* injection into a venous plexus) of local anesthetics containing epinephrine may cause an appreciable rise in the pressure. In hypertensive patients, adequate preoperative sedation and short appointments may be necessary; it may be advisable to eliminate epinephrine or reduce the amount used (*i.e.,* 1:100,000 instead of 1:50,000). If the patient regularly sees his physician, rechecking blood pressure in the dental office is not likely to provide additional information. On the other hand, if a patient is receiving treatment for hypertension or if the patient does not regularly visit his physician, be sure to determine his blood pressure before instituting dental treatment.

A compelling reason, other than dental treatment, for taking the pressure of a patient who does not regularly visit his physician is that it is a valuable method of medical case finding that the dentist can perform. Anyone who has seen the irreversible ravages of a cerebrovascular accident (stroke) due to hypertension can readily appreciate the service to the patient that the dentist performs by taking a few minutes of his or his assistant's time to take the patient's blood pressure and, if the pressure is significantly elevated, to refer him to the physician for further diagnosis and treatment.

Use of symptoms alone to determine whether a patient is hypertensive is unreliable inasmuch as many patients are asymptomatic until they have a stroke or develop irreversible renal disease. If the patient is a known hypertensive, determine the blood pressure just before each dental appointment to ascertain that it is adequately controlled at acceptable levels for the dental procedure to be performed.

Method

Blood pressure determination is easily accomplished and is well within the capabilities of every dentist. The cost of the simple equipment required (stethoscope and sphygmomanometer) is low. Seat the patient and place his right arm on a table or a desk so that the forearm is adequately supported at elbow level—about the level of the heart. Center the rubber balloon of the cuff over the brachial artery. This artery is usually palpable about three quarters of the way across the arm going in a lateral-to-medial direction (*i.e.,* in the medial one fourth of the arm). Wrap the pressure cuff smoothly and *snugly* around the upper arm with its lower border 1 to 2 inches above the elbow crease in the antecubital fossa.

Palpate the patient's radial pulse and pump the cuff up to about 20 to 30 mm Hg *above* the point at which the pulse is no longer palpable. (This is the best way to determine how high to pump up the cuff, since choosing an arbitrary height may not be high enough in hypertensive patients. Conversely, if the arbitrary height chosen is too high, it would result in unnecessary pain to the patient and probably cause an iatrogenic elevation of the blood pressure.) It is essential to always record the systolic pressure by palpation to avoid missing the occasional occurrence in hypertensives of a silent gap (the *auscultatory gap,* a region of variable magnitude between the systolic and diastolic pressures where Korotkoff's sounds temporarily disappear during auscultation of the partially occluded brachial artery), which can give a falsely low reading on auscultation alone.

Apply either the bell or the diaphragm of the stethoscope over the artery just distal to the elbow crease and slowly deflate the cuff—about 3 mm Hg per heartbeat—until the first sound appears. Record this first sound as the systolic pressure. Further lower the pressure in the cuff until the sounds disappear. Record this point as the diastolic pressure. The point of muffling of the sounds is generally taken as the diastolic reading.

Usually the sound will disappear completely within about 5 mm Hg of the point of its muffling. In cases of wide disparity between the point of disappearing and muffling, record both points. For example, if the patient's systolic pressure (point of appearance of the sound) were 120, the sound muffled at 80 mm Hg and disappeared at 40 mm Hg, the pressure should be recorded as 120/80/40 or 120/80–40. With wide disparity between points of muffling and disappearance, the true diastolic pressure is usually about halfway between the two points.

If unsure about the determination of the pressure or the patient appears to be unduly anxious, repeat the procedure several times in sequence at one sitting. In such cases, carefully lower the cuff pressure to 0 mm Hg before retaking the pressure. Failure to do so will cause venous congestion, pain, and iatrogenic elevation of the patient's pressure.

A number of digitally recording syphgmomanometers are now marketed as are smaller electronic devices capable of recording pulse and blood pressure from an electrode attached to a patient's finger. In general, these types of equipment perform equally as well as the manual equipment, although differences in diastolic readings occur depending on the particular signal used to record the diastolic pressure. Electronic devices should be calibrated from time to time against a manual sphygmomanometer to detect mechanical problems.

Factors Influencing Results

Faulty technique in taking the blood pressure may induce error. If the cuff is applied too loosely, if it is not completely deflated before applying, or if it is too small for the patient's arm size, the pressure readings obtained will be erroneously high and will not represent the pressure in the artery at the time of determination. The one factor above that is not within the province of the practitioner to change is the arm size. The width of the cuff should be about 20% greater than the diameter of the patient's arm. In patients who have unusually large arms, it may be appropriate to use a "thigh" cuff. If a thigh cuff is not available, keep in mind that the readings will be somewhat higher than are correct. If the cuff is deflated too rapidly (more than 2 to 3 mm Hg per heartbeat), the recorded systolic pressure will be erroneously low and the diastolic pressure too high.

Careful attention to the proper techniques does not require a great deal of effort, and after some experience, the pressure will be as easily determined correctly as by using sloppy techniques that lead to error.

Anxiety and pain are factors that may

cause an elevation of the blood pressure of the patient above his true resting level. Pain and anxiety must not be induced in the procedure of taking the pressure and must be accounted for in interpretation of the pressure.

Normal Range

The normal median blood pressure is about 150/90. With increasing age, the systolic pressure may increase, probably as a result of arteriosclerosis. This systolic elevation is approximately equal to 100 plus the patient's age. Less elevation is expected in the diastolic pressure with advancing age, and it is sustained elevation of the diastolic pressure that is primarily responsible for the adverse renal effects of hypertension. Refer patients whose pressure is consistently greater than 160/95 (after several readings, alleviating pain, and allaying anxiety) to their physician for further diagnosis and treatment.

Examination of the Head, Neck, and Oral Cavity

The ability to perform a thorough physical examination of the superficial structures of the head, neck, and oral cavity is essential for all dentists and any clinician involved in diagnosing and treating oral disease.

NORMAL ANATOMIC STRUCTURES THAT MAY BE IDENTIFIED BY SUPERFICIAL PHYSICAL EXAMINATION OF THE HEAD, NECK, AND ORAL CAVITY*

Head—Extraoral Structures
- Face
  - Skin
  - Nose (alae, external nares, nasal mucosa)
  - Eyes (pupils, palpebral and bulbar conjunctivae, irises, lacrimal caruncle, lacrimal glands and duct orifices, orifice of the nasolacrimal duct, eyebrows, eyelashes, commissures)
  - Jaws (mandibular border, angle, symphysis, condyle and coronoid processes; malar process, maxilla, infraorbital foramen, lingual notch, maxillary sinuses)
  - Masticatory muscles (temporalis, masseter, buccinator)
  - Parotid gland
  - Muscles of expression (obicularis oris, depressor and levator anguli oris, obicularis oculi)
  - Distribution of branches of the facial nerve
  - External carotid, lingual, and temporal pulses
- Scalp and Cranium—frontal, occipital, and temporal bones; mastoid process; nuchal point; frontal sinuses; cranial aponeurosis; insertion of temporal muscle
  - Ears (pinna, external auditory meatus and canal, tragus, helix)

Head—Intraoral Structures
- Lips—skin and mucosal surfaces, vermilion border, commissures, oral vestibule, minor salivary glands, labial frenum
- Cheeks—buccinator muscle, buccal fat pad, buccal frenum, occlusal line, orifice and papilla of parotid gland duct (Stensen's duct), minor salivary glands, Fordyce's granules, buccal vestibule, mental foramen
- Tongue—dorsum (anterior two thirds and posterior one third; filiform, fungiform, vallate, and foliate papillae; foramen cecum; lymphoid follicles of posterior one third); ventral surface (mucosa, fimbriated folds, superficial veins and varicosities, anterior lingual glands and ducts [Blandin and Nuhn])
- Floor of Mouth—plica submandibularis, submandibular duct, and orifice of submandibular and sublingual gland ducts (Wharton's duct); lingual vestibule, genial tubercles, mylohyoid ridge, lingual nerve
- Palate—hard and soft palates, reflecting line, foveae pterygoidae, maxillary tuberosity, pterygoid hamulus, tensor palati muscle, anterior and posterior palatine canals, uvula

---

* No attempt is made during a routine head and neck examination to identify each structure; however, the ability to recognize all of them is basic to performing a physical examination of this region in which asymmetries, swellings, discolorations, changes in texture, and tender areas may have to be differentiated from normal structures.

- Gingivae—marginal gingivae, attached keratinized (alveolar) and nonkeratinized (areolar) gingivae, gingival sulcus, interdental papillae
- Retromolar Region—retromolar pad, external oblique ridge, palatoglossal arch (anterior pillar of fauces), pterygomandibular ligament, retromolar triangle, stylohyoid ligament
- Pharynx—palatine tonsils, palatopharyngeal arch (posterior pillar of fauces), tonsillar crypts, posterior pharyngeal wall, lateral pharyngeal wall, orifice of eustachian tube and posterior nares, larynx, pyriform fossa, epiglottis, internal pterygoid muscle, Waldeyer's ring, lingual tonsils, adenoids
- Teeth—chart designation and name of each

Neck—anterior triangle, posterior triangle, submaxillary triangle, sternocleidomastoid, platysma, digastric and mylohyoid muscles, thyroid and cricoid cartilages, trachea, wings of hyoid bone, thyroid gland, anterior and posterior cervical lymph nodes, submandibular lymph nodes, sternal notch and clavicles, first cervical vertebra (Atlas), carotid pulse

Relationships—mesial, distal, anterior posterior, buccal, labial, lingual, palatal, coronal, sagittal, lateral, interproximal, gingival

Such examination should be carried out on all new patients and repeated at least yearly on patients of record. To perform this examination procedure successfully, the following are necessary:

- Adequate *knowledge* of the *anatomy* of the region to be able to recognize normal structures and their common variations
- A *well-practiced technique* for displaying all of the skin and mucosal surfaces of the head, neck, and oral cavity with minimal discomfort to the patient; a *routine* that ensures systematic examination of all the tissues that can be approached in this way
- *Knowledge* of the *variety* of *disease* processes that can affect the superficial structures of the head, neck, and oral cavity
- *Ability to succinctly record (in writing)* both normal and abnormal findings noted during the examination

The order of examination is a matter of individual choice, but it is more effective to develop and follow an established routine. Ideally, necessary intraoral and bite-wing radiographs should be available when the systematic examination of the oral cavity is carried out.

Equipment. Tongue blades or dental hand mirrors, gauze pads, dental chair, and a lamp or flashlight for illuminating the oral cavity

Examination Sequence. A suggested sequence of examination includes the inner surfaces of the lips, the mucosa of the cheeks, the maxillary and mandibular mucobuccal folds, the palate, the tongue, the sublingual space, the gingivae, and then the teeth and their supporting structures. Examine last the tonsillar and the pharyngeal areas and any lesion, particularly if it is painful. Complete visualization of the smooth mucosal surfaces of the lips, cheeks, tongue, and sublingual space can be obtained by using two tongue depressors. These permit excellent examination of these mucosal surfaces and more important, enable determination of whether possible contagious lesions are present before placing one's fingers within the mouth. Make a more detailed examination of the teeth and supporting tissues with the mouth mirror, the explorer, and the periodontal probe. After the general examination of the oral cavity has been completed, make the detailed study of the lesion or the area involved in the chief complaint. Give special attention to the location, appearance, size, physical character, and distribution of all lesions.

Examine the teeth for dental caries, occlusal relations, possible prematurities, inadequate contact areas or restorations, evidence of food impaction, gingivitis, periodontal disease, or fistulae. Have the patient protrude the tongue for examination of the dorsum and then raise it to the palate to permit good visualization of the sublingual space. The patient should then extend the tongue forcibly out of the right and left sides of the mouth to permit good visualization of the sublingual space and to permit careful examination of the left and right margins. Examine the tonsillar fossae and the oropharynx.

Palpate for adenopathy after the intraoral examination has been completed and the exact location and the nature of the lesion have been determined. Give special attention to the lymph nodes draining the areas where lesions are present. The superficial and the deep lymph nodes of the neck are best examined from behind the patient with the head inclined forward sufficiently to relax the tissues overlying the lymph nodes. Look for distention of the superficial veins as well as for evidence of thyroid enlargement (see also the next section).

Use bimanual or bidigital palpation for examination of the tongue, cheeks, and floor of the mouth. Use rubber gloves or rubber finger cots when these structures are palpated if there is any doubt concerning the infectious nature of the lesion. Palpation is also useful in determining the degree of tooth movement. Two resistant instruments, such as mirror handles or tongue depressors, placed on the buccal and the lingual surfaces of the tooth furnish more nearly accurate information than when fingers alone are directly employed.

Note the general appearance of the individual; evaluate his emotional reactions and note the general nutritional state. Record the character of the skin and the presence of petechiae or eruptions, as well as the texture and the quality of the hair. Examine the conjunctiva and skin for petechiae and the sclera and skin for evidence of jaundice. Determine the reaction of the pupils to light when observable.

Abnormalities

The following abnormalities should be specifically sought and noted in the regions covered by the oral examination.

Facial Structures. Observe the patient's skin for color, blemishes, pigmentation abnormalities, vascular abnormalities such as angiomas, telangiectiasias, nevi and tortuous superficial vessels; asymmetry, ulcers, pustules, nodules, and swellings; note the color of the conjunctiva. Palpate the jaws and superficial masticatory muscles for tenderness or deformity. Note any scars.

Lips. Note lip color, texture, and any surface abnormalities, angular or vertical fissures, lip pits, cold sores, ulcers, scabs, nodules, ker-

atotic plaques, and scars; palpate upper and lower lips for any thickening, induration, or swelling; note orifices of minor salivary glands and the presence of Fordyce's granules.

Cheeks. Note any changes in pigmentation and movability of the mucosa, a pronounced linea alba, leukoedema, hyperkeratotic patches, intraoral swellings, ulcers, nodules, scars, other red or white patches, and Fordyce's granules. Observe openings of Stensen's ducts and establish their patency by first drying the mucosa with gauze and observing character and extent of salivary flow from duct openings with and without milking of the gland. Palpate muscles of cheek.

Maxillary and Mandibular Mucobuccal Folds. Observe color, texture, any swellings or fistulae; palpate for swellings and tenderness over the roots of the teeth and for tenderness of the buccinator insertion by pressing laterally with a finger inserted over the roots of the upper molar teeth.

Hard and Soft Palate. Illuminate the palate and inspect for discoloration, swellings, fistulae, papillary hyperplasia, tori, ulcers, recent burns, hyperkeratinization, asymmetry of structure or function, and orifices of minor salivary glands; palpate for swellings and tenderness.

Tongue. Inspect the dorsum of the tongue while it is at rest for any swelling, ulcers, coating, or variation in size, color, and texture. Observe and note the distribution of filiform and fungiform papillae, margins of the tongue, crenations and fasciculations, depapillated areas, fissures, ulcers, and keratotic areas. Note any deviations as patient protrudes tongue and attempts to move it to the right and left. Wrap a piece of gauze (4×4 cm) around the tip of the protruded tongue to steady it, and lightly press a warm mirror against the uvula to observe the base of the tongue and vallate papillae; note any ulcers or significant swellings. Holding the tongue with the gauze, gently guide the tongue to the right and retract the left cheek to observe the entire lateral border of the tongue for ulcers, keratotic areas, red patches, and the foliate papillae. Repeat for the opposite side, and then have patient touch the tip of the tongue to the palate to display the ventral surface of the tongue and floor of the mouth; note any varicosities, tight frenal attachments, stones in Wharton's ducts, ulcers, swellings, and red or white patches. Gently palpate the muscles of the tongue for nodules and tumors, extending the finger onto the base of the tongue and pressing forward if this has been poorly visualized or any ulcers or masses are suspected. Note tongue thrust on swallowing.

Floor of the Mouth. With the tongue still elevated, observe the openings of Wharton's ducts, the salivary pool, and the character and extent of right and left secretions and any swellings, ulcers, and red or white patches. Gently explore and display the extent of the lateral sublingual space, again noting ulcers and red or white patches.

Gingivae. Observe color, texture, contour, frenal attachments, ulcers, marginal inflammation, resorption, festooning, Stillman's clefts, hyperplasia, nodules, swellings, and fistulae.

Teeth and Periodontium. Note missing or supernumerary teeth, mobile or tender teeth, caries, defective restorations, dental arch irregularities, orthodontic anomalies, abnormal jaw relationships, occlusal interferences, extent of plaque and calculus deposits, dental hypoplasia, and discolored teeth.

Tonsils and Pharynx. Note the color, size, and surface abnormalities of tonsils and ulcers, tonsilloliths, and inspissated secretion in tonsillar crypts. Palpate tonsils for discharge or tenderness; note restriction of the oropharyngeal airway. Observe the faucial pillars for nodules, red and white patches, lymphoid aggregates, and deformities. Observe the postpharyngeal wall for swellings, nodular lymphoid hyperplasia, hyperplastic adenoids, postnasal discharge, and heavy mucus secretions.

Submandibular Triangle and Neck. See next section.

Temporomandibular Joint. Observe deviations in the path of the mandible on opening and closing. Palpate the joints and listen for clicking and crepitus during opening and closing; note any tenderness over the joint or masticatory muscles while palpating. Explore the anterior wall of the external auditory meatus for tenderness and pain. Reinspect occlusion for "slips," occlusal interferences, and limitations of movement.

After the routine examination has been completed, additional questioning may be indicated. With the information obtained from the history and the physical examination, a definite diagnosis can usually be made, or at least the possibilities will have been greatly limited. More specialized clinical examinations such as palpation of the major salivary glands, dental pulp vitality testing, and detailed examination of the masticatory muscles and temporomandibular joint are appropriate at this time to confirm a suspected diagnosis.

Special radiographic studies and a variety of laboratory aids to diagnosis (such as hematologic or bacteriologic studies, blood serologic findings, or biopsy studies, if needed) can also now be requested more intelligently.

Examination of the Neck and Lymph Nodes

Examination of the neck is a natural extension of a routine dental examination. It may be performed with little difficulty in a dental chair and can yield important medical information to the examining dentist. For example, a patient without a history of heart disease may have distention of the neck veins, suggesting right-sided heart failure; the trachea may deviate from the midline suggesting pulmonary or mediastinal pathology; there may be enlargement of the thyroid gland, salivary glands, or lymph nodes. A clinician who does not examine the neck overlooks these important signs of disease, decreasing his skill as a diagnostician.

A normal cervical lymph node is not palpable on routine examination. Palpable nodes are the primary sign of past or current lymph node disease and may indicate one of a large number of infectious, immune, or neoplastic diseases. The diseases that most commonly cause enlargement of the cervical lymph nodes include acute bacterial or viral infection of the head and neck region such as acute abscesses, infectious mononucleosis, and cat-scratch disease; chronic bacterial infections such as syphilis or tuberculosis; leukemia; lymphoma; metastatic carcinoma; collagen disease; allergic reactions (especially serum sickness); and sarcoidosis. A less well-known entity affecting the cervical lymph nodes is the recently recognized mucocutaneous lymph node syndrome. This disease, thought to be a rickettsial infection, affects children under 5 years of age and is characterized by cervical lymphadenopathy, rash, fever, stomatitis, and conjunctivitis.

In order to examine the neck the clinician must be familiar with its normal anatomy. The neck is divided into two triangles by the sternocleidomastoid muscle (Fig. 2-2). The anterior triangle is bordered by the inferior border of the mandible, the anterior border, and the sternomastoid muscle. The posterior triangle of the neck is bordered by the trapezius muscle, the clavicle, and the sternomastoid muscle.

The important landmarks at the midline of the neck are the hyoid bone, thyroid cartilage, cricoid cartilage, and trachea (Fig. 2-3).

Soft tissue structures that can be observed include the external jugular veins, which cross the sternomastoid muscle. These veins may be distended due to congestive failure of the right side of the heart, obstruction of the vena cava, or constrictive pericarditis. When examining the neck veins, the back of the dental chair should be placed at a 45° angle to the floor. If the jugular vein is observed to be distended over 2 cm above the

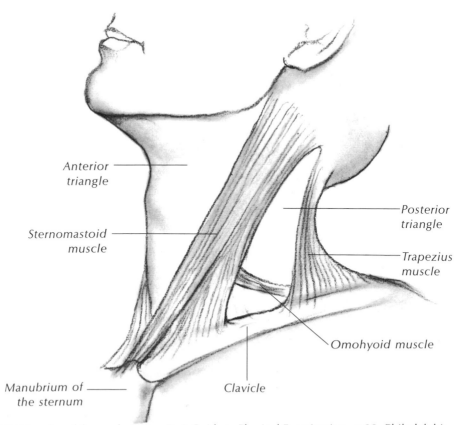

Fig. 2-2 Triangles of the neck. (Bates B: A Guide to Physical Examination, p 28. Philadelphia, JB Lippincott, 1974)

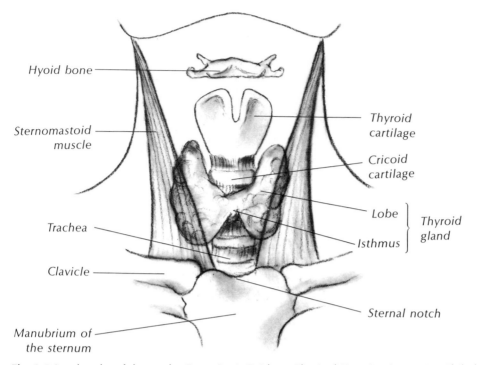

Hyoid bone

Sternomastoid muscle

Trachea

Clavicle

Manubrium of the sternum

Thyroid cartilage

Cricoid cartilage

Lobe

Isthmus

} Thyroid gland

Sternal notch

Fig. 2-3 Landmarks of the neck. (Bates B: A Guide to Physical Examination, p 28. Philadelphia, JB Lippincott, 1974)

sternum, it is a sign of disease. In severe cases of right-sided heart failure, neck veins may be distended up to the angle of the mandible.

Other soft tissue structures include the salivary glands and the thyroid gland. Salivary gland enlargement is discussed in Chapter 11. The *thyroid gland* is examined in the lower portion of the neck. The isthmus of the gland crosses the trachea just above the manubrium, and the two lobes lie below the sternomastoid muscles. Enlargement of the gland may be detected by placing the fingers between the sternomastoid muscle and the trachea below the region of the thyroid cartilage. If a mass is palpated, the patient should be asked to swallow. If thyroid enlargement is present, the mass will move up and down with the trachea as the patient swallows.

The dentist should be familiar with the lymphatic drainage of the head (Fig. 2-5) and the proper technique for lymph node examination. The patient is first observed for any obvious asymmetries or enlargements of the neck. The clinician then follows a routine procedure for examining lymph nodes so that regions of the neck are not excluded.

One good method of examining lymph nodes is to begin with the most superior nodes and work down to the clavicle. Using this method, the clinician first palpates just anterior to the tragus of the ear for the preauricular nodes then to the mastoid process and base of the skull for the posterior auricular and occipital nodes. Just under the chin are the submental nodes; further posterior along the mandible are the submandibular nodes. The superficial cervical nodes lie superficial to the sternomastoid muscle; the deep cervical nodes lie deep to the same muscle. In order to examine the deep cervical nodes properly, the head should be turned to the side opposite the nodes to be examined. The posterior cervical nodes are located in the posterior triangle of the neck and lie at the border of the trapezius muscle. The supraclavicular nodes are just above the clavicle, lateral to the sternomastoid muscle (Fig. 2-4).

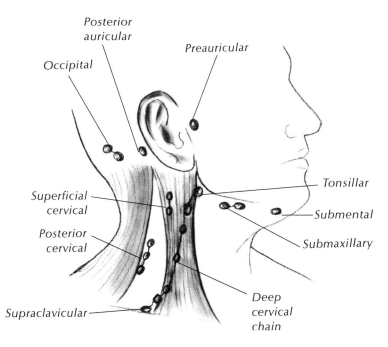

Posterior
auricular

Preauricular

Occipital

Tonsillar

Superficial
cervical

Submental

Posterior
cervical

Submaxillary

Supraclavicular

Deep
cervical
chain

Fig. 2-4 Lymph nodes of the head and neck. (Bates B: A Guide to Physical Examination, p 29. Philadelphia, JB Lippincott, 1974)

The technical aspect of locating enlarged lymph nodes is relatively simple. Understanding the clinical significance of the enlarged node requires more knowledge and clinical experience. If a clinician examines all his patients for enlarged cervical lymph nodes, he will notice that many have palpable nodes. A majority of these will be old, fibrotic nodes from past oral or pharyngeal infections. Clinically, it is important to distinguish old, fibrotic nodes from nodes enlarged due to active disease.

Lymph nodes enlarged from infection are relatively easy to distinguish from fibrotic nodes. The patient may give a history of recent rapid enlargement. The nodes will be tender to the touch, and the overlying skin may be red and warm.

Neoplastic nodes are more difficult to distinguish from fibrotic nodes. They are usually not painful, and when they are small the patient will be unaware of their presence. Classically, nodes enlarged due to cancer are described as "fixed to underlying tissues." This is true in advanced disease when the malignant cells break out of the lymph node capsule and send out projections tying the nodes to the surrounding connective tissue. Unfortunately, patients diagnosed using this

criterion are usually terminal and have large untreatable lesions. More subtle, earlier changes include gradually enlarging lymph nodes with no signs or symptoms of localized infection. This is especially important in the detection of lymphoma, in which the first sign is often enlargement of the cervical nodes. The 5-year survival rate for Hodgkin's lymphoma approximates 90% if the diagnosis is made when only one lymph node chain is involved. Early detection gives an excellent chance for cure, and the dentist who routinely examines the neck considerably increases the chances of survival of a patient with early Hodgkin's disease.

Some clinicians discount any significance to the finding of gradually enlarging nodes if the patient gives no history of systemic symptoms. Systemic symptoms rarely occur in early lymphoma. A patient with recently enlarging nodes and systemic symptoms most likely has a self-limiting infection. Asymptomatic patients with enlarging nodes should raise a strong suspicion of lymphoma or other malignancy.

Diseases other than lymphoma may cause gradually enlarging nodes. Hodgkin's lymphoma is emphasized here because it is curable and may be suspected on the basis of a

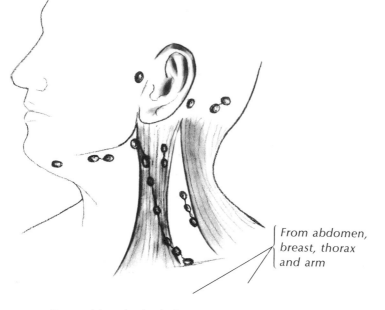

External lymphatic drainage

Internal lymphatic drainage (*e.g., from mouth and throat*)

Fig. 2-5 Lymphatic drainage of the head and neck. (Bates B: A Guide to Physical Examination, p 29. Philadelphia, JB Lippincott, 1974)

lymph node examination and history only. Metastatic carcinoma, detected as enlarging neck nodes, may be the first sign of disease in patients with primary carcinoma. This is especially true in cases of primary carcinoma in difficult to detect primary sites such as the nasopharynx or base of the tongue. Sarcoidosis, collagen diseases, and immune diseases may also cause gradual lymph node enlargement. These diseases are discussed in detail in Chapters 18 and 24.

The dentist who includes examination of the neck as part of a routine dental examination provides an important service to his patients. The examination aids in detecting undiagnosed systemic disease, which may affect dental treatment as well as increase the possibility of early diagnosis of cancer.

Examination of Cranial Nerve Function

In evaluating patients with oral sensory or motor complaints, it is important to know whether there is any objective evidence of abnormality of cranial nerve function that might relate to the patient's oral symptoms. A definitive answer to this question usually comes from specific testing of cranial nerve function as part of a routine general physical examination carried out either by the patient's general physician, an internist, or neurologist. Although the value of such a detailed examination of cranial nerve function cannot be questioned, there are certainly occasions when the dentist needs to know whether cranial nerve function is intact, yet the results of the physician's careful examination may not be immediately available. On these occasions, a superficial examination of cranial nerve function carried out by the dentist himself may help direct diagnostic efforts until the neurologist's or internist's report is available. The following schema (Table 2-1) is provided with such circumstances in mind and not as a substitute for a thorough neurologic examination carried out by a skilled specialist.

On the other hand, as described earlier, more and more dentists and oral surgeons

Table 2-1. A Summary of Cranial Nerve Examinations

CRANIAL NERVE	FUNCTION	USUAL COMPLAINT	TEST OF FUNCTION	PHYSICAL FINDINGS
I (Olfactory)	Smell	None or loss of "taste" if bilateral	Sense of smell with each nostril tested individually	No smell
II (Optic)	Vision	Loss of vision	Visual acuity Visual fields of each eye	Decreased visual acuity or loss of visual field
III (Oculomotor)	Eye movement Pupillary constriction	Double vision	Pupil and eye movement	Failure to move eye in field of motion of muscle Pupillary abnormalities
IV (Trochlear)	Eye movement	Double vision, especially on down and medial gaze	Ability to move eye down and in	May be difficult to detect anything if 3rd nerve intact
V (Trigeminal)	Facial, nasal and oral sensation Jaw movement	Numbness Paresthesia	Pinprick sensation on face Corneal reflex Masseter contraction	Decreased pin and absent corneal reflex, weakness of masticatory muscles
VI (Abducens)	Eye movement	Double vision on lateral gaze	Move eyes laterally	Failure of eye to abduct
VII (Facial)	Facial movement	Lack of facial movement, eye closure Dysarthria	Facial contraction Smiling	Asymmetry of facial contraction
VIII (Auditory and vestibular)	Hearing Balance	Hearing loss Tinnitus Vertigo	Hearing test Nystagmus Balance	Decreased hearing Nystagmus Ataxia
IX (Glossopharyngeal)	Palatal movement	Trouble with swallowing	Elevation of palate	Asymmetric palate
X (Vagus)	Palatal movement Vocal cords	Hoarseness Trouble swallowing	Elevation of palate Vocal cords	Asymmetric palate Brassy voice
XI (Spinal accessory)	Turns neck	None	Contraction of sternocleidomastoid and trapezius	Paralysis of sternocleidomastoid muscle
XII (Hypoglossal)	Moves tongue	Dysarthria	Protrusion of tongue	Wasting and fasciculation or deviation of tongue

(Adapted from Tyler HR: A summary of cranial nerve examinations. In Sonis S, Jandinski J [eds]: The neurological examination In symposium on physical and laboratory diagnosis. Dent Clin North Am 18:25, 1977)

working in hospitals are being called upon to take responsibility for the admitting history and physical examination of their patients. In view of the focus of interest of dentists and oral surgeons, it is logical that the physical examination they carry out should be complete as far as the head and neck are concerned. Under such circumstances, examination of neurologic function in other regions of the body would also be performed. If confronted with such situations, or if one is interested to learn more about the evaluation and interpretation of cranial nerve function than this brief section can provide, a variety of texts on both the general physical and neurologic examination are available, representative examples of which are included in the bibliography.

In addition to the detailed evaluation of cranial nerve function performed by the neurologist, several techniques of special interest in oral sensory and motor evaluation may provide special information about cranial nerve function in the orofacial region. These approaches have been discussed by Bosma in an excellent review, and when used by the dentist in the evaluation of various oral dysfunctions, it is likely that the information gained can be superior to that provided by the neurologist's routine examination. In other words, the dentist's professional training and experience give him a specialized knowledge of the range of normal oral function that provides a dimension of accuracy and refinement not available to one less experienced in examination of the mouth. For this reason, instruction and experience in the evaluation of cranial nerve function, particularly as it relates to the oral cavity (*e.g.,* cranial nerves V, VII, IX, X, and XII), is fully justified as part of a dentist's education.

The routine cranial nerve evaluation is systematically carried out according to the sequence of cranial nerves from I to XII. Each examiner will develop his own routine for this procedure, but it should always be standardized so that the results of repeated examinations carried out at different times will be comparable and that all functions are tested on each occasion. Similar considerations apply to the evaluation of spinal nerve functions, and the cranial nerve examination is often integrated into a standardized routine of the general neurologic examination.

Olfactory Nerve (I)

Olfactory nerve function is traditionally tested by closing one of the patient's nostrils with a finger and asking him if he can smell a strongly scented volatile substance such as coffee or lemon extract. The test is then repeated for the other nostril. The patient should sniff strongly to draw the volatile molecules well into the nose. Such a procedure tests for olfactory nerve function only when the nasal airway is patent to the olfactory receptors and when the substance being tested does not produce a response from the patient solely on the basis of chemical irritation of nonspecific somatic sensory receptors in the nasal mucosa. Such responses are due to stimulation of branches of the trigeminal nerve. For this reason, substances such as ammonia, perfumes (because of alcoholic content), and onions, although strongly scented, cannot be used to test for olfactory function. A compact "scratch and sniff" test (suitable for clinical use) that uses 50 different microencapsulated olfactory stimulants (UPSIT) has recently been developed by the University of Pennsylvania Clinical Smell and Taste Research Center for more accurate and comprehensive testing of olfactory function (see also Chap. 16).

Optic Nerve (II)

Optic nerve function is tested by investigation of visual acuity and the visual fields. In addition, those trained in the use of the ophthalmoscope can use this instrument to examine the ocular fundus directly for lesions. Visual acuity is tested with the familiar wall chart but can also be evaluated by asking the patient to read print of various sizes in a book or newspaper held at various distances from the patient's eyes.

Gross defects in the field of vision can be detected by having the patient indicate how close to the midline a pencil held in the observer's hand must be brought before it can be seen. For this test, known as the *confrontation test,* hold the pencil 2 to 3 feet to one side of the patient's face while the patient covers the other eye. Move the pencil in turn along the main axes of the field of vision until the patient can see it.

Ocular Nerves (III, IV, VI)

The three ocular nerves are concerned with the pupillary reflex (III), accommodations (III), and eye movements (III, IV, and VI), and they are tested simultaneously by examining the size, outline, and reaction of each pupil to light and dark and to accommodation for near and far vision. Conjugate eye movements, individual eye movements, and convergent vision (all under the control of bilateral extraocular eye muscles) are tested by having the patient follow the path of a pencil held at a distance and close up, as it traverses right to left and up and down movements.

Trigeminal Nerve (V)

The trigeminal nerve is tested for both motor and sensory function. The small *motor* branch of this nerve supplies the muscles of mastication, and the strength of these muscles is used as a measure of the intactness of their motor supply. The force of contraction and muscle bulk (motor loss leads to laxity and muscle atrophy) of the masseter and temporal muscles are noted by external palpation of these muscles bilaterally while the patient clenches. Lateral movement of the jaw against the examiner's finger is one test of pterygoid function. Weakness of temporalis, masseter, and pterygoids may also manifest itself in deviation of the jaw when the patient opens his mouth. (Disorders of the temporomandibular joint may produce similar signs, however, with instability of the jaw to passive displacement at the temporomandibular joint resulting in easy subluxation of the joint.)

Another useful test of motor power of the masticatory muscles is their ability to carry out voluntary displacement of the jaw against the imposed resistance of the examiner's hand. Place your thumb on the molar table with fingers externally about the body and ramus. The patient moves the jaw forward, sideways, and upward, his head steadied by your other hand.

Abnormalities of the jaw jerk may indicate muscular weakness or an abnormality of the proprioceptive reflex arc controlling jaw movements. Press your index finger downward and posteriorly above the mental eminence, and lightly strike the finger with a percussion hammer or with one or two fingers of the other hand. A single reflex response can usually be discerned by palpation in normal subjects. The principle is the same as that underlying the more familiar knee-jerk test.

Sensory function of the trigeminal nerve should logically be tested for all three divisions (ophthalmic, maxillary, and mandibular), but testing is often focused on the corneal reflex to touch (ophthalmic division), rather cursory testing of touch and pinprick sensation on the facial skin, and often no testing of the intraoral mucosa. The dentist's interest in orofacial problems will often require more detailed evaluation of intraoral sensitivity and skin sensitivity for the lower half of the face; however, complete evaluation of all sensory modalities subserved by branches of the 5th cranial nerve (pain, touch, temperature, two-point discrimination, and taste—*i.e.,* gustatory fibers of 7th cranial nerve traveling with the lingual branch of the 5th nerve) is rarely possible and is usually attempted only as part of a thorough research investigation.

A variety of instruments are available as aids in sensory evaluation, and many can be adapted for testing of trigeminal sensory function: (graded von Frey hairs, a series of fine hairs or nylon fibers calibrated according to the force required to bend the filament when it is placed against skin, mucosa, or tooth; two-point esthesiometers often designed with a pistol grip to facilitate placement of the points of the instrument on the oral mucosa (similar testing can be carried out with a simple caliper); calibrated thermal devices for application of hot and cold; discs of sandpaper of various grades for evaluation of textural differences; stereognostic forms for evaluation of oral stereotactic ability; and two-dimensional maps of the oral mucosa on which sensory response about a lesion or area of paresthesia can be accurately recorded. (Taste testing techniques are described in Chap. 16.) Abnormalities in any of these various modalities of trigeminal sensory function may be taken as evidence of an abnormality of the affected branch of the 5th cranial nerve and provide additional evidence for the diagnosis of neuropathy that may be suggested by the patient's subjective report of paresthesia, pain, numbness, or other unusual sensation.

Facial Nerve (VII)

The facial nerve is tested for abnormalities of motor function involving the "mimetic" muscles of facial expression and also for gustatory disorders (see Chap. 16). A gustosalivary reflex involves facial nerve gustatory stimuli and increased salivary function, and affections of the chorda tympani may be associated with failure of salivary flow to increase following application of lemon juice or citric acid to the affected side of the mouth.

Motor function of the 7th cranial nerve is tested by observing facial muscle function in response to requests to wrinkle the forehead, frown, close the eyelids tightly, wink, open the mouth, retract the mouth, blow out the cheeks, pucker the lips, screw up the nose, whistle, and speak. Close observation and comparison of the right and left sides may be necessary to detect minor degrees of facial paralysis; in other patients the defect will be obvious and disfiguring.

Acoustic Nerve (VIII)

Acoustic nerve function includes both cochlear (hearing) and vestibular (balance) components, which are physiologically distinct and tested separately. Hearing may be tested at three levels of sophistication:

1. By observing the patient's ability to hear normal speech and a whisper, or the ticking of a watch held at varying distances from each ear
2. With one or more tuning forks held near each ear, on the mastoid process, and on the forehead (allowing separation of nerve and conduction deafness as well as identification of unilateral defects)
3. Most precisely, by means of audiometric testing

Simple tests for vestibular function include the past-pointing test and observation for the eye movements characteristic of nystagmus (a fast jerk to the direction indicated followed by a slow return to the midline, with or without rotary movements of the eyeball) when the patient is asked to look to one side and then upward. More elaborate studies of vestibular function involve tests for the occurrence of past-pointing, nystagmus and vertigo, and nausea when cold water or a blast of cold air is injected into the external auditory canal of the upright patient.

Glossopharyngeal Nerve (IX)

The glossopharyngeal nerve provides taste fibers to the posterior aspect of the tongue (tests are described in Chap. 16), somatic sensory fibers to the same area of the tongue as well as pharynx and soft palate (tested along with 10th nerve sensory function, see below), and motor fibers to the stylopharyngeus muscle that plays only a minor role in palatal function, preventing any accurate testing of 9th cranial nerve motor function.

Vagus Nerve (X)

The vagus nerve is the chief motor nerve of the pharynx and larynx and also provides sensory fibers to the pharyngeal and faucial mucous membrane. Routine testing is carried out by observation of pharyngeal movements (e.g., symmetrical elevation of the soft palate and shortening of the uvula when the patient says "ah") and the pharyngeal or gag reflex (i.e., contraction of the palate and faucial muscles in response to touching the mucosa of the posterior pharynx). (With the use of a topical analgesic spray the gag reflex may be temporarily eliminated and the soft palate and pharynx palpated manually for masses and muscular tonus.) Since the major clinical problem associated with 10th cranial nerve dysfunction is dysphagia, more detailed evaluation of this nerve's function can include careful observation of swallowing. The laryngeal component of the vagus nerve is studied by inspection of laryngeal function with indirect laryngoscopy (head lamp and dental mirror with tongue extended) and by various vocal tests of phonation. Pulse and respiratory rates are measures of the visceral component of the vagus nerve, although a variety of other factors also affect these rates.

Spinal Accessory Nerve (XI)

The spinal accessory nerve is tested through its motor supply to the trapezius and sternomastoid muscles. For the trapezius, ask the patient to shrug his shoulders against the resistance of your hands; for the sternomastoid, to turn and flex his head against the same resistance.

Hypoglossal Nerve (XII)

The hypoglossal nerve provides motor supply to the tongue; hypoglossal paralysis causes deviation of the tongue when the patient extrudes it. Atrophy of the tongue musculature may be noted on oral examination and its muscular tonus by the force with which the patient can push the tongue against either cheek or by evaluation of the tongue jerk. Dyskinesia such as may occur in parkinsonism and amyotrophic lateral sclerosis is observed on the dorsal surface of the tongue, particularly when the tongue comes to the rest position after vigorous or forceful activity. Crenation of the margin of the tongue caused by forceful and persistent molding of the organ against irregular lingual surfaces of the dental arch is frequently seen in neurologically normal patients and is difficult to evaluate as a sign of lingual atrophy. More often than not, crenation is the result of muscle tension that may also be manifest in other parts of the body or may accompany severe malocclusion. Occasionally, it may be due to true macroglossia. (See Chapter 10.)

Special Examination of Other Organ Systems

The compact anatomy of the head and neck and the close relationship between oral function and that of the contiguous nasal, otic, laryngopharyngeal, and ocular structures require that evaluation of an oral problem must often be combined with evaluation of one or more of these related organ systems. For detailed evaluation of these extraoral systems, the dentist should request that the patient consult the appropriate medical specialist who is informed of the reason for the consultation. The usefulness of this consultation will usually depend on the dentist's knowledge of the interaction of the oral cavity with adjacent organ systems as well as the ability to recognize symptoms and signs of disease in the extraoral regions of the head and neck. Superficial inspection of these extraoral tissues is therefore a logical part of the dentist's examination for the causes of certain oral problems.

Disorders of the temporomandibular joint, referred pain, oropharyngeal and skin cancer screening, dysgeusia, salivary gland disease, postsurgical oropharyngeal and oronasal defects, and various congenital syndromes affecting the head and neck are all conditions that frequently are brought to the dentist's attention and require him to look beyond the oral cavity in his examination of the head and neck. The details of special examination of the ears, nose, eyes, pharynx, larynx, and facial musculature and integument are beyond the scope of this chapter, but the reader concerned with the evaluation of any of the problems listed above is advised to consult texts dealing with physical examination of these organs and to obtain training in the use of the head lamp, otoscope, and ophthalmoscope as well as techniques such as indirect laryngoscopy and the inspection of the nasal cavity. Knowledge of disease processes affecting these organ systems is also a prerequisite.

The dentist's initial evaluations of extraoral tissues do not infringe on the rights of, or reduce the professional activities of other medical specialists, and they can contribute significantly to collaboration of dentist and physician in the management of many oral problems. Provided the patient's permission is obtained before these nonsurgical procedures are carried out, there would seem to be no legal bar to the dentist's examining these extraoral organ systems, *although, in general, he is prohibited by law from making a specific diagnosis for, and treating extraoral problems.* In all cases where there is any concern about the presence of disease in any of these extraoral organ systems, of course, seek referral and treatment for the patient from the appropriate medical service. To clearly indicate the preliminary nature of your examination of extraoral tissues and that your area of legal diagnostic competency is restricted to the oral cavity, record and describe the results of the extraoral examination as *impressions* and not as *diagnosis;* moreover, carefully record attempts at making appropriate referral to a physician when the presence of systemic disease is suspected.

A useful compendium summarizing commonly used physical and laboratory examinations for these various organ systems, as well as some discussion of diseases of dental and oral significance affecting these tissues is provided by Sonis and Jandinski.

Laboratory Studies

Laboratory studies are an extension of the physical examination in which tissue, blood, urine, or other specimens are obtained from the patient and subjected to microscopic, biochemical, microbiological, or immunologic examination. With increasing knowledge concerning the variety of diseases affecting the oral cavity, greater use can be made of information obtained from such laboratory tests in identifying the nature of a patient's disease. A laboratory test alone rarely establishes the nature of an oral lesion, but when interpreted in conjunction with information obtained from the history and the physical examination, the results of laboratory tests will frequently establish or confirm a diagnostic impression. Specimens obtained directly from the oral cavity (*e.g.*, scrapings of oral mucosal cells, tissue biopsy, and swabs of exudates) as well as the specimens more commonly submitted to the clinical diagnostic laboratory (*e.g.*, blood, urine) may provide information of value in the diagnosis of oral lesions: demonstration of yeasts and mycelia in a Gram-stained scraping of the oral mucosa is necessary to confirm a diagnosis of oral candidiasis (thrush); demonstration of a significant titer of serum heterophil antibody and of the characteristic changes in the numbers and types of circulating leukocytes is necessary to establish a diagnosis of infectious mononucleosis as an explanation for oral lesions attributed to this disease.

Since lesions of the oral cavity are often either complicated by or the result of coexistent systemic disease, many of the laboratory studies needed in dental practice are those widely used in medicine. The systemic disease that the dentist suspects is usually of greater significance to the patient than the oral lesion with which he presented, and in investigating a problem of this type, the dentist is in effect investigating a medical problem. For this reason, it has been argued that the patient in whom systemic disease is suspected should be referred to a physician without further tests being ordered by the dentist. This procedure is clearly the correct one under some circumstances, and professional judgment is required. However, in the following situations, laboratory studies made by the dentist prior to medical referral are appropriate and may be necessary if the nature of the patient's problem is to be identified.

1. Diseases affecting the oral cavity often exhibit features peculiar to this region, and a dentist trained in the management of diseases of the oral cavity may well be better equipped to select appropriate laboratory tests and evaluate their results than is a physician with no specific knowledge of the region. For example, a dentist is unlikely to submit a swab of the oral mucosa for routine microbiological testing because he knows that this procedure rarely provides any information of diagnostic significance in reference to the mouth. A physician, however, who is accustomed to obtaining valuable information by similar testing of pharyngeal swabs will frequently carry out such a test. Similarly, biopsy specimens of lesions peculiar to the oral cavity (*e.g.*, median rhomboid glossitis and the calcifying odontogenic tumor of Pindborg) may be misdiagnosed by a pathologist who is unfamiliar with lesions of the oral cavity.

2. Referral of a patient to a physician can solve the dentist's diagnostic problem only when the patient accepts the referral. If the lesion is only minor or if the patient is unwilling to admit to himself that the lesion may be of systemic origin, then he may reject the dentist's advice, delay in following up the referral, or even seek treatment elsewhere. Failure to follow up a referral may sometimes stem from the patient's belief that the dentist is straying beyond his area of competence, but is more often the result of anxiety created by the dentist's suggesting that the patient may have an undiagnosed medical problem.

Referral to a physician is therefore often possible only when confidence is firmly established between dentist and patient. Patients who seem unwilling to accept referral to a physician often agree to a simple laboratory test (urine sugar, blood sugar, hematocrit) carried out in the dentist's office. When the results of such tests are positive, they strengthen the dentist's recommendation and often achieve the desired referral. In modern society the results of a test (*i.e.*, "science") sometimes carry more weight than the advice of a professionally trained individual.

3. A dentist will usually refer a patient to a physician only when he has a strong conviction that the patient has a systemic problem. Such conviction may be based on failure of a patient's gingival tissues to respond to a periodontal treatment that is usually effective or on some other unusual sign or symptom observed. If the patient otherwise appears well, the dentist may lack the courage of his convictions and delay referral, hoping that the problem is only transitory. The results of simple laboratory tests carried out by the dentist can often confirm suspicions that the patient has an undiagnosed medical problem and thus strengthen belief that a referral is necessary.

4. When a patient presents to a dentist with a specific oral diagnostic problem, the dentist can easily introduce laboratory tests as a necessary part of his diagnostic procedure, provided that he explains the need for the tests to the patient. If the patient elects to have the tests performed by his own physician or by a clinical diagnostic laboratory, then the dentist has already achieved his goal. If the patient prefers to have the dentist perform a simple test, the dentist will find that the procedure will be tolerated as long as it is carried out as competently and skillfully as he performs his usual dental procedures. When a dentist suspects a medical problem, even though the patient is unaware of it and does not have any unusual oral problems, the introduction of laboratory testing and even medical referral may be more difficult. Problems of this type can be solved by introducing *screening examination of selected groups of patients* into the practice.

Epidemiologic study of disease has shown that some diseases (*e.g.,* diabetes, anemia, tuberculosis, tertiary syphilis, coronary heart disease, and certain cancers) may be present for many years without the patient being aware that he is ill. Studies that have been well summarized in a World Health Organization (WHO) monograph have also shown that simple laboratory tests (*e.g.,* measurement of blood sugar concentration, hematocrit, chest x-rays) may detect these diseases at this early stage when they are presumably easier to treat and less likely to progress to incapacitating disease. Although screening tests of this type have usually been carried out by physicians or public health authorities, they are applicable to any defined population with a high degree of susceptibility to one or more of these diseases. Patients regularly attending dental clinics or private dental offices constitute such a population. Screening programs for hyperglycemia (detection of diabetes) as described by Pride and Demp, hypertension, and carriers of beta-hemolytic streptococci (rheumatic fever prevention; as described by Franchi and colleagues) have been carried out by groups of dentists in cooperation with public health authorities. Many of these tests do not require a trained medical technologist and are well within the abilities of a dentist and assistants. Table 2-2 lists a few simple tests that can be incorporated into the routine work-up of patients attending dental clinics and offices and indicates the population sample to which they might profitably be applied. (Details of these tests are included in Chap. 3.)

It must be stressed that screening tests of this type and, in fact, the majority of studies carried out by dentists for detection of systemic diseases do not themselves constitute a diagnosis. For example, a dentist who finds sugar in the urine of a patient should *not* tell him that he has diabetes, but should inform him that the results of the test indicated an abnormality and that he should seek medical consultation. Abnormal results for any of the tests should be sent directly to the patient's physician, and the diagnosis of diabetes, hypertension, or other disease should be made by the physician on the basis of physical examination, history, and possibly further laboratory tests. Management of any systemic problem detected is also within the province of the physician, and the dentist should not consider prescribing medication or other treatment for systemic disease detected in this way, even though he might be required to provide local care for the oral manifestations. The physician may decide that in the latent stage of the disease only surveillance and advice to the patient are required.

The success of all screening for systemic disease, whether carried out by the public

Table 2-2. Screening Tests Used In Dentistry to Determine Latent Systemic Disease

TEST	DISEASE	SUITABLE POPULATION SAMPLE
Blood pressure and pulse rate	Hypertension Cardiovascular disease	All adult patients
Microhematocrit	Anemia	All patients over 50 All patients scheduled for general anesthesia or multiple dental extractions
Urine sugar and 2-hour postprandial blood sugar (Dextrostix)	Diabetes	Obese patients All patients over 50 Patients with strong family history of diabetes
Bleeding time and tourniquet test	Bleeding problems	Patient with history of excessive bleeding after oral surgery Patients with history of frequent bruising
Hepatitis B$_s$ antigen	Hepatitis B carrier state	Patients with history of hepatitis, renal dialysis; male homosexuals; travelers from areas of endemic infection; patients from mental institutions and prisons; patients with Down's syndrome; immunocompromised patients

health authorities or by dentists, depends upon the availability of physicians willing to accept such referrals. When ordering or carrying out a laboratory test for detection of systemic disease, always consider what can practically be done with the results of the test. Laboratory testing without follow-up is not only futile but can lead to serious anxiety in the patient. (Specific laboratory tests are discussed in detail in the next chapter.)

FINAL DIAGNOSIS

The final diagnosis can usually be reached following chronologic organization and critical evaluation of the information obtained from the patient's history, the physical examination, and the results of the radiologic and laboratory examinations. A critical evaluation of the assembled data obtained from the various aids to diagnosis represents the most important phase of all the diagnostic procedures.

For medicolegal reasons, the final diagnosis, as well as details of the history and the physical, radiographic, and laboratory examinations should be entered into the pa-

tient's record, and the patient or a responsible member of the patient's family informed of the diagnosis. The final diagnosis usually identifies the diagnosis for the patient's primary complaint first (*i.e.*, the stated problem for which he sought dental or medical advice), with subsidiary diagnoses of concurrent problems following, numbered 2, 3, 4, and so on. Previously diagnosed conditions that remain as actual or potential problems are also usually included, with the comment "by history," "previously diagnosed," or "treated" to indicate their status. Other problems that were identified but not clearly diagnosed during the current evaluation can also be listed with the qualification "to be ruled out" (R/O). Because oral medicine is concerned with regional problems that may or may not be modified by concurrent systemic disease it is common for final diagnoses to include both oral lesions and systemic problems of actual or potential significance in the etiology or management of the oral lesion. For example, a diagnosis might read as follows:

1. Rampant dental caries secondary to radiation-induced xerostomia

2. Carcinoma of tonsillar fossa, by history, excised and treated with 6500 rad 2 years ago
3. Cirrhosis and prolonged bleeding time, by history
4. Hyperglycemia; R/O diabetes

Following a careful review of all historical, clinical, and laboratory findings and repeated examination of the patient, a definite diagnosis cannot always be made. In such cases, use a descriptive term for the patient's symptom or lesion instead of a formal diagnostic term, with the added comment of "idiopathic" or "unexplained," or "functional" or "symptomatic" in the case of symptoms without apparent physical abnormality (see Chap. 17). The clinician must decide what terminology to use in conversing with the patient and his family and whether to clearly identify this diagnosis as a "undetermined diagnosis." Irrespective of the decision, it is important that the dentist recognize the equivocal nature of the patient's problem and the need for additional evaluation, either by referring the patient to another consultant, by additional testing, or by placing the patient on recall for follow-up studies.

In formulating a final diagnosis, one of the most difficult problems is to determine whether the chief complaint of the patient is organic or "functional," that is, a manifestation of the patient's emotional state. In making this evaluation, attempt to determine the meaning that the patient attaches to his symptoms and, more important, what possible advantage he gains from the symptoms.

Emotional reactions may be manifest during the interview by unusual concern or anxiety exhibited by the patient, such as obvious or excessive perspiration, lip-biting, and so on. The kind of language or the tone of the voice used by the patient may be significant. He may present manifestations of both organic and emotional factors, in which event the historian should determine whether the emotional factor is of major significance or whether it preceded the organic symptoms. In many instances, the evidence for local organic diseases is equivocal. If painful lesions are present, they should be treated symptomatically during the time required to complete the diagnostic procedures. The patient will have little respect for the most capable clinician if he does not alleviate pain, and with relief of pain the patient's attitudes change, anxiety subsides, and the nature of the patient's problem becomes clearer.

Patients should also be clearly informed of the results of the various examinations and tests, where they correlate with the patient's signs and symptoms, and where they clearly establish that a particular diagnostic concern of the clinician or patient has not been confirmed. Because patients' anxieties frequently emphasize the possibility of a potentially serious diagnosis, it is important to point out, when the facts allow, that the biopsy revealed no evidence of a malignant growth, the blood test revealed no abnormality, and that no evidence of diseases such as diabetes, leukemia, syphilis, or cancer was found. The patient has a right to information of this nature and is almost as grateful for it as for a specific diagnosis. Equally important is the need to explain to the patient the nature, significance, and treatment of any lesion or disease that has been clearly diagnosed.

If additional studies or consultations are required, the dentist is responsible for arranging the appointment (or giving the patient adequate instructions to enable him to make the appointment) and furnishing the consultant with a resume of the patient's history and physical findings, as well as the results of the radiologic and laboratory studies to date.

The results of diagnostic studies are confidential information and not released or discussed with anyone other than the patient without the patient's specific permission. Local or institutional custom will guide the clinician in deciding when this permission should be obtained in writing and when verbal consent is adequate. Exceptions to this general rule are made in the case of minors, where with few exceptions it is expected that the results of diagnostic findings will be discussed with the parents, and in the case of reportable infectious diseases, where the results of certain laboratory tests are public information and made available by the public health authorities to qualified individuals. When records are subpoenaed for legal use, a signed consent from the patient usually accompanies the court order.

MEDICAL RISK ASSESSMENT FOR DENTAL PATIENTS

The medical history and physical examination procedures as just described are oriented primarily toward establishing a diagnosis for a particular symptom or problem for which a patient is seeking medical or dental consultation. Equally well, these procedures are applicable to the overall *routine history and physical*, which should be carried out periodically on apparently healthy individuals as well as on patients known to have medical problems. In both of these situations the end point of the process is the formulation of a diagnosis followed by a decision whether specific treatment is required. The same history and physical examination procedures are also used to evaluate the medical status of patients scheduled to undergo general anesthesia or more elaborate diagnostic or surgical procedures (*e.g.*, the routine history and physical examination customarily carried out on all hospital inpatients usually within 24 hours of their admission). In this case, the end point of the process is an evaluation of any special risks posed by the patient's compromised medical status in the circumstance of the planned anesthetic, diagnostic, or surgical procedure. To achieve this end point, a step beyond formulation of a diagnosis is required and is referred to as *medical risk assessment*.

Medical risk assessment is the responsibility not only of physicians and dentists who admit patients to hospitals for specific anesthetic, diagnostic, or surgical procedures but also of any clinician who plans to carry out even a minor procedure of any type on an ambulatory patient basis. A routine of initial history and physical examination thus becomes essential for all dental patients because even the apparently healthy patient may on evaluation be found to have historical or examination findings of sufficient significance to cause the dentist to reevaluate the plan of treatment, modify a medication, or even postpone a particular treatment until additional diagnostic data are available. To respect the familiar medical axiom *"primum non nocere"* (first do no harm), all procedures carried out on a patient and all prescriptions or instructions given to a patient should be pre-ceded by a conscious consideration by the clinician as to the risk of the particular procedure to the patient. Medical risk assessment, by establishing a formal summary in the chart of specific risks likely to occur in treating a particular patient, ensures that continuous self-evaluation will be carried out by the clinician without his becoming paralyzed by unrealistic concerns.

Medical risk assessment in the context of dental medicine thus refers to the process of obtaining the medical history, performing a physical examination, and ordering and interpreting the laboratory, radiographic, and other data necessary to knowledgeably plan and carry out dental therapy for both inpatients and ambulatory patients. Medical risk assessment presumes the following abilities:

- To recognize significant deviations from normal health status that may affect dental management
- To make informed judgments on the risk of dental procedures to both ambulatory patients and inpatients
- To identify the need for medical consultation

Recognizing Significant Deviations from Normal Health Status that May Affect Dental Treatment

Signs and symptoms of previously undiagnosed medical problems may influence dental management as well as the assessment of the current status of patients with known medical problems. The field of oral medicine developed at a time when the use and availability of preventive medical care was much more limited than it has been in recent decades. The likelihood that routine evaluation of a patient before dental treatment will reveal a major undiagnosed medical problem is now decreased, although the dentist should always be alert to the possibility. More often now, the dentist finds himself evaluating a patient who carries one or more medical diagnoses and is under treatment for at least one chronic disease as well as other intercurrent problems. In this circumstance, the dentist must also evaluate the current status of the particular problem and assess the extent of concomitant specific organ damage and compromised physiologic function that have resulted. For example, simply knowing that a patient is diabetic provides relatively little information about his response to dental or oral surgery. The dentist must also have information concerning blood sugar levels, current medication, any recent changes of medication, hospitalizations, or other acute problems resulting from the diabetes, blood pressure levels, any evidences of arrhythmias, peripheral or cerebral vascular occlusions, evidences of delayed healing or recent infections, and the patient's anxieties about dental care.

Many patients who are under treatment for specific medical problems will also have had a recent period of hospitalization during which more extensive evaluation of these problems may have been carried out. Review of the hospital admission records (which are available to the dentist or physician who requests them from the hospital record room, enclosing a signed release from the patient) often provides a more objective measure of the extent of the patient's medical problem as well as a yardstick by which to assess any subsequent improvement or deterioration. Hospital records may also indicate any untoward events associated with surgery, anesthetic, or particular medications. The results of earlier physical and laboratory examinations are available for comparison with current findings.

In assessing the health status of any patient, the dentist may need to order additional laboratory tests to obtain current information on either the presence or severity of a given disorder. In the United States, current (1983) Joint Commission on the Accreditation of Hospitals' policies regarding the privileges of dentists who are medical staff members in hospitals allow qualified attending oral surgeons the privilege of carrying out an admission history and complete physical examination for patients without medical problems who are admitted for oral surgical care. Included is the responsibility for a physical examination that encompasses skin, head and neck, thorax and lungs, lymph nodes, heart, blood pressure and pulse, and neurologic and mental status, as well as the responsibility for ordering laboratory, radiographic, or other diagnostic procedures pertinent to particular abnormalities detected in the history or on physical examination.

When patients with known medical problems are admitted for dental care or when medical problems are detected by the dental staff or oral surgeon carrying out a physical examination, current policies assign the responsibility for medical evaluation and medical risk assessment to a physician approved by the hospital staff (see below under identifying the need for medical consultation).

Making Informed Judgments on the Risk of Dental Procedures to Both Ambulatory Patients and Inpatients

A decision to provide dental treatment or not for a medically compromised patient is traditionally arrived at by the dentist requesting the patient's physician to "clear the patient for dental care." Unfortunately, in many cases, the physician is provided with little information about the nature of the dental treatment to be carried out and may have little other than his own personal experience with dental care on which to judge the stress likely to be associated with the proposed dental treatment. The response of a given patient even to specific dental treatment situations may also be unpredictable, particularly when the patient has a number of disease processes and is maintained on a variety of medications. In addition, the practitioner identified by the patient as his physician may not have adequate or complete data from previous evaluations that are needed to make an informed judgment about the patient's likely response to dental care. All too frequently, the dentist receives the brief comment, "OK for dental care," and the absence of responses that indicates uncertainty on the part of the physician suggests that clearances are often given casually and subjectively rather than being based on objective physiologic data.

More important, the practice of having the patient "cleared" for dental care confuses the issue of responsibility for untoward events occurring during dental treatment. While in many situations the dentist must rely on the physician or other consultant for expert diagnostic information and for an opinion about the advisability of dental treatment or the need for special precautions, *the dentist retains the primary responsibility for the proce-dures actually carried out and for the immediate management of any untoward complications.* The dentist is most familiar with the procedures he is carrying out as well as their likely com-plications, but he must also be able to assess patients for medical or other problems likely to set the stage for development of compli-cations.

Identifying the Need for Medical Consultation

In the preceding sections, the occasions on which a dentist may need to obtain medical consultation on one of his patients are briefly outlined: the patient with known medical problems who is admitted to the hospital for dental treatment (or who will have similar dental treatment on an outpatient basis), the patient in whom abnormalities are detected during history-taking or on physical or labo-ratory examination, and the patient who has a high risk for development of particular medical problems. Numerous examples of situations of this type are also given through-out this text.

When there is need for a specific consul-tation, the consultant should be selected for his appropriateness to the particular prob-lem, and the problem and specific questions to be answered should be clearly transmitted to the consultant, preferably in writing. Full details of the planned dental procedure with an assessment of time, stress to the patient, and expected period of posttreatment disa-bility should be given, as well as details of the particular symptom, sign, or laboratory abnormality that occasioned the consultation.

Medical risk assessment of patients before dental treatment offers the opportunity for greatly improving dental services for patients with compromised health. It does require considerably more clinical training and un-derstanding of the natural history and clinical features of systemic disease processes than have been customarily taught in undergrad-uate dental education programs; however, partial solution to this problem has been achieved through undergraduate assign-ments in hospital dentistry and most impor-tant, through hospital-based dental general practice and oral surgery residency pro-grams. The privileges recently accorded to oral surgeons in many hospitals that have assigned them the responsibility for carrying out the history, complete physical examina-tion, and medical risk assessment of many of their patients is an indication of the achieve-ment that has been made. It is to be hoped that revisions in dental undergraduate curri-cula will recognize this need and provide greater emphasis on both the pathophysiol-ogy of systemic disease and the practical clin-ical evaluation and management of these problems in the dental student's program. More information must also be collected on the effects of particular dental treatments as well as anesthetic procedures on physiologic processes, both in health and with particular disease states.

BIBLIOGRAPHY

Alpers BJ, Mancall EL: Essentials of the Neurolog-ical Examination. Philadelphia, FA Davis, 1971

Ballinger JT, et al: Diseases of the Nose, Throat and Ear, 11th ed. Philadelphia, Lea & Febiger, 1969

Barness LA: Manual of Pediatric Physical Diag-nosis. Chicago, Year Book Medical Publishers, 1957

Barrett RA: Diagnostic laboratory test—Who needs it? J Am Soc Prev Dent 3:26, 1973

Berglund G, et al: Prevalence of primary and sec-ondary hypertension: Studies in a random pop-ulation sample. Br Med J 2:554, 1976

Berman CL, van Stewart A, Ramazzotto LT, et al: High blood pressure detection; A new public health measure for the dental profession. J Am Dent Assoc 92:116, 1976

Bird B: Talking with Patients, 2nd ed. Philadel-phia, JB Lippincott, 1973

Boies LR, Hilger JA, Priest RE: Fundamentals of Otolaryngology, 4th ed. Philadelphia, WB Saun-ders, 1967

Bosma JF: Sensorimotor examination of the mouth and pharynx. Front Oral Physiol 2:78, 1976

Chapman WE: Automated multitest laboratories. Needs and potential. Postgrad Med 52:41, 1972

Cobb S: Technic of interviewing a patient with psychosomatic disorder. Med Clin North Am 28:1210, 1944

Falace DA: Physical evaluation of the dental pa-tient. Current practices and opinions. J Dent Educ 42:537, 1978

Franchi GJ, Rennquist KC, Yarashus DA: The den-tist's role in the primary prevention of rheumatic fever. Report of the Stickney Public Health District's 3-year dental study on throat cultures. J Am Dent Assoc 75:1389, 1967

Goepfert H: The diagnosis of neck mass. Continuing Educ :31, 1981

Greene DA: Localized cervical lymphadenopathy induced by diphenylhydantoin sodium. Arch Otolaryngol 101:446, 1975

Halstead CL, et al: Physical Evaluation of the Dental Patient. St Louis, CV Mosby, 1982

Hussey HH: Lymphadenopathy induced by diphenylhydantoin. JAMA 233:61, 1975

Joint Commission on Accreditation of Hospitals: Medical staff privileges. In Accreditation Manual for Hospitals, p 97, 1982

King GE: Taking the blood pressure. JAMA 209:1902, 1969

Kirkendall WM, et al: Recommendations for human blood pressure determination by sphygmomanometers. Circulation 36:980, 1967

Krupp MA, Chatton MJ: Current Medical Diagnosis and Treatment. Los Altos, Lange Medical Publishers, 1973

Land M: Management of emotional illness in dental practice. J Am Dent Assoc 73:631, 1966

Langen D: Diagnoses based on verbal expressions. Dtsch Med Wochenschr 82:1006, 1957

Leadingham RS: The medical history. Ann Intern Med 27:929, 1948

Mann GV: The influence of obesity on health. N Engl J Med 291:178, 226, 1974

Mitchell DF: Recent developments and advances in oral diagnosis. Prac Dent Mono, January, p 30, 1965

Morris AL: The medical history in dental practice. J Am Dent Assoc 74:129, 1967

Overly TM: Discovering the functional illness in interview. JAMA 186:116, 1963

Pickney ER: Role of the dentist in the detection of non-dental diseases. J Am Dent Assoc 50:185, 1955

Pillsbury DM: A Manual of Dermatology. Philadelphia, WB Saunders, 1971

Pride TA, Demp SD: The incidence of patients with diabetes seen in a dental outpatient clinic. Pa Dent J 32:144, 1965

Romriell GE, Streeper SN: The medical history. Dent Clin North Am 26:3, 1982

Russell AS, Taragoza AJ, Shea R: Mucocutaneous lymph node syndrome in Canada. Can Med Assoc J 112:1210, 1975

Sabes WR, Blozis GG: The clinical laboratory—What it means to you and your patients. J Am Soc Prev Dent 3:33, 1973

Scheie HG, Albert DM: Adler's Textbook of Ophthalmology, 8th ed. Philadelphia, WB Saunders, 1969

Sonis ST, Jandinski JJ (eds): Symposium on physical and laboratory diagnosis. Dent Clin North Am 18: Jan, 1974

Stamler J: High blood pressure in the United States—An overview of the problem and the challenge. Proc Nat Conf High Blood Pressure Education. DHEW Pub # NIH 73-486, 1973

Stevenson I: The Diagnostic Interview, 2nd ed. New York, Harper & Row, 1971

Suomi JD, Horowitz HS, Barbano JP: Self-reported systemic conditions in an adult study population. J Dent Res 54:1092, 1975

Trieger N, Goldblatt L: The art of history taking. J Oral Surg 36:118, 1978

Veterans Administration Cooperative Study on Antihypertensive Agents: Effects of treatment on morbidity in hypertension. II. Results in patients with diastolic blood pressure averaging 90 through 114 mm Hg. JAMA 213:1143, 1970

Vidic B, Melloni BJ: Applied anatomy of the oral cavity and related structures. Otolaryngol Clin North Am 12:3, 1979

Weider A, et al: Cornell medical index: A method for quickly assaying personality and psychosomatic disturbances in men in the armed forces. War Med 7:209, 1945

Woodworth JV: Interrelationship of medicine and dentistry. JADA 68:259, 1964

3

Diagnostic Laboratory Procedures

VERNON J. BRIGHTMAN

Microbiology, Serology, and Immunology
   Demonstration of Microorganisms in
      Oral Tissues Sampled by Means of
      Smears
   Caries Activity Test
   Phase-Contrast and Dark-Field Micro-
      scopic Examination of the Micro-
      bial Flora from Plaque and Gingival
      Crevice
   Bacterial Cultures in Endodontics

Microbial Isolation and Antibiotic Sen-
   sitivity Testing
Laboratory Tests for Syphilis
Tests for Beta-Hemolytic Streptococ-
   cal Infections
Serologic Tests for Chronic Candidal
   Infections
Virus Isolation and Serology
Laboratory Procedures in Suspected
   Collagen Autoimmune Diseases

The role of diagnostic laboratory procedures in the evaluation of the dental patient was outlined in Chapter 2 and is referred to in many sections of this text dealing with particular oral and systemic diseases. This chapter describes in detail laboratory tests of interest to the dentist, as well as specific indications for these tests in situations that are likely to arise in dental practice. No attempt has been made to cover the full range of tests used in the evaluation of systemic disease, but those that are often used as indices of the presence or severity of systemic disease of dental interest have been included. For further information, the reader should consult standard references on clinical laboratory diagnostic procedures.

Diagnostic laboratory procedures include simple tests that can be carried out conveniently in the office or the clinic and those that require the services of a trained medical technician working in a specially equipped laboratory. Depending on the circumstances and the particular information needed about a patient, one of these approaches may be more appropriate. With the variety of procedures now available from diagnostic laboratories and the routine use in laboratories of quality controls to ensure the accuracy of tests, greater emphasis is usually placed on tests performed in licensed diagnostic laboratories. Office procedures have not been entirely superseded, however. A number of tests must still be carried out in the office or at the bedside, and selected office procedures are still important in the diagnosis and management of some conditions.

Office tests (also referred to as *chairside tests* in the dental literature) require only simple and relatively inexpensive equipment and can usually be performed with an acceptable degree of accuracy without extensive specialized training. In tests of this type, simplicity and rapidity are more important than accuracy, and the results should be interpreted with this in mind. Positive findings should usually be confirmed before the patient is told of any abnormality. Conversely, in the face of strong clinical evidence of a systemic abnormality, a single negative test should not bar further medical evaluation.

Diagnostic laboratory technology has changed considerably over the past 20 years, and many procedures, such as blood counts and blood chemistry determinations that were previously performed manually, are now being provided by automated multitest machines that provide as many as 20 separate determinations on a single sample of blood. This automation and increased speed have been matched with an increased demand for accuracy and quality control by both clinicians and third-party payors and a need to control the costs of laboratory tests. Many specimens currently submitted to a licensed diagnostic laboratory are analyzed with sophisticated equipment often with on-line connections to a computer that scans the test results and maintains them within a high level of accuracy before storing the information for immediate or subsequent retrieval. Diagnostic laboratories in hospitals and communities are now often large facilities that may process tens of thousands of specimens daily (to offset costs of the equipment) under the supervision of a pathologist and a small staff of highly trained technicians.

Under these circumstances, problems usually arise from errors in sampling and handling of specimens and improper labeling of containers, rather than from technical laboratory errors. When using a diagnostic laboratory, a clinician must be aware of not only the particular laboratory value needed but also of the recommended method for obtaining and handling the specimen, the laboratory's requirements regarding submission of specimens for testing, and the need for accurate labeling of specimens.

Even when all precautions are observed, the result of a single laboratory examination should be accepted judiciously, especially when it is at variance with the clinical history and physical findings. The result of a single laboratory test is always less significant than the study of a series of examinations made at appropriate intervals. In many circumstances it is still considered important to confirm an abnormal laboratory test result by subsequently obtaining a second specimen, although the need for second specimens clearly decreases as laboratory testing becomes more accurate. Rarely, conflicting data from clinical examination and laboratory tests may result from the coexistence of two separate diseases.

Automated multitest laboratory procedures offer additional advantages of being able to handle small specimen volumes, providing updated ranges of normal values, and keeping the cost of routine hematologic and blood chemistry tests low. A clinician may initially be confused by the plethora of data contained on a multitest report, but developments in the design of data printouts and "starring" of significant abnormalities have made analysis of these data easier.

Multitest laboratory reports often draw attention to the presence of significant systemic abnormalities that may have been undetected by the history and clinical examination. The information about individual patients that is obtained in this way should not be looked on as a waste product of the age of automation because evidence shows that certain chronic diseases can be predicted through laboratory tests before they are clinically apparent. Tests

carried out at an American Medical Association (AMA) convention indicated that of men between 30 and 65 years of age whose living habits and stress parallel those of physicians, 20% showed abnormalities of carbohydrate metabolism that should be investigated for diabetes mellitus; 30% showed abnormalities of cholesterol that could be indicative of coronary and thrombotic vascular disease; 10% to 15% showed abnormalities of uric acid metabolism, and 15% showed urine and blood abnormalities pointing to renal disease. Routine serum electrophoresis on all hospital admissions in one study has also resulted in detection of an unexpected number of patients with multiple myeloma, amyloidosis, and other dysglobulinemias.

A variety of automated systems are available commercially. The Technicon Instruments Corporation,* a pioneer in this field, is probably the best known supplier of automated diagnostic laboratory equipment, although other manufacturers share the market. The 1981 *Guide to Scientific Instruments* listed 15 manufacturers of electronic blood-cell counters and 33 manufacturers of automatic clinical chemical analyzers. Whereas some of these automated systems are concerned with multiple tests run on the same blood specimen, others are semiautomatic and others carry out a single test on multiple samples. Commercially available prepackaged and proportioned reagents minimize the amount of preparation needed for operation of most automated systems and contribute to the consistency of results obtained. Examples of automated diagnostic laboratory equipment in fairly general use are described in many of the following sections of this chapter together with a description of those office procedures that have an acceptable level of accuracy or special use in patient management. Automated laboratory equipment varies from laboratory to laboratory, and the packaging of tests is determined by the particular equipment in use. Clinicians must be familiar with the general outline of procedures in the laboratory they customarily use. For the most part, in this chapter we describe procedures appropriate to the equip-

---

* Technicon Instruments Corporation, Tarrytown, NY 10591

ment we are familiar with through the hospital and commercial laboratories we currently use, with the knowledge that changes in procedure, technique, and equipment are to be expected as this field develops further.

Organization of the Diagnostic Laboratory Service. In the following sections, indications, collection of specimens, equipment, procedures, and interpretation of results are described for office procedures (smaller type). For tests to be carried out in a diagnostic laboratory, indications, specimen collection, and interpretation of results are stressed with a limited description of the laboratory procedures and equipment as needed for an understanding and interpretation of test results. For convenience, laboratory procedures are usually grouped together according to the division of the hospital laboratory service that performs a particular group of tests: hematology, blood chemistry, urinalysis, histopathology and cytology, microbiology, and immunology. This arrangement is followed in both the text and bibliography for this chapter.

Hematology refers to counting and microscopic examination of the formed elements of blood (erythrocytes, leukocytes, and platelets) as well as measurement of hemoglobin concentration and the chemical constituents of plasma that are concerned in the process of hemostasis and clot formation. *Blood chemistry* refers to individual measurement of the large number of enzymes and other chemical substances dissolved and transported in the blood serum. Similar analyses are also carried out on urine, saliva, and other body fluids. A number of important constituents of the erythrocyte as well as substances bound to the erythrocyte are also measured in the clinical chemistry laboratory. *Toxicology* refers to a rapidly expanding field devoted to the detection and measurement of medications, drugs, other abused substances, and environmental toxins in body fluids. *Histopathology and cytology* (also referred to as surgical pathology) include the microscopic examination of tissue sections and individual cells, respectively. (Microscopic examination of blood cells and bone marrow specimens is included under hematology.) *Microbiology* refers to the isolation and identification of viruses, bacteria, fungi, and protozoan and metazoan parasites obtained from infected tissues and body fluids, as well as from the skin and body orifices, which also have their own normal microbial flora. *Immunology* (serology) is the detection and quantitation of antibodies and similar substances that appear in the serum, tissues, and other body fluids in response to antigenic stimulation of both exogenous and endogenous origin; it also includes assay of both the fluid (humoral) and cellular components involved in the immune response. Because of the specificity of the antigen–antibody reaction, an increasing number of immunologic techniques are also used to assay specific protein and protein-bound chemical constituents of blood in the blood chemistry and toxicology laboratories.

Interpretation of Diagnostic Laboratory Test Results. Laboratory test results generated by automated equipment are usually returned to the clinician on a computer printout that lists the results of determinations run on the specimen and the range of normal values for each determination. This service is particularly useful because the range of normal values often differs from laboratory to laboratory, depending on the exact techniques used and the source of the specimens usually analyzed in a particular laboratory. The service also helps eliminate errors caused by a clinician's failure to accurately remember a long list of normal values. On the other hand, to be fluent in the language of medicine, a clinician still needs to commit to memory the normal adult values for the commonly used diagnostic laboratory tests. A list of normal values is provided in Table 3-1.

Many diagnostic laboratory printouts also group together the determinations that lie outside the normal range, mark them with an asterisk, or otherwise tag these results to draw them to the clinician's attention. In many cases, particular determinations require action on the part of the physician or dentist, who must interpret the particular laboratory test result in light of current clinical findings. Based on experience with a particular laboratory, a clinician learns which tagged results have clinical significance and which represent only "noise" from an automated system that of necessity is more rigid

Table 3-1. Normal Adult Values for Some Common Diagnostic Laboratory Tests

Test	Normal Value
Total RBC count	4–5.5 million/mm³ blood
Total WBC count	4–10,000/mm³ blood
Differential WBC count	Neutrophils 43–77% Lymphocytes 17–47% Monocytes 0–9% Eosinophils 0–4% Basophils 0–2%
Hemoglobin concentration	14–18 g/dl for males 12–16 g/dl for females
Hematocrit	40–50%
Platelet count	150,000–450,000/mm³ blood < 50,000, spontaneous bleeding likely
Sedimentation rate	0–20 mm/hr
Bleeding time	< 5–6 minutes
Prothrombin time	12–15 sec (80–100%) Values > 2–3 × normal (30%–50%) indicate bleeding tendency
Blood sugar	fasting 70–100 mg/dl 2-hr postprandial < 120 mg/dl
Urine (qual)	negative for sugar and protein
Serum calcium	8.8–10.5 mg/dl
Serum inorganic phosphorus	2–5 mg/dl
Serum alkaline phosphatase	1–4 Bodansky units 3–13 King–Armstrong units 30–110 IU
Serum uric acid	2–8 mg/dl
Blood urea nitrogen (BUN)	< 25 mg/dl
Serum creatinine	0.7–1.4 mg/dl
Serum protein	6–8 g/dl
Serum cholesterol	< 300 mg/dl
Serum triglycerides	< 175 mg/dl
Serum bilirubin (total)	0–1.5 mg/dl
Serum potassium	3.5–5.5 mEq/liter
Serum sodium	135–148 mEq/liter
Serum chloride	96–110 mEq/liter
Serum carbon dioxide	18–32 mEq/liter

in its interpretations of laboratory test data than is the clinician, who has additional information about the patient.

HEMATOLOGY

Collection of Blood Specimens

Capillary, venous, and arterial blood specimens are all used at times for the performance of hematologic and blood chemistry determinations; the choice depends on what values are needed. *Capillary blood specimens* are convenient for office and chairside procedures. The specimen is usually obtained by pricking the patient's finger (an earlobe or ankle pad may also be used). *Venous blood specimens* are used for the majority of determinations performed in a clinical diagnostic laboratory. Venipuncture is usually performed on an antecubital vein. In general, venipuncture provides a more representative sample that is less likely to be affected by admixture of tissue fluid or by stasis than are capillary blood samples. *Arterial blood specimens* are obtained by puncturing the radial artery (it is usually necessary to obtain superficial skin anesthesia before probing for this vessel) or through a catheter or other arterial line inserted for a diagnostic or therapeutic purpose.

Providing reasonable care is taken to preserve and handle blood specimens, the majority of tests can be performed on specimens transported to the laboratory in appropriate tubes. A few tests (*e.g.,* blood sedimentation rate and some blood clotting measurements) must be carried out on freshly drawn specimens, and some have special handling requirements.

Capillary Blood Specimens

Equipment Jar of sponges soaked in 70% alcohol; jar of dry sponges; sterile blood lancet

Procedure The palmar surface of the patient's index finger or second finger is gently rubbed with a sponge soaked with 70% alcohol, excess alcohol is wiped off, and the alcohol is allowed to evaporate. The prepared area is rapidly punctured with a blood lancet, with care taken not to squeeze the finger. The patient's hand is held at about waist level, and the first drop of blood that wells up is wiped away with a dry sponge. The next drops that appear are allowed to flow into a capillary tube appropriate for the procedure planned or are collected on a glass slide. Capillary blood samples collected in this way are usually nonsterile. An automatic spring-loaded lancet (*e.g.*, Autoclix*) may be used in place of the conventional hand-held lancet.

Venipuncture

Although a number of laboratory tests can be performed on capillary (finger-prick) blood, most hematologic and chemical determinations are performed on samples of venous blood. For this purpose, blood is obtained from a superficial antecubital vein that can be conveniently dilated by occlusion of the veins of the upper arm with a tourniquet. Blood can usually be obtained from this location with a minimum of trauma and without complication, provided an acceptable technique is learned and strictly followed.

Equipment A 10-ml or 20-ml sterile disposable syringe with a 20-gauge needle or Vacutainer,[†] needle, adaptor, and evacuated collection tubes, Velkret tourniquet or approximately 20 in of soft rubber tubing less than ½ in diameter, jar of sponges soaked in 70% alcohol, jar of dry sponges

Procedure Detailed directions for performing a venipuncture are provided in many texts. In outline, all techniques follow the same sequence, which must be kept in mind whenever a venipuncture is being carried out.

1. Prepare the patient and equipment.
2. Apply a tourniquet and select the vein to be punctured.
3. Prepare the puncture site with 70% alcohol; air dry.
4. Insert the needle through the skin and into vein.
5. Aspirate blood into a syringe or Vacutainer tube.
6. Remove the tourniquet.
7. Place a dry cotton swab over the puncture and withdraw the needle; bring patient's forearm back against his upper arm while he

maintains finger pressure on cotton at the puncture site with the other hand.

Evacuated tubes containing prepared amounts of anticoagulants or preservatives are available commercially. Blood may be collected directly into these tubes with the Vacutainer technique or injected through the stopper if the blood is collected in a syringe. Vacutainer tubes containing various anticoagulants and preservatives are identified by the stopper color. The laboratory should be consulted as to the appropriate tube to use when collecting blood for a specific test. For example, the lavender-stopper tube contains ethylenediaminetetraacetic acid (EDTA) anticoagulant, the anticoagulant of choice for preservation of formed elements of blood and for most hematologic procedures. The red-stopper tube contains no anticoagulant or preservative and is used for specimens of clotted blood. The clear, straw-colored fluid (serum) obtained by centrifuging clotted blood in the red-stopper tube is used routinely in serologic procedures (titration of antibodies) and for measurement of substances transported in the serum (*e.g.*, enzymes, calcium, phosphorus).

Changes occur in blood even when it is mixed with a preservative, and if possible, all specimens should be delivered to the laboratory within 1 to 2 hours. Clotted blood for serologic procedures may be sent by mail provided the tube is well sealed and protected from breakage; all other specimens should be hand delivered. If delivery will be delayed, blood specimens may be stored in a household refrigerator provided they are protected from freezing. Freezing and thawing of whole blood causes rapid lysis of red blood cells with release of the cellular contents (including hemoglobin) into the serum; such hemolyzed specimens are unsuitable for the majority of hematologic and blood chemistry procedures.

Many clinical diagnostic laboratories prefer to perform the differential white cell count and examination of red cell morphology on a smear of blood prepared at the time the specimen is obtained rather than from a specimen preserved some hours with EDTA or oxalate. The smear may be made either from finger-prick blood or from a drop of blood discharged from the venipuncture needle. In either case, a drop of blood is placed at one end of a clean microscope slide (1" × 3") and the slide placed on the bench. The end of a second or "pusher slide" is placed at an angle of 45 degrees to the first and gradually drawn toward the drop of blood until contact is made, and the drop spreads along the junction of the two slides. Then the tilted slide is pushed

---

* Biodynamics, Boehringer Mannheim Company, 9115 Hague Road, Indianapolis, Indiana 46250
† Becton, Dickinson & Company, Rutherford, NJ 07070

smoothly and rapidly away from the drop, producing an even film of blood. The smear is allowed to air dry and is labeled and submitted to the laboratory. When Wright's stain or other Romanovsky-type stain is used, no extra fixative is needed before staining, and if necessary, the smear may be left safely in the air-dried state for some hours before staining.

All specimens submitted to the laboratory should be clearly labeled with the patient's name and address and the date and be accompanied by a written request for the required tests. Most laboratories require that specimens be submitted only in specified containers and be accompanied by the laboratory's test request slip. Laboratories handling tens of thousands of specimens daily are unable to give special attention to improperly labeled or packaged specimens and will often simply discard them.

The Microhematocrit and Detection of Anemia in the Office

Anemia is defined as a decrease in the amount of oxygen-carrying substance per unit volume of blood and may result from a reduction in the number of red cells per cubic millimeter of blood, a reduction in hemoglobin concentration, or both. Anemia may therefore be detected by several laboratory procedures: total red cell count, hemoglobin concentration, and hematocrit. Of these procedures, only the hematocrit can be performed accurately without special training and with simple equipment. When performed on capillary blood obtained from a finger prick, this procedure is known as the *microhematocrit* and measures the percentage volume occupied by the red cells in relation to the total volume of blood in a centrifuged capillary tube. The microhematocrit is a rapid and accurate means of detecting anemia in the office or clinic setting when the services of a diagnostic laboratory are not readily available.

Indications The classic signs and symptoms of anemia are dyspnea, pallor, or tachycardia. The classic signs are not always present, and the following should also suggest to the examining clinician that anemia may be present: a history of excessive blood loss; pallor, especially of the oral mucous membrane, palate, conjunctiva, nail beds, and palms; unexplained syncope; excessive fatigue; glossitis and atrophy of lingual papillae; recurrent or persistent gingivitis and

stomatitis; gingival hemorrhage out of proportion to recognized local factors; petechial hemorrhages; and unexplained bruising. None of these signs, however, is specifically related to anemia alone and each may have other explanations.

A variety of procedures, in addition to those measures of reduced oxygen-carrying substance described above, are used in evaluating a patient suspected of being anemic to ensure that other conditions leading to a similar clinical picture are not overlooked (*e.g.*, a complete medical history and physical examination and total and differential white cell counts are usually necessary). If the patient is unwilling to accept this referral or if these procedures are not readily available, the hematocrit will indicate the presence or absence of anemia. The hematocrit is consequently a valuable initial test.

The hematocrit may also be determined as part of the evaluation of a patient's ability to tolerate a general anesthetic or oral surgical procedure, even when there is no clinical reason to suspect the presence of anemia. In an anemic patient, reduction in the amount of oxygen transported in the blood as a result of anoxia or hemorrhage will have more serious consequences than will similar reductions in the nonanemic patient. When general anesthesia for oral surgery is performed on an outpatient emergency basis, determination of the microhematocrit provides a necessary index of the patient's ability to tolerate the procedure without delaying the referral of the patient to a diagnostic laboratory.

Equipment Equipment for obtaining blood sample (see preceding section), two heparinized microhematocrit capillary tubes;* a box of matches; a microhematocrit centrifuge* equipped with reader and magnifier (Fig. 3-1)

Procedure Blood obtained by finger prick or venipuncture is allowed to flow by capillary attraction into two microhematocrit tubes until each is about three fourths full. The column of blood should be free from air bubbles. If inadequate blood is obtained from the first punc-

---

* The technique described here is that used with the Clay–Adams Hemofuge (Clay–Adams, Division of Becton, Dickinson & Company, 299 Webro Road, Parsipany, NJ 07054). A variety of other models are available, some using 32-mm tubes, others 75-mm tubes. Many benchtop clinical centrifuges can also be modified with a microhematocrit head for this purpose. Separate microhematocrit tube readers are required with many models.

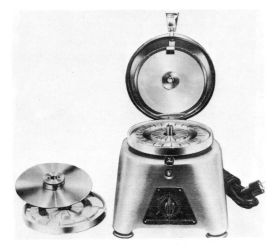

Fig. 3-1 Clay–Adams microhematocrit centrifuge.

and increase in hematocrit above the normal levels indicates the presence of erythrocytosis (polycythemia). Minor degrees of anemia and erythrocytosis may also result from hemodilution or concentration. The presence of anemia may likewise be masked if fluid is lost from the intravascular compartment (*e.g.,* in dehydration).

Anemia itself is not one specific disease but a symptom or sign that can indicate some abnormality in formation of red cells or their loss by hemorrhage or destruction. Any patient with a significantly reduced (or increased) hematocrit should be further investigated to establish the etiology of the condition before treatment. In many cases, administration of iron, folic acid or vitamin B_{12} *before* the etiology of an anemia is recognized may prevent the true nature of the disease from being discovered.

ture, a second finger should be prepared and the procedure repeated.

The end of each tube away from the column of blood is sealed by melting the glass in the flame of a match or small gas jet, without heating the blood. The tubes are cooled and placed opposite each other in the slots of the head of the centrifuge with the sealed ends pointing outward. The centrifuge head covers are closed, and the centrifuge timer is set for 5 minutes. The centrifuge is started and it accelerates to 12,500 rpm and stops automatically at the end of the required time; the centrifuge head covers are then removed. With the aid of a magnifying lens for greater accuracy, the hematocrit is read by means of the scale incorporated in the head of the instrument.

Interpretation The normal ranges of values for hematocrit in adults and children are given in Table 3-2. Reduction in hematocrit below the normal levels indicates the presence of anemia,

The Complete Blood Count

The complete blood count is a series of tests commonly run as a unit, and the results are valuable in determining the systemic response to oral infections and in ruling out systemic diseases as the cause of oral lesions. The complete blood count provides qualitative and quantitative information about the formed elements of the blood—erythrocytes (RBC), leukocytes (WBC), and platelets—which are subject to physiologic variation as well as more dramatic changes with diseases such as anemia, leukemia, neutropenia, and agranulocytosis; bacterial, viral, and parasitic infections; immunologic abnormalities; bleeding problems; and other blood dyscrasias. The complete blood count is performed on automatic equipment with additional microscopic evaluation of abnormal specimens; it provides an accurate and very frequently used screening evaluation of the hematopoietic system.

The complete blood count includes the following:

1. The *total red cell count* (*i.e.,* the total number of RBC/mm³ of blood)*
2. The *hemoglobin concentration* (Hb) expressed in g/dl of blood†

Table 3-2. Normal Range of Values for Hematocrit

AGE	VALUES
Birth	54
2 months	42
1–2 years	36
4 years	37
8 years	39
12 years	40
Adult male	42–50
Adult female	40–48

* mm³ = cubic millimeter (10^{-6} liter)
† g/dl = grams per deciliter (100 ml or 10^{-1} liter); also referred to as "grams %."

3. The *hematocrit* (Hct) or packed-cell volume (PCV) expressed as a percentage
4. The *red cell indices* (MCV, MCHC, and MCH; see below)
5. The *total white cell count* (*i.e.*, the total number of WBC/mm³)
6. The *differential white cell count*
7. *Examination of a stained blood smear*

The term *CBC* is often used to designate a complete blood count that includes all of the seven items listed above and is equivalent to a "complete blood count with white cell differential." Because in the past the platelet count had to be performed as a separate step with special equipment, it was usually not included in the complete blood count and was ordered and billed as a separate procedure. With some newer automated equipment (*e.g.*, the Technicon H6000 System),‡ however, the platelet count is performed and reported along with the red and white cell analyses as part of the complete blood count. When ordering a complete blood count, the clinician should determine beforehand exactly which tests are included by the particular laboratory he is using.

While some of the components of the complete blood count (*e.g.*, hematocrit, hemoglobin, differential white cell count, and examination of a stained blood smear) can be carried out manually by simple, nonautomated procedures or by direct microscopic visualization of a thin, stained film of blood, the tendency has been for automated procedures to supersede manual procedures to a large extent because of the cost saving and greater accuracy provided by the automated procedures. Indications for selecting manual techniques are described in the following sections where appropriate; otherwise, the procedures described refer to automated approaches.

The seven or eight different values reported as the complete blood count include some values that are actually measured by the equipment and others (referred to as derived values) that are calculated from one or more of the measured values. Depending on the particular equipment and technique used, a given component of the complete

‡ Technicon Instruments Corporation, Dept. 4, Tarrytown, NY 10591

blood count may be measured directly or calculated from other values. The mean corpuscular volume (MCV) and hematocrit are examples of values that frequently change from direct measurement to derived value (and vice-versa) as technology changes. Because a derived value is only as accurate as the direct measurements it is based on, the clinician who wishes to check one value against another, as is often done with complete blood counts, must be aware of which of the reported values are directly measured. Some details of automated hematologic equipment currently in use are given in the following sections to illustrate this point.

Total Erythrocyte Count and Mean Corpuscular Volume

The RBC count in the normal adult varies from approximately 4 to 5.5 million cells per cubic millimeter of blood. Alterations in the count are found in anemia and erythrocytosis (polycythemia) and in changes in circulating blood volume following shock or dehydration. A total RBC count is usually performed at least once during each hospitalization, including dental admissions, but is not usually repeated unless the progress of an anemia or other abnormality is being followed.

Office and Chairside Procedures. Inaccuracies in the total RBC count are numerous and include both human errors in diluting, mixing, and counting and errors inherent in the equipment used. Historically, the test was performed manually under a microscope by direct counting of the number of cells in a diluted sample of blood contained in a calibrated chamber of a special glass microscope slide (*hemocytometer technique*). Errors with this technique frequently exceeded the changes that occur in the number of RBCs with many diseases, and the technique has been discarded in favor of electronic counting methods. Where automated electronic equipment is not available, reliance must be placed on either the hemoglobin or hematocrit determinations as a measure of the RBC.

Automated Procedures. Electronic counting of erythrocytes is usually carried out with equipment such as the Coulter Counter

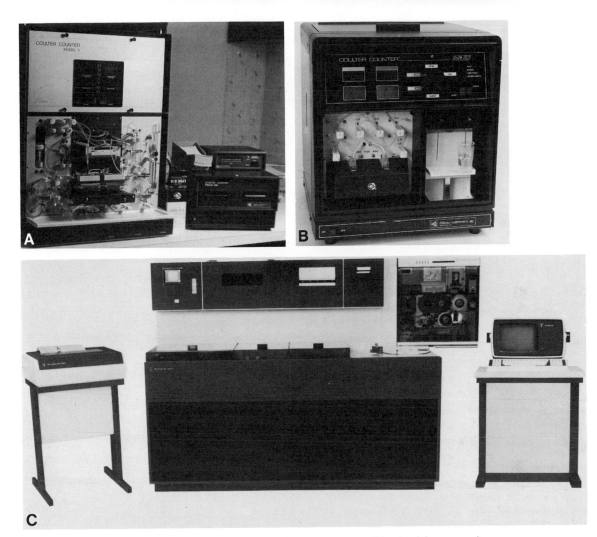

Fig. 3-2 (A, B & C) Some examples of automated equipment used in the laboratory determination of the complete blood count. See text for additional details. (A) Coulter Counter Model S, used in larger laboratories. (B) Coulter Counter M430, a semiautomated analyzer designed for the smaller laboratory, and providing the four most widely requested hematology parameters: total WBC count, hemoglobin concentration, total RBC count, and the hematocrit. (A & B, courtesy Coulter Electronics Inc, Hialeah, Fl 33012) (C) The Technicon H6000 Hematology System, a computer controlled blood cell analyzer providing all components of the complete blood count. Total RBC, WBC and platelet counts are obtained by light interference measurements, and the differential WBC count by the Hemalog D 3-channel automated Flow Cytometer (Automated Leukocyte Differential Counter) incorporated in the machine. A thin smear of blood suitable for manual microscopic examination or automated optical scanning is automatically prepared on Mylar tape from each specimen processed through the Autoslide unit attached to the upper right hand side of the cabinet. Numerical test result data and histograms of RBC and platelet numbers, a scatter plot for the three WBC channels, and performance curves for the major parameters measured are displayed electronically and printed out for hard copy. (See also Figure 3-4). (Courtesy Technicon Instruments Corporation, Tarrytown, NY, 10591). (A & B) are bench-top units; (C) is a large freestanding system.

Model S* (see Fig. 3-2) which also *measures* the erythrocyte mean cell volume (MCV) the total WBC count, and hemoglobin concentration. The hematocrit and the other two RBC indices—mean corpuscular hemoglobin (MCH) and mean corpuscular hemoglobin concentration (MCHC)—are automatically *calculated* at the same time as derived values (see following sections for a discussion of MCV, total WBC count, hemoglobin concentration, MCH, and MCHC).

For this electronic RBC counting technique, a sample of whole blood preserved with EDTA is used. One milliliter of blood is aspirated into the machine and automatically diluted with modified Eagle's solution before being drawn through three narrow channels equipped with electrodes (aperture tubes). As each cell passes through an aperture, its presence and dimensions are accurately recorded by a drop in voltage across the electrodes. The results of the three aperture tubes are averaged, and an average RBC count and MCV (calculated electronically from the record of RBC dimensions) are displayed and printed out by the machine. The sensitivity of the machine is set such that particles the size of platelets are not recorded. White cells are included in the RBC total but are of no significance because of the usual 1000:1 ratio of RBC to WBC in the peripheral blood.

The error with this technique is less than ±10%, although problems are encountered when the total WBC is over 20,000/mm³, or when RBCs agglutinate in the presence of abnormal antibodies (cold agglutinins), and the clumping of RBCs causes spuriously low RBC counts and high MCVs. With automated techniques, deviations in RBC count from normal that are greater than 0.5 million/mm³ are considered significant. The normal range of RBC (and other values reported by the Coulter Counter Model S) are illustrated in Figure 3-3 as they appear on the printout provided by the machine. Values below the normal range are referred to as *anemic* and those above as *polycythemic*.

The numbers of circulating RBCs are also significantly altered by such physiologic factors as exertion, emotion, meals, and extremes of temperature. Serial studies of the

RBC count should therefore be run on specimens obtained at roughly the same time each day.

In other electronic techniques (*e.g.*, Technicon H6000 System; see Fig. 3-2C), RBCs are enumerated and measured by light interference techniques, and a histogram of RBC numbers and size is displayed on the printout (see Fig. 3-4).

Measurement of Hemoglobin Concentration

The hemoglobin concentration, expressed as *grams* of hemoglobin per deciliter of blood, is commonly measured to obtain information about circulating RBCs and the amount of oxygen-carrying substance they contain, thereby providing information similar to that given by the total RBC count and hematocrit. The hemoglobin concentration is also used for the calculation of MCHC and MCH, which are used in determining the nature of a patient's anemia.

The hemoglobin concentraton is usually measured on anticoagulated venous blood by reacting the sample with a reagent that converts the hemoglobin to a stable, colored product; the concentration of this colored compound is measured in a photoelectric colorimeter in comparison with a standard. It is important that the equipment be regularly and accurately calibrated, and the most satisfactory techniques are those for which stable standards are commercially available (*e.g.*, the Drabkin technique, in which hemoglobin is converted to the stable pigment cyanmethemoglobin). Certified standards and the test reagent, Drabkin's solution (potassium cyanide and ferricyanide and sodium bicarbonate), are both commercially available. Other techniques using 0.1N hydrochloric acid (Sahli method) or 0.1N sodium carbonate (oxyhemoglobin method) are still used in smaller laboratories; these latter methods are often used on samples of capillary blood drawn into a special hemoglobin-diluting pipette and mixed with the reagent. Errors with these less sophisticated procedures may be ±10% or greater in comparison with an error of less than ±5% with automated photoelectric determination on venous specimens.

---

* Coulter Electronics, Inc., Hialeah, FL 33012

Fig. 3-3 One example of an automated hematology print-out sheet for the complete blood count used with the Coulter Counter Model S, which measures total RBC count, RBC mean cell volume (MCV), total WBC count and hemoglobin concentration, with the hematocrit and other two RBC indices (MCH and MCHC) automatically calculated at the same time, as derived values. The differential white cell count and platelet count are measured manually, or on other automated equipment as appropriate. The test results illustrated are all in the normal range. With a more advanced model, the Coulter Counter S-Plus II, a platelet count and a graphic display of cell size on a data terminal can also be obtained. With computer-linked systems, additional hard copy listing the results of specific tests run on the patient's blood sample and the range of normal values is usually provided for the patient's records. (Courtesy Coulter Electronics, Inc., Hialeah, Fla. 33012).

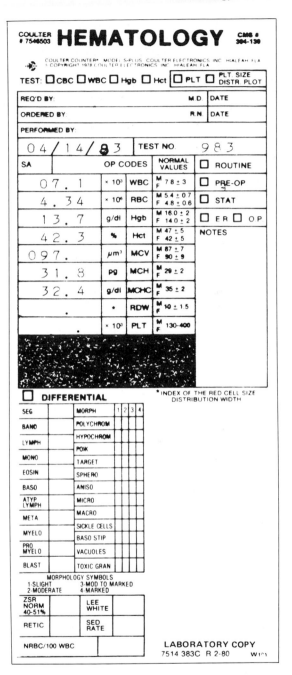

Hemoglobin concentration is now usually measured as one unit of an automated multitest system such as the Coulter Counter Model S or the Technicon H6000 System. It can also be measured with equal accuracy in smaller automatic chemical analyzers that incorporate a spectrophotometer, such as the Model 368 analyzer combined with the Clin-icard System,* or the Digecon System† used in some office laboratories and many large hospitals for "stat" specimens.

For adult males, the normal range of hemoglobin concentration is 14 g/dl to 18 g/dl

* Instrumentation Laboratory, Inc, Lexington, MA 02173
† Sherwood Medical Industries, Inc, Bridgeton, MO 63042

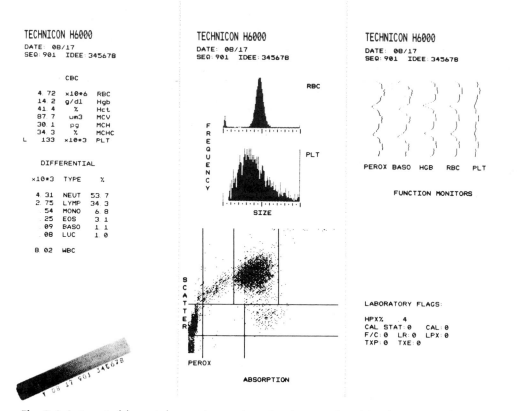

Fig. 3-4 Automated hematology printout sheet for the complete blood count used with the Technicon H6000 System. This computer-generated comprehensive patient data report includes test results (left-hand column), histograms and *x,y* display (middle column), and performance curves (right-hand column). The stained blood film automatically prepared by the instrument on Mylar tape is also illustrated. See text for additional details. (Courtesy of Technicon Instruments Corporation, Dept. 4, Tarrytown, NY, 10591)

of blood; adult females usually have slightly lower values, 12 g/dl to 16 g/dl; and children vary from a high of 17 g/dl to 20 g/dl in the newborn to a low of 10 g/dl to 12 g/dl during the first year of life, with a gradual increase to adult values by the age of 10 years. Values of 10 g/dl or less detected in ambulatory dental patients should be confirmed by repeating the test, and the patient should then be referred for medical evaluation.

Hematocrit

Both office and automated techniques provide accurate measurement of the hematocrit (the percentage of the blood occupied by the RBC). Both micro- (see previous section) and macrotechniques are available for measuring the hematocrit as the packed-cell volume (*i.e.*, the percentage volume occupied by the RBC in a centrifuged column of anticoagulated blood). With the advent of automated cell counters, the hematocrit is now usually calculated from the flow rate of cells through an aperture tube and the distribution of cell size (as in the Technicon H6000 System), or simply obtained as a derived value from the total RBC count and the MCV (Coulter Counter Model S). Because the packed RBC volume can be measured with considerable accuracy, the hematocrit was once accepted as an absolute standard against which a clinician could compare other RBC measurements that were at variance with clinical findings. Because of the greater degree of accuracy now obtained for both RBC counts and hemoglobin measurements with automated equipment and the uncertainty whether on a given laboratory report the hematocrit represents a measured or derived value, the hematocrit is accorded less importance.

Erythrocyte Indices and Classification of Anemias

In evaluating the nature of anemia, assistance is obtained by calculating standard indices relating to the size of the RBC and its hemoglobin content. Historically, these indices were derived from values for the three basic RBC measurements: total RBC count, hemoglobin concentration, and hematocrit. Currently, the RBC indices are either routinely calculated as derived values by the automated equipment used for the complete blood count or in the case of MCV (see preceding section), may be calculated from actual cell measurements performed by the Coulter Counter.

The following are the three most commonly used RBC indices:

1. The hemoglobin content of the erythrocyte, referred to as the *mean corpuscular hemoglobin* (MCH), expressed in picograms of hemoglobin per cell and calculated as

$$MCH = \frac{\text{hemoglobin concentration in g/dl of blood} \times 10}{\text{RBC in millions/mm}^3}$$

2. The concentration of the hemoglobin in the erythrocyte, referred to as the *mean corpuscular hemoglobin concentration* (MCHC), expressed as a percentage and calculated as

$$MCHC = \frac{\text{hemoglobin concentration g/dl of blood} \times 100}{\text{hematocrit}}$$

3. Average red cell volume, referred to as the *mean corpuscular volume* (MCV), expressed as cubic microns per cell and measured directly or calculated as

$$MCV = \frac{\text{hematocrit} \times 10}{\text{RBC in millions/mm}^3}$$

The changes seen in the red cell indices in the three morphologic types of anemia are illustrated in Table 3-3. Because the indices represent an average value, their usefulness is somewhat decreased in anemias having mixed populations of RBCs (*e.g.,* a mixed normocytic and microcytic population).

Once the presence of anemia (or conversely, erythrocytosis) has been confirmed by an abnormal hematocrit, total RBC count, or hemoglobin concentration, investigation of the patient should proceed to the stage where an accurate diagnosis of the cause of the anemia is established. This is accomplished by means of a thorough history and physical examination, consideration of the possible causes of anemia in the patient (differential diagnosis), followed by a logical sequence of laboratory tests designed to identify the type of anemia present and specify its pathogenesis.

One important classification of anemia that is of help in determining its cause is based on the morphologic abnormality of the RBC that divides anemias into *microcytic, normocytic,* and *macrocytic.* Morphologic abnormality is usually recognized in the stained smear of peripheral blood (see below) but is also accurately specified by electronic counting and calculation of RBC indices. Further subdivision into hypochromic and normochromic is also possible, depending on the

Table 3-3. Changes Seen in Red Cell Indices in the Three Morphologic Types of Anemia

TYPE OF ANEMIA	MCV	MCH	MCHC
Microcytic, hypochromic	↓	↓	↓
Macrocytic, normochromic	↑	↑	Normal
Normocytic, normochromic	Normal	Normal	Normal

average amount of hemoglobin in the RBC. (Hyperchromia, which is often noted in stained smears of macrocytic anemias, is an artifact caused by the increased thickness of macrocytes, which causes them to appear more densely colored by transmitted light.) The causes of each type of anemia are discussed in Chapter 22.

The laboratory studies used to evaluate an anemia may include one or more of the following hematologic procedures: reticulocyte count, gastric analysis and the Schilling test, serum iron and total iron-binding capacity, serum vitamin B_{12} and folate, occult blood in feces, bone marrow aspiration and biopsy, sickle cell preparation and hemoglobin electrophoresis, and RBC sedimentation rate.

The Total White Blood Cell Count

The white cell count in the normal adult varies from approximately 4,000 to 10,000 leukocytes per cubic millimeter of circulating blood. An increase in the number of leukocytes (leukocytosis) is the most common alteration observed, usually as a response to an infectious process or a large area of tissue necrosis. Leukocytosis also occurs in leukemia, in polycythemia, and as a physiologic response to exercise, fear, pain, and digestion. A decrease in the number of leukocytes (leukopenia) may be associated with depression of the bone marrow, agranulocytosis, aplastic anemia, allergic and toxic reactions to drugs, certain infections (usually viral), cirrhosis, and collagen diseases (Table 3-4).

In the management of dental patients, the total WBC count is used as one index of the presence of a systemic infectious process and to rule out the possibility of leukemia or ma-

lignant neutropenia in patients with oral lesions compatible with these diagnoses.

The total WBC count is performed on the same blood specimen as is used for the total RBCs, and like the latter, it may be performed manually with a hemocytometer or with an automated cell counter. Although the automated technique is more accurate, the difference in accuracy between the two techniques is less important than in the RBC count because the changes in WBCs commonly encountered in disease are proportionally greater, and errors are therefore less significant. To count WBCs in the presence of RBCs, RBCs are lysed by diluting the blood sample with dilute acetic acid or equivalent reagent supplied by the manufacturer of the automated equipment, leaving the WBCs intact.

The Differential White Blood Cell Count

Because the WBCs of circulating blood are of several types and of varied origin, the total leukocyte count is of limited use without a differential count of the various types of cells present. Five types of WBC are commonly present in circulating blood, and the relative percentages of each as well as the range for the absolute count of each per cubic millimeter of blood are listed in Table 3-5 and illustrated in Figures 3-5 and 3-6.

Neutrophils (polymorphonuclear leukocytes), eosinophils, and basophils are all derived from precursor cells in the red bone marrow. Because these three cell types and their precursors also have prominent cytoplasmic granules, as a group they are referred to as cells of the granulocyte or myeloid (bone

Table 3-4. Common Conditions Associated with Leukocytosis and Leukopenia

Leukocytosis	Leukopenia
Physiologic leukocytosis—exercise— digestion—fear and pain	Influenza—measles—respiratory tract infections
Acute and chronic infections	Malignant neutropenia
Polycythemia	Catarrhal jaundice
Leukemia	Reaction to certain drugs—amidopyrine, barbiturates, sulfonamides
	Typhoid—paratyphoid fevers

Table 3-5. Average Percentage and Absolute Values for Differential Leukocyte Count

Type of Cell	Percent	Absolute Numbers per mm^3
Neutrophils	43–77	3,000 to 7,000
Basophils	0–2	0 to 100
Eosinophils	0–4	50 to 300
Lymphocytes	17–47	1,000 to 3,500
Monocytes	0–9	100 to 600

marrow-derived) series.* Monocytes and lymphocytes (this designation includes both B and T cell types) are grouped separately and referred to as nongranular cells or mononuclear cells, partly on morphologic grounds and partly because their response to a variety of pathologic processes differs from that of the granulocytes.

Traditionally, the differential WBC count is performed on an air-dried smear (film) of blood stained with Wright's or other Romanovsky-type stain to differentiate RBCs from WBCs and the different types of WBCs from each other (see Figs. 3-5 and 3-6). The relative percentages of each type of WBC are obtained by counting a minimum of 100 to 200 cells per slide, and the fields counted are selected in such a way that the effect of uneven distribution of the WBCs in the smear is overcome.

This manual technique requires considerable skill and experience and is an expensive procedure considering the number of differential WBC counts performed each day by most diagnostic laboratories and the staff of skilled technicians needed to perform them. A variety of approaches have therefore been made to automation of the differential WBC count in recent years. This development has

lead to the introduction not only of new technologies but also of new concepts of WBC classification that involve different cytochemical characteristics than those revealed by the conventional Romanovsky-type stains used in the manual procedure. The three currently used counting and classification approaches—manual microscopic examination of a stained smear, automated pattern recognition systems for screening stained smears, and automated flow cytochemistry staining systems—will therefore each be discussed separately. Large laboratories currently use a combination of methods, relying on an automated system to screen specimens for abnormals and manually checking abnormals and a predetermined sample of normals. Smaller laboratories may still use manual techniques with or without automated blood film preparation and staining equipment to provide more uniform slides.*

Manual Technique for Differential White Blood Cell Count. The air-dried smear of blood used for this technique may be prepared either from a drop of capillary blood obtained by finger prick, from a drop of venous blood discharged from the Vacutainer needle after venipuncture, or from the unclotted whole blood samples preserved with EDTA that are usually submitted for a complete blood count. Laboratories' requirements vary in this regard because both the quality of the smear and the ability of preservatives to produce artifactual changes in WBC morphology must be considered. A recent innovation has been the addition to existing automated equipment of a unit capable of automatically preparing high-quality stained blood films on Mylar tape as the other components of the complete blood count are processed.†

Once stained, the blood smear is examined microscopically, and the proportion of each type of WBC is calculated as a percentage of the first 100 or 200 cells examined. When performed in this manner, the differential

---

* Current knowledge indicates that monocytes and lymphocytes are also produced in the bone marrow and cannot be designated as *nonmyeloid*. The use of the terms *myelo-* and *myeloid* for neutrophilic, eosinophilic, and basophilic leukocytes and their bone marrow precursor cells persists however, and distinction between these myeloid cells and the nongranular mononuclear cells still forms the basis for separation of a variety of hematologic disorders (*e.g.*, myelocytic versus lymphocytic leukemia; myeloid metaplasia, etc)

* Hemaprep, Geometric Data Corporation, Wayne, PA 19087
† Technicon Autoslide; also incorporated in the Technicon H6000 System. Technicon Instruments Corp, Dept 4, Tarrytown, NY 10591

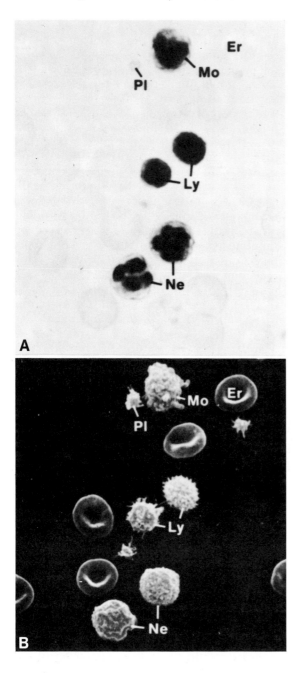

Fig. 3-5 The appearance of erythrocytes (RBC), leukocytes (WBC), and platelets in a stained wet-mount preparation observed by light microscopy (*A*) and scanning electron microscopy (*B*) to illustrate nuclear configuration and cytoplasmic staining reaction as well as surface configuration. The appearance of RBC, WBC, and platelets, as observed with light microscopy in dried thin smears of peripheral blood stained with Wright's stain or other Romanovsky-type stain and traditionally used in hematology, is similar to that illustrated in *A* for a stained wet-mount preparation. (x2260; Er = erythrocyte; pl = dendritic form of an activated platelet; Mo = monocyte; LY = B lymphocytes; and Ne = neutrophils; Kessel RG, Kardon RH: Tissues and Organs: A Text-Atlas of Scanning Electron Microscopy. San Francisco, WH Freeman, 1979. Copyright © 1979)

phocytes in the peripheral blood, for example, has no direct physiological effect on the number of cells of the myeloid series in the peripheral blood. It is the *absolute* or actual number of cells of a given type that has physiological and diagnostic significance. To avoid misinterpretation, the differential count obtained by microscopic examination of a stained smear is best expressed as an absolute figure that may be obtained by calculating the percentage of the total WBC count made up by each cell type. Because laboratory reports customarily report only the relative count, the absolute count for each cell type must be derived by multiplying the total WBC count by the percent figures given on the report. The range of normal for each cell type expressed as an absolute count is listed in Table 3-5.

Absolute counts of neutrophils and lymphocytes may be calculated by this method, but those cells present in small numbers (*e.g.*, eosinophils) are represented by so few cells in the 100 to 200 counted that an accurate estimate is impossible by this method. Where an accurate absolute *eosinophil count* is required (and only manual techniques are available), the blood specimen is stained with a dye that selectively stains the granules of the eosinophils red, lyses other WBCs, and renders RBCs invisible, allowing the eosinophils to be counted in a hemocytometer.

As a rule, one type of cell is responsible for an elevation in the total WBCs, and the leukocytosis is usually designated according

count of each WBC type is expressed *relative* to the other cell types, and changes in one cell type are inevitably associated with changes in other cell types because the sum of percentages of all cell types reported in a differential WBC count must always add up to 100%. This inverse relationship does not in fact occur; a change in the number of lym-

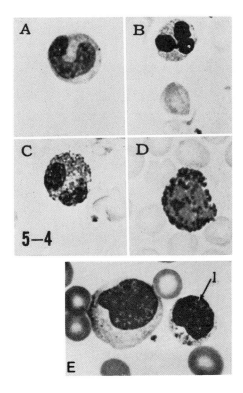

Fig. 3-6 Granular (*A–D*) and nongranular (*E*) leukocytes from peripheral blood smear from a normal subject; Wright's stain, oil immersion. *A,* stab (band) neutrophil; *B,* segmented neutrophil; *C,* bilobed eosinophil; *D,* mature basophil; *E,* monocyte and a large lymphocyte (1) with azurophilic granules in the cytoplasm. (Piliero SJ, Jacobs MS, Wischnitzer S, et al: Atlas of Histology, pp 61, 63. Philadelphia, JB Lippincott, 1965)

to the cell most markedly increased (*e.g.,* a patient with a total WBC count of 12,000/mm³, and with 50% of the differential composed of lymphocytes, is usually said to have a lymphocytic leukocytosis. Because the maximum number of lymphocytes is normally about 3,500/mm³, this would be an *absolute lymphocytic leukocytosis*; on the other hand, a patient with a total WBC of 6,000 and the same differential would have only a *relative lymphocytic leukocytosis*, possibly because of a decrease in neutrophils).

Automated Pattern Recognition Systems for Screening Stained Smears. A number of automated, optical differential cell counters that scan and classify cell types on conventional stained smears of blood (wedge smears) or the more randomly distributed smears prepared by centrifugal distribution of blood in a special apparatus* (spun smears) have been developed and tested in recent years. Comparison of these automated scanners[†] and routine manual methods reveal that both approaches are equally accurate and precise and able to identify abnormal smears for more detailed review. Because the manual differential counting technique is known to be of limited accuracy and reproducibility, the automated scanning of smears is likely to replace the manual technique as a means of screening the large number of blood smears processed in larger laboratories. The automated scanners have the additional advantages of screening a large number of cells per slide (500 or more) and of recognizing and classifying RBC and platelet abnormalities as well as those of the WBC.

Automated Flow Cytochemistry Staining Systems. A new technology to detect and differentiate WBCs in suspension using a flow system and cytochemical staining was introduced in the early 1970s and is currently in use in many larger diagnostic laboratories equipped with the Hemalog D series of Automated Leukocyte Differential Counters.[‡] These instruments measure the angle and intensity of light-scattering of single cells in suspension and differentiate cells on the basis of cell size, index of refraction between the cell and the suspending medium, and light absorption of the varied cell types enhanced by dye-coupled enzyme-substrate reactions. Granulocytes are detected by means of their myeloperoxidase, which produces a dark precipitate in the cells; a lipase in the monocytes (alphanaphthol butyrate esterase) dyes them brown-red with fuschin; and alcian blue stains the heparin-containing granules of basophils blue-green. Eosinophils are counted as a subset of the stained granulocytes on the basis of their more intense myeloperoxidase staining reaction. Lymphocytes

*The Abbott Spinner, Abbott Laboratories, North Chicago, IL 60064
† Hematrak, Technicon Instruments Corporation, Dept. 4, Tarrytown, NY 10591
‡ Technicon Instruments Corporation, Dept. 4, Tarrytown, NY 10591, also incorporated in the H6000 System

are identified as a group of small cells that give poor peroxidase reactions.

Each of the three enzyme–dye reactions is analyzed by a different channel of the machine, which provides a visual display of an x,y scatter plot (where x = absorption and y = size) of the cells counted in each channel (see Fig. 3-7). Each point on the display represents a cell, and the points distribute in such a way that one may define clusters of many cells that are related to one of the cell types defined morphologically on the conventional Wright-stained blood smear. A total of up to 10,000 cells is analyzed in each channel, the machine separating and counting the cell clusters by computer to produce the differential white cell count as illustrated in Figure 3-4.

This new technology offers considerable advantage over the conventional manual technique, including the ability to screen a large number of specimens and save considerable time and labor, increased precision of counting as a result of the large number of cells analyzed in each specimen, and differential counts based on absolute rather than relative counts. Despite the different biophysical principles used in detecting and differentiating WBCs with this approach, counts performed in this manner closely approximate those performed optically with Wright-stained smears, particularly in regard to neutrophil, lymphocyte, and eosinophil counts. Like other automated hematology techniques, automated flow cytometry is designed primarily to identify normal WBC differentials, separating out the abnormal specimens for detailed manual, optical examination. In standard operation, an instrument of the Hemalog D series flags approximately 20% of all specimens as outside the normal range and requiring further examination; extreme accuracy in identifying atypical cells and immature RBC and WBC is not required. Because of its unique way of classifying cells and the increased sensitivity it provides for detecting small numbers of leukemic cells, this technology is considered of great value in the diagnosis and treatment of leukemic patients. Some of the artifacts associated with manual differential WBC counts on blood that has been held in preservatives too long do not occur with the flow cytometry technique. Accurate differentials

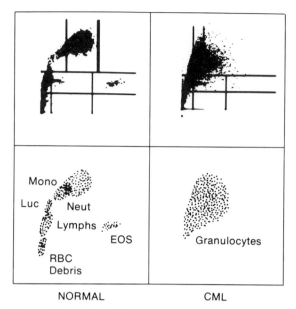

Fig. 3-7 Examples of the x, y myeloperoxidase scatter plots obtained by automated flow cytochemistry in a normal person (left hand panels) and in a patient with chronic myelogenous leukemia (CML; right-hand panels). Each point in the upper panels represents a measurement of size (y-axis) and myeloperoxidase reaction (x-axis) of a single cell. The lower panels schematically demonstrate how the measurements on 10,000 cells form clusters that correlate with traditional cell types. Data such as these are generated for each channel of the Hemalog D series Automated Leukocyte Differential Counter and illustrate the fact that the traditional WBC types have been independently rediscovered by this new biophysical approach and are shown to be separate classes of cells rather than artifacts of a morphologic taxonomy. (Mono, monocytes; Neut, neutrophils; Lymphs, lymphocytes; Luc, large unstained cells; EOS, eosinophils; RBC debris, ghosts of lysed RBC; see text for additional discussion.) (From Ross DW, Bardwell A: Automated cytochemistry and the white cell differential in leukemia. Blood Cells 6:455, 1980; Courtesy Springer–Verlag, New York, NY)

may now be performed on specimens preserved as long as 48 hours, allowing specimens that correlate poorly with clinical diagnosis to be re-run on the original blood sample.

Interpretation of White Blood Cell Counts. Total and differential WBC counts are usually obtained together and interpreted as a unit. Because significant changes in the differential

WBC count rarely occur without some changes in the total WBC count, changes over time can usually be monitored adequately by serial total WBC counts. The WBC count is influenced by diurnal changes and a number of physiological variables, in addition to pathologic states. Care should therefore be taken to draw blood samples for serial blood counts at the same time each day; small variations noted in either total or differential WBC counts should not be considered significant.

Of increases in the number of circulating WBCs, neutrophilic leukocytosis is the most common; it is a somewhat nonspecific reaction to tissue destruction (compare fever) of infectious, traumatic, or other cause. When the leukopoietic stimulus to the bone marrow is strong enough, immature leukocytes also increase in number in the circulating blood. Immature leukocytes exhibit less segmentation of the nucleus (band forms), and the relative percentages of immature and mature types making up the neutrophil count are often expressed as percent *bands* and percent segmented forms (*segs*) respectively. Segmented neutrophils usually constitute about 45% to 75% of the total differential count in health. In dental patients, neutrophilic leukocytosis may accompany an acute alveolar abscess, pericoronitis, or acute necrotizing ulcerative gingivostomatitis.

Because the percentage of immature neutrophils and the total neutrophil count represent an index of the patient's ability to defend against a disease, elaborate differential counts such as the Schilling and Arneth counts have been used to predict a favorable or unfavorable prognosis to an infectious process. These counts have largely disappeared in the antibiotic era, but the term *shift to the left*, to indicate an increase in the more immature forms of the neutrophils, is still used.

The disease processes commonly associated with changes in the numerical values for the different leukocyte series are listed in Table 3-6. Very large increases in the neutrophil count characteristically occur in myelogenous leukemia (*e.g.*, 25,000 and greater) but may also occur as an exceptional response to an

Table 3-6. Diseases Commonly Associated with Numerical Variations of Different Leukocytes

POLYMORPHONUCLEARS	LYMPHOCYTES
Increase	*Increase*
Myelogenous leukemia	Lymphocytic leukemia
Acute infectious disease	Mumps—German measles
Erythroblastosis fetalis	Whooping cough
Intoxications by drugs and poisons	Chronic infections
	Convalescence from acute infections
Decrease	*Decrease*
Malignant neutropenia	Aplastic anemia
Aplastic anemia	Myelogenous leukemia
Lymphocytic leukemia	

MONOCYTES	EOSINOPHILS
Increase	*Increase*
Monocytic leukemia	Eosinophilic leukemia
Infectious mononucleosis	Allergic diseases
Hodgkin's disease	Scarlet fever
Gaucher's disease	Hodgkin's disease
Malaria—kala-azar	Some skin diseases
Tuberculosis	Protozoan diseases—trichinosis
Subacute bacterial endocarditis	*Decrease*
Decrease	Typhoid fever
Aplastic anemia	Aplastic anemia

infectious agent. Such nonneoplastic increases in neutrophils are referred to as a *leukemoid reaction*.

Lymphocytosis in dental patients usually results from a viral upper respiratory illness. The leukocytosis that accompanies infectious mononucleosis is characterized by the appearance of unusual mononuclear cells that are usually listed in the differential WBC as "atypical" lymphocytes (or lymphocyte variants).

Eosinophilia of any significant degree may result from an allergic process, parasitic infection, or a lymphoma such as Hodgkin's disease.

Decreases in the number of circulating WBCs most commonly affect the neutrophils and are referred to as a *neutropenia*. Neutropenias are often detected in patients with severe periodontal lesions, recurrent mouth ulcers, and other evidences of delayed healing of the oral mucosa. In screening patients with such problems for hematologic abnormalities it is important to calculate the absolute neutrophil count because minor degrees of neutropenia may not be reflected in the relative differential count if the total WBC count is low. A particularly severe form of neutropenia in which both relative and absolute differential WBC counts usually reveal severe reduction in the numbers of all circulating granulocytes is referred to as *agranulocytosis*. In order to detect *cyclic neutropenia* (a fairly rare condition characterized by repeated 3-day to 7-day episodes of marked reduction in circulating neutrophils alternating with longer periods with a normal white cell count and characteristically associated with episodes of mouth ulceration, gingivitis, poor healing, and progressive periodontal destruction), it may be necessary to repeat differential and total WBC counts two to three times a week for up to 1 to 2 months.

Examination of a Stained Blood Smear

Examination of a Wright's-stained smear of blood is a long established component of the complete blood count that provides information about morphologic abnormalities of RBCs and platelets in addition to the differential WBC count. The value of this procedure lies in the fact that a trained hematology technician examines the stained blood smear microscopically and provides a description of any abnormal cells that is included on the laboratory report. The differential WBC count actually has little diagnostic validity unless the figure lies well outside the normal range,* and it is the morphologic description of abnormal cells that constitutes the important diagnostic information that can be obtained from the stained blood smear.

The stained blood smear is usually examined only if abnormalities are detected in the total RBC, total WBC, or differential WBC counts. Automated optical scanning techniques provide information on abnormal RBCs and a platelet estimate (see following section), in addition to a WBC differential, but abnormal smears detected in this way are also usually examined manually. The various manual and automated methods used to prepare the stained blood smear are described in earlier sections of this chapter.

The stained blood smear provides a variety of information about the RBC: size (*macrocytes* and *microcytes*), shape (*anisocytosis, poikilocytosis, spherocytosis*), and hemoglobin content (*hyperchromia* and *hypochromia*). Immature RBC, WBC, and other abnormal cells that appear in the bloodstream in some disease states may also be observed and are recorded on the report of the stained smear.

Of the immature red and white cells that occasionally appear in the peripheral blood, the following are likely to be reported in the examination of a stained smear (usually in patients with leukemia, a leukemoid reaction or severe anemia).

The Red Blood Cell Series. *Normoblast,* a nucleated red-cell precursor (NRBC), is slightly larger than an erythrocyte and contains a small round pyknotic nucleus and a basophilic or eosinophilic cytoplasm depending on its degree of maturity.

The White Blood Cell Series. In the *myelocyte,* a nucleated precursor of a granulocyte,

---

*75% of the variance in the differential WBC count is accounted for by analytical and sampling variability plus physiological changes rather than by disease processes, irrespective of whether manual or automated techniques are used

the nucleus is still round and oval, finely structured, and without obvious nucleoli, and the cytoplasm is basophilic, with few of the granules that distinguish the three types of mature granulocyte. The *metamyelocyte*, a smaller and more mature cell, has an indented nucleus more like that of the mature granulocyte and a less basophilic cytoplasm with definite granules. *Prolymphocytes* (large lymphocytes, transitional cells or atypical lymphocytes), *proplasmocytes*, and *promonocytes*, immature precursors of lymphocytes, plasma cells, and monocytes, respectively, are larger than the mature cells and show varying degrees of nuclear and cytoplasmic immaturity reflected in the texture of the nuclear chromatin, presence of nucleoli, cytoplasmic granules, and staining. The more immature cells of the granulocytic and nongranulocytic series are called *blast cells*.

The Platelet Count

Platelets are small 2 μ to 5 μ particles released from the cytoplasm of large multinucleated cells (megakaryocytes) located in the red bone marrow. Because of the platelets' small size and tendency to aggregate (an important phenomenon related to their function in the hemostatic mechanism), platelet counts on peripheral blood have a large technical error. Counts are performed manually using a special hemocytometer counting chamber and a phase-contrast microscope or by means of an automated cell counter such as the Technicon Autoanalyzer or H6000 System. Counts are also carried out on the stained blood smear, and the calculation is based on the ratio of platelets to RBC in the smear. This optical technique, which is referred to as a *platelet estimate*, is performed manually or with an automated optical scanner (*e.g.*, Technicon Hematrak) and is as accurate as counts of platelets in suspension.

The normal platelet count ranges from 150,000/mm^3 to 450,000/mm^3. When the count is low, the bleeding time can be expected to be prolonged, the tourniquet test positive, and clot retraction abnormal (see section on Bleeding and Clotting Abnormalities). When the count is below 50,000/mm^3 to 60,000/mm^3, spontaneous bleeding and petechiae may appear. Diseases commonly associated with an increase (thrombocytosis) or decrease (thrombocytopenia) in circulating platelets are listed in Table 3-7.

Other Commonly Used Hematology Procedures

Reticulocyte Count

As the RBCs mature in the bone marrow, losing their nuclei and accumulating hemoglobin before entering the bloodstream, the amount of nucleoprotein in their cytoplasm also decreases. An RBCs thus changes from a nucleated cell with a basophilic cytoplasm

Table 3-7. Platelet Changes Associated with Some Common Diseases of Dental Interest (Normal values 150,000–450,000/mm^3 of blood)

INCREASE IN PLATELETS (THROMBOCYTOSIS)	DECREASE IN PLATELETS (THROMBOCYTOPENIA)
Polycythemia vera Hemolytic anemias Chronic myelocytic leukemia Acute rheumatic fever	Thrombocytopenic purpura Symptomatic purpura hemorrhagica due to 　Chemical or physical agents 　Acute and chronic leukemias 　Aplastic anemia 　Pernicious anemia 　Hemolytic jaundice 　Banti's disease 　Gaucher's disease 　Bacterial endocarditis

to a nonnucleated cell with an eosinophilic cytoplasm. Approximately 0.5% to 1.5% of the circulating RBC in health retain evidence of the cytoplasmic nucleoprotein reticulum that can be stained by mixing freshly drawn blood with saturated cresyl blue, preparing a fixed smear, and examining the cells with a microscope. During periods of active erythropoiesis, the number of cells that stain in this fashion (reticulocytes) increases as does the number of polychromatophilic cells, and cells containing nuclear remnants in the usual Wright-stained smear of blood. Anemia without reticulocytosis is an index of exhaustion of iron stores or inability of the bone marrow to respond to the anemia.

Gastric Analysis and the Schilling Test

Several types of megaloblastic macrocytic anemia of different etiology are caused by vitamin B_{12} deficiency. Of fundamental importance in the differentiation of this group of anemias is the Schilling test, a measure of the patient's ability to absorb orally administered radioactive vitamin B_{12} labeled with ^{60}Co. Following oral administration of the radioactive vitamin B_{12}, unlabeled vitamin is given intramuscularly as a flushing dose to induce urinary excretion of the labeled vitamin, which is measured in a 24-hour urine specimen. The flushing dose is the essence of the Schilling test, which allows vitamin B_{12} absorption measurements to be made with acceptable doses of radioactivity. Patients with pernicious anemia (who are unable to absorb orally administered vitamin B_{12}) excrete less than 5% of the orally administered dose in comparison with excretion of 8% to 25% by normal individuals. In patients with pernicious anemia, repetition of the test 3 days later together with administration of gastric intrinsic factor will result in normal levels of urinary excretion of the orally administered radioactive vitamin B_{12}.

The presence of free hydrochloric acid in the gastric contents is incompatible with a diagnosis of pernicious anemia, and measurement of gastric acidity (*gastric analysis*) is also used in the differentiation of this group of anemias. Absolute achlorhydria strongly suggests the presence of pernicious anemia, but only if the gastric analysis is carried out following administration of histamine to provide the greatest possible stimulation for acid secretion. A variety of techniques of gastric analysis are used; for details, the reader is referred to a textbook of clinical pathology.

Sprue, another cause of megaloblastic anemia associated with malabsorption in the small intestine and fatty stools (steatorrhea), is differentiated on the basis of abnormal absorption of D-xylose, estimation of fecal fat, radiographic examination of the lower gastrointestinal tract, and occasionally, jejunal biopsy.

Serum Iron and Total Iron-Binding Capacity

Iron deficiency is the most common cause of anemia; however, anemia occurs only after depletion of iron stores, and iron deficiency (sideropenia) may exist for some time before the appearance of anemia and is responsible for a number of clinical problems. Iron is an important structural component of muscle protein (myoglobin), the cytochromes, and other electron transport proteins, as well as a cofactor for several enzymes. Ultrastructural defects have been demonstrated in the cells of iron deficient animals, and iron deficiency probably affects resistance to a variety of infectious agents. Chronic fatigue and impaired exercise tolerance occur in iron deficiency as well as in anemia. Iron deficiency without anemia (sideropenia) also has been demonstrated in 20% of patients with chronic mouth ulcers from a variety of causes, but is probably secondary to chronic iron loss through the denuded epithelium rather than an etiologic factor for any one type of mouth ulcer.

The major portions of the body iron stores are contained in RBC hemoglobin (60% of total body iron) or stored as ferritin or hemosiderin in liver, spleen, and bone marrow (30% of total body iron; usually less in females). Less than 0.1% circulates in the blood-stream bound to a beta-globulin plasma protein (transferrin), the form in which available iron stores are transported in the body. Iron deficiency is usually detected on the basis of the amount of iron bound to transferrin in the plasma (referred to as *serum iron*) and the total amount of iron that can be bound to the plasma transferrin *in vitro* (referred to as *total iron-binding capacity* or TIBC). The ratio of serum iron divided by TIBC, expressed as a percentage, gives the *percentage saturation.* Values for serum iron and TIBC under different conditions are illustrated in Figure 3-8. The range for normal serum iron is 55 μg/mm^3 to 185 μg/mm^3; for TIBC, 250 μg/mm^3 to 425 μg/mm^3; and percent saturation, 20% to 55%. In iron deficiency, serum iron falls but TIBC increases; in anemias associated with chronic infection and malignancy, both serum iron and TIBC are decreased. Oral contraceptives may also decrease the percent unsaturation. Iron stores may also be demonstrated and roughly measured by staining of bone marrow smears for iron.

Iron deficiency (sideropenia or hypochromic microcytic anemia) is corrected by administration of iron supplements; however, as iron supplements produce a number of changes in the hematopoietic picture, they should be withheld following detection of iron deficiency, at least until an adequate diagnostic evaluation has been carried out to determine the cause of iron deficiency.

The mean corpuscular hemoglobin (MCH) level is a good predictor of iron deficiency; at MCH levels greater than 30 pg per cell, the probability of diminished iron saturation is low; below 27 pg, the probability increases rapidly.

Vitamin B$_{12}$ and Folate Assays

Most megaloblastic anemias (MCV greater than 95 μ^3) are caused by a deficiency of vitamin B$_{12}$ or folic acid. A small but significant group result from administration of drugs that impair DNA metabolism and are used as cancer chemotherapeutic agents (*e.g.,* 6-mercaptopurine; 5-fluorouracil). Vitamin B$_{12}$ and folate are crucial in the synthesis of DNA but not for RNA and protein synthesis; hence, cells with a rapid turnover (notably cells of the erythrocyte series and epithelial cells of the mouth and gastrointestinal tract) continue to grow without dividing, resulting in megaloblastic changes that have been demonstrated in the mouth but are most evident in the bone marrow. An intact gastric mucosa with functional parietal cells to produce intrinsic factor, adequate pancreatic enzymes to degrade the B$_{12}$ intrinsic factor–R factor complex, and a functional terminal ileum for binding and absorption of the B$_{12}$ intrinsic factor complex are needed for optimal B$_{12}$ absorption. Vitamin B$_{12}$ deficiency thus may be suspected on the basis of dietary deficiency and malabsorption in the upper gastrointestinal tract (pernicious anemia, gastrectomy) or the lower gastrointestinal tract (sprue, intestinal resection, neoplasms, regional ileitis). Folate deficiency may be sus-

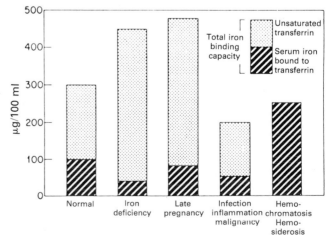

Fig. 3-8 Serum iron and iron-binding capacity in various disorders (Thorn GW et al: Harrison's Principles of Internal Medicine, 9th ed, p 1516. New York, McGraw–Hill, 1980)

pected on the basis of dietary deficiency, increased requirements (pregnancy, hemolysis, and hemodialysis), malabsorption in the lower gastrointestinal tract (as above), or as a side-effect of drugs (phenytoin, alcohol, isoniazid, and possibly, oral contraceptives). Vitamin B_{12} and folate deficiencies have been identified as the cause of anemia noted in 5% of patients with recurrent aphthous ulcers (sometimes referred to as pseudoaphthae in these circumstances). Atrophic glossitis and other oral mucosal changes also occur characteristically with vitamin B_{12} and folate deficiencies.

There are thus a number of situations in which a clinician may suspect vitamin B_{12} or folate deficiency and request measurement of serum levels. In general, however, there is no justification for these measurements unless the MCV is greater than 95 μ^3 or significant macrocytosis (in the case of a mixed nutritional anemia) is noted on examination of a stained smear.

Occult Blood in Feces

Bleeding into the gastrointestinal tract is a common cause of chronic blood loss leading to significant degrees of anemia in both males and females. Rapid loss of large amounts of blood leads to either the passage of obvious blood with the stools or to passage of partially digested blood (classically described as black tarry stools or melena). Dilated and thrombosed veins in the rectoanal mucosa (hemorrhoids) may also be the cause of blood mixed with stools. More often, however, blood loss into the gastrointestinal tract is slow and persistent, such that a severe degree of anemia may occur without any sign of blood appearing in the feces. For this reason, one of the first procedures performed on a patient with an anemia of unknown origin is intended to rule out the possibility of slow and persistent gastrointestinal hemorrhage by looking for occult blood in the feces. This test has little place in the usual dental practice, but in a hospital an initial screening test such as this may become the responsibility of the dentist in charge of a patient in whom an anemia has been detected.

Most of the methods for clinical determi-

nation of occult blood in stool (or urine) employ phenolic compounds such as gum guaiac, benzidine, or orthotoluidine, which are oxidized to colored compounds by peroxidase activity contained in the heme portion of hemoglobin. Many of the tests are unsatisfactory in that they are either relatively insensitive or more often too sensitive and may give false positive tests. The latter is the case with the commercially available Occultest or Hemotest reagent tablets. A positive test obtained with this technique can be interpreted as indicative of gastrointestinal hemorrhage only if the patient has been on a meat-free diet for some days and the possibility of swallowed blood originating from mouth, gums, or nose has been ruled out. Unfortunately, the most satisfactory tests for occult blood depend on the use of freshly constituted reagents, which is often impractical for a test to be used in clinic or hospital ward (as distinct from a laboratory).

Following dental extractions, all tests for occult blood in feces may be positive for several days.

Bone Marrow Aspiration and Biopsy

Detailed evaluation of patients with anemia, leukemia, multiple myeloma, metastatic malignancy, and other space-occupying lesions frequently involves study of the immature erythropoietic and leukopoietic cells of the bone marrow. This is usually accomplished by aspiration of red bone marrow cells through a large-bore needle inserted through a trochar into the iliac crest or sternal marrow space. The aspirate is then smeared thinly on a glass slide or coverslip, stained with Wright's stain, and examined in the same way as a smear of capillary or venous blood. Bone marrow biopsy is also used where an indication of the spatial relationship and degree of hyperplasia or hypoplasia of the cellular elements in the marrow is needed. The specimen is usually obtained from the crest of the ilium. Histologic sections are prepared from these specimens and stained by Wright's stain.

In patients with macrocytic anemia, bone marrow aspiration is used to demonstrate the megaloblastic changes that affect the precursors of the red cells (as well as leukocytes and platelets) in the bone marrow. For example, in both vitamin B_{12} and folic acid deficiency anemias, all stages of red cell precursors become enlarged and develop a characteristic sievelike appearance of their nuclear chromatin with prominent nucleoli. These cells, which do not occur in normal RBC maturation, are referred to as *megaloblasts*. They rarely appear in the circulating bloodstream.

Bone marrow aspirates may also be stained selectively to demonstrate the extent of iron stores in this hemopoietic tissue.

Sickle Cell Preparation and Hemoglobin Electrophoresis

The red blood cells of patients with sickle cell disease (homozygous form of a genetic abnormality common in blacks) or sickle cell trait (heterozygous condition) contain an abnormal hemoglobin molecule that alters the shape of the red cell when the oxygen tension is decreased. This abnormal molecule is the basis of the sickling phenomenon that occurs intravascularly in these patients and can also be demonstrated *in vitro* by observing the cells in a drop of blood diluted with sodium bisulfite and sealed on a microscope slide. This is commonly known as *sickle cell preparation*. In a positive test, microscopic examination of the preparation after 10 to 15 minutes reveals elongated, curved cells with multiple pointed extrusions.

The presence and relative concentration of this abnormal hemoglobin (hemoglobin S) as well as the abnormal hemoglobins characteristic of other inherited hemoglobinopathies such as hemoglobin C disease, are measured more accurately by electrophoresis of hemoglobin contained in the red cells. Because the majority of patients with sickle cell trait (as distinct from patients with sickle cell disease) have no symptoms or signs of disease but may be poor surgical and anesthetic risks, screening of susceptible populations by hemoglobin electrophoresis has been proposed.

In sickle cell disease (hemoglobin SS disease) 75% to 95% of the hemoglobin on electrophoresis is found to be an abnormal hemoglobin S, and the remainder fetal hemoglobin F. In sickle cell trait (heterozygous AS condition) 20% to 45% of the hemoglobin is S and the remainder normal adult hemoglobin A.

Erythrocyte Sedimentation Rate

The erythrocyte sedimentation rate (ESR) is not part of the work-up for an anemia but is included here because it is usually performed in the hematology section of the clinical laboratory. The ESR measures the rate at which RBCs sediment in a tube of plasma. The rate is accelerated when changes in plasma proteins cause the RBCs to aggregate or when there are changes in the physicochemical properties of plasma or the red cell surface. The test is helpful in following the progress of some chronic infections (tuberculosis and osteomyelitis) as well as diseases characterized by altered globulins such as the collagen diseases, nephritis, rheumatic fever, and the dysproteinemias. It is claimed to be more sensitive than temperature, WBC count, weight, and subjective symptoms as an indication of progress of some diseases. Marked elevations usually indicate the presence of disease, the exact nature of which should be investigated.

In the Westergren method a graduated sedimentation tube is filled with oxalated blood and placed in an absolutely vertical position. The erythrocyte level is read at 10-minute intervals and at the end of the hour. The generally accepted normal sedimentation rates in 60 minutes for this method are males, 0 to 15 mm; females, 0 to 20 mm. The sedimentation rate may be increased in women with intrauterine contraceptive devices (IUDs) and women taking anovulatory steroids (oral contraceptives). This test is also of considerable importance in the diagnosis of giant cell arteritis (*temporal arteritis;* see Chap. 16) and a closely related disease, *polymyalgia rheumatica,* which are uncommon but clearly defined causes of recurrent facial pain.

Office Procedures for the Detection of Abnormalities of Bleeding and Clotting

When a patient who is scheduled for dental surgery (local anesthetic injections, scaling, periodontal, and oral surgery) gives a convincing and reasonably well-documented history of a bleeding abnormality (*e.g.*, prolonged bleeding following previous dental surgery, spontaneous bruising, petechial hemorrhages, multiple transfusions following surgery), the dental surgery should be deferred until medical consultation can be obtained. In most cases this consultation would include a medical history and physical examination as well as the following laboratory work-up for bleeding abnormalities: complete blood count; measurement of bleeding time, prothrombin time, and partial thromboplastin time; and a platelet count. With the exception of the hematocrit and bleeding time, these procedures require specialized equipment and a trained technician.

On other occasions the history of bleeding given to the dentist is equivocal and open to several explanations. The stimulus for obtaining a full hematologic work-up as listed above would then be weaker for both patient and dentist. Under these circumstances, detection of an abnormal hematocrit, a prolonged bleeding time, or an abnormal capillary fragility test (all simple screening tests the dentist can perform himself) may provide the necessary stimulus for referral of the patient for a more detailed work-up. It should be stressed, however, that *negative findings on these screening tests do not rule out the possibility of a bleeding abnormality in the patient.*

When blood tests are performed outside the office, the bleeding time and capillary fragility test must be performed as office (chairside) procedures by the clinician unless the patient goes in person to the laboratory to have blood drawn.

Bleeding Time—Ivy Technique

Indications Combined with determination of the hematocrit, the bleeding time is a useful screening test in a patient with a history of prolonged bleeding following previous surgery. It is important to remember that although the bleeding time is elevated in many disorders of the hemostatic mechanism, other patients may have severe and potentially life-threatening bleeding abnormalities and still have normal bleeding times. In other words, detection of an elevated bleeding time is usually indicative of a disorder of the hemostatic mechanism, but *a*

normal bleeding time does not exclude the possibility that the patient may have a bleeding abnormality.

This test should not be carried out on a patient with strongly suggestive evidence of a bleeding abnormality. Casual performance of the test is not justified where there is a risk of prolonged bleeding resulting from the test, and nothing is gained by delaying the referral of such a patient for a full hematologic evaluation.

Equipment Sphygmomanometer and cuff; jar of sponges soaked in 70% alcohol and a jar of dry sponges; blood lancet; three or four pieces of filter paper about 1-inch square; watch with second hand.

Procedure The patient is seated comfortably with his arm supported on the chair arm or the thigh. The sphygmomanometer cuff is applied to the patient's upper arm and inflated to 40 mm pressure. An area on the palmar (inner) surface of the forearm about halfway between elbow and wrist that is free of superficial veins is located and prepared by scrubbing with an alcohol-soaked swab. After the area has air-dried, the skin of the prepared area is tensed and punctured with a blood lancet cutting deep enough such that the hilt is firmly pressed against the skin of the arm. The lancet is immediately removed and the time noted on a watch equipped with a second hand. Every 30 seconds by the watch, an edge of filter paper is touched against the drop of blood that wells up. The length of time until the bleeding ceases is the bleeding time in minutes. The area is finally cleansed with a swab slightly moistened in 70% alcohol. With experience, the bleeding time and hematocrit can be determined simultaneously with a single finger prick.

Interpretation The upper limit of normal for the bleeding time performed by the Ivy technique is usually given as 5 to 6 minutes. (With other techniques such as the Duke earlobe methods, values as high as 7 to 8 minutes are normal.) If an abnormal value is obtained, the test should be repeated on a different area of the same arm or the opposite arm.

An abnormal bleeding time is usually the result of abnormalities in the structure or ability of the capillary blood vessels to contract (*e.g.*, von Willebrand's disease) or abnormalities in the number or functional integrity of platelets. Tissue thromboplastins released by the trauma of the incision are usually adequate to mask any deficiencies in the intrinsic coagulation scheme. In severe hemophilia of different types and deficiencies of prothrombin and fibrinogen, however, the bleeding time may be increased. An abnormal bleeding time is therefore not diagnostic of any one type of hemostatic disorder, and a dental patient with an abnormal bleeding time requires a more detailed hematologic work-up.

A bleeding time of 5 minutes does not mean that a patient will stop bleeding from any type of wound in 5 minutes. The time for bleeding to stop is related to the way in which the wound was produced, the caliber of the vessel involved in the hemorrhage, the amount of tissue damage adjacent to the wound, and systemic factors such as blood pressure and individual response to the type of anesthetic. A patient with thrombocytopenia may have a bleeding time of 15 minutes but may bleed continuously from areas of chronically inflamed gingival tissue.

Capillary Fragility Test—Tourniquet Test, Rumpel Leede Test

Indications The capillary fragility test is used to screen for a bleeding abnormality, especially where there is suspicion of a deficiency of platelets (thrombocytopenia), abnormal platelet function (thrombasthenia), a deficiency of prothrombin (*e.g.*, with Dicumarol therapy), or damaged or poorly supported capillary walls (*e.g.*, in purpura, scurvy, and some collagen diseases). The microhematocrit and bleeding time are often run concurrently.

The capillary fragility test is a test of the ability of the superficial capillaries of the skin of the forearm and hand to withstand an increased intraluminal pressure and a certain degree of hypoxia, developed over a 5-minute period by occlusion of the veins of the upper arm with a blood pressure cuff. The blood vessels of normal individuals withstand these conditions, and petechial hemorrhages will not appear on the forearm and hand from rupture of superficial capillaries.

The discovery of petechiae in the oral cavity or on the skin is the most common indication for the capillary fragility test, especially where the petechiae are confined to the oral cavity and could also conceivably have resulted from local trauma or denture irritation. If these petechiae (or ecchymoses—areas of spontaneous bruising) are easily and accurately identifiable, nothing is to be gained by performing the capillary fragility test rather than a planned hematologic work-up. In fact, the test may result in a dramatically positive result, with large numbers of

petechiae disfiguring the hand and forearm for some days. It is important, therefore, to perform a medical history including a drug history and an examination of the patient's mouth, arms, and hands for petechiae before proceeding with this test. The capillary fragility test should not be confused with the measurement of erythrocyte fragility (determination of the lowest concentration of sodium chloride that will hemolyze a patient's red blood cells).

Equipment Sphygmomanometer and cuff; microscope slide

Procedure The patient is seated with one arm supported on the chair arm or thigh. The dentist should explain to the patient that his blood pressure will be taken and that the cuff will be left on a little longer than the patient may be used to. He should explain further that the procedure may make the patient's arm a little numb and even painful, but that the discomfort will quickly disappear once the cuff is removed. During this time the dentist examines the patient's forearm and hands for any petechiae and records their location with an ink spot. The blood in a petechial hemorrhage lies extravascularly and should not disappear upon pressure with the surface of a glass microscope slide. Other small lesions likely to be confused with petechiae are telangiectasias (blood is intravascular, and the lesion should blanch upon pressing with the slide) and insect bites (the history often indicates this).

The blood pressure cuff is applied in the customary manner, and the patient's systolic and diastolic arterial blood pressures are recorded. The pressure in the cuff is reduced to 0, and the cuff is reinflated to a point halfway between systolic and diastolic pressures. This pressure is maintained for 5 minutes, during which the forearm and hand are examined for development of new petechiae. The patient's hand should not be moved vigorously while the cuff is in place because movement will increase anaerobic muscular glycolysis, lactate accumulation, and pain. After 5 minutes, the cuff is removed and the patient allowed to exercise his arm to restore the circulation.

Interpretation If any unequivocal petechiae develop distal to the cuff (toward the hand) after the cuff has been applied, the test is recorded as positive. If only one or two petechiae are seen, or if those seen are not convincing in their appearance, a negative test is recorded; retesting at another time then depends upon the dentist's impression of the nature of the problem that he is investigating.

In mild states of "capillary fragility," it is possible to record a positive test at one time and a negative test at another. Because of the variability in this test, it is not advisable to draw definite conclusions about the significance of the results when a single positive test is elicited in a dental patient. A positive test does, however, justify the need for consultation with the patient's physician if the patient is already receiving medical care, or the need for referral for further medical work-up if such is not the case. In addition to those conditions listed in the indications for this test, the test is also positive on occasion in an otherwise healthy person who is convalescing from a recent infection, commonly an upper respiratory infection, or who has a history of allergy. False-positive tests are also said to be more common in red-haired persons and in infants and in the elderly.

Perhaps the most important use of this test in dental practice is as a screening test for scurvy, which is a known though very uncommon etiologic factor in periodontal disease and hemorrhagic gingivitis. The tourniquet test is always positive in scurvy. A diagnosis of scorbutic gingivitis or periodontal disease is very difficult to support if the patient has a negative tourniquet test.

Since the bleeding time and capillary fragility test are carried out directly on the patient, they are sometimes referred to as *clinical tests* of platelet function, to distinguish them from other *laboratory tests* of platelet function (such as the platelet count) in which a sample of the patient's blood is studied in the laboratory.

Laboratory Evaluation of Bleeding and Clotting Abnormalities

To evaluate bleeding and clotting abnormalities, the following group of tests are the accepted minimum: the complete blood count, the bleeding time and the platelet count (as described above), the prothrombin time, and the partial thromboplastin time. Abnormalities in any of these tests usually indicate the need for further evaluation by more sophisticated tests. Since the history remains the single most important screening device for clotting abnormalities, these procedures are usually carried out on patients who report one or more of these abnormalities: a clear history of excessive bleeding on more than one occasion; a history of excessive and unex-

plained blood loss after circumcision, tonsillectomy, adenoidectomy, appendectomy, extraction or deciduous tooth exfoliation, as well as gross bleeding or hematoma formation after surgery or parturition (blood loss requiring transfusion or a large hematoma developing within 12 to 24 hours after any of these surgical procedures is significant); frequent hematoma or persistent bleeding after minor injury; recurrent epistaxis; and even abnormal menstrual flow.

An outline of the blood coagulation pathway necessary to the understanding and interpretation of these tests is illustrated in Figure 3-9, and the International Nomenclature for Blood Coagulation Factors and Their More Common Synonyms is given in Table 3-8.

Prothrombin Time

Prothrombin time (one-stage method of Quick) is performed by measuring the time required for development of a clot in a patient's citrated or oxalated plasma to which have been added known amounts of tissue thromboplastin and calcium. Since the last two reagents are present in excess, any delay in clotting in this test suggests an abnormality of the prothrombin complex or a very severe fibrinogen deficiency. The tissue thromboplastin used in the test does not require Factors VIII, IX, or XI, so deficiencies of these factors cannot be detected with this procedure; however, deficiencies of Factors V, VII, and X do cause lengthening of the prothrombin time.

The prothrombin time is used as a screening test for the evaluation of suspected clotting abnormalities and also as an index of the degree of clotting abnormality in patients with deficiencies of prothrombin and Factors VIII and X as a result of liver disease, malabsorption, or therapy with coumarin drugs. Doses of coumarin are usually maintained to give prothrombin times that are two to two and a half times longer than normal. A prothrombin time greater than three times the normal time indicates a hemorrhagic tendency.

The results of this test are expressed in two ways: as the number of seconds required for clot formation in the test and as *prothrombin*

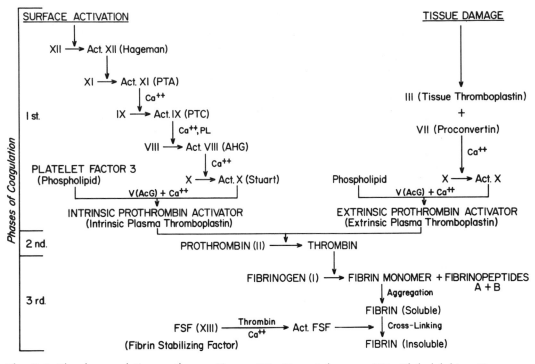

Fig. 3-9 Blood coagulation pathway. (Avery GB: Neonatology, p 406. Philadelphia, JB Lippincott, 1975)

concentration (activity) percent. The latter is derived from a curve of the length of time for clot formation in the test as related to the concentration of prothrombin. This curve is constructed by repetitive performance of the test with serial saline dilutions of normal plasma. Because of the asymptotic nature of this curve in the range of 50% to 100%, variations of a few seconds in the time for clotting cause a large variation in prothrombin concentration percent, which is not necessarily significant of a clinical abnormality. The accuracy of the test increases below 50%. Prolongation of the prothrombin time to two to three times normal corresponds to a prothrombin concentration percent of 30% to 50%.

Since the normal prothrombin time is subject to considerable variation as a result of differences in testing technique, the prothrombin time for a specimen should always be reported along with the day's normal value for the test. Specially designed instruments (prothrombin meters) have made the performance of this test much easier, but it is still subject to considerable experimental error, except in the hands of an experienced technician. The normal prothrombin time is usually reported as 12 to 15 seconds.

Partial Thromboplastin Time and Factor Assays

Partial thromboplastin time is carried out in much the same way as is the prothrombin time except that a crude phospholipid extract known as *partial thromboplastin* is used instead of tissue thromboplastin (both tissue thromboplastin and partial thromboplastin are available commercially for these tests). Partial thromboplastin, which is free of Factors V, VIII, IX, X, XI, and XII, contains mainly the platelet factor 3 responsible for producing plasma thromboplastin. This test thus reproduces the "intrinsic" coagulation mechanism (compare with prothrombin time which uses extrinsic system thromboplastin) and is a very sensitive measure of plasma factor deficiencies. Deficiencies of Factors V and VIII through XII are detected by this procedure (only the absence of Factor VII is not de-

Table 3-8. International Nomenclature for Blood Coagulation Factors and Their More Common Syndromes

FACTOR	SYNONYM
I	Fibrinogen
II	Prothrombin
III	Tissue Thromboplastin
IV	Calcium
V	Labile Factor, Proaccelerin, Accelerin, Ac Globulin
VII	Stable Factor, Proconvertin, Serum Prothrombin Conversion Accelerator (SPCA)
VIII	Antihemophilic Globulin (AHG), Antihemophilic Factor (AHF)
IX	Plasma Thromboplastin Component (PTC), Christmas Factor
X	Stuart-Prower Factor
XI	Plasma Thromboplastin Antecedent (PTA)
XII	Hageman Factor
XIII	Fibrin-Stabilizing Factor

tected). The normal partial thromboplastin time may vary from laboratory to laboratory, and the specific laboratory being used should be consulted for its normal value.

The bleeding time, tourniquet test, platelet count, clot retraction (see below), prothrombin time, and partial thromboplastin time form a group of screening tests that will identify the presence of almost all abnormalities of both extrinsic and intrinsic clotting mechanisms. These tests may not provide a definite diagnosis of the exact nature of a deficiency, but they will allow localization of the abnormality to several possibilities that can be investigated more closely with the aid of the *thromboplastin generation test, prothrombin consumption test,* and tests for the presence of *anticoagulants* and *inhibitors.*

In general, the bleeding time will identify thrombocytopenia and other defects in vascular permeability; the platelet count will identify thrombocytopenia, the prothrombin time defects in phase III of the coagulation scheme, and the partial thromboplastin time defects in phase II. Coagulation defects are also sometimes identified by correction experiments; because fresh normal serum contains Factors VII, IX, X, XI, and XII, the ad-

dition of this to a patient's serum will correct a coagulation defect due to one of these factors. Similar procedures utilizing other blood fractions and purified factor preparations may allow the defect in the patient to be pinpointed. These are discussed in more detail in Chapter 23. The test for capillary fragility may also be useful particularly in the diagnosis of vascular defects.

Coagulation or Clotting Time (Lee White) and Clot Retraction

One milliliter of venous blood is placed in each of four dry test tubes of standard size, maintained in a water bath. The first is tilted at 30-second intervals until the blood no longer flows. The next tube is tilted until clotting occurs, after which the third and fourth tubes are similarly treated. The average time between venipuncture and clotting in the last three tubes is expressed in minutes as the clotting time. The normal range is 10 to 25 minutes. The whole procedure including venipuncture should be performed by a trained technician with standardized procedures. Many variations of the test use tubes and syringes coated with nonwettable solutions in an attempt to make the test more sensitive. Because of the risk of addition of tissue thromboplastin during venipuncture, this is at best a crude test, and it correlates poorly with platelet count, bleeding time, tourniquet test, and clot retraction. It is frequently omitted from a routine work-up for a suspected clotting problem, although it is frequently used to monitor the degree of anticoagulation produced by treatment with heparin. The effects of heparin are too variable for its dose to be monitored by the prothrombin time (which is used to monitor anticoagulation produced by coumadin-type drugs) or the partial thromboplastin time.

Coagulation or clotting time has also been measured by a *capillary tube method,* using blood obtained by finger prick. The possibilities for admixture of tissue thromboplastins in variable amounts with this technique are so great that it is generally considered to be too unreliable a test to be worth performing. Its use is restricted to infants and in other situations in which a venipuncture cannot be obtained. Irrespective of the procedure used, the coagulation time cannot be relied upon as a screening procedure, since all too often the test fails to give an abnormal result, even with known hemophiliacs.

Clot retraction is a phenomenon observed following formation of a clot; fibrin contracts, and serum is exuded from the clot, which visibly shrinks. This phenomenon occurs both *in vivo* and *in vitro* and is very important in sealing of a wound against continued hemorrhage. Clot retraction largely depends on the presence and functional integrity of the platelets; however, when the character of the *in vitro* clot is observed following the Lee White coagulation time procedure, variations in clot retraction are also noted in patients with diseases involving fibrinogen deficiency, anticoagulants, prolonged coagulation times, and abnormal globulins.

Platelet Survival Time

The platelet survival time is measured in thrombocytopenic purpura and other diseases in which rapid destruction of platelets occurs (usually from immunologic reactions involving antiplatelet antibodies). A sample of autologous or isologous (compatible) platelets labeled with radioactive ^{51}Cr is added to a sample of the patient's blood and reinjected intravenously. The amount of radioactivity is then measured in blood samples taken at intervals over the next few days, depending on the design of the experiment. The normal platelet survival time (time for the circulating radioactivity to drop to 10% of its peak value after injection of ^{51}Cr-labeled platelets) is between 8 and 9 days. Even in a normal individual, only a fraction of the injected radioactivity is recovered in the circulating platelets; the remainder is sequestered in the cells of the reticuloendothelial system. The results of this test are, therefore, sometimes expressed as the peak percentage of platelets recovered in the day following the transfusion of ^{51}Cr-labeled platelets. The normal range for platelet recovery is 20% to 30%.

Fibrinolysis, Clot Lysis, and Fibrin Split Products

Blood contains an intrinsic mechanism for the breakdown of fibrin (the fibrinolytic system), which is catalyzed by the enzyme, *plasmin*, normally present in blood as an inactive precursor, *plasminogen*. Plasminogen may be activated by a streptococcal enzyme (*streptokinase*) and by endogenous mechanisms.

Circulating fibrinolysis may be detected by the clot lysis test in which the patient's plasma is added to a fresh blood clot from a normal person and the clot observed for lysis. Alternatively, in mildly affected patients whose blood will clot in a tube, the patient's own clot is observed for lysis (compare with the clot retraction test in which the clot shrinks and exudes serum, but does not lyse). Where fibrinolysis is extensive, plasma can be shown to be low in fibrinogen and rich in the breakdown products of fibrin (*fibrin split products*), using a specific test for blood fibrinogen levels. In the most common cause of hypofibrinogenemia, a disease called *disseminated intravascular coagulation* (DIC), which may complicate pregnancy, cancer, septicemia, blood transfusion reactions, and other shocklike syndromes, fibrinolysis is a prominent change that takes place secondary to intravascular coagulation, leading to accumulation of fibrin split products in the serum. Fibrin split products are demonstrated definitively by immunoassay and are screened for by special blood coagulation tests.

Fibrinolysis in the alveolar process surrounding an extraction socket has been implicated in the pathogenesis of dry socket; however, tests of fibrinolytic activity in serum or saliva are of no value in screening for this complication of dental extractions.

Current textbooks of clinical pathology or hematology should be consulted for further details of tests used in the detection of blood clotting abnormalities, as well as the variations likely to be observed in the many hemorrhagic states now recognized. These are also discussed in Chapter 23, Bleeding and Clotting Disorders.

Ascorbic Acid Assay

Deficiency of ascorbic acid (vitamin C) leads to scurvy, one component of which is a hemorrhagic gingivitis. Although scurvy is largely unknown in Western countries except in poorly nourished infants, a condition known as *subclinical scurvy* is still considered widely as a component in the etiology of gingivitis. As pointed out earlier, in the absence of other symptoms of scurvy, a negative capillary fragility test and failure to respond to a diet enriched with vitamin C should cast serious doubt on this possibility in a given patient; however, measurement of blood levels of ascorbic acid is requested from time to time. This is usually accomplished by measurement of levels in the buffy coat (the layer of fibrin, white cells, and platelets that remains on the surface of the specimen after centrifuging clotted blood) or by measuring the amount excreted in the urine in a given period following ingestion of a test dose of ascorbic acid.

BLOOD, URINE, AND SALIVA CHEMISTRY

Many of the blood chemistry determinations commonly used in the evaluation of systemic disease are described in this section. In general, evaluation of a suspected systemic abnormality is best handled by referral of the patient to a physician, but in the circumstances outlined below, a dentist may find it more appropriate to order certain blood chemistry tests himself. A dentist working in a hospital may also be requested to order many of these as screening tests for his patients before seeking consultation from the medical staff about a suspected systemic problem. The dentist may also be treating a patient with a known systemic disease, and an understanding of the results of blood chemistry determinations that have already been carried out on that patient is often essential in planning dental treatment.

Urinalysis and salivary analysis are discussed at the end of this section. Many of the determinations carried out on these body fluids are chemical in nature, and these analyses are usually handled by the chemistry division of the laboratory service.

The requirements for submission of specimens for various chemical analyses may vary from laboratory to laboratory, depending on the equipment and procedures used. General directions covering standard requirements are discussed in the section on Automation in Clinical Chemistry that follows and in a number of the sections dealing with specific tests.

Office Procedures for the Detection of Hyperglycemia, Glucosuria, and Other Abnormal Urinary Constituents

Detection of diabetes mellitus in a dental patient can be important for the following reasons:

1. The response of diabetic patients to periodontal therapy may be much less satisfactory than what might be expected of a nondiabetic under similar conditions.
2. The healing of oral tissues following surgery in the diabetic may be slower and subject to more complications (tissue necrosis and secondary infection) than that experienced by a nondiabetic.
3. Certain oral diseases are predisposed to occur in association with diabetes mellitus (*e.g.,* thrush, denture sore mouth).
4. The systemic effects of acute localized oral infections may be much greater in the diabetic than in the nondiabetic.
5. Diabetes mellitus is a disease of insidious onset that is not infrequently complicated by serious tissue changes leading to permanent cardiovascular, renal, cerebral, and optic damage.

In 1975, the National Commission on Diabetes ranked diabetes and its complications the third leading cause of death by disease in the United States. For this reason, it is recommended that any member of a health profession who suspects that a patient may be diabetic should take necessary steps to determine if this is so (*e.g.,* further testing or referral for medical consultation). In the final analysis, a diagnosis of diabetes mellitus should be made only by a physician; however, it may not always be possible or appropriate for a dentist to refer a patient for medical consultation at the first suspicion of diabetes. Under these circumstances further testing of the patient by the dentist is desirable and appropriate.

Since many diabetics excrete glucose in their urine, testing the urine with a commercially available reagent strip (TesTape,* Clinistix,† Chemstrip‡) is the most convenient

* Eli Lilly & Co, Box 618, Indianapolis, IN, 46206
† Ames Co, Division of Miles Laboratories, Inc, Elkhart, IN 46515
‡ Bio-Dynamics Division of Boehringer Co, Indianapolis, IN 46250

though not a very sensitive means of screening for diabetes. Unfortunately, mild diabetics and diabetics with raised thresholds for urinary excretion of glucose may not exhibit glucosuria unless they have recently ingested large quantities of carbohydrate. False positive urine sugar tests also occur in individuals with renal glucosuria (a familial condition characterized by a lowered renal threshold for glucose and normal blood glucose levels) and as a result of other reducing sugars in the urine (*e.g.*, lactose in the urine of nursing mothers) if a specific glucose oxidase containing reagent strip is not used. Determination of the blood glucose concentration provides a more sensitive diagnosis of diabetes especially if it is performed at a fixed time after a standard meal.

Three schedules for determination of blood glucose concentration are used:

1. Determination of fasting blood glucose is frequently used as a screening test for hyperglycemia in hospitalized patients. On an outpatient basis, however, maintenance of the fasting state from the evening meal until the next morning is difficult to ensure and may lead to a degree of hypoglycemia that an outpatient cannot tolerate without fainting.
2. Determination of the blood glucose 2 hours after a meal containing 75 g of carbohydrate (2-hour postprandial blood glucose) is a more sensitive measurement of the hyperglycemia associated with diabetes. Both fasting and 2-hour postprandial blood glucose measurements can be carried out on capillary blood using the Dextrostix,* Visidex,* or Chemstrip bG† reagent strips. Because of its convenience, simplicity, and sensitivity, this test is recommended as the best screening procedure for a dentist to use if he suspects a patient may be diabetic and feels that he must explore the problem further himself prior to medical referral.
3. The glucose tolerance test is one of the procedures used for the definitive diagnosis of diabetes mellitus. It is performed on a series of blood samples by a laboratory and is used to confirm a diagnosis of diabetes in patients who do not exhibit consistently elevated fasting blood glucose levels (see following section for details).

Two-Hour Postprandial Blood Glucose—Dextrostix, Visidex, or Chemstrip bG Techniques

The 2-hour blood glucose test should ideally be programmed for a particular appointment and the patient prepared with an explanation of the test and the diet instructions, as outlined below. However, the test can be performed immediately, if on questioning the patient the dentist can satisfy himself that the patient has ingested approximately 75 g of carbohydrate approximately 2 hours earlier. A sample of urine should also be collected and checked for glucose whenever the test is performed. Directions for the detection of glucosuria are therefore also included in this section.

Indications

1. For evaluation of a patient suspected of having diabetes mellitus. The initial manifestations of diabetes mellitus are quite varied, but its presence should be suspected whenever any of the following are found: history of weight loss in the presence of adequate or excessive dietary intake; history of excessive thirst and attendant excessive and frequent urination; history of repeated episodes of boils, skin infections, and periodontal abscesses; presence of severe periodontitis with excessive bone loss. The suspicion should also be greater where there is a family history of diabetes or where the patient has been obese for some time.
2. As a screening test for diabetes mellitus where the dentist is interested in examining his patients for the presence of this disease even in the absence of characteristic signs and symptoms. Yearly testing of all patients over 50, all patients with a family history of diabetes, and all obese‡ patients has been proposed.

---

* Ames Co. Division of Miles Laboratories, Inc., Elkhart, In 46515

† Bio-dynamics Division of Boehringer Co., Indianapolis, In 46250

‡ A useful index of obesity based on easily obtainable data is the Ponderal index:

height (in) $\div \sqrt[3]{\text{weight (lbs)}}$

A patient with a ratio of 12.4 or less on this scale is categorized as obese (see also Fig. 3-10 and Table 3-9).

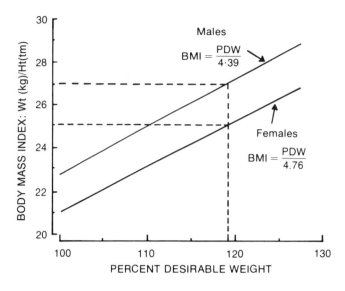

Fig. 3-10 Comparison of body mass index (BMI) and percent desirable weight (PDW) for men and women. The definition of obesity is complex, and no satisfactory index of obesity has been devised. It has been shown that of measures using height and weight, the body mass index (BMI) has the highest correlation with both skinfold thickness and body density. In addition, BMI is linearly related to the index of percent desirable weight (PDW). The latter is derived from the medium frame ideal body weight estimates of the Society of Actuaries, which have been endorsed by several conferences on obesity as recommended standards for weight in relation to height. A PDW of 120% corresponds to a BMI of 25 for men and 27 for women, and it is recommended that obesity be defined as those values equal to or greater than these criteria. Table 3-9 lists weights for heights that correspond to these criteria. The BMI is not a satisfactory method for assessing obesity in children because BMI increases with age in nonobese children up to about age 15. (National Diabetes Data Group: Classification and diagnosis of diabetes mellitus and other categories of glucose intolerance. Diabetes 28:1039, 1979)

3. As a measure of the degree of control of the disease in a patient who is known to be a diabetic, but who is not under regular medical care and is unwilling to accept referral to a physician for reevaluation of this disease.

Equipment Diet instructions (see below); blood lancet; jar of sponges soaked in 70% alcohol; jar of dry sponges; Dextrostix, Visidex, or Chemstrip bG reagent strips; wash bottle; urine jar; reagent strips to test for glucosuria

Diet Instructions for a 50- to 100-g Carbohydrate Meal.* If the test will be done in the morning, the patient may select one of the following groups of food for breakfast at 8 o'clock a.m., eating everything listed in the group, plus anything else he desires:

* Current recommendations for the 2-hour postprandial blood sugar specify a 75-g dose of carbohydrate administered either as a glucose solution or commercially prepared carbohydrate meal. If either of these is not available for testing in the office, one of the meals given above will provide an approximate dose of 50 g to 100 g carbohydrate.

1. 1 serving of fruit juice
   1 bowl of cereal with 2 teaspoons of sugar
   1 cup of milk
   coffee or tea with sugar, or milk
2. 1 serving of fruit or fruit juice
   3 pancakes with syrup
   coffee or tea with sugar, or milk
3. 3 slices of bread or rolls
   3 teaspoons of jelly, jam, preserves or syrup,
   coffee or tea with sugar or milk
4. 2 glazed doughnuts or sweet rolls
   coffee or tea with 2 teaspoons of sugar

If the patient will be retested in the afternoon, he may eat one of the following meals for lunch at 1 o'clock p.m., eating everything listed in the meal, plus anything else he wishes:

1. 1 sandwich
   1 piece of cake or pie
   coffee or tea with sugar, or milk
2. 1 serving of potatoes or dried beans or corn
   2 slices of bread or rolls
   1 piece of cake or pie
   coffee or tea with sugar, or milk

Table 3-9. Standards for Obesity Based on Body Mass Index (BMI) and Percent Desirable Weight (PDW)

	MEN		WOMEN	
Height* (m)	Average[†] weight (kg)	Weight for body mass index of 27 and for percent desirable weight of 120% (kg)	Average[†] weight (kg)	Weight for body mass index of 25 and for percent desirable weight of 120% (kg)
1.45			46.0	54
1.48			46.5	55
1.50			47.0	56
1.52			48.5	58
1.54			49.5	59
1.56			50.4	61
1.58	55.8	68	51.3	62
1.60	57.6	69	52.6	64
1.62	58.6	71	54.0	66
1.64	59.6	73	55.4	67
1.66	60.6	75	56.8	69
1.68	61.7	77	58.1	71
1.70	63.5	78	60.0	72
1.72	65.0	80	61.3	74
1.74	66.5	82	62.6	76
1.76	68.0	84	64.0	77
1.78	69.4	86	65.3	79
1.80	71.0	87		81
1.82	72.6	89		83
1.84	74.2	91		84
1.86	75.8	94		86
1.88	77.6	95		88
1.90	79.3	97		90
1.92	81.0	99		92
(ft) (in)	(lb)	(lb)	(lb)	(lb)
4 10			102	119
4 11			104	123
5 0			107	128
5 1			110	132
5 2	123	149	113	138
5 3	127	153	116	142
5 4	130	158	120	146
5 5	133	162	123	150
5 6	136	167	128	155
5 7	140	173	132	160
5 8	145	178	136	165
5 9	149	184	140	170
5 10	153	189	144	175
5 11	158	194	148	180
6 0	162	200	152	185
6 1	166	205		190
6 2	171	211		195
6 3	176	216		200
6 4	181	222		206

* Based on height without shoes and weight without clothes.
[†] Recommended weight in relation to height derived from the medium-frame ideal body weight estimates of the Society of Actuaries, Fogarty International Center, NIH, Conferences on Obesity, 1973 and 1978.

Procedure A sample of capillary blood is obtained as described under Collection of Blood Specimens. The first few drops that well up are wiped away, and the next few drops freely applied to the *entire* reagent area on the printed side of a *blood glucose* reagent strip. The blood is allowed to permeate and react with the reagents contained in the strip (glucose oxidase and an indicator system) for exactly 1 minute. The blood is then washed from the strip as completely as possible with a sharp stream of water from the wash bottle or faucet. (With Chemstrip bG no water is used; excess blood is wiped off with a tissue.) The test area of the strip is immediately compared with the color chart on the side of the bottle, matching the strip by placing it at the top of the appropriate color block and reading from color block to test strip. If the color obtained is intermediate between two color blocks, the result is interpolated; otherwise, the value for a matching block is read directly. Visidex and Chemstrip bG strips are specially manufactured for visual color matching; for accurate use, Dextrostix must be read with a colorimeter. Special equipment is available for this purpose in the office or laboratory (Dextrometer[†]) and in the home (Glucometer Reflectance Photometer[†]). A new reflectance photometer (Accu-ChekbG[‡]) is also available for patients who are unable to read Chemstrip bG results accurately from a color chart.

The patient is requested to void a sample of urine in the specimen jar provided; this is tested for the presence of glucose by using the appropriate reagent strip (Tes-Tape, Clinistix, Chemstrip; see following section), dipping a piece of strip into the urine, and waiting 1 minute before matching it with the color chart on the package.

Interpretation

Blood Glucose. The normal range of blood glucose in the fasting state is approximately 70 to 100 mg/dl. The concentration rises to about 160 mg/dl following a meal in the normal person but returns to the fasting level within 2 hours. In the diabetic of moderate severity, fasting levels may reach 200 mg/dl; postprandial levels are greater than this and may persist for longer than

[†] Ames Co, Division of Miles Laboratories, Elkhart, IN, 46515
[‡] Bio-dynamics Division of Boehringer Co., Indianapolis, IN 46250

2 hours after a meal (Fig. 3-11). Within the range of 40 to 250 mg/dl, Dextrostix, Visidex, and Chemstrip bG give estimates of blood glucose concentration that agree fairly well with those obtained with more elaborate techniques. These reagents can therefore be used to measure the range of values that are likely to be experienced in dental outpatients. Beyond this range, Dextrostix, Visidex, and Chemstrip bG tend to underestimate the blood glucose concentration to a varying degree, a fact that must be considered in evaluating patients in hospital emergency rooms where severely hyperglycemic (and often comatose) patients are usually seen. The test does usually differentiate between hypoglycemia and hyperglycemia and is also useful as a gross approximation of blood glucose control for diabetic outpatients. Glucose oxidase in Dextrostix, Visidex, and Chemstrip bG is inhibited by fluoride commonly used as a preservative of venous blood samples submitted to the clinical laboratory for accurate measurement of blood glucose concentration by one of the standard reducing (nonenzymatic) techniques. Dextrostix, Visidex, Chemstrip bG or other glucose oxidase estimations cannot be used on such samples.

The diagnosis of diabetes mellitus should be made only after a complete medical history, physical examination, and appropriate laboratory tests have been carried out by a physician; however, when the 2-hour postprandial blood glucose concentration is below 120 to 140 mg/dl, it is unlikely that the patient will be found to have previously undetected diabetes mellitus. When the 2-hour postprandial concentration is above 140 mg/dl, the patient is clearly metabolizing glucose in an abnormal fashion, and he may have diabetes. The patient with fasting blood glucose above 100 mg/dl or a 2-hour postprandial concentration above 140 mg/dl as measured by this technique should be referred to a physician for further evaluation.

Urine Glucose. When the blood level of glucose exceeds 160 to 180 mg/dl, the normal renal threshold for glucose, glucose appears in the urine, and the urine will give a positive test for glucose. The renal threshold for glucose may become elevated as a result of kidney disease, and this phenomenon is an important cause of false-negative tests for glucosuria in diabetes and a number of other diseases that may be associated with hyperglycemia.

Glucosuria secondary to hyperglycemia is very frequently caused by diabetes mellitus, but may also be associated with hyperthyroidism,

Fig. 3-11 Three glucose tolerance curves. The normal glycemic response to the oral administration of 100 gm of glucose (A). The rise in blood-sugar level is rapid, but a normal value is restored in 2 hours. In B, the glycemic response is slower, and normal values are not restored until the third hour, as found in mild diabetes. The fasting hyperglycemia and the continued increase in the blood-sugar level, even at the third hour, are seen in severe diabetes (C). Glycosuria usually occurs when the blood-sugar level is maintained (for several hours) at about 160 mg/dl, as depicted by the heavy black line. (Duncan: Diseases of Metabolism. Philadelphia, WB Saunders)

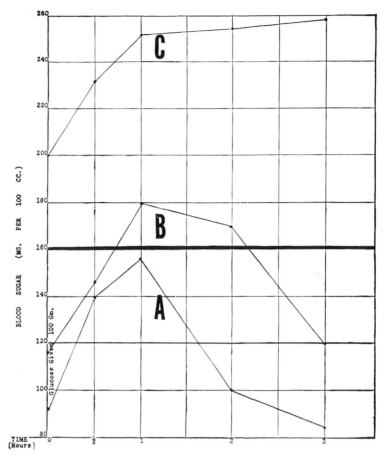

general anesthesia, and intracranial lesions such as a stroke. Glucosuria without hyperglycemia is seen in patients with renal glucosuria (patients in whom glucose spills into the urine at normal levels), in 10% to 15% of normal pregnancies and in other nondiabetic patients under stress or following ingestion of a high-carbohydrate meal.

Detection of Glucose and Other Abnormal Urinary Constituents

The group of tests commonly referred to as *urinalysis* is described in detail in a following section. Urinalysis in this sense requires the services of a diagnostic laboratory. Some components of the urinalysis, however, may be of immediate interest to the dentist, and in order to screen for the presence of certain systemic diseases, it is common practice to test for these while the patient remains in the clinic. Paper or plastic strips or tapes impregnated with reagents and indicator are available* † for this purpose. Various strips may test for some or all of the following urinary constituents in addition to glucose: protein, ketones, blood, *p*H, bilirubin, urobilinogens, and nitrate.

Indications The indications for testing for glucosuria were outlined at the beginning of this section. A test for proteinuria is sometimes included as a screening test in the medical evaluation of a dental patient. Ketonuria is an uncommon finding except in very poorly controlled diabetics, or as a result of a low-carbohydrate weight-reducing diet. A patient who is

* Ames Co, Division of Miles Laboratories, Inc, Elkhart, IN 46515
† Bio-Dynamics, Division of Boehringer Co, Indianapolis, IN

clinically jaundiced might have this observation confirmed by testing for bilirubinuria.

Equipment Urine jar; reagent strips

Procedure Detailed procedures are included with each product and should be followed carefully. Urine strips are not washed before matching.

Interpretation

Glucosuria. Urine normally should be free of glucose unless the blood level exceeds the renal threshold as a result of an excessively large meal, lowered renal threshold, or some pathologic state. Positive tests for urinary glucose are therefore always potentially significant and if positive on repeated testing, should be followed by measurement of blood glucose under controlled conditions (see next section).

Both false-negative and false-positive results occur with strip tests for urinary glucose: Glucose oxidase in most urinary test strips is inhibited by a variety of reducing metabolites sometimes present in urine. Such inhibitory substances, which give rise to false-negative tests for urinary sugar, have been identified in the urine of patients receiving 2.4 g or more of aspirin daily, patients under treatment with levodopa for Parkinson's syndrome, and patients with carcinoid syndrome or alcaptonuria. These false negative reactions may be minimized by dipping only the lower part of the glucose oxidase-impregnated strip in the urine and estimating the color change in the narrow band of color at the advancing edge of the moistened section of the strip, where glucose migrates ahead of the inhibitory molecules. Urine collected in jars contaminated with chlorhexidine antiseptic will give a false-positive test. Dextrostix, Visidex and Chemstrip bG should not be used to detect glucosuria.

Proteinuria. Urine from a healthy person contains only a very small amount of protein, about 50 mg in a 24-hour excretion (about 1200 ml to 1500 ml). This is not enough protein to be detected by ordinary chemical means in a single specimen and will not be found without concentration of a 24-hour specimen. Therefore, any proteinuria detected in a single specimen is usually a sign of a pathologic condition, with the following exceptions. *Functional proteinuria* is the occurrence of protein in the urine without the presence of any known disease complex; it

may be associated with unusual muscular exertion, prolonged exposure to cold, pregnancy, or orthostatic proteinuria. *False-positive* readings for proteinuria may also occur, especially at the "trace" level, if the specimen is stale or has been stored in a contaminated container or if the patient is taking alkalinizing medications.

Proteinuria due to pathologic change may be the result of a variety of diseases. In general, these may be classified as *prerenal* proteinuria (not due to primary kidney disease), *renal* proteinuria (due to primary kidney disease) and *postrenal* or *false* proteinuria (due to addition of protein to the urine at some point distal to the kidney tubules). When proteinuria is detected in a dental patient who is not known to be suffering from a disease likely to be responsible for the finding, the patient should be requested to repeat the test himself several times over the next few days, varying the time of testing. If the proteinuria persists, the patient should be referred to a physician for evaluation of the finding.

Reaction (*p*H). The extremes of *p*H consistent with health cover a wide range from 4.7 to 8.0; hence the *p*H of urine is of little use as a diagnostic aid except in relation to the acid–base metabolism of a patient. Where this is in question, as in seriously ill, hospitalized patients, urine *p*H must be correlated with diet, blood electrolyte levels, medications, and other variables in order to be meaningful. There is no value in checking the *p*H of urine as part of a routine outpatient urinalysis, even though this test remains a component of most urinalysis tapes.

Hematuria. Detection of occult blood in urine is a valuable additional test provided by several urine test strips. Although hematuria may be produced by a wide variety of conditions, in most cases it is indicative of a condition requiring medical treatment even when the hematuria is only of microscopic extent and the patient is unaware of it. False-positive reactions are common in urine obtained during menstruation, but otherwise a positive test for hematuria, especially if obtained on repeated specimens, is significant. False negatives may be encountered when the red cells in the urine have not hemolyzed. Diseases commonly giving rise to hematuria are nephritis, kidney stones, kidney and urinary tract infections, urethritis and prostatitis, tumors of the urinary tract, collagen diseases, leukemia, blood dyscrasias, and hemorrhagic states. Clearly, detailed medical work-up is needed to determine the cause of hematuria, in the same way that it is needed for proteinuria and glycosuria.

Bilirubinuria. When the total blood bilirubin is elevated, primarily at the expense of the direct reacting bilirubin, the direct reacting bilirubin is spilled over in the urine, giving a positive test with an appropriate reagent strip. The significance of bilirubinuria is discussed more fully in a following section.

Laboratory Measurement of Venous Blood Sugar Concentration, Oral Glucose Tolerance Test, Plasma Insulin, and Glycosylated Hemoglobin

Venous Blood Sugar Measurement

Screening office procedures that a dentist may use for detection of glucosuria and hyperglycemia are outlined in the preceding section where the use of urinary test tapes, Dextrostix, Visidex, and Chemstrip bG is discussed. Since these reagents provide only a range of glucose concentration rather than an exact figure, the facilities of a diagnostic laboratory are needed for more accurate measurement. Because elective periodontal and oral surgery procedures on diabetics are usually performed only when the patient is under good metabolic control, an accurate blood glucose concentration is often needed. This may be obtained through referral of the patient to a physician or to a clinical diagnostic laboratory. Alternatively, the necessary blood specimens can be obtained in the dental office or clinic and shipped to the laboratory. The specimen should be collected according to the directions of the laboratory being used and should be transported there as soon as possible and should not be frozen.

Test results are quoted in terms of plasma glucose or venous whole blood glucose. While a variety of enzymatic and chemical procedures (*e.g.,* glucose oxidase, hexokinase, O-toluidine, Somogyi–Nelson, Auto-Analyzer ferricyanide, and neocuproine techniques) are used by different laboratories, comparable figures for both plasma and whole blood glucose are obtained by all techniques when adequate quality-controlled procedures are followed. In general, values for whole blood glucose are approximately 0.86 times values for plasma glucose.* Table 3-10 lists normal glucose values for nonpregnant adults and children. As described in the preceding section, the fasting blood sugar or 2-hour postprandial levels can be measured, or a glucose tolerance test can be performed as a more definitive procedure.

The Oral Glucose Tolerance Test

For many years, the glucose tolerance test has been the accepted procedure for making a definitive diagnosis of diabetes mellitus and for distinguishing diabetes from other causes of hyperglycemia such as hyperthyroidism. While the glucose tolerance test is both expensive and demanding of a patient's time, especially when performed as a 3- or 5-hour test, and a number of other laboratory determinations such as measurement of plasma insulin or glycosylated hemoglobin have been proposed as alternative criteria for the diagnosis of diabetes, *the validity of the oral glucose tolerance test (OGTT) in the diagnosis of diabetes was reaffirmed at an international meeting held in 1978 under the sponsorship of the National Diabetes Data Group of the USPHS National Institutes of Health.* The recommendations of this meeting regarding the OGTT (which were subsequently endorsed by the American, Australian, British, and European diabetes societies as well as the World Health Organization) are followed in this section. Because other methods of performing and interpreting the glucose tolerance test will no doubt continue in use for some time, a brief outline of other methods of interpreting a

---

* Blood glucose determinations carried out as part of an automated multitest blood chemistry profile (*e.g.,* SMA-12, SMAC, "Chemzyme Evaluation") are usually measured on serum derived from a sample of clotted blood ("red-topped tube" or Serum Separator tube). Such serum glucose concentrations are essentially equivalent to plasma glucose concentrations determined on a sample of blood preserved with sodium fluoride and anticoagulated with potassium oxalate. These plasma specimens (for "quantitative measurement of blood glucose") are usually used for the 2-hour postprandial or glucose tolerance tests, and the term *plasma glucose* is therefore used throughout the following discussion.

Table 3-10. Normal Blood Glucose Levels in Nonpregnant Adults and Children* (National Diabetes Data Group of the National Institutes of Health, 1979)

	NONPREGNANT ADULTS	CHILDREN
Fasting Value		
venous plasma	< 115 mg/dl	< 130 mg/dl
venous whole blood	< 100 mg/dl	< 115 mg/dl
capillary whole blood	< 100 mg/dl	< 115 mg/dl
2-Hour Oral Glucose[†]		
Tolerance Test Value		
venous plasma	< 140 mg/dl	< 140 mg/dl
venous whole blood	< 120 mg/dl	< 120 mg/dl
capillary whole blood	< 140 mg/dl	< 140 mg/dl
Oral Glucose Tolerance Test[†]		
Values at ½, 1, or 1½ hours		
venous plasma	< 200 mg/dl	
venous whole blood	< 180 mg/dl	
capillary whole blood	< 200 mg/dl	

* Glucose values above these concentrations, but below the criteria for diabetes or impaired glucose tolerance (see text), should be considered nondiagnostic for these conditions (Diabetes, 28:1039, 1979)

[†] Based on 75 g oral glucose dose

series of blood glucose values recorded after a test meal are included at the end of the discussion on the OGTT, preceding the sections on plasma insulin and glycosylated hemoglobin.

Current recommendations for the diagnosis of diabetes mellitus in nonpregnant adults base the diagnosis on (1) unequivocal elevation of plasma glucose concentration together with the classic symptoms of diabetes, *or* (2) elevated *fasting* plasma glucose concentration equal to or greater than 140 mg/dl on more than one occasion, *or* (3) sustained elevated plasma glucose concentration equal to or greater than 200 mg/dl after an oral glucose challenge of 75 g on *more than one* occasion (OGTT).

Thus, in the absence of obvious diabetes symptoms such as polyuria, polydipsia, ketonuria, and rapid weight loss and without gross and unequivocal elevation of plasma glucose, quantitative measurement of plasma glucose under carefully standardized conditions is the prescribed method for making a clinical diagnosis of diabetes. The prescribed methods are first, measurement of fasting plasma glucose; and if fasting plasma glucose is not elevated on more than one occasion, then performance of the OGTT.

Elevated levels for fasting plasma glucose in this context include any concentrations equal to or greater than 140 mg/dl (or greater than 120 mg/dl for venous or capillary *whole blood* glucose). The OGTT is not necessary for the diagnosis of diabetes mellitus if the fasting plasma glucose is greater than 140 mg/dl because virtually all patients with fasting plasma glucose greater than 140 mg/dl have OGTT's that meet or exceed criterion number 3 above. To meet criterion number 3 (*i.e.*, sustained elevated plasma glucose concentration after an oral glucose challenge), values equal to or greater than 200 mg/dl (or greater than 180 mg/dl for venous *whole blood*) must be obtained *both* at times 2 hours after the ingestion of the glucose challenge *and* at some other point between time 0 and 2 hours. While separate criteria are used for children, no adjustment for age is made in the case of adults evaluated by these criteria.

The oral glucose challenge traditionally used in the glucose tolerance test has varied from 50 g to 100 g, administered either as a glucose solution, commercially prepared carbohydrate load, or a meal equivalent to this glucose dose, but the current recommendations for the OGTT as defined above specify a *75-g dose*. The test should also be performed on the morning after at least 3 days of unrestricted diet (greater than 150 g carbohydrate daily) and physical activity, and the subject should have fasted for at least 10 hours but not more than 16 hours before the test (water is permitted during this period). The subject should remain seated and should not smoke throughout the 2-hour test period.

A fasting blood sample should be collected, after which the glucose dose in a concentration no greater than 25 g/dl of flavored water should be drunk in about 5 minutes (nausea is reported to be less common with the 75-g rather than the 100-g dose). Zero time is the beginning of the drink, and blood samples are then collected at 30-minute intervals for 2 hours (a total of five blood samples per test). Venous rather than capillary blood samples are preferred, and unless concentrations are to be measured immediately with a rapid glucose analyzer, the blood sample should be collected in a tube containing sodium fluoride to inhibit glycolysis and potassium oxalate to prevent clotting. The blood sample should be centrifuged and separated within 4 hours, and the plasma frozen unless glucose levels are to be determined immediately.

The OGTT should be administered only to healthy ambulatory patients who are known to be taking no drugs that interfere with the laboratory determination of glucose (see Table 3-11). Abundant evidence shows that otherwise normal subjects will on occasion exhibit transient elevations in the fasting plasma glucose and impaired glucose tolerance as a result of numerous factors other than diabetes. It is imperative, therefore, that elevated fasting plasma glucose or OGTT values be demonstrated on more than one occasion (as specified in the criteria for diagnosis of diabetes mellitus given above) before a clinical diagnosis of diabetes is made.

The term *impaired glucose tolerance* (IGT) is used to describe patients who fail to satisfy the criteria for diabetes stated above, but who fulfill all three of the following: the fasting blood glucose concentration must be below the value that is diagnostic of diabetes; the glucose concentration 2 hours after a 75-g oral glucose challenge must be between normal and diabetic values; and a value obtained ½, 1, or 1½ hours after the test dose must be unequivocally elevated (see Table 3-10). Glu-

cose values above the concentrations listed in Table 3-10 but below the criteria for diabetes or IGT should be considered nondiagnostic for either diabetes or IGT.

In appropriate circumstances, the dentist can and should use the fasting blood glucose and the OGTT to evaluate blood glucose levels obtained on a patient whom he is called upon to treat, and form his own impression of the patient's diabetic status (normal, impaired glucose tolerance, or diabetic). The variety of criteria available, however, on occasion leads to conflicting interpretations, and the decision whether to inform a patient that he is diabetic or not should properly be left to the individual who has the responsibility for managing and treating the patient's systemic disease (*i.e.*, the patient's physician). Although diabetes is a recognized serious hazard to health, recent studies have shown that the methods of treatment that have been used often do not halt the progression of the disease. A controversy therefore exists as to whether individuals with mild degrees of glucose intolerance should be treated with hypoglycemic agents and dietary control or whether the patient should be spared the attendant anxiety of such a diagnosis until it is more firmly established or other methods of treatment become available. There is no doubt that use of the term *diabetic* to describe a patient invokes unjustified social, psychologic, economic, and medical sanctions except when glucose intolerance is severe enough to warrant treatment.

Other Procedures that Have Been Used for the Diagnosis of Diabetes specify varied test doses of carbohydrate and conditions for carrying out the glucose tolerance test, as well as varied criteria for interpreting the blood glucose values obtained. Of these, the following are still used with sufficient frequency to warrant description of the criteria of interpretation. With the criteria proposed by *Fajans and Conn* (one of the few sets of criteria that is based on statistical interpretation of data rather than on a consensus of experts), the diagnosis of diabetes mellitus is made if any two of the following are abnormally high: fasting blood sugar > 100 mg/dl, 1 hour > 160 mg/dl, and 2 hour > 120 mg/dl. In the *Wilkerson point system*, a score of 2.0 or more

Table 3-11. Drugs Reported to Interfere with Laboratory Tests for Serum Glucose

DRUG	EFFECT ON SERUM GLUCOSE VALUE	LABORATORY TEST
Acetaminophen	Increase	SMA 12/60
Aminosalicylic acid	Increase	Alkaline ferricyanide method
Ascorbic acid	Increase	O-toluidine procedure; alkaline ferricyanide procedure; neocuproine procedure
	Decrease	Glucose oxidase dianisidine procedure, coupled glucose oxidase method; glucomatic method
Chloropropamide	Decrease	Boehringer GOD-PERID method
Dextran	Increase	Alkaline ferricyanide method; HBAH procedure; O-toluidine procedure; glucose oxidase methods
Epinephrine	Increase	SMA 12/60 (at 10 mg/dl); alkaline ferricyanide method
Hydralazine	Increase	SMA 12/60
	Decrease	Glucose oxidase method of Boehringer
Iron dextran	Increase	Glucose oxidase method; O-toluidine method; p-HBAH procedure; alkaline ferricyanide method
Iron sorbitex	Increase	O-toluidine method; p-HBAH procedure; alkaline ferricyanide procedure; glucose oxidase methods
Isocarboxazid	Decrease	Glucose oxidase method of Boehringer
Isoniazid	Decrease	Glucose oxidase method of Boehringer
Isoproterenol	Increase	SMA 12/60
Levarterenol	Increase	Alkaline ferricyanide method
Levodopa	Increase	SMA 12/60; alkaline ferricyanide method
Mercaptopurine	Increase	SMA 12/60
Methyldopa	Increase	SMA 12/60
Nalidixic acid	Increase	Copper reduction methods
Nitrazepam	Decrease	Glucose oxidase method of Boehringer
Phenacetin	Decrease	GOD-PERID procedure
Phenazopyridine	Decrease	Delays coupled glucose oxidase reaction
Phenformin	Decrease	Boehringer GOD-PERID method
Propylthiouracil	Increase	SMA 12/60
Tetracycline	Increase	Hexokinase reaction; O-toluidine method; MBTH procedure of Neeley
Tolbutamide	Increase	Glucose oxidase methods

National Diabetes Data Group, Classification and Diagnosis of Diabetes Mellitus and other Categories of Glucose Intolerance. Diabetes 28:1039, 1979 (Courtesy of American Diabetes Assoc, Inc, NY 10016)

indicates diabetes, the score being assigned on the basis of fasting blood sugar > 110 mg/dl, 1 point; 1 hour > 170 mg/dl, 0.5 point; 2 hour > 120 mg/dl, 0.5 point; and 3 hour > 110 mg/dl, 1 point. The *University Group Diabetes Program (ΣS00) criteria* are based on the sum of the 1-, 2-, and 3-hour levels of blood sugar. If the sum of these is 500 or more, a diagnosis of diabetes is made.

Other variations of the glucose tolerance test, such as tests prolonged to 5 or 7 hours,

or the use of intravenous glucose or cortisone challenges are not currently recommended as criteria for the diagnosis of diabetes mellitus.

The fasting blood glucose and the 2-hour postprandial blood glucose remain the most useful measures of plasma glucose for monitoring control in a previously diagnosed diabetic. Alternatively, the glycosylated hemoglobin concentration provides a useful indicator of the plasma glucose level averaged over time. The OGTT should not be used to monitor blood glucose control in a known diabetic.

Measurement of Plasma Insulin

The concentration of plasma insulin (immunoreactive insulin, IRI) can be measured using a radioisotope immunoassay, a procedure now available in many hospitals and larger diagnostic laboratories. Controversy exists as to whether plasma insulin levels alone, or in combination with oral glucose tolerance levels, should be used for the diagnosis of diabetes. Plasma insulin levels range between 10 μU/ml and 100 μU/ml in both normal and diabetic individuals. The response of plasma insulin with time following a test meal rather than the actual level of insulin is the important diagnostic feature of the test. In obese subjects the level may exceed 200 μU/ml.

Glycosylated Hemoglobin

Glycosylated hemoglobin is normally formed in the circulating blood by the nonenzymatic addition of hexose molecules to the N-terminal valine of the beta chains of hemoglobin A. A number of these glycohemoglobins (referred to in this case as hemoglobin A_{1a-c}, or minor hemoglobins) are formed in the blood, depending on the particular hexose molecule involved. The more commonly measured glycohemoglobin, HbA_{1c}, contains one or two molecules of glucose attached to each hemoglobin A molecule. Cation-exchange column chromatography, isoelectric focusing, and spectrophotometric techniques are used to measure glycosylated hemoglobin, and radioimmunoassay allows specific measurement of HbA_{1c} in the presence of high concentrations of other hemoglobins (*e.g.*, fetal hemoglobin).

The degree of glycosylation of HbA directly depends on the concentration of blood glucose. As expected, the concentration of these minor hemoglobins is known to be two to three times greater in poorly controlled diabetics than in nondiabetics, with the concentration being reduced to near normal levels when blood glucose is well controlled. Because the glycosylated hemoglobin level reflects the blood glucose level averaged over time rather than at the time of venipuncture

only, it is considered to be a better indicator of diabetic control than are individual blood glucose levels.

A number of studies have been carried out to determine whether assay of HbA_{1c} is useful in diagnosing diabetes, the value of repeated measurements of HbA_{1c} in monitoring diabetic control, and the relationship of "glucose control," as measured by HbA_{1c} concentrations, to sequelae of diabetes. In general, if a patient has an increased HbA_{1c} or HbA_{1a-c} concentration *and* an increased fasting glucose concentration, diabetes is present, and additional testing by means of a glucose tolerance test is unnecessary. This combination of tests identifies persons in need of treatment because the increased glucose concentration indicates a problem at the time of testing and the increased HbA_{1c} indicates that the problem has persisted for some time. Repeated measurement of HbA_{1c} has also been confirmed as a sensitive monitor of glucose control in both type I and type II diabetes and in insulin-dependent diabetic pregnant women.

Correlations between HbA_{1a-c} concentrations and a number of abnormalities associated with diabetes (*e.g.*, RBC, WBC, platelet, and coagulation abnormalities; hormonal profiles; lipid profiles; and both micro- and macrovascular disease) are also stronger than those between blood glucose levels, and many of these abnormalities responsible for the unfortunate long-term sequelae of diabetes.

The normal range of total glycosylated hemoglobin ($HbA_{1a + b + c}$) is 5.5% to 9.0% of total hemoglobin. Values as high as 16.6% $\pm$ 7.6% are seen in untreated diabetics. The presence of other abnormal hemoglobins interferes with the assay.

Automation in Clinical Chemistry

The development over the last two decades of a large number of automatic* and automated† methods of performing chemical analyses on blood and other body fluids for clin-

---

* A mechanical device that performs in accordance with a manually preset set of conditions
† A mechanical device that is regulated by feedback of information such that the apparatus is self-adjusting.

ical purposes has increased the number of chemical assays available to the clinician and improved precision and reproducibility of individual test results. Despite the high initial costs of more sophisticated *multitest computer-controlled systems* installed in larger laboratories and the increasing costs of reagents, the cost of assaying the more frequently studied chemical constituents of blood has been maintained at a low level by corresponding reductions in the number of laboratory personnel needed. Smaller automatic instruments suited to the limited specimen load of an individual office or clinic but using automatic procedures and prepackaged reagents to provide accurate chemical assays for a number of the more commonly measured values (*dedicated single-test instruments*) have also been developed. While measurement of some chemical constituents may still be very expensive, the cost of the more commonly used tests has remained quite low, and determination of blood sugar, blood electrolytes, and some 15 or so other "blood chemistries" is still only a minor component of either outpatient or inpatient costs. To a large extent this low cost has been achieved by grouping and packaging together a number of more commonly used tests (usually referred to as a *profile* or *evaluation*), by programming automatic chemical analyzers to perform large numbers of these tests routinely (in some cases, as many as 250 or more tests per hour), and by conserving reagents by using only microaliquots of a specimen for each test.

The term *screening test*, which previously referred to the testing of a group of apparently healthy individuals with inexpensive and crude tests, now more frequently refers to a blood chemistry profile performed with a high level of accuracy but not necessarily individualized to a patient's specific diagnostic problem. With the exception of the small number of dip-stick techniques described in the preceding section (dealing with office procedures for detecting hyperglycemia, glycosuria, and other abnormal urinary constituents), very few manual procedures are accepted for blood chemistry as far as the more commonly measured values are concerned.

Under these circumstances, it is important for the clinician to have at least elementary knowledge of the type of equipment and procedures used in the laboratory to which the specimens are submitted, as well as some understanding of the automatic single and multitest instruments currently available for use in offices and clinics. A brief review of this topic is provided here without attempting to cover the full range and variety of instruments that are currently available or under development by numerous manufacturers.

Multitest Systems Used in Larger Laboratories

The *Technicon SMA 12/60* and *SMA 6/60* are prototype multichannel biochemical analyzers, many of which are still in use in hospital and community laboratories. They carry out repeated chemical determinations on aliquots of each specimen by pumping the sample into plastic tubing where it is mixed with proportioned volumes of reagents, allowed to react, and then replaced successively by a washing fluid and a new sample. These continuous-flow reaction units require a relatively small sample volume, and several reaction units can be combined in parallel to allow simultaneous determination of several chemical components. Multiple sample centrifuges, samplers, dialyzers, and timed reagent packs are also essential components. The SMA 12/60 (see Fig. 3-12) carries out 12 simultaneous determinations that usually include blood urea nitrogen (BUN), total bilirubin, lactate dehydrogenase (LDH), serum glutamic-oxaloacetic transaminase (SGOT), alkaline phosphatase, calcium, inorganic phosphorus, total protein, uric acid, albumin, glucose, and cholesterol. Other tests such as serum creatinine, sodium, potassium, and bicarbonate can be interchanged with these, depending on the needs of the population being studied. The SMA 6/60 is commonly programmed to provide analyses of chloride, bicarbonate, potassium, sodium, BUN, and creatinine.

Computerized data processing was found to be essential to handle the volume of data and reports generated by these analysers and similar instruments and to ensure the rapid distribution of reports to the clinician ordering the tests. Computerized programming of the machine is also made possible by continuous monitoring of the results with rejection of data, reprocessing of specimens, and au-

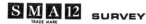 **SURVEY**

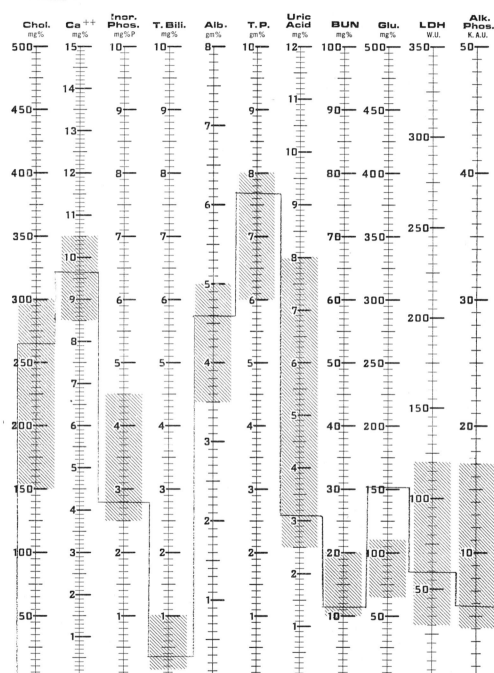

Fig. 3-12 Automated blood chemistry printout, Technicon SMA-12. Shaded bars represent the normal range for each test; the continuous line tracing out a bar graph represents values for a particular blood specimen. (Courtesy of Technicon Instruments Corporation, Dept. 4, Tarrytown, NY, 10591)

tomatic shutdown of the machine when results lying outside a predetermined range are obtained. These developments, together with improvements in chemical operation, graphic display, and printout of results are incorporated in the *Technicon SMAC* (Sequential Multiple Analyzer plus Computer; see Figs. 3-13 and 3-14), which is in operation in many large laboratories. The SMAC is a 24-channel system that allows 20 tests and a number of calculations (derived values) to be run simultaneously using only 450 μl serum. Positive specimen identification can be maintained throughout the analytic process, and continuous monitoring of the data generated provides a high level of quality control and ensures compliance with professional, state, and federal licensing requirements in this regard. The *Technicon SMA II* is a more recent version intended for the laboratory with a smaller work load; it uses many of the same components developed for the SMAC, can handle up to 24 tests on a single specimen, and allows the operator to select for reporting only the tests requested by the clinician. It is also equipped with a computer that allows storage of up to 1,000 completed chemistry reports and various quality insurance programs for monitoring performance. Unlike the SMAC, it is flexible enough to allow insertion of an emergency specimen into a sequence of routine specimens.

Comparable multitest systems include the *American Monitor* KDA and *Parallel* instruments, the latter equipped with the familiar bar-code method of positive specimen identification that is affixed to each specimen on receipt and identifies it throughout processing; the *Hycel*[†] M and *SKS 60* systems, which copy the manual process of chemical analysis more closely by utilizing conveyor systems of test tubes, automatic pipettors, and heaters; and the more recently developed *Kodak*[‡] *EKTACHEM*, which uses a novel concept of multilayer thin film analysis derived from Kodak instant film technology (a metering system dispenses a precisely measured volume of serum onto an analytical slide that contains

the appropriate dry test reagents distributed through several thin layers of film). The reaction takes place on the slide under controlled conditions, and the end product is measured colorimetrically by reflectometry (see Fig. 3-15). Other multiple test equipment (Electro-Nucleonics[§] *GEMSAEC* and the Union Carbide" *CentrifiChem*) uses centrifugal force to mix samples and reagents in special curvettes that rotate past a light beam to measure the results of the chemical reaction; this type of equipment is particularly suited to serum enzyme analysis.

Other manufacturers[*] have marketed systems that provide a limited battery or profile, usually representing the most common tests required for acute patient care management (glucose, electrolytes, BUN, creatinine, and protein). Results from these instruments are equally reliable as a result of their automatic operation, calibration, and standardization procedures.

General Purpose Analyzers and Dedicated Single-Test Instruments

General purpose and single-test analyzers are also standard equipment in large laboratories for handling single tests ordered in large numbers and frequently repeated on the same patient (*e.g.*, blood glucose, BUN, and uric acid). The *Technicon Auto Analyzer* is the most familiar of these, although other manufacturers[†] have introduced instruments with

§ Electro-Nucleonics Inc, Separation & Analytical Systems Division, 368 Passaic Ave, Fairfield, NJ 07006
" Union Carbide Corp, Clinical Diagnostics, 270 Marble Ave, Pleasantville, NJ 10570

* For example, Instrumentation Laboratory Inc, 9 Galen St, Watertown, MA 02171—IL643 and 446 analyzers for electrolytes; IL504 and 508 for electrolytes and the four standard acute care "blood chemistries." Beckman, Clinical Instruments Div, 200 S. Kraemar Blvd, Brea, CA 92621—ASTRA four and eight systems covering similar values.
† For example, Abbott Laboratories, North Chicago, IL 60064—ABA50, ABA100 and VP models; Beckman, Clinical Instruments Div, 200 S Kraemar Blvd, Brea, CA 92621—Trace I and III models; Ames Co, Division of Miles Laboratories, Inc, Elkhart, IN 46514—PACER and AutoPACER models; DuPont Instruments Division, DuPont Co, Wilmington, DE 19898—aca series I, II, and III, which among other special features include prepackaged reagents in special plastic packs that serve both as reaction chamber and curvette for photometric analyses

* American Monitor Corp, 5425 W. 84th St, Indianapolis, IN 46268
† Hycel Inc, 7920 Westpark Dr, Houston, TX 77063
‡ Eastman Kodak Co, Kodak Apparatus Division, 901 Elmgrove Rd, Rochester, NY 14650

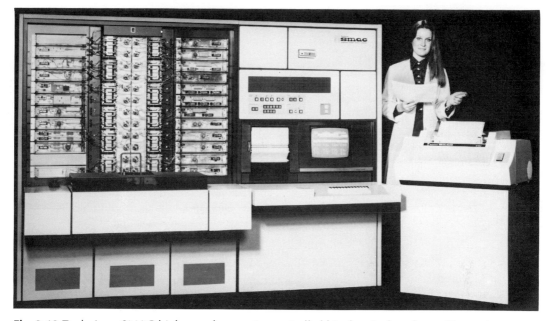

Fig. 3-13 Technicon SMAC high-speed computer-controlled biochemical analyzer. (Courtesy of Technicon Instruments Corporation, Dept. 4, Tarrytown, NY, 10591)

SmithKline Clinical Laboratories, Inc.

1075 FIRST AVENUE
KING OF PRUSSIA, PA. 19406

JOHN M. DOLPHIN, M.D.
PATHOLOGIST - LABORATORY DIRECTOR
HELEN C. OELS, M.D., PH. D.
DIRECTOR ANATOMICAL PATHOLOGY

PATIENT NAME	AGE	SEX	SPECIMEN DATE	DATE RECEIVED	DATE REPORTED	LAB NO	CLIENT NO
	39	F	03/10/83	03/10/83	03/11/83		

TEST NAME	RESULTS	NORMAL RANGE
CHEMZYME EVALUATION	PAGE NO. 1 OF 1	
* DUPLICATE REPORT *		
* TRIGLYCERIDES	184 MG/DL	30-39 YR 20-150MG/DL
CHOLESTEROL, TOTAL	255 MG/DL	30-39YR 140-270MG/DL
* ALKALINE PHOSPHATASE	119 U/L	20-39 YEARS
		FEMALE: 35-110 U/L
LDH	164 U/L	80-250 U/L
SGO-TRANSAMINASE	28 U/L	8-50 U/L
* SGP-TRANSAMINASE	61 U/L	0-45 U/L
BILIRUBIN, TOTAL	.8 MG/DL	0.0-1.5 MG/DL
PROTEIN, TOTAL	7.0 GM/DL	6.0-8.2 GM/DL
ALBUMIN	4.3 GM/DL	3.5-5.5 GM/DL
GLOBULIN	2.7 GM/DL	1.5-3.6 GM/DL
A/G RATIO	1.6 /1	1.1/1 TO 2.2/1
SODIUM	140 MEQ/L	135-148 MEQ/L
POTASSIUM	4.5 MEQ/L	3.5-5.5 MEQ/L
CHLORIDE	107 MEQ/L	96-110 MEQ/L
CO2 CONTENT	22 MEQ/L	18-32 MEQ/L
* CALCIUM	11.8 MG/DL	8.8-10.7 MG/DL
PHOSPHORUS-INORGANIC	2.5 MG/DL	ADULT: 2.0-5.0 MG/DL
URIC ACID	7.1 MG/DL	FEMALE: 2.8-7.5MG/DL
GLUCOSE	90 MG/DL	
FASTING NORMALS:		
	LESS THAN 50 YRS OF AGE: 75-115MG/DL	
CREATININE	.9 MG/DL	0.7-1.4 MG/DL
UREA NITROGEN	12 MG/DL	5-25 MG/DL
BUN/CREATININE RATIO	13.3	3.5-35.0

* ALL TESTS PER THIS REQUEST ARE COMPLETED *

JOHN M DOLPHIN MD-PATHOLOGIST-LABORATORY DIRECTOR

P-008

SmithKline Clinical Laboratories, Inc.

P.O. BOX M
KING OF PRUSSIA, PENNSYLVANIA 19406

UNIV OF PENN   ORAL MED

4019 IRVING ST
PHILA PA   19104

Fig. 3-14 Example of a computer-generated printout of results for a single blood specimen run on the Technicon SMAC biochemical analyzer or comparable instrument. The results of 20 separate chemical analyses and two derived values)A/G ratio and BUN/creatinine ratio) are reported together with specimen identification data and age-specific range of normal values for each component analyzed. * indicates a result that falls outside a predetermined range of normality and is flagged by the computer for retesting and drawn to the clinician's attention in this fashion. This group of tests would be ordered as a single evaluation on the blood specimen submitted and is here referred to as a *chemzyme analysis.* (Courtesy of Technicon Instruments Corporation, Dept. 4, Tarrytown, NY, 10591)

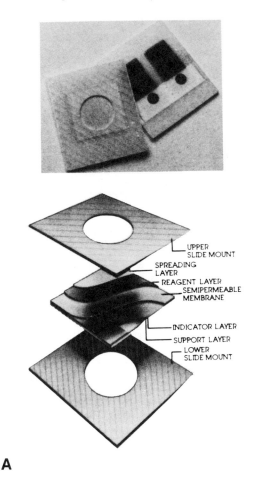

Fig. 3-15. The Kodak EKTACHEM Clinical Chemistry Analyzer makes use of a unique dry chemistry process that uses postage-stamp size slides (*A*) that contain in layers of dry film all the reagents required for a particular test. Slides for colorimetric tests contain a white, microscopically porous spreading layer and one or more reagent layers where typically an enzymatic reaction occurs. This produces a dye proportional to the quantity of analytic in the patient sample, which is measured by the EKTACHEM analyzer's reflectance spectrometer (*B*). *A*, Components of the Kodak EKTACHEM Clinical Chemistry Slide for BUN/urea. *B*, Key operations inside the Kodak EKTACHEM. (Reproduced with permission of the Eastman Kodak Company, Rochester, NY 14650)

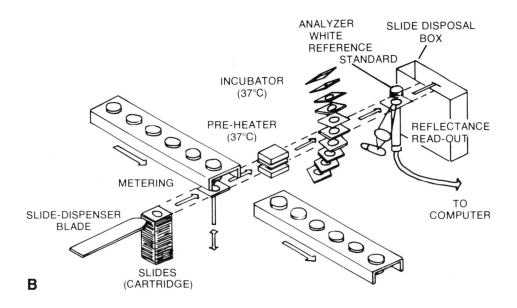

similar capabilities, some of which can analyze over 100 specimens an hour.

Automatic Blood Chemistry Analyzers for the Smaller Laboratory

The accuracy of blood chemistry determinations carried out in the office, clinic, and small laboratory has been improved considerably by the availability of automatic instruments that incorporate a photoelectric colorimeter or spectrophotometer and use a programmed sequence of procedures for calibration and measurement of control and test specimens, as well as prepackaged and proportioned reagents. In general because small unlicensed diagnostic units usually do not participate in established quality control programs, the data they generate are often considered to be less reliable than those produced by licensed laboratories, and the costs of tests run in this fashion are often not directly reimbursed by third-party payors. However, many instruments of this type are capable of accurate analyses that are far superior to those carried out manually under similar circumstances 10 or more years ago. Standard equipment of this type includes the *Clinical Analyzers* that use a series of prepunched program cards for each of the available analyses, the *Bausch and Lomb Spectronic 400** and the *LKB† Reaction Rate Analyzer*.

Of particular interest in this regard is the more recently marketed *Ames‡ Seralyzer* (see Fig. 3-16), which like the Kodak EKTACHEM and the Eyetone Reflectance Colorimeter uses solid-phase chemistry and reflectance spectrophotometry for the manual analyses of a number of blood components, including glucose, BUN, bilirubin, uric acid, and the enzyme LDH. Reagents are contained in a stable form in a porous matrix strip similar to those used in the more familiar blood and urinary glucose test strips, and special reaction modules are inserted in the machine for each separate analysis. A complete profile of

tests is projected, suggesting the possibility that rapid, accurate, and low-cost blood chemistry analyses may eventually be available as manual office and chairside procedures using relatively inexpensive equipment.

Submission of Specimens for Blood Chemistry Analyses

Although the majority of blood chemistry procedures are now carried out on 0.5 ml or less of serum, venipuncture remains the method of choice for obtaining blood specimens for this purpose. Unless otherwise determined by the requirements of a particular test, fasting blood specimens are needed because this reduces the number of substances circulating in the blood that might interfere with the chemical analyses (*e.g.*, lipid droplets transported in the blood after a meal or even after a cup of coffee with cream) and provides some standardization with regard to those components whose concentration alters significantly after meals or on a diurnal basis. Depending on the requirement specified by the laboratory receiving the specimen, blood for chemical analysis is submitted either as whole blood anticoagulated with EDTA, centrifuged clotted blood ("serum on the clot"), or serum aspirated or pipetted from the clot after centrifugation. Special tubes (Serum Separator tubes) allow for submission of "serum on the clot" under conditions that prevent remixing of serum and cells.

Interpretation of Blood Chemistry Reports

The results of blood chemistry tests are now usually reported by means of computer-generated printouts that list both the values obtained on the submitted specimen and the range of normal values. Values lying outside the normal range are usually grouped together or tagged with an asterisk to alert the clinician. The clinician also often needs to rearrange the data on the printout in his mind, so that groups of tests relating to a particular organ system or physiological function are compared. This arrangement is also used in the following discussion of in-

---

* Bausch and Lomb Inc, Instruments and Systems Div, P.O. Box 743, Rochester, NY 14603

† LKB Instruments, Inc, 9319 Gaither Rd, Gaithersburg, MD 20877

‡ Ames, Division of Miles Laboratories, Inc, Elkhart, IN 46515

dividual blood chemistry procedures. Tables listing differential diagnoses suggested by particular patterns of abnormalities noted on blood chemistry profiles have been published, but in most circumstances prove too lengthy for everyday use.

Serum Calcium, Phosphorus, Alkaline Phosphatase, and Leukocyte Alkaline Phosphatase

When lesions of the jaw bones are discovered on dental radiographic examination and systemic bone diseases such as Paget's disease, fibrous dysplasia, primary or secondary hyperparathyroidism, osteoporosis, multiple myeloma, osteogenic sarcoma, or metastatic malignancy are suspected, it is customary to order serum calcium, phosphorus, and alkaline phosphatase determinations as initial screening procedures. These three determinations are also included in the standard SMA 12/60, SMAC, or equivalent blood chemistry profiles, and abnormal values may be discovered in the absence of signs or symptoms suggestive of bone disease. Some of the other conditions (*e.g.*, kidney and liver disease) likely to be associated with such abnor-

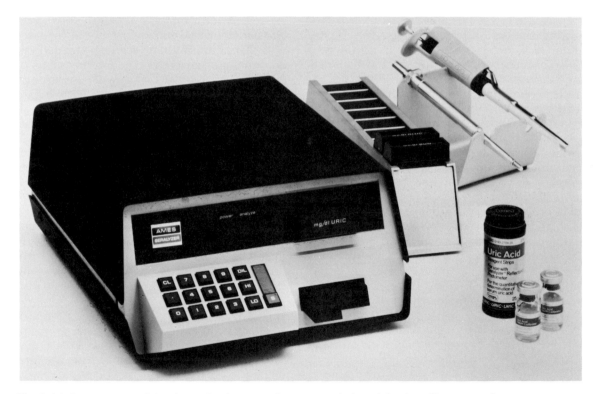

Fig. 3-16 Components of the Ames Seralyzer, an instrument designed for the office or small laboratory with a limited work load. Illustrated are micropipettes, prepackaged reagent strips and control samples module for blood glucose analysis, and the automatic Seralyzer Reflectance Photometer with analysis of blood uric acid in progress. (Courtesy of Ames Co, Division of Miles Laboratories, Inc, Elkhart, IN, 46514)

malities are also discussed in the following paragraphs. The commonly observed changes in these values that occur in these systemic bone diseases are described in Table 3-12.

Serum calcium as reported usually refers to total serum calcium, and about one half of this is usually present in an ionized form. The normal range varies somewhat with the technique used, and ranges quoted by the laboratory performing the test should always be consulted. The value quoted in texts is usually 8.5 mg/dl to 10.5 mg/dl (*or* 5 mEq/liter). The concentration of calcium in serum and body fluids tends to vary inversely with the concentration of *inorganic phosphorus* (2 mg/dl to 5 mg/dl *or* 1.8 mEq/liter). The product of serum calcium concentration × serum phosphorus concentration (both expressed in mg/dl serum) is constant at about 30 to 40 in normal adults, but may be as high as 50 to 60 in growing children. At serum calcium levels below 7 mg/dl (such as may occur in patients with hypoparathyroidism), signs of tetany (neuromuscular excitability, positive Chvostek's sign) appear. General anesthetic and surgical procedures may lead to cardiac arrhythmia and heart block under these circumstances. Decreased serum calcium levels are also seen when there is hypoproteinemia (due to decreased binding by serum protein) and in renal disease.

Patients with histologically diagnosed giant cell lesions of the jaw bones are frequently referred for serum calcium, phosphorus, and alkaline phosphatase determinations to rule out the possibility of hyperparathyroidism. This is probably a worthwhile procedure, but the frequency with which cases of hyperparathyroidism are detected is not known. Current reviews of hyperparathyroidism indicate that cystic bone lesions are probably the end stage of hyperparathyroidism and that discovery of chemical abnormalities (increased serum alkaline phosphatase or calcium) and subtler bone changes (subperiosteal resorption of the bony cortex in the fingers and possibly loss of the dental lamina dura) are better clues. Discovery of cases of hyperparathyroidism is even more rewarding if the population sampled is restricted to persons with a history of multiple calcific renal calculi, or the clinical syndrome that accompanies hypercalcemia, since hypercalcinuria and hypophosphatemia are generally present in the early stages of hyperparathyroidism. Radioassay techniques for parathormone are now available and allow for more specific diagnosis of increased parathyroid activity. Elevated serum

Table 3-12. Comparison of Calcium, Phosphorus, and Alkaline Phosphatase Values in the More Common Disorders of Bone and Calcium Metabolism

	SERUM CALCIUM	SERUM PHORPHORUS	SERUM ALKALINE PHOSPHATASE
Normal	8.8 to 10.5 mg Ca/dl blood	2 to 5 mg P/dl blood	1 to 4 units/dl blood in adult (Bodansky)
Rickets	Usually normal except in tetany	Decreased	Increased 20 to 40 × normal
Osteomalacia	Decreased	Decreased	Little if any change
Hyperparathyroidism	Marked increase	Usually decreased	Increased 2 to 50 × normal
Paget's disease	Usually normal	Usually normal	Occasionally elevated
Osteogenesis imperfecta	Usually normal	Usually normal	Usually normal—at times slightly increased
Solitary bone cysts	Normal	Normal	Normal
Metastatic osseous neoplasms	May be elevated	Normal	Normal or may be slightly elevated
Tetany	7 mg Ca/dl blood or less	Normal or elevated	Normal

calcium levels are also seen in association with carcinoma metastatic to bone and as a result of some dietary deficiencies.

Alkaline phosphatase occurs in many tissues of the body but notably in osteoblasts. Increases in the serum concentration of this enzyme are seen primarily as a result of increased osteoblastic activity but also in association with obstructive liver disease and a variety of miscellaneous conditions such as malignancy or abscess of the liver, amyloid disease, leukemia, and sarcoidosis. In the absence of evidence of liver disease, the rise is usually assumed to be the result of increased osteoblastic activity.

It should be remembered that increased osteoblastic activity is not restricted to sclerosing (radiopaque) bone lesions but may be quite high in lytic (radiolucent) bone lesions also, as a result of the remodeling of the surrounding bone that accompanies a lytic lesion. Increases are also observed in periods of rapid bone growth in infancy and childhood, during pregnancy, and in healing fractures. In general, alkaline phosphatase is raised in obstructive liver disease of both intra- and extrahepatic origin. It is not increased in acute A, B, or non-A, non-B hepatitis except during brief phases of the disease in which obstruction to bile flow may occur.

As with other enzyme assays (see Serum Enzymes, this section), direct measurement is not possible, and values are expressed as "units" in terms of the level of enzyme activity (*e.g.*, by measuring changes in substrate or some product of the reaction) and not in micrograms. The normal values for serum alkaline phosphatase are 1 to 4 Bodansky units or 3 to 13 King–Armstrong units/dl and 30 to 110 IU (International units) per milliliter in the current SMA12/60 or SMAC, automated analyses.

Alkaline phosphatase has been shown to exist as several isozymes, originating respectively in bone, liver (biliary duct epithelium), placenta, and intestine. These isozymes vary in heat stability as well as electrophoretic mobility, but attempts to separate them on this basis have not been universally successful, partly because of overlap of the normal and abnormal ranges. More than 30% heat stable alkaline phosphatase suggests a liver origin for the increased enzyme, less than 30% suggests a bone origin.

Another alkaline phosphatase is present in the granulocytes of circulating blood, and a histochemical technique is used to demonstrate this enzyme (*leukocyte alkaline phosphatase*—LAP) as a diagnostic aid in the differentiation of myelogenous leukemia from the florid leukocytosis (leukemoid reaction; total WBC may be as high as 100,000 cells/mm^3) seen in some pyogenic infections, tuberculosis, drug intoxications, and malignant disease encroaching on the bone marrow. In acute and chronic leukemias, LAP is usually low; the enzyme is absent from normal and malignant cells of the lymphocytic series; it is increased in mongolism. This test for LAP should not be confused with that for serum alkaline phosphatase as described above.

Serum Uric Acid

Serum uric acid concentration normally lies in the range of 4 mg/dl to 8.5 mg/dl for males and 2.8 mg/dl to 7.5 mg/dl for females. Uric acid is a metabolic end product of nucleoprotein metabolism derived from the purine molecule. Increases may result from increased dietary intake (in patients with renal insufficiency), but are usually evidence of gout or acute phases of diseases such as leukemia, lymphomas, anemia, or lobar pneumonia, in which there is rapid destruction of large numbers of DNA-rich leukocytes. Elevations of serum uric acid also frequently occur in patients taking diuretic medications and constitute one of the most commonly observed abnormalities detected on blood chemistry profiles.

Measurement of serum uric acid is important in the evaluation of intrinsic disease of the temporomandibular joint, particularly when nodules consistent with gouty tophi (subcutaneous deposits of urates) are noted about the face or ears. In gout, values of 8 mg/dl to 15 mg/dl for serum uric acid are usually observed. Some medications for gout and salicylates tend to lower serum uric acid levels. Uric acid is also excreted in the saliva, and cases of uric acid-containing salivary calculi have been reported. Where this is suspected, the calculus can be submitted to a diagnostic laboratory for identification of the sodium biurate crystals.

Serum Albumin and Globulin, Total Serum Protein, Serum Protein Electrophoresis, and Immunodiffusion

The concentrations of serum albumin and globulin as well as the total serum protein concentration* are routinely measured as part of the standard blood chemistry profile. Serum albumin and a number of proteins involved in coagulation (*e.g.,* fibrinogen) are synthesized in the liver; globulins are produced by cells of the plasma cell series. Because albumin and globulin constitute the major proteins of serum (fibrinogen is removed with the clot), liver dysfunction may be detected by a change in the relative concentrations of serum albumins and globulins. This abnormality, which is referred to as a *reversal of the albumin/globulin (A/G) ratio,* is automatically calculated by the analyzer from the chemical measurements of these two serum components.

Elevations of *total serum protein* most commonly occur as a result of diseases affecting the production of globulins by the plasma cells, such as multiple myeloma, amyloidosis, and the collagen diseases. Raised serum protein also occurs with the nephrotic syndrome. In the majority of these conditions, abnormal serum proteins are produced along with the elevation in total protein, and these abnormal proteins are detected by the technique of serum protein electrophoresis (see Fig. 3-17 and Table 3-13).

In *serum protein electrophoresis* a small volume of serum is subjected to a low-voltage electric current, causing the proteins of the serum to migrate at different rates. When the serum proteins are distributed across a piece of filter paper or a block of starch or other gelled supporting medium in this way, they may be separated and stained as relatively distinct bands and the concentration of each serum protein component calculated. By this technique, albumins and fibrinogen may be

* Note that the concentration of serum proteins, like the concentration of hemoglobin, is expressed in g/dl, rather than in mg/dl, the unit used for most other blood chemistry determinations.

separated from the globulins, and the globulins separated into four main groups: alpha-1, alpha-2, beta, and gamma globulins.

Serum protein electrophoresis will also demonstrate the presence of abnormal serum proteins such as the macroglobulins that occur in multiple myeloma (myeloma proteins), amyloidosis, collagen diseases, and the nephrotic syndrome. This procedure is therefore a useful screening test in patients with suspected oral lesions of multiple myeloma or systemic lupus erythematosus. Because of the ease with which this test detects abnormal serum proteins, it has been suggested as a screening test for use in selected populations for the detection of multiple myeloma before bone lesions develop.

In dental practice, it is recommended that serum protein electrophoresis (to rule out the presence of multiple myeloma) be carried out in patients with radiolucent defects detected in radiographic examination of the cranium and jaws (especially where they are not associated with pulpal or periodontal disease), patients with atypical facial neuralgia, patients with soft-tissue or intrabony lesions of the oral cavity diagnosed by biopsy as plasmacytoma, and all patients with serum protein levels greater than 8.5 g/dl as determined by automated chemical analysis.

Antibodies as a group move as part of the gamma globulin fraction, but the changes that occur with the development of immunity following a specific infectious disease are too small to be reflected in changes in the serum protein electrophoresis when it is performed as a clinical laboratory procedure. Deficiencies of various fractions of gamma globulin that occur in a group of fairly rare and usually congenitally acquired diseases known as the agammaglobulinemias may be detected with serum protein electrophoresis, but are usually recognized by the technique of *immunodiffusion* performed alone or in conjunction with electrophoresis. By this technique, four major components of gamma globulin (immunoglobulins IgA, IgM, IgG, and IgE) are determined. Normal values for the serum protein fractions obtained by electrophoresis and immunodiffusion are illustrated in Tables 3-13 and 3-14. Excessive production of gamma globulin (Fig. 3-17) is referred to as a gammopathy with the qualifying term, *mon-*

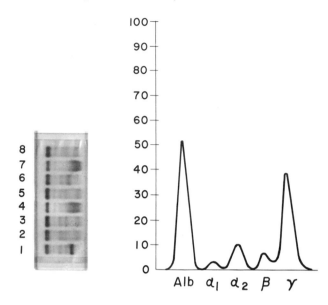

Fig. 3-17 Cellulose acetate electrophoresis of serum from a patient with a monoclonal gammopathy. The actual stained strip (*left*) shows the eight serums that were separated simultaneously. Normal serum is shown at 8; the patient's serum is at 1. The other numbers represent various other serums, including two (4 and 7) with a diffuse increase in immunoglobulins. A plot of the densitometer readings is shown on the right. The various serum proteins are in the same relative positions on both the strip and the graph. The patient's monoclonal increase in immunoglobulin is shown as a sharp spike in the gamma region. (Halstead JA [ed]: The Laboratory in Clinical Medicine, Interpretation and Application. Philadelphia, WB Saunders, 1976)

Table 3-13. Normal Adult Values for Electrophoretic Fractionation of Serum Proteins by the Cellulose Acetate Method

PROTEINS	G/DL
Total proteins	6.5 to 8.2
Albumin	3.3 to 5.0
α1-globulin	0.2 to 0.4
α2-globulin	0.6 to 0.8
β2-globulin	0.6 to 1.1
γ-globulin	0.9 to 1.9

oclonal or *polyclonal,* depending on whether the cells producing the abnormal gamma globulin (paraprotein) stem from a single clone or from multiple clones of plasma cell precursors.

Serum Cholesterol, Triglycerides and Lipoprotein Electrophoresis

Studies of the development of diseases of the cardiovascular system such as atherosclerosis, arteriosclerosis, coronary heart disease, and hypertension have demonstrated that age, physique (especially obesity), elevated blood glucose, triglycerides, and serum cholesterol are all related. Although the correlation of serum cholesterol with increased blood pressure appears to be due to a correlation between serum cholesterol and obesity, it nevertheless has become a common practice to measure the serum cholesterol and triglycerides and to attempt to control the level by diet as a prevention for these diseases. Screening clinics for arteriosclerotic cardiovascular disease therefore usually offer this measurement in addition to measurement of blood pressure and an electrocardiogram. Total serum cholesterol normally ranges from 160 mg/dl to 300 mg/dl depending on the patient's age. At levels over 300 mg/dl, patients are usually cautioned to reduce their dietary intake of animal fat, eggs, and other foods likely to increase the serum cholesterol level. Total serum cholesterol is also elevated in hypothyroidism, in obese and elderly diabetics, and in patients with the nephrotic syndrome. Patients with serum triglycerides above 175 mg/dl are also usually given dietary counseling.

Determination of these components is included as part of the usual blood chemistry profile to screen the risk factors for arteriosclerotic cardiovascular disease and is an important component of the evaluation of patients with unusual facial and oral nodules confirmed as xanthomas by biopsy.

Since lipids in general are water insoluble, they are transported in serum as lipoproteins in combination with alpha and beta globulins. A variety of lipoproteins have been identified in serum by *lipoprotein electrophoresis* (a variant of the technique of serum protein electrophoresis) in which the lipoproteins are stained selectively and quantitatively esti-

Table 3-14. Range of Immunoglobulin Levels in the Sera of Normal Subjects at Various Ages

AGE	IgG (MG/DL)	IgM (MG/DL)	IgA (MG/DL)
Newborn	750–1650	2–30	0–10
1 to 3 months	275–750	10–70	5–60
4 to 6 months	200–1150	10–80	10–90
7 to 24 months	250–1500	20–150	15–125
2 to 3 years	400–1500	20–150	20–250
3 to 8 years	550–1500	20–150	20–300
9 to 16 years	600–1600	35–150	20–400
Adults	600–1600	60–200	20–500

(Freedman SO: Clinical Immunology. New York, Harper & Row, 1971)

mated (as in routine serum protein electrophoresis) by optical scanning with a densitometer and integration of the isolated components on the paper or cellulose acetate electrophoresis strip. With this technique, several major abnormalities of serum lipoproteins that are usually identified as (Fredrickson) types I to V have been described. Of these, the most common are type II—an inherited disorder usually manifested during childhood or adolescence that features fat-containing nodules (xanthomas) of the tendons of the feet, legs, and elbows and soft yellow plaques on the eyelids (xanthelasma)—and type IV—an adult onset disorder often associated with obesity, maturity onset diabetes, and a high incidence of premature ischemic heart disease. It is characterized by excessive levels of pre-beta lipoproteins (triglycerides), and the chemical determination of serum triglycerides (but not cholesterol) usually shows very high levels of 300 mg/dl or greater. Abnormalities of lipoprotein may be either primary or secondary to other causes such as liver disease, diabetes mellitus, the nephrotic syndrome, alcoholism, and pancreatitis and abnormalities of serum globulins.

Serum Bilirubin Concentration and Liver Function Tests

Jaundice (clinically evident hyperbilirubinemia) can be recognized by examination of the color of the skin, oral mucous membrane, and sclera (whites) of the eyes. It is a significant finding in that it may indicate, among other things, the presence of hepatitis, which can constitute an infectious hazard for a dentist and his patients; the presence of other liver disease, which may be complicated by a deficiency of prothrombin and other clotting factors, or a decreased tolerance to anesthetics and other medications. Jaundice is usually not evident until the total serum bilirubin (derived from red blood cells, broken down at the end of their normal 120-day life span) rises from a normal range of 0.1 mg/dl to 0.8 mg/dl to above 2 mg/dl to 3 mg/dl. Patients may therefore report symptoms suggestive of liver disease or a history of contact with patients with hepatitis without being jaundiced. In either case, where direct referral of the patient to a physician is not possible, determination of total serum bilirubin (usually as a component of a blood chemistry profile) may be a valuable screening procedure, since this serum component may be raised in the preicteric phase of the disease.

In hepatitis, the hyperbilirubinemia is the result of hepatocellular damage, but in other diseases it may result from either overproduction of bilirubin from broken down red blood cells (e.g., hemolytic anemia) or obstruction to flow of bile from the liver cells to the duodenum (e.g., intrahepatic cholestasis in cirrhosis or extrahepatic cholestasis due to mechanical blockage of the bile duct from a gallstone). Diagnosis of mild degrees of liver damage is usually made on the basis of a battery of *liver function tests,** which include measurement of alkaline phosphatase, transaminases, lactic dehydrogenase, 5'-nucleotidase (see following section on Serum Enzymes), cholesterol, prothrombin time, and in special instances, Bromsulphalein (BSP) retention.

Direct and Indirect Reacting Bilirubin

Hemoglobin is released from the red blood cells and converted to bilirubin in the reticuloendothelial system of the body (reticuloendothelial cells are found in the interstitial connective tissues and lymph nodes and in greater concentration in liver, spleen, and bone marrow) from where it is transported in the blood and combined with serum proteins. Such bilirubin (referred to as *unconjugated bilirubin*) cannot be filtered by the renal glomerulus and is taken up from the blood by the hepatic parenchyma, which conjugates the bilirubin with glucuronic acid. The *conjugated bilirubin,* bilirubin glucuronide, is excreted into the bile canaliculi and passes from the bile duct into the small intestine where it is modified by bacterial action, partially resorbed, and excreted in the urine and feces.

When jaundice is caused by increased formation of bilirubin (*e.g.,* in hemolytic anemias) or by decreased uptake and conjugation of bilirubin by the liver (*e.g.,* in nonobstructive liver disease), the bilirubin accumulating in the blood will be largely unconjugated. In obstructive jaundice where the problem lies primarily with excretion of conjugated bilirubin from the liver, the bilirubin in the blood will be largely conjugated. Unconjugated bilirubin is soluble only in alcoholic solvents, whereas conjugated bilirubin is water soluble. This distinction between conjugated and unconjugated bilirubin is the basis of tests specifying the proportion of *conjugated (direct or 1-minute)* and *unconjugated (indirect,* reacting to form a colored complex in the test only after extraction with alcohol) bilirubins making up the total serum bilirubin.

Since conjugated bilirubin is water soluble, it will pass the glomerular barrier and appear in the urine once the renal threshold for bilirubin is exceeded in the blood. (Compare with unconjugated bilirubin, which cannot pass the glomerulus and gains entrance to urine only after passage through the lower intestine and conversion to urobilinogen. The usual yellow color of urine is due to urobilinogen and various bacterial modifications of it, but not to bilirubin.) In hyperbilirubinemia, the presence of bilirubin in the urine may precede for some time the appearance of clinical jaundice and may be noticed by the patient as a darkening of the urine. Testing of urine with the characteristic deep yellow to dark brown in the jaundiced patient is probably unnecessary, especially when the same color is imparted to the foam developed on shaking the specimen ("foam test"). However, where there is uncertainty, one of the paper strip tests discussed earlier in this chapter can be used to indicate the presence or absence of bilirubin.

Tests of Renal Function

Impairment of renal function may be explored by a variety of laboratory tests in addition to clinical procedures such as blood pressure measurement, intravenous and retrograde pyelography, ultrasound examination, and renal biopsy. These laboratory tests include the following:

1. Tests of glomerular function—urea and creatinine clearance
2. Tests indicating severe glomerular or tubular damage—blood urea nitrogen (BUN) or nonprotein nitrogen (NPN), serum creatinine, and proteinuria (see under Urinalysis)
3. Tests of tubular function—specific gravity of urine (see under Urinalysis) and phenolsulfonphthalein concentration and dilution.

---

* Note that the presence of normal liver function tests does *not* exclude the possibility of persistent or chronic hepatitis that may be associated (in the case of hepatitis B infection) with the presence of infectious virus in the bloodstream and saliva. Rigorous testing in this regard is based on the presence or absence of hepatitis B_s antigen in the blood rather than on evidence of liver damage—see discussion in Chapter 20 and under hepatitis B surface antigen elsewhere in this chapter.

Blood Urea Nitrogen

As a result of deamination of amino acids primarily in the liver, the soluble nitrogenous end product of protein catabolism (urea) is produced, transported in the blood, and excreted by the kidneys. In advanced renal failure the ability of the kidney to excrete urea is impaired, and the BUN may rise. With some few exceptions, a raised BUN is evidence of impaired renal function, but many patients with renal impairment do not show a raised BUN. The normal value for the BUN is 5 mg/dl to 25 mg/dl. Values as high as 100 mg/dl to 200 mg/dl may occur in the terminal stages of renal failure; these values are sometimes associated with tissue changes characteristic of uremia. Lower levels are referred to as *azotemia* and may or may not be associated with uremic changes.

In a patient with impaired renal function, the BUN can be raised significantly by ingestion of protein. Since blood is a protein-rich substance, hemorrhage into the upper gastrointestinal tract, as from dental extractions, hemorrhagic gingivitis, or peptic ulcer, may also raise the BUN in such patients.

In general, the majority of renal diseases are readily diagnosed on information obtained from clinical history, physical examination, and urinalysis. Although the BUN will probably remain as a standard screening test for renal disease, its sensitivity in early renal disease is open to serious question, and it is usually supplemented with the measurement of serum creatinine (see below). The dentist who questions the possibility of undiagnosed renal disease in a patient is likely to obtain better information from referral to an internist.

Two methods for detecting increased blood urea are available commercially as office-screening procedures (Urograph* and Azostix†). Both involve a strip impregnated with urease, which splits urea [$(NH_2)_2CO$], with formation of carbon dioxide and ammonia (detected by change in an indicator). This technique does not quantitate blood urea and does not detect early renal disease.

Serum Creatinine

Creatinine is a metabolic product of creatine phosphate dephosphorylation in muscle. It is produced at a fairly constant rate, is maintained at a stable level, and is excreted in the urine by a combination of glomerular filtration and tubular resorption. *Creatinine clearance* is probably the most frequently used measure of renal function. Serum creatinine levels, like the BUN, tend to be raised only in the later stages of renal disease, and a raised serum creatinine is sometimes taken to be an indication of chronic renal damage. Measurement of serum creatinine is preferable to that of urea because dietary protein and protein catabolism in the body do not influence serum creatinine concentration as they do the urea concentration. (Do not confuse measurement of serum creatinine with that of *serum creatine* and *creatine phosphokinase [CPK,* another muscle enzyme], which are also frequently measured in the laboratory, but as indicators of muscle disease and not as renal function tests—see section on Serum Enzymes.)

Both BUN and serum creatinine are included in most acute care and routine blood chemistry profiles. Values of BUN over 25 mg/dl are considered abnormal, but are difficult to interpret as an isolated value unless in the range of 40 mg/dl to 50 mg/dl or over. A concentration of serum creatinine over 15 mg/dl indicates impairment of urine formation; minor changes are significant. Usually the BUN level is about 10 times greater than the serum creatinine; a lower level (decreased *BUN/creatinine ratio*) is generally associated with severe disease or a low-protein diet. A higher ratio reflects excessive nitrogen intake, hypercatabolic state, upper gastrointestinal hemorrhage, or renal failure. Absolute values, particularly the serum creatinine, are more important than the ratio. Because creatinine is eliminated almost entirely in the urine, its concentration in serum rises when there is either insufficient formation or excretion of urine.

---

* General Diagnostics, Division of Warner Lambert, Morris Plains, NJ 07950

† Ames Co, Division of Miles Laboratories Inc, Elkhart IN 46515

Serum Enzymes

Destruction or alteration of cellular function in various parts of the body affects the enzymatic content of serum. A number of enzymes are therefore measured in serum for diagnosis of medical problems. The majority of these have no functional activity in serum and are simply being transported as a result of leakage from damaged or injured cells, increased metabolic activity, or decreased rate of destruction. Measurement of serum enzymes is usually carried out as a diagnostic procedure in patients suspected of disease of the myocardium, liver, and pancreas and hematologic disorders such as megaloblastic anemia, leukemia, and lymphomas. However, alkaline phosphatase, LDH, and SGOT are also provided as part of the usual screening blood chemistry report by many laboratories.

SGOT (AST) and SGPT (ALT)

Two transaminases (glutamic-oxaloacetic, SGOT; and glutamic-pyruvic, SGPT) are present in large amounts in liver, heart, kidney, and skeletal muscle.* Acute destruction of any of these tissues, especially liver, leads to an increase of serum concentration above the normal value of 8 U/liter to 50 U/liter to values as high as 100 U/liter to 2000 U/liter for SGOT, and above 25 U/liter for SGPT. SGOT concentration is also a sensitive indicator of myocardial necrosis, significant rises occurring with infarction of as little as 10% of that organ, but not with angina pectoris or coronary insufficiency.

In hepatitis and other forms of liver disease with associated liver necrosis, serum levels of SGOT and SGPT both rise, even before clinical symptoms appear. Values in the range of 1000 U/liter to 2000 U/liter are frequently seen. Serum transaminase levels are included with determination of specific antigen and antibody for hepatitis B virus and antibody for hepatitis A virus in screening evaluations for viral hepatitis. As there are

---

* The nomenclature for specific transaminases varies. SGOT is also known as aspartate transaminase (AST), and SGPT is alanine transaminase (ALT)

no specific immunologic tests currently available for hepatitis non-A, non-B, elevation of SGPT in particular is considered important in screening for evidence of this infection after blood transfusion.

SGOT and less frequently, SGPT are also elevated in muscular dystrophy and some inflammatory disorders of skeletal muscle. Smaller elevations also occur following crushing muscle injuries and with metastasis of tumors to the liver.

LDH and CPK

Lactate dehydrogenase (LDH) is distributed in the same tissues as SGOT, as well as in the erythrocytes. Tissue levels are normally $1000\times$ those found in serum, and leakage of the enzyme into serum from even a small mass of damaged tissue will increase the serum level concentration to a detectable level. The normal value for LDH varies from laboratory to laboratory and in the literature; as a general rule, values of 200 U/liter to 400 U/liter can be considered normal. Values as high as 1000 U/liter to 2000 U/liter are seen in myocardial infarction.

Each tissue has its own pattern of *isoenzymes* or isozymes (enzymes with similar or identical substrate activity but with minor distinguishable differences in protein composition), and diffusion from a given tissue may impress its pattern onto the pattern found in serum. Five isozymes of LDH have been identified on the basis of either heat stability or electrophoretic mobility and are routinely measured in some diagnostic laboratories. LDH_{1-2} (the "heart" fractions) are the fastest moving fractions on electrophoresis, are also heat stable, and increase selectively with myocardial necrosis. LDH_5 (the "liver" fraction) is the slowest moving fraction and a more sensitive indicator of liver cell damage than total LDH.

In acute myocardial disease, changes in LDH are similar to those of SGOT. LDH activity (especially LDH_5) is also greatly increased in patients with vitamin B_{12} and folic acid deficiency anemias, apparently as a result of intramedullary destruction of cells of the erythrocyte series. Changes in LDH activity are used as an index of recovery following therapy for these diseases. LDH$_{2-3-4}$ increase in acute leukemias, chronic myelogenous leukemia, infectious mononucleosis, and in some lymphomas.

From the preceding discussion, it should be apparent that no single serum enzyme determination is specific for the diagnosis of myocardial infarction. Sequential changes in serum enzymes, however, can be of considerable value in the evaluation of a patient with suspected infarction. For this purpose, the most commonly used laboratory procedures (which supplement clinical evaluation and an increasing battery of cardiac diagnostic procedures) are LDH, SGOT, and creatine phosphokinase (CPK). Repeated determinations are usually made throughout the week following the suspected infarct. These repeated determinations allow a kinetic analysis (change in serum enzyme concentration with time) to be made, this being considered more accurate than a single determination of each enzyme. The characteristic sequence of enzyme elevation is illustrated in Figure 3-18: an increase in CPK within 4 hours after the heart attack, followed by a rise in SGOT by 12 hours and increased LDH 1 to 2 days later. Of these, only the LDH increase may persist for any length of time, and an increased LDH may be the only laboratory evidence of an otherwise "silent" infarct. The value of LDH isozyme fractionation thus becomes apparent, since an increase in total LDH unaccompanied by other serum enzyme increases could also be explained by necrosis occurring in a variety of organs (e.g., lungs) and by red blood cell hemolysis.

Amylase and Lipase

Serum amylase is derived both from the parotid gland and the pancreas. Enzymes derived from each source have been shown to be different but are not distinguished in the usual test. Small increases may occur with parotid hyperplasia seen in cirrhosis, but raised levels are usually due to pancreatitis. In patients with acute pancreatitis, *serum amylase levels* generally rise to values greater than 550 Somogyi units/dl and even as high as 2000 to 4000 units. Any acute disease process affecting the gastrointestinal tract adjacent to the pancreas, the bile duct, or pancreatic duct may result in elevation of this serum enzyme, as will surgical procedures on the pancreas or adjacent tissues. *Lipase* may also be increased in acute pancreatitis; in chronic pancreatitis, values range from normal (20 units/ml to 75 units/ml to about 250 units/ml to 400 units/ml. Morphine and cholinergic drugs cause a temporary rise in serum lipase and amylase as a result of contraction of the sphincter of Oddi. Mumps and other acute infections of the parotid gland, by blocking the secretion of amylase, are associated with a mild elevation of serum amylase to about 250 units/ml to 600 units/ml.

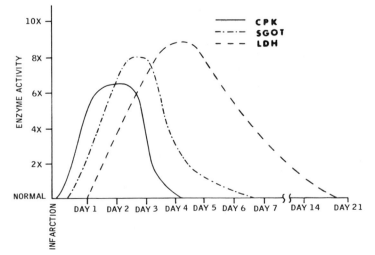

Fig. 3-18 Temporal relationships of SGOT, CPK, and LDH elevations in myocardial infarction. (Raslavicus PA, Shen EM: Laboratory diagnosis by chemical methods. Dent Clin North Am 18:169, 1974)

Acid Phosphatase

Acid phosphatase occurs in large quantities in the prostate and erythrocytes. Elevated serum levels are found in about three fourths of patients with metastatic prostatic carcinoma and in about one fourth of these before metastasis occurs. The serum level also rises as a result of prostatic massage or biopsy and may also be increased in metastatic breast carcinoma as a result of production of this enzyme by the neoplastic tissue.

Alkaline Phosphatase and 5'-Nucleotidase

The causes of raised serum alkaline phosphatase and the dual origin of this enzyme from liver and bone cells are described in the previous section dealing with abnormalities of serum calcium and phosphorus. In the presence of increased serum alkaline phosphatase, determination of serum 5'-nucleotidase, which is elevated in obstructive biliary disease but not in bone disease, can be helpful in identifying the site of origin of the alkaline phosphatase.

Blood Electrolytes

Oral surgeons undertaking the care of severely traumatized patients are trained in the management of patients with dehydration and other disorders of acid–base balance that are likely to be seen in surgical patients. In these circumstances it is customary to use information gained from measurement of blood electrolyte concentration as well as information gained from clinical examination of the patient, fluid intake and output, a urinalysis, and a hematocrit. Plasma levels of sodium, potassium, chloride, and bicarbonate are usually measured. Interpretation of these values requires thorough knowledge of acid–base equilibrium, and attempts to alter the levels observed should not be undertaken without such knowledge.

Changes in blood electrolyte concentrations in ambulatory patients are most commonly associated with use of diuretic medications prescribed for control of hypertension or weight loss. Hypokalemia (serum potassium below 3.5 mEq/liter) may be seen secondary to the use of diuretics and adreno-corticosteroids, but also following prolonged vomiting and diarrhea, or renal disease. Small degrees of hypokalemia are significant and often are associated with muscle weakness and tremors, as well as an increased susceptibility to digitalis intoxication. Hyponatremia (serum sodium below 120 mEq/liter) occurs in a variety of conditions, usually as a result of combined water and sodium depletion (*e.g.,* severe hemorrhage, heatstroke). Chloride depletion usually accompanies hypokalemia.

Thyroid Function Studies

Thyroid function is currently measured either by uptake of a radioisotope by the thyroid gland (a well-established technique in nuclear medicine, which is outside the scope of this chapter and is described only briefly at the end of this section) or by direct measurement of thyroid hormones, triiodothyronine (T_3) and thyroxine (T_4), in serum. Developments in these laboratory techniques in recent years have displaced older methods of assaying thyroid function such as the *basal metabolic rate* (BMR—an inaccurate and elaborate technique for measuring thyroid function by its effect on total body metabolism) and *protein-bound iodine* (PBI—a very reliable test for thyroid function with a clinical accuracy of 90% to 95% that unfortunately is often affected by contaminating substances ingested by the patient in food or drugs and by trace amounts of iodide in the reagents and atmosphere of the laboratory). Careful preparation of the patient for thyroid function studies is still necessary, however, since iodides administered in drugs (notably cough expectorants), x-ray contrast media, various thyroid medications, and other drugs (lithium, large doses of aspirin, estrogens, steroids, phenytoin [Dilantin], and warfarin [Coumadin]) do interfere with the T_3 and T_4 assays, which have replaced the PBI. The newer assays are, however, more specific in their measurement of thyroid hormone activity and are not interfered with by various iodine-containing proteins with little hormonal activity that are synthesized by the thyroid gland in some diseases.

T_4 levels in serum are currently measured

either by protein displacement techniques or by radioimmunoassay (RIA). Numerous kits are available commercially for performing these tests and the special laboratory facilities formerly required for the PBI are no longer necessary. The range of normal varies considerably depending on the particular kit or technique used, but an even greater source of confusion results from the lack of direct correlation between serum T_4 as currently measured and the amount of free T_4 that is active in the tissue. Serum T_4 levels measured in this way depend on the availability of thyroxine-binding sites on plasma proteins and on the serum level of such proteins. When estrogen levels increase (*e.g.*, premenstrually, during pregnancy, or with use of anovulatory steroids), thyroxine-binding sites increase in serum and serum T_4 levels increase, unfortunately without any alteration in the amount of free T_4 accessible to the tissues. Raised serum T_4 levels may be found in a completely euthyroid person as a result of increased protein binding caused not only by estrogens but by other substances as well.

Some solution to this problem has been achieved with the T_3 *resin uptake test.* This test is a measure of the available protein-binding sites for both T_3 and T_4 in serum, a low T_3 resin uptake test indicating an increase in binding sites for T_3 and T_4. (Despite its name, this test does *not* measure T_3 serum concentration.) The T_3 resin uptake test has no meaning alone, but when interpreted in conjunction with the serum T_4 level, it provides a more accurate estimate of effective T_4 serum concentration (*e.g.*, a high T_3 resin uptake test and a high serum T_4 mean an increase in the secretion rate of thyroxine and therefore hyperthyroidism); a low T_3 resin uptake and high serum T_4 represent a euthyroid state.

The results of the T_3 resin uptake and the serum T_4 are often multiplied together to calculate the *effective thyroxine level** (also referred to as the T_7 level or free thyroxine index, depending on the units in which the T_3 resin uptake is expressed). Using these procedures an euthyroid patient might give the following results: T_3 resin uptake, 24.3% (normal range 25% to 35%); serum T_4, 9.5 μg/dl (5.3 μg/dl to 14.5 μg/dl); and T_7, 2.31 (1.32 to 5.08). In some laboratories the *serum T_3 concentration* is measured by radioimmunoassay and expressed in μg/dl, but in most cases where a figure designated T_3 appears in a laboratory report it still refers to the T_3 resin uptake test and will be expressed as a percentage.

Some solution to the chaos that has resulted because of the multiplicity of new (and badly named) thyroid function tests introduced in the past decade is promised by the test referred to as the *effective thyroxine ratio*, which simultaneously accounts for T_4 concentration and the binding capacity of plasma proteins for T_4, without actually calculating serum levels of T_4 in micrograms.

Other new procedures that may occasionally help in elucidating the etiology of a thyroid problem include *radioimmunoassay of plasma thyrotropin* (TSH, the pituitary hormone-regulating thyroid activity) and the use of synthetic thyrotropin-releasing hormone (TRH—the hypothalamic component of pituitary–thyroid interaction) in clinical tests.

Radioisotopic studies of the thyroid gland include *radioactive iodine (^{131}I) scans* for determining the size and function for all or part of the thyroid gland and ^{99m}Tc-*pertechnetate uptake* studies to measure the ability of the thyroid to concentrate iodinelike compounds. In a thyroid scan, the distribution of radioactivity in a flat plane corresponding to the gland is plotted by means of multiple measurements of radioactive emission sys-

---

* The T_7 value is calculated as follows:

$$T_7 = \frac{\%T_3 \text{ uptake}}{100} \times \text{Total } T_4 \text{ value (μg/dl)}$$

Normal T_7 values vary with the laboratory and the methods used to determine T_3 and T_4 values. In general, the following rules apply:

When both T_3 uptake and serum T_4 are increased, the most likely diagnosis is hyperthyroidism.

When both T_3 uptake and serum T_4 are decreased, the most likely diagnosis is hypothyroidism.

When T_3 uptake is low but T_4 is high, serum protein binding of hormone (due to estrogens or pregnancy, for example) increases.

When T_3 uptake is high but T_4 is low, serum protein binding of hormone (due to nephrosis or testosterone, for example) decreases.

tematically determined in this plane. Areas of increased radioactivity or areas of little uptake can be detected and the extent and nature of nodular lesions of the thyroid evaluated. Such scans are not restricted to the thyroid. With use of appropriate isotopes, scans can be carried out on all the major organs including bone, liver, brain, and salivary glands (see section on Salivary Analyses). More than one isotope may be used on a given patient in order to separate malignant from benign nodules in an organ on the basis of isotope uptake. ^{131}I, ^{99m}Tc-pertechnetate and ^{75}Se-selenomethionine are all used for thyroid scans for this purpose. Otherwise "cold," thyroid nodules that show uptake of ^{75}Se-selenomethionine are most likely thyroid carcinoma.

For radioisotope uptake studies of the thyroid gland, ^{99m}Tc-pertechnetate is usually preferred over ^{131}I because pertechnetate is not incorporated into thyroid hormones (organically bound) even though it is concentrated by the gland (compare with uptake of ^{99m}Tc-pertechnetate by the salivary glands). Its physical half-life is only 6 hours, and uptake studies can therefore be repeated on successive days without interference from radioactivity retained from the earlier studies. ^{99m}Tc-pertechnetate is a gamma ray emitter and special gamma ray cameras are needed to record its concentration in (over) the thyroid gland. ^{99m}Tc-pertechnetate is an artificially produced isotope manufactured daily in nuclear medicine laboratories by the passage of water through a column of more stable radioactive molybdenum obtained commercially from a reactor. By appropriate laboratory manipulation, pertechnetate can be incorporated into a variety of physical forms that enhance its uptake by one organ system over another. In hyperthyroidism, values greater than 50% are found for both ^{131}I and ^{99m}Tc-pertechnetate uptake; in hypothyroidism, values are less than 15%.

Urinalysis

A routine urine examination consists of a report of the macroscopic appearance of the specimen, the reaction (pH), the specific gravity, the qualitative test for sugar and al-bumin (protein), and microscopic examination of the sediment for casts, cells, or organisms.

The examination should be made on the first urine voided in the morning. If the urine cannot be examined within an hour or so, a few drops of toluene added to the specimen will avoid glycolysis and the deterioration of casts and cells. The color and the clarity of the specimen are noted, and its reaction is determined by means of litmus or nitrazine paper. Unless the urine is freshly voided, the reaction is of little significance. The specific gravity is read with a urinometer.

Microscopic examination of the urinary sediment will reveal the presence of urinary casts, red and white blood cells, and bacteria. Cells and casts are reported in "numbers per high power field" (hpf) or "numbers per low power field" (lpf). More than five white blood cells or two red blood cells per high power field is considered abnormal, provided the specimen is not contaminated with vaginal secretions. White or red cell casts constitute an abnormal finding, usually indicative of urine stasis and concentration within the kidney. If the urine is obtained under sterile conditions, the sediment may be stained and examined for bacteria. Squamous epithelium from the bladder, urethra, and vagina is a normal finding. Red cell casts indicate an active glomerular lesion. Increased numbers of hyaline casts, other casts from the renal tubules and oval fat bodies (usually very pronounced in nephrosis), are all seen in a variety of disease states.

Data provided by a urinalysis that cannot be obtained by testing with paper strip reagents are of use in detecting renal dysfunction and pathologic changes in the renal parenchyma, collecting system, or bladder.

Chemical analyses are also carried out on urine as a measure of various systemic metabolic reactions that may be indicative of disease. Since individual samples of urine vary greatly in concentration due to diurnal variations in fluid intake and metabolic activity, such analyses usually need to be performed on an aliquot of pooled samples of urine collected over a 24-hour period, rather than on a single randomly collected sample. The following analyses are of interest.

Urine Calcium Determination— Sulkowitch Test

In this easily performed semiquantitative test for urinary calcium, urine and Sulkowitch reagent (oxalate and acetic acid) are mixed and allowed to stand for 2 to 3 minutes. A trace of precipitate is normal. Increased precipitation is reported as 1, 2, 3, or 4+.

The test is usually positive in conditions in which osteolytic lesions are present, such as hyperparathyroidism and other conditions with hypercalcemia. It is negative in rickets, sprue, and tetany. Since the test is roughly quantitative, in patients subject to tetany a negative test following on a series of positive tests is indicative of hypocalcemia (serum calcium less than 7.5 mg/dl) and may herald an attack of tetany.

5-Hydroxyindoleacetic Acid Assay

Carcinoid syndrome, an uncommon cause of *episodes* of severe hypertension with flushing that result from secretion of a vasopressor agent (serotonin) from a specific type of tumor in the gastrointestinal tract (carcinoid tumor), is detected by measurement of an excretory end product of serotonin metabolism (5-hydroxyindoleacetic acid) in the urine. This procedure has special application for this unusual type of episodic hypertension, however, and is not generally used in the evaluation of patients with persistently raised blood pressure levels.

Vanillylmandelic Acid Assay

Two potent vasopressor agents (epinephrine and norepinephrine) are produced not only by the normal adrenal medulla but also by tumors of this tissue and certain tumors (pheochromocytoma, neuroblastoma and ganglioneuroma) that occur outside the adrenal, but like the adrenal medulla, are also embryologically of neural crest origin. Increased serum levels of these vasopressors are reflected in increased urinary concentration of the catecholamines themselves, as well as in their metabolic excretory end products, vanillylmandelic acid (VMA) and the metanephrines. Urinary concentration of VMA (the usual screening test for pheo-

chromocytoma and related problems) is measured on an aliquot of a 24-hour urine collection, care being taken in the preparation of the patient to have him avoid coffee and other drugs and foods that may give falsely elevated VMA levels. The normal range of urinary VMA is 2.0 to 10 mg per 24 hours.

Determination of Metal Cations in Serum and Urine

Provided samples of serum, urine, (and saliva) are first freed of protein and polysaccharide, the concentration of various heavy metals (such as Hg, Pb, Cu, Zn) in the sample can be measured by atomic absorption spectrophotometry. This technique allows detection of small amounts of these cations by means of special equipment that measures the degree of absorption of characteristic bands of the electromagnetic spectrum by a vaporized sample containing a given heavy metal. More recently the technique of anodic stripping voltammetry has been introduced and may replace atomic absorption spectrophotometry for the assay of metallic cations.

Mercury

Blood and urinary concentrations of *mercury* are frequently measured in the evaluation of individuals who may have been exposed to mercury vapor over an extended period of time (*e.g.*, dentists and their staffs working in poorly ventilated areas contaminated by mercury spills and aerosols). Normal values for blood mercury are less than 2.0 μg/ml; and less than 20 μg/liter for urine collected over a 24-hour period. Acceptable levels of safety for individuals with occupational exposure are usually listed somewhat higher.

Although there is a relationship between occupational exposure and mercury levels in the urine as demonstrated in group studies, an accurate relationship does not exist for single determinations on an individual. There is considerable daily variation in urinary excretion of mercury, and it is important that repeated assay of urinary mercury be carried out before a diagnosis of chronic mercury intoxication is made. In general, levels above 20 μg/liter of urine (based upon a 24-hour urine collection) are considered abnormal and evidence of unusual exposure to mercury and its absorption and excretion. Studies of dentists and their office assistants have usually shown that levels greater than 20 µg/liter are fairly common, one such study reporting a level of 40 µg/liter in 50 urban dentists. Although over 10% of the dental offices included in this study had atmospheric concentrations of mercury vapor over 0.1 mg/m³, this raised level of urinary excretion is not always accepted as evidence of chronic mercury intoxication. It should, however, serve as a warning of this potential hazard in dental practice, and it is hoped that improved practices of mercury hygiene, which become essential when dental operatories are carpeted, will lead to decreased levels of urinary mercury excretion being found among dentists in further years.

Screening tests for the level of mercury vapor in dental offices have also been developed in recent years. These allow detection of as little as 0.01 mg of mercury per cubic meter of air over a 4-week exposure period, the threshold limit value for humans exposed over long periods of time being 0.05 mg/m³ of air. Monitors that can be worn by the dentist and his office assistants are also available commercially.*

Although the concentration of mercury in blood and urine is generally accepted as an index of exposure, inherent limitations in the assay techniques frequently produce inaccurate and unreliable results; moreover, the mercury content of blood and urine is not an indicator of *total body burden of mercury*. Because the blood mercury level declines as soon as exposure ceases, mercury concentrations in blood, urine, and hair (another commonly used specimen for analyses of mercury and other metallic ions) are only a measure of recent or current exposure. When mercury exposure has been low but chronic, it is difficult to relate these values to the body burden. Direct measurement of mercury in bone samples and more recently, an x-ray fluorescence technique that can measure mercury levels *in situ* in bone and head tissues, have been used for this purpose. The prevalence of neurologic electrodiagnostic abnormalities (both polyneuropathies and

mononeuropathies such as carpal tunnel syndrome) has been shown to be higher in dentists with high mercury body burdens. Mercury accumulation following short-term exposure can also be measured by this technique.

Lead

In suspected chronic *lead poisoning*, urine and blood lead levels are sometimes measured in addition to evaluation for hematologic anomalies commonly associated with this problem (raised reticulocyte count, anemia, and basophilic stippling of the RBC). For children under 5 years of age, blood lead levels up to 40 µg/dl are considered normal. Lead interferes with the biosynthesis of hemoglobin, and the detection of heme precursors can be useful in detecting lead poisoning. Tests for these precursors include determination of delta-amino-levulinic acid in urine (ALA), coproporphyrin in urine and zinc protoporphyrin in serum, RBC's and urine. Of these determinations, measurement of urinary zinc protoporphyrin is currently considered the most important screening test. Evidence of past levels of lead absorption has also been found in the dentine of exfoliated deciduous teeth, although the technique has not been widely used clinically and has been supplanted by x-ray fluorescence measurements of bone lead.

Copper and Zinc

Serum and urinary levels of *copper and zinc* are altered in a variety of disease states (*e.g.,* cirrhosis) and following therapy with penicillamine and other medications. An association between these levels and alterations in taste sensitivity (dysgeusia) has not been confirmed, however (see Chap. 16). There is also considerable controversy as to the normal ranges for these cations in serum and urine.

Representative values for metallic cations are as follows: *blood lead*—normal < 30 µg/dl, asymptomatic 30–60 µg/dl, symptomatic > 60 µg/dl; *urinary lead*—normal < 80 µg/L, acceptable level in exposed workers < 150 µg/L, dangerous level of exposure > 150 µg/L. *Plasma Zinc*—60–120 µg/dl; *urinary zinc*—150–300 µg/24 hours; *serum copper*—70–150 µg/dl, with increases to as high as 300 µg/

* 3M Company, St. Paul, MN 55101

dl during the third trimester of pregnancy; *urinary copper*—20–65 μg/24 hours.

Toxicology

As a result of a number of technologic advances, the science of toxicology has developed in recent years from its original concern with forensic problems to include the assay of medications in the bloodstream (therapeutic drug monitoring) as well as the measurement of poisons and other abused substances in the blood and urine of patients (medical toxicology). To some extent, development of medical toxicology has gone hand in hand with the epidemic of the abuse of drugs and other substances that has occurred in the developed countries of the world in the last 25 years. Therapeutic drug monitoring has developed with the realization that the circulating blood level of a medication is frequently a better indicator of the effective dose than is the size of the dose administered periodically by mouth or parenterally. The use of atomic absorption spectroscopy and gas chromatography equipment and developments in microchemical analysis have helped reduce the cost of many toxicologic assays to a point where measurement of a large number of individual drugs and poisons can be obtained at a price comparable to that of other diagnostic tests. Screening evaluations of blood and urine to search for illicit drug use have also been developed, partly as an aid in the diagnosis of the comatose patient (comprehensive drug overdose evaluations) but also as a means of monitoring compliance of addicts on methadone or other drug treatment programs.

A large number of tests are currently available for common poisoning agents, and in many cases rapid but highly accurate and reliable assays can be obtained to assist with the treatment of a potential accidental poisoning fatality (*e.g.,* alcohol, barbiturates, carbon monoxide, salicylates, heavy metals, digitoxin, digoxin, quinidine, pesticides, hypnotics, and tranquilizers). Computer-linked assays of methadone as well as a variety of other commonly abused narcotics and drugs are used in methadone treatment centers for analysis of urinary specimens to check that each methadone dose is consumed by the patient and not sold and to check for continuing use of other illicit drugs. Screening evaluations have also proved of considerable help in detecting the problem of multiple drug abuse that has become prevalent (*e.g.,* alcohol taken with other drugs is implicated in 20% of accidental deaths and suicides each year in the United States).

Therapeutic drug monitoring provides a means of using potentially toxic medications with greater safety and efficacy, effective drug levels often being achievable with lower but more accurately timed doses than were possible before chemical monitoring (versus monitoring by means of clinical response and side-effects) became possible. Unexplained therapeutic failures of an otherwise effective drug have also been traced to individual metabolic differences affecting the blood level of the drug that is produced by a given dose regimen. This approach has been successful in many cases in determining the cause of seizures in epileptics who were thought to be adequately treated with phenytoin and in reducing the gingival hyperplasia produced by this drug without allowing the blood concentration to fall below a level that will prevent seizures. Poor response to tricyclic antidepressant medications has also been associated with a "therapeutic window" effect, in which clinical response can be achieved only by maintaining blood levels in a relatively narrow zone of concentration. A partial listing of some of the more commonly used medications for which blood level monitoring is available and often beneficial is given in Table 3-15. Most institutions and commercial laboratories with toxicology divisions now list well over 100 medications, abused substances, heavy metals, and commonly available poisonous substances for which assays in blood and urine are available on a routine basis. Through collaboration with larger toxicologic reference laboratories, an even more extensive list of assays is available.

Interpretation of toxicologic assays requires knowledge of the timing of blood or urine collection, the elimination characteristics of the particular drug being monitored, and the effects of concurrent disease and other drugs on these parameters. Close collaboration between clinician and laboratory both before and after the specimen is collected is essential.

Table 3-15. Drugs for Which Blood Level Monitoring May Be Beneficial*

	GENERIC NAME	TRADE NAME
Antiepileptics	Primidone	Mysoline
	Phenobarbital	Luminal
	Phenytoin	Dilantin
	Carbamazepine	Tegretol
	Clonazepam	Clonopin
	Ethosuximide	Zarontin
	Valproic Acid	Depakene
Cardiac Drugs	Digoxin	Lanoxin
	Digitoxin	Digitoxin
	Procainamide	Pronestyl
	Quinidine	Quinidine Sulfate
	Lidocaine	Xylocaine
	Disopyramide	Norpace
	Thiocyanate	Nitroprusside
Antibiotics	Chloramphenicol	Chloromycetin
	Gentamicin	Garamycin
	Tobramycin	Nebcin
	Amikacin	Amikin
Psycho-therapeutic Agents	Lithium	Lithane
	Amitriptyline	Elavil
	Nortriptyline	Aventyl
	Imipramine	Tofranil
	Desipramine	Norpramin
Miscellaneous	Acetaminophen	Tylenol
	Theophylline	Aminophylline
	Acetylsalicylic acid	Aspirin
	Methotrexate	Methotrexate

Substances commonly screened for in a comprehensive drug overdose evaluation are as follows:*

- Alcohols and volatiles—acetone, ethyl alcohol, isopropyl alcohol, methyl alcohol
- Amphetamines—amphetamine and methamphetamine
- Barbiturates—amobarbital (Amytal), butabarbital (Butisol), butalbital, pentobarbital (Nembutal), phenobarbital (Luminal), secobarbital (Seconal)
- Benzodiazepines—chlordiazepoxide (Librium), diazepam (Valium), oxazepam (Serax)

* Service Manual and Fee Schedule, Smith-Klein Clinical Laboratories—Philadelphia, Inc, January, 1982, 1075 First Ave, King of Prussia, PA 19406

- Cocaine and its metabolites
- Codeine
- Morphine and its derivatives—heroin, meperidine (Demerol), methadone (Dolphine)
- Other tranquilizers and antidepressants—amitriptyline (Elavil), carisprodol (Soma), desipramine (Norpramin), doxepin (Sinequan), ethchlorvynol (Placidyl), imipramine (Tofranil), meprobamate (Miltown), nortriptyline (Aventyl)
- Other sedatives and analgesics—acetaminophen (Tylenol), glutethimide (Doriden), pentazocine (Talwin), propoxyphene (Darvon), methaqualone (Quaalude), salicylates
- Miscellaneous—methyprylon (Nodular), phencyclidine (PCP), phenothiazines, phenylpropanolamine, quinine

Salivary Analyses

In recent years, through the adaptation of standard laboratory procedures to the analysis of parotid and submaxillary gland secretions, a large body of data on the composition of saliva has become available. Little use seems to have been made of this information in the diagnostic evaluation of patients with possible salivary gland disease, although sialography, for example, has become a readily available procedure. To some extent, the high mucopolysaccharide content of saliva prevents its analysis by the current routine automated multitest systems, but following dialysis both conventional and automated methods of analysis can be used.

Requests for collection and analysis of saliva usually come from internists who are interested in the evaluation of patients with such varied diseases as cystic fibrosis, Addison's disease, primary aldosteronism as a cause of hypertension, heavy metal intoxication, and renal failure. The salivary sodium/potassium ratio is the most commonly measured variable, but urea concentration and flow rate are also measured. Research scientists studying exfoliative cytology, virus isolation, immunoglobulin concentrations, and taste dysfunction are also developing diagnostic procedures.

Assistance is often requested from the dentist in obtaining these specimens. Both total mixed whole saliva specimens and the secretions collected directly from individual parotid and submaxillary–sublingual glands are used. Cannulation of the duct is usually avoided, and specimens of parotid and mixed submaxillary–sublingual salivas are collected with small cups held to the orifice by light suction. Curby or Carlsson–Crittenden cups are used for the parotid secretion, and Truelove and colleagues have described a soft rubber cup suitable for the submaxillary–sublingual secretions. Since the salivary secretions are affected by many factors such as anxiety, the time of day, and the state of hydration, experience with the technique is required of both the patient and dentist if consistent results are to be obtained. The concentration of most substances excreted in saliva is flow-rate dependent, and concentrations are usually corrected to a standard flow rate.

Salivary function studies include measurement of total salivary flow (mixed saliva), rate of flow of saliva from the cannulated or cupped parotid orifices, rate of discharge of radiopaque dye from the salivary gland following retrograde sialography, and rate of uptake and secretion of ^{99m}Tc-pertechnetate by the salivary glands following injection of the isotope into an antecubital vein (sequential salivary scintigraphy). Special gamma cameras are needed to measure pertechnetate concentration over salivary glands, and the small size of the glands usually prohibits adequate scanning (compare thyroid and brain scans); however, the function of the four major salivary glands can be studied independently, and large nodules that do not take up the isotope can be noted. The greatest value of salivary scintigraphy lies in its ability to detect mild degrees of suppression of salivary gland function as may occur in Sjögren's syndrome, drug-induced xerostomia, and other chronic sialadenites. Further details of these salivary function tests are given in Chapter 11.

The concentration of Na and K in parotid saliva may be conveniently measured in the SMA 6/60 autoanalytic procedure in which all specimens are routinely dialyzed to remove protein before their electrolyte concentration is measured, or in other equipment, once the specimen has been dialyzed. A sample of approximately 1.0 ml of parotid saliva is needed for the procedure. Normal values for unstim-ulated parotid saliva are 25 mEq/liter for K, and < 10 mEq/liter for Na and 15 mEq/liter to 18 mEq/liter for Cl. In inflammation of the parotid, the Na concentration may rise to twice the normal value; the K concentration may rise to 35 mEq/liter to 50 mEq/liter in various sialadenoses.

In Sjögren's syndrome, the major functional abnormality in the parotid gland is in luminal transport in the ductal region, and leakage of serum components into the parotid saliva is minimal. Flow rate is markedly reduced, salivary phosphate concentration is reduced, and sodium and chloride concentrations are greatly elevated; salivary IgA concentration increases moderately and abnormal protein bands can be distinguished by electrophoresis; urea and potassium concentration are unchanged. In parotid enlargement accompanying cirrhosis, parotid flow rate, and parotid salivary concentrations of potassium, calcium, protein, and amylase increase; immunoglobulin levels remain normal.

HISTOPATHOLOGY AND CYTOLOGY

Biopsy Examination

Histologic study of the tissue from an oral lesion is often required to make a definite diagnosis. Tissue removed for diagnostic purposes is known as a biopsy. In the oral cavity, biopsy examination is used to confirm a diagnosis of malignancy in a clinically suspicious lesion and as a diagnostic aid in the evaluation of nonneoplastic lesions such as mucosal nodules and papillomas, erosive lichen planus, erythema multiforme, lupus erythematosus, pemphigus, and pemphigoid and desquamative gingivitis. Because of the rare occurrence of carcinoma arising in the wall of a dental cyst, it has been recommended that all tissue removed from periapical lesions should be submitted for histologic examination.

To many the term *biopsy* is synonymous with *cancer,* and the use of some euphemism such as "removal of tissue for examination" may be more acceptable to some patients.

The oral surgeon is well equipped and experienced to perform a biopsy; however, the

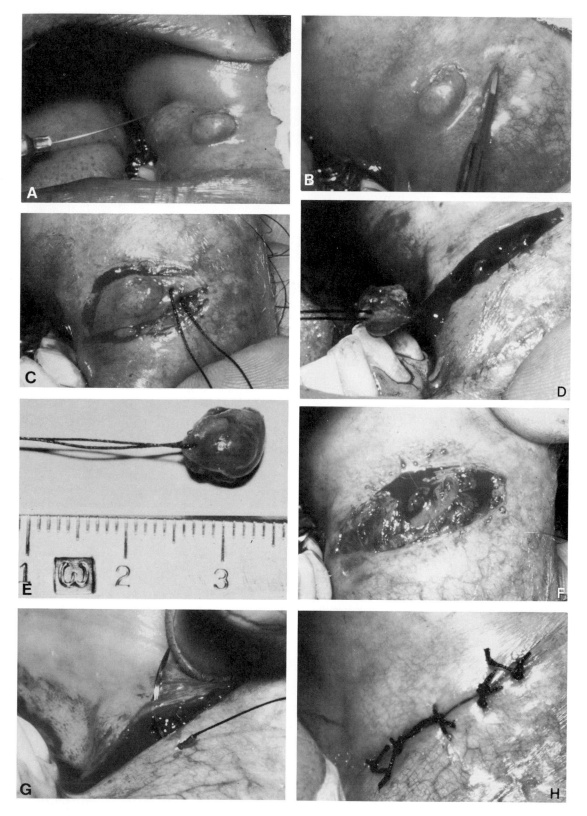

general practitioner who performs exodontia can also perform routine biopsies of most oral lesions. Tissue can be removed readily for diagnosis if a few general rules are observed.

The following data should accompany the specimen: the date of the biopsy; the name, age, and sex of the patient; the area of the biopsy specimen; and a brief description of the clinical appearance of the lesion and the associated symptoms, along with the tentative clinical diagnosis.

Iodine-containing surface antiseptics should be avoided, since they have a tendency to stain certain tissue cells permanently. The type of anesthetic used and a statement whether the tissue was removed with the scalpel (generally preferred) or with the electrocautery should be noted. In suspected malignant lesions the electrocautery is the method of choice of some surgeons, particularly when the entire growth cannot be removed.

The biopsy specimen should include not only some of the lesion but also clinically normal tissue (see Fig. 3-19). Small lesions should be removed completely when the biopsy is taken (excisional biopsy, compare with incisional biopsy, when only a portion of the lesion is removed). In all instances sufficient tissue should be obtained. In the case of suspected granulomatous lesions (e.g., ulcers or lymph nodes possibly infected with tuberculosis or other chronic infectious agent), it may be desirable to use a part of the biopsy for animal inoculations, injections, or other bacteriologic procedures.

The portion of the biopsy to be used for routine (formalin-fixed, paraffin-embedded, hematoxylin-and-eosin-stained sections) histologic study should be placed at once in a suitable fixing solution—usually 10% neutral buffered formalin—and sent to the pathology laboratory. Most laboratories will provide specimen jars with appropriate fixative as well as mailing tubes and requisition sheets for the dentist's use.

Special fixation procedures and fixatives are normally required for specimens that are to be studied by special techniques (e.g., electron microscopy, fluorescent or other labeled antibody staining, histochemical demonstration of enzymes and other cell components), and the clinician should inquire from the collaborating laboratory about any special requirements before proceeding with the biopsy. In some cases, fresh, unfixed tissue is required and should be delivered to the laboratory as soon as possible after the surgical procedure, either in a vial of sterile saline or covered with gauze moistened with saline. In cases of suspected lymphoma, *touch preparations* of the cut surface of the excised lymph node are made before fixation of the specimen. This is achieved by pressing the cut surface against a cleaned microscope slide, and immediately fixing the cells adherent to the slide with 95% alcohol or Spraycyte.* Where *fresh frozen tissue* is required, *small* fragments of the excised tissue may be quick-frozen satisfactorily by placing them in a small glass or plastic vial and immersing the vial in an acetone (or alcohol) and dry-ice freezing mixture and transporting the vial

* Clay–Adams, Division of Becton–Dickinson and Co, 299 Webro Road, Parsippany, NJ 07054

Fig. 3-19 Technique of excisional biopsy. *A*, Anesthetic solution is delivered around the periphery of a dome-shaped nodule in the cheek, avoiding distortion of the involved tissues. *B*, A #15 blade is used to create an eliptical incision including a margin of normal mucosa. The incision is carried to a depth that includes normal tissue beyond the border of the lesion. *C*, A traction suture is placed at one end of the ellipse of tissue, and tension is applied by way of the suture while dissection continues using a scalpel. This eliminates accidental crushing or injury of the specimen with forceps or other instruments. *D*, Dissection is completed. *E*, Close-up of excised lesion including surrounding margin of normal tissue; *F*, Surgical site before suture closure. *G*, First suture is applied in the midpoint of the surgical site in order to coapt the mucosal margins, and *H*, The incision is closed with interrupted silk sutures (4/0). (Courtesy of Snyder MD, Rosenberg ES: Quintessence International, 9:25, 1980)

of frozen tissue to the laboratory in dry ice. Slow freezing of tissues, particularly at temperatures above $-60°C$ causes serious disruption of cells and tissues and often renders the specimen useless for microscopic examination. In general, where frozen sections are to be prepared, it is preferable to perform the biopsy close to the collaborating laboratory so that the fresh, unfixed tissue can be delivered promptly to the laboratory where more satisfactory rapid freezing techniques are available.

Special procedures are needed for the histologic examination of teeth. If routine (hematoxylin-and-eosin-stained) sections of the dental pulp are required, the apex of the root of the tooth should be clipped with a pair of pliers, or a small hole should be drilled into the radicular pulp with a dental bur to allow penetration of fixative. If sections of the undecalcified tooth (hard sections, ground sections) are required for the demonstration of abnormalities of the enamel and dentin, the tooth should be submitted either intact or in several longitudinal slices stored in sterile saline. (This last type of preparation is usually available only by special arrangement with a laboratory specializing in studies of teeth or bones.)

For routine (hematoxylin-and-eosin-stained) sections, the pathologist's report will require from 3 days to a week. If the specimen contains calcified tissue, a longer time is required. Even after biopsy study, it is not always possible to make a definitive diagnosis, but the pathologist may be able to suggest certain diagnostic possibilities. Repeated biopsy studies may be required before a final diagnosis can be made.

Biopsy examination of selected oral tissues may also be used in the diagnosis of some systemic disease processes. In sarcoidosis and amyloidosis, many organs are affected including the soft tissues of the oral cavity, which can provide an easily accessible site for biopsy. Biopsies of the tongue, gingivae, palate, and cheek mucosa have been used for this purpose, and they provide at least as much information as biopsies of the liver, lymph nodes, or rectal mucosa in these conditions. Since the major salivary glands are relatively inaccessible for biopsy, a useful estimate of the nature and extent of any pansialadenitis (*e.g.*, Sjögren's syndrome) can be obtained by biopsy of the minor salivary glands of the palate or cheek. Palatal biopsies for this purpose are usually carried out with a 5-mm diameter cylindrical trephine punch, whereas cheek and lip biopsies are usually incisional and allow dissection of a cluster of small glands. The latter technique is more certain to provide glandular tissue, and an entire gland lobule can usually be serially sectioned to obtain a count of the number of areas of lymphoid infiltration. (This can be helpful in diagnosing early Sjögren's syndrome.) Cheek and lip biopsies do, however, carry the hazard of damage to branches of the trigeminal nerve with paresthesia and deformity of the lip. Patients should also be cautioned about the development of extraoral bruising when minor salivary glands are dissected from the lip.

Granulomas have been demonstrated in biopsies of normal appearing palatal mucosa in 38% of patients with sarcoidosis. In one study, focal lymphocytic sialadenitis of the buccal minor salivary glands was reported in approximately 60% of patients with Sjögren's syndrome with or without rheumatoid arthritis, and in 27.5% of patients with rheumatoid arthritis; and in another series, lymphocytic aggregates were demonstrated in 82% of punch biopsies of the palate of patients with various connective tissue diseases, but only 6% of control patients. Criteria for the diagnosis of Sjögren's syndrome based on biopsy of the minor salivary glands have been recently reviewed in several publications in the dental literature. Biopsies of the minor salivary glands that are taken to search for evidence of systemic disease should be serially sectioned, since granulomas and lymphoid infiltration may be only focal changes not present throughout the specimen.

Biopsies of the tongue and mucobuccal fold have been reported to be positive in over 90% of cases of primary amyloidosis and may be more sensitive than gingival biopsies in this form of the disease; secondary amyloidosis may be diagnosed by gingival biopsy in about 60% to 75% of cases provided light (congo red stain), polarizing, and fluorescent (thioflavine T stain) microscopy are used. Formalin-fixed tissue is satisfactory for these studies.

Procedures for Specimens to be Examined in the Electron Microscope

A number of special reagents and procedures are used for fixation and processing of tissue to be examined for ultrastructural detail in the electron microscope. For this level of magnification, the excellent preservation of cellular detail required is obtained by cutting the specimen into tiny blocks before fixation (to allow rapid penetration of fixative) by use of special fixatives that preserve cellular detail with minimum disruption from rapid dehydration or osmotic shock and by further postfixation and processing of tissue in the laboratory after the initial period of prefixation. Techniques vary from laboratory to laboratory and from tissue to tissue, and the special fixatives required, together with directions for handling the specimen, are usually supplied by the collaborating laboratory. Formalin-fixed specimens are unsatisfactory for high-resolution electron microscopy, although some of the intracellular markers used in diagnostic electron microscopy are adequately preserved in formalin-fixed and deparaffinized tissues. The decision to use ultrastructural studies should preferably be made at the time the biopsy specimen is obtained. In the absence of specific directions from a laboratory, the following fixation procedure gives good results for a wide variety of tissues.

As soon as possible after the surgical procedure, carefully section the biopsy specimen with fresh scalpel or razor blades into pieces no larger than 0.5 cm diameter, identifying each fragment in relation to the overall specimen and lesion. Immerse the pieces in Karnovsky's fixative (4% paraformaldehyde and 5% glutaraldehyde in 0.1 M sodium cacodylate buffer at pH 7.2) for 2 to 4 hours, and deliver promptly to the laboratory. If there is to be any delay in delivering the specimen, the pieces of the biopsy specimen should be sectioned further into fragments approximately 1 mm in diameter, once the initial 2 to 4 hours of prefixation has occurred. When the specimens reach the laboratory they are rinsed in sodium cacodylate buffer and postfixed in 2% s-collidine-buffered osmic acid and subsequently stained in alcoholic uranyl acetate. Following dehydration, the tissue fragments are embedded in blocks of epon (methyl methacrylate) and sections cut at 0.7 to 0.8 μ, stained with toluidine blue and methylene blue, and examined in the light microscope. Suitable blocks are then re-oriented, and thin sections for electron microscopic examination are prepared on an ultramicrotome with subsequent additional staining with uranyl acetate and lead hydroxide as required before observation.

Ultrastructural examination of biopsies has been shown to be useful in the diagnosis of a number of tumors occurring in or adjacent to the oral cavity. This approach is particularly useful in the differential diagnosis of malignant neoplasms that are composed largely of spindle-shaped cells (e.g., fibrosarcoma, leiomyosarcoma, rhabdomyosarcoma and malignant schwannoma) or undifferentiated round cells (e.g., lymphoma, anaplastic carcinoma, melanoma, Ewing's sarcoma, neuroblastoma, esthesioblastoma, paraganglioma and embryonic rhabdomyosarcoma). Since the electron microscope highlights plasma membranes and junctional complexes between cells, ultrastructural study can be very useful in separating poorly differentiated adenocarcinoma and squamous cell carcinoma. By identifying functional cell products, this technique assists in the recognition of a number of tumors of both exocrine and endocrine gland origin, as well as mast cell tumors and tumors arising from neural crest derivatives. Ultrastructural study also assists in the classification of tumors composed of cells with granular eosinophilic cytoplasm: those in which the granular character results from a large number of mitochondria (e.g., oncocytoma and Warthin's tumor in the salivary glands) and those in which it results from many lysosomal granules (e.g., granular cell myoblastoma and inborn lysosome disorders such as Fabry's disease). It is also an important research tool that in most cases is now needed to complement and optimize the information obtained through structural study of excised tissue.

Intraoral Exfoliative Cytology

Cytologic study, although eliminating many of the disadvantages of the biopsy, by no means supplants the usual biopsy study. Over the last 25 years considerable experience has been gained with the exfoliative cytologic techniques in oral diagnosis that were originally developed by Silverman and Sandler. A variety of oral diseases have been studied with this technique, but the procedure is of most value in the evaluation of suspected malignancies, especially when these present as ulcerated or red nonkeratinized lesions. (See Chapter 6)

Oral cytology should never be relied on for diagnosis of an oral lesion simply because it may be easier to obtain than a biopsy. If a dentist sees a lesion that he feels has even the slightest chance of being malignant, he should work to his utmost to see that the lesion is biopsied adequately at the earliest opportunity. With these considerations in mind, Papanicolaou-stained smears of oral mucosal lesions are indicated in the following circumstances in clinical dentistry:

1. For rapid laboratory evaluation of an oral lesion that on clinical grounds is thought to be malignant. Approximately 1 week is required under most circumstances for processing and reporting on a biopsy. In the case of advanced malignancies where delay or preliminary incision of the lesion is not warranted, laboratory confirmation of the clinical impression often can be obtained by a Papanicolaou-stained smear in 1 to 2 days.
2. For laboratory evaluation of an oral lesion that on clinical grounds is thought to be premalignant and for which the dentist is unable to obtain permission for a biopsy.
3. In patients with multiple premalignant lesions. Biopsy of multiple lesions or entire removal of extensive lesions may not be feasible, and cytology may be a very practical adjunct to biopsy.
4. For sequential laboratory evaluation of an area of mucosa that has previously been treated by excision or radiation to remove a malignancy. Successive biopsies are often not possible, and cytology provides something better than simple clinical observation, especially where previous treatment has led to scarring or other tissue change.
5. For evaluation of vesicular lesions (herpes simplex, pemphigus, pemphigoid) where facilities for rapid evaluation of a Tzanck smear (see section on Microbiology) are not available or where more detailed cytology is required.

The clinical value of exfoliative cytology is directly related to the skill of the cytologist and his experience with oral smears. A dentist who proposes to use this laboratory procedure should first determine which laboratories available to him routinely handle oral smears. The laboratory will frequently provide a kit (slides, cytoscraper, mailing tube) with instructions for obtaining, fixing, and transporting the specimen. In general, the preparation of the smear is similar to that used to obtain oral smears for other purposes (see section on Microbiology) with the exception that firm pressure with a wooden or steel scraper must be used to ensure that adequate numbers of cells are obtained, and the smear must be fixed immediately. For this purpose, an aerosol fixative such as Spraycyte or 95% alcohol may be used.

Oral exfoliative cytology has been used for the study of other nonmalignant changes in the oral cavity (*e.g.*, studies of buccal mucosa in various anemias and of the maturation of the buccal mucosa with the menstrual cycle) but these studies, like exfoliative cytology of cells secreted from the major salivary ducts, remain in the experimental stage. Oral cytology is generally most helpful in evaluation of nonkeratinized "red patches" or ulcerative lesions of the oral mucosa. Specimens obtained from heavily keratinized "white patches" are composed mainly of superficial squames, and the more immature basal cells are not represented on the smear.

The standard classification used in oral cytology reports is as follows: class I, normal cells; class II, some atypical cells, but no evidence of malignancy; class III, changes in nuclear pattern of indeterminate nature; no definite evidence of malignancy, but clearly aberrant cells are present; class IV, suggestive of malignancy; class V, obvious malignant changes. A report of class III, IV, or V changes should always be followed by a biopsy of the lesion.

Immunofluorescence Procedures

Fluorescent dyes such as fluorescein isothiocyanate (FITC) and rhodamine can be chemically linked (conjugated) with antibody globulin without destroying the specificity of the antibody. Such fluorescent-labeled antibody is used to detect specific antigen–antibody reactions and can be used to locate either antigens or antibodies of known specificity in tissue sections. When tissue sections labeled in this fashion are illuminated with ultraviolet light in an ultraviolet microscope, specific labeled tissue components can be identified by their bright apple-green fluorescence against a dark or counterstained background. This technique is used to identify a number of tissue structures and abnormal deposits of antibody globulin and other macromolecules, as well as bacteria and viruses in infected tissues and smears.

Fluorescent antibody procedures are carried out in one of three ways (see Fig. 3-20):

Direct Immunofluorescence. Fluorescent-labeled antiserum directed against a particular tissue component* is applied directly to a thin, unfixed smear or tissue section mounted on a slide, and the slide is incubated at 37°C to allow the antigen and labeled antibody to react. Following incubation, the slide is washed in buffered normal saline to remove unreacted labeled antibody, and the slide examined in the ultraviolet microscope. Nonspecific reactions are common with this technique, which requires a separate *labeled* antibody preparation for each component to be located. It has largely been superseded by either the indirect or sandwich techniques.

Indirect Immunofluorescence. Unlabeled specific antiserum directed against a partic-

ular tissue component is applied directly to the smear or tissue section, allowed to react, and followed by a FITC-conjugated antiglobulin antiserum.[†] Following incubation and washing to remove unreacted reagents, the slide is examined in the ultraviolet microscope. Similar staining reactions to those observed with the direct technique are obtained, but the technique has several advantages. In general, the fluorescence is brighter because several fluorescent antiglobulin molecules bind onto each of the antibody molecules in the specific antiserum. Because the process of conjugation is lengthy, there is considerable cost saving and versatility to the indirect technique, which requires only one labeled antiserum (antiglobulin antiserum). Staining of more than one tissue component per slide can also be accomplished, but usually with some loss of specificity. A variation of this technique uses complement as an additional reagent that binds the specific antigen–antibody complex and a FITC-labeled anticomplement antiserum to locate the complex.

Both the direct and indirect techniques may be used to detect either antigen or antibody molecules located in a tissue section. A third method, the sandwich technique, is specifically designed for demonstration of specific antibody.

Sandwich Technique of Immunofluorescence. Appropriately fixed tissue sections are reacted with a solution of the antigen for which specific antibody is to be identified in the section. Following incubation and washing, FITC-labeled antiserum with the same specificity as that to be identified in the section is applied to the section. The labeled antiserum again identifies the location of the tissue component (in this case a specific antibody). The name *sandwich technique* refers to the fact that antigen is sandwiched between two layers of the same specific antibody, one labeled and one not.

In addition to these procedures using flu-

---

* Prepared by immunizing another animal species with this tissue component, bleeding the animal to obtain antiserum (containing antibody globulin directed against the tissue component), and purifying and labeling the globulin molecules in the antiserum with FITC (or other fluorochrome as appropriate).

† An antiserum prepared by injecting another animal species with purified globulins obtained from the species in which the specific antiserum was prepared and labeled as above with FITC.

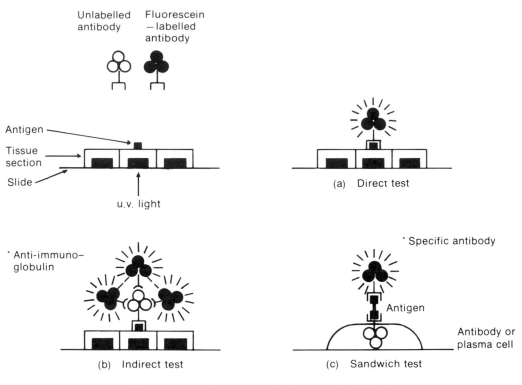

Fluorescent antibody tests. * = fluorescein labelled.

Fig. 3-20 Diagrammatic illustration of the direct, indirect, and sandwich techniques used in the immunofluorescence staining procedure. (Courtesy of Roitt IM, Lehner T: Immunology of Oral Diseases. Oxford, Blackwell Scientific Publications, 1980)

orescent markers, use is made of other diagnostic immunologic procedures in which enzymes such as peroxidase or phosphatase are coupled to antibody and visualized by conventional histochemical rather than fluorescence methods, using either the light or electron microscope.

Techniques of immunofluorescence should be distinguished from other nonimmunologic techniques of fluorescence microscopy that are used to locate microorganisms or tissue components rich in lipids or nucleic acids, which specifically bind with a variety of fluorochromes (*e.g.*, auramine–rhodamine in the case of lipids, and acridine orange in the case of nucleic acids; see section dealing with staining of smears and sections for *Mycobacterium tuberculosis*).

Special techniques of fixation or frozen sections of unfixed tissue, which leave specific antigen and antibody molecules intact, are required for immunofluorescence proce-

dures. Details vary from laboratory to laboratory, and it is essential that the clinician determine whether the collaborating laboratory requires unfixed, quick frozen, or specially fixed tissue for the proposed study. A buffered-sucrose transporting medium that gives good preservation of tissue for immunofluorescent studies has been devised, and allows mailing of specimens from a distance in the case of laboratories that use prefixed tissue blocks (rather than quick frozen, unfixed tissue) for preparation of slides for this purpose. It is customary to submit a specimen of normal tissue from the same anatomic location and a tube of clotted blood or serum with the specimen for immunofluorescence studies so that appropriate controls to check for nonspecific reactions can be run simultaneously. Likewise, a specimen taken from the lesion and fixed in neutral buffered-formalin is also submitted to allow orientation of specific immunofluorescent-labeled components in the overall hematoxylin-and-eosin-stained picture.

Cytogenetics and Chromosome Analysis

All normal human somatic cells contain 46 chromosomes, which are the morphologic units of organization of the nuclear DNA coding for the genetic information in the cell. Unless a cell is actively dividing by mitosis, the chromosomes cannot be demonstrated. However, during the stage in the mitotic cycle known as metaphase, the chromosomes are distinct, stainable structures, and they can be counted and classified.

A study of the gross features of an individual's genetic makeup therefore can be made by examining cells from an area of the body (e.g., bone marrow, testis, tumors) where rapid division is occurring and mitoses are plentiful, or by stimulating mitosis in explanted cells maintained in tissue culture. This latter approach is the one more commonly used, and it depends on the discoveries of Nowell, and Moorhead and colleagues, who showed that the small lymphocytes of blood can be stimulated to divide by phytohemagglutinin (a plant extract used to separate red from white blood cells) and that preparations rich in metaphase cells can be obtained by culturing these cells with colchicine or vinblastine sulfate.

Giemsa-stained preparations with the chromosomes well separated are made from the treated cells, and the number and morphology of these units are recorded as the karyotype or idiogram of the cell. Cytologists have agreed on a standard nomenclature for karyotypes. An analysis is recorded as 46 XY for a normal male and 46 XX for a normal female, X and Y referring to the sex chromosomes and the preceding digits to the total number of chromosomes (autosomes and sex chromosomes).

Even if it is assumed that the answer to the observable differences among individuals and their susceptibility to various diseases lies in the genetic makeup of the individual, chromosome analysis is only a gross tool with which to investigate these problems. Without doubt there are many genetic differences among individuals that are observable by chemical analysis of body tissues, but are too small to be visualized as morphologic alterations in chromosomes (e.g., sickle cell disease).

There are a growing number of diseases in which genetic abnormalities are reflected in chromosome abnormalities. The most readily detected abnormality is aneuploidy, in which an error in meiosis during production of a sperm or an ovum leads to an abnormal number of chromosomes in all the cells of an individual. For example, males with Klinefelter's syndrome (a complex of anomalies including hypogonadism, a characteristic build and facies, bony anomalies, and often mental retardation) have a 47 XXY or even 48 XXXY karyotype; patients with Turner's syndrome (another complex anomaly that includes hypogonadism, a spadelike chest, webbed neck, and mandibular hypoplasia) have a 45 XO karyotype.

Abnormalities of number may also affect the autosomes, for example, Down's syndrome (mongolism), in which there is an extra chromosome 21 (trisomy 21) with a karyotype of 47 XY for a male. Lack of an autosome is quite rare. These abnormalities may affect all or only a percentage of cells of any one type. This latter situation is referred to as chromosome mosaicism. Structural variations in chromosomes can also be detected and are referred to, for example, as translocations, deletions, inversions, and rings.

Information regarding abnormalities in the number and size of the X chromosome is also obtained by counting Barr bodies. The Barr body is a mass of sex chromatin corresponding to one of the two female X chromosomes. It is about 1μ in size and can be visualized with oil immersion microscopy in about 30% to 60% of the cells of a female. It is seen only when at least two X chromosomes are present and is not seen in the cells of a male. Barr bodies are usually observed in stained smears of the buccal mucosa; the technique is used in the preliminary diagnosis of abnormalities of the X chromosome, such as Turner's syndrome.

Although the medical literature contains many references to the use of chromosomal analysis in human disease, the dental literature contains few references, even though there are a large number of chromosomal abnormalities associated with oral anomalies, such as facial and oral clefts, palatal vaulting, mandibular hypoplasia, or prognathism and dental agenesis. Gorlin and colleagues, Barr, Nasjleti, and Shear and Wilton have provided reviews and case reports of oral disease associated with chromosomal abnormalities.

Chromosome analysis is most useful in evaluating dental patients in whom oral developmental abnormalities (clefts; dental or jaw agenesis) are associated with other physical developmental abnormalities. The procedure is available in many referral clinics frequently located in pediatric hospitals, and the patient should be referred to the clinic once the need for the study has been established by prior consultation with the clinic. The technique requires considerable skill and experience in interpretation of preparations, and until computerized methods of analyzing smears are perfected, the procedure will remain expensive.

The discovery that trisomy 21 (Down's syndrome) is associated with a high frequency of chronic myelogenous leukemia and that patients with this extra (Philadelphia) chromosome survive better than do other patients with chronic myelogenous leukemia has suggested that chromosome analysis may be a valuable screening tool for indicating predisposition to certain malignancies. The recognition of other chromosomal anomalies in association with other leukemias, lymphomas, and malignancies and as a result of infection with herpes simplex and other viruses suggests that increasing use will be made of this technique.

MICROBIOLOGY, SEROLOGY, AND IMMUNOLOGY

The association of microbial agents with oral disease may be demonstrated either by recognizing characteristic microorganisms in smears prepared from the lesions, by isolating the agent in pure culture, by measuring the concentration of specific antibodies to the microorganism in serum or saliva, or by recognizing characteristic tissue changes or microorganisms in biopsies.

Microbiologic procedures of interest to the dentist include stained smears, microbial cultures, serology, and immunologic techniques.

Demonstration of microorganisms in oral tissues sampled by means of *smears* or biopsy. (Bacteria and fungi may be demonstrated in routine formalin-fixed, paraffin-embedded sections by use of a number of special staining techniques as described in the section on Histopathology and Cytology. Viruses may likewise be demonstrated by electron microscopy in appropriately fixed and stained tissue sections and body fluids. Simple office and chairside procedures for the demonstration of microorganisms in smears prepared from the oropharyngeal mucosa and other oral tissues are described in this section.)

Microbial culture techniques. Despite the complex endogenous oral bacterial flora, isolation of microorganisms from an oral lesion and their growth and identification in the laboratory can on occasion provide useful information concerning the etiology of the lesion. This procedure is of most help when specimens are obtained during the acute phase of an infection (*i.e.*, usually within 1 to 2 days of onset of symptoms) and where exogenous pathogens are involved. It is particularly useful in determining the etiology of viral infections, in which a group of viruses may produce very similar clinical manifestations.

Serology refers to the measurement of antibodies and other substances that increase in concentration in serum (and in saliva and other body fluids) following contact with infectious agents (or other noninfectious foreign antigenic substances). Serologic procedures are particularly applicable to the diagnosis of infectious processes when acute phase specimens are either not available or fail to reveal an etiologic agent for the disease. They are also used routinely to confirm that a suspected infectious agent (or some of its antigens) actually penetrated the patient's tissues and elicited a humoral antibody response, and they may be of help in distinguishing the "carrier state" from an infection. Since some infectious processes are accompanied by a rise in certain serum components that are not true antibodies (gamma globulins), titration of serum for such substances as C-reactive protein is also referred to as a serologic procedure.

In dental practice, serology is used as an aid in the diagnosis of syphilis, infectious mononucleosis, herpes simplex, and other virus infections affecting the oral cavity. Serologic tests are also useful in diagnosing beta-hemolytic streptococcal infections, the sequelae of which (*e.g.,* rheumatic cardiac valvular damage) are of significance in planning dental treatment. The level of specific salivary and serum antibody to *Candida* has also been shown to be of diagnostic value in chronic oral candidiasis.

Other immunologic procedures. The specific interaction of antigen and antibody is utilized in a variety of laboratory tests, some of which have already been referred to in other sections of this chapter (*e.g.,* radioimmunoassay for various hormones, immunodiffusion techniques for the separation and quantitation of gamma globulins, and fluorescent antibody techniques) as well as others that are beyond the scope of this text (*e.g.,* cross-matching and typing of donors' and recipients' blood for transfusion; immunohematology). In addition clinical use is being made of an increasing number of procedures concerned with lymphocyte (T cell)-mediated immune processes in which humoral (serum or tissue fluid) antibody may play little or no part. Tests for lymphocyte transformation and macrophage migration-inhibition factor, for example, are carried out with samples of peripheral blood from which cells (lymphocytes and macrophages) are isolated and studied in cell culture. Laboratory tests for cell-mediated immunity are becoming particularly important in the study of hypersensitivity reactions, and are already being used in specialized laboratories to supplement the classical clinical procedure of skin testing.

Microbial culture techniques and serologic procedures are described in some detail in the following pages. In general, specimens for all these procedures should be obtained with an aseptic technique. A 10-ml sample of clotted venous blood (no preservative) is required for all serologic tests. After separation of the clot by centrifugation, the serum may be stored frozen at −5° to −10°C for many months (or even transported safely unfrozen by mail), since antibody gamma globulins are relatively heat stable.

Other immunologic procedures are covered only briefly, with emphasis on fairly long-established techniques concerned with the diagnosis of collagen (autoimmune) diseases. For additional information on the increasing number of procedures designed to measure cell-mediated immune reactions, the reader is referred to Chapter 24 and to recent texts on clinical immunology that provide comprehensive coverage of these topics.

Demonstration of Microorganisms in Oral Tissues Sampled by Means of Smears

Smears of oral mucosal cells and exudates are usually studied in dental patients for one of three reasons: (1) to determine the morphology of microorganisms present in an oral lesion, (2) to detect premalignant and malignant changes in the oral mucosa, and (3) to detect giant cells and other unusual cells that occur in vesicular virus infections (herpes simplex, varicella, and herpes zoster) and pemphigus. For (1) the smear is usually air dried, heat fixed, and Gram stained; for (2) and (3) the smear may be immediately fixed with 95% alcohol or Spraycyte and stained by the Papanicolaou technique. This staining procedure requires the services of a diagnostic laboratory and is described more fully in the section on Histopathology and Cytology. For (3) the smear may also be air dried, fixed with methanol, and Giemsa stained. This procedure requires no elaborate apparatus or special skill and can be completed in 1 hour.

Gram-Stained Smears for Bacteria and Fungi

Indications Gram-stained, heat-fixed smears are used in four specific situations in the evaluation of dental patients:

1. Whenever a specimen (exudate, swab, scraping) is submitted to a diagnostic laboratory for isolation and identification of microorganisms associated with an oral lesion, a heat-fixed smear should accompany it. Only a proportion, and sometimes none, of the organisms seen in the smear may grow on routine microbiologic culture media. The smear is then a valuable piece of information.
2. Endodontists frequently advise preparation of a smear from paper points, removed from

the root canal, for evaluation of the micro-biologic status of the canal prior to filling.

3. A scraping or swab of an oral lesion is needed to confirm a diagnosis of thrush.

4. A scraping of a gingival lesion or mucosal ulcer is sometimes used to confirm a diagnosis of acute necrotizing ulcerative stomatitis.

Equipment Clean glass microscope slides (1 in × 3 in), cotton swab, tongue blade or swab stick; gas burner or alcohol lamp; six Coplin jars containing 50 ml of each of the following Gram-stain reagents* in sequence—crystal violet, Gram's iodine, absolute ethanol (three jars), safranin; microscope with oil immersion lens, immersion oil.

Smears made from the oral cavity, unlike those prepared from *in vitro* bacterial cultures, contain large amounts of mucosal cells, polymorphonuclear leukocytes, mucus, and oral debris. Decolorization of oral smears by the "dropping technique" is usually unsatisfactory, and the Bartholomew technique, in which slides are dipped into the various reagents of the Gram stain for fixed periods of time without using a visual end-point of decolorization, usually gives better results.

Procedure The material for the smear is obtained by firmly scraping a cotton swab or tongue blade over the area of mucosa under study or by scraping deeply into ulcerated tissue with a sterilized wire loop. The material obtained is smeared over the surface of a slide, covering as large an area as possible, thinning the specimen with a drop of tap water, if necessary. The smear is allowed to air dry, after which it is fixed by passing the slide through a flame several times. The smear is stained by dipping the slide in the following sequence of stains: crystal violet, 1 minute, rinse under running tap water; Gram's iodine, 1 minute, rinse; dip in and out of each of the three jars of ethanol, rinse; safranin, 1 minute, rinse; blot and air dry.

The stained smear is examined under the microscope. The slide is scanned at low power (× 100), and the nature of the smear is determined.

Fragmented and smeared cells, which are common, are of no significance because the heat fixation used frequently damages many cells. Unidentified debris, strands of fibrin, and food particles may also be seen. Final examination is made under oil immersion at × 1,000.

* Available from medical supply houses

Interpretation Smears of the gingival crevice will show large numbers of bacteria of varied morphologic forms lying for the most part outside the tissue cells. These microorganisms will be seen in all mouths whether they are healthy or diseased. When a picture such as this is seen, the smear is reported as *mixed oral bacterial flora*. Two characteristic pictures that are of diagnostic value are smears from lesions of thrush and from lesions of acute necrotizing ulcerative gingivostomatitis.

The smear from the *lesions of thrush* will show large numbers of yeasts and fungal mycelia and frequently only small numbers of the usual mixed oral bacterial flora. Two morphologic forms of the causative agent of thrush (*Candida*) will be seen in these lesions (Figs. 3-21 to 3-23).

Yeasts are large ovoid, deeply gram-positive structures like large cocci, but frequently they have buds rising from their surface. *Pseudomycelia* are long, gram-positive rods with only one or two side branches, occasionally with a yeast cell budding from one of the branches.

Both yeasts and pseudomycelia may be seen lying free in the smear in tangled masses associated with debris, tissue cells, and bacteria or attached to the surface of desquamated epithelial cells. Suspected mycelia should always be checked under oil immersion (× 1,000) to differentiate them from chains of bacteria, strands of fibrin, and other filamentous structures.

The smear from the *lesions of acute necrotizing ulcerative gingivostomatitis* will usually show large numbers of the mixed oral bacterial flora, plus easily recognized fusiforms and *Borreliae* (spirochetes). In some smears as many as half of all bacteria seen are fusiforms or spirochetes.

The presence of the fusospirochetal complex indicates that the ulcerative process has been secondarily infected with Vincent's organisms. It does not give any information on the reason for this secondary infection, which may have been any one or more of a variety of predisposing factors (*e.g.*, virus infection, heavy smoking, emotional stress, agranulocytosis, chronic gingivitis, and irritation from calculus or an opposing tooth).

Fusiforms and spirochetes are frequently seen in small numbers in the gingival crevice of patients who do not have acute necrotizing ulcerative gingivostomatitis. In acute infections, however, they are found in greatly increased numbers and often to the exclusion of other oral microbial forms (Fig. 3-24). (See also the following discussion on the use of dark-field and phase-contrast microscopy for the evaluation of gingival scrapings in determining the status of periodontal lesions.)

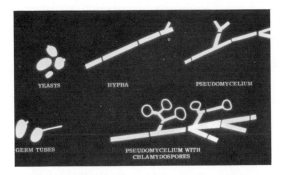

Fig. 3-21 Diagram of morphologic forms of *Candida*.

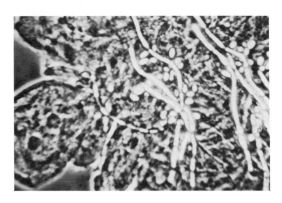

Fig. 3-22 Phase-contrast photomicrograph of yeasts and pseudomycelia of *Candida* attached to oral epithelial squames. (Sumter Arnim, M.D. and Martin Lunin, M.D.)

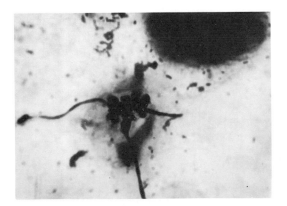

Fig. 3-23 Yeast and pseudomycelia of *Candida* in a Gram-stained preparation from the oral mucosal lesions of thrush. (×900)

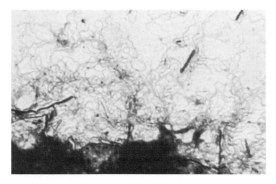

Fig. 3-24 Fusiform bacteria and treponemes (*Borrelia*) in a Gram-stained smear of an ulcer in a patient with necrotizing ulcerative stomatitis. (×900)

Where a full set of Gram's reagents is not available, satisfactory slides can be made by following the same technique for preparing the smear and then staining with crystal violet alone. This procedure is adequate for differentiation of yeasts and the fusospirochetal complex. Other microbiologic staining techniques can of course be carried out on heat-fixed smears (*e.g.*, the Ziehl–Neelsen stain or fluorochrome stain for acid-fast bacilli used in the recognition of *Mycobacterium*. The etiologic agent of tuberculosis, *M. tuberculosis*, has been demonstrated in oral ulcers by this technique.)

Smears for Suspected Actinomycotic Lesions

One criterion for the diagnosis of an infection with *Actinomyces* is the demonstration of characteristic sulfur granules in the purulent exudate. Sometimes these granules (which are in fact colonies of the fungus) can be readily identified by the naked eye in the pus itself, but the following procedure may be necessary to demonstrate and differentiate them from particles of inspissated pus. Several drops of the exudate are added to 2 to 3 ml of sterile saline in a test tube or Petri dish; the fluid is agitated and then allowed to stand for a few minutes. Sulfur granules will not dissolve even with vigorous shaking and will settle to the bottom of the vessel. The granules are washed in this fashion with several changes of saline, and then a granule is removed with a loop or pipette and placed on a microscope slide. Another slide is placed on top of the granule, and it is crushed with firm pressure. The slides are separated and covered with a coverslip for wet-mount observation of radiating mycelia and clubs (examine under subdued light under the low-power objective of the microscope). Because special procedures are usually needed to culture these organisms, the dentist should indicate to the laboratory when he suspects an infection with *Actinomyces*.

Giemsa-Stained Smears and the Tzanck Smear

Indications These smears are used for identification of the giant cells that accompany vesicular virus infections (herpes simplex, varicella and herpes zoster) and are commonly known as *viral giant cells*; and for identification of acantholysis, a characteristic tissue change occurring in pemphigus. In both diseases the smear is made from the cells making up the floor of the lesion. The technique of obtaining a smear from this location and staining it is known as the *Tzanck smear*.

Equipment Jar of sponges soaked in 70% alcohol; sterile hypodermic needle or blood lancet; microscope slides; Coplin jar of methanol, Coplin jar of Giemsa stain;* microscope; immersion oil.

Procedure An oral vesicle of recent origin is selected and the area isolated and dried or cleansed gently with an alcohol swab, if it is on the skin. The vesicle is then punctured with a sterile needle or lancet and the roof peeled back to expose the base of the lesion. The fluid contents of the vesicle are absorbed onto a cotton swab, and cells are obtained from the base of the vesicle by scraping it with the tip of the needle or lancet. The material thus obtained is smeared over a small area on a glass microscope slide, allowed to air dry, and then fixed by dipping in methanol for 10 minutes. The slide can then be sent to a laboratory or it can be stained by immersing in dilute Giemsa stain for 50 minutes.

The fluid from a vesicle is frequently also a valuable specimen for recovery of viruses. If a virus infection is suspected, the fluid contents absorbed onto the swab should be transferred to appropriate transport media, as described in a following section.

Interpretation In a Giemsa-stained smear the cells are similar in appearance to those seen in a Wright's-stained smear of peripheral blood. In addition to clumps of epithelial cells, a Tzanck smear will contain a variety of inflammatory cells, erythrocytes, and fibrin strands.

Vesicles from herpes simplex and varicella infections also contain a variable number of large multinucleate cells known as viral giant cells (Fig. 3-25). These are distinguished from clumps of epithelial cells by the lack of granularity in the cytoplasm and absence of intercellular membranes in the giant cells. Inclusion bodies are not revealed by Giemsa staining and can be seen only if the smear is stained by the more elaborate Papanicolaou or hematoxylin and eosin techniques. Tzanck smears should be scanned first at low power ($\times 100$) and any large cells "spotted" with the oil immersion objective ($\times 1,000$) for identification of viral giant cells. If a vesicle is ruptured, there is little chance of recovering recognizable giant cells from the ulcerated surface. Similarly, in herpes simplex infections, the cells at the base of the vesicle begin to disintegrate within 12 to 24 hours after the vesicle appears.

Vesicles from pemphigus contain inflammatory elements as well as epithelial cells that have become separated from adjacent cells by the process of acantholysis, the characteristic pathologic change that produces the intraepithelial vesicles of pemphigus.

When either viral giant cells or acantholytic cells are seen in a Tzanck smear, it is referred to as a positive Tzanck smear. In the case of suspected pemphigus, a positive Tzanck smear should always be followed by referral (usually to a dermatologist) so that the diagnosis can be confirmed by biopsy.

Caries Activity Tests

Well over a dozen different types of tests have been devised to measure the cariogenic potential of the oral cavity. Some are only of

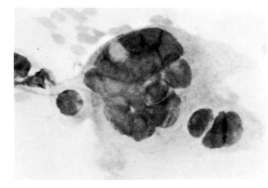

Fig. 3-25 "Viris" giant cell in Giemsa-stained Tzanck smear from vesicle of primary herpes simplex virus infection. ($\times 900$)

---

* Available as a 50-fold concentrate from medical supply houses; 1 ml is added to the Coplin jar, which is then filled with water and the contents mixed.

historical interest, since the variables they were designed to measure have been shown to play little or no role in caries production. Those that remain of interest rely on the acidogenic and aciduric properties of the oral bacterial flora, activity being measured either by means of bacterial growth (*e.g.*, the *Lactobacillus* count) or a change in an acid–base indicator (*e.g.*, the Snyder test). In addition, the buffer capacity of saliva is sometimes measured. These tests were devised to provide a measure of caries activity in populations being studied for the anticaries effects of dentifrices, etc., and to identify individuals with high cariogenic potential well before they develop rampant caries.

Both the *Lactobacillus* count and Snyder test continue to be used in population studies, and both measures show fair correlation with the *overall* caries experience of a study population. A fall in buffer capacity can also be a valuable predictor of new caries activity, which will only appear clinically some months in the future. However, even in population studies, caries activity tests show less than the 0.9% coefficient of correlation that is desirable for such statistical estimates. *The prognostic value of these tests for the individual patient is considerably less*, with the likelihood of the *Lactobacillus* count as a predictor of caries activity being in error by a factor of 20% (or more) in any one patient. The failure of both the *Lactobacillus* count and Snyder test as diagnostic vehicles when applied to individuals needs to be stressed, since in recent years, various caries prevention programs have again encouraged the use of the Snyder test in dental practice, and the equipment needed to perform the test in the dental office has been widely marketed.

The chief value of the Snyder test is that it can provide an objective demonstration of caries activity that may be more convincing to the patient than the threat of future carious cavities. In like manner, the *Lactobacillus* count has been used in some dental schools as a measure of the success of dietary (and caries) control in patients maintained on the Combined Caries Control Program (*Lactobacillus* counts and dietary restriction of carbohydrate) originally described by Becks. Provided no specific prognosis regarding future dental caries experience is made to an individual patient based on the results of these tests, use of both the *Lactobacillus* count and the Snyder test for these limited purposes seems justified.

A significant correlation has also been shown in group studies between the average count of *Streptococcus mutans* in plaque and dental caries experience during the ensuing year; however, no data exist to show that counts of this species, which has been implicated as a causative agent of dental caries, provide any greater predictive accuracy for future caries activity than do counts of *Lactobacillus* or other acidogenic/aciduric species.

Snyder Test

Kits are available commercially for carrying out the Snyder test in the dental office. In brief, the test consists of the incubation of a sample of paraffin-stimulated saliva mixed with pH 5.0, bromocresol green, dextrose agar at 37°C for 3 days. A change of the indicator to yellow (green is no longer the predominant color, pH 4.2 or less) in 24 hours indicates high caries activity; no change in 72 hours, low activity.

Lactobacillus Count

Five milliliters of paraffin-stimulated mixed saliva is collected in a screw-cap bottle and shaken by machine for 2 minutes. The saliva sample is diluted 1/100 with distilled water, and duplicate 1.0 ml and 0.1 ml aliquots, respectively, of the diluted sample are added to Petri dishes containing 20 ml of cooled liquified agar. The solidified media is incubated for 3 days at 37°C, at which time characteristic colonies of *Lactobacillus* are counted, the count expressed as the average number of colonies per milliliter of the original saliva sample.

Salivary Buffer Capacity

The volatile bicarbonate anion is an important component of the salivary buffer system, and collection and titration of saliva in this test must be carried out under a layer of paraffin oil to prevent loss of this anion. Two milliliters of saliva collected under paraffin oil are added to 4 ml of distilled water under a paraffin seal. The delivery end of a microburet and a microglass electrode are introduced under the seal, and the amount of 0.5N hydrochloric acid required to bring the saliva to *pH* 5.0 is measured. Saliva samples requiring less than 0.45 ml of standard hydrochloric acid in this test have *low buffer capacity;* those requiring 0.45 ml or more have *high buffer capacity.*

Phase-Contrast and Dark-Field Microscopic Examination of the Microbial Flora from Plaque and Gingival Crevice

Special techniques to demonstrate the morphology and motility of microorganisms in wet mounts of scrapings from dental plaque and the gingival crevice are used in dentistry for two purposes: to educate patients regarding the effectiveness of home care procedures, and more recently in a number of research laboratories and periodontal offices, to estimate the proportions of subgingival spirochetes and motile bacteria as a predictor of continuing periodontal deterioration. With regard to plaque specimens, no predictive data exist to correlate the numbers or types of microorganisms noted in plaque by phase microscopy (the most commonly used equipment for this purpose) with future caries activity on an individual tooth or patient basis. Better correlations have been documented for subgingival specimens between the proportions of spirochetes with or without motile rods noted in the specimen and the progression of periodontal destruction with deepening of the crevice or periodontal pocket.

In one study by Listgarten, using dark-field microscopy, spirochetes and motile rods on the average constituted 16% and 28%, respectively, of the crevice flora in those mouths in which periodontal destruction was progressing. By contrast, spirochetes and motile rods made up only 2% and 7% of the crevice flora in patients in whom periodontal destruction had been halted. Research is continuing to determine whether such semiquantitative estimations of the subgingival microbial flora have predictive value in determining the effectiveness of home-care procedures, the optimal frequency for professional curettage and prophylactic procedures, the prognosis of individual periodontally involved teeth, and the need for surgical treatment.

Specimens required for both educational demonstration and semiquantitative estimates are obtained on the tip of a small curette either inserted into the gingival crevice or pocket, or used to collect supragingival deposits, in the case of dental plaque studies. The material removed on the curette is suspended in 0.85% sodium chloride containing 1% gelatin, dispersed well by aspirating and expelling the material three times through a disposable tuberculin syringe and a 23-gauge needle, and a drop expelled onto a glass microscope slide, which is then covered with a coverslip. Examples of spirochetes, motile bacteria, and coccal forms are illustrated in Figure 3-26. For demonstrations to patients, the phase-contrast and dark-field microscopes can be equipped with a television

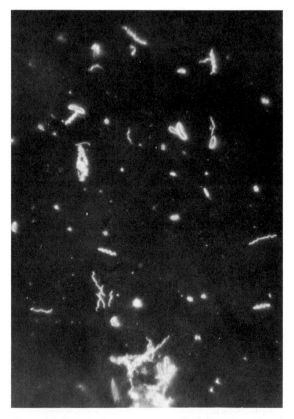

Fig. 3-26 Gingival crevice microbial flora examined by darkfield microscopy. Spirochetes, cocci, and rods can all be distinguished and enumerated. Motility can also be examined directly in this darkfield microscopic preparation and a count of motile versus nonmotile forms obtained. (Courtesy of Dr. Max Listgarten, Philadelphia)

camera that transmits an enlarged image of the microscope field to a monitor.

A similar technique may be used to demonstrate the presence of oral trichomonads, but does not allow differentiation of the saprophytic oral species (*Trichomonas tenax*) from the genital species (*Trichomonas vaginalis*). Electron microscopic observation is needed for accurate determination of the size of the organism and the attachment of the undulating membrane, the two morphologic features that distinguish these two species.

Bacterial Cultures in Endodontics

Culturing of paper points inserted into root canals prior to sealing became a routine step in endodontic therapy 30 to 40 years ago, at a time when the concept of focal infection was commonly used to explain a variety of diseases of unknown etiology. The development of endodontic therapy and its acceptance by the medical profession were due in large part to the dentist's ability to show that no microorganisms were cultured from the canal prior to sealing it. In recent years, the safety of endodontic therapy has not been challenged, and various authors have already questioned whether the procedure is necessary as a routine and whether it is even a useful predictor of a successful outcome to endodontic treatment. Since no attempt is usually made to detect anaerobic bacteria* present in the canal and since the presence or absence of bacteria in the canal shows little relationship to the bacteriologic status of the periapical tissue, the validity of the procedure as an index of sterility of the canal and periapical tissues is open to criticism.

Although there is no question of the usefulness of the procedure in cases that show a persistent active, apical infectious process requiring careful selection of an antibiotic, the results of surveys of diplomates of the American Board of Endodontics reveal that fewer than one half routinely cultured root canals. Fewer than one third used the procedure only "when indicated" in the endo-

---

* Procedures for submitting specimens for anaerobic culture are described in the following section, Microbial Isolation and Antibiotic Sensitivity Testing.

dontic treatment of nonvital teeth, teeth with persistent pain or discomfort, and those which had an exudate in the canal or an area of periapical pathosis. Other authors justify the procedure as a check on the dentist's aseptic technique and as a definite aid in the management of problem cases.

Undoubtedly, some of this controversy is due to the fact that great care has to be taken both in obtaining a sample from the apical portion of the canal and in the method of culturing. Leakage of saliva into the canal through an inadequate temporary seal and contamination of the paper point or the canal while obtaining the specimen will give rise to false-positive results; and contamination of the paper point with antiseptics or residual inhibitory medicaments, failure to use both aerobic and anaerobic culture techniques, and inability to sample organisms located in accessory canals will lead to false-negative results.

Full details of the technique commonly used in endodontic practice are described by Grossman and in other endodontic texts. Other authors have used somewhat more elaborate techniques that are necessary, if critical judgments are to be made about the success or failure of a particular endodontic procedure. Failure to inactivate residual antimicrobial medicaments retained in the canal from a previous visit is probably one of the greatest hazards leading to false-negative results. The reference in the bibliography by Möller should be consulted by those interested in critical studies of root canal infections.

In those studies in which a comparison has been made between teeth that were sealed after negative cultures from the root canal, and those that were sealed while the canal still contained culturable microorganisms (or those sealed without any cultures being obtained), the success rate was on the average 10% higher after negative cultures (range of 2% to 15% in various studies with an average success rate of 80% even in the presence of culturable microorganisms in the canal prior to sealing). Problems in the selection of cases in these two groups and the short period of time over which endodontic success is commonly measured underline the fact that the controversy, "to culture or not to culture," has probably not yet been solved. The current status of the debate has been extensively recorded in a number of symposia.

Microbial Isolation and Antibiotic Sensitivity Testing

Isolation of the Oral Microbial Flora

Because the oral cavity possesses its own extremely heavy microbial flora and because the majority of infectious processes about the mouth are mixed endogenous infections derived from this flora, bacterial isolation procedures are of limited value in diagnosing oral disease. In certain specific situations, however, they are indicated in the management of suppurative lesions around the mouth, to aid in the diagnosis of candidiasis, and to identify pathogens among throat flora.

In the management of suppurative lesions around the oral cavity (excluding the throat; see following section.) Identification of the microorganisms present in pus aspirated from these lesions can provide information on the nature of the infectious process. Since the majority of these lesions are treated by surgical drainage coupled with systemic use of one of the antibiotics effective against both gram-negative and gram-positive organisms, this information is usually available only in retrospect.

Should the lesion fail to respond to the initial treatment, the results of bacterial isolation procedures together with the antibiotic sensitivity testing of the isolates will provide a rational basis for further antibiotic treatment. Interpretation of the results of bacterial culture of pus is possible only where the lesion has no demonstrable connection with the oral cavity. If the pus or the specimen is contaminated with oral flora, the more rapidly growing members will appear on the inoculated medium to the exclusion of more fastidious organisms. Not infrequently, cultures inoculated with aspirated pus will fail to grow, and it is important to submit a heat-fixed smear of the pus along with the specimen to determine whether failure to produce growth indicates sterility of the pus or the presence of any organism unlikely to grow on the media used.

Since the majority of oral suppurative lesions are mixed infections derived from the patient's own oral flora, a mixture of microorganisms easily recognizable as members of the normal oral flora will usually be reported when these lesions are studied bacteriologically. Isolation of the commonly acknowledged pathogens (*e.g.*, *Clostridium tetani*, coagulase-positive *Staphylococcus*, beta-hemolytic *Streptococcus*) in pure culture from oral lesions is less common. When the pathogens occur in mixed culture in a suppurative lesion, their presence is probably no more significant than it is when they are occasionally found in the normal oral cavity.

This generalization does not apply in regard to interpretation of the results of swabs taken from the throat (*i.e.*, the posterior pharyngeal wall and tonsillar fossa). In that location (see text), even small numbers of beta-hemolytic streptococci are always considered exogenous pathogens. Gram-negative enteric bacteria are often isolated from the mouths of patients under treatment with antibiotics, sometimes to the exclusion of other oral flora. No specific oral lesions are associated with this change in the oral microbial flora (compare with overgrowth of yeasts with production of thrush), although various degrees of coated tongue and pseudomembranous stomatitis are common in hospitalized and seriously ill patients who characteristically exhibit such gram-negative bacterial overgrowths. Various coliforms, *Proteus*, and *Bacteroides* are usually found in small numbers even in healthy mouths, provided a search is made for them with selective media. Overgrowth of these microorganisms, usually following suppression of antibiotic-sensitive gram-positive species, presumably accounts for their appearance in large numbers in some patients' mouths.

The complete list of genera that have been reported from the oral cavity is extensive, and many of them can be identified and isolated only by special culture methods. In general, those organisms reported by clinical diagnostic laboratories represent a sampling of the less fastidious and more prevalent members of the oral flora (Table 3-16). The frequency with which organisms are isolated by routine cultural methods roughly correlates with their concentration in mixed saliva (Ta-

Table 3-16. Major Groups of Microorganisms in Human Saliva*

High count group

Total anaerobes	1×10^8
Total aerobes	4×10^7
Total streptococci	1.8×10^7
Veillonella	1.7×10^7
Streptococcus salivarius	1.1×10^7
Neisseria	
Micrococci	2×10^6
Diphtheroids	

Intermediate count group

Fusobacterium	5.6×10^4
Lactobacillus	3.5×10^4
Staphylococcus	5.0×10^3
Leptotrichia	3.0×10^3
Bacteroides	3.0×10^3

Low count group

Candida	2.0×10^2
Coliforms	1.0×10^2
Actinomyces	
Proteus	
Spirochetes	< 100
Nonhemolytic streptococci	

* Numbers per milliliter of mixed saliva. (Adapted from Richardson RL, Jones M: J Dent Res 37:697, 1958)

ble 3-17). The organisms associated with some common oral infectious processes such as acute necrotizing gingivitis are not recovered by standard isolation procedures.

Specimens intended for bacterial isolation should be obtained with an aseptic technique so that the organisms collected on the swab are representative of the lesion under study. Swabs should not be allowed to dry out once the specimen is collected and should either be inoculated directly when they are obtained or taken immediately to the laboratory. If any delay is expected, the specimen should be inoculated into a suitable transport medium, such as any nutrient broth or fluid thioglycollate medium (available commercially in individual tubes). Since transport medium for virus specimens contains antibacterial antibiotics, it is unsuitable for bacterial specimens, although it is satisfactory for specimens for isolation of yeasts and fungi.

No one bacteriologic medium or culture technique will allow the isolation of all mi-

Table 3-17. Frequency of Isolation of Different Bacterial Species and Yeasts from the Pulp Canals of Infected Molar Teeth

MICROORGANISM	FREQUENCY OF ISOLATION (%)	
	(I)*	(II)†
Streptococcus salivarius (α)	70	76.6
Streptococcus mitis (α)	10	20
Streptococcus hemolyticus (β)	10	23.3
Staphylococcus albus	23	16.6
Staphylococcus aureus	5	6.6
Neisseria catarrhalis and other nonpathogenic *Neisseria*	3	20
Lactobacilus	13	26
Enterobacteriaceae	17	6.6
Yeasts	3	20

* (Cohen MM, Joress SM, Calisti LP: Bacteriologic study of infected deciduous molars. Oral Surg 13:1382, 1960)
† (Tomić K, Jelinek E: Comparative study of the bacterial flora in the surroundings, the root canals and sockets of deciduous molars. Int Dent J 21:375, 1971)

croorganisms. When an infection with organisms that require special handling is suspected (*e.g.*, *Mycobacterium tuberculosis*, *Actinomyces*, *Neisseria gonorrheae*, *Candida*, and other fungi or anaerobic species of bacteria), the laboratory should be informed so that appropriate procedures can be used. Blood agar and Sabouraud's agar (for yeasts and fungi) are generally used for primary inoculation of oral specimens.

As an aid in the diagnosis of candidiasis. The yeast *Candida* is listed as a member of the normal oral microbial flora, and in some populations, such as hospitalized patients, 70% of individuals may be asymptomatic carriers. Even in populations where the carrier rate is lower, isolation of *Candida* from the oral cavity is of little diagnostic value unless the organism has been demonstrated in large numbers in smears obtained from the suspected lesion or where a raised titer of serum or salivary fluorescent antibody is present. Isolation of yeasts from an oral specimen is requested on occasion, however, simply to confirm the findings obtained by microscopic examination of the smear or to obtain precise identification of the species involved.

The various causes of overgrowth of *Candida* in the oral cavity, as well as the characteristic lesions associated with oral candidiasis, are described in Chapter 6. Masses of yeastlike fungi can be demonstrated in the surface layers of the lesions of acute candidiasis by microscopic examination of biopsy specimens stained with hematoxylin and eosin or special fungal stains (*e.g.*, Brown and Brenn, or periodic acid-Schiff [PAS], and Gram-stained smears of the lesions contain yeasts and pseudomycelia (see preceding section, Gram-stained Smears for Bacteria and Fungi). The risk of inducing a fungemia by biopsy of the lesions of acute oral candidiasis is unknown, although probably low. However, since the Gram-stained smear on the surface of the lesion usually confirms the nature of the lesion adequately (see Fig. 3-23), biopsy is rarely indicated.

The throat, like the oral cavity, has its own normal flora, and throat swabs will usually contain large numbers of alpha-hemolytic streptococci, diphtheroids, and pneumococci whether or not the mucosa is inflamed. Throat swabs are therefore of diagnostic value only where a pathogen not normally found in that location (*e.g.*, beta-hemolytic *Streptococcus*) is present in large numbers. Since the eradication of carriers of beta-hemolytic streptococci and the prompt treatment of streptococcal sore throat are important ways of preventing rheumatic fever and glomerulonephritis, the dentist can contribute to preventing these diseases by referring patients with acute exudative pharyngitis and tonsillitis to a physician for adequate medical diagnosis and treatment. The dentist himself may also wish to submit throat swabs for isolation of beta-hemolytic streptococci in patients with pharyngitis, exudative tonsillitis, fever over 37.7°C, sore throat with or without fever, tender cervical nodes, or previous history of rheumatic fever. In a 2-year period in one health district in Illinois where dentists were encouraged to participate in a screening program for beta-hemolytic streptococcal infection, 213 patients (14% of all throat swabs) were found to have beta-hemolytic streptococci in their throats.

Neisseria gonorrhoeae, the causative agent of gonorrhea, is not part of the normal throat flora, although several closely related species, *N. catarrhalis (Branhamella catarrhalis)*, *N. pharyngis (N. sicca)*, and possibly *N. meningitidis* (a causative agent of bacterial meningitis when it penetrates the pharyngeal mucosa and invades the bloodstream and meninges), are commonly found in normal throat swabs. However, cases of pharyngitis following orogenital intercourse have been reported in which *N. gonorrhoeae* was isolated from throat swabs, this finding indicating that this species can also persist for some time in this location.

N. gonorrhoeae is an especially fastidious species and special transport media and culture techniques are needed for its isolation from throat or genitourinary secretions. Differentiation of this species from other endogenous pharyngeal *Neisseria* depends largely on the results of *in vitro* sugar fermentation tests and growth on blood agar, and unequivocal identification of a throat isolate such as *N. gonorrhoeae* may not always be possible. Because of the large number of saprophytic *Neisseria* and *Veillonella* in both the throat and oral cavity, a diagnosis of gonorrheal pharyngitis or stomatitis *cannot* be made on the basis of a finding of intracellularly located gram-negative cocci in a pharyngeal smear (although this criterion is commonly used for the presumptive diagnosis of gonococcal infection of the genitourinary tract, based on smears of genitourinary secretions).

Ideally, specimens for the isolation of *N. gonorrhoeae* should be inoculated onto appropriate media at chairside to ensure optimal recovery of this fastidious species. For this purpose, special Petri dishes known as *Jembec plates* are available. These contain a selective medium (Thayer–Martin medium [see Table 28-4], or less satisfactorily, chocolate agar, which inhibits growth of saprophytic *Neisseria*, yeasts, and many other oropharyngeal bacterial species) and a well into which a CO_2-releasing tablet can be placed before sealing the plate in a "zip-loc" bag or other airtight container to ensure that the organisms are maintained in a CO_2-enriched atmosphere during transport to the laboratory. Because genital and pharyngeal gonorrhea, like syphilis and hepatitis B, are reportable diseases, all confirmed positive isolations of *N. gonorrhoeae* are routinely reported by the laboratory to the local health authority. Serologic tests are not available for the diagnosis of gonorrhea.

Bacterial Antibiotic Sensitivity Testing

Antibiotic sensitivity is usually carried out once the various bacteria in the specimen have been isolated in pure culture. Since this requires a delay of at least 24 hours in obtaining the results, testing of a mixed culture is sometimes used. This method allows some opportunity for *in vitro* interaction between the various organisms involved, similar though not identical to those occurring *in vivo*, and it has been advocated for oral specimens, the majority of which contain a mixed flora. In most circumstances, however, antibiotic sensitivity and determination of the minimal inhibitory concentration (MIC) of particular antibiotics are carried out on pure culture isolates.

Whatever the method of testing used, the results are only a guide to the selection of an antibiotic. All oral lesions that fail to respond to antibiotic therapy are not caused by antibiotic-resistant strains. A decision to change antibiotics should be based not only on the results of the antibiotic sensitivity test but also on an examination of the possibilities that dense fibrous tissue or necrotic bone is preventing adequate penetration of the antibiotic, that oral fluids are continuously reinfecting the lesion, and that suppuration or evidence of infection will continue until bony sequestrum or necrotic root tissue is removed.

The normal oral flora contains many organisms, such as alpha- and nonhemolytic streptococci, yeasts, staphylococci, and gram-negative bacilli, which are either naturally resistant to the more common antibiotics or rapidly develop resistance under treatment. Systematic testing of bacteria isolated from saliva and the gingival crevice has revealed that among patients attending dental clinics, at least 94% have some penicillin-resistant oral microorganisms, 25% have penicillin-resistant streptococci, and 20% or more have some erythromycin-resistant bacteria. Since many oral suppurative lesions respond to treatment with penicillin, erythromycin, and tetracyclines, however, it is apparent that all antibiotic-resistant organisms reported in a specimen from the usual mixed oral infection do not require specific antibiotic treatment.

Antibiotic treatment of the majority of oral infections is largely empirical, but in most cases it appears to be successful. In the rare case that does not respond, assistance can sometimes be obtained by antibiotic sensitivity testing of organisms isolated from the lesion. For example, penicillin-resistant enterococci (as well as *Escherichia coli* and *Pseudomonas* species) are commonly isolated from persistently infected pulp canals and probably contribute to the failure of these canals to heal. Although many of these enterococcal species are sensitive to ampicillin and erythromycin, there is enough species variation in this regard to justify antibiotic sensitivity testing of these isolates as a guide to selecting an antibiotic that will eradicate them from the canal.

The choice of an antibiotic for treatment of an oral infection thus usually depends only partly on the results of microbial isolation and antibiotic sensitivity testing in the laboratory. In general, the dictum that it is preferable to prescribe from a limited armamentarium of drugs that have limited and relatively well-understood side effects, is a valuable one, especially for a dentist who might administer antibiotics only rarely. Resistant oral infections will be encountered from time to time, however, and an alternative antimicrobial or one suggested by the results of antibacterial sensitivity testing of selected isolates may be needed.

Longitudinal studies of pyogenic bacteria isolated in clinical diagnostic laboratories over the last two to three decades have shown changes in the type of bacteria associated with infections in a particular anatomic region, as well as changing patterns of antibiotic sensitivity. To some extent, these changes are certainly associated with patterns of antibiotic use. Similar changes have been noted with bacteria isolated from dental pyogenic infections (see Tables 3-18 and 3-19).

The total proportion of streptococci isolated has decreased, mainly because of a reduction in the number of division I (pyogenic group) and division II (viridans group) of streptococci; division III (enterococci) have remained stable. Conversely, the proportion

Table 3-18. Types of Bacteria Isolated from Dental Pyogenic Infections in Four Studies, 1966 to 1979, per cent

	DATES OF SURVEYS			
TYPE OF BACTERIA	1966–7[†]	1973–4	1975–7	1978–9
Streptococci				
Division I (Pyogenic group*)	18	29	27	21
Division II (Viridans groups*)	38	46	45	36
Division III (*Enterococcus* group*)	25	6	8	9
All streptococci	81	81	80	66
Staphylococci	5	10	14	12
Escherichia coli	11	5	4	10
Genus *Pseudomonas*		3	1	5
Genus *Klebsiella*	2	1	1	7
All gram-negative bacteria	12	9	6	22

* Previous classification.
[†] Bacteria classified as species of gaffkya accounted for 1% of bacteria isolated during this period.
(Woods R: The changing nature of pyogenic dental infections. Aust Dent J 23:107, 1978)

Table 3-19. Antibiotic Sensitivity, per cent, of Bacteria Isolated in Four Studies, 1966-1979

		DATES OF SAMPLES STUDIED			
BACTERIA	ANTIBIOTIC	1966–7	1973–4	1975–7	1978–9
All cases studied	Penicillin	63	75	73	55
	Tetracycline	92	73	42	56
	Erythromycin	95	96	92	90
	Ampicillin		85	78	65
Streptococci (all Divisions)	Penicillin	76	92	91	84
	Tetracycline	91	75	43	52
	Erythromycin	100	98	97	96
	Ampicillin		97	94	92
Staphylococci	Penicillin	0	0	0	0
	Tetracycline	100	50	21	40
	Erythromycin	100	100	84	73
	Ampicillin		38	16	7
	Co-trimoxazole			100	73
Gram-negative bacteria	Penicillin	0	0	0	0
	Tetracycline	91	71	78	76
	Erythromycin	64	71	44	79
	Ampicillin		29	11	17

(Woods R: The changing nature of pyogenic dental infections. Aust Dent J 23:107, 1978)

of gram-negative bacteria (*Escherichia, Pseudomonas* and *Klebsiella*) isolated from dental infections has increased quite significantly. These changes represent an overall reduction in the penicillin-sensitive portion of the oral pyogenic flora.

The penicillins (including semisynthetic penicillins such as ampicillin and amoxicillin) are probably still the most commonly used antibiotics for the treatment of dental pyogenic infections, when no clinical differentiation or antibiotic testing of bacterial isolates is attempted. The continued sensitivity of most streptococci (which are still the organisms most likely to be associated with a dental pyogenic infection) to this group of antibiotics provides a rationale for continuing this practice, although tetracycline and erythromycin for the most part are excellent alternatives, despite evidence of decreasing sensitivity of streptococci and staphylococci to tetracycline. In response to the knowledge of an increased frequency of isolation of gram-negative species, use of a cephalosporin is reasonable and probably fairly frequent.

Alternatively, selection of an appropriate antibiotic can be based on consideration of a table such as Table 3-20, which lists antibiotics of first choice, as well as alternative drugs for a wide range of microbial species likely to be encountered in oral infections. Table 3-21 provides a list of antibiotics grouped according to their general mode of action and as they are used in bacterial antibiotic sensitivity testing. These tables should be of use to the dentist in the selection of an antibiotic for treatment of an oral infection. In any case, *administration of an alternative antibiotic that is suggested by these tables or as a result of antibiotic sensitivity testing should not be commenced until the dentist is fully aware of the nature of the drug, its complications, and the means of detecting and treating such complications.* Extreme caution should always be used in prescribing antibiotics with frequent toxic side-effects (*e.g.,* chloramphenicol, streptomycin, and sulfonamides) but particularly in the case of children and patients with compromised renal and hepatic function.

Since antibiotics such as methicillin, cloxacillin, and carbenicillin have an important place in the management of life-threatening infections that may not be amenable to other treatment, unnecessary use of them for the treatment of localized oral infections is unjustified, particularly where the resistant bacterial strain of concern to the dentist is only part of the total flora cultivated from the oral lesion. Where a persistent oral infection is shown to contain a relatively pure culture of a bacterial species that is susceptible only to one of the more rarely used antibiotics, consultation with the patient's physician or (in the hospital) with a member of the hospital's Division of Infectious Disease is highly desirable.

All candidal species are resistant to antibacterial antibiotics and sensitive to the two commonly used antifungal antibiotics, nystatin and amphotericin B, as well as the newer antifungal agents (see Chapter 6); routine sensitivity testing of these isolates is not necessary.

Routine antimicrobial prophylaxis for the control of wound infections is not recommended for minor oral surgical or nasopharyngeal procedures because the wound infection rate is low (less than 2%), the extensive normal oropharyngeal flora notwithstanding. Radical head and neck procedures (*e.g.,* excision of oropharyngeal cancers, jaw resections, open reduction of jaw fractures) have a higher wound infection rate that is probably related to prolonged duration of surgery, previous radiation treatment, poor nutrition, age, and staphylococcal carrier state. In these cases, a cephalosporin or a penicillinase-resistant penicillin given 1 hour before surgery and continued for 24 hours or less postoperatively is recommended. Recommendations for administrations of antibiotics for prophylaxis against bacterial endocarditis in patients with organic or surgically induced cardiac valvular defects are given in Chapter 19.

Bacterial Cultures of Tooth Apices

Cultures made from the apical region of extracted teeth by any of various techniques must be interpreted with caution because of the technical difficulties involved in removing teeth without contamination with the oral flora.

From the standpoint of the bacteriologic technique, an external approach or a root amputation method of culturing is preferable. Because of the additional surgical procedures required in this culturing technique, it is seldom agreed to by the patient. This method is best applied to anterior teeth and single-rooted teeth, especially those in the maxilla.

The difficulty in obtaining bacteriologically significant cultures does not arise because of the inability to maintain an aseptic operating technique but because of the difficulty in rendering the operative field, particularly the gingival sulcus, sterile. The repeated application of the usual topical medicaments is

Table 3-20. Current Use of Antimicrobial Agents in the Therapy of Infections

Organisms	Drug of First Choice	Alternative Drugs†
*Streptococcus pyogenes**	Penicillin G or V	An erythromycin, a cephalosporin, vancomycin
*Streptococcus viridans**	Penicillin G with or without streptomycin	A cephalosporin, vancomycin
Streptococcus faecalis†	Penicillin G with an aminoglycoside	Vancomycin with an aminoglycoside
Anaerobic streptococci†	Penicillin G	A cephalosporin, clindamycin, chloramphenicol, erythromycin
*Streptococcus pneumoniae**	Penicillin G	A cephalosporin, erythromycin, chloramphenicol, clindamycin
*Staphylococcus aureus** Penicillin G-sensitive Penicillin G-resistant	Penicillin G	A cephalosporin, vancomycin, clindamycin Methicillin, cloxacillin or dicloxacillin, a cephalosporin, vancomycin, or erythromycin with rifampin
Neisseria† sp	Penicillin G	A sulfonamide, a tetracycline
Neisseria gonorrhoeae	Penicillin G	Ampicillin or amoxicillin, erythromycin, a tetracycline, spectinomycin
Bacillus†	Penicillin G	An erythromycin, a tetracycline
Clostridium	Penicillin G	A tetracycline, a cephalosporin, erythromycin, chloramphenicol, clindamycin
Corynebacterium†	Penicillin G with or without an aminoglycoside	Vancomycin, rifampin with or without penicillin G
Escherichia†	Ampicillin or gentamicin	A cephalosporin, a tetracycline, chloramphenicol
Aerobacter† (Enterobacter)	Cefamandole, gentamicin tobramycin	Carbenicillin, ticarcillin
Klebsiella†	A cephalosporin	Gentamicin, tobramycin, chloramphenicol
Proteus mirabilis	Ampicillin, gentamicin	A cephalosporin
Proteus sp	Gentamicin, tobramycin	Ticarcillin
Pseudomonas	Carbenicillin, ticarcillin with or without gentamycin or tobramycin	Gentamicin, tobramycin
Hemophilus†	Ampicillin, amoxicillin	Trimethoprim-sulfamethoxazole
Bacteroides†	Penicillin G	Chloramphenicol, clindamycin
Serratia	Gentamicin	Amikacin, cefoxitin

Table 3-20 (*continued*)

ORGANISMS	DRUG OF FIRST CHOICE	ALTERNATIVE DRUGS[†]
Fusobacteria[†]	Penicillin G	Chloramphenicol, clindamycin, a cephalosporin, erythromycin, a tetracycline
Actinomyces[†]	Penicillin G	A tetracycline, a cephalosporin, chloramphenicol
Nocardia	A sulfonamide with or without ampicillin	A sulfonamide with or without minocycline, a tetracycline, and trimethoprim-sulfamethoxazole
Treponema pallidum	Penicillin G	A tetracycline, erythromycin
Mycoplasma[†] sp	Erythromycin, a tetracycline	
Histoplasma capsulatum	Amphotericin B	
Candida[†]	Nystatin, amphotericin B, ketoconazole	
Blastomyces	Amphotericin B	

* Many of the organisms listed, especially those marked † are often present in oral specimens, but probably only rarely as pathogens requiring specific antibiotic treatment. Antibiotics listed under First Choice and as Alternative Drugs are those currently prescribed for the treatment of severe or life-threatening infections that are consistently associated with particular organisms. The less common antibiotics or antibiotic combinations listed here should not be used routinely for dental and oral infections, but only where there is evidence that a particular organism or group of organisms are etiologically related to an otherwise resistant infection, where the orofacial infection is severe or even life-threatening (*e.g.,* progressive cellulitis and infection of fascial spaces), and where adequate doses of the First Choice antibiotic have failed to control the infection (see text for more detailed discussion).

† Alternative drugs are indicated in patients hypersensitive to equally effective or more effective agents. In general, these alternative drugs are potentially more dangerous than equally active drugs and likely to be less effective in many cases.

(Adapted from Goodman L S, Gilman A (eds): The Pharmacological Basis of Therapeutics, 6th ed., p 1087–1093, 1980. Consult for further details.)

ineffective in sterilizing this area. Actual cauterization of the gingival crevice by heat immediately before the extraction is the most effective method of sterilizing the gingival sulcus.

Requests for elimination of dental foci of infection are far less common than some 10 to 20 years ago. Cultures of tooth apices are usually required only in those rare cases in which a clinician (allergist, ophthalmologist, or dermatologist, in most cases) seeks to prepare an endogenous bacterial vaccine for the treatment of a resistant problem thought to result from dental focal infection.

The old procedure of seeding the gingival sulcus with a culture of *Serratia marcescens* to check on contamination of the root apex by the oral flora during extraction is not acceptable because this organism is a potential pathogen.

Blood Cultures

Since transient bacteremia can be demonstrated in 70% to 90% of patients during dental extractions or periodontal surgery, bacterial endocarditis may occur as a complication of dental surgery in patients with rheumatic valvulitis, congenital heart disease, or cardiac surgery. Bacterial endocarditis also occurs as a complication of infectious processes and surgical manipulation elsewhere in the body.

Table 3-21. Antibiotic Groups

GENERIC GROUP FOR SUSCEPTIBILITY TESTS	ANTIBIOTIC GENERIC NAMES	SOME COMMON TRADE NAMES
Penicillin G (inactivated by penicillinase)	Penicillin G (aqueous, Na, K salts)	Bicillin, Wycillin
	Procaine penicillin G	Crysticillin
	Benzathine penicillin G (phenoxymethyl)	Bicillin, Permapen,
	Penicillin V	PenVee, V-Cillin, Penicillin VK
Penicillins not inactivated by penicillinase. All *Staphylococcus* susceptible, except a few resistant to methicillin	Methicillin	Staphcillin, Celbenin
	Oxacillin	Prostaphlin, Bactocill
	Cloxacillin	Tegopen, Cloxacillin
	Dicloxacillin	Dynapen, Veracillin, Pathocil
	Nafcillin	Unipen, Nafcil
(Broad-spectrum) penicillins* (also effective against some gram-negative bacteria)	*Hemophilus, Escherichia,* and *Proteus mirabilis*	
	Ampicillin	Amcill, Amcap, Omnipen, Polycillin, Principen, Totacillin
	Amoxicillin	Amoxil, Larotid, Polymox
	Hetacillin	Versapen
	Pseudomonas, Enterobacter and *Proteus* spp.	
	Carbenicillin	Geocillin, Geopen, Pyopen
	Ticarcillin	Ticar
Cephalosporins*	Cefamandole	Mandol
	Cefoxitin	Mefoxin
	Cephalexin	Keflex (oral)
	Cephaloglycin	Kafocin (urinary tract infections only)
	Cephalothin	Keflin
	Cephradine	Anspor, Velosef
(Third-generation cephalosporins)	Cefotaxime	Claforan
	Moxalactam	Moxam
	Cefoperazone	Cefobid
Other antistaphylococcal antibiotics		
Complex sugar--	Lincomycin[†]	Lincocin
Complex sugar--	Clindamycin[†]	Cleocin
Glycopeptide--	Vancomycin[†]	Vancocin
Complex sugar--	Novobiocin[†]	Albamycin
Aminoglycosides	Amikacin	Amikin
	Gentamicin	Garamycin, Gentamicin
	Kanamycin	Kantrex
	Neomycin	Mycifradin and Myciquent, Neobiotic, Neosporin (topical use only)
	Paromomycin	Humatin
	Streptomycin (Dihydrostreptomycin)	Seldom used alone; not used because of neurotoxicity
Tetracyclines	Tetracycline	Achromycin, Panmycin, Sumycin, Tetracyn, Tetrex

Table 3-21. *(continued)*

GENERIC GROUP FOR SUSCEPTIBILITY TESTS	ANTIBIOTIC GENERIC NAMES	SOME COMMON TRADE NAMES
Tetracyclines, cont.	Chlortetracycline	Aureomycin
	Oxytetracycline	Terramycin
	Demethyl chlortetracycline	Declomycin
	Methacycline	Rondomycin
	Doxycycline	Vibramycin
	Minocycline	Minocin
Chloramphenicol	Chloramphenicol	Chloromycetin
(Macrolides) Erythromycin group	Erythromycin	Erythrocin, Ilosone, Ilotycin, Pediamycin, E-Mycin, Bristamycin
	Triacetyloleandomycin	Tao
Polypeptides	Colistin (Polymyxin E)	Coly-Mycin
	Polymyxin B	Aerosporin
	Bacitracin	Bacitracin and Baciquent (topical use only)
Spectinomycin	Spectinomycin	Trobicin
Sulfonamides	Sulfisoxazole	Gantrisin
	Sulfamethoxazole	Gantanol
	Trimethoprim-sulfamethoxazole	Bactrim, Septra
	Sulfadiazine	Suladyne
	Sulfasalazine	Azulfidine (ulcerative colitis)
Antituberculosis preparations	Aminosalicylic acid	Pamisyl, Parasal, Teebacin
	Cycloserine	Seromycin
	Isoniazid (isonicotinic acid hydrazide, INH)	Hyzyd, Niconyl, Nydrazid
	Rifampin	Rifadin, Rimactane
Miscellaneous antibacterial agents	Nitrofurazone	Furacin (topical use only)
	Nitrofurantoin	Furadantin, Macrodantin (urinary tract use only)
	Furazolidone	Furoxone (intestinal tract only)
	Nalidixic acid	Neg-Gram
Antifungal agents	Amphotericin B	Fungizone
	Clotrimazole	Lotrimin, Mycelex
	Flucytosine	Ancobon
	Griseofulvin	Fulvicin, Grifulvin V, Grisactin, Gris-Peg
	Ketaconazole	Nizoral
	Nystatin	Mycostatin, Nilstat
Antiprotozoal preparations	Metronidazole	Flagyl
	Chloroquine	Aralen

* Cross-allergenic with penicillin
† No cross-allergenicity in penicillin-sensitive individuals

Unlike the transient bacteremia that accompanies dental surgery, the bacteremia seen in patients with bacterial endocarditis persists and may be detected by inoculating 5 to 10 ml of venous blood into appropriate culture media. Except for situations in which a blood culture is positive as a result of contamination of the specimen or surgical manipulation at the time the specimen was obtained, a positive blood culture is an indication of septicemia or bacterial endocarditis. Because bacteremia may not be continuously present, repeated testing over several days may be necessary before a positive culture is obtained. In patients suspected of having bacterial endocarditis, antibiotic therapy is contraindicated until a positive diagnosis based on blood culture is made, since serum levels of antibiotics will reduce the chance of obtaining a positive blood culture even when inhibitors are used in the medium.

An automated system for the detection of bacteria in normally sterile fluids has been developed and applied in the diagnosis of bacteremias. The instrument (BACTEC System)* detects isotopically labeled $^{14}CO_2$ released by the metabolism of bacteria utilizing ^{14}C-labeled substrates added to the blood sample. Both aerobic and anaerobic cultures are possible, and single-sample and multiple-sample models are available, as is an identification system for a limited range of bacterial species. Modifications of the technique in which other metabolites are measured by gas chromatography and used as an index of the growth of particular bacterial species have been introduced. This highly sensitive technique for detecting bacterial metabolism obviates the need for tedious subculture of bottles that appear visually to have no bacterial growth and reduces the risk of laboratory-introduced contamination of the specimen.

Anaerobic Cultures

The oral microbial flora normally contains a large number of anaerobic and microaerophilic species that undoubtedly play an important role in many orofacial infections, as well as infected human bites, traumatic wounds, and lung abscesses contaminated with saliva, dental plaque, and gingival aggregates. With standard methods of isolating bacteria from clinical specimens, the majority of anaerobic species are inhibited and overgrown by the aerobic species, and special methods for submitting and culturing oral specimens must be adhered to if these anaerobic species are to be isolated and identified. From a practical point of view, isolation and identification of anaerobic species is possible only when a limited number of different bacteria are present in the specimen, and the ratio of anaerobic to microaerophilic species is high, permitting slower growing anaerobic species to flourish. For this reason, anaerobic culture techniques are usually applied only to specimens of pus or other exudates aspirated from deep wounds and abscesses and where there is little likelihood of a persistent sinus or opening allowing continuous contamination of the site with surface bacteria.

In general, specimens for anaerobic culture should be obtained with a sterile syringe and needle, although surgical specimens obtained under aseptic conditions and free from surface contaminants are acceptable. Throat and saliva swabs, sputum, feces, and voided urine are *unacceptable,* as are extracted teeth, subgingival scrapings, cultures from tooth apices (except those obtained under the rigorous conditions described in the preceding section), swabs of pus draining into the oral cavity or onto the skin, and swabs of superficial wounds. The rate of success for isolation of anaerobic species in these circumstances is so low that specimens of this type submitted for anaerobic cultures are usually discarded by the laboratory.

Special anaerobic transport systems are needed for submitting specimens for anaerobic cultures consisting of an evacuated rubber-stoppered vial containing a gelled transport medium. To inoculate the vial, all remaining air is expelled from the syringe and needle in which the specimen has been obtained, the rubber stopper sterilized by rubbing with 70% ethanol or suitable disinfectant, and the specimen inoculated through the rubber stopper. The transport medium contains an oxidation–reduction (eH) indicator that should exhibit the color of the fully reduced state before inoculation. Fluid thioglycollate medium and other media containing an excess of reduced-sufhydryl groups to

* Johnston Laboratories, Cockeysville, MD 21030

lower the oxidation–reduction potential are also used as transport media, but are less satisfactory, particularly if the specimen is to be transported some distance before inoculation into a definitive medium. Portable anaerobic culture systems (*e.g.*, Gas Pak) are also available for direct inoculation of "reduced" blood agar plates or other solid medium at the chairside, after which the plates are sealed in an airtight container in which the oxygen content is quickly reduced by means of prepackaged reagents placed in the container. *Fusobacterium, Bacteroides melaninogenicus, Eubacterium*, and anaerobic cocci represent the anaerobic species most commonly isolated from abscesses around the mouth and orofacial area.

Anaerobic culture and isolation procedures require considerably longer than aerobic procedures because of the slower growth rate of anaerobic species. Antibiotic sensitivity testing similar to that carried out on aerobic species can be provided for anaerobic isolates as well. The special procedures required for isolation and propagation of anaerobic bacteria increase the cost of these procedures compared with the more standard aerobic procedures. A specimen for aerobic culture and a smear prepared from the specimen should always be submitted along with the specimen for anaerobic culture as a necessary check should no organisms be isolated on anaerobic or aerobic cultures.

Laboratory Tests for Syphilis

Syphilis is an infectious disease that can be a potential hazard for the dentist and his assistants and a source of persistent and permanent tissue damage for the patient because of its potential for progressive subclinical infection. The causative agent of syphilis (*Treponema pallidum*) cannot be readily isolated and grown in laboratory culture, and a diagnosis of syphilis rests very heavily on serologic procedures. Demonstration of *T. pallidum* in exudates from some suspected syphilitic lesions is possible, utilizing a fluorescent antibody technique (see next section—Dark-field and Fluorescent Microscopy in the Diagnosis of Syphilis), but the results of such procedures must also be confirmed by study of the patient's serum.

STS, TPI, and FTA-ABS

Serologic tests are indicated in the patient with lesions suggestive of primary or secondary syphilis to confirm the clinical diagnosis; and in the patient with a history of previously treated syphilis, for evidence of persistent and progressive infection. Since venereal disease control is a matter of community interest, serologic tests for syphilis are usually performed free of charge by public health laboratories. Screening tests for syphilis are also performed by private laboratories, although in all states the results of positive tests must be reported to the public health authorities. All screening tests for syphilis measure an antibodylike substance called *reagin*, which develops in serum following infection with *T. pallidum* and cross-reacts with certain extracts of heart muscle that are used as antigen in the test. Reagins are thought to be produced as a result of spirochetes combining with the patient's tissues and are probably antibodies to altered tissue components, rather than antibodies to the *Treponema*.

These screening tests for syphilis are referred to as the *serologic test for syphilis* (STS) or by specific names associated with the technique used (*e.g.*, Wassermann; Kolmer, complement fixation tests; Venereal Disease Research Laboratory test [VDRL]; Hinton; Kahn and Kline, flocculation tests; and RPR, rapid plasma reagin test, a microflocculation test performed on a card impregnated with reagents). Since reagin is not a specific antibody produced only by infection with *T. pallidum*, false-positive reactions are seen with some frequency. Referred to as *biologic false-positive reactions*, these findings may be significant in themselves since they may be found in association with other treponemal infections (yaws, relapsing fever), the collagen vascular diseases (*e.g.*, lupus erythematosus and rheumatoid arthritis), in sarcoid, infectious mononucleosis, lymphomas, and following smallpox and tetanus vaccinations.

False-positive reactions are distinguished from positive serologic tests caused by syphilis by means of the *Treponema immobilization test* (TPI). Laboratory strains of *T. pallidum* can be maintained alive and virulent for 5 to 10 days on artificial media, and serum containing antibody developed as a result of infection with this organism will specifically inhibit the motility of these laboratory cultures. The TPI is based on this procedure and is available in large venereal disease reference laboratories as a follow-up test for checking the specificity of positive tests detected by the usual screening STS. The test is expensive to maintain and is not available as a primary screening test.

In some laboratories the *fluorescent treponemal antibody absorption test* (FTA-ABS test) is also used. This is somewhat easier to perform in that slides coated with dead organisms of the laboratory strain of *T. pallidum* can be prepared beforehand and subsequently reacted with the patient's serum and an antiserum to human globulin coupled to a fluorescent dye. The slide is then examined in ultraviolet light; with sera containing specific antitreponemal antibody, the organisms fluoresce (see earlier section on Immunofluorescence Procedures for more detailed explanation of this technique). The FTA-ABS test is said to be less specific, but more specific than the TPI test, particularly in late syphilis. It is also less costly and hazardous to perform, since it utilizes heat-killed smears of *Treponema* rather than live, virulent, motile cultures.

Because of the frequency with which false-positive tests are associated with serious underlying disease and because of the possibility that a persistent positive serologic test may represent progressive syphilitic involvement of the heart, central nervous system, and other vital structures, it is recommended that all patients with positive screening STS detected during dental evaluation should be referred for further medical evaluation. More detailed investigation of these patients by, for example, the TPI or FTA-ABS tests, quantitative STS, or examination of the spinal fluid, and the decision whether treatment is necessary are ultimately the responsibility of the physician rather than the dentist. Since almost half of the patients who have latent syphilis may have a negative STS, tests for specific treponemal antibody (TPI or FTA-ABS) are also recommended in patients who have clinical signs strongly suggestive of syphilis, even if they have a negative STS.

The STS, TPI, and FTA-ABS are negative immediately after infection has occurred but may become positive while the primary lesion is still present. Up to 85% of patients will have a positive FTA-ABS (most sensitive test) during the primary stage. Reagin and specific antibodies to *T. pallidum* begin to appear 2 to 3 weeks after infection, and in secondary-stage syphilis all three tests are usually positive. In most cases adequate treatment of the disease results in disappearance of positive serologic tests. However, low titers may persist, and a decision as to whether these persistent positive reactions indicate a "serologically fast" state or progressive (latent) infection may be very difficult to make; such decisions should be referred to a dermatologist or public health clinic.

The newest treponemal test in general clinical use is the microhemagglutination assay for *T. pallidum* (MHA-TP). In this procedure, absorbed patient serum (as in the FTA-ABS test) is mixed with erythrocytes previously tagged with treponemal antigen. The presence of antibody to *T. pallidum* causes agglutination of the red cells. The test has been modified to use small volumes and is thus termed microhemagglutination.

The FTA-ABS was previously performed only in larger hospitals and in reference or state laboratories. The test is now more widely used because it is available in commercial kit form; however, adequate quality control may be a problem in those laboratories where the test is performed infrequently.

The technically simple MHA-TP is gaining popularity. Many laboratories confirm nontreponemal test results with the MHA-TP and obtain an FTA-ABS only if the MHA-TP results are questionable.

Dark-field and Fluorescent Microscopy in the Diagnosis of Syphilis

Since serologic tests are of little value early in the primary stage of syphilis, a positive diagnosis can be made only by demonstration of the *Treponema* in the lesions. Dark-field microscopy has long been the technique used for this purpose, motile spiral organisms being easily distinguished when they refract light in an otherwise dark microscope field. Unfortunately, the oral cavity generally contains other nonpathogenic, motile, spiral bacteria, and accurate identification of the type of organism seen becomes impossible when the specimen is derived from a lesion in or adjacent to the oral cavity.

With the availability of syphilitic antiserums specifically absorbed to remove cross-reactions with treponemas other than *T. pallidum*, it is possible to identify the presence of this organism in smears from the oral cavity by use of the fluorescent labeling technique. Where this test is available in reference laboratories, the smear prepared by scraping the lesion should be air dried and transported to the laboratory as soon as possible or stored frozen in an airtight package. Routine hematoxylin-and-eosin-stained sections prepared from biopsied tissue may also fail to provide a clear-cut diagnosis of a suspected syphilitic lesion unless special staining is used to detect the microorganism in the tissue section.

Tests for Beta-Hemolytic Streptococcal Infections

Isolation of beta-hemolytic streptococci from throat swabs is usually possible during the acute stage of streptococcal pharyngitis and tonsillitis. Since infection with this organism is often recognized only in retrospect as the patient develops symptoms of rheumatic fever or subacute glomerulonephritis as a sequel to the development of hypersensitivity to products of tissues damaged in the original infection, in many instances recourse has to be made to immunologic methods for diagnosing the infection.

Beta-hemolytic streptococci isolated from the pharynx or other locations are usually grouped initially by bacitracin sensitivity (group A organisms inoculated on a blood agar plate fail to grow around a paper disc impregnated with bacitracin) and then by Lancefield serologic precipitin reactions (utilizing the organism's group-specific carbohydrate). Typing of group A strains on the basis of the M protein (Griffith typing) may also be carried out. Rheumatic fever may occur as a complication of infection with any group A strain; subacute glomerulonephritis usually results from infection with specific strains: types 12 (most frequent), 4, 18, 25, and Red Lake.

Serum Antistreptolysin O

The most commonly used serologic test is measurement of *serum antistreptolysin O titer (ASO)*, a specific antibody formed in response to antigenic stimulation by a soluble hemolysin produced by the beta-hemolytic streptococcus.

The ASO titer is usually raised in patients with acute rheumatic fever, levels greater than 200 Todd units generally being accepted as indicative of recent beta-hemolytic streptococcal infection. The level of the ASO titer is not correlated with the presence or absence or cardiac damage in rheumatic fever.

The ASO titer is positive in 90% to 95% of patients with acute rheumatic fever in the third week after infection with beta-hemolytic streptococci, the titer gradually falling thereafter, so that at the end of 2 months only 70% to 75% are positive; at 6 months, 35% and at 12 months, 20%.

Serologic Tests for Chronic Candidal Infections

Investigators have shown that whereas the majority of individuals have low serum and salivary titers of antibody to *Candida albicans*, the titer of antibody capable of reacting with this organism and binding a fluorescent labeled antihuman globulin increases in both saliva and serum with chronic candidal infection of the oral cavity (see earlier section on Immunofluorescence Procedures for more detailed explanation of this technique). The procedure is indicated in patients suspected of having chronic atrophic candidiasis (denture sore mouth, angular cheilitis) and candidal leukoplakia, in both of which demonstration of fungi and yeasts by microscopy may be less satisfactory than in acute candidal infection (thrush, antibiotic sore mouth). For the procedure, approximately 50 ml of whole saliva collected while the patient chews paraffin or gum and 10 ml of clotted blood are needed.

Because salivary antibody is present in low concentration, titers in saliva are expressed in terms of a concentration rather than a dilution. Patients with candidiasis usually have serum titers from 1:32 to 1:512, and whole neat saliva (1×) gives a positive reaction without concentration. Carriers of *Candida* have titers below 1:16 in serum and 16× or more concentrated saliva gives a positive reaction. Patients who do not have yeasts in their saliva may have serum levels as high as 1:8, but a positive reaction in saliva is seen only with saliva concentrated 64× or more. Although some overlap of titers is seen between the group with candidiasis and the carrier group, the procedure is of definite value in separating patients with chronic oral candidiasis from carriers.

Some controversy exists concerning the significance of serum agglutinin titers to *Candida*. Extremely high titers (1:10,000 or >) are often found in patients with systemic candidiasis and the endocrine candidiasis syndrome, but the level of serum agglutinins among patients with mucous membrane candidiasis and apparently uninfected individuals has usually been considered too variable to be of any diagnostic significance. Careful investigation of the mouths and serum of individuals with and without full dentures has indicated that the levels are not entirely random and that a considerable number of the raised serum agglutinin titers to *Candida* may be due to denture stomatitis associated with chronic candidiasis (see Chap. 6). In general, higher serum agglutinin titers occur among oral carriers of *Candida* than among those whose oral cavity is free of *Candida,* and patients with the "generalized simple" and "granular" varieties of palatal stomatitis have higher titers than those with "localized simple" palatal stomatitis or no stomatitis. Otherwise, severity of the palatal inflammation does not correlate with the serum titer, except that the highest titers are seen in patients with angular cheilitis and rhomboid glossitis in association with palatal denture stomatitis. It is recommended that patients with high titers whose oral candidiasis shows poor response or frequent relapse with topical antifungal therapy be considered as possibly having systemic candidiasis. Unfortunately, some infected individuals also are found with zero or very low titers, and the presence or absence of a serum agglutinin titer alone cannot be used to make a diagnosis of oral candidiasis. Live suspensions of *Candida* are preferred to formalin-inactivated suspensions for these *in vitro* agglutinin tests, since some sera react only with the former.

Virus Isolation and Serology

A variety of viral agents are involved either directly or indirectly as causative agents of oral disease (Table 3-22). As with other infectious diseases, clear diagnosis of a virus infection is possible only where the infectious agent is demonstrated or a rise in specific antibody to the virus is detected following the infection. With the exception of the Tzanck smear used in the diagnosis of herpes simplex and varicella infections (see earlier section), all laboratory procedures for viral diagnosis require special facilities that are usually provided only by regional laboratories and in the past often established by state health departments concerned with the epidemiology of viral infections, but more and more also by private laboratories providing a comprehensive diagnostic service.

Consideration of Table 3-22 indicates that viral diagnostic studies can be useful in patients with the following lesions: acute pharyngitis and tonsillitis; acute stomatitis (ulcerative stomatitis, gingivostomatitis, vesicular stomatitis, and oral exanthems); vesicular and ulcerative lesions of the lip and perioral tissues; acute parotitis; erythema multiforme, and Stevens–Johnson syndrome following an upper respiratory or gastrointestinal infection. A virus infection should also be suspected if any of the following signs and symptoms are noted: a relative lymphocytosis with absence of significant leukocytosis; atypical lymphocytes; malaise and muscle pain; acute gastrointestinal disturbance; rash or vesicular skin lesions; lymphadenopathy out of proportion to the extent of the oral lesions and not restricted to nodes draining the lesion.

Some common acute lesions of the mouth and throat are of multiple etiology. In many cases the emergency treatment of these lesions is the same irrespective of the etiology, but a clear definition of the etiology is necessary if understanding and treatment of these problems are to advance. In some situations a clear definition of the etiology may also be necessary to prevent recurrences and serious complications. Fusospirochetal gingivitis (Vincent's gingivitis) and acute sore throat are both acute lesions of multiple etiology. A diagnosis of Vincent's gingivitis does not exclude the possibility of a recent

Table 3-22. Viral Agents Associated with Oral Disease

AGENT	CHARACTERISTIC ORAL FINDINGS
Herpes simplex	1. Acute ulcerative gingivostomatitis and/or pharyngitis 2. Recurrent herpes labialis
EB virus[†]	Oral lesions of infectious mononucleosis: tonsillitis and pharyngitis, palatal exanthem or petechiae, submandibular and cervical lymphadenopathy.
Coxsackie A* (Types 2, 3, 4, 6, 8, 9, 10)	Herpangina
Coxsackie A* (Type 10)	Lymphonodular pharyngitis
Coxsackie A* (Types 5, 16)	"Hand, foot, and mouth disease" (Toronto epidemic)
Coxsackie B* (Types 3, 5)	Oral ulcers, frequently associated with epidemic pleurodynia
Rubella	Oral ulcers, palatal exanthem
Mumps	Acute parotitis
Adenovirus (Types 1, 2, 3, 5, 6, 14)	Acute febrile pharyngitis and pharyngoconjunctival fever
ECHO* (Type 16)	Herpangina (Boston exanthem)
ECHO* (Type 9)	Oral ulcers and rubelliform lesions
Influenza Parainfluenza Respiratory syncytial Adenovirus Reovirus* ECHO*	1. Oral ulceration and erythema multiforme in convalescent period 2. Acute ulcerative gingivitis in convalescent period
Vaccinia	Perioral ulcers in unvaccinated individuals from contact with recent vaccination site

* Virus isolation and serologic studies are available for all of these virus infections; however, for those marked (*) serologic tests can be done only if the viral agent is first isolated from the patient.

[†] Also associated (probably as a causative agent) with Burkitt's lymphoma and nasopharyngeal carcinoma.

viral infection that predisposed to overgrowth of the fusospirochetal complex of oral microorganisms. In fact, herpes simplex virus frequently can be isolated from patients with Vincent's gingivitis, and without facilities for virus isolation and serology, the differentiation of Vincent's gingivitis from primary herpes simplex gingivostomatitis may be impossible. An acute sore throat may be the result of a virus infection, an infection with beta-hemolytic streptococci (strep throat), allergy, infectious mononucleosis, or even diphtheria or Vincent's angina, and careful studies have shown that in many instances the appearance of the throat gives little clue to the etiology. In these and other lesions of multiple etiology, accurate diagnosis is possible only where routine bacterial and viral diagnostic procedures are used to supplement the findings of history, examination, and hematologic tests.

Routine viral diagnostic studies (virus isolation and serology) are presently unavailable for the majority of colds and upper respiratory infections (usually caused by rhinoviruses), acute gastrointestinal disturbances, or lesions caused by varicella virus (chickenpox, herpes zoster). Although the causative agent of infectious mononucleosis is now known to be the Epstein–Barr virus, routine diagnosis for this condition still rests on the heterophil antibody titration, supplemented in some cases by titration of specific antibody to the Epstein–Barr virus.

Recent Developments in Diagnostic Virology

The high cost of reagents and cell cultures used in virus isolation procedures, the fact that both virus isolation and serologic techniques can usually provide only a retrospective diagnosis that is mainly of epidemiologic value, and the limited applicability of automated or other rapid techniques to virus diagnosis have severely restricted the availability of virus diagnostic laboratory services in recent years and have caused them to become some of the most costly clinical laboratory procedures. At the same time, a number of antiviral chemotherapeutic agents have been licensed for clinical use for specific viral infections, emphasizing the need for rapid virus diagnostic procedures. At the moment, immunofluorescence and related procedures (e.g., RIA and ELISA—see below) for the detection of viral antigens in infected tissues offer the best hope in this regard, and a number of laboratories feature this approach, sometimes in combination with electron-microscopy. In the United States, however, general use of this technique of viral diagnosis has been hampered by lack of a wide range of commercially available specific antiviral antisera.

Where appropriate reagents and virologists experienced with the use of immunofluorescence techniques for virus diagnosis are available, influenza A and B, respiratory syncytial virus, parainfluenza, mumps, adenovirus, and measles can be found in respiratory secretions with equal or greater sensitivity with this approach than with traditional tissue culture procedures. The technique is also applicable to the rapid diagnosis of herpes simplex, cytomegalovirus, varicella, and rubella virus infections. Electron-microscopy has been most helpful in identifying cytomegalovirus in urine, herpes simplex virus in vesicular fluid, as well as multiple viral agents in feces.

Other methods for augmenting a reaction between viral antigen and specific antibody to make the reaction more easily measurable include counterimmunoelectrophoresis and the linking of the antibody to a larger particle (latex spheres or erythrocytes). The latter, referred to as *immune adherence hemagglutination*, forms the basis for rapid diagnosis in stool of a relatively new group of viral agents (rotaviruses) implicated in the etiology of childhood diarrhea. A number of solid-phase immunoassays in use for the rapid detection of viral antigens in clinical specimens use specific antiviral antibody that is attached covalently or electrostatically to a plastic surface, where it combines with viral antigen and abstracts it from the clinical specimen.

The viral antigen linked in this way is then detected by introduction of a second antiviral antibody that has been labeled in some way. In *radioimmunoassays (RIA)*, ^{125}I is used as the label, and antigen is measured in a gamma counter. In *enzyme-linked immunosorbent assays (ELISA)*, either peroxidase or alkaline phosphatase is used as the label, and antigen is measured spectrophotometrically after incubation with a color-producing substrate specific for the enzyme. The analogy between these sandwich techniques and those described under Immunofluorescence Procedures (see earlier section) is clear, and the limitation resulting from a limited range of specific antiviral antisera also exists.

RIA and ELISA are used for the detection of hepatitis A and B viruses in stool and for diagnosis of rotavirus; ELISA is used to detect herpes simplex in infected fluids as has been described. RIA and ELISA also have a wide range of applicability in the measurement of circulating hormones, in immunology, bacteriology, and in assays of other proteins or substances that attach to proteins. Because ELISA does not use radioactivity (c.f. RIA), the reagents are relatively stable, and tests may be carried out on a sporadic basis with relatively inexpensive equipment and without the hazards and disposal problems associated with use of radioactive isotopes. Results can be read within 24 hours, in time to be clinically useful.

Routine* Procedures for Specimens for the Virus Diagnostic Laboratory

Identification of viral agents associated with oral lesions will be most successful when the following group of specimens is obtained: a swab or preferably scrapings from the suspected lesion; a throat swab; a rectal swab or preferably a stool specimen; and two samples of venous blood, one drawn as soon as possible after the onset of illness (*acute* specimen) and the other drawn 1 to 2 months later (*convalescent* specimen). In some cases other spec-

* With the development of newer and often more rapid methods of virus diagnosis in recent years (see preceding section), modifications of these traditional tissue culture and serologic procedures described in this section should be expected, depending on those used by a particular laboratory.

imens may be especially valuable—*e.g.*, fluid removed from an intact vesicle (recurrent herpes labialis), a swab of freshly secreted saliva (mumps), or a throat gargle (influenza).

All material obtained directly from a lesion or by swabbing a mucosal surface should be mixed with a small volume (about 1.0 ml) of any sterile liquid bacteriologic or tissue culture medium (except soybean medium) and the swab discarded. Narrow-mouthed specimen jars containing tissue culture medium (such as lactalbumin and Hank's complete tissue culture medium) with penicillin and streptomycin added to control bacterial growth can often be obtained from virus diagnostic laboratories. After mixing, the cap of the jar should be tightly screwed on and the jar labeled with the usual identifying information, preferably with lead pencil on Zo adhesive tape, and the cap of the jar sealed with a piece of the same tape. Where possible, the specimen should be delivered immediately to the virus diagnostic laboratory. If this is not possible, the specimen should be packed in dry ice and maintained at this temperature (less than $-60°$ C) until it is delivered to the laboratory. Storage for a few hours unfrozen in a household refrigerator is preferable to allowing the specimen to freeze slowly by storing it in a household freezer.

Stool specimens are an important source of virus, especially in the latter stages of some infections, and the patient should be strongly encouraged to provide this specimen. For this purpose, a wide-mouthed jar with a few milliliters of medium should be provided, together with a tongue blade. The patient is instructed to collect stool on toilet paper after his next bowel movement and to transfer a portion to the jar. Once obtained, stool specimens should be labeled and stored as described above for specimens obtained from a lesion.

Ten milliliters of blood should be obtained for both the acute and convalescent specimens and stored in tubes with no anticoagulant or preservative. After labeling, the specimen should be allowed to clot and then stored at refrigerator temperature (unfrozen) until it is sent to the virus diagnostic laboratory. Blood specimens should never be frozen and may be mailed to the laboratory without significant loss of antibody titer.

Interpretation of Laboratory Diagnostic Studies for Virus Infections

Possible Interpretations. Whenever a virus is isolated from an individual with oral lesions, the following possible interpretations should be considered.

1. *The virus is the direct etiologic agent of the oral lesions.* When the lesions represent a primary infection (the patient's first experience with this virus), this relationship will usually be confirmed by a fourfold or greater increase in titer of specific serum antibody to the virus in the convalescent blood specimen as compared with the acute specimen. However, if the acute blood specimen is drawn more than 7 to 10 days after the onset of the illness, this increase may not be detected, and reliance may have to be placed on the presence of a high titer in the acute and convalescent specimens, which may wane 3 to 6 months later (see Fig. 3-27).

2. *The virus is the direct etiologic agent of a current or recent infection that has predisposed the patient to the development of oral lesions.* Virus may be found on some occasions in the throats, stools, or saliva of individuals with clinical and microbiologic evidence of necrotizing ulcerative gingivitis and stomatitis. These oral lesions and other less specific stomatitides may also occur in individuals convalescing from a virus infection. In each case, serologic confirmation of the relationship between the virus isolation and the clinical symptoms of the virus infections (and not the oral lesions) may be as described in interpretation (1).

In other cases of necrotizing ulcerative gingivitis and in cases of erythema multiforme, Stevens–Johnson syndrome, and generalized stomatitis, a relationship between recent virus infection and the development of the oral lesions can often be established. Virus isolation will usually be negative, but serologic studies with standard viral antigens (herpes simplex, influenza, parainfluenza, respiratory syncytial, adenovirus) may show a high titer to one virus, which wanes 3 to 6 months later.

3. *The virus is the direct etiologic agent of a current or recent infection that is unrelated to the development of the oral lesions.* This interpretation must always be borne in mind when the oral lesions observed do not correspond with

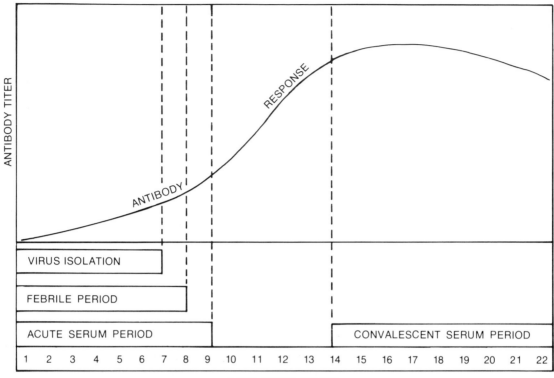

Fig. 3-27 Suggested times for collecting specimens for virus isolation and serology in relation to period of clinical illness. (Courtesy of Laboratory Procedures, Inc, Division of Smith, Kline & French Clinical Laboratories, Inc, 600 Park Ave, King of Prussia, PA 19406)

the lesions known to result from direct oral infection with the isolated virus. A decision between interpretations (2) and (3) in these situations can only be made when there is an accurate record of the illness and the oral lesions available.

In certain virus infections (herpes simplex, adenovirus, echovirus, and reovirus), virus may persist in the mouth, throat, or gastrointestinal tract of an infected individual without signs or symptoms of clinical disease (carrier state). The coexistence of the carrier state and oral lesions can lead to a false association of supposed infectious agent and oral lesions. Isolation of herpes simplex virus from the saliva of an individual with recurrent aphthous ulcers (canker sores) is a not uncommon example of this phenomenon.

4. *The virus was introduced as a contaminant during the handling or processing of the specimen.* Unidentified myxoviruses and reoviruses are common contaminants of tissue cultures and laboratory animals used for the isolation of human viruses.

Herpes Simplex Virus Infections

The virus most frequently isolated from oral lesions is herpes simplex virus type I. Where the clinical findings are those of an acute ulcerative gingivostomatitis and pharyngitis, the results of virus isolation and serologic studies in the majority of cases will be as described in interpretation (1) above. Virus is usually found in gingivae, saliva, and throat swabs and less frequently in the stool: a complement-fixing serum antibody titer (CF) of less than 1:8 is usually found in the acute serum and a titer of 1:16 to 1:64 in the convalescent serum. Where virus isolation and serologic studies provide no evidence of virus infection accompanying the clinical state, the possibility remains that some other viral agent undetectable by current techniques is involved or that the lesions are nonviral.

Herpes simplex virus is rapidly inactivated under a variety of conditions, and the details of the procedure used to obtain and handle the specimen for virus isolation should always be checked where negative results are obtained. The titer of antibody to herpes virus in the acute and convalescent serums will often be a useful guide in these circumstances.

The vesicles of recurrent herpes labialis (cold sores) contain herpes simplex virus, but the amount present is less than that in the saliva of an individual during the acute stage of a primary infection, and infectious virus usually remains for only 24 to 48 hours after the appearance of the lesions. Virus can rarely be obtained from a ruptured vesicle or from the saliva, throat, or stools of an individual with recurrent herpes labialis. This recurrent form of herpes simplex infection always occurs in individuals with a significant titer of herpes antibody (CF titer > 1.8), and there is no increase of titer during an episode.

Type II, the genital strain of herpes simplex virus, is rarely isolated from oral lesions, and typing of oral isolates is necessary only where there is a suggestion that a primary oral lesion may have been acquired by orogenital contact. Serum titers to herpes simplex are routinely measured against a standard type I strain (usually the HF strain or a recently isolated strain), and anti-type II titers are not usually available as routine clinical laboratory studies.

Coxsackievirus Infections

Because of the multiplicity of types of coxsackieviruses, serologic studies are not usually carried out until a virus has been isolated from the patient. Both coxsackie A and B viruses are excreted in the feces and can be readily isolated from that source. Isolation of coxsackie A from the oral cavity, however, is not always possible even when the patient has oral ulcerations concomitantly with other evidences of coxsackie A infection. Some workers have reported that inoculation of the salivary sediment obtained by centrifuging saliva is more likely to give positive isolation of the virus, suggesting that the coxsackie A virus is closely associated with the desquamating oral mucosal cells and is not free in the saliva.

Serologic Tests for Infectious Mononucleosis and Other Epstein–Barr Virus Infections

Patients with infectious mononucleosis develop an increased serum titer of an antibody that cross-reacts with red blood cells from other species (heterophil or Forssman antibody). Whenever a patient is suspected of having infectious mononucleosis because of symptoms, examination findings, or hematologic abnormalities, the titer of heterophil antibody is used to confirm the diagnosis. The traditional test for heterophil antibody is based on agglutination of sheep red cells and is known as the Paul-Bunnell test. The (Davidsohn) differential test is a modification of the Paul-Bunnell test, in which the serum titer of sheep agglutinins is measured before and after absorption of the patient's serum with beef or guinea pig red cells to make the test more specific for detecting infectious mononucleosis. More recently it has been shown that horse red cells that have been treated with formalin will also react with antibody in the serum of patients with infectious mononucleosis and that the reaction is more specific than the reaction with sheep red cells. Rapid qualitative slide agglutination tests (e.g., Mono-Test*) based on this new reagent are therefore now used as screening tests for this infection.

The qualitative slide agglutination test is claimed to be more sensitive than the Paul–Bunnell and differential tests in that it often gives a positive result earlier in the disease. The type of test for heterophil antibody is therefore always specified when reporting the results of these procedures. Positive tests for heterophil antibody may also be seen in patients with serum sickness, acute viral hepatitis, multiple myeloma, and malignant lymphomas. Ten milliliters of clotted blood are required for both the rapid slide agglutination and the Paul–Bunnell and differential tests.

In recent years, the causative agent of infectious mononucleosis has been identified as the Epstein–Barr virus (EBV), a herpes-type virus with a predilection for cells of the lymphoid series. This virus can be maintained in

* Wampole Laboratories, 35 Commerce Road, Stamford, CN 06902

the laboratory only in continuous cultures of lymphocytes that are transformed to lymphoblasts by the virus. Isolation procedures for this virus are, therefore, presently limited to a small number of laboratories with the capability for such studies, but the availability of laboratory cultures of the virus has allowed the development of serologic tests for virus-related antigens. Such tests provide far more specific information on the etiology of suspected cases of infectious mononucleosis than does the heterophil titration.

As a result of these developments, it has been shown that in about 10% of adults, more frequently in children and almost uniformly in children undergoing primary EBV infections, heterophil antibodies do not develop. Since infectious mononucleosislike illnesses, unaccompanied by heterophil antibody responses, can also be caused by cytomegalovirus, adenovirus, *Toxoplasma*, and probably other, as yet unknown agents, the value of EBV-specific serologic tests is readily apparent.

The availability of these new diagnostic procedures has also resulted in the demonstration that EBV is associated (probably as the etiologic agent) with both Burkitt's lymphoma and nasopharyngeal carcinoma. Both epidemiologic data and evidence obtained from the transforming ability of EBV on lymphocyte cultures strongly implicate EBV as an oncogenic agent. Serologic surveys for virus-specific antibodies also have confirmed the existence of widespread infection with this virus in many communities.

Hepatitis B$_s$ Antigen and Other Tests for Hepatitis B Infection

Hepatitis B surface antigen (HB$_s$Ag*) refers to a particulate substance consisting of 20-nm diameter spheres and tubules that occur in the serum of individuals infected with hepatitis B virus. Hepatitis B virus itself is also present in the serum of infected individuals as a larger, 42-nm diameter, coated particle

---

* Also referred to in the older literature as HAA (hepatitis-associated antigen) or Australian antigen (because of its original discovery in the serum of an Australian aboriginal in a study of immunologic responses to multiple transfusions).

(the Dane particle) containing an inner core with virus specific DNA polymerase activity and a coating of HB$_s$Ag (see Fig. 3-28A). The Dane particle is infectious; purified HB$_s$Ag (see Fig. 3-28B), however, is not infectious. Because excess HB$_s$Ag is produced and discharged into the bloodstream and is readily detected in serum by routine laboratory diagnostic procedures, the presence of HB$_s$Ag is used as a marker of *current* hepatitis B virus infection in both patients and blood products used for transfusions. The antigens present in the core of the Dane particle and the surface antigens both produce specific antibody in the infected individual, and these antibodies (anti-HB$_c$ & anti-HB$_s$) are used as markers of prior infection.

Various techniques have been used for detecting and measuring the level of HB$_s$Ag in serum and other blood products; of these, radioimmunoassay is more sensitive than immunodiffusion, immunoelectrophoresis, and complement-fixation methods. HB$_s$Ag can be detected in serum as early as 30 to 40 days after exposure to the virus and 2 to 4 weeks before a rise in SGOT or SGPT, the earliest laboratory evidence of liver damage in hepatitis. HB$_s$Ag usually disappears from the bloodstream within 1 to 6 weeks after the infection becomes apparent. However, infected individuals can also carry the surface antigens and remain asymptomatic (though infectious) during the incubation period and after clinical infection for 1 month to 25 years. HB$_s$Ag has also been detected in the saliva and genital secretions of infected individuals, and there is no doubt that the virus can be transmitted by the oral and genital routes as well as parenterally.

The carrier state is not uncommon and some concern has been raised that dentists (and other health professionals with a high risk of exposure) may sometimes acquire the infection through contact with infected patients and even become chronic carriers. In the absence of detectable HB$_s$Ag in the serum of a patient suspected of having active serum hepatitis, the patient is considered to be noninfectious. Similar criteria are applied in the evaluation of blood and blood products destined for transfusion, and FDA regulations now require that HB$_s$Ag titers be run on all banked blood products. The titer of serum

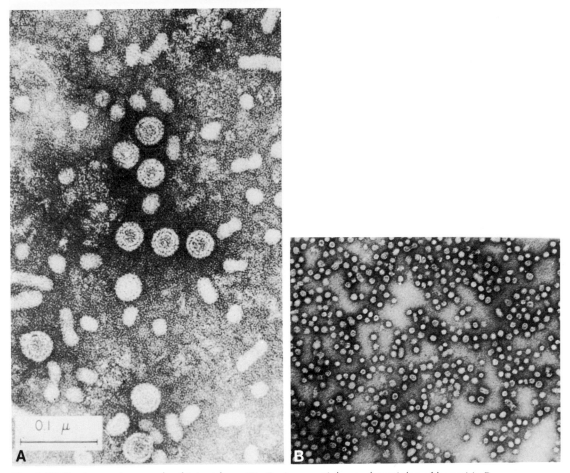

Fig. 3-28 Electron micrograph of intact hepatitis B virus particles and particles of hepatitis B surface antigen (HB$_s$Ag). *A,* Viral particles (Dane particles) and HB$_s$Ag particles (both spheres and rods are seen) present in plasma of a human hepatitis B carrier. *B,* Purified (noninfectious) particles of HB$_s$Ag in a sample of hepatitis B vaccine (MSD Heptavax B). (Courtesy of Merck, Sharp & Dohme, Division of Merck & Co, Inc, West Point, PA, 19486)

antibody to HB$_s$Ag (anti-HB$_s$Ag) is sometimes used as an index of immunity to hepatitis B virus and evidence of recovery from the infection. However, since both HB$_s$Ag and anti-HB$_s$Ag can occur simultaneously in the one serum sample, there is controversy as to whether a titer of anti-HB$_s$Ag can be used as evidence that a previously infected individual is no longer infectious.

There is still no one test that allows the contagious patient in whom virus replication and secretion are actively proceeding to be clearly distinguished from one who is convalescing from hepatitis B or from the chronic carrier of HB$_s$Ag. All may be HB$_s$Ag-positive,

but all are not necessarily contagious. One of the antigenic specifications of HB$_s$Ag that has been separated by precipitation reactions following immunodiffusion, the *e-antigen,* also appears to have prognostic value as to the chronicity of the infection. HB$_s$Ag-positive individuals who are e-antigen-negative are less likely to be contagious than those who are e-antigen-positive.

While individual responses to the virus may vary on occasion, the general pattern of development and waning of serum titers of HB$_s$Ag, anti-HB$_c$ and anti-HB$_s$, and serum transaminases in relation to the clinical illness in acute hepatitis B infection is illustrated in

Figure 3-29. Where the chronic carrier state develops (persistent hepatitis B infection or chronic active hepatitis B), HB$_s$Ag titers are maintained usually with detectable levels of anti-HB$_c$ and rarely anti-HB$_s$. Because hepatitis B vaccine* is free of infectious virus and contains only purified HB$_s$Ag, actively immunized individuals have titers of anti-HB$_s$ but neither anti-HB$_c$ (which is produced only in response to infectious virus) nor HB$_s$Ag. The amount of HB$_s$Ag in each dose of vaccine is inadequate to produce a detectable serum titer of HB$_s$Ag even immediately following a dose of vaccine.

Prepackaged reagents for carrying out HB$_s$Ag (AUSTRIA-II),† anti-HB$_s$ (AUSAB)† and anti-HB$_c$ (CORAB)† titrations by means of radioimmunoassay are customarily used. In most states, hepatitis B infection is a reportable disease, and positive tests for HB$_s$Ag must be reported by the laboratory to the local public health authority.

Antibody to hepatitis A virus (anti-HAV) can also be detected by means of radioimmunoassay. A positive test for anti-HAV can result either from recent infection with this virus or from infection sometime in the past. (Chronic infection with this virus has not been identified.) Measurement of acute phase antibody (I$_g$M) to HAV can also be carried out and indicates recent infection (within the last 3 to 4 months), if the test is positive.

Virus isolation procedures for both HAV and hepatitis non-A, non-B infections are not available. A diagnosis of hepatitis non-A, non-B is made in the recently transfused patient on the basis of appropriate clinical signs and symptoms, elevated bilirubin and SGPT (ALT) levels, and negative tests for HB$_s$Ag, anti-HB$_s$, anti-HB$_c$, and anti-HAV.

Laboratory Procedures in Suspected Collagen Autoimmune Diseases

The group of diseases that includes systemic lupus erythematosus (SLE), scleroderma, dermatomyositis, thyroiditis, rheumatoid arthritis, and Sjögren's syndrome as well as immune hemolytic anemias and neutropen-

* Heptavax-B, Merck, Sharp, & Dohme, Division of Merck & Co, Inc, West Point, PA 19486
† Lederle Laboratories, Pearl River, NY 10965

ias is characterized by unusual immunologic reactions (*e.g.,* autoantibody, hypergammaglobulinemia, and dysproteinemia). In addition to routine laboratory tests such as urinalysis and complete blood count, tests used in the diagnosis of these diseases include those for the presence of lupus erythematosus (LE) factor, antinuclear antibodies, rheumatoid factor, and other antibodies directed against various cellular components of the patient's tissues. These unusual antibodies result from the exposure of previously sequestered cellular components to the antibody-forming mechanism, with or without subtle alteration in antigenic structure.

LE Test. In this test, patient serum suspected of containing LE factor (an antinuclear antibody) is mixed with the patient's granulocytes obtained from the buffy coat of the blood. In the presence of the LE factor, the LE cell develops as a large phagocytic cell with the nucleus flattened to one side by an amorphous cytoplasmic inclusion derived from phagocytosed granulocyte nuclei. The test is positive in 75% to 80% of patients with systemic lupus erythematosus, but negative in patients with the discoid form of the disease.

The LE factor is only one of several different antinuclear and anticytoplasmic antibodies that develop in this disease and may be demonstrated in serum from the patient with lupus by a variety of complement fixation, immunofluorescent, hemagglutinating, and flocculation reactions. Because the LE factor is not specific for a diagnosis of lupus erythematosus and also occurs in some patients with other collagen diseases, it has been superseded as a routine clinical test by more direct measurement of antinuclear antibodies, which can also be tested for conveniently and accurately with indirect immunofluorescence techniques.

Antinuclear Antibody Test (ANA). Four types of antinuclear antibodies that produce characteristic patterns of immunofluorescence can be identified by this technique. Both the titer of the serum (or joint fluid) and the magnitude of fluorescence are taken into consideration in reporting positive results. Tests that are scored as only 1+ or 2+ (on a 1+

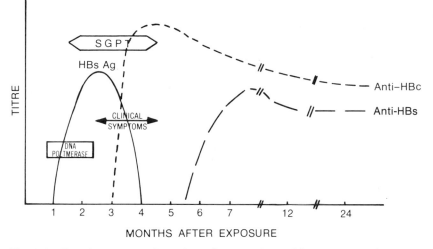

Fig. 3-29 Development and waning of serum titers of hepatitis B surface antigen (HB$_s$Ag), antibodies to hepatitis B core antigen (anti-HB$_c$) and surface antigen (anti-HB$_s$), and serum transaminases (SGPT) in relation to clinical illness in acute hepatitis B infection. (Hribar DLA: Aust Dent J 22:471, 1977)

to 4+ scale) on undiluted serum are usually not reported as positive. The four patterns of nuclear fluorescence detected by this technique are caused by differences in the distribution of antigens in the cell nucleus. These four patterns are characteristically described as follows:

- *Diffuse*–Homogenous distribution of specific fluorescence throughout the nucleus; produced by antinuclear protein antibody bound to nucleoprotein; especially characteristic of SLE but also seen in rheumatoid arthritis, Sjögren's syndrome and scleroderma
- *Shaggy*–Peripheral distribution of fluorescence; produced by anti-DNA antibody and usually seen only in SLE, especially with active nephritis
- *Speckled*–Discrete particulate staining of the nucleus; produced by an antibody against a nuclear glycoprotein; seen most commonly in rheumatoid arthritis, liver disease, ulcerative colitis, Sjögren's syndrome and scleroderma; nonspecific reactions of this type also occur in elderly normal individuals
- *Nucleolar*–A relatively rare pattern seen most often in scleroderma and Sjögren's syndrome

Anti-DNA Binding Activity. Anti-DNA antibodies to both double-stranded and single-stranded DNA are measured even more accurately by means of a radioactive assay technique. Anti-DNA binding activity, as measured by this technique (*i.e.,* > 25 units/ml) is usually found only in patients with SLE and active nephritis. Levels between 15 units/ml and 25 units/ml may occur in a number of diseases including rheumatoid arthritis, scleroderma, chronic active hepatitis, erythema multiforme, purpura, dermatomyositis, and carcinoma. Levels up to 15 units/ml are normal.

When ANA or anti-DNA antibody titers are high, the LE test is usually positive. With lower antinuclear antibody titers, the LE test may be negative, hence current preference for antinuclear antibody testing. If serologic tests for antinuclear antibodies are negative, a diagnosis of SLE can be ruled out.

Other serologic abnormalities in patients with autoimmune disorders include positive tests for rheumatoid factor, latex fixation, antitissue antibodies, and anti-RBC antibodies. A brief description of these tests follows.

Rheumatoid factor, an antibody reacting with gamma globulin, is detected by the ability of serum containing this factor to agglutinate particles coated with human gamma globulin. Different types of particles (*e.g.*, latex spheres and clays) have been used as the carrier of the gamma globulin, and the names of the procedures are derived from the carrier. *Latex fixation* at a 1:160 or greater is considered a positive test, and this is likely to be found in about 90% of sera from patients with rheumatoid arthritis, and in about 70% and 25% of sera from patients with Sjögren's syndrome and lupus erythematosus, respectively.

Patients with rheumatoid arthritis, Sjögren's syndrome, and lupus erythematosus often have raised complement and serum gammaglobulin levels (polyclonal hypergamma-globulinemia), marked by elevated total gammaglobulin, IgA, and IgM levels, as well as a variety of *antitissue antibodies* detectable in serum by immunofluorescence techniques. These antitissue antibodies are to some extent specific for the particular organ involved in the autoimmune disorder, and are therefore of considerable diagnostic importance; they include antithyroglobulin and antithyroid microsomal antibodies in Hashimoto's thyroiditis, antisalivary duct epithelium antibody in Sjögren's syndrome, antiparietal cell antibodies in pernicious anemia, antiskeletal muscle antibodies in dermatomyositis, antiglomerular basement membrane antibodies in lupus nephritis, and antimyelin antibodies in a number of demyelinating diseases. Antitissue antibodies may also result from diverse inflammatory disorders affecting specific organs with release of modified tissue antigens into the blood-stream and subsequent *autoantibody* production.

The immune hemolytic anemias often occur in association with the collagen diseases, but also as a result of lymphoproliferative diseases, virus infections, and Rh and other blood group incompatibilities. Characteristically, antibodies directed against surface antigens of the red cell can be demonstrated in the immune hemolytic anemias by use of the Coombs' (antiglobulin) test. The *direct Coombs' test* is carried out by mixing antihuman globulin with the patient's washed red cells, a positive test (agglutination) demonstrating the presense on the red cell surface of incomplete or blocking antibody (*i.e.*, monovalent antibody directed against and com-

bined with the surface antigens of the red cell, but incapable of agglutinating then without a "bridge" of antiglobulin). The *indirect Coombs' test* detects incomplete anti-red cell antibody that is free in the patient's serum, and capable of agglutinating isologous erythrocytes in the presence of antihuman globulin.

Antibodies directed against red cells may be either of the "warm" type resulting in red cell agglutination at usual incubation temperatures of 30°C to 37°C, or of the "cold" type with maximal reactivity at refrigerator (4°C to 20°C) temperatures. Antibodies of this latter type, referred to as *cold agglutinins,* may occur in patients with collagen diseases, as well as following some virus infections (infectious mononucleosis, influenza) and primary atypical pneumonias due to *Mycoplasma pneumoniae* and in patients with lymphomas and cirrhosis. Titers below 1:64 are found frequently in normal individuals and are believed to be due to past infection with organisms having antigenic determinants similar to those of the red blood cell. Intravascular agglutination of red cells does not usually manifest itself in patients with cold agglutinins, even when they are exposed to wintry conditions. However, in one disease (paroxysmal cold hemoglobinuria) that may complicate tertiary syphilis and in which a special type of complement-fixing, autohemagglutinating serum antibody of the cold variety occurs (DC antibody), episodes of pain and intense hemolysis with jaundice and hemoglobinuria may follow exposure of the patient to cold.

In Vitro Evaluation of Lymphocyte Function

Clinical laboratory evaluation of suspected *cellular* immune deficiency states currently includes the following:

1. Enumeration of lymphocyte subpopulations (T cells and B cells) using *immunofluorescence techniques* to identify immunoglobulin receptors on B cells and *rosetting techniques* (fractionation of circulating human lymphocytes by specific binding with sheep RBC) for T cells
2. Assessment of the ability of lymphocytes to proliferate, produce mediators, and exhibit cytotoxicity

3. Measurement of rates of phagocytosis, bacterial ingestion, and bacterial killing by sequential microscopic or bacteriologic study of mixtures of inert particles, bacteria, and leukocytes (polymorphonuclear leukocytes or macrophages) incubated *in vitro*

4. Use of nitroblue tetrazolium stain to identify leukocytes with decreased bacterial inactivating properties. (In normals, 10% of leukocytes give a positive test, reducing the soluble dye by means of peroxidase enzymes to an insoluble blue precipitate that identifies the active cells. In chronic granulomatous disease, few leukocytes will stain; the difference between normal and abnormal cell populations is also enhanced by the addition of endotoxin.)

For comprehensive clinical evaluation of cellular immune deficiency, these *in vitro* procedures are combined with a number of *in vivo* approaches such as measurement of delayed hypersensitivity to a battery of standard antigens (*Candida*, coccidioidin, *Staphylococcus*, purified protein derivative (PPD), streptokinase–streptodornase, and trichophyton); development of sensitivity to dinitrochlorobenzene (DNCB) or phytohemagglutinin (PHA); and measurement of chemotactic migration of polymorphonuclear leukocytes from abraded skin across a porous membrane attached to the patient's wrist by means of a Boyden chamber. These *in vivo* clinical procedures are not included within the purview of the diagnostic laboratory, and the interested reader should consult a textbook of clinical immunology for additional details.

Lymphocyte Transformation and Migration Inhibitory Factor: Of the various laboratory procedures available for study of the ability of lymphocytes to proliferate, produce mediators, and exhibit cytotoxicity, *lymphocyte transformation* and assay of *migration inhibitory factor* are the two most widely used *in vitro* correlates of cell-mediated immunity.

Lymphocyte transformation (i.e., stimulation and transformation of both B and T lymphocytes to lymphoblasts following exposure to mitogenic agents) is assayed by means of DNA or protein synthesis in the transforming cells. Mitogenic stimulants used include PHA

and concanavalin A (Con A), which primarily stimulate T cells; pokeweed mitogen, which stimulates both T and B cells; and lipopolysaccharide endotoxins (LPS), which stimulate B cells. Results are expressed as a comparison of radioactivity uptake in cultures derived from the patient versus "normally reacting" cultures exposed simultaneously to the mitogen. Statistical analysis of the data is necessary to normalize data resulting from differential growth rates in the tissue cultures of lymphocytes being studied.

Sensitized lymphocytes, when activated *in vitro* by a specific antigen, produce a soluble factor, *migration inhibitory factor* (MIF), which retards the migration of macrophages or monocytes from capillary tubes. The production of MIF for macrophages *in vitro* correlates with the *in vivo* state of cellular hypersensitivity in the donor of the lymphocytes for the test. Assay of MIF is based on either a direct technique in which sensitized human lymphocytes are mixed with guinea pig macrophages or human monocytes in a capillary tube and exposed to selected antigens or indirectly, in which sensitized lymphocytes and antigen are allowed to react separately for 1 to 2 days, and the cell-free supernatant from this culture is tested for its effect on macrophages or monocytes in capillary tubes. The direct technique is used as a screening procedure, a positive test being taken as an indication of normal function; the indirect test allows examination of the various components involved when a negative response is obtained.

Lymphocyte transformation has a wide range of application in assessing and monitoring immunodeficiency states and the results of various therapies applied to correct them. It is also a very useful diagnostic tool for determining host components that do not elicit strong humoral responses and hence cannot be detected by more conventional serologic techniques. As far as oral disease is specifically concerned, lymphocyte transformation has been used to detect autoimmune responses in severe aphthous ulceration and Behçet's syndrome and together with leukocytoxic reactions, in the investigation of the role of *Actinobacillus actinomycetemcomitans* (strain Y4) in periodontal disease.

Assay of MIF is also used for the general

evaluation of lymphocyte function and for the detection of sensitized lymphocyte populations responding to various tissue antigens and drugs and hence presumably of etiologic significance in autoimmune and allergic inflammatory conditions. Skin testing to various antigens always carries the hazard of untoward reactions and the possibility of sensitizing the patient to a new substance. *In vitro* tests, such as assay of MIF in response to the selected antigens, are free of these problems and correlate well with the *in vivo* state of cellular hypersensitivity of the lymphocyte donor.

Radioallergosorbent Test for Antigen-Specific IgE

Allergic reactions of the immediate type (*e.g.*, asthma, eczema, allergic dermatitis, and anaphylactic shock) are mediated by reactions between circulating IgE (produced by previously sensitized lymphocytes) and specific allergen, with resulting basophil degranulation and release of vasoactive substances of the histamine class. Traditionally, susceptibility to these abnormal responses is measured by immediate skin test reactions of the "wheal and flare type," induced by intradermal injection or pricking of the substance into the skin. A number of clinical diagnostic laboratory approaches to this problem are now available including measurement of total serum IgE levels by solid-phase radioimmunoassay (RIST*) or other immunologic procedures and measurement of antigen-specific IgE by another solid-phase radioimmunoassay referred to as the radioallergosorbent test or RAST.* In the latter, allergen-coated particles are incubated in the patient's serum, allowing binding of all classes of specific immunoglobulin to the particles. These coated particles are then reacted with a radiolabeled anti-IgE antibody, and the amount of radioactivity uptake is measured. Good correlation exists between the results of skin testing and RAST for a number of allergens, and though relatively more expensive, RAST provides an opportunity for detection of allergic reactivity for patients who cannot be taken off antihistamines or other medications that interfere with the skin reaction, in patients for whom

skin testing is contraindicated because of dermatologic disease or the likelihood of extreme responses such as anaphylactic shock, and possibly for substances such as food allergens and directly vasoactive amine releasers, such as aspirin and iodinated contrast media, which do not give positive skin tests.

It should be noted that for the two major groups of potential sensitizing agents commonly encountered in dentistry, local anesthetic drugs and eugenol, methyl methacrylate, and various plastics and metals used in dental restorations and prostheses, laboratory evaluation currently provides little assistance in the identification of the allergic patient.

For local anesthetic drugs and many other drugs such as penicillin, there is poor correlation between either laboratory measures of cellular immunity or skin test reactivity and the likelihood of untoward clinical response. Evaluation of allergic responsiveness in these cases still depends on clinical challenge carried out with gradually increasing doses of the suspected offending agent under circumstances where an untoward reaction can be quickly and safely controlled.

In the case of methyl methacrylate, dental medicaments, and restorative and prosthetic materials, reactions of the allergic contact dermatitis type are usually involved, rather than local swelling or systemic responses of the anaphylactic type. Diagnosis of such reactivity is still carried out clinically by means of patch tests.

The reader interested in more details of these clinical diagnostic procedures is referred to textbooks of clinical immunology and dermatology, and in the case of patch testing, to publications of the North American Contact Dermatitis Group.

BIBLIOGRAPHY

Bennington JL: Cost control of laboratory testing. In The Laboratory in Clinical Medicine, Interpretation and Application, 2nd ed. Philadelphia, WB Saunders, 1981

Benson ES, Rubin M (eds): Logic and Economics of Clinical Laboratory Use. New York, Elsevier/North Holland Biomedical Press, 1978

Beutner EH et al: Immunopathology of the Skin, 2nd ed. New York, John Wiley, 1979

Bryant NJ: Laboratory Immunology and Serology. Philadelphia, WB Saunders, 1979

---

* Pharmacia, Piscataway, NJ

Castleman B (ed): Case records of the Massachusetts General Hospital weekly clinicopathological exercises. Normal laboratory values. N Eng J Med 283:1276, 1970

Court Brown WM: Human Population Cytogenics. New York, John Wiley & Sons, 1967

Fitzpatrick TB et al (eds): Dermatology in General Medicine, 2nd ed. New York, McGraw-Hill, 1979

Frankel S, Reitman S, Sonnenwirth AC: Gradwohl's Clinical Laboratory Methods and Diagnosis. St. Louis, CV Mosby, 1970

Fudenberg HH (eds): Basic and Clinic Immunology, 3rd ed. Los Altos, CA, Lange Medical Publication, 1980

Gell PGH, Coombs RRA, Lachmann PT: Clinical Aspects of Immunology, 3rd ed. Oxford, Blackwell Scientific Publications, 1975

Grossman LI: Endodontic Practice, 8th ed. Philadelphia, Lea & Febiger, 1974

Haeckel RJ: Future perspectives of automation in clinical chemistry. J Clin Chem Clin Biochem 18:455, 1980

Halstead JA, Halstead CH: The Laboratory in Clinical Medicine, Interpretation and Application, 2nd ed. Philadelphia, WB Saunders, 1981

Henry JB: Todd-Sanford-Davidsohn Clinical Diagnosis and Management by Laboratory Methods, 16th ed. Philadelphia, WB Saunders, 1979

Johnson RH: Clinical laboratory tests of interest to the dentist. In Mitchell DF (ed): Symposium on oral medicine. Dent Clin North Am. p 203, March 1968

Lennette EH, Schmidt NJ (eds): Diagnostic Procedures for Viral and Rickettsial Diseases, 3rd ed. New York, American Public Health Association, 1964

Miller SE, Weller JM: A Textbook of Clinical Pathology. Baltimore, Williams & Wilkins, 1971

Northan BE: Whether automation. Ann Clin Biochem 18:189, 1981

Pribor HC, Altschuler CH: The laboratory's role in cost containment. Lab Management 17:20, 1979

Quick AJ: Bleeding Problems in Clinical Medicine. Philadelphia, WB Saunders, 1970

Quick AJ: Hemorrhagic Disease and the Pathology of Hemostatis. Springfield, IL, Charles C Thomas, 1974

Raslavicus PA, Shen EM: Laboratory diagnosis by chemical methods. Dent Clin North Am 18:155, 1974

Reiner M et al (ed): Standard Methods of Clinical Chemistry, Vols 1-7. New York, Academic Press, 1953-1972

Rose NR, Friedman H (eds): Manual of Clinical Immunology. Washington, DC, American Society Microbiology, 1980

Sabes WR et al: Value of medical diagnostic screening tests for dental patients. J Am Dent Assoc 80:133, 1970

Sherlock S: Diseases of the Liver and Biliary System, 6th ed. St. Louis, CV Mosby, 1981. Oxford, Blackwell Scientific Publications, 1975

Sonis ST, Jandinski JJ (eds): Symposium on physical and laboratory diagnosis. Dent Clin North Am 18: January, 1974

Wintrobe MM et al: Clinical Hematology, 8th ed. Philadelphia, Lea & Febiger, 1981

Hematology

Barberi T et al: Spectrum of von Willebrand's disease: A study of 100 cases. Br J Haematol 35:101, 1977

Bartels PH, Wied GL: Automated image analysis in clinical pathology. Am J Clin Pathol 75:489, 1981

Brecher G et al: When to do differentials. How often should differential counts be repeated? Blood Cells 6:431, 1980

Bull B, Korpman RA: Characterization of the WBC differential count. Blood Cells 6:411, 1980

Challacombe SJ et al: Haematological features and differentiation of recurrent oral ulceration. Br J Oral Surg 15:37, 1977–78

Chanarin I: The Megaloblastic Anemias, 2nd ed. Oxford, Blackwell Scientific Publications, 1979

Diamond LK, Porters FS: The inadequacies of routine bleeding and clotting times. N Eng J Med 259:1025, 1958

Drenick E et al: Bypass enteropathy. Intestinal and systemic manifestations following small bowel bypass. JAMA 236:269, 1976

Griner PF, Oranbury PR: Predictive values of erythrocyte indices for tests of iron, folic acid and vitamin B_{12}. Am J Clin Pathol 70:748, 1978

Gulati GL: Hematrak Model 480 Automated Differential System: Clinical evaluation. J Clin Lab Auto 2:41, 1982

Hardison CS: The sedimentation rate. JAMA 204:257, 1968

Jacobs A: The non-haematological effects of iron deficiency. Clinical Science 53:105, 1977

Lee GR et al: Iron-deficiency anemia and the sideroblastic anemias. In Harrison's Textbook of Medicine, 9th ed. Chap 310. New York, McGraw-Hill, 1980

Leithold SL, Friedman IA: Laboratory aids in the recognition of bleeding disorders. Med Clin North Am 53:61, 1969

Lessin LS, Jensen WN: Sickle cell symposium. Arch Intern Med 133:529, 1974

Martel A: Coagulation investigations in patients bleeding after tooth extraction. Sven Tandlak Tidskr 64:795, 1971

Miller RE: Hematology: Automated white blood

cell differential counting by flow-analysis. Clin Lab Med 1:127, 1981

Nye SW et al: The partial thromboplastin time as a screening test for the detection of latent bleeders. Am J Med Sci 243:279, 1962

Pierre RV: Automation of blood film preparation and staining utilizing the Technicon Autoslide. Blood Cells 6:471, 1980

Ross DW, Bardwell A: Automated cytochemistry and the white cell differential in leukemia. Blood Cells 6:455, 1980

Wray D et al: Recurrent aphthae: Treatment with vitamin B_{12}, folic acid and iron. Br Med J 2:490, 1975

Blood, Urine and Saliva Chemistry

ADA Council on Dental Materials and Devices: Recommendations in mercury hygiene. J Am Dent Assoc 88:391, 1974

Asplund J et al: Long-term insulin treatment in two non-diabetic patients. JAMA 246:870, 1981

Avioli LW, Krane SM (eds): Metabolic Bone Disease. New York, Academic Press, 1979

Berris RF, Huttner WA, Le Rogers R: Routine postprandial blood glucose determinations in a general hospital. JAMA 198:135, 1966

Clements RS et al: Comparison of various methods for rapid glucose estimation. Diabetes Care 4:392, 1981

Editorial: Diagnosis of thyroid diseases. Can Med Assoc J 110:1001, 1974

Ellul DA: Glycosylated hemoglobin: A literature review. Am J Med Tech 46:657, 1980

Fairney A: The use of biochemical tests in the diagnosis of disorders of calcium metabolism. Ann Chem Biochem 17:161, 1980

Feldman JM, Kelley WN, Lebovitz HE: Inhibition of glucose oxidase paper tests by reducing metabolites. Diabetes 19:337, 1970

Florey C du V, Acheson RY: Blood pressure as it relates to physique, blood glucose and serum cholesterol. U.S.P.H.S. National Center for Health Statistics, Series II, No. 34, October 1969

Gabbay K et al: Glycosylated hemoglobins and long-term blood glucose control in diabetes mellitus. J Clin Endocrinol Metab 44:859, 1977

Gutman A: The past four decades of progress in the knowledge of gout, with an assessment of the present status. Arthritis Rheum 16:431, 1973

Jacobs MB, Ladd AC, Goldwater LJ: Absorption and excretion of mercury in man. VI. Significance of mercury in urine. Arch Environ Health 9:454, 1964

Jarrett RJ, Keen H, Hardwick C: "Instant" blood sugar measurement using Dextrostix and a reflectance meter. Diabetes 19:724, 1970

Jorgensen KD: A semi-quantitative test for mercury in air. Acta Odontol Scand 32:305, 1974

Jovanovic L, Peterson CM: The clinical utility of glycosylated hemoglobin. Am J Med 70:331, 1981

Karl MM: The serum alkaline phosphatase. JAMA 203:591, 1968

Kassirer JP: Clinical evaluation of kidney function. N Engl J Med 285:385, 499, 1971

Kassirer JP: Clinical assessment of the kidneys. Prog Clin Pathol 7:33, 1978

Levin WC: Multiple myeloma. Arch Intern Med 135:27, 1975

Levy RI (ed): Nutrition, Lipids and Coronary Heart Disease. New York, Raven Press, 1979

Lowman RM, Cheng CK: Diagnostic roentgenology—radioisotope studies. In Rankow RM, Polayes IM (eds): Diseases of the Salivary Glands, Chap 4, p 90. Philadelphia, WB Saunders, 1976

Lueg MC: Asymptomatic primary hyperparathyroidism. Hosp Prac p 29, July 1982

Mandel ID: Sialochemistry in diseases and clinical situations affecting the salivary glands. CRC Crit Rev Clin Lab Sci 12:321, 1980

Mandel ID, Baurmash H: Sialochemistry in Sjögren's syndrome. Oral Surg 41:182, 1976

Maugh TH: Diabetes Commission: Problem severe, therapy inadequate. Science 191:272, 1976

National Diabetes Data Group: Classification and diagnosis of diabetes mellitus and other categories of glucose intolerance. Diabetes 28:1039, 1979

Pribor HC, Bates HM: Clinical value of the BUN/creatinine ratio. Lab Management p 23, 1976

Reece RL: What you should know about automated chemical screening. Resident Staff Physician 15:128, 1969

Schneider PB: Laboratory examination of the thyroid. I. In vitro tests. II. In vivo tests. Postgrad Med 56:91, 101, 1974

Schneyer LH, Schneyer CA: Secretory Mechanisms of Salivary Glands. New York, Academic Press, 1967

Shannon IL et al: Modified Carlson-Crittenden device for the collection of parotid fluid. J Dent Res 41:778, 1962

Shapiro IM, Block P: Summary of International Conference on Mercury Hazards in Dental Practice. J Am Dent Assoc 104:489, 1982

Sialadenosis and sialadenitis. Pathophysiological and diagnostic aspects. Adv Otorhinolaryngol 26:1, 1981

Skyler J: Symposium on home blood glucose monitoring. Diabetes Care 3:57, 1980

Vanderberger J et al: Blood serum mercury test report. J Am Dent Assoc 94:1155, 1977

Whitehouse FW: The diagnosis of diabetes: How to determine which patients to treat. Med Clin North Am 62:627, 1978

Yam LT: Clinical significance of the human acid phosphatases. Am J Med 56:604, 1974

Young DS, Tracy RP: Instrumental development in clinical chemistry. Prog Clin Pathol 8:123, 1981

Histopathology and Cytology

Alling CC, Secord RT: A technique for oral exfoliative cytology. Oral Surg 17:668, 1964

Barr ML: Sex chromatin and phenotype in man. Science 130:679, 1959

Barr RN: Public Health: Cytogenetics laboratory services. North-West Dent 44:169, 1965

Blozis GG: Parotid cytology. IADR Preprinted Abstracts, 43:Abstract No. 367, p 129, 1965

Chang T, Coursin DB, Hauck M: Leukocyte chromosome study of 22 families with cleft lip and/or cleft palate members. Cleft Palate J 7:402, 1974

Chaudnry AP et al: Electron microscopy: Its application in diagnostic pathology. NY State J Med 80:1809, 1980

Chisholm DM et al: Lymphocytic sialadenitis in the major and minor glands: A correlation in postmortem subjects. J Clin Pathol 23:690, 1970

Cooke BED: Biopsy procedures. Oral Surg 11:750, 1958

Daniels TE et al: The oral component of Sjögren's syndrome. Oral Surg 39:875, 1975

Fejerskov O et al: The oral cavity and salivary glands. In Johannessen JV: Electron Microscopy in Human Medicine in Digestive System. Part I, New York, McGraw-Hill, 1980

Folsom TC et al: Oral exfoliative study. Review of the literature and report of a three-year study. Oral Surg 33:61, 1972

Gardner DG, Lim H: The oral and dental manifestations of trisomy D syndrome. Oral Surg 34:87, 1972

Golbus MS: The current scope of antenatal diagnosis. Hosp Pract 17:179, 1982

Goldsby JW, Staats OJ: Nuclear changes of intraoral exfoliated cells of six patients with sickle-cell disease. Oral Surg 16:1042, 1963

Gorlin RJ, et al: Effect of X-chromosome aneuploidy on jaw growth. J Dent Res 44:269, 1965

Greenspan JS et al: The histopathology of Sjögren's syndrome in labial salivary gland biopsies. Oral Surg 37:217, 1974

Hampar B: Possible implications of virus-induced chromosomal aberrations. J Dent Res 45:561, 1966

Hayes RL et al: Oral cytology: its value and its limitations. J Am Dent Assoc 79:649, 1969

Janczuk Z et al: Cytologic studies on the secretion of the parotid gland in healthy subjects. Czas Stomat 19:387, 1966

Knudson AG: Genetics and etiology of human cancer. In Harris H, Hirschorn K (eds): Advanced Human Genetics, p 1–51. New York, Plenum Press, 1977

Kyle RA, Spencer RJ, Dahlin DC: Value of rectal biopsy in the diagnosis of primary systemic amyloidosis. Am J Med Sci 251:501, 1966

Lehner T: Oral biopsy in the diagnosis of amyloidosis. Isr J Med Sci 4:1000, 1968

Lustenberger AA, Shapiro LR: An introduction to cytogenetics in medicine and dentistry. J Oral Med 29:64, 1974

McKusick VA: Mendelian Inheritance in Man, 5th ed. Baltimore, John's Hopkins University Press, 1978

Mendelsohn ML et al: Computer-oriented analysis of human chromosomes: I. Photometric estimation of DNA content. Cytogenetics 5:223, 1967

Moorhead PS et al: Chromosome preparations of leukocytes cultured from human peripheral blood. Exp Cell Res 20:613, 1960

Nasjleti CE: Possible supernumerary chromosome associated with hypodontia. J Dent Res 45:973, 1966

Nowell PC: Phytohemagglutinin: An initiator of mitosis in cultures of normal human leukocytes. Cancer Res 20:462, 1960

Rowley JD: The clinical usefulness of chromosome studies in patients with leukemia. Compr Ther 6:57, 1980

Rowley JD: Do all leukemic cells have an abnormal karyotype. N Eng J Med 305:164, 1981

Sandler HC: Reliability of oral exfoliative cytology for detection of oral cancer. J Am Dent Assoc 68:489, 1964

Sandler HC et al: Exfoliative cytology for detection of early mouth cancer. Oral Surg 13:994, 1960

Savery EB: Human cytogenetics with special regard to oral changes in chromosome abnormalities. Tandlaegebladet 76:28, 1972

Seymour AE et al: Electron microscopy in surgical pathology: A selective review. Pathology 13:111, 1981

Shear M, Wilton E: Cytogenetic studies of the basal cell carcinoma syndrome. J Dent Assoc Africa 23:99, 1968

Silverman S et al: The diagnostic value of intraoral cytology. J Dent Res 37:195, 1958

Silverman S Jr: Early detection of oral cancer; A simple screening technic. Practical Dent Monogr p 3, July 1959

Snyder MB: Indications and method for oral soft tissue biopsy. Comp Contin Educn III:63, 1982

Stahl SS: Correlation of cytodiagnosis and biopsy in the evolution of an experimentally induced carcinoma 16:985, 1963

Tarpley TM et al: Minor salivary gland involvement in Sjögren's syndrome. Oral Surg 37:64, 1974

Tzanck A: Le cytodiagnostic immédiate en dermatologie. Bull Soc Franc Dermatol Syph 2:68, 1947

Tzanck A et al: Immediate cytologic examination in dermatology. Ann Dermatol Syph 8:205, 1948

Umiker W et al: Exfoliative cytology in radiotherapy of oral cancer. Radiology 75:107, 1960

Umiker W et al: Oral smears in the diagnosis of carcinoma and premalignant lesions. Oral Surg 13:897, 1960

Vassar PS, Culling CFA, Taylor HE: Fluorescent stains with special reference to amyloid and connective tissue. Arch Pathol 68:487, 1959

Yunis JJ (ed): New Chromosomal Syndromes. New York, Academic Press,1977

Microbiology and Immunology

ADA Council on Dental Therapeutics: Type B (serum) hepatitis and dental practice. J Am Dent Assoc 92:153, 1976

Aldrete JA, Johnson DA: Allergy to local anesthetics. JAMA 207:356, 1969

August DS, Levy BA: Periapical actinomycosis. Oral Surg 36:588, 1973

Baer H: In vitro methods in allergy. In Samter, M (ed): Symposium on Allergy in Adults: Review and Outlook, Med Clin North Am 58:85, 1974

Bender IB, et al: To culture or not to culture. Oral Surg 18:527, 1964

Blumberg, BS: Bioethical questions related to hepatitis B antigen. In Supplement on Viral Hepatitis; Present Status of Basic Clinical and Laboratory Studies. Am J Clin Pathol 65:848, 1976

Buchbinder M: A statistical comparison of cultured and non-cultured root canal cases. J D Res 20:93, 1941

Budtz-Jorgensen E: Denture stomatitis. V candida agglutinins in human sera. Acta Odontol Scand 30:313, 1972

Burnham TK, Bank PW: Antinuclear antibodies: I. Patterns of nuclear immunofluorescence. J Invest Derm 62:526, 1974

Davenport JC: The oral distribution of candida in denture stomatitis. Br Dent J 129:151, 1970

DiPiro JT et al: Antimicrobial prophylaxis in surgery. Am J Hosp Pharm 38:320, 487, 1981

Dmochowski L: Viral Type A and Type B hepatitis. Morphology, biology, immunology and epidemiology—A review. In Supplement on Viral Hepatitis; Present Status of Basic Clinical and Laboratory Studies. Am J Clin Pathol 65:741, 1976

Evans AS: Clinical syndromes in adults caused by respiratory infection. Med Clin North Am 51:803, 1967

Fisher AA: Contact Dermatitis, 2nd ed. Philadelphia, Lea & Febiger, 1973

Fisher AA: Contact stomatitis, glossitis and cheilitis. In Symposium on Allergy in Otorhinolaryngology. Otolaryngol Clin North Am 7:827, 1974

Franchi GJ, Rehnquist KC, Yarashus DA: The dentist's role in the primary prevention of rheumatic fever. Report of the Stickney Public Health District's 3-year dental study on throat cultures. J Am Dent Assoc 75:1389, 1967

Freedman SO: Clinical Immunology, Chap 22. Laboratory Tests. New York, Harper & Row, 1971

Gardner AF: The odontogenic cyst as a potential carcinoma: A clinicopathologic appraisal. J Am Dent Assoc 78:746, 1969

Goldberg RJ: Use of antibiotics in the treatment of infectious diseases in dentistry, Penna Dent J Sept-Oct 1982

Goldman L, Goldman B: Contact testing of the buccal mucous membrane for stomatitis venenata. Arch Dermatol Syph 50:79, 1944

Grossman LI (ed): Transactions Fifth International Conference on Endodontics. University of Penna., 1973

Harding SA: Microbiology: Microbial antigen detection. Clin Lab Med 1:49, 1981

Henle W, Henle G: The Epstein-Barr virus (EBV) in Burkitt's lymphoma and nasopharyngeal carcinoma. Ann Clin Lab Sci 4:109, 1974

Henle W, Henle GE, Horwitz CA: Epstein-Barr virus specific diagnostic tests in infectious mononucleosis. Human Pathol 5:551, 1974

Herrmann EC, Jr et al: Diagnosis of viral diseases and the advent of antiviral drugs. Pharm Ther 7:35, 1979

Hochstein HD, Kirkham WR, Young VM: Recovery of more than 1 organism in septicemias. N Eng J Med 273:468, 1965

Hoff G, Bauer, S: A new raid slide test for infectious mononucleosis. JAMA 194:351, 1965

Hooks JJ, Jordan GW (eds): Viral infections in oral medicine. Procedural Institute Symposium on Viruses and Oral Diseases, National Institute Health, Bethesda, Maryland. 1980, New York, Elsevier, 1982

Hsiung GD et al: The use of electron microscopy for diagnosis of virus infections: An overview. Prog Med Virol 25:133, 1979

Kalnins V: Actinomycotic granuloma. Oral Surg 32:276 1971

Keyes PH et al: The use of phase-contrast microscopy and chemotherapy in the diagnosis and treatment of periodontal lesions: An initial report. Quintessence Int 1:51; 2:69, 1978

Khairat O: The non-aerobes of post-extraction bacteremia. J Dent Res 45:119, 1966

Lane AJ, Grossman LI: Culturing root canals by endodontic diplomates: a report based on a questionnaire. Oral Surg 32:461, 1971

Larato DC: The antibiotic sensitivity test in dental practice. Oral Surg 22:682, 1966

Lehner T: Immunofluorescent investigation of Candida albicans antibodies in human saliva.

Arch Oral Biol 10:975, 1965

Lehrer T: Immunofluorescence study of Candida albicans in candidiasis, carriers and controls. J Pathol Bacteriol 91:97, 1966

Lennette EH (ed): Manual of Clinical Microbiology. Washington, DC, American Society of Microbiologists, 1980

Listgarten MA, Levin S: Positive correlation between the proportions of subgingival spirochetes and motile bacteria and susceptibility of human subjects to periodontal deterioration. J Clin Perodontal 8:122, 1981

Littner MM et al: Acute streptococcal gingivostomatitis. Oral Surg 53:144, 1982

MacKinney AA, Cline WS: Infectious mononucleosis. Br J Haematol 27:367 1974

Marlay E: The relationship between dental caries and salivary properties at adolescence. Aust Dent J 15:412, 1970

Martin RS et al: Assessment of expectorated sputum for bacteriological analysis based on polymorphs and squamous epithelial cells: Six-month study. J Clin Microbiol 8:635, 1978

McHenry MC, Gavan TL: Selection and use of antibacterial drugs. Progr Clin Pathol 6:205, 1975

McIntosh K: Recent advances in viral diagnosis. Arch Pathol Lab Med 104:3, 1980

Miller A, Niederman JC, Andrews L: Prolonged oropharyngeal excretion of Epstein-Barr virus after infectious mononucleosis. N Engl J Med 288:229, 1973

Möller AJR: Microbiological examination of root canals and periapical tissues of human teeth. Methodological studies. Odontol Tidsk 74[Suppl.]:1, 1966

Morse DR: Does culturing contribute to endodontic success? Transactions Fifth International Conference on Endodontics. pp 91-100. University of Pennsylvania, 1973

Mosley JW, et al: Hepatitis B virus infection in dentists. N Engl J Med 293:729, 1975

Naidorf IJ: Is culturing contributory to endodontic success? Transactions Fifth International Conference on Endodontics, pp 101–7. University of Pennsylvania, 1973

Niederman JC, et al: Infectious mononucleosis: clinical manifestations in relation to EB virus antibodies. JAMA 203:205, 1968

Nielsen JO, Dietrickson O, Juhl E: Incidence and meaning of the "e" determinant among hepatitis B antigen positive patients with acute and chronic liver disease. Report from Copenhagen Hepatitis Acuta Programme. Lancet 2:913, 1974

Norkraus G, Magnius L, Iwarson S: "e"—antigen in acute hepatitis B. Br Med J 1:740, 1976

North American Contact Dermatitis Group: The Role of Patch Testing in Allergic Contact Dermatitis, 4th ed. New York, American Academy Dermatology, 1978

Olgart LG: Rationalized endodontic treatment by a bacteriologic direct sampling technique. J Dent Res 49:1427, 1970

Oliet S (ed): Symposium on endodontics. Dent Clin North Am 18[2]:April, 1974

Peterson LR, Balfour HH, Jr: Advances in clinical virology. Prog Clin Pathol 8:239, Chap 10, 1981

Ribaux CL: Etude du protozoaire buccal Trichomonas tenax en microscopie electronique á balayage et en transmission. J Biol Buccale 7:157, 1979

Richardson RL, Jones M: A bacteriologic census of human saliva. J Dent Res 37:697, 1958

Rogosa M et al: Selective medium for the isolation and enumeration of oral lactobacilli. J Dent Res 30:682, 1951

Rogosa M et al: Blood sampling and cultural studies in the detection of post-operative bacteremias. J Am Dent Assoc 60:171, 1960

Rosenberg WE, Fischer RW: Improved method for intraoral patch testing. Arch Dermatol 87:155, 1963

Slatkin M: Trends in the diagnosis and treatment of syphilis. Med Clin North Am 49:823, 1965

Stolpe JR: Chemical and bacteriological tests for determining susceptibility to, and activity of dental caries: A review. J Public Health Dent 30:141, 1970

Sutter VL, Finegold SM: Anaerobic bacteria: Their recognition and significance in the clinical laboratory. Prog Clin Pathol 5:219, 1973

Taichman NS, et al: Leukotoxicity of an extract from Actinobacillus actinomycetem comitans for human gingival polymorphonuclear leukocytes. Inflammation 5:1, 1981

Thayer HH: Contraindication for use of Serratia marcescens as tracer organisms in research. J Dent Res 45:853, 1966

Voller A et al: The enzyme-linked immunosorbent assay (ELISA). Alexandria, VA Dynatech Labs, 1979

Watkins BJ: Viral hepatitis B.: A special problem in prevention. J Am Soc Prevent Dent 6:8, 1976

Weismer PJ et al: Clinical spectrum of pharyngeal gonococcal infection. N Engl J Med 288:181, 1973

Woods R: A dental caries susceptibility test based on the occurrence of Streptococcus mutans in plaque material. Aust Dent J 16:116, 1971

Woods R: Antibiotic treatment of pyogenic infections of dental origin. Aust Dent J 13:151, 1968

Woods R: The changing nature of pyogenic dental infections. Aust Dent J 23:107, 1978

Zukerman AJ, Taylor PE: Persistence of the serum hepatitis (SH-Australia) antigen for many years. Nature 223:81, 1969

4

Oral Medicine in the Hospital

MARTIN S. GREENBERG

The hospital dental department should serve as a community referral center where dental treatment for patients with severe systemic disease and evaluation of diagnostic problems of the mouth and jaws are practiced at the highest level. These two disciplines of oral medicine are best performed in the hospital because of the availability of sophisticated diagnostic and life-sustaining equipment as well as the proximity of expert consultants in all areas of health care.

Hospital oral medicine problems may be seen by the dentist in three ways:

1. The patient may be admitted as an inpatient to the dental service. This is done most frequently for patients requiring dental care who have severe medical problems.
2. The patient may be seen as a hospital outpatient. This is the common procedure for a majority of patients with diagnostic problems of the oral mucosa, jaws, and salivary glands.
3. The patient may be seen on consultation at the request of another department of the hospital. Some of the most difficult and unusual problems evaluated by the hospital dentist are seen as consultations.

Examples of problems rarely seen in outpatient practice, but commonly seen in hospitalized patients are oral ulcers, oral bleeding, and oral infection secondary to blood dyscrasias or chemotherapy; acute parotitis in debilitated patients; dental care to prevent osteoradionecrosis prior to radiotherapy; and dental care to prevent infection prior to organ transplant or open heart surgery.

In order to handle consultations properly, the dentist must be familiar with the proper method of requesting and answering consultants. Hospitals may differ in the form used, but there is a universally accepted method that should be followed.

REQUESTING INFORMATION

The standard format used to request medical information from other departments is simple. The difficulty arises in deciding what medical information is necessary for a partic-

ular patient. This requires experience as well as knowledge of how a medical problem may change dental treatment.

When requesting information from other departments, it is necessary to write only two or three sentences containing the following data: age and sex of the patient, dental treatment to be performed, and medical information required. A typical consultation request follows:

> The patient is a 35-year-old male who requires multiple dental extractions under local anesthesia. A history of a possible heart murmur was elicited. Is a murmur present, and if so, is it functional or organic?

Several points should be made concerning the above theoretical consultation request to a cardiologist. *The request is brief.* Detailed descriptions of the nuances of dental therapy are unnecessary, but information regarding surgery or extensive treatment should be included.

The request is specific. The cardiologist is asked for medical information concerning the presence of an organic heart murmur. He is not asked to give "clearance" for treatment. When vague requests are sent to physicians asking questions such as "Is it all right to treat the patient?" the physician may not understand the information required and send a vague or noncommittal reply. These vague replies are often stored in a patient's chart as alleged legal protection, but they rarely assist the dentist in treating the patient effectively. The chief rule in requesting a consultation is to be aware of what medical information is required and request that information, not "clearance."

ANSWERING CONSULTATIONS

There is a standard format that should be followed when answering consultations from other hospital departments. Consultations that are only answered by short phrases such as "denture adjusted" or "tooth extracted" are unsatisfactory, since the physician who hospitalized the patient for a medical problem is not given sufficient information. This information may be important in the management of the patient. Below is an uncomplicated consultation concerning a patient who developed dental pain while hospitalized for a medical problem:

> The patient is a 55-year-old male who was hospitalized 5 days ago because of an acute onset of severe chest paints. A diagnosis of acute myocardial infarction was made, and the patient is now being treated with complete bedrest and heparin. The patient began complaining of pain in the maxillary left molar region yesterday. He states that the pain is made worse when cold fluids are placed in his mouth. Examination at bedside shows no asymmetries, masses, or lesions of the neck, skin of the face, or of the salivary glands. There are two marble-sized left submandibular lymph nodes that are not tender and are freely movable. The patient states that they have been present, unchanged in size, for many years. The temporomandibular joint is normal. The left buccal mucosa has a small 5 mm × 3 mm shallow ulcer opposite the maxillary first molar. There is no induration present around the ulcer. This same tooth has a large carious lesion and a sharp edge of enamel. No other dental or oral mucosal lesions are noted.

IMPRESSIONS

1. Dental pain secondary to pulpitis of a maxillary molar. There is no indication that this is referred chest pain, especially since cold locally applied exacerbates the pain.
2. Traumatic ulcer of buccal mucosa secondary to sharp tooth.

RECOMMENDATIONS

1. Place sedative temporary filling in tooth and smooth rough edge at bedside to minimize stress to patient at this time.
2. Follow oral ulcer for healing; should see significant healing within 1 week or will reevaluate to exclude carcinoma.
3. After acute phase of myocardial infarction, permanently treat tooth. Follow patient to ascertain whether pain disappears with above management, or whether further treatment is necessary. Recommend minimal treatment at this time because of medical condition and anticoagulant therapy.

Note that the following outline was used in answering the above sample consultation:

1. Brief summary of pertinent information from the patient's medical chart
2. History of oral complaint
3. Examination findings
4. Impressions and/or differential diagnosis
5. Recommendations for treatment

A brief summary has several functions. First, the consultation becomes a complete entity. When another clinician reads the consultation he will immediately understand the case. Second, a consulting dentist must read the medical chart before making a diagnosis or recommending treatment. A patient with oral lesions may also have skin, genital, anal, or eye lesions that will make the diagnosis easier. The chart will often have information such as physical or laboratory findings that will affect the type of dental treatment that should be recommended.

Having to write an intelligent opening statement encourages a rushed clinician to read the entire chart before writing the consultation. A good medical summary makes it clear to the physician who requested it that the dentist has read the chart and taken its contents into consideration when making recommendations.

The second portion of the consultation is a summary of examination findings. It should contain comments regarding the neck, face, salivary glands, temporomandibular joint, oral mucosa, gingiva, and teeth. A description of abnormalities should be made in this section, not a diagnosis. The diagnosis may be wrong, but at least an accurate description is available to refer to when examining the patient at a later date. It is also important to remember not to use dental jargon or symbols when writing consultations; it is easier, but the physician may not understand their meaning.

The last portion of the consultation is labeled "Recommendations," and is an important procedure in hospital etiquette. All treatment for a hospitalized patient must be approved by the admitting clinician. He is the person ultimately responsible for the patient. Therefore, recommendations for treatment are made by the dentist, but the admitting physician has the authority to accept or reject them.

HOSPITAL DENTISTRY FOR PATIENTS WITH SEVERE MEDICAL PROBLEMS

A dentist may choose to hospitalize a patient with severe medical problems for several reasons including the availability of emergency resuscitation supplies, of nursing care before and after the dental procedure, of consultants in other medical disciplines, of clinical laboratory facilities before and after the dental procedure, and of operating room and anesthesiologists. Several medical insurance plans now cover hospitalization for patients with severe medical problems admitted for dental treatment.

Once the dentist decides that a patient should be treated in a hospital, he should consider whether the dental procedure should be done on an inpatient or outpatient basis. The reason for utilizing the hospital determines this choice. For example, if the hospital is being utilized for a patient with severe heart disease because of the resuscitation equipment available, hospitalization before and after the procedure may be unnecessary, and outpatient hospital management will accomplish the objectives. Conversely, a patient with hemophilia may require cryoprecipitate to elevate Factor VIII levels prior to oral surgery. In this case the hospital is more important for preoperative management and postoperative observation than for the procedure.

The dentist may choose to hospitalize patients with the following disorders for dental treatment:

- bleeding disorders due to hereditary disease, bone marrow suppression, extensive liver disease, or anticoagulant therapy
- susceptible to shock due to adrenocortical insufficiency or uncontrolled diabetes
- severe cardiovascular disease including those with prosthetic heart valves
- susceptible to infection due to primary or secondary immune deficiency

- require heavy sedation or general anesthesia
- neuromuscular or other physical disability requiring special dental equipment for proper management.

Many hospitals allow single-day admissions. This is convenient for patients requiring heavy sedation or general anesthesia who do not require extensive pre- or postoperative care.

Dental patients admitted to the hospital should have a complete medical history and a head and neck examination noted on the chart by a member of the dental staff. Most hospitals require a physical examination by a physician, but this does not excuse the dentist from writing his history and regional exam findings on the chart. Dentists admitting patients to a hospital may not be able to perform a complete physical examination, but they must be competent to understand the implications of the physician's examination and its relationships to the dental procedure to be performed. If the physician writes under heart examination "PMI 6th ICS AAL gr iv/vi systolic (m) in mitral region radiating to axilla," the dentist should understand that the heart is enlarged and a probable organic murmur is present. Further evaluation such as a cardiology consultation may be necessary before dental surgery is performed.

The hospital dentist should write the necessary orders for patients he admits including diet, frequency of vital signs, bedrest, medications and laboratory tests. He should be able to interpret the results of the tests he orders.

In summary, the hospital dentist is in charge of the total welfare of the hospitalized patients he admits. He may not be able to treat all problems that arise, but he must know who to consult in order to treat these problems. He must also be trained to answer complex consultations regarding oral disease that are sent from other departments.

Hospital general practice residency programs in dentistry train residents in physical diagnosis, laboratory diagnosis, and advanced oral medicine to help them manage dental patients with severe medical problems. The future of dentistry and oral medicine in the hospital rests with the men and women being trained in these programs. Their training will not only benefit the dental profession, but more important, will also raise the level of oral health care available for patients with compromised health.

Part II

ORAL DISEASE

5

Ulcerative, Vesicular and Bullous Lesions

MARTIN S. GREENBERG

A clinician attempting to diagnose ulcerative and vesiculobullous disease of the mouth is confronted with many diseases having a similar clinical appearance. The oral mucosa is thin, causing vesiculae and bullae to break rapidly into ulcers and ulcers are easily traumatized from teeth as well as food and become secondarily infected by the oral flora. These factors may cause lesions that have a characteristic appearance on the skin to have a nonspecific appearance on the oral mucosa.

Mucosal disorders may occasionally be correctly diagnosed from a brief history and rapid clinical examination, but this approach is usually insufficient and leads to incorrect diagnosis and improper treatment. The history is frequently underemphasized, but when correctly performed it gives as much information as does the clinical examination. A detailed history of the present illness is of particular importance when attempting to diagnose oral mucosal lesions. A complete review of systems should be obtained for each patient, including questions regarding the presence of skin, eye, genital, and rectal lesions. Questions should also be included regarding symptoms of diseases associated with oral lesions; therefore, each patient should be asked about the presence of symptoms such as joint pains, muscle weakness, dyspnea, diplopia, and chest pains.

The clinical examination should include a thorough inspection of the exposed skin surfaces, and the diagnosis of oral lesions requires knowledge of basic dermatology because many disorders occurring on the oral mucosa also affect the skin. Dermatologic lesions are classified according to their clinical appearance and include the following basic lesions:

- *Macules*—well-circumscribed, flat lesions that are noticeable because of their change from normal skin color. They may be red due to the presence of vascular lesions or inflammation, or pigmented due to the presence of melanin, hemosiderin, and drugs.
- *Papules*—solid lesions raised above the skin surface that are smaller than 1 cm in diameter. Papules may be seen in a wide variety of diseases including erythema multiforme simplex, rubella, lupus erythematosus, and sarcoidosis.

- *Plaques*—solid raised lesions that are over 1 cm in diameter; they are large papules.
- *Nodules*—these lesions are present deep in the dermis, and the epidermis can be easily moved over them.
- *Vesicles*—elevated blisters containing clear fluid that are under 1 cm in diameter.
- *Bullae*—elevated blisterlike lesions containing clear fluid that are over 1 cm in diameter.
- *Erosions*—moist, red lesions often caused by the rupture of vesicles or bullae as well as trauma.
- *Pustules*—raised lesions containing purulent material.
- *Ulcer*—a defect in the epithelium; it is a well-circumscribed depressed lesion over which the epidermal layer has been lost.
- *Purpura*—reddish to purple, flat lesions caused by blood from vessels leaking into the subcutaneous tissue. Classified by size as petechiae or ecchymoses, these lesions will not blanch when pressed.
- *Petechiae*—purpuric lesions 1 mm to 2 mm in diameter. Larger purpuric lesions are called ecchymoses.

A detailed history of the present illness is essential in making the diagnosis of oral mucosal disease. Three pieces of information that should be obtained early in the history will help the clinician rapidly categorize a patient's disease and simplify the diagnosis: length of time the lesions have been present (acute or chronic lesions), past history of similar lesions (primary or recurrent disease), and number of lesions present (single or multiple). In this chapter, the diseases are grouped according to the information obtained above. This information serves as an excellent starting point for the student who is just learning to diagnose these disorders, as well as experienced clinicians who are aware of the potential diagnostic difficulties.

The first section of this chapter deals with acute multiple lesions that tend to occur only once, the second portion of the chapter deals with recurring oral mucosal syndromes, and the third portion deals with the patient with chronic multiple lesions. The final section describes diseases that present as chronic single lesions. It is hoped that classifying the disorders in this way will help the clinician avoid the common diagnostic problem of confusing viral infections with recurring oral syndromes, such as recurrent aphthous stomatitis, or disorders that present as chronic progressive disease, such as pemphigus and pemphoid.

THE PATIENT WITH ACUTE MULTIPLE LESIONS

Acute Viral Stomatitis

Three viruses may cause an infection that primarily involves the oral mucosa: herpes simplex virus (herpesvirus hominis), coxsackievirus, and varicella zoster virus. Primary herpes simplex infections will be discussed below; recurrent herpes simplex infections and chronic herpes simplex infections are described later in the chapter under recurring and chronic oral lesions.

Primary Herpes Simplex Virus Infections

There has been a renewed interest in herpes simplex virus (herpesvirus hominis) among clinicians and researchers. Once thought to cause only a mild childhood infection and recurrent herpes labialis, the virus is now known to cause encephalitis, dermatitis, keratoconjunctivitis, genitourinary infection, and disseminated disease in newborns and is suspected as a cause of cancer of the cervix, mouth, and pharynx.

There are now over 50 known herpes viruses. Four of these infect man, including herpes simplex virus (HSV), varicella zoster virus, and EB virus (Epstein-Barr virus), which causes infectious mononucleosis and Burkitt's lymphoma.

A major cause of the renewed interest in HSV followed the finding of two types of HSV in man, HSV 1 and HSV 2 with different biologic and serologic properties. HSV 1 is responsible for a majority of cases of oral and pharyngeal infection, meningoencephalitis, and dermatitis above the waist. HSV 2 is implicated in a majority of genital infections, infections of the newborn, and dermatitis below the waist.

Nahmias studied 89 cases of primary herpetic gingivostomatitis: 86 cases were caused by HSV 1; 3 cases were caused by HSV 2. Primary oral herpes with HSV 2 has been related to oral sex with patients having genital HSV 2 lesions.

Primary HSV infection of the newborn is related more frequently to HSV 2 and is usually caused by contact of the newborn with vaginal lesions of the mother during birth. These infections of the newborn result in viremia and disseminated infection of the brain, liver, adrenals, and lungs. Some cases may be prevented by cesarean section to avoid direct contact of the neonate with the lesions. Bloodborne virus may also infect some fetuses.

HSV 2 is considered a venereal disease, and evidence is accumulating relating HSV 2 to carcinoma of the uterine cervix. The evidence is a result of epidemiologic studies that related increased incidence of HSV 2 serum antibodies to patients who develop invasive cervical carcinoma. There is also some evidence relating HSV 1 to oral carcinoma, but these are preliminary reports.

Primary oral infection with HSV occurs in patients with no prior infection with HSV 1. Transmission of the virus occurs during close personal contact. Infection of the fingers (herpetic whitlows) of health professionals may occur during treatment of infected patients. Dentists may experience primary lesions of the fingers from contact with lesions of the mouth or saliva of patients who are asymptomatic carriers of HSV (see Fig. 5-1). Physicians, nurses, and other hospital personnel may contract the infection during handling of tracheal catheters.

Newborns of mothers with antibody titers are protected by placentally transferred antibodies during the first 6 months of life. After 6 months of age the incidence of primary HSV 1 infection increases. Incidence of primary HSV 2 infection does not increase until after 14 years of age when sexual activity begins. The incidence of primary HSV 1 infection reaches a peak between 2 to 3 years of age. Studies of neutralizing and complement-fixing antibodies to HSV have shown a continual rise in percentage of patients who have had contact with the virus until 60 years of age, demonstrating that although the primary infection with HSV 1 is chiefly a disease of infants and children, new cases continue to appear during adult life. This is consistent

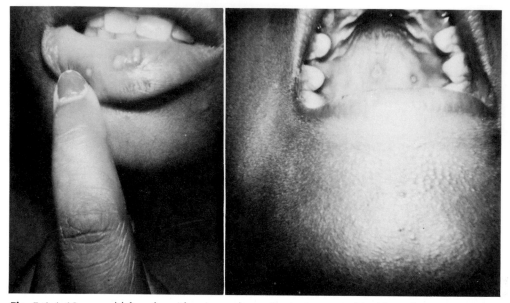

Fig. 5-1 A 12-year-old female with primary herpetic gingivostomatitis. Note discrete, round, shallow ulcers surrounded by inflammation as well as marginal gingivitis of palatal gingiva.

with the many reports of adults with primary herpetic gingivostomatitis.

The incidence of primary herpes infection has been shown to vary according to socioeconomic group. This was first reported in 1939 by Burnett and Williams, who studied the incidence of antibodies to HSV in various social classes. They found that 37% of college graduates had antibody to HSV, whereas 93% of patients in a city hospital had antibody. This has been confirmed by others including Greenberg and colleagues, who found 70% of ward patients in a city hospital with antibody to HSV, whereas Ship and colleagues reported 31% of professional school students with HSV antibody. MacCallum found that 96% of pregnant women in a working class London district had antibody to HSV, whereas 41% of pregnant women in a wealthier district had HSV antibody.

The incidence of primary herpetic gingivostomatitis is unknown, although the number of patients with a history of primary herpes is low even among those with serum antibody to the virus. Blank and Rake thought that 99% of the cases of primary herpes were subclinical, although the apparently low incidence of a history of classical primary herpetic gingivostomatitis is also in-

fluenced by the young age of patients who develop the infection, by the improper diagnosis of some cases, and by the cases of primary herpetic pharyngitis that cannot be clinically distinguished from other causes of viral pharyngitis. Evans and Dick reported HSV as a common cause of pharyngitis in a group of hospitalized college students.

Clinical Manifestations of Primary Oral Herpes The patient usually presents to the clinician with a full-blown oral and systemic disease, but a history of the mode of onset will be helpful in differentiating lesions of primary HSV infection from other types of acute, multiple lesions of the oral mucosa.

The patient will have a history of generalized prodromal symptoms that precede the local lesions by 1 to 2 days. This is helpful in differentiating this viral infection from allergic stomatitis or erythema multiforme, in which local lesions and systemic symptoms appear together. These generalized symptoms include fever, headache, malaise, nausea, and vomiting. A negative past history of recurrent herpes labialis and a positive history of close contact with a patient with primary or recurrent herpes is also helpful in making the diagnosis.

Approximately 1 to 2 days after the pro-dromal symptoms, small vesicles appear on the oral mucosa (Fig. 5-2). The vesicles quickly rupture leaving shallow, round, dis-crete ulcers surrounded by inflammation. The lesions occur on all portions of the mu-cosa. As the disease progresses several le-sions may coalesce, forming some larger ir-regular lesions.

An important diagnostic criteria in this dis-ease is the appearance of a generalized acute, marginal gingivitis. The entire gingiva is edematous and inflamed. Several small gin-gival ulcers are often present (Fig. 5-3). Ex-amination of the posterior pharynx will re-veal inflammation, and the submandibular and cervical lymph nodes are characteristi-cally enlarged and tender.

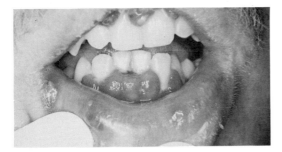

Fig. 5-2 Severe gingivitis in patient with primary her-petic gingivostomatitis.

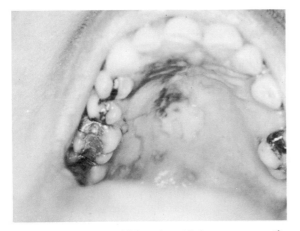

Fig. 5-3 A 43-year-old female with large nonspecific ulcers of the palate. A careful history and laboratory studies demonstrated that these were coalesced ul-cers in an adult with a primary herpes simplex infec-tion.

Primary HSV in otherwise healthy children is a self-limiting disease. The fever ordinarily disappears within 3 or 4 days, and the lesions begin healing in a week to 10 days, although HSV may continue to be present in the saliva for up to a month after the onset of disease.

Laboratory Diagnosis Patients with a typical clinical picture of generalized symptoms fol-lowed by oral vesicles, round shallow sym-metrical oral ulcers, and acute marginal gin-givitis, but who do not have a history of recurrent herpes are easily diagnosed as hav-ing primary herpetic gingivostomatitis, and laboratory tests are rarely used (Fig. 5-4). Other patients, especially adults, may have a less typical clinical picture, making the diag-nosis more difficult (Fig. 5-5). This is espe-cially important when distinguishing primary herpes from erythema multiforme. The treat-ment of extensive erythema multiforme in-cludes the use of systemic corticosteroids, whereas use of corticosteroids in primary herpes is contraindicated.

The following laboratory tests are helpful in the diagnosis of a primary herpes infec-tion.

Cytology. A fresh vesicle can be opened and a scraping made from the base of the lesion and placed on a microscopic slide. The slide may be stained with Giemsa and searched for multinucleated giant cells, synctium, and ballooning degeneration of the nucleus. This is helpful in distinguishing HSV lesions from erythema multiforme, allergic stomatitis, and recurrent aphthous stomatitis, but not vari-

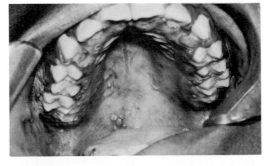

Fig. 5-4 Primary herpes infection in a 17-year-old male. Note unruptured palatal vesicles and intense marginal gingivitis.

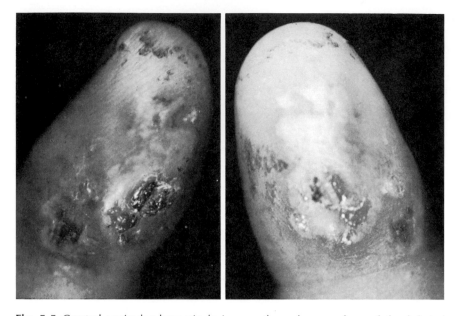

Fig. 5-5 Crusted vesicular herpetic lesion on the palmar surface of the left index finger. Primary infection associated with intraoral tissues of a patient with primary infection or a carrier by a dental student. (Blechman, Pascher: Oral Surg 12:186)

cella zoster lesions, which also contain multinucleated giant cells. Fluorescent staining of cytology smears has been used by Griffin to differentiate lesions of HSV from other lesions. Silverman took cytology specimens from 25 adults with primary herpes infection; 92% had positive results.

HSV Isolation. Isolation and neutralization of a virus in tissue culture is the most positive method of identification. Primary rabbit kidney and human amnion are both sensitive to HSV, but the chorioallantoic membrane of chick embryos has also been used.

A clinician must remember that isolation of HSV from oral lesions does not necessarily mean that HSV caused the lesions. Patients who have lesions from other causes may also be carriers of HSV. Studies have indicated that between 2% to 4% of the population are asymptomatic carriers of HSV and serve as a continual reservoir of virus for new primary infection.

Antibody Titers. Conclusive evidence of a primary HSV infection includes testing for complement-fixing or neutralizing antibody in acute and convalescent sera. An acute serum

specimen should be obtained within 3 or 4 days of the onset of symptoms. The absence of detectable antibodies plus the isolation of HSV from lesions is compatible with the presence of a primary HSV infection. Antibody to HSV will begin to appear in a week and reach a peak in 3 weeks. A convalescent serum can confirm the diagnosis of primary HSV infection by demonstrating at least a fourfold rise in anti-HSV antibody. If anti-HSV antibody titers are the same in both the acute and convalescent sera, the lesions from which HSV was isolated were recurrent lesions.

Treatment The treatment of acute herpetic gingivostomatitis in healthy children and adults remains primarily supportive, although experimental use of antiviral agents has taken place in recent years.

Routine supportive measures include aspirin or acetaminophen for fever and fluids to maintain proper hydration and electrolyte balance. If the patient has difficulty eating and drinking, a topical anesthetic may be administered prior to meals. Dyclonine hydrochloride, 0.5%, has been shown to be an excellent topical anesthetic for the oral mucosa.

If this medication is not available, a solution of diphenhydramine hydrochloride (Benadryl), 5 mg/ml, mixed with an equal amount of milk of magnesia also has satisfactory topical anesthetic properties. Infants who are not drinking because of severe oral pain should be referred to a pediatrician for maintenance of proper fluid and electrolyte balance.

Antibiotics are of no help in the treatment of primary herpes infection, and use of corticosteroids is contraindicated. Antiviral agents have been utilized with success in newborns or in immunosuppressed patients with primary herpes infections. Idoxuridine (IUDR), cytosine arabinoside (Ara-C), and adenine arabinoside (Ara-A) have been used systemically, although severe side-effects including hepatic and renal toxicity have been reported. Chien and colleagues reported minimal side-effects with use of Ara-C in the treatment of HSV infection in neonates and immunosuppressed patients. Further details regarding use of antiviral agents are discussed with sections on recurrent and chronic HSV.

Coxsackievirus Infections

Coxsackieviruses are RNA enteroviruses, which are named for the town in upper New York State where they were first discovered. Coxsackieviruses have been separated into two groups, A and B. There are 24 known types of coxsackie group A and 6 types of coxsackie group B. These viruses cause hepatitis, meningitis, myocarditis, pericarditis, and acute respiratory disease. Three clinical types of infection of the oral region that have been described are usually caused by group A coxsackieviruses: herpangina, hand-foot-and-mouth disease, and acute lymphonodular pharyngitis. Types of coxsackie A have also been described as causing a rare mumps-like form of parotitis.

Herpangina Coxsackie A4 has been shown to cause a majority of cases of herpangina, but types A1 to A10 as well as types A16 to A22 have also been implicated. Because many antigenic strains of coxsackievirus exist, herpangina may be seen more than once in the same patient. Unlike herpes simplex infections, which occur at a constant rate, herpangina frequently occurs in epidemics that have their highest incidence from June to October. The majority of cases affect young children, but infection of adolescents and adults has also been reported.

Clinical Manifestations The infection begins with generalized symptoms of fever, chills, and anorexia. The fever and other symptoms are generally milder than those experienced with primary HSV infection. The patient will also complain of sore throat, dysphagia, and occasionally, sore mouth. Examination of the mouth and posterior pharyngeal wall show bilateral discrete small vesicles most commonly involving the posterior pharynx, tonsils, faucial pillars, and soft palate. Lesions are found less frequently on the buccal mucosa, tongue, and hard palate (Fig. 5-6). Within 24 to 48 hours the vesicles rupture, forming small 1-mm to 2-mm ulcers. The disease is usually mild, and will heal without treatment in 1 week.

Herpangina may be clinically distinguished from primary HSV infection by several criteria:

1. Herpangina occurs in epidemics; HSV infections do not.
2. Herpangina tends to be milder than HSV infection.
3. Lesions of herpangina occur on the pharynx and posterior portions of the oral mucosa, whereas HSV primarily affects the anterior portion of the mouth.

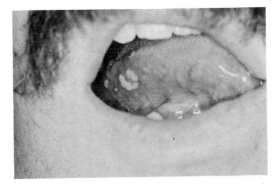

Fig. 5-6 A cluster of vesicles on the tongue in a patient with herpangina. The patient had lesions of the posterior pharyngeal wall and tonsils, but there was no gingivitis. Coxsackie A$_4$ was isolated in tissue culture.

4. Herpangina does not cause a generalized acute gingivitis like that associated with primary HSV infection.
5. Lesions of herpangina tend to be smaller than those of HSV.

Laboratory Studies A smear taken from the base of a fresh vesicle and stained with Giemsa will *not* show ballooning degeneration or multinucleated giant cells. This will help to distinguish herpangina from herpes simplex and herpes zoster, which do show these changes.

Coxsackievirus is harder to isolate in tissue culture than are the herpes viruses and is best identified by isolation in monkey kidney tissue culture or propagation and neutralization in suckling mice.

Treatment Herpangina is a self-limiting disease, and treatment is supportive, including proper hydration and topical anesthesia when eating or swallowing is difficult.

Hand-Foot-and-Mouth Disease Hand-foot-and-mouth disease is caused by infection with coxsackie A16 in a majority of cases, although instances have been described in which A5, A10, B2, or B5 have been isolated. The disease is characterized by low-grade fever, oral vesicles and ulcers, and nonpruritic macules, papules, and vesicles particularly of the extensor surfaces of the hands and feet. The oral lesions are more extensive than those described for herpangina, and lesions of the hard palate, tongue, and buccal mucosa are common.

Adler and colleagues studied 20 cases of hand-foot-and-mouth disease. The patients ranged in age from 8 months to 33 years, with 75% of cases occurring below 4 years of age. The clinical manifestations lasted 3 to 7 days. The most common complaint of the 20 patients was sore mouth, and clinically, all of the 20 patients had lesions involving the oral mucosa. Because of the more frequent oral involvement, dentists are more likely to see patients with this disease than with herpangina, and they should remember to examine the hands and feet for maculopapular and vesicular lesions when patients present with an acute stomatitis and fever. Treatment is the same as for herpangina.

Acute Lymphonodular Pharyngitis In 1962, Steigman, Lipton, and Braspinick described a previously undocumented disorder caused by coxsackie A10, which was seen in 15 patients around the vicinity of Louisville, Kentucky. The clinical picture differed from other types of coxsackie A infection in the oropharyngeal region.

The early clinical picture is similar to that of herpangina in several aspects in that it occurs most frequently in children and starts with fever, anorexia, sore throat, and mild lymphadenopathy. The clinical appearance of the lesions differs from those seen in herpangina and hand-foot-and-mouth disease. Instead of vesicles and ulcers, raised whitish yellow nodules on an erythematous base present on the posterior pharyngeal wall; these lesions are aggregates of lymphocytes. No oral lesions are present. The disease is self-limiting with symptoms and signs disappearing in 1 to 2 weeks. Treatment is symptomatic.

Varicella Zoster Virus Infection

Varicella zoster virus (VZ) is a DNA virus that is similar to herpes simplex virus, causes both a primary and a recurrent infection, and remains latent in nerve tissue. VZ is responsible for two major clinical infections of man: chickenpox (varicella) and shingles (herpes zoster). The current theory accepted by most investigators is that chickenpox is a generalized primary infection that occurs the first time an individual contacts the virus. This is analogous to the acute herpetic gingivostomatitis of herpes simplex virus. After the primary disease is healed, the VZ virus becomes latent in the dorsal root ganglia of spinal nerves or extramedullary ganglia of cranial nerves. Cheatham has demonstrated intranuclear viral inclusions in the dorsal root ganglia of nerves supplying areas affected with zoster; and Esiri and Tomlinson have demonstrated viral particles in Schwann cells.

The VZ virus becomes reactivated in some individuals causing lesions of localized herpes zoster (HZ). These lesions are considered similar in pathogenesis to recurrent herpes labialis with HSV. Cases have been reported in which the clinician suspected transmission of zoster by contact with chickenpox, although these cases are disputed. It is not disputed that a child without prior contact with VZ virus can develop chickenpox after contact with a patient with HZ. Patients with leukemia, lymphoma, or taking immunosuppressive drug therapy have an increased susceptibility to severe HZ. These HZ infections may be deep-seated and disseminated, causing pneumonia, meningoencephalitis, and hepatitis; however, apparently normal patients who develop HZ do not appear to have a significant incidence of underlying malignancy. Juel–Jensen studied over 800 HZ patients and found the rate of malignant disease no higher than in the general population.

Clinical Manifestations *General Findings*
Chickenpox is a childhood disease characterized by mild systemic symptoms and a generalized, intensely pruritic eruption of maculopapular lesions that rapidly develop into vesicles on an erythematous base. Oral vesicles that rapidly change to ulcers may be seen, but the oral lesions are not an important symptomatic, diagnostic, or management problem. HZ lesions may be confined to the mouth and face; therefore, this is a more important diagnostic problem for dentists (see Fig. 5-7).

HZ commonly has a prodromal period of 2 to 4 days, when shooting pain, paresthesia, burning, and tenderness appear along the course of the affected nerve. Unilateral vesicles on an erythematous base then appear in clusters, chiefly along the course of the nerve, giving the characteristic clinical picture of single dermatome involvement. Some lesions probably spread by viremia occur outside the dermatome. The vesicles turn to scabs in 1 week, and healing takes place in 2 to 3 weeks. The nerves most commonly affected with HZ are C3, T5, L1, L2 and the first division of the trigeminal nerve.

When the full clinical picture of HZ is present with pain and unilateral vesicles, the diagnosis is not difficult. Diagnostic problems arise during the prodromal period, when pain is present without lesions. Unnecessary surgery has been performed because of the diagnosis of acute appendicitis, cholecystitis, or dental pulpitis. A more difficult clinical problem is pain caused by VZ virus without

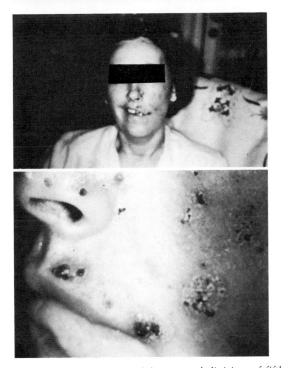

Fig. 5-7 Herpes zoster of the second division of fifth nerve.

lesions developing along the course of the nerve (herpes sine herpes; zoster sine eruption). Diagnosis in these cases is based on clinical symptoms and the serologic procedures described under primary herpes simplex infection.

The disease becomes more severe and complications more common in elderly and immunosuppressed patients. The complications include generalized HZ with involvement of internal organs and postherpetic neuralgia. Postherpetic neuralgia has been shown to be caused by inflammation and fibrosis of the affected nerve and may cause severe pain months or years after the skin lesions have healed.

HZ may also affect motor nerves. HZ of the sacral region often causes paralysis of the bladder. The extremities and diaphragm have also been paralyzed during episodes of HZ.

Oral Findings Twenty percent of HZ cases affect the cranial nerves. The trigeminal nerve is most commonly involved, but lesions of the eye and forehead caused by involvement of the first division are much more common than oral involvement because of infection of the second and third divisions. Hall studied 22 patients with HZ of the trigeminal nerve; 18 involved the first division, 2 the second, and 2 the third. This is consistent with findings of other workers who found the first division involved 15 to 20 times more frequently than the second and third divisions.

The individual oral lesions of HZ are similar to those seen with herpes simplex. The diagnosis is made on the basis of a history of pain and the unilateral nature and segmental distribution of the lesions (see Fig. 5-8). When the clinical appearance is typical and vesicles are present, oral HZ is easily differentiated from other acute multiple lesions of the mouth, which are bilateral and not preceded or accompanied by severe neurologic pain.

Because oral lesions occurring alone are rare, isolated oral lesions can be misdiagnosed particularly when erythema, edema, and nonspecific ulceration is seen without the presence of vesicles. In these cases, a cytology smear (preferably from the base of an intact vesicle), viral culture, or biopsy is necessary for diagnosis.

The pain of HZ may be localized to the tongue, palate, or teeth and may be misdiagnosed as pulpitis. The lesions may become confluent and necrotic, especially in immunosuppressed patients who may experience necrosis of underlying bone. HZ of the geniculate ganglion is a rare form of the disease causing Bell's palsy, unilateral vesicles of the external ear, and vesicles of the oral mucosa.

Laboratory Findings Giemsa-stained scrapings from the base of a fresh vesicle will show multinucleated giant cells and intranuclear inclusions. This can help differentiate HZ infection from other vesicular eruptions such as herpangina but not from herpes simplex virus infection, which has similar cytologic findings. Immunofluorescence may be used when proper laboratory equipment is available. VZ virus may be isolated in a variety of primary human tissue cultures including amnion. Demonstration of a rising antibody titer is rarely necessary for diagnosis except in

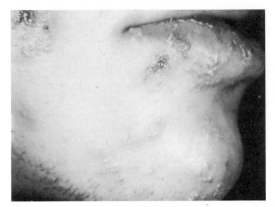

Fig. 5-8 Herpes zoster of the third division of fifth nerve, right side.

cases of herpes sine eruption, in which it is the only means of confirming suspected cases.

Treatment Treatment of HZ is symptomatic in uncomplicated cases of skin or mouth involvement. Disseminated HZ in immunosuppressed patients should be treated with vidarabine (Ara-A) or acyclovir. In patients over 60, corticosteroids should be administered to prevent or minimize the occurrence of postherpetic neuralgia. Keczkes in a controlled trial showed a significant reduction in the incidence of postherpetic neuralgia in patients taking steroids. No incidence of dissemination occurred. The management of postherpetic neuralgia is often difficult and unsatisfactory. Phenytoin (Dilantin) or carbamazepine (Tegretol) controls some cases, while alcohol block or nerve section may be necessary for intractable pain.

Erythema Multiforme

Erythema multiforme (EM) is an acute disease of the skin and mucous membranes that may cause several types of skin lesions, hence the name, *multiforme*. The oral lesions, typically rapidly rupturing vesicles and bullae, are often an important component of the clinical picture and are occasionally the only component. Erythema multiforme may occur once or recur and should be considered in the diagnosis of multiple acute oral ulcers whether or not there is a past history of similar lesions.

Etiology

There is evidence that EM is mediated by deposition of immune complexes in the superficial microvasculature of the skin and mucosa. Kazmierowski and Wuepper studied specimens of lesions less than 24 hours old from 17 patients with EM; 13 of the 17 had deposition of IgM and C3 in the superficial vessels. Safai and colleagues detected elevated levels of immune complexes and decreased complement in fluid samples taken from vesicles. Specific factors that trigger the immune complex vasculitis include food allergy, drug allergy, reactions to microorganisms, radiotherapy, underlying systemic disease, and neoplasia. The drugs most commonly related to an erythema multiforme reaction include antibiotics, barbiturates, phenylbutazone, and carbamazepine.

EM reactions have been related to a wide variety of bacterial, fungal, and viral infections, including *Mycoplasma*. Especially interesting are the reports of EM related to episodes of recurrent herpes labialis. Shelley reported that 15% of patients with recurrent EM have a preceding recurrent herpes simplex virus infection. The same author used herpes simplex antigen to skin test one of these patients, and EM lesions resulted.

Episodes of EM have been related to leiomyoma of the stomach and uterus as well as fibroma of the ovary. Other diseases related to EM include Crohn's disease of the bowel, Addison's disease, sarcoidosis, and carcinoma.

The majority of EM cases have no obvious related allergy or disease; many of these patients are extensively tested for underlying systemic disease and allergy with no positive result. Some cases are attributed to emotional causes; most are labeled *idiopathic*. Lazada and Silverman reported on the characteristics of 50 EM patients seen in an oral medicine clinic. Just over 50% of the cases were of unknown etiology, with stress or emotional factors the second largest category. Other significant categories included reactions to recurrent herpes simplex infection and allergy.

Clinical Manifestations

General Findings EM is seen most frequently in children and young adults. It has an acute or even an explosive onset; generalized symptoms such as fever and malaise appear in severe cases. A patient may be asymptomatic and in less than 24 hours have extensive lesions of the skin and mucosa. EM simplex is the least severe form of the disease and is characterized by macules and papules 0.5 cm to 2 cm in diameter, appearing in a symmetrical distribution. The vesiculobullous form of the disease is more severe and can cause extensive sloughing of skin leading to severe disability or occasionally death caused by secondary infection or fluid and electrolyte imbalance.

The most common cutaneous areas involved are the hands, feet, and the extensor surfaces of the elbows and knees. The face and neck are commonly involved, but only severe cases will affect the trunk. Generalized vesiculobullous EM of the skin, mouth, eyes, and genitals is called Stevens–Johnson syndrome, named after the two who described this clinical picture in 1922. The skin lesions of EM take many forms, but the pathognomonic target or iris lesion should be looked for in each case (Fig. 5-9). These lesions consist of a central bulla or pale area surrounded by edema and bands of erythema. Sometimes the lesions contain several concentric red bands.

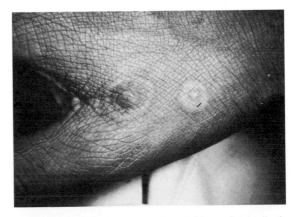

Fig. 5-9 Target lesions in patient with erythema multiforme.

Oral Findings Oral lesions commonly appear along with skin lesions (see Fig. 5-10). In some cases oral lesions are the predominant or single sign of disease. When the oral lesions predominate and no target lesions are present on the skin, EM must be differentiated from other causes of acute multiple ulcers, especially primary herpes simplex infection. This distinction is important because corticosteroids may be the treatment of choice in EM but they are specifically contraindicated in primary herpes simplex infections. A single oral lesion is not characteristic. When there are no skin lesions and the oral lesions are mild, diagnosis may be difficult and is usually made by exclusion of other diseases. Cytologic smears and virus isolation may be done to eliminate the possibility of primary herpes infection. Biopsy may be taken when acute pemphigus is suspected. The histologic picture of oral EM is not considered specific, but the finding of a perivascular lymphocytic infiltrate and epithelial edema and hyperplasia is considered suggestive of EM.

The diagnosis is made on the basis of the total clinical picture, including the rapid onset of lesions. The oral lesions start as bullae on an erythematous base, but intact bullae are rarely seen by the clinician, because they break rapidly into irregular ulcers (Figs. 5-11 and 5-12). Viral lesions are small, round, symmetrical, and shallow, but EM lesions are larger, irregular, deeper, and often bleed. Lesions may occur anywhere on the oral mucosa with EM, but involvement of the lips is especially prominent, and gingival involvement is rare. This is an important criterion for distinguishing EM from primary herpes simplex infection, in which generalized gingival involvement is characteristic. Kennett studied 9 cases of EM; 7 of the 9 patients had extensive labial lesions. Shklar studied 16 cases of EM in children; 8 had intraoral lesions, but all had lip lesions.

In full-blown clinical cases, the lips are extensively eroded, and large portions of the oral mucosa are denuded of epithelium. The patient cannot eat or even swallow and drools blood-tinged saliva. Within 2 or 3 days the labial lesions begin to crust. Healing occurs within 2 weeks in a majority of cases,

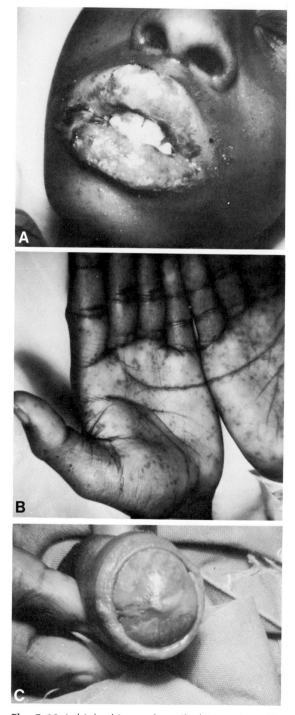

Fig. 5-10 Labial, skin, and penile lesions in a 17-year-old with erythema multiforme. The lesions began less than 12 hours before the pictures were taken.

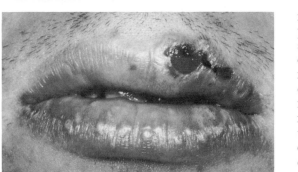

Fig. 5-11 Early vesicular lesions in a patient who develops erythema multiforme after each episode of recurrent herpes labialis.

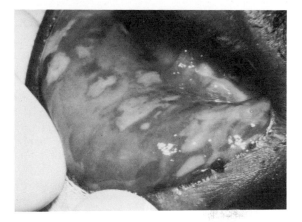

Fig. 5-12 Intraoral lesions of erythema multiforme in an 18-year-old male.

but in some severe cases extensive disease may continue for several weeks.

Treatment

Mild cases of oral EM may be treated with supportive measures only, including topical anesthetic mouthwashes and a soft or liquid diet. Patients who require intravenous fluid therapy to prevent electrolyte imbalance should be treated in consultation with a physician. Moderate to severe EM may be treated with a short course of systemic corticosteroids in patients with no contraindications to their use. Systemic corticosteroids should only be used by clinicians familiar with the side-effects, and in each case potential benefit should be carefully weighed against potential

risk. The protein-wasting and adrenal-suppressive effects of systemic steroids are not significant when their use is for a short-term effect, and the clinical course of the disease may be shortened. An initial dose of 30 mg/day to 50 mg/day prednisone or methylprednisolone for several days and then slowly reduced is considered helpful in shortening the healing time, particularly when started early in the course of the disease. Higher doses of steroids are necessary for severe cases. It should be noted that the efficacy of this treatment has not been proven by controlled clinical trials and is questioned by some authors.

Allergic Stomatitis

Antibody–antigen reactions may cause clinical diseases of the mouth and face. Anaphylactic or immediate type hypersensitivity reactions characterized by edema, such as urticaria and angioneurotic edema, are discussed in detail in the chapter on immunology. Allergic reactions may also cause acute multiple vesicles and ulcers of the oral mucosa. These reactions may result from a systemically administered antigen that causes a reaction either on both mucosa and skin or on the mucosa alone. Oral allergic reactions to systemically administered antigens, especially drugs, have had a variety of names in the literature, such as stomatitis medicamentosa. The lesions are characterized by inflammation, ulcers, and vesicles and are the same as in erythema multiforme localized to the oral mucosa. Separation of these two entities leads to unnecessary confusion, and the term stomatitis medicamentosa should be discarded.

Other oral vesicles and ulcers of allergic etiology should be distinguished from erythema multiforme: the fixed drug eruption and contact allergy. The fixed drug eruption is characterized by a localized area of erythema, edema, and vesiculation in a specific area of the skin or mucosa whenever a specific allergen is administered. This reaction is rare on the oral mucosa but has been reported as a reaction to barbiturates.

Contact allergy is caused by a delayed-type hypersensitivity reaction to topical antigens.

On the skin it is referred to as contact allergic dermatitis or dermatitis venenata, and the oral lesions are referred to as stomatitis venenata or contact stomatitis. The skin reaction may be caused by poison ivy, leather, rubber, nickel, medications, or other chemicals. The skin lesions are typically an itching, erythematous area with superficial vesicles directly at the site where the allergen contacted the skin (Fig. 5-13). The oral lesions are thought to occur less frequently than skin lesions, even when the same allergen has contacted both skin and oral mucosa. The reason for the decreased rate of oral contact allergy is most likely saliva, which dilutes allergens, washes them from the surface of the mucosa, and digests them with enzymes. Some investigators believe that the thick keratin layer of skin serves as a better source of protein for combination with haptens than the relatively thin layer of keratin present on some areas of the oral mucosa.

Clinical Manifestations

Stomatitis venenata, like other allergic reactions, can be caused by a wide variety of substances including chrome cobalt dentures, gold crowns, denture soft-lining material, chewing gum, dental amalgam, acrylic

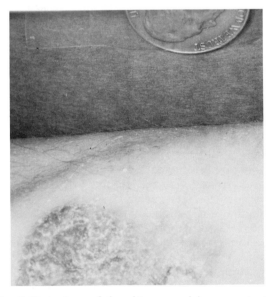

Fig. 5-13 Lesions of the skin caused by a contact allergy to nickel. Note inflammation and ulceration.

dentures, temporary fixed bridges, toothpaste, and orthodontic elastics.

Contact allergy to dental amalgam is usually caused by mercury, which is released during condensation. In most cases condensed amalgam will not cause a reaction even in patients with known sensitivity to mercury. Toothpaste contact allergy is rare but does occur. Most recently, Kirton reported 10 patients with an allergy to a highly flavored toothpaste (Close-Up); Millard reported three cases of allergy to the same toothpaste. The allergy was thought to be caused by the cinnamon oil present in the toothpaste. The clinical features included swelling, cracking, and fissuring of the lips, perioral desquamation and edema, angular cheilitis, swelling of the gingiva, and oral ulcers. All lesions disappeared within a week after discontinuing use of the toothpaste.

Allergy to acrylic is rare and usually caused by free monomer. This allergy is relatively common in dentists and dental technicians. Occasional reports of allergy to denture bases have been characterized by inflammation and angular cheilitis. Some of these reports were poorly documented and may have been denture sore-mouth secondary to chronic atrophic candidiasis rather than allergy. Bradford and Nealy reported cases confirmed by patch tests.

The clinical appearance of stomatitis venenata is difficult to differentiate from trauma. Erythema, edema, and in severe cases, ulceration at the site of contact is the hallmark of the disease. Although itching is a characteristic complaint of the skin, burning is the common complaint on the oral mucosa.

Kerr reported 12 cases of allergy secondary to gum chewing. The patients complained of burning of the tongue and gingiva. Examination showed erythema and ulceration of the buccal mucosa, atrophy of the lingual filiform papillae, and edema of the tongue. The lesions cleared when the gum chewing stopped. Skin tests were not performed to confirm the allergy.

Diagnosis

The patch test is the only test that can be used to distinguish contact allergy from other lesions. In this test the suspected allergen is placed on normal nonhairy skin. The best test site is the upper portion of the back. The test substance is covered in most instances and allowed to remain in contact with the skin for 48 hours. The patch is removed, and 2 to 4 hours later the area examined for persistent erythema. Further details of this technique can be obtained from Maxey, Adams, and Fisher.

Patch testing of the skin may not be reliable in diagnosis of hypersensitivity reactions confined to the oral mucosa. Patch testing directly on the oral mucosa has been attempted by incorporating the test substance in Orabase, by use of a prosthetic appliance to hold the substance in place, or by use of a rubber cup attached to the teeth.

Treatment

Management of stomatitis venenata depends on the severity of the lesions. In mild cases removal of the allergen will suffice. In severe cases with extensive erythema or ulceration, application of a topical corticosteroid preparation is helpful.

Oral Ulcers Secondary to Cancer Chemotherapy

Chemotherapeutic drugs are frequently used to cause remission of both solid tumors and hematologic malignancies. The four major types of anticancer drugs are as follows:

1. Alkylating agents (cyclophosphamide, chlorambucil)
2. Antimetabolites (methotrexate, 6-mercaptopurine)
3. Antibiotics (adriamycin, actinomycin D, bleomycin)
4. Alkaloids (vincristine, vinblastine). These drugs are used singly or in combination to treat a wide variety of malignant diseases.

One of the common side-effects of the anticancer drugs is multiple oral ulcers. Dentists who practice in hospitals where these drugs are used extensively may see oral ulcers secondary to such drug therapy more frequently than any other lesion described in this chapter.

Anticancer drugs may cause oral ulcers directly or indirectly. Drugs that cause stomatitis indirectly depress the bone marrow and immune response leading to invasive infections of the oral mucosa. Others, such as methotrexate, cause oral ulcers by direct effect on the replication and growth of oral epithelial cells by interfering with nucleic acid and protein synthesis and leading to thinning and ulceration of the oral mucosa. Oral ulcers may be an early sign of drug toxicity and in some cases may warrant reduction of drug dosage or complete cessation of therapy.

Drugs that commonly cause oral ulcers include methotrexate, 5-fluorouracil, actinomycin D, adriamycin, bleomycin, and daunorubicin. Drugs that occasionally cause oral ulcers include 6-mercaptopurine, hydroxyurea, vinblastine, and procarbazine.

Jaffee and colleagues treated 10 patients with methotrexate. The most frequent side-effect was ulceration of the lips and buccal mucosa. Metzger and colleagues studied 22 patients taking methotrexate. Stomatitis severe enough to require reducing the dose of the drug was present in eight patients.

Bleomycin is an antitumor antibiotic used to treat squamous cell carcinoma of the head and neck. Huntington and colleagues found oral ulcers to be the most distressing side-effect. The oral ulcers began within 2 weeks after initiation of therapy and lasted for 2 weeks after therapy was completed. Nutrition was impaired during the period of oral disease. Cohen, as well as Halnan, found ulcers of the lips, buccal mucosa, and tongue in their patients taking bleomycin.

Cortes and co-workers studied 31 patients taking adriamycin for bronchogenic carcinoma; 23 developed severe stomatitis, characterized by ulceration of the buccal mucosa, palate, and tongue. Blum and Carter observed stomatitis in 80% of their patients taking adriamycin. The stomatitis began as a burning sensation with erythema and ulceration following in 2 to 3 days.

Dreizen and co-workers reviewed the records of 570 patients receiving chemotherapy for leukemia; 20% developed stomatitis. The severity of stomatitis was not drug or dose specific. The dentist may examine patients taking chemotherapy for either diagnosis or management. He may be asked to give his opinion concerning whether the stomatitis results from chemotherapy or other causes such as allergy or viral infection. The oral lesions secondary to chemotherapeutic drugs are characteristically deep, large, necrotic ulcers with no tissue tags and a minimal inflammatory base that may affect all mucosal surfaces (see Fig. 5-14). They may be distinguished clinically from other types of acute, multiple ulcers both by a history of recent chemotherapy and by clinical appearance of the lesions (see Fig. 5-15). Acute viral lesions are shallow, round, symmetrical, and surrounded by inflammation and have tissue tags from ruptured vesicles. Lesions from allergic reactions and erythema multiforme show evidence of an acute inflammatory reaction. They are surrounded by inflammation, may bleed, and have tissue tags from ruptured bullae. Recurrent aphthous lesions are also smaller, more symmetrical, and demonstrate clinical signs of an inflammatory rather than an atrophic process.

Severe oral lesions secondary to chemotherapy requires reduction of the dose or stopping medication. This is often not possible, and oral ulcers like alopecia and myelosuppression are the price that must be paid for successful tumor remission. All ulcers should be cultured because they are often infected with gram-negative bacilli and may lead to fatal septicemia. Ulcers should be biopsied when chronic fungal infection is suspected.

To increase patient comfort, topical anesthetic mouthrinses such as dyclonine (Dyclone) or diphenhydramine hydrochloride (Benadryl) may be used. Oral hygiene rinses with bland mouthwashes should be prescribed to cleanse the lesions. Tetracycline mouthrinses or 0.5% povidone iodine solu-

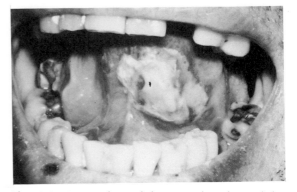

Fig. 5-15 Large ulcer of the ventral surface of the tongue in a leukemic patient receiving chemotherapy with daunorubicin.

tions can be used to attempt to reduce the incidence of secondary infection. A potent antimicrobial agent, chlorhexidine, has been used with success but has not been approved for use as a mouthrinse in the United States.

Patients taking antimetabolites are often mentally depressed due to the terminal nature of their disease. Dentists not accustomed to managing terminal patients may tend to spend as little time with these patients as possible. This impulse should be resisted. Words of kindness and friendly conversation are often considerably more helpful than a prescription for a topical anesthetic mouthrinse.

Acute Necrotizing Ulcerative Gingivitis

A gingivitis associated with large numbers of fusospirochetal organisms and other microbial forms may vary from an extremely acute reaction in which painful ulcerative, necrotic, and membranous lesions predominate, to chronic infections with few symptoms. The extent of involvement of the gingival and oral tissues and the accompanying systemic reactions vary greatly.

Acute necrotizing ulcerative gingivitis (ANUG) is found most often in the adolescent and young adult, and although poor oral hygiene is common and an important predisposing cause, the disease may occur in individuals with relatively good oral hygiene (see Fig. 5-16). Inadequate nutrition, hematologic disorders, insufficient rest, and heavy smok-

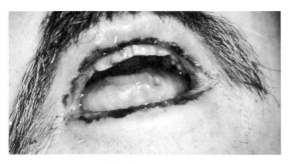

Fig. 5-14 Ulcers of the lips and tongue in a cancer patient receiving methotrexate.

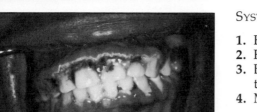

Fig. 5-16 Acute necrotizing ulcerative gingivitis.

ing may predispose to this disease. Pindborg found ANUG in 10.7% of those smoking over 10 cigarettes per day, compared with 1.5% in nonsmoking subjects.

The actual prevalence of this disease in the United States is not known. Giddon and colleagues studied the prevalence of ANUG in 12,500 students served by the Harvard University Dental Health Service. About 0.9% of the total sample developed ANUG during the period of study. A 4% prevalence in those students who made use of the dental clinic was observed. Members of the junior class were most often affected. A relation to stress was noted as evidenced by an increased frequency related to examination and vacation periods.

A characteristic symbiosis of the fusospirochetal organisms is observed in the clinical lesions of this condition. The *Borrelia vincentii* and the *Fusobacterium dentium* are predominant with respect to numbers, but other organisms of the oral flora are also present.

Predisposing factors of major importance in determining the clinical onset of this disease include the following:

LOCAL FACTORS

1. Pericoronitis
2. Overhanging margins of restorations, ill-fitting crowns, inlays, or prosthetic appliances; inadequate contact areas resulting from dental caries or faulty restorations and food impaction
3. Any local area of poor oral hygiene
4. Preexisting marginal gingivitis
5. Smoking

SYSTEMIC FACTORS

1. Emotional stress
2. Fatigue
3. Blood dyscrasias, including depression of the bone marrow and leukemia
4. Malnutrition

The importance of fusospirochetal microorganisms in the clinical development of ANUG is questioned by some clinicians, since these organisms frequently are found in small numbers in mouths with poor oral hygiene in which neither subjective nor objective manifestations of this disease are present. This should not be disturbing. The fusospirochetal organisms are present in such overwhelming numbers in ANUG that it is unlikely that they are merely "innocent bystanders." In contrast with the large numbers of these microbial forms in the lesions of ANUG, there are relatively few of these microbial forms in oral decubital, oral herpetic, and aphthous ulcerations.

Nutritional deficiencies *per se* are not the chief systemic predisposing cause of this disease, nor is ANUG the result of nicotinic acid deficiency, as has been suggested by several clinicians. Fields found many and varied manifestations of deficiency diseases among the prison-camp inmates in the Philippines, but ANUG was rare. Two important predisposing factors have been observed: smoking or recent extractions—the majority of the smokers used more than 1 pack of cigarettes per day—and a history of acute anxiety, which was usually experienced 1 or 2 weeks before the onset of the disease.

Kardachi and Clarke reviewed the literature regarding the etiology of ANUG. They noted that the known predisposing factors such as stress and smoking may influence the gingival circulation and postulated that the lesion of ANUG is due to aseptic necrosis of the gingival epithelium secondary to inadequate blood flow.

The preponderance of evidence indicates that ANUG is an endogenous infection and is therefore not communicable. During World War II, Dean and Singleton made careful epidemiologic studies on U.S. Coast Guard and U.S. Maritime personnel. There was no evidence that ANUG was easily transmissible. There is no justification requiring the reporting of this disease and negative smear findings as criteria of cure.

Clinical Manifestations

The onset of acute forms of the disease is usually sudden, with pain, tenderness, profuse salivation, a peculiar metallic taste, and spontaneous bleeding from the gingival tissues. The patient commonly experiences a loss of the sense of taste and a diminished pleasure from smoking. The teeth are frequently thought to be slightly extruded, sensitive to pressure, or to have a "woody sensation." At times they are slightly movable. Barnes and associates studied 218 cases of ANUG. The signs they noted most frequently were gingival bleeding and blunting of the interdental papillae.

The typical lesions of ANUG consist of necrotic, punched-out ulcerations, developing most commonly on the interdental papillae and the marginal gingivae (see Fig. 5-16). This ulceration can be most easily observed on the interdental papillae (see Fig. 5-17), but ulceration may develop on the cheeks, the lips, and the tongue where these tissues come in contact with the gingival lesions or following trauma. Ulcerations also may be found on the palate and in the pharyngeal area (Fig. 5-18). When the lesions have spread beyond the gingivae, blood dyscrasias should be ruled out by ordering a total and differential white blood cell count.

The ulcerative lesions may progress to involve the alveolar process, with sequestration of the teeth and bone (see Figs. 5-19 and 5-20). When gingival hemorrhage is a prominent symptom, the teeth may become superficially stained a brown color, and the mouth odor is extremely offensive.

The tonsils should always be examined, since these organs may be affected. The regional lymph nodes usually are slightly enlarged, but occasionally the lymphadenopathy may be marked, particularly in children.

The constitutional symptoms in primary ANUG are usually of minor significance when compared with the severity of the oral lesions. Significant temperature elevation is unusual even in severe cases, and when it exists other accompanying or underlying diseases should be ruled out, including blood dyscrasias and primary herpetic gingivostomatitis.

Treatment

The therapy of ANUG uncomplicated by other oral lesions or systemic disease is local debridement. At the initial visit the gingivae should be debrided with both irrigation and periodontal curettage. The extent of the debridement depends upon the soreness of the gingivae. The clinician should remember that the more quickly the local factors are removed the faster will be the resolution of the lesions. Special care should be taken by the clinician to debride the area just below the marginal gingivae. Complete debridement may not be possible on the first visit because of the soreness. The patient must return, although the pain and other symptoms disappear, to remove all remaining local factors.

Treatment of ANUG is not finished until

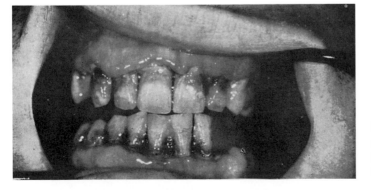

Fig. 5-17 Extensive necrosis of the interdental papillae; marginal and attached gingivae are caused by extensive fusospirochetal gingivitis.

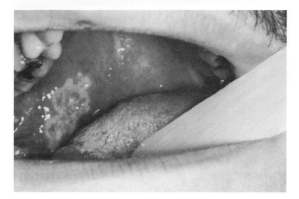

Fig. 5-18 Palatal ulceration in a 21-year-old male with fusopirochetal stomatitis that began as a necrotizing lesion of a pericoronal flap.

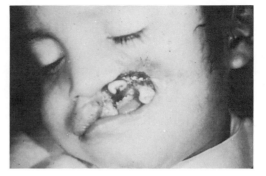

Fig. 5-19 Cancrum oris or noma. (Courtesy of Dr. Gustavo Berger, Guatemala City, Guatemala)

there has been a complete gingival curettage and root planing including removing overhanging margins and all other predisposing local factors. After the first visit, careful home care instruction must be given to the patient regarding vigorous rinsing and gentle brushing with a soft brush. Patients should be made aware of the significance of such factors as poor oral hygiene, smoking, and stress.

Antibiotics are usually not necessary for routine cases of ANUG confined to the marginal and interdental gingivae. These cases can be successfully treated with local debridement, irrigation, curettage, and home care instruction including hydrogen peroxide (approximately 1.5% to 2% in water) mouth rinses three times a day.

With extensive gingival involvement, lymphadenopathy, or other systemic signs and cases in which mucosa other than the gingivae is involved, antibiotics should be considered. Penicillin is the drug of choice in patients with no history of sensitivity to the drug. Patients whose lesions have extended from the gingivae to the buccal mucosa, tongue, palate, or pharynx should be placed on antibiotics and should have appropriate studies to rule out systemic diseases such as blood dyscrasias. After the disease is resolved the patient should return for a complete periodontal evaluation. Periodontal treatment should be instituted as necessary. The patient must be made aware that unless the local etiologic factors of the disease are removed ANUG may return.

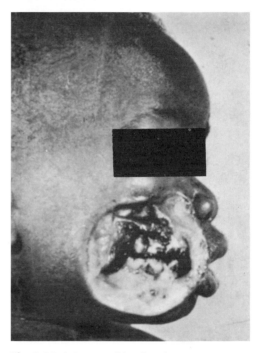

Fig. 5-20 A 3-year-old girl with cancrum oris. Slough has separated, exposing much of the bone of lower and upper jaw. (Emslie RD: Oral Pathol Child 90:105, 1952)

THE PATIENT WITH RECURRING ORAL ULCERS

Recurring oral ulcers are among the most common clinical problems seen by clinicians who manage diseases of the oral mucosa. There are several diseases that should be included in the differential diagnosis of a patient who presents with a history of recurring ulcers of the mouth including recurrent aphthous stomatitis, Behçet's syndrome, recurrent HSV infection, recurrent erythema multiforme, and cyclic neutropenia.

Recurrent Aphthous Stomatitis

Recurrent aphthous stomatitis (RAS) is a disorder characterized by recurring ulcers confined to the oral mucosa in patients with no other signs of disease. Many specialists and investigators in oral medicine no longer consider RAS to be a single disease but rather several pathologic states with similar clinical manifestations. Immunologic disorders, nutritional deficiencies, and hormonal abnormalities have all been implicated in cases of RAS.

Patients with RAS are classified in three categories depending on the clinical presentation of the lesions: minor ulcers, major ulcers (Sutton's disease; periadenitis mucosa necrotica recurrens) and herpetiform ulcers. Minor ulcers are less than 1 cm in diameter and heal without scars. Major ulcers are over 1 cm in diameter and scar on healing. Herpetiform ulcers are considered a distinct clinical entity that manifest as recurrent crops of dozens of small ulcers that appear throughout the oral mucosa.

Etiology

It was once assumed that RAS was a form of recurrent HSV infection, and there are still clinicians who mistakenly refer to RAS as "herpes." In the early 1950s, studies performed by Blank and associates and Stark and colleagues as well as by Dodd and Ruchman, demonstrated by use of viral isolation techniques, antibody studies, and biopsies that herpes simplex virus was not the etiologic agent of RAS. These studies were confirmed by Ship and associates in 1961 and by Griffin in 1963 and reconfirmed by MacFarlane in 1974. Investigations are still underway to determine whether another virus, particularly a latent virus, is a cause of RAS. These studies are particularly active in the area of herpetiform ulcers, where inclusion bodies suggestive of virus infection have been detected in biopsy specimens. The majority of current investigators regard RAS as

an abnormality of the immune response. Some investigators categorize RAS with the autoimmune diseases; others consider it an abnormal immunologic reaction to antigens of oral bacteria, particularly *Streptococcus sanguis* 2A.

Evidence for the autoimmune nature of the disease includes studies by Lehner, who demonstrated binding of immunoglobulins and complement in the cytoplasm of oral mucosal cells of RAS patients. Another study by Lehner showed an increase in hemagglutinating antibody to an extract of fetal oral mucosa in RAS patients. Both of these studies suggest a role for antibody in the formation of RAS lesions. In another study, Lehner's results suggest a possible role for cellular immunity in the formation of RAS. The lymphocytes of 28 RAS patients, 12 control patients, and 13 patients with other oral ulcers were tested for cellular immune reaction to oral mucosa using the lymphocyte transformation test. Twelve of the RAS patients were positive reactors; none of the controls was positive. One RAS patient was tested during lesions and during remissions; lymphocyte transformation was positive during lesions and negative during remissions.

Other experimental work that supports an autoimmune hypothesis for RAS includes work by Dolby, who demonstrated that lymphocytes from RAS patients decrease the survival time of oral epithelial cells, and Rogers, who found an increased lymphocytotoxicity for oral mucosal cells in RAS patients.

Evidence implicating an immunologic reaction to S. sanguis 2A has been accumulating since 1963 when Barile and then Stanley and colleagues isolated this organism from RAS lesions. These initial studies met with skepticism, because S. sanguis is a normal component of the oral flora and could be a secondary containment of the lesions. Evidence that has strengthened the theory includes work by Graykowski and associates, which showed an increased delayed hypersensitivity reaction to S. sanguis among RAS patients. *In vitro* evidence has been added to the clinical studies since 1972, when Donatsky and Bendixen demonstrated cellular hypersensitivity to S. sanguis 2A in RAS patients using the leukocyte migration test.

In 1974 Donatsky and Dabelsteen studied

humoral immunity to *S. sanguis* 2A by the immunofluorescent technique. RAS patients had antibody to *S. sanguis* 2A but not to *Neisseria,* another normal component of the oral flora. These results support the concept that the immune reaction to *S. sanguis* 2A is specific, rather than a general reaction to the oral flora. This experimental evidence is confused somewhat by the results of an experiment by Francis and Oppenheim in 1970, which showed a decreased immune reactivity to *S. sanguis* 2A in RAS patients. In summary, considerable evidence shows that RAS is accompanied by an altered immune response. Whether this response is the primary cause of the disease awaits further investigation.

The relationship of RAS to psychological and social factors has been studied extensively. Epidemiologic studies by Ship and others were designed to study logically the possible effects of these factors on the occurrence of RAS. A major relationship was found between socioeconomic groups and RAS. Patients with higher social status had a considerably higher incidence of RAS. The personality of RAS patients was characterized as rigid, striving, and inflexible.

An inherited predisposition to RAS has also been described. Miller and co-workers studied 1,303 children from 530 families and demonstrated an increased susceptibility to RAS among children of RAS-positive parents. A study by Ship and associates showed that patients with RAS-positive parents had a 90% chance of developing RAS whereas patients with no RAS parents had a 20% chance of developing the lesions. Further evidence for the inherited nature of this disorder results from studies in which genetically specific HLA antigens have been identified in RAS patients.

Nutritional deficiency may be a contributing factor to RAS in a small percentage of patients. Wray and co-workers found that approximately 15% of RAS patients studied had a deficiency of serum iron, folate, or vitamin B_{12}. A majority of these deficient patients benefited from specific replacement therapy. Challacombe and colleagues found nutritional deficiency in approximately 7% of RAS patients. Ferguson reported that celiac disease is a contributing factor in a small percentage (5%) of patients with RAS and rec-

ommended that RAS patients with decreased whole blood folate have a jejunal biopsy to rule out celiac disease.

Clinical Manifestations

The first episodes of RAS most frequently begin during the second decade of life. The lesions are confined to the oral mucosa and begin with prodromal burning anytime from 2 to 48 hours before an ulcer appears. During this initial period a localized area of erythema develops. Within hours, a small white papule forms, ulcerates, and gradually enlarges over the next 48 to 72 hours. The individual lesions are round, symmetrical, and shallow (similar to viral ulcers), but no tissue tags are present from ruptured vesicles (see Fig. 5-21; this helps to distinguish RAS from disease with irregular ulcers such as EM, pemphigus, and pemphigoid). Multiple lesions are often present, but the number, size, and frequency of them vary considerably (Fig. 5-22). The

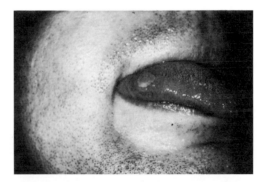

Fig. 5-21 Recurrent aphthous stomatitis of the tongue.

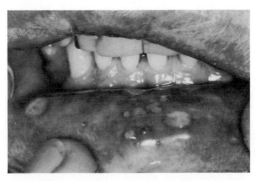

Fig. 5-22 Recurrent aphthous stomatitis of the lip in a 45-year-old female.

buccal and labial mucosa are most commonly involved. Lesions are less common on the heavily keratinized palate or gingiva. In mild RAS, the lesions reach a size of 0.3 cm to 1.0 cm and begin healing within a week. Healing without scarring is usually complete in 10 to 14 days.

Most patients with RAS have between two and six lesions at each episode and experience several episodes a year. The disease is an annoyance for the majority of patients with mild RAS, but it can be disabling for patients with severe, frequent lesions especially those classified as major aphthous ulcers. Patients with major ulcers develop deep lesions that are larger than 1 cm in diameter and may reach 5 cm (see Fig. 5-23). Large portions of the oral mucosa may be covered with large, deep painful ulcers that can become confluent. The lesions are extremely painful and interfere with speech and eating (Fig. 5-24). Many of these patients continually go from one clinician to another looking for a "cure." The lesions may last for months causing confusion with squamous cell carcinoma, chronic granulomatous disease, or pemphigoid. The lesions heal slowly leaving scars that may result in decreased mobility of the uvula and tongue and destruction of portions of the oral mucosa.

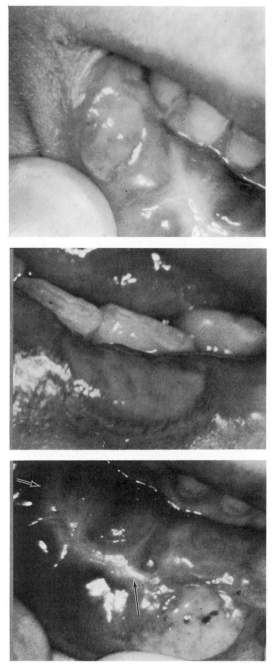

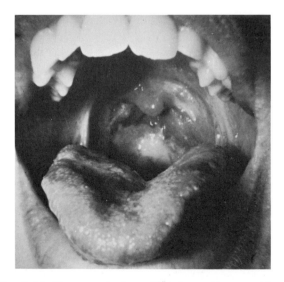

Fig. 5-23 Pharyngeal ulcerations in a 17-year-old patient with continuous recurrent aphthous stomatitis for 5 years.

Fig. 5-24 Recurrent aphthous stomatitis of the lower lip of a 23-year-old woman with a 14-year history of periodic mucosal ulcerations. Lesions are large, extremely painful, and persist for several months, characteristic of major aphthous stomatitis. Note the extensive scarring of the lip in adjacent areas.

Diagnosis

The diagnosis of RAS in both the minor and major forms is basically one of exclusion. Characteristic is the patient with round symmetrical recurring ulcers confined to the oral mucosa that heal spontaneously with no other signs or symptoms. The history and examination should exclude lesions of the skin, conjunctiva, genitalia, or rectum. Laboratory tests should be performed to rule out blood dyscrasias.

Treatment

Proper management of RAS includes more than the application of medication. Clinicians are often surprised that the intensity of the complaint is not matched by the severity of the clinical lesions. Patients may complain of severe pain, and the clinician may see only two or three relatively small lesions causing him to dismiss the patient with a quick home remedy. This management often leads to multiple consultations, myriad remedies, and confusion. Time should be spent reassuring the patient of the local nature of the disease and informing him that there are no sure, quick cures, only palliative therapy.

Medications prescribed should depend on the severity of the disease. In mild cases with two or three small lesions, the application of a topical protective emollient such as Orabase is all that is necessary. In more severe cases the use of topical corticosteroid preparations is helpful in decreasing the healing time of the lesions. Preparations such as triamcinolone or fluorometholone may be applied topically to the lesions four times daily, after eating and at bedtime.

In cases of severe RAS, treatment with topical tetracycline should be considered, but the potential benefits must always be weighed against the risk of allergic reaction and oral candidiasis. Guggenheimer and associates demonstrated that tetracycline mouthrinses reduced the healing time of RAS lesions by 50%, but noted that erythema multiforme, hives, and candidiasis occurred in a small number of patients. Graykowski and Kingman carried out a double-blind controlled study of tetracycline in patients with RAS; tetracycline decreased the severity, pain, and healing time of the lesions.

One method of using the topical tetracycline is to dissolve the contents of one capsule (250 mg) in 50 ml of water and use this mixture as an oral rinse four times a day. Increased contact of the medication with larger lesions can be obtained by placing the antibiotic solution on a gauze pad and using this as a compress directly on the lesion. In refractile cases of major RAS, steroid lozenges may be helpful. Recently, several double-blind controlled studies have been carried out examining the effect of levamisole, an immunomodulating drug thought to have promise in the treatment of RAS. It was not proven effective, and up to one third of the patients experienced side-effects of nausea, dysgeusia, or hyperosmia.

Behçet's Disease

Behçet's disease, described by the Turkish dermatologist Hulushi Behçet, was classically described as a triad of symptoms including recurring oral ulcers, recurring genital ulcers, and eye lesions. As more cases are reported in the literature, the concept of the disease has changed from a triad of signs and symptoms to the concept of a multisystem that remains elusive. The highest incidence of Behçet's disease has been reported in Japan and the eastern Mediterranean, but cases have been reported worldwide including North America. The incidence of the disease in Japan appears to have increased severalfold in the last 20 to 25 years; the reason is unclear.

Etiology

Behçet's disease is currently considered to be caused by circulating immune complexes that lead to vasculitis of small and medium-sized blood vessels. These complexes have been detected in areas of active disease. Studies of the immune abnormalities associated with Behçet's disease have included findings described above in patients with recurrent aphthous stomatitis (RAS). This has led some investigators to believe that Behçet's disease and RAS are both manifestations of a similar disorder of the immune response.

Another area of investigation of Behçet's syndrome is its relationship to environmental pollutants. In Japan some evidence relates Behçet's to presence of polychlorinated biphenyls (PCBs) and DDT (chlorophenothane).

Clinical Manifestations

The most common single site of involvement of Behçet's disease is the oral mucosa (see Fig. 5-25). Recurring oral ulcers appear in over 90% of patients; these lesions cannot be distinguished from RAS. Some Behçet's patients experience mild recurring oral lesions; others have the deep, large scarring lesions characteristic of major RAS. These lesions may appear anywhere on the oral or pharyngeal mucosa. The genital area is the second most common site of involvement and includes ulcers of the scrotum and penis in males and ulcers of the labia in females. The eye lesions consist of uveitis, retinal vasculitis, optic atrophy, conjunctivitis, and keratitis.

Generalized involvement occurs in over half of Behçet patients. Skin lesions are common and usually manifest as large pustular lesions. These lesions may be precipitated by trauma, and it is common for Behçet's patients to have a cutaneous hyperreactivity to minor trauma (pathergy). The finding of a pustule forming 24 hours after a needle puncture is considered diagnostic. Arthritis, usually involving one or two large joints, is common. The affected joint may be red and swollen as in rheumatoid arthritis, but involvement of small joints of the hand does not occur, and permanent disability does not result.

In some patients central nervous system involvement is the most distressing component of the disease. This may include brainstem syndrome, involvement of the cranial nerves, or neurologic degeneration resembling multiple sclerosis. Other reported signs of Behçet's syndrome include thrombophlebitis, intestinal ulceration, venous thrombosis, and psychiatric disease. Laboratory changes may include leukocytosis, eosinophilia, hypergammaglobulinemia, and an increased erythrocyte sedimentation rate.

Diagnosis

An international symposium on Behçet's disease was held in Istanbul, Turkey in 1977, but one universally accepted definition was not possible. One set of criteria for the diagnosis of Behçet's disease was published by Mason and Barnes, who described four major diagnostic criteria and six minor criteria. The major criteria included: recurring oral ulcers, recurring genital ulcers, eye lesions, and skin lesions. The minor diagnostic criteria included: gastrointestinal lesions, vascular lesions, cardiovascular lesions, arthritis, central nervous system involvement, and a positive family history. Using this system a positive diagnosis is made when three major criteria or two major and two minor criteria are present. These criteria appear to be a reasonable guideline for diagnosis, but the clinician should be aware that they do not exclude all other inflammatory diseases, which explains why a universally acceptable definition remains elusive.

Treatment

Management of Behçet's disease depends on the extent of its clinical manifestations. Patients with severe systemic involvement are treated with systemic corticosteroids and an immunosuppressive agent such as azathioprine or cyclophosphamide. Treatment for oral lesions is similar to that for RAS lesions. Use of fibrinolytic agents, transfer factor, and colchicine have been advocated, but no controlled studies have been performed, and even preliminary reports have been inconclusive.

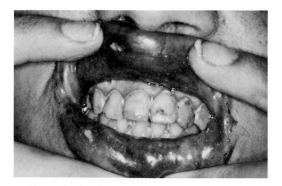

Fig. 5-25 Ulcers of the labial mucosa in a 22-year-old female with Behçet's syndrome. (Courtesy of Dr. Robert Arm)

Recurrent Herpes Simplex Virus Infection

Recurrent herpes infection of the mouth (recurrent herpes labialis; recurrent intraoral herpes simplex infection) occurs in patients who have experienced a previous herpes simplex infection and who have serum antibody protection against another exogenous primary infection. In otherwise healthy individuals, the recurrent infection is confined to a localized portion of the skin or mucous membranes. The weight of evidence suggests that recurrent herpes is not a reinfection but a reactivation of virus that remains latent in nerve tissue between episodes in a nonreplicating state. Herpes simplex has been cultured from the trigeminal ganglion of human cadavers, and recurrent herpes lesions commonly appear after surgery involving the ganglion. The virus travels down the nerve trunk to infect epithelial cells spreading from cell to cell causing a lesion.

The published evidence demonstrating that RAS is not caused by herpes virus induced many to believe that recurrent herpes infection of the oral region occurred only on the lips and not on the oral mucosa; this has been shown to be false. RAS and intraoral herpes can both exist intraorally and are two separate and distinct disease processes. In 1965, Griffin documented four cases of recurrent intraoral herpes (RIH) using fluorescent antibody-staining of cytology smears. In 1969, Greenberg and colleagues carried out a controlled study of 140 hospitalized patients; five of these patients developed RIH, which was identified by virus isolation, cytology, and antibody studies. As a result of this study, clinical criteria for distinguishing RIH from RAS were suggested (see below). These clinical distinctions were confirmed by Weathers and Griffin.

All patients who experience primary herpes infection do not experience recurrent herpes. Tokumaru suggested that a decrease in serum IgA may be associated with the lesions, but this has not been confirmed by others. Greenberg and Brightman tested levels of serum immunoglobulins in 78 patients susceptible to recurrent herpes infection. They found that low levels of serum IgA may be related to the development of RIH but not recurrent herpes labialis (RHL). Wilton and others related the development of RHL to a decrease in cell-mediated immunity, particularly lymphokin activity, while Heineman and Greenberg found a relationship between cell-protective antiherpes activity in saliva and RHL. Cell-protective activity was significantly higher in susceptible patients who did not develop RHL, and this same salivary activity fell sharply during episodes of RHL.

Patients with T lymphocytic deficiencies such as kidney transplant patients taking immunosuppressive drugs or patients with hematologic malignancies may develop disseminated recurrent herpes infection; chronic herpes may also develop in immunosuppressed patients (see chronic oral ulcers).

Clinical Manifestations

RHL, the common cold sore or fever blister, may be precipitated by fever, menstruation, ultraviolet light, and perhaps emotional stress. The lesions are preceded by a prodromal period of tingling or burning. This is accompanied by edema at the site of the lesion, followed by formation of a cluster of small vesicles (Fig. 5-26). Each vesicle is from 1 mm to 3 mm in diameter with the size of the cluster ranging from 1 cm to 2 cm. Occasionally, the lesions may be several centimeters in diameter, causing discomfort and disfigurement (these larger lesions are more common in immunosuppressed individuals). Frequency of recurrences varies.

RIH lesions are similar in appearance to RHL lesions, but the vesicles break rapidly to form ulcers. The lesions are typically a cluster of small vesicles or ulcers, 1 mm to 2

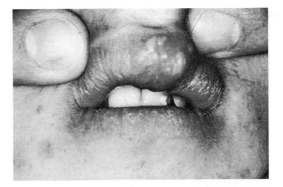

Fig. 5-26 Multiple vesicles of recurrent herpes labialis.

mm in diameter, clustered on a small portion of the heavily keratinized mucosa of the gingiva, palate, and alveolar ridges (see Fig. 5-27). In contrast, lesions of recurrent aphthous stomatitis tend to be larger, spread over a larger area of mucosa, and have a predilection for the less heavily keratinized buccal mucosa, labial mucosa, or floor of the mouth.

Diagnosis

If laboratory tests are desired, RIH can be distinguished from RAS by cytology smears taken from the base of a fresh lesion. Smears from herpetic lesions will show cells with ballooning degeneration and multinucleated giant cells; RAS lesions will not. Viral cultures will distinguish herpes simplex from varicella zoster infections.

Treatment

Recurrent herpes infections of the lips and mouth are seldom more than a temporary annoyance in otherwise normal individuals and should be treated only symptomatically. Some patients with severe RHL are so uncomfortable or disfigured during episodes that they seek professional consultation.

Many forms of RHL treatment have been advocated, but most have not withstood the scrutiny of well-controlled clinical trials, including photodynamic inactivation, smallpox vaccinations, and topical ether.

The placebo effect must be considered when evaluating drug activity against RHL. Terezhalmy and associates carried out a double-blind controlled study of a bioflavinoid ascorbic acid complex. They reported a decrease in healing time from 10 to 4 days and speculated that the decrease in healing time resulted from decreased capillary permeability. Preliminary studies also report beneficial results with intradermal injections of influenza virus vaccine and AMP. The studies were not controlled.

Idoxuridine (IDU) has been used parenterally in the treatment of generalized herpes and topically for ocular herpes. It has not been shown effective when used topically to treat RHL.

Vidarabine (Ara-A) is less toxic than is IDU and has been used successfully when administered parenterally for patients with neonatal herpes and topically for ocular herpetic infection. Ara-A and Ara-AMP, a water-soluble derivative of Ara-A, were tested in placebo-controlled, double-blind trials in the

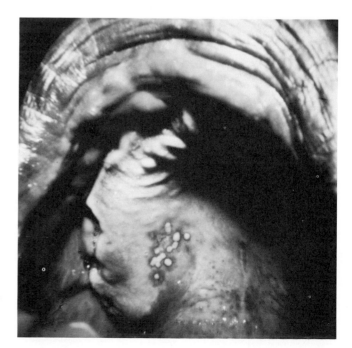

Fig. 5-27 Typical lesions of recurrent intraoral herpes simplex virus infection. A cluster of small vesicles and ulcers of the heavily keratinized oral mucosa.

treatment of RHL. Both were ineffective, presumably because skin penetration of the medication was inadequate. The results on intraoral ulcers or opened skin vesicles may differ.

Encouraging results have been published regarding the antiherpes effect of acyclovir, a drug that produces its antimetabolic activity only in cells infected with herpes virus. Normal cells are not affected. The drug has already been approved for topical use in patients with primary genital herpes and for immunosuppressed patients with herpes infections. Intravenous acyclovir has been tested on immunosuppressed patients and was shown to be a potent, nontoxic, antiherpes agent that appeared more effective than IDU or vidarabine.

THE PATIENT WITH CHRONIC MULTIPLE LESIONS

This group of disorders is frequently misdiagnosed for weeks to months. Because they may be confused with recurring oral mucosal disorders, the clinician will avoid misdiagnosis by carefully questioning the patient on the initial visit. In recurring disorders such as lesions seen in patients with aphthous stomatitis, the patient may experience continual ulceration of the oral mucosa, but individual lesions heal and new ones form. In the category of disease described below, the same lesions are present for weeks to months. The major diseases in this group are pemphigus vulgaris, pemphigus vegetans, bullous pemphigoid, cicatricial pemphigoid, and erosive lichen planus.

Pemphigus Vulgaris

Pemphigus is a potentially fatal bullous disease of the skin and mucosa. Pemphigus is now classified by most investigators as an autoimmune disease in which antibody against intercellular substance of the epithelium acting with complement causes loss of cell-to-cell adhesion, resulting in acantholysis. The four variations of pemphigus are pemphigus vulgaris, pemphigus vegetans, pemphigus foliaceus, and pemphigus erythematosus. Pemphigus vegetans is a variant of pemphigus vulgaris and pemphigus erythematosus is a variant of pemphigus foliaceus. Oral mucosal involvement is of little consequence in the foliaceus and erythematosus forms of the disease; therefore, this discussion will be confined to pemphigus vulgaris and vegetans.

Pemphigus vulgaris is the most common form of pemphigus (80% of cases). Circulating antibodies, mostly IgG immunoglobulins, cause separation of cells by destruction of the intercellular substance. Pemphigus has also been reported coexisting with other autoimmune diseases, particularly myasthenia gravis. Patients with thymoma have a higher incidence of pemphigus. Several cases of pemphigus have been reported of patients with all three disorders. Several reported cases of pemphigus were induced by penicillamine, a drug used in the treatment of Wilson's disease and rheumatoid arthritis. Most cases disappeared after penicillamine was discontinued, but some patients required extended therapy. The incidence of pemphigus is highest among Jews, with an increased susceptibility also reported among Italians, Greeks, and Arabs. The peak incidence of pemphigus occurs in the fourth and sixth decade of life, but cases have been reported at all ages including occasional cases occurring before puberty. The mortality for patients with pemphigus has dropped dramatically since the introduction of treatment with corticosteroids in the 1950s. The death rate is presently approximately 10%, occurring most frequently in elderly patients and in patients requiring high doses of corticosteroids. Patients in this latter group often die from infection with *Staphylococcus aureus*.

Clinical Manifestations

The lesions of pemphigus vulgaris result from destruction of the intercellular substance in the prickle cell layer. This causes the upper layers of epithelium to pull away from the basal cell layer, resulting in acantholysis (see Fig. 5-28). The classical lesion of pemphigus is a thin-walled bulla arising on otherwise normal skin or mucosa. The bulla rapidly breaks but continues to extend peripherally, eventually leaving large areas denuded of skin. A characteristic sign of the

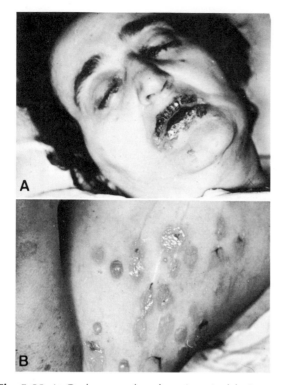

Fig. 5-28 *A,* Oral mucosal and conjunctival lesions of pemphigus. *B,* Bullae on skin showing unruptured bullae, ruptured bullae, and early scab formation in same patient.

disease may be obtained by application of pressure to an intact bulla. In patients with pemphigus vulgaris the bulla will enlarge by extension to an apparently normal surface. Another characteristic sign of the disease is that pressure to an apparently normal area will result in formation of a new lesion. This phenomenon, called the Nikolsky sign, results from the upper layer of the skin pulling away from the basal layer. The Nikolsky sign is most frequently associated with pemphigus, but may also occur in epidermolysis bullosa and Ritter's disease.

Some patients with pemphigus develop acute fulminating disease, but in most cases the disease develops more slowly, usually taking months to develop to its fullest extent.

Oral Manifestations. Eighty to ninety percent of patients with pemphigus vulgaris develop oral lesions sometime during the course of the disease, and in 60% of cases the oral lesions occur first. Pisanti studied 76 patients with pemphigus vulgaris: 56% had the initial lesions only in the mouth; 32% had initial lesions in the mouth and on one skin site; only 12% had skin lesions alone as the initial sign. Hashimoto and Lever studied electron microscope specimens of oral mucosa from patients with pemphigus vulgaris. They theorized that initial lesions of pemphigus vulgaris most frequently occurred in the oral mucosa because the epithelium demonstrated less intercellular substance and fewer intercellular junctions, making the area most susceptible to acantholysis.

The oral lesions may begin as the classic bulla on a noninflamed base (Fig. 5-29); more frequently, the clinician will see shallow ulcers because the bullae break rapidly (Fig. 5-30). Most commonly the lesions start on the buccal mucosa, often areas of trauma along the occlusal plane (Fig. 5-31). The palate and gingiva are other common sites of involvement. A thin layer of epithelium peels away in an irregular pattern leaving a denuded base. The edges of the lesion continue to extend peripherally over a period of weeks until they involve large portions of the oral mucosa (see Fig. 5-32).

It is common for the oral lesions to be present from 4 months before the skin lesions appear. If treatment is instituted during this time, the disease will be easier to control and the chance for an early remission of the disorder enhanced. Frequently however, the initial diagnosis is missed and the lesions misdiagnosed as herpes infection, Vincent's

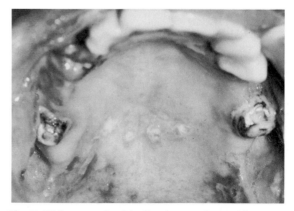

Fig. 5-29 Intact palatal bullae in a patient with pemphigus vulgaris.

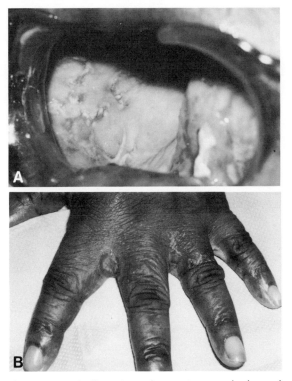

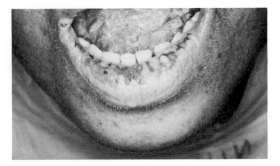

Fig. 5-31 Chronic labial lesions in a patient with pemphigus vulgaris.

Fig. 5-30 *A,* Shallow, irregular erosions on the buccal mucosa and ventral surface of the tongue caused by pemphigus. *B,* Bullae between the fingers of the same patient.

infection, or candidiasis. Zegarelli studied 26 cases of intraoral pemphigus vulgaris. The average time from onset of the disease to diagnosis was 6.8 months. He also noted that several patients had coexisting candidiasis, which sometimes masked the typical clinical picture of the pemphigus lesions.

Diagnosis

With a proper history the clinician should be able to distinguish the lesions from those caused by acute viral infections or erythema multiforme because of the acute nature of the latter diseases. It is also important for the clinician to distinguish pemphigus lesions from those in the aphthous stomatitis (RAS) category. RAS lesions may be severe, but individual lesions heal and recur. In pemphigus the same lesions continue to extend peripherally over a period of weeks to months. Lesions of pemphigus are not round and symmetrical like RAS, but are shallow and

irregular and often have detached epithelium at the periphery. In early stages of the disease, the sliding away of the oral epithelium resembles skin peeling after a severe sunburn. In some cases the lesions may start on the gingiva and be called *desquamative gingivitis.* It should be remembered that desquamative gingivitis is not a diagnosis in itself; these lesions must be biopsied to rule out the possibility of pemphigus vulgaris, as well as pemphigoid, cicatricial pemphigoid, and erosive lichen planus.

Laboratory Tests

Any patient with chronic multiple oral lesions must be questioned regarding the presence of skin bullae. If a skin lesion is present the patient should be referred to a dermatologist for a biopsy. Biopsies are best taken of intact vesicles and bullae less than 24 hours old, but because these lesions are rare on the oral mucosa, the biopsy should be taken from the advancing edge of the lesion where areas of characteristic acantholysis may be observed by the pathologist. Biopsies taken from the center of a denuded area are nonspecific histologically as well as clinically. Sometimes several biopsies are necessary before the correct diagnosis can be made. If the patient shows a positive Nikolsky sign, pressure can be placed on the mucosa to produce a new lesion, and this fresh lesion may then be biopsied.

Cytologic examination as described by Tzanck may also be of help in the diagnosis of pemphigus vulgaris, although the results are not as definitive as biopsy. Cytology has

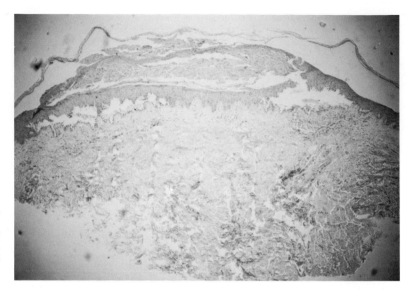

Fig. 5-32 Histologic picture of pemphigus vulgaris. The bulla is intraepithelial because of acantholysis (×32). (Courtesy of Margaret Wood, M.D.)

been a successful aid in the diagnosis of oral pemphigus although more difficult in the mouth than skin because intact bullae rupture so rapidly. The technique described is as follows: a fresh lesion is scraped with the end of a spatula; the material is spread over two slides; the slides are fixed in methyl alcohol and stained with Giemsa or Papanicolaou stain. On a positive smear, many separate acantholytic, rounded, epithelial cells will be seen with large deeply staining nuclei and prominent nucleoli.

Indirect immunofluorescent antibody tests have been described that are helpful in distinguishing pemphigus from pemphigoid and other chronic oral lesions. In this technique, serum from a patient with bullous disease is placed over a prepared slide of an epidermal structure such as guinea pig esophagus. The slide is then overlaid with fluorescein-tagged antihuman gamma globulin. Patients with pemphigus vulgaris will have antibodies against intercellular substance that will show up under a fluorescent microscope. The titer of the antibody has been directly related to the level of clinical disease. A direct test for the presence of antibodies against intercellular substance using specimens of the patient's own skin or mucosa has also been described. This direct test is more sensitive during the early stages of pemphigus when the lesions are confined to the oral mucosa. In this technique, fluores-

cein-tagged antihuman gamma globulin is placed over the patient's tissue specimen. In cases of pemphigus vulgaris, this antibody will bind the immunoglobulin deposits in the intercellular substance and show a positive fluorescence under the fluorescent microscope. A complement component (C3) is also found and may be the only evidence of disease in early lesions. This test is in common use in many medical center laboratories and should be routinely used when the diagnosis of pemphigus is suspected by taking a specimen of apparently normal tissue around the site of a lesion.

Treatment

An important aspect of patient management is early diagnosis. If treatment is instituted when the oral lesions are present before the skin lesions start, lower doses of medication can be used for shorter periods of time to control this disease. The mainstay of treatment remains systemic corticosteroids. When the lesions are confined to the mouth, the initial dose of prednisone to suppress the lesions is approximately 100 mg daily. After the lesions have been controlled the dose should be very slowly lowered. Because steroid therapy may be necessary for long periods of time, the patient should be managed by a clinician experienced in the use of long-term high-dose steroid therapy. Since the advent of the use of steroids to treat pemphigus, the death rate from this disease has dropped to approximately 10%. These deaths usually occur in elderly debilitated patients or patients who require hundreds of milligrams of prednisone daily to control their disease.

Lever recently published a long-term follow-up of 63 cases of patients with pemphigus: 10% of the patients died, usually as a complication of high-dose corticosteroid therapy; 40% of the patients were cured requiring no medication; 20% required maintenance on low doses of corticosteroids; and 30% continued to have recurrent disease. Successful attempts have been made to combine antimetabolites with corticosteroids in order to reduce the complication of high-dose corticosteroid therapy. Methotrexate, cyclophophamide, and azathioprine have been used successfully to reduce the level of anti-intercellular substance antibody in the serum resulting in control of the disease. Others have used gold salts, a treatment commonly used for management of rheumatoid arthritis. Auerbach and Bystryn have used a combination of plasmapheresis and antimetabolites in patients resistant to other forms of treatment.

Pemphigus Vegetans

Pemphigus vegetans is a relatively benign variant of pemphigus vulgaris in which the patient demonstrates the ability to heal the denuded areas. Two forms of pemphigus vegetans are recognized, the Neumann type and the Hallopeau type. The Neumann type is more common, and the early lesions are similar to those seen in pemphigus vulgaris with large bullae and denuded areas. These areas attempt healing by developing vegetations of hyperplastic granulation tissue. In the Hallopeau type, pustules, not bullae, are the initial lesion. These pustules are followed by verrucous, hyperkeratotic vegetations.

Oral Manifestations

Oral lesions are common in both forms of pemphigus vegetans and may be the initial sign of disease. Rice described a case of pemphigus vegetans in which the initial lesions were on the gingiva. The gingival lesions were described as lacelike ulcers with a purulent surface on a red base. Baer described the gingival lesions as having a granular or cobblestone appearance. Schweers reported oral lesions of the buccal and sublingual mucosa. The lesions were on an erythematous base and had a shaggy surface with white patches. As in pemphigus vulgaris, the chronic nature of the multiple oral lesions suggests pemphigus and makes biopsy a necessity.

Bullous Pemphigoid

Bullous pemphigoid occurs chiefly in children under 5 years of age and adults over 60; it is self-limited and rarely lasts over 5 years. In pemphigoid, the initial defect is not intraepithelial as in pemphigus vulgaris, but is rather subepithelial in the region of the basement membrane. There is no acantholysis and no Nikolsky sign. The disease is rarely life threatening because the bullae do not extend at the periphery to form large denuded areas as in pemphigus. The lesions of bullous pemphigoid remain localized and heal spontaneously. The etiology of this disease is unknown, but circulating antibodies against a basement membrane zone antigen have been detected. No sexual or racial predisposition has been demonstrated.

Oral Manifestations

Oral involvement in bullous pemphigoid is less common than in pemphigus and is less likely to occur before the skin lesions, which are often relatively mild. Lever reported 33 patients with bullous pemphigoid. Oral lesions were present in 11. In three cases the oral lesions occurred prior to the skin lesions. The oral lesions most frequently occurred on the buccal mucosa. The oral lesions of pemphigoid are smaller, form more slowly, and are less painful than those seen in pemphigus vulgaris. The extensive labial involvement seen in pemphigus is not present. Shklar reported a case of bullous pemphigoid with skin lesions and desquamative gingivitis. The gingival lesions consisted of generalized edema, inflammation, and desquamation with localized areas of discrete vesicle formation. This is similar to the oral lesions characteristic of benign mucous membrane pemphigoid.

Diagnosis

A biopsy should be performed to distinguish this disease from pemphigus, especially in the early stages of the disease when clinical differences are not as apparent. Histology will show subepithelial bulla formation in contrast to the intraepithelial lesions seen in pemphigus (see Fig. 5-33). Indirect immunofluorescent antibody testing will demonstrate circulating IgG antibody against basement membrane antigens (in contrast to the anti-intracellular substance antibodies seen in pemphigus). This can distinguish it from pemphigus. Tzanck smears are negative for acantholytic cells. The direct immunofluorescent test is more reliable in bullous pemphigoid as well as pemphigus, and a biopsy specimen should be taken for direct immunofluorescence testing of IgG and complement whenever the diagnosis of bullous pemphigoid is suspected. Positive specimens will demonstrate IgG and complement in the basement membrane zone.

Treatment

The use of systemic corticosteroids is usually necessary in the treatment of bullous pemphigoid, although the doses are lower and

are given for a shorter period of time than with pemphigus. Good results have also been reported with low-dose corticosteroids combined with immunosuppressive drugs. Use of sulfones or sulfapyridine has controlled the disease in some patients.

Cicatricial Pemphigoid

Cicatricial pemphigoid (CP), also called benign mucous membrane pemphigoid, is a chronic disease that chiefly occurs in patients over 50 years of age. The lesions are subepithelial vesicles that occur on any mucosal surface and may lead to scarring of the affected region. This scarring is most serious when the eyes are involved. Adhesions may develop between the bulbar and palpebral conjunctiva, and corneal damage is common. Blindness results in close to 15% of patients. Lesions may also occur in the mucosa of the genitals, esophagus, larynx, and trachea. Involvement of the esophagus and trachea may cause strictures leading to difficulty in swallowing or breathing and require emergency surgery. Skin involvement has been described in approximately one quarter of CP patients.

Diagnosis

At one time it was theorized that immunofluorescent testing could be used to distinguish CP from bullous pemphigoid because anti-

Fig. 5-33 Histologic picture of bullous pemphigoid. The bullae is subepithelial. (Courtesy of Margaret Wood, M.D.)

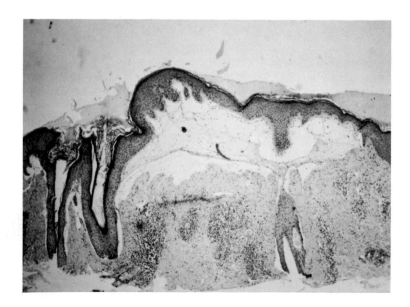

bodies against the basement membrane zone were detected in patients with bullous pemphigoid and not in patients with CP. As immunofluorescent testing techniques improved, anti-basement membrane zone antibodies were detected in serum specimens obtained from CP patients with extensive disease. Using the direct immunofluorescent technique (see pemphigus section for description), biopsy specimens taken from CP patients will demonstrate positive fluorescence for immunoglobulin and complement in the basement membrane zone in 50% to 80% of patients. The direct immunofluorescent technique is excellent for distinguishing CP from pemphigus, where specimens obtained will show immunoglobulin and complement deposition in the intercellular substance of the prickle-cell layer of the epithelium. CP is distinguished from bullous pemphigoid by clinical manifestations.

Oral Manifestations

Oral lesions are the most common finding in CP, and the mouth may be the only site involved. Lever reported 30 patients with CP: oral lesions were present in 27 of the 30 patients; conjunctival involvement was present in 23 patients; and the average age of onset of the disease was 60 years. In a recent review article Lever summarized the findings in 261 cases. Ninety-one percent of the patients had oral lesions and 66% had eye lesions. The oral lesions of CP may start as nonspecific

erosions similar to pemphigus, or as intact vesicles.

The chance of observing intact vesicles is greater in CP than in pemphigus because the lesions are thicker walled, being subepithelial rather than intraepithelial (see Fig. 5-34). In this observer's experience, it is not uncommon to see erosions on the cheeks and vesicles on the palate. CP is a more slowly developing disease than is pemphigus, and the lesions are smaller and extend less by peripheral extension. Pemphigus patients may have a majority of the oral mucosa denuded, but only localized areas are commonly involved in CP.

Gingival lesions have been described as a form of desquamative gingivitis. Some cases are restricted to the gingiva, and all cases of desquamative gingivitis should have CP ruled out as a possible cause (see Fig. 5-35). Whenever CP is suspected as a cause of chronic oral ulcers or desquamative gingivitis, a biopsy must be taken. The specimen should be studied by both routine histopathology and direct immunofluorescence.

Treatment

Management of CP depends on the severity of symptoms. When the lesions are confined to the oral mucosa, systemic corticosteroids will suppress their formation, but the clinician must weigh the benefits against the hazards from side-effects of the drug. Unlike pemphigus, CP is not a fatal disease, and long-term use of steroids for this purpose

Fig. 5-34 Intact palatal bullae in a patient with cicatricial pemphigoid.

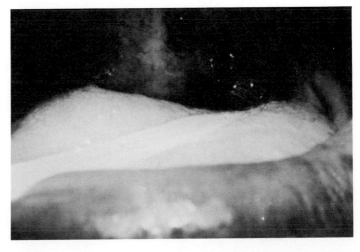

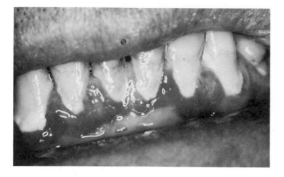

Fig. 5-35 Chronic desquamative gingival lesions of cicatricial pemphigoid.

must be carefully evaluated particularly because most cases are chronic and treatment will be required for a long period of time. Patients with mild disease should be treated with topical and intralesional steroids. In severe cases, systemic steroids may be necessary. Forty to 60 mg of prednisone will usually control the disease, and the dose should be slowly tapered to the lowest dose necessary to control symptoms. Topical and intralesional steroids may be used to minimize the dose of systemic steroids. Alternate-day steroid therapy should be used whenever feasible to reduce the risk of side-effects. In some cases, systemic steroids may be discontinued for months at a time and only used for short periods during acute flare-ups. In cases where high doses of steroids are necessary for long periods of time, the clinician should consider combining prednisone with an immunosuppressant such as azathioprine or cyclophosphamide. In all cases patients taking these drugs must be followed closely with appropriate laboratory tests to detect complications of drug therapy.

Dapsone (Avlosulfon), an antileprosy drug, has been used alone or with prednisone to treat CP. Good results have been reported in some cases. All clinicians must remember that CP patients must be evaluated periodically for possible eye involvement.

Erosive and Bullous Lichen Planus

The majority of cases of lichen planus present as white lesions (discussed in detail in Chap. 6). An erosive and bullous form of this disease presents as chronic multiple oral mucosal ulcers and will be considered here. Ero-

sive and bullous lesions of lichen planus occur in the severe form of the disease when extensive degeneration of the basal layer of epithelium causes a separation of the epithelium from the underlying connective tissue. In some cases the lesions will start as vesicles or bullae and have been classified as *bullous lichen planus;* in other cases the disease is characterized by ulcers and is called *erosive lichen planus.* Both of these disorders are variations of the same process and should be considered together.

The relationship of erosive lichen planus to squamous cell carcinoma has been debated by several authors for many years. Zegarelli reported six cases of cancer developing in patients with pre-existing lichen planus. In this study of 450 patients, all carcinomas developed in patients with the erosive form of the disease. Silverman detected a cancer rate of 2.5% in 200 lichen planus patients; four of the five cases of carcinoma occurred in patients with the erosive form of the disease. Andreasen detected no cases of cancer in 115 patients. He as well as Shklar believes that the purported relationship between lichen planus and cancer is either coincidental or a confusion of lesions of lichen planus with leukoplakia. A large-scale study of this question is warranted.

Clinical Manifestations

Erosive lichen planus is characterized by the presence of vesicles, bullae, or irregular shallow ulcers of the oral mucosa. The lesions are usually present for weeks to months and can be distinguished from those of aphthous stomatitis because lesions of aphthous stomatitis form and heal in a period of 10 days to 2 weeks. The disease is difficult to distinguish from cicatricial pemphigoid unless the characteristic white papular or lacy lesions characteristic of lichen planus are present (see Figs. 5-36 and 5-37). A significant number of cases of erosive lichen planus present with a picture of desquamative gingivitis (see Fig. 5-38). It is important to remember that desquamative gingivitis is not a disease entity but a sign of disease that can be caused by erosive lichen planus, pemphigus vulgaris, or cicatricial pemphigoid. Biopsy should be performed in all cases to make the diagnosis.

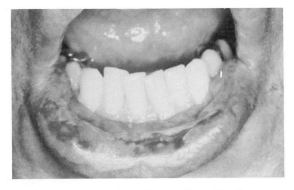

Fig. 5-36 Erosive lichen planus of the labial mucosa.

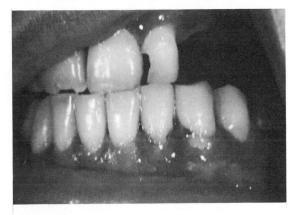

Fig. 5-38 Desquamative gingival lesions in a patient with erosive lichen planus.

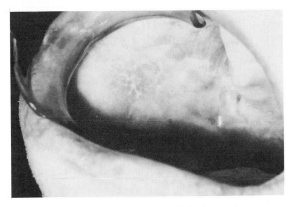

Fig. 5-37 Erosive lichen planus of the buccal mucosa. Note the large, shallow ulcers with adjacent white striae typical of lichen planus.

Diagnosis

A clinical diagnosis may be made when the erosive or bullous lesions are accompanied by the typical white lesions of lichen planus. Definitive diagnosis, however, is done by biopsy. Biopsy of the erosive lesions will show hydropic degeneration of the basal layer of epithelium. This can distinguish it from cicatricial pemphigoid, which is also a subepithelial lesion but which shows an intact basal layer, or pemphigus vulgaris, in which acantholysis will be demonstrated.

Treatment

The bullous and erosive form of lichen planus can be distressingly painful. The treatment of choice is topical corticosteroids. Betamethasone aerosal spray was shown to be effective by Greenspan. Intralesional steroids can be used for indolent lesions, and in cases of se-

vere exacerbation, systemic steroids may be considered for short periods of time. Recent reports of oral griseofulvin therapy have shown favorable results and further clinical trials are indicated.

Because the debate regarding the occurrence of squamous cell carcinoma in areas of erosive lichen planus has not been completely resolved, it would be prudent to periodically evaluate all patients with erosive and bullous forms of lichen planus for the presence of suspicious lesions.

THE PATIENT WITH SINGLE ULCERS

The most common cause of single ulcers on the oral mucosa is trauma. Trauma may be caused by teeth, food, dental appliances, dental treatment, heat, chemicals, or electricity (see Fig. 5-39). The diagnosis is usually simple and is based on the history and physical findings. The most important differentiation is to distinguish trauma from squamous cell carcinoma. The dentist must examine all single ulcers for significant healing in 1 week; if healing is not evident in this time a biopsy should be taken to rule out cancer. (Cancer of the mouth is discussed in detail in Chapter 9.)

In this section four infections that may cause a chronic oral ulcer are discussed, including histoplasmosis, blastomycosis, mucormycosis, and chronic herpes simplex infection. Syphilis, another infection that may cause a single oral ulcer in the primary and

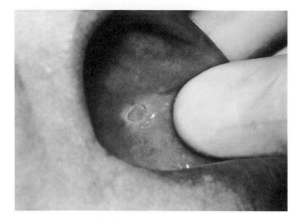

Fig. 5-39 Traumatic ulcer of the buccal mucosa secondary to cheek biting.

tertiary stages is described in the chapter on sexually transmitted diseases.

Histoplasmosis

Histoplasmosis is caused by the fungus *Histoplasma capsulatum*, a dimorphic fungus that grows in the yeast form in infected tissue. Infection results from inhaling dust contaminated with droppings, particularly from infected birds or bats. An African form of this infection is caused by a larger yeast, which is considered a variant of *H. capsulatum* and is called *Histoplasma duboisii*.

In endemic areas such as the Mississippi and Ohio River valleys, serologic evidence of previous infection may be found in up to 75% to 80% of the population. In most cases, particularly in children, primary infection is mild, manifesting as a self-limiting pulmonary disease that heals leaving fibrosis and calcification similar to tuberculosis. In a small percentage of cases, progressive disease results in cavitation of the lung and dissemination of the organism to the liver, spleen, adrenals, and meninges. The African form of the infection is more likely to occur in the subcutaneous tissues, bones, and joints. Patients with the disseminated form of the disease show evidence of bone marrow involvement by anemia and leukopenia. Immunosuppressed or myelosuppressed patients are more likely to develop the severe disseminated disease.

Oral Manifestations

Oral involvement is usually secondary to pulmonary involvement and occurs in a significant percentage of patients with disseminated histoplasmosis. Oral mucosal lesions may appear as a papule, a nodule, an ulcer, or a vegetation. If a single lesion is left untreated it will progress from a firm papule to a nodule, which ulcerates and slowly enlarges. The cervical lymph nodes are enlarged and firm. The clinical appearance of the lesions, as well as the accompanying lymphadenopathy, often resembles squamous cell carcinoma, other chronic fungal infections, or even Hodgkin's disease. Mayes reported a case of oral lesions presenting in the African form of the disease. The patient had an expansile osteolytic lesion involving the alveolar bone and gingiva.

Diagnosis

Definitive diagnosis of histoplasmosis is made by culture of infected tissues or exudates on Sabouraud's or other appropriate media. Biopsy of infected tissue will show small oval yeasts within macrophages and reticuloendothelial cells, as well as chronic granulomas, epithelioid cells, giant cells, and occasionally caseation necrosis. Skin tests and serology are not definitive because of significant numbers of false-negative and false-positive reactions.

Treatment

Histoplasmosis may be successfully managed with the use of intravenous amphotericin B for 10 to 12 weeks. The patient should be managed by a clinician experienced in the use of amphotericin B and familiar with its potential side-effects.

Blastomycosis

Blastomycosis is a fungal infection caused by *Blastomyces dermatitidis*. This dimorphic organism can grow in either a yeast or mycelial phase. The organism is found as a normal inhabitant of soil, and therefore the highest incidence of this infection is found in agricultural workers, particularly in the middle

Atlantic and southeastern portions of the United States. This geographic distribution of the infection has led to the designation by some as *North American blastomycosis.* Infection by the same organism, however, has also been found in Mexico as well as Central and South America.

Infection with blastomyces begins in a vast majority of cases by inhalation, causing a primary pulmonary infection. Although an acute self-limiting form of the disease exists, the infection commonly follows a chronic course beginning with mild symptoms such as malaise, low-grade fever, and mild cough. If the infection goes untreated the symptoms will worsen to include shortness of breath, weight loss, and production of blood-tinged sputum. Infection of the skin, mucosa, and bone may also occur, resulting from metastatic spread of organisms from the pulmonary lesions through the lymphatic system. The skin and mucosal lesions start as subcutaneous nodules, progressing to well-circumscribed indurated ulcers.

Oral Manifestations

Oral lesions are rarely the primary site of infection. When oral lesions have been reported as a first sign of blastomycosis, they have occurred in patients with mild pulmonary symptoms that have been overlooked by the patient or his physician. Most cases of oral involvement will demonstrate concomitant pulmonary lesions on chest x-ray.

The most common appearance of the oral lesions of blastomycosis is a nonspecific, painless verrucous ulcer with indurated borders, often mistaken for squamous cell carcinoma. Occasionally this mistake is perpetuated by an inexperienced histopathologist who confuses the characteristic pseudoepitheliomatous hyperplasia with malignant changes.

Other oral lesions that have been reported include hard nodules and radiolucent jaw lesions. Page reported two cases of painless oral mucosal ulcers as the first sign of blastomycosis; in both cases a careful history revealed mild respiratory symptoms. Bell reported seven cases of oral lesions occurring in patients with blastomycosis; four presented as chronic oral ulcers and three as

radiolucent bone lesions. Chest x-rays showed concomitant pulmonary involvement in all cases. Oral and facial lesions do not appear to be unusual in patients with blastomycosis. Witorsch and Utz studied 40 cases of blastomycosis; ten of the patients had either oral or nasal lesions.

Dentists should include the diagnosis of blastomycosis in the differential diagnosis of a chronic oral ulcer. The diagnosis cannot be made on clinical grounds alone. The index of suspicion should increase when a chronic painless oral ulcer appears in an agricultural worker or when the review of systems reveals pulmonary symptoms. Diagnosis is made on the basis of biopsy and on culturing the organism from tissue. The histologic appearance will show pseudepitheliomatous hyperplasia, with a heavy infiltrate of chronic inflammatory cells, and microabscesses.

Treatment

Treatment for blastomycosis is antifungal medication. Intravenous amphotericin B for 8 to 10 weeks causes resolution of the disease. Amphotericin B is a toxic medication that can cause abnormal renal function, cardiac arrhythmias, and bone marrow supression. It should be administered only by clinicians experienced in detecting and managing side-effects associated with the drug. Another medication, ketoconazole, has fewer side-effects but is still in the experimental stage.

Mucormycosis

Mucormycosis (phycomycosis) is caused by an infection with a saprophytic fungus that normally occurs in soil or as a mold on decaying food. The fungus is nonpathogenic for healthy individuals and can be cultured regularly from the human nose, throat, and oral cavity. (The organism represents an opportunistic rather than a true pathogen.) Infection occurs in individuals with decreased host resistance such as those with poorly controlled diabetes or hematologic malignancies, or those undergoing cancer chemotherapy or immunosuppressive drug therapy. In the debilitated patient, mucormycosis may appear as a pulmonary, gastrointestinal, disseminated, or rhinocerebral infection.

The rhinomaxillary form of the disease, a subdivision of the rhinocerebral form, begins with the inhalation of the fungus by a susceptible individual. The fungus invades arteries and causes damage secondary to thrombosis and ischemia. The fungus may spread from the oral and nasal region to the brain causing death in a high percentage of cases. Symptoms include nasal discharge caused by necrosis of the nasal turbinates, ptosis, proptosis secondary to invasion of the orbit, fever, swelling of the cheek, and paresthesia of the face.

Oral Manifestations

The most common oral sign of mucormycosis is ulceration of the palate, which results from necrosis due to invasion of a palatal vessel. The lesion is characteristically large and deep causing denudation of underlying bone (Fig. 5-40). Ulcers from mucormycosis have also been reported on the gingiva, lip, and alveolar ridge. The initial manifestation of the disease may be confused with dental pain or bacterial maxillary sinusitis caused by invasion of the maxillary sinus. The clinician must include mucormycosis in the differential diagnosis of large oral ulcers occurring in patients debilitated from diabetes, chemotherapy, or immunosuppressive drug therapy.

Early diagnosis is essential if the patient is to be cured of this infection. Negative cultures do not rule out mucormycosis because the fungus is frequently difficult to culture from infected tissue, so a biopsy must be taken when mucormycosis is suspected. The histopathologic specimen will show necrosis and nonseptate hyphae, which are best demonstrated by a periodic acid-Schiff stain.

Treatment

When diagnosed early, mucormycosis may be cured by a combination of surgical debridement of the infected area and systemic administration of amphotericin B for 1 to 3 months. Proper management of the underlying disorder is an important aspect affecting the final outcome of treatment. All patients given amphotericin B must be closely followed for renal toxicity by repeated measurements of the blood urea nitrogen and creatinine.

Chronic Herpes Simplex Virus Infection

Herpes simplex virus infections have customarily been divided into primary and recurrent form. Immunosuppressed patients may develop a chronic form of herpes infection; therefore, chronic herpes simplex infection should be included in the differential diagnosis when immunosuppressed patients develop chronic oral ulcers. The chronic form of herpes appears to be a variation of recurrent herpes simplex infection rather than a primary infection. Kidney transplant patients taking immunosuppressive drug therapy, patients on high doses of corticosteroids, and patients with leukemia or lymphoma or other disorders that alter the T-lymphocyte response are those most susceptible to this disease.

Lesions appear on the skin or the mucosa of the mouth, rectal, or genital area. They begin as an ordinary recurrent herpes infection but remain for weeks to months developing into a deep ulcer that may measure up to several centimeters in diameter. Chronic herpes simplex infection has been reported with both Type 1 and Type 2 herpes viruses. The major problem associated with this disease is progression from the mucocutaneous

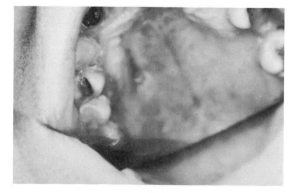

Fig. 5-40 Mucormycosis of the palate in a kidney transplant patient taking immunosuppressive drugs (azathioprine and prednisone).

form to the disseminated form which is a frequent cause of death in immunosuppressed patients.

Oral Manifestations

Lesions of chronic herpes may occur on the lips or intraoral mucosa. Shneidman reviewed 18 cases of chronic herpes infection; seven cases occurred in renal transplant patients and eight in patients with hematologic malignancies. Fourteen of the 18 patients had oral or perioral lesions. The oral lesions may resemble the small, round, symmetrical lesions associated with recurrent herpes infection, or they may be large, deep lesions that are often confused with other diseases (see Fig. 5-41). The lesions last from weeks to months and may reach several centimeters in

diameter. The larger lesions often have raised margins (see Fig. 5-42). If the lesions are undiagnosed or improperly treated they may lead to disseminated fatal disease.

Diagnosis

Ulcers caused by chronic herpes infection may be differentiated from the other chronic multiple oral mucosal lesions by a Tzanck preparation made from the base of a lesion. Specimens positive for herpes infection will demonstrate multinucleated giant cells. In older lesions, false-negative cytology smears may occur. If chronic herpes infection is still suspected, a biopsy should be taken from the margin of the lesion, which will show intranuclear inclusion bodies and multinucleated giant cells. Viral cultures must be used to distinguish infection with herpes simplex virus from infection with varicella zoster virus. If chronic herpes infection is diagnosed in a patient without known systemic disorder, the patient should be referred for a complete medical evaluation to rule out the possibility of an underlying malignancy or immunosuppressive disease.

Treatment

Mild cases of chronic herpes should be treated with topical acyclovir. In severe cases where dissemination is possible, parenteral acyclovir should be considered.

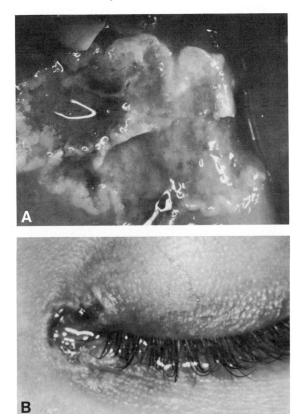

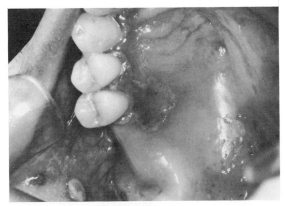

Fig. 5-41 *A,* Large ulcer of the buccal mucosa caused by a chronic herpes simplex infection in a kidney transplant patient. *B,* Herpetic ulcer near the eye of the same patient.

Fig. 5-42 Chronic herpes simplex infection of the palate in a patient taking chemotherapy for acute leukemia.

BIBLIOGRAPHY

Herpes Simplex Infections

Baringer JR, Swoveland P: Recovery of herpes simplex virus from human trigeminal ganglions. N Engl J Med 288:648, 1973

Bart BJ, Fisher I: Primary herpes simplex infection of the hand. Report of a case. J Am Dent Assoc 71:74, 1965

Bastian FO et al: Herpesvirus hominis: Isolation from human trigeminal ganglion. Science 178:306, 1972

Becker WB, Kipps A, McKenzie D: Disseminated herpes simplex virus infection—Its pathogenesis based on virological and pathological studies in 33 cases. Am J Dis Child 115:1, 1968

Berg JW: Esophageal herpes: Complication of cancer therapy. Cancer 8:731, 1955

Breeden CJ, Hall TC, Tyler RH: Herpes simplex encephalitis treated with systemic 2-iodo 5'deoxyuridine. Ann Intern Med 65:1050, 1966

Brightman VJF et al: Herpes simplex virus in ocular, nasal and oral secretions of patients with herpetic keratitis. J Dent Res 45:178, 1966

Brightman VJ, Guggenheimer JG: Herpetic parenchyma—Primary herpes simplex infection of the finger. J Am Dent Assoc 80:112, 1970

Burnet FM, Williams SW: Herpes simplex—A new point of view. Med J Aust 1:637, 1939

Carton CA, Kilbourne ED: Activation of latent herpes simplex by trigeminal sensory-root section. N Engl J Med 246:172, 1952

Chien LT et al: Effect of adenine on severe herpesvirus hominis infections in man. J Infect Dis 128:658, 1973

Deforest A, Klein M: The immunoglobulin response in recurrent herpes simplex infection in man. Fed Proc 27:734, 1968

Douglas RG, Couch RB: A prospective study of chronic herpes simplex virus infection and recurrent herpes labialis in humans. J Immunol 104:289, 1970

Evans AS, Dick EC: Acute pharyngitis and tonsillitis in University of Wisconsin students. JAMA 190:699, 1964

Felber TD et al: Photodynamic inactivation of herpes simplex—Report of a clinical trial. JAMA 223:289, 1973

Goldman L: Reactions of autoinoculation for recurrent herpes simplex. Arch Dermatol 84:1025, 1961

Greenberg MS, Brightman VJ, Ship II: Clinical and laboratory differentiation of recurrent intraoral herpes simplex infections following fever. J Dent Res 48:435, 1969

Griffin JW: Fluorescent antibody study of herpes simplex virus lesions and recurrent aphthae. Oral Surg 16:945, 1963

Jaffe EC, Lehner T: Treatment of herpetic stomatitis with idoxuridine. Br Dent J 124:392, 1968

Juel–Jensen BE: Severe generalized primary herpes treated with cytarabine. Br Med J 2:154, 1970

Juel–Jensen BE: Treatment of herpes simplex lesions of the face with idoxuridine—Results of a double blind controlled trial. Br Med J 2:987, 1964

Juel–Jensen BE: Herpes simplex lesions of the face treated with idoxuridine applied by spray gun—Results of a double blind controlled trial. Br Med J 1:901, 1965

Juel–Jensen BE, MacCallum FO: Herpes Simplex, Varicella and Zoster. Philadelphia, JB Lippincott, 1972

Kern AB, Schiff BL: Smallpox vaccinations in the management of recurrent herpes simplex—A controlled evaluation. J Invest Dermatol 33:99, 1959

Kilbrick S, Katy AS: Topical idoxuridine in recurrent herpes simplex. Ann NY Acad Sci 173:83, 1970

Kvasnička A: Relationship between herpes simplex and lip carcinoma in selected cases. Neoplasma 12:61, 1965

Lindgren KM, Douglas RC Jr, Couch RB: Significance of herpesvirus hominis in respiratory secretions of man. N Engl J Med 278:517, 1968

Lodmell DL et al: Prevention of cell-to-cell spread of herpes simplex virus by leukocytes. J Exp Med 137:706, 1973

Logan WS, Tindall JP, Elson ML: Chronic cutaneous herpes simplex. Arch Dermatol 103:606, 1971

Medak H et al: Cytopathologic study as an aid in the diagnosis of vesicular dermatoses. Oral Surg 32:204, 1971

Muller SA, Hermann EC Jr, Winkelmann RK: Herpes simplex infections in hematologic malignancies. Am J Med 52:102, 1972

Nahmias AJ: Disseminated herpes simplex virus infections. N Engl J Med 282:684, 1970

Nahmias AJ: Infections caused by herpesvirus hominis. In Hoeprich P (ed): Infectious Diseases, pp 841–852. New York, Harper & Row, 1972

Nahmias AJ, Alford CA, Korones SB: Infection of the newborn with herpesvirus hominis. Adv Pediatr 17:185, 1970

Nahmias AJ, Roizman B: Infection with herpes simplex viruses 1 and 2. N Engl J Med Part I, 289:667; Part II, 289:719; Part III, 289:781, 1973

Nahmias AJ et al: Genital infection with herpesvirus hominis types 1 and 2 in children. Pediatrics 42:659, 1968

Najjar TA et al: The use of 5-iodo-2'deoxyuridine

(IUDR) in orabase and plastibase for treatment of oral herpes simplex. J Oral Med 24:53, 1969

Nash G, Foley FD: Herpetic infection of the middle and lower respiratory tract. Am J Clin Pathol 54:857, 1970

Porter PS, Baughman RD: Epidemiology of herpes simplex among wrestlers. JAMA 194:998, 1965

Rapp F, Duff R: Transformation of hamster embryo fibroblasts by herpes simplex viruses type 1 and type 2. Cancer Res 33:1527, 1973

Rollins TG: Smallpox vaccination for chronic herpetic ulcers. JAMA 214:762, 1970

Rosato FE et al: Herpetic paronythia—An occupational hazard of medical personnel. N Engl J Med 283:804, 1970

Scott TFM et al: Pathology and pathogenesis of the cutaneous lesions of variola, vaccinia, herpes simplex, herpes zoster and varicella. In Kidd JG (ed): The Pathogenesis and Pathology of Viral Diseases, pp 74–98. New York, Columbia University Press, 1950

Scott TFM, Tokumaru T: The herpesvirus group. In Horsfall FL, Tamm I (eds): Viral and Rickettsial Infections of Man, pp 892–914. Philadelphia, JB Lippincott, 1965

Shelley WB: Herpes simplex virus as a cause of erythema multiforme. JAMA 201:153, 1967

Ship II: The oral and perioral manifestations of herpes simplex virus. In Rowe NH (ed): Symposium on Oral and Perioral Ulcerations, p 17, 1974

Ship II, Brightman VJ, Laster LL: The patient with recurrent aphthous ulcers and the patient with recurrent herpes labialis—a study of two population samples. J Am Dent Assoc 75:645, 1967

Ship II et al: Recurrent aphthous ulcerations and recurrent herpes labialis in a professional school student population. Oral Surg 13:1191, 1960

Silverman S, Beumer J: Primary herpetic gingivostomatitis of adult onset. Oral Surg 36:496, 1973

Tarro G, Sabin AB: Virus—Specific labole, nonvirion antigen in herpes virus-infected cells. Proc Natl Acad Sci USA 65:753, 1970

Terni M: Infection with the virus of herpes simplex, the recrudescence of the disease and the problem of latency. G Mal Infett Parassit 23:433, 1971

Tokumaru T: A possible role of αA-immunoglobulin in herpes simplex virus infection in man. J Immunol 97:248, 1966

Weinstein L, Chang T: The chemotherapy of viral infections. N Engl J Med 289:725, 1973

Wilton JMA, Ivanyi L, Lehner T, Notkins AL: Cell mediated immunity in herpesvirus hominis infections. Br Med J 1:723, 1972

Workshop on the Treatment and Prevention of Herpes Simplex Virus Infections. J Infect Dis 277:117, 1973

Wyburn–Mason R: Malignant changes following herpes simplex. Br Med J 2:615, 1957

Coxsackie Virus Infections

Adler JL et al: Epidemiologic investigation of hand-foot-and-mouth disease. Am J Dis Child 120:309, 1970

Lennette EH, Magoffin RL: Virologic and immunologic aspects of major oral ulceration. J Am Dent Assoc 87:1055, 1973

Steigman AJ, Lipton MM, Braspennick H: Acute lymphonodular pharyngitis: A newly described condition due to coxsackie A virus. J Pediatr 61:331, 1962

Varicella Zoster Virus Infection

Cheatham WJ et al: Varicella—A report of two fatal cases with necropsy, virus isolation and serologic studies. Am J Pathol 32:1015, 1956

Eisenberg E: Intraoral isolated herpes zoster. Oral Surg 45:214, 1978

Esiri MM, Tomlinson AH: Herpes zoster. Demonstration of virus in trigeminal nerve and ganglion by immunofluorescence and electron microscopy. J Neurol Sci 15:35, 1972

Feldman S, Hughes WT, Daniel CB: Varicella in children with cancer: Seventy-seven cases. Pediatrics 56:388, 1975

Hall HD, Jacobs JS, O'Malley JP: Necroses of maxilla in patient with herpes zoster. Oral Surg 37:657, 1974

Hatziotis J: Herpes zoster of the maxillary nerve. Report of a case. Dent Digest 78:242, 1972

Hope–Simpson RE: The nature of herpes zoster—A long-term study and a new hypothesis. Proc R Soc Med 58:9, 1965

Hudson CD, Vickers RA: Clinicopathologic observations in prodromal herpes zoster of the fifth cranial nerve. Oral Surg 31:494, 1971

Juel–Jensen BE: Herpes simplex and zoster.. Br Med J 1:406, 1973

Kelly A: Ramsay Hunt with contralateral Bells. N Engl J Med 288:266, 1973

Muller SA, Winkleman RK: Cutaneous nerve changes in zoster. J Invest Dermatol 52:71, 1969

Nally FF, Ross JH: Herpes zoster of the oral and facial structures. Oral Surg 32:221, 1971

Slack PM, Taylor–Robinson D: "Catching" shingles. Lancet 1:369, 1973

Smith JH: Dermal transmission of virus as a cause of shingles. Lancet 1:267, 1973

Verben RS, Heineman HS, Stiff RH: Localized odontalgia occurring during herpes zoster of the maxillary division of the fifth cranial nerve. Oral Surg 26:441, 1968

Weisengreen HH: Postherpetic (trigeminal) neuralgia—Report of case. J Am Dent Assoc 85:139, 1972

Erythema Multiforme

Ackerman AB, Penneys NS, Clark WH: Erythema multiforme exudativum: distinctive pathological processes. Br J Dermatol 84:554, 1971

Al–Ubaidy SS, Nally FF: Erythema multiforme: Review of twenty-six cases. Oral Surg 41:601, 1976

Basler RSW: Bullous erythema multiforme with benign neoplasm. JAMA 225:995, 1973

Brenner SM, Delany HM: Erythema multiforme and Crohn's disease of the large intestine. Gastroenterology 62:479, 1972

Buchner A, Lozada F, Silverman S: Histopathologic spectrum of oral erythema multiforme. Oral Surg 49:221, 1980

Carswell WA: A case of sarcoidosis presenting with erythema multiforme. Am Rev Respir Dis 106:462, 1972

Dawber RPR: Idoxuridine and erythema multiforme after herpes simplex. Br Med J 4:300, 1972

D'Onofrio ED: A case report: Erythema multiforme with oral lesions only. J Oral Med 29:25, 1974

Erythema multiforme. [Editorial]. Br Med J 1:63, 1972

Huff C, Weston WL: The photodistribution of erythema multiforme. Arch Dermatol 116:477, 1980

Jensen JL: Acute episodic inflammatory lesions of the mucous membrane and skin. J Am Dent Assoc 100:896, 1980

Kazmierowski JA, Wuepper KD: Erythema multiforme: Immune complex vasculitis of the superficial cutaneous microvasculature. J Invest Dermatol 71:366, 1978

Kennett S; Erythema multiforme affecting the oral cavity. Oral Surg 25:366, 1968

Lighterman I: Erythema multiforme limited to the oral cavity. Report of a case. Oral Surg 11:1237, 1958

Lozada F, Silverman S, Jr: Erythema multiforme: Clinical characteristics and natural history of fifty patients. Oral Surg 46:628, 1978

Moschella SL, Pillsbury DM, Hurley HJ: Dermatology, pp 387–390. Philadelphia, WB Saunders, 1975

Rasmussen JE: Erythema multiforme in children. Br J Dermatol 95:181–186, 1976

Safai B, Good RA, Day NK: Erythema multiforme: Report of two cases and speculation on immune mechanism involved in the pathogenesis. Clin Immunol Immunopathol 7:379, 1977

Shelley WB: Herpes simplex virus as a cause of erythema multiforme. JAMA 201:153, 1967

Shklar G: Oral lesions of erythema multiforme; Histologic and histochemical observations. Arch Dermatol 92:495, 1965

Shklar G, McCarthy PL: Oral manifestations of erythema multiforme in children. Oral Surg 21:713, 1966

Smith RG: Erythema multiforme exudativum: Recurrent oral lesions. J Dent 1:223, 1973

Stevens AM, Johnson FC: A new eruptive fever associated with stomatitis and ophthalmia. Am J Dis Child 24:526, 1922

Webster GM, Simon JF: Erythema multiforme limited to the oral cavity—Report of a case. J Am Dent Assoc 83:1106, 1971

Wermut W, Kubasik A: Erythema multiforme, Addison's disease, and Stevens-Johnson syndrome. Br Med J 3:531, 1972

Allergic Stomatitis

Adams RM: Occupational Contact Dermatitis, pp 52–63. Philadelphia, JB Lippincott, 1969

Bradford EW: Case of allergy to methyl methacrylate. Br Dent J 84:195, 1948

Brendlinger DL, Tarsitano JJ: Generalized dermatitis due to sensitivity to a chrome-cobalt removable partial denture. J Am Dent Assoc 81:395, 1970

Crissey JT: Stomatitis, dermatitis and denture materials. Arch Dermatol 92:45, 1965

Davenport JC: An adverse reaction to a silicone rubber soft lining material. Report of a case. Br Dent J 128:545, 1970

Elgart ML, Higdon RS: Allergic contact dermatitis to gold. Arch Dermatol 103:649, 1971

Everett FG, Hice TL: Contact stomatitis resulting from the use of orthodontic rubber elastics—Report of case. J Am Dent Assoc 88:1030, 1974

Fisher AA: Contact Dermatitis, 2nd ed, pp 307–324. Philadelphia, Lea & Febiger, 1973

Fisher AA, Lipton M: Allergic stomatitis due to "Baxin" in a dentifrice. Arch Dermatol Syph 64:640, 1951

Frykholm KO: On mercury from dental amalgam—Its toxic and allergic effects and some comments on occupational hygiene. Acta Odontol Scand 15(Suppl):22, 1957

Gaul EL: Immunity of the oral mucosa in epidermal sensitization to mercury. Arch Dermatol 93:45, 1966

Hale JE, Barnardo DE: Ulceration of mouth due to emepronium bromide. Lancet 1:1973

Johnson HH, Schonberg IL, Bach NF: Chronic atopic dermatitis with pronounced mercury sensitivity—Partial clearing after extraction of teeth containing mercury amalgam fillings. Arch Dermatol Syph 63:279, 1951

Juhlen L, Ohman S: Allergic reaction to mercury in red tattoos and in mercury adjacent to amalgam fillings. Acta Dermatol 48:103, 1968.

Kennett S: Stomatitis medicamentosa due to barbiturates. Oral Surg 25:351, 1968

Kerr DA, McClatchey KD, Regezi JA: Allergic gingivostomatitis (due to gum chewing). J Periodont 42:709, 1971

Kirton V, Wilkerson DS: Contract sensitivity to toothpaste. Br Med J 2:115, 1973

Kowitz G, Lucatorto F, Bennett W: Effects of dentifrices on soft tissues of the oral cavity. J Oral Med 28:105, 1973

Maxey LW: Dental allergy patch testing in dentistry and the allergic patient. In Frazier CA (ed): Dentistry and the Allergic Patient, pp 227–238. Springfield, IL, Charles C Thomas, 1973

Millard LG: Contact sensitivity to toothpaste. Br Med J 1:676, 1973

Nealey ET, del Rio CE: Stomatitis venenata—Reaction of a patient to acrylic resin. J Pros Dent 21:480, 1969

Shea JJ, Gillespie SM, Waldbott GL: Allergy to fluoride. Ann Allergy 25:388, 1967

Strain JC: Reactions associated with acrylic denture base resins. J Pros Dent 18:465, 1967

Cancer Chemotherapy

Blum RH, Carter SK: Adriamycin, a new anticancer drug with significant clinical activity. Ann Intern Med 80:249, 1974

Cohen IS et al: Cutaneous toxicity of bleomycin therapy. Arch Dermatol 107:553, 1973

Cortes EP, Takita H, Holland JF: Adriamycin in advanced bronchogenic carcinoma. Cancer 34:518, 1974

Dreizen S, Bodey GP, Rodriquez V: Oral complications of cancer chemotherapy. Postgrad Med 58:75, 1975

Dreizen S, McCredie KB, Keating MJ: Chemotherapy induced oral mucositis in adult leukemia. Postgrad Med 69:103, 1981

Halnan KE et al: Early clinical experience with bleomycin in the United Kingdom in a series of 105 patients. Br Med J 4:635, 1972

Huntington MC, du Priest RW, Fletcher WS: Intraarterial bleomycin therapy in inoperable squamous cell carcinomas. Cancer 31:153, 1973

Jaffe N et al: Favorable response of metastatic osteogenic sarcoma to pulse high-dose methotrexate with citrovorum rescue and radiation therapy. Cancer 31:1367, 1973

Metzger AL et al: Polymyositis and dermatomyositis, combined methotrexate and corticosteroid therapy. Ann Intern Med 81:182, 1974

Mulley G: Proguanil and mouth ulcers. Lancet 2:177, 1974

Recurrent Aphthous Stomatitis

Barile MF et al: L-form of bacteria isolated from recurrent aphthous stomatitis lesions. Oral Surg 16:1395, 1963

Blank H et al: Recurrent aphthous ulcers. JAMA 142:125, 1950

Brugmans J, DeCree J, Verhagen H: Treatment of aphthous stomatitis. Lancet 2:842, 1973

Challacombe SJ, Barkhan P, Lehner T: Hematologic features and differentiation of recurrent oral ulceration. Br J Oral Surg 15:37, 1977

Cohen L: Etiology, pathogenesis and classification of aphthous stomatitis and Behçets syndrome. J Oral Pathol 7:347, 1978

Cunliffe WJ et al: Behçets syndrome and oral fibrinolytic therapy. Br Med J 2:486, 1973

Dodd K, Ruchman I: Herpes simplex virus not the etiologic agent of recurrent stomatitis. Pediatrics 5:883, 1950

Dolby AE: Recurrent aphthous ulceration—effect of sera and peripheral blood lymphocytes upon oral epithelial tissue culture cells. Immunology 17:709, 1969

Donatsky O, Bendixen G: In vitro demonstration of cellular hypersensitivity to Strep 2A in recurrent aphthous stomatitis by means of the leukocyte migration test. Acta Allergol 27:137, 1972

Donatsky O, Dabelsteen E: An immunofluorescence study on the humoral immunity to Strep 2A in recurrent aphthous stomatitis. Acta Pathol Microbiol Scand 82:107, 1974

Drinnan AJ, Fischman SL: Randomized, double-blind study of levamisole in recurrent aphthous stomatitis. J Oral Pathol 7:414, 1978

Ferguson MM et al: Progeston therapy for menstrually related aphthae. Int J Oral Surg 7:463, 1978

Ferguson MM et al: Coeliac disease associated with recurrent aphthae. Gut 21:223, 1980

Francis TC: Recurrent aphthous stomatitis and Behçet's disease. Oral Surg 30:476, 1970

Francis TC, Oppenheim JJ: Impaired lymphocyte stimulation by some streptococcal antigens in patients with recurrent aphthous stomatitis and rheumatic heart disease. Clin Exp Immunol 6:573, 1970

Garcia–Goday F: Therapy for aphthous lesions reviewed. J Pedol 4:74, 1979

Gier RE et al: Evaluation of the therapeutic effect of levamisole in treatment of recurrent aphthous stomatitis. J Oral Pathol 7:405, 1978

Gordon N: Aphthous stomatitis and foreign bodies. Lancet 1:565, 1974

Graykowski EA et al: Recurrent aphthous stomatitis—Clinical, therapeutic, histopathologic, and hypersensitivity aspects. JAMA 196:637, 1966

Graykowski EA, Hooks JJ: Summary of workshop on recurrent aphthous stomatitis and Behçets syndrome. J Am Dent Assoc 97:599, 1978

Graykowski EA, Kingman A: Double/blind trial of tetracycline in recurrent aphthous ulceration. J Oral Pathol 7:376, 1978

Griffin JW: Fluorescent antibody study of herpes simplex virus lesions and recurrent aphthae. Oral Surg 16:945, 1963

Guggenheimer J, Brightman VJ, Ship II: Effect of chlortetracycline mouthrinses on the healing of recurrent aphthous ulcers—a double blind controlled trial. J Oral Ther Pharmacol 4:406, 1968

Hooks JJ: Possibility of a viral etiology in recurrent aphthous ulcers and Behçets syndrome. J Oral Pathol 7:353, 1978

Kaplan B, Cardarelli C, Pinnell SR: Double-blind study of levamisole in aphthous stomatitis. J Oral Pathol 7:400, 1978

Lehner T: Stimulation of lymphocyte transformation by tissue homogenates in recurrent oral ulceration. Immunology 13:159, 1967

Lehner T: Immunological aspects of recurrent oral ulceration and Behçets syndrome. J Oral Pathol 7:424, 1978

Lehner T, Matteo A: Acute phase proteins, C9, factor B, and lysozyme in recurrent oral ulceration and Behçets syndrome. J Clin Pathol 33:269, 1980

Lennette EH, Magoffin RL: Virologic and immunologic aspects of major oral ulcerations. J Am Dent Assoc 87:1055, 1973

MacFarlane TW, Ross CA, Cohen BJ: Oral ulceration and infective agents. Br Med J 30:643, 1974

Miller MF et al: Effect of levamisole on the incidence and prevalence of recurrent aphthous stomatitis. J Oral Pathol 7:387, 1978

Miller MF, Garfunkel AA, Ram CA, Ship II: The inheritance of recurrent aphthous stomatitis observations on susceptibility. Oral Surg 49:409, 1980

Olson JA, Silverman S: Double-blind study of levamisole therapy in recurrent aphthous stomatitis. J Oral Pathol 7:393, 1978

Oppenheim JJ, Francis TC: The role of delayed hypersensitivity in immunological processes and its relationship to aphthous stomatitis. J Periodontol 41:205, 1970

Rogers RS, Sams M, Shorter RG: Lymphocytotoxicity in recurrent aphthous stomatitis. Arch Dermatol 109:361, 1974

Sallay K et al: Adenovirus isolation from recurrent oral ulcers. J Periodontol 44:712, 1973

Segal AL et al: Recurrent herpes labialis, recurrent aphthous ulcers and the menstrual cycle. J Dent Res 4:797, 1971

Ship II: Socioeconomic status and recurrent aphthous ulcers. J Am Dent Assoc 73:120, 1966

Ship II: Epidemiologic aspects of recurrent aphthous ulcerations. Oral Surg 33:400, 1972

Ship II, Ashe WK, Scherp HW: Recurrent "fever blister" and "canker sore" tests for herpes simplex and other viruses with mammalian cell cultures. Arch Oral Biol 3:117, 1961

Ship II, Brightman VJ, Laster LL: The patient with recurrent aphthous ulcers and the patient with recurrent herpes labialis—A study of two population samples. J Am Dent Assoc 75:645, 1967

Stanley HR, Graykowski EA, Barile MF: The occurrence of microorganisms in microscopic sections of aphthous and nonaphthous lesions and other tissues. Oral Surg 18:335, 1964

Stark MM, Kibrick S, Weisberger D: Studies on recurrent aphthae—Evidence that herpes simplex is not the etiological agent with further observations on the immune responses in herpetic infections. J Lab Clin Med 44:261, 1954

Sutton RL: Periodenitis mucosa necrotica recurrens. J Cutan Dis 29:65, 1911

Wilson CWM: Food sensitivities, taste changes, aphthous ulcers and atopic symptoms in allergic disease. Ann Allergy 44:302, 1980

Wray D et al: Recurrent aphthae. Treatment with vitamin B12, folic acid, and iron. Br Med J 2:490, 1975

Wray D et al: Nutritional deficiencies in recurrent aphthae. J Oral Pathol 7:418, 1978

Behçets Syndrome

Gamble CN et al: The immune complex pathogenesis of glomerulonephritis and pulmonary vasculitis in Behçet's disease. Am J Med 66:1031, 1979

Graham–Brown RAC, Sarkany I: Failure of colchicine and fibrinolytic therapy in Behçet's disease. Clin Exp Dermatol 5:87, 1980

Lavalle C et al: Behçet syndrome and palate perforation. Arth Rheum 22:308, 1979

Lehner T: Behçet's syndrome and auto-immunity. Br Med J 1:465, 1967

Lehner T: Pathology of recurrent oral ulceration and oral ulceration in Behçet's syndrome—light, electron, and fluorescence microscopy. J Pathol 97:481, 1969

Mason RM, Barnes CG: Behçet's syndrome with arteritis. Ann Rheum Dis 28:95, 1969

O'Duffy JD, Carney JA, Deodhar S: Behçet's disease—Report of 10 cases, 3 with manifestations. Ann Intern Med 75:561, 1971

O'Duffy JD, Taswell HF: Blood transfusion therapy in Behçet's disease. Ann Intern Med 80:279, 1974

O'Duffy JD: Summary of international symposium on Behçet's disease. J Rheum 5:229, 1978

Recurrent Herpes Simplex Virus Infection

Bierman SM: The mechanism of recurrent infection by herpes virus hominis. Arch Dermatol 112:1459, 1976

Caron GA: Carcinoma at the site of herpes simplex infection. JAMA 243:2396, 1980

Embil JA, Manuel R, McFarlane S: Concurrent oral and genital infection with an identical strain of herpes simplex Type I. Sex Transm Dis 8:70, 1981

Greenberg MS: Salivary activity against herpes simplex virus. I.A.D.R. 52nd Annual Meeting, 1974. Atlanta, March 1974

Greenberg MS, Brightman VJ: Serum immunoglobulins in patients with recurrent intraoral herpes simplex infections. J Dent Res 50:781, 1971

Greenberg MS, Brightman VJ, Ship II: Clinical and laboratory differentiation of recurrent intraoral herpes simplex virus infections following fever. J Dent Res 48:385, 1969

Greenberg MS, Heineman H: Salivary protection against recurrent herpes labialis. (Abstr). 29th Annual Meeting, Am Acad Oral Path, Kansas City, 1975

Griffin JW: Recurrent intraoral herpes simplex virus infection. Oral Surg 19:209, 1965

Guinan ME et al: Topical ether and herpes simplex labialis. JAMA 243:1059, 1980

Juel–Jensen BE, MacCullum FO: Herpes simplex lesions of the face treated with idoxuridine applied by spray gun—results of a double blind control trial. Br Med J 1:901, 1965

MacCullum FO, Juel–Jensen BE: Herpes simplex virus skin infection in man treated with idoxuridine in dimethyl sulphoxide—results of double blind controlled trial. Br Med J 2:805, 1966

Mayne DG: Possible treatment for cold sores (letter). Br Med J 2:1368, 1979

Miller JB: Treatment of active herpes virus infections with influenza virus vaccine. Ann Allergy 42:292, 1979

Myers MG et al: Failure of neutral-red photodynamic inactivation in recurrent herpes simplex virus infections. N Engl J Med 293:945, 1975

Neils RE et al: Chronic herpes simplex in a patient with leukemia treated with parenteral Vidarabine. Arch Dermatol 115:1449, 1979

Nugent GR, Chou SM: Treatment of labial herpes. JAMA 224:132, 1973

Overall JC: Persistent problems with persistent herpes viruses (Editorial). N Engl J Med 305:97, 1981

Park NH et al: Acyclovir in oral and ganglionic herpes simplex virus infections. J Infect Dis 140:802, 1979

Park NH et al: Topical therapeutic efficacy of 9-(2-hydroxyethoxymethyl) guanine and 5-iodo-5'-amino-2', 5'dideoxyuridine on oral infection with herpes simplex virus in mice. J Infect Dis 141:575, 1980

Rapp F, Li JLH, Jerkofsky M: Transformation of mammalian cells by DNA containing viruses following photodynamic inactivation. Virology 55:339, 1973

Saral R et al: Acyclovir prophylaxis of herpes simplex virus infections: A randomized double-blind, controlled trial in bone-marrow transplant recipients. N Engl J Med 305:63, 1981

Selby PJ et al: Parenteral acyclovir therapy for herpes virus infections in man. Lancet 2(8155):1267, 1979

Sklar SH, Buimouvici–Klein E: Adenosine in the treatment of recurrent herpes labialis. Oral Surg 48:416, 1979

Stalker WH: Facial neuralgia associated with recurrent herpes simplex. Oral Surg 49:502, 1980

Terezbalmy GT, Bottomley WK, Pellen GB: The use of water-soluble bioflavinoid-ascorbic acid complex in the treatment of recurrent herpes labialis. Oral Surg 45:56, 1978

Tokumaru T: A possible role of gamma A-immunoglobulin in herpes simplex virus infection in man. J Immunol 97:248, 1966

Weathers DR, Griffin JW: Intraoral ulcerations of recurrent herpes simplex and recurrent aphthae—two distinct clinical entities. J Am Dent Assoc 81:81, 1970

Pemphigus

Auerbach R, Bystryn J: Plasmopheresis and immunosuppressive therapy. Arch Dermatol 115:728, 1979

Baer PN et al: Pemphigus vegetans. Oral Surg 28:282, 1969

Bennett CG, Shulman ST, Baughman RA: Prepubertal oral pemphigus vulgaris. J Am Dent Assoc 100:64, 1980

Beutner EH et al: Autoantibodies in pemphigus vulgaris. JAMA 192:682, 1965

Elias PM et al: Childhood pemphigus vulgaris. N Engl J Med 287:758, 1972

Eversole LR et al: Oral lesions as the initial sign in pemphigus vulgaris. Oral Surg 33:354, 1972

Gilmore HK: Early detection of pemphigus vulgaris. Oral Surg 46:641, 1978

Hashimoto K, Lever WF: An electron microscope study on pemphigus vulgaris of the mouth and the skin with special reference to the intercellular cement. J Invest Dermatol 48:540, 1967

Hasler JF: The role of immunofluorescence in the diagnosis of oral vesiculobullous disorders. Oral Surg 33:362, 1972

Lever WF: Pemphigus and Pemphigoid. Charles C Thomas. Springfield, IL, 1965

Lever WF, Goldberg HS: Treatment of pemphigus vulgaris with methotrexate. Arch Dermatol 100:70, 1969

Lever WF, Schaumburg–Lever G: Immunosuppressants and prednisone in pemphigus vulgaris: therapeutic results obtained in 63 patients between 1961 and 1975. Arch Dermatol 113:1236, 1977

McQueen A, Campbell HD: Pemphigus vulgaris—Cytodiagnosis of the oral lesion. Br J Oral Surg 10:69, 1972

Meurer M, Millins JL, Rogers RS, Jordan RE: Oral pemphigus vulgaris: A report of ten cases. Arch Dermatol 113:1520, 1977

Neumann–Jensen B et al: Pemphigus vulgaris and pemphigus foliaceus coexisting with oral lichen planus. Br J Dermatol 102:585, 1980

Peck SM et al: Studies in bullous diseases, immunofluorescent serologic tests. N Engl J Med 279:951, 1968

Pisanti S et al: Pemphigus vulgaris—incidence in Jews of different ethnic groups according to age, sex and initial lesion. Oral Surg 38:382, 1974

Razzaque A et al: Pemphigus: Current concepts. Ann Intern Med 92:396, 1980

Rice JS et al: Pemphigus vegetans. Oral Surg 16:1383, 1963

Savin JA: The events leading to the death of patients with pemphigus and pemphigoid. Br J Dermatol 101:521, 1979

Schweers CA et al: Further observations on phemphigus vegetans. Oral Surg 28:442, 1969

Shklar G: The oral lesions of pemphigus vulgaris. Oral Surg 23:629, 1967

Shklar G: Recent research on oral mucous membrane diseases. Oral Surg 30:242, 1970

Shklar G, Cataldo E: Histopathology and cytology of oral lesions of pemphigus. Arch Dermatol 101:635, 1970

Wilgram GF, Caulfield JB, Lever WF: An electron microscope study of acantholysis in pemphigus vulgaris. J Invest Dermatol 36:373, 1961

Zegarelli DJ, Zegarelli EV: Intraoral pemphigus vulgaris. Oral Surg 44:384, 1977

Pemphigoid

Brody HJ, Pirozzi DJ: Benign mucous membrane pemphigoid. Arch Dermatol 113:1598, 1977

Foster ME, Nally FF: Benign mucous membrane pemphigoid (cicatricial mucosal pemphigoid): A reconsideration. Oral Surg 244:697, 1977

Hardy KM, Perry HO, Pingrie GC, Kirby TJ: Benign mucous membrane pemphigoid. Arch Dermatol 104:467, 1971

Lever WF: Pemphigus and pemphigoid. J Am Acad Dermatol 1:2, 1979

McCarthy PL: Benign mucous membrane pemphigoid. Oral Surg 33:75, 1972

Nieboer C, Roeleveld CG, Kalsbeek GL: Localized chronic pemphigoid. Dermatologica 156:24, 1978

Shklar G, McCarthy PL: Oral manifestations of benign mucous membrane pemphigus (mucous membrane pemphigoid). Oral Surg 12:950, 1959

Shklar G, Meyer I, Zacarian SA: Oral lesions in bullous pemphigoid. Arch Dermatol 99:663, 1969

Erosive Lichen Planus

Andreasen JO: Oral lichen planus I. A clinical evaluation of 115 cases. Oral Surg 25:31, 1968

Aufdemorte TB, Devillez RL, Gieseker DR: Griseofulvin in the treatment of three cases of oral erosive lichen planus. Oral Surg 55:459, 1983

Fulling H: Cancer development in oral lichen planus. Arch Dermatol 108:667, 1973

Goldstein BH, Katz SM: Immunofluorescent findings in oral bullous lichen planus. J Oral Med 34:8, 1979

Greenspan JS, Yeoman CM, Harding SM: Oral lichen planus. Br Dent J 144:83, 1978

Haseldon FG: Bullous lichen planus. Oral Surg 24:472, 1967

Rogers R, Sheridan PJ, Jordon R: Desquamative gingivitis. Oral Surg 42:316, 1976

6

Red and White Lesions of the Oral Mucosa

VERNON J. BRIGHTMAN

TERMINOLOGY

White Lesion, Red Lesion, Leukoplakia, and Erythroplakia

White lesion is a nonspecific term used to describe any abnormal area of the oral mucosa that on clinical examination appears whiter than the surrounding tissue and is usually slightly raised, roughened, or otherwise of a different texture from adjacent normal tissue. White lesions result from a variety of pathologic changes and have miscellaneous etiologies. On closer inspection, some can be further categorized on the basis of particular clinical features, such as their history, location, texture, and the ease with which they can be dislodged from the mucosa. For the most part, however, microscopic examination of scrapings or tissue biopsied from these lesions is needed for accurate diagnosis.

A variety of factors have been suggested as the cause of these areas of whitish mucosa: increased thickness of the epidermal covering with increased production of keratin (hyperkeratosis) or production of abnormal keratins and imbibition of fluid by the upper layers of the mucosa. Of these, the production of abnormal keratins, which imbibe fluid far more readily than does normally keratinized oral mucosa, is probably the most important factor. In other situations, the white appearance is explained by coagulation of surface tissue, such as occurs in a burn, and formation of a pseudomembrane composed of desquamating epithelial cells, fibrin, inflammatory cells, microorganisms, and food debris that remain attach to the mucosal surface. In general, white lesions result from injury to the mucosa or are a consequence of racial or other genetically determined characteristics of the mucosa.

Despite the heterogeneity of the disease processes included under the heading of *white lesions*, the term is well established in the dental literature, and in the case of hyperkeratotic white lesions, for many years has implied a lesion that must be biopsied and carefully examined for any malignant change. More recently, however, the frequency with which hyperkeratotic white lesions lead to oral cancer has been questioned, and other clinically detectable changes, referred to as *red lesions*, have been shown to have a far greater precancerous potential. *Red lesion* in this context refers to an area of reddened mucosa that may be smooth and "atrophic looking" or exhibits a granular, velvety texture. Such lesions occur alone or with areas of hyperkeratosis and are generally found only by more careful examination than is required for demonstration of most white lesions.

The majority of both red and white lesions are asymptomatic. In terms of oral cancer screening, white lesions and red lesions are now often discussed together to emphasize the varied appearance of precancerous oral mucosal changes and the fact that lesions that most often undergo malignant change exhibit mixed red and white areas. This concept is reflected in the title of this chapter and is discussed more fully in the last section of the chapter, entitled Red and White Lesions with Defined or Uncertain Precancerous Potential.

The term *leukoplakia* is also used clinically to refer to white lesions of the oral mucosa, particularly those that appear leathery and cannot be dislodged easily. As currently used, *leukoplakia* implies no specific histologic lesion and no particular precancerous potential and signifies little else than nonspecific white lesion. This usage differs from that found in the literature before about 1960, when *leukoplakia* was used with a variety of specific connotations (e.g., for a white lesion with particular clinical features that were believed to signal precancerous change; for any lesion with histologically established precancerous changes (epithelial dysplasia) and often irrespective of its clinical appearance, or simply for a leathery white patch that does not rub off easily).

In recent years, there has been a growing acceptance of the definition for leukoplakia proposed by the World Health Organization (WHO) Collaborating Reference Center for Oral Precancerous Lesions:* "a white patch

* In 1978, as an interim report on the development of an internationally accepted system for classification of oral precancerous lesions, the WHO Collaborating Reference Center published definitions and illustrations of leukoplakia and nine related lesions (carcinoma *in situ*, stomatitis nicotina, erythroplakia, lichen planus, candidiasis, habitual cheek biting, discoid lupus erythematosus,

or plaque that cannot be characterized clinically or pathologically as any other disease." As such, the term specifically excludes white lesions that can be identified as lichen planus, syphilitic mucous patches, white sponge nevus, candidiasis, lupus erythematosus, chemical burns, and other stomatitides and makes no reference to the presence or absence of epithelial dysplasia. *Leukoplakia* thus remains an acceptable diagnostic term but only for lesions that have been biopsied and show no specific histologic or clinical diagnostic features.

The WHO Reference Center uses the term *erythroplakia,* analogously to *leukoplakia,* to designate lesions of the oral mucosa that present as bright red, velvety plaques and cannot be characterized clinically or pathologically as being caused by any other condition. Epithelial dysplasia is described as a more constant feature of erythroplakia but is not essential to the definition.

Nonkeratotic and Keratotic White Lesions

Clinically, a basic distinction is made between white lesions that are easily dislodged with gentle rubbing or scraping and those that resist such attempts. Those that dislodge easily and often leave a slightly reddened or raw patch of mucosa are either simply debris or a pseudomembranous inflammation and are referred to as *nonkeratotic.* Those that resist rubbing and scraping are considered to involve thickening of the mucosal epithelium, possibly as a result of increased thickness of the keratinized layers (hyperkeratosis), and are referred to as *keratotic.* Histologic examination for the most part confirms these features, although the presence or absence of specific epithelial changes, such as acanthosis, spongiosis, and ortho- and parahyperkeratosis cannot be judged accurately from the clinical appearance of the lesion and should not be assumed from the designation of a

white sponge nevus, and submucous fibrosis). These definitions have been incorporated into the appropriate sections of this chapter in the hope of "encouraging a uniform system of terms and definitions to facilitate comparability of data," in what still remains a difficult and uncertain area of oral medicine.

particular white lesion as nonkeratotic or keratotic.

Pseudomembranous inflammation of the oral mucosa is associated with a variety of physical, chemical, and microbial agents (see following discussion of nonkeratotic white lesions); of these, lesions caused by acute infection with the endogenous oral fungus *Candida* are sufficiently common and characteristic of the pseudomembranous type of white lesion that *Candida* infection is often thought of only in this regard. More detailed study of other oral white lesions, however, have demonstrated that *Candida* is also frequently associated with hyperkeratotic white lesions and may play an etiologic role in the development of hyperkeratosis and in the clinical appearance of the hyperkeratotic lesion. Despite this broader concept of the role of *Candida* infection in oral white lesions, the distinction between white lesions that are easily dislodged (nonkeratotic) and those that are not (keratotic) is still used clinically and has been retained in this chapter. The character of a particular white lesion (nonkeratotic versus keratotic), however, cannot be used as a certain guide to whether infection with *Candida* species is involved. The ubiquitous nature of *Candida* as an endogenous oral infectious agent also supports the use of antifungal agents as adjuncts in the management of both keratotic and nonkeratotic white lesions (see subsequent sections), rather than restricting them to the treatment of acute candidiasis.

Classification of Red and White Lesions

It will be clear from these introductory comments and the text that follows that our understanding of red and white lesions is far from complete and that clinical and histologic criteria alone do not always provide a firm basis for classifying this heterogeneous group of disorders. Studies of cell kinetics and long-term computerized analyses of clinical and histologic data (two newer ways of approaching this topic) may in the future suggest different schemes of classification. More than fifty disorders are discussed in this chapter, and for this purpose, they are organized into five major groups:

1. *Variations in structure and appearance of the normal oral mucosa*
   Leukoedema
   Fordyce granules
   Linea alba and other areas of frictional cornification
2. *Nonkeratotic white lesions*
   Habitual cheek-biting
   Burns (thermal burns; those caused by aspirin, dental medicaments, and other iatrogenic causes; radiation mucositis; uremic stomatitis)
   Those caused by specific infectious agents (Koplik's spots, syphilitic mucous patches)
3. *Candidiasis*
   Acute pseudomembranous candidiasis (thrush)
   Acute atrophic candidiasis (antibiotic sore-mouth)
   Chronic atrophic candidiasis (denture sore-mouth and angular cheilitis)
   "Id" reactions
   Median rhomboid glossitis
   Chronic hyperplastic candidiasis
   Oral candidiasis in association with extraoral lesions (orificial and intertriginous sites, gastrointestinal candidiasis, chronic mucocutaneous candidiasis, systemic candidiasis)
4. *Keratotic white lesions with no increased potential for the development of oral cancer*
   Stomatitis nicotina
   Traumatic keratoses
   Intraoral skin grafts
   Focal epithelial hyperplasia
   Psoriasiform lesions (psoriasis, Reiter's syndrome, geographic tongue, "ectopic geographic tongue")
   Oral genodermatoses
5. *Red and white lesions with defined or uncertain precancerous potential*
   Leukoplakia (homogenous, nodular or speckled, and verrucous)
   Erythroplakia
   Oral lesions associated with use of tobacco and alcohol (cigarette, cigar, and pipe smoking; snuff dipping; tobacco and betel-nut chewing; reverse smoking)
   Electrogalvanically induced oral white lesions
   Carcinoma *in situ*
   Bowen's disease
   Oral submucous fibrosis
   Actinic keratosis, elastosis, and cheilitis
   Discoid lupus erythematosus
   Dyskeratosis congenita
   Lichen planus
   Oral lichenoid reactions (erythema multiforme, lupus erythematosus and dermatomyositis, drug-induced lichenoid reactions, secondary syphilis, graft-versus-host reactions)

This grouping provides a practical schema for the clinician faced with making decisions about particular lesions but also retains the various clinicopathologic entities that are currently included under the topic of red and white lesions.

Miscellaneous Other Oral Mucosal Lesions with Red or White Appearance

By custom, the terms *white lesion* and *red lesion* do not include localized inflammatory changes of the oral mucosa or lesions such as benign migratory glossitis (geographic tongue) and erythema circinata migrans, despite their mixed red and white appearance. These lesions and those of hairy tongue, which is occasionally mistaken for an extensive white patch on the tongue, are described in Chapter 10. Vesiculobullous lesions and oral ulcers are also discussed as a separate category (see Chap. 5) even though the desquamating sheets of epithelium over ruptured bullae, the mixed red and white patches of mucosa in erythema multiforme, and even the pseudomembrane covering isolated oral ulcers are from time to time mistaken for white lesions. (In general, vesiculobullous lesions and ulcerative lesions are quite painful, even when covered with a pseudomembrane, allowing them to be easily distinguished from white lesions, which as a group are relatively painless).

The lesions of lichen planus and other lichenoid keratoses, however, are included among the white lesions as well as in the discussion of vesiculobullous lesions because of the variable manifestations of lichen planus, which occurs in bullous and erosive forms as well as a nonerosive keratosis. Uncertainty about the precancerous potential of lichen planus also requires that it be considered along with other white lesions that have increased potential for malignant transformation.

Where there is thus a well-established tradition for describing particular categories of oral lesions as white or red, lack of firm definition for either category has led to problems in classification and in some instances to uncertainty about the meaning of a particular diagnosis. Much might be gained, therefore, by eliminating such descriptive terms as *red lesion* and *white lesion* and replacing them with terms that refer to the general category of pathologic change involved: atrophic, hyperkeratotic, ulcerative vesiculobullous. This approach has been in use in the field of gynecologic pathology for some years to describe analogous lesions of the vulvovaginal mucosa and has gained wide acceptance.

VARIATIONS IN STRUCTURE AND APPEARANCE OF THE NORMAL ORAL MUCOSA

Leukoedema

In some individuals, the buccal mucosa retains its normal softness and flexibility but exhibits a grayish white, slightly folded, opalescent appearance that has been variously described as epithelium covered with a diffuse, edematous film or velvetlike veil. This appearance is referred to as *leukoedema;* similar changes may affect the mucosa of the lips. This change can be temporarily eliminated by stretching or scraping the mucosa, but re-establishes itself almost immediately. Underlying melanin pigment appears to enhance the opalescence, making these changes more prominent. Histologically, the epithelium in these situations is rather thicker than normal, with broad rete processes. The cells in the superficial part of the stratum spinosum appear vacuolated in hematoxylin-and-eosin-(H&E) stained sections because they contain considerable quantities of glycogen (see Fig. 6-1). The cells at the surface may be flattened, but they retain pyknotic nuclei, and there is usually no obvious keratinization.

This phenomenon has long been considered a normal variant; however, a number of epidemiologic studies have demonstrated a correlation between leukoedema and the use of tobacco. Clinically, leukoedema is at times mistakenly identified as leukoplakia, although the histologic appearance of tissue biopsied from such areas will indicate its true nature. Because of the innocuous nature of leukoedema, biopsy examination is rarely included in epidemiologic investigations. Clinical criteria for identifying leukoedema are also rather diffuse, although a clinical grading system has been used in some studies. Conclusions based on comparison of data

Fig. 6-1 Leukoedema, histologic section. Note vacuolated cells in the superficial part of the stratum spinosum (×120; from WHO Collaborating Centre for Oral Precancerous Lesions: Definition of leukoplakia and related lesions: An aid to studies on oral precancer. Oral Surg 46:518, 1978; courtesy CV Mosby Co., St. Louis, MO 63141)

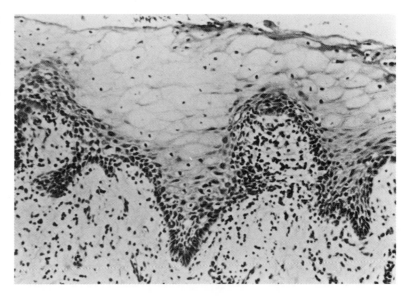

from different studies thus must be viewed with caution. The available data suggest that leukoedema occurs most often in the 15 to 35 age group, affects males almost twice as frequently as females, and is correlated with tobacco use (pipe more than cigarette, and cigarette more than snuff) and amount of smoking. The highest prevalence is reported in blacks in the United States (50% to 90%) and the lowest (<2%) in native peoples of India, Africa, and New Guinea. Prevalences of 5% to 40% have been reported for whites in several US and European studies. An in-

teraction between racially determined predisposing factors and smoking is postulated as the etiology of this phenomenon. There is no evidence to suggest that leukoedema predisposes or progresses to keratosis of the buccal mucosa.

Fordyce Granules

The oral mucosa normally contains a number of both small and large tubuloacinar sebaceous glands (referred to as *Fordyce granules*), especially in the lip and buccal mucosa, but also occasionally on the palate, gingivae, and tongue (see Fig. 6-2). Histologically, they are identical with the sebaceous glands of the skin except for the absence of associated hair follicles. They occur in 80% to 95% of the adult population as well as in adolescents, and they are neither ectopic structures nor adenomas. They are normal oral mucosal adnexal glands that vary in frequency with age and between individuals. No specific function has been ascribed to these glands or to their lipase-containing secretion. They rarely appear to undergo histopathologic change, although small keratin-filled pseudocysts of the intraoral sebaceous gland ducts, analogous to milia occurring on the skin, have been described. Isolated examples of sebaceous cell adenoma of the oral mucosa have been reported, but it is not clear that these arise from Fordyce granules.

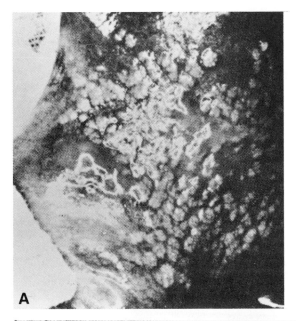

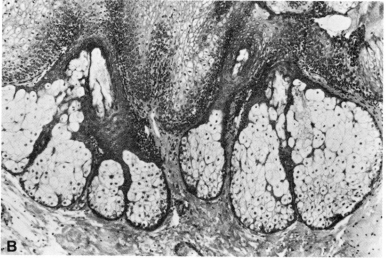

Fig. 6-2 *A,* Fordyce granules on the internal surface of the cheek of a 70-year-old man. *B,* Histologic section of Fordyce granules reveals tubuloacinar sebaceous gland as appendages to an acantholitic buccal epithelium. (From Monteil RA: Fordyce granules: Disease, heterotopia or adenoma? An histologic and ultrastructural study. J Biol Buccale 9:109, 1981; courtesy Societé Nouvelle des Publications Médicales et Dentaires, Paris 75009 France)

Clinically, the nature of these small, white or yellowish submucosal plaques is apparent on close inspection, and it is only when they are particularly large or almost confluent that they are considered of diagnostic interest. Occasionally, collections of these glands on the keratinized external mucosal vermilion border of the lips are considered disfiguring and are surgically removed. Otherwise, no treatment is indicated. The number of Fordyce granules is stated to increase with age and is not correlated with systemic atherosclerosis or smoking. Adenoma sebaceum, the characteristic facial lesion of tuberous sclerosis, is a form of angiokeratoma and unrelated to sebaceous gland tissue. As might be expected, tuberous sclerosis is not associated with increased numbers of Fordyce granules even though angiokeratomas of the oral mucosa have been described in this condition. Epidemiologic studies of intraoral sebaceous glands (which were at one time inappropriately referred to as Fordyce *disease*) have been carried out by Halperin, Miles, and Sewerin, and their ultrastructural characteristics recently described by Monteil.

Linea Alba and Other Areas of Normal Frictional Cornification

Variations in structure of the mucosa in different parts of the mouth reflect variation in function. Where the mucosa overlies bone as in the hard palate and gingiva and there is frequent frictional contact with food, the epithelium is keratinized under normal conditions and exhibits a stratum granulosum, well-developed rete processes, and a densely collagenous lamina propria that merges with the periosteum (see Fig. 6-3A). These features are consistently found on the hard palate and somewhat more irregularly on the gingiva, possibly owing to variation in dietary and oral hygiene practices. Depending on the degree of keratinization and thickness of the stratum corneum in these areas, the palate and gingivae appear whiter than the adjacent nonkeratinized mucosa of the soft palate, areolar gingiva, and buccal and lingual sulci. The mucosa that does not overlie bone (soft palate, cheeks, lips, floor of the mouth, and ventral surface of the tongue) is generally nonkeratinized, with shallow or few rete pro-

cesses and a relatively noncollagenous lamina propria (see Fig. 6-3B).

One exception to this generalization is that in most individuals a line of keratinization can be found on the buccal mucosa parallel to the line of occlusion and expanding to a triangular area just inside each labial commissure. Referred to as the *linea alba*, this zone also indicates an area of normal frictional cornification and may appear whiter and more distinct in some individuals, when it is highly cornified. Variable degrees of keratinization of these different zones are compatible with normal, although the effects of smoking, food texture, and other oral environmental irritants are certainly reflected in the range of cornification observed. In general, increased frictional cornification in one area is accompanied by similar changes in other normally keratinized areas of the mouth and is a diffusely distributed rather than a patchy phenomenon.

NONKERATOTIC WHITE LESIONS

Habitual Cheek-Biting

Masticatory trauma can be responsible for a variety of white lesions. For example, sudden inadvertent biting of the cheek, tongue, or lip mucosa produces an ulcer of variable severity, usually with characteristic contused margins to identify its traumatic etiology (see Chap. 5); transient whitish tags of necrotic tissue are common around such ulcers (see Fig. 6-4). With repeated biting, the chronically traumatized area may become thickened, scarred, and paler than the surrounding mucosa. Chronic lesions of this type usually occur well back in the cheeks, in association with areas of traumatic or tobacco-induced keratosis that will justify biopsy, as discussed in a subsequent section of this chapter.

The term *habitual cheek-biting* (sometimes referred to as *morsicato buccarum*), however, is generally used for a more superficial lesion produced by frequently repeated rubbing, sucking, or chewing movements that abrade the surface of a wide area of the lip or cheek mucosa without producing discrete ulcera-

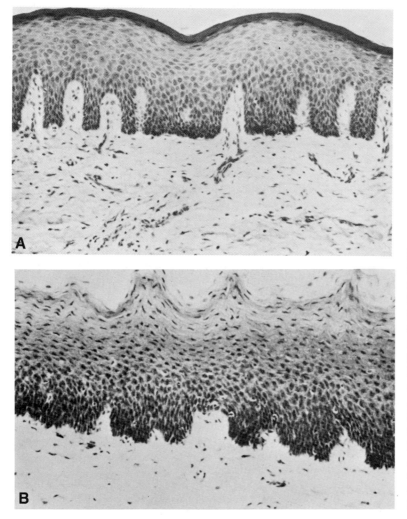

Fig. 6-3 Variations in structure of the normal oral mucosa. *A,* Normal hard palate; keratinized epithelium with well-developed rete processes. (Hematoxylin & eosin [H&E], ×96) *B,* Normal mucosa from the floor of the mouth; nonkeratinized epithelium, shallow rete processes, and delicate lamina propria (H & E, ×120). (From WHO Collaborating Centre for Oral Precancerous Lesions: Definition of leukoplakia and related lesions: An aid to studies on oral precancer. Oral Surg 46:518, 1978; courtesy CV Mosby Co., St. Louis, MO 63141)

tion (see Fig. 6-5). Such lesions feel rough to the examiner's fingers and appear as poorly outlined, macerated, and reddened areas, usually with whitish patches of partly detached surface epithelium. Histologic examination is not helpful and rarely indicated, although long-established lesions may be associated with areas of keratosis and increased thickness of the epithelium.

Habitual cheek-biting usually occurs as an unconscious nervous habit or in association with uncontrolled tongue thrusting or chewing and grinding jaw movements in individuals with neuromuscular disorders such as tardive dyskinesia. Awareness of a habit is often all that is needed for a patient to elim-

inate these lesions, although medical attention to food packs, occlusal discrepancies, or rough tooth surfaces that encourage a habit may be needed. Prescription of a small dose of diazepam (5 to 10 mg at bedtime) or a plastic occlusal nightguard may be necessary when the habit occurs mostly during sleep.

Prevalence studies in a sample of Scandinavians of all ages (0.5% had evidence of either lip- or cheek-biting) and institutionalized South African school children (4.6%) support the role of stress and anxiety in producing this self-induced lesion. Differential diagnosis includes white sponge nevus, chemical burns, reaction to locally applied medicaments, and candidiasis.

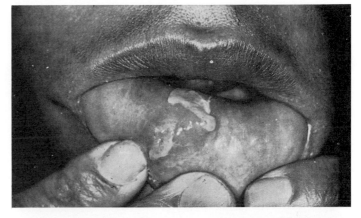

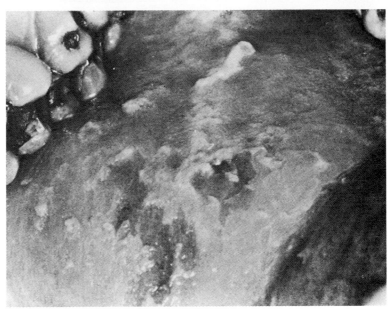

Fig. 6-4 Traumatic injury to the lip resulting from a fall. The sudden onset, severe pain, swelling, and irregular margins aid in differentiating the lesion from a more chronic white lesion. Transient whitish tags of necrotic tissue are common around such traumatic lesions.

Fig. 6-5 Lesions of habitual cheek biting. Irregular white flakes alternating with superficial erosion. (From WHO Collaborating Centre for Oral Precancerous Lesions: Definition of leukoplakia and related lesions: An aid to studies of oral precancer. Oral Surg 46:518, 1979; courtesy CV Mosby Co., St. Louis, MO 63141)

Burns

Burns of the oral mucosa are a frequent cause of transient nonkeratotic white lesions, the white appearance of the mucosa being attributable to a superficial pseudomembrane composed of coagulated tissue with an inflammatory exudate. Except in xerostomic individuals, the normal coating of saliva protects the oral mucosa from many physical and chemical agents, and significant damage occurs only when there is prolonged contact or a severe insult. For the same reason, injuries to the oral mucosa of xerostomic individuals are likely to be more severe, even from otherwise minor burns such as those caused by hot cigarette smoke. Superficial necrosis and scarring of the oral mucosa from a burn is rare except for burns caused by a very hot object (*e.g.*, a hot dental instrument or molten impression compound; see Fig. 6-6), anesthetic gas explosions, or electrical burns (see Chap. 14). Oropharyngeal and esophageal burns from ingestion of caustic liquids such as lye usually affect the pharynx and esophagus more severely than the oral cavity.

Mild *thermal burns* of the oral tissues are common as a result of the accidental ingestion of hot food or beverages. These are usually of little consequence because the symp-

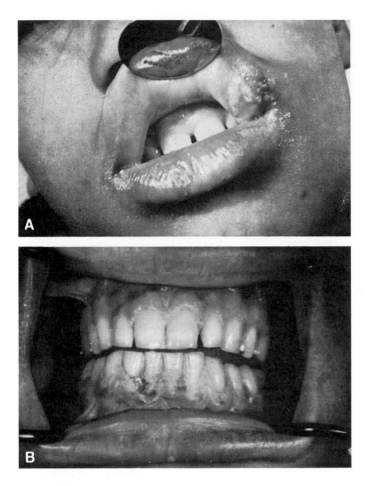

Fig. 6-6 *A*, Thermal burn of the lips resulting from contact with hot dental forceps. *B*, Thermal burn of the mandibular gingiva caused by hot hydrocolloid impression material.

toms are of relatively short duration and involve a comparatively small area. The burn may be difficult to detect on clinical examination unless the surface layers of epithelium have desquamated. The anterior third of the tongue and the palate are common sites of burns caused by hot foods and beverages. Central palatal burns associated with the eating of pizza, fondue, or other hot cheese dishes are often more severe, although the patient is usually unaware of the cause of the lesion until a careful history is taken. These "pizza burns" usually appear as centrally located, whitish gray or ulcerated lesions of the middle third of the hard palate (see Fig. 6-7). The superficial necrosis and ulceration result from a combination of the heat of the cheese and its adhesion to the blistered epithelium.

A severe slough of the soft oral tissues will result from holding CO_2 snow, or "dry ice"

in the mouth, a practice indulged in occasionally by children. The tongue and lips are usually most seriously affected. Frostbite of the lips with a complaint of persistent swelling and redness can occur from prolonged contact of a child's lips with ice-cream and other frozen confections ("popsicle panniculitis") or very cold metal or glass objects. After thawing, the frozen epithelium may look dry and rougher than the surrounding tissue but rarely blisters or develops a pseudomembrane.

Aspirin and *aspirin-containing* compounds are a common source of burns of the oral mucosa (see Fig. 6-8). They occur when an acetylsalicylic acid-containing analgesic compound is placed in the mucobuccal fold for the relief of pulpitis, periostitis, or a periapical abscess. Irregularly shaped, white, pseudomembranous, painful lesions develop

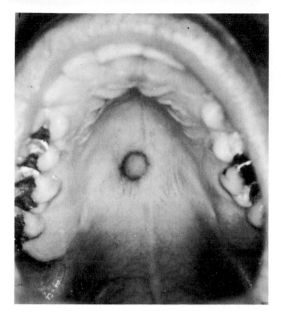

Fig. 6-7 "Pizza" burn. Burn of palatal mucosal tissues caused by melted cheese and hot sauce. (Courtesy Drs. D.W. Cohen and J.L. Dannenberg, Philadelphia, PA)

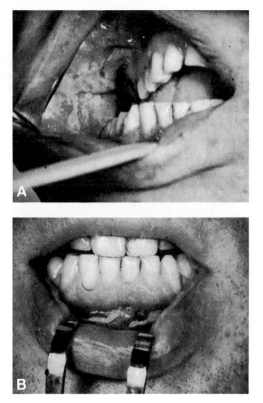

Fig. 6-8 Acetylsalicylic acid (aspirin) burns of the oral mucosa resulting from placing a crushed aspirin tablet in the mucobuccal fold opposite the molars (*A*) and the lower anteriors (*B*).

where the medicament touches the oral mucosa and the gingival tissues. The entire cheek mucosa may be diffusely involved. The tissues are painful, and the white cauterized areas may be easily removed, leaving a painful, raw, bleeding area. Similar but milder burns can be produced by prolonged use of aspirin-containing chewing gum, and the margins of ulcers exposed to this topical analgesic often become white and thickened (*see Fig. 10-23*).

Other commercially available *toothache drops* contain creosote, guiacol, or a related phenol derivative that also has a caustic action on the oral mucosa. Because these toothache-relieving agents are rarely confined to the carious lesion, gingival and mucosal burns are the rule when these agents are used by the patient. Many of the *medicaments* traditionally used in dental practice also cause painful burns and white lesions of the gingivae and the oral mucosa when they accidentally come in contact with dry oral tissues. Chromic acid, trichloroacetic acid, silver nitrate, beechwood creosote, eugenol, paraformaldehyde, phenol, and tincture of iodine should not be allowed to come in contact with the mucous membranes of the mouth unless cauterization of tissue is desired.

In some patients, application of a 70% ethyl alcohol solution will result in a sloughing of the oral mucosa. Chronic topical application of isopropyl alcohol has also been shown to produce a *coagulative hyperkeratosis* and *acanthosis* of the oral mucosa. Maceration and sloughing of nonkeratinized mucosa may occur with excessive use of *proprietary mouthrinses*, some of which contain 25% ethyl alcohol as well as detergents, astringents, essential oils, and other antiseptic agents. *Cotton roll burns* (Fig. 6-9) and burns from a variety of medications in compressed tablet form (*e.g.*, vitamin C tablet burns) are other examples of transient iatrogenic burns of the oral mucosa caused by dehydration, pseudomembrane formation, and stripping of superficial tissue.

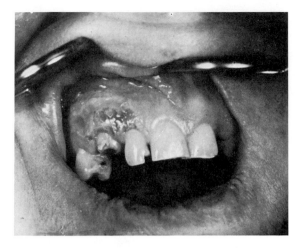

Fig. 6-9 "Cotton roll" burn. The denudation of the epithelium from the buccal gingiva in the maxillary right second incisor, cuspid, and premolar area resulted from the rapid removal of a cotton roll.

Radiation mucositis secondary to therapeutic radiation of head and neck cancer develops towards the end of the first week of therapy as a diffuse redness most apparent on the poorly keratinized areas of the oral mucosa. Pseudomembrane formation follows with large areas of the mucosa covered with a grayish white slough alternating with areas of more severe ulceration.

The term *uremic stomatitis* is given to the extensive pseudomembranous white lesions that are sometimes seen in seriously ill patients with renal failure and blood urea nitrogen (BUN) levels in excess of 50 mg/dl. This lesion is traditionally explained as a chemical burn resulting from increased ammonia levels in saliva secondary to the action of urease-containing microorganisms on salivary urea. While uremia is often associated with a marked ammoniacal odor to the breath, the unexplained appearance of uremic stomatitis in only a small proportion of patients with renal failure and raised BUN levels, and the fact that the lesions often resolve despite a persistently raised BUN, suggest that other abnormal metabolites, xerostomia, and secondary bacterial or fungal infection may account for the extensive white lesions of uremic stomatitis. With the greater availabil-

ity of renal dialysis, uremic stomatitis appears to have become a relatively uncommon complication of renal failure.

Nonkeratotic White Lesions Caused by Specific Infectious Agents

Thrush or acute pseudomembranous candidiasis, which is described in the following section, is the classical example of a nonkeratotic white lesion resulting from invasion of the superficial layer of the oral mucosa by an endogenous oral infectious agent. Similar though usually less dramatic lesions may result from blood-borne infection of patches of the oral mucosa with other and usually exogenously acquired infectious agents. *Koplik's spots* caused by measles virus and *syphilitic mucous patches* (see Chap. 28) are examples of this phenomenon. Erythema and inflammation of localized areas of the oral mucosa are followed by exudation of fibrin and inflammatory cells that coagulate to form a pseudomembrane. Attempts at removal of the characteristic white spots or patches in both cases reveal a reddened, raw mucosal surface.

Similar white lesions may be seen as a result of infection of the oral mucosa with a variety of other exogenous and endogenous microorganisms, but are not usually specifically described other than as a localized stomatitis or mucositis. *Klebsiella pneumoniae* infection has been associated with the presence of white pseudomembranous lesions superimposed on a denudative gingivitis following therapeutic radiation.

Treatment of Nonkeratotic White Lesions

Nonkeratotic white lesions associated with underlying erosion and inflammation of the mucosa are often painful and when extensive (*e.g.*, radiation mucositis) will require prescription of topically applied analgesic agents (0.5% aqueous antihistamine rinses, lidocaine gel). Otherwise, treatment includes elimination of the physical, chemical, or microbial agent involved and prescription of bland saline or bicarbonate mouthrinses. Antibiotic treatment is rarely needed. With the exception of habitual cheek-biting, these le-

tively short lived, and *Candida* s no part in their etiology. Section of the macerated mucosa s also not a feature of habitual

CANDIDIASIS

Candida infection is associated with both nonkeratotic and keratotic oral white lesions. In one series of patients, *Candida* was isolated from 84% of patients with thrush, 75% with antibiotic sore mouth, 77% with angular cheilitis, 69% with denture sore mouth, as well as 84% with chronic hyperplastic candidiasis (*Candida* leukoplakia) and 100% with chronic mucocutaneous candidiasis. *Candida* is usually referred to as an opportunistic* infectious agent that despite a battery of proteases is poorly equipped to invade and destroy tissue, unless it is provided with an opportunity to rapidly reproduce and a portal of entry. The role of *Candida* as an opportunistic invader versus etiologic agent in either keratotic or nonkeratotic oral white lesions has not been clearly established, although recent ultrastructural and microbiologic studies may provide information in this regard. In the same way, the significance of this organism as an oral carcinogen or co-carcinogen is uncertain; however, the almost constant association of *Candida* with the speckled red and white type of leukoplakia and the hyperplastic effects of *Candida* demonstrated *in vitro* suggest that it may not be solely an

---

* A number of fungi, protozoa, and bacteria are not pathogenic in healthy humans but may behave as virulent pathogens in those suffering from a variety of apparently unrelated systemic disorders (leukemias, lymphomas, diabetes); those treated intensively with broad-spectrum antibiotics, antimetabolites, and other cytotoxic agents; those with inborn or acquired immune-deficiencies; and those with defects in the structure of skin and mucous membranes. These opportunistic organisms include *Candida*, as well as *Aspergillus, Cryptococcus,* and other fungi; the protozoae *Pneumocystis carinii , Cryptosporidium* and *Isospora;* the *Mycobacterium avium/intracellulare* group of atypical mycobacteria; and cytomegalovirus, Epstein Barr virus, and herpes simplex virus. (See also discussion of factors involved in chronic mucocutaneous candidiasis and systemic candidiasis, at end of this section on candidiasis.)

innocuous opportunistic infectious agent and that treatment of chronic oral white lesions should include efforts to control oral candidiasis.

Both nonkeratotic and keratotic white lesions associated with *Candida* infection are discussed in this section to provide an overview of oral lesions associated with this organism. It will be clear, however, that some of these lesions could also be discussed under Nonkeratotic White Lesions and others under the section dealing with Red and White Lesions with Defined or Uncertain Precancerous Potential. Oral candidiasis is very often only one manifestation of a more generalized infection that may involve other mucosal and skin surfaces as well as deeper tissues; a brief outline of the extraoral manifestations of *Candida* infection is included at the end of this section as a necessary background for consideration of red and white oral mucosal lesions associated with *Candida*.

Thrush

Clinical Features

Thrush (acute pseudomembranous candidiasis) is the prototype of oral infections with the yeastlike fungus *Candida*. It is a superficial infection of the upper layers of the oral mucosal epithelium and results in the formation of patchy white plaques or flecks on the mucosal surface that are composed of desquamated epithelial cells, inflammatory cells, fibrin, yeasts, and mycelial elements. The surrounding mucosa may or may not be reddened, but removal of the plaques by gently rubbing or scraping usually reveals an area of erythema or even shallow ulceration. Because of their prevalence, rather characteristic appearance, and ease of removal, the lesions of thrush are often cited as representative of the nonkeratotic group of white lesions.

A diagnosis of thrush is commonly made on the basis of the appearance of the lesion, with or without confirmation by smear or culture of *Candida*. (Strictly speaking, a firm diagnosis of thrush should be made only when the organism is demonstrated in a stained smear or imprint culture prepared from the characteristic clinical lesion. Similar appearing oral mucosal lesions can also result from other causes, for example, medications, food debris, other infectious agents, chemical burns.)

Candida species are a normal component of the oral microbial flora and become established there during or soon after birth, usually by direct spread from the mother's genital tract. Lesions of thrush are seen in children and adults of all ages, whenever the number of *Candida* in the oral cavity increases significantly, or oral environmental conditions alter and promote colonization of the surface epithelium by this opportunistic organism. When the number of *Candida* are reduced or eliminated by administration of antifungal agents, the lesions of thrush rapidly disappear. Transient episodes of thrush may occur as isolated phenomena that disappear spontaneously with minimum or no treatment and are unrelated to any recognized predisposing factor (infections of this type are common in neonates and young children as their oral flora becomes established). Alternatively, the lesions may promptly recur following treatment, suggesting the persistence of a predisposing factor. A clinical presentation of this type is more common in adult candidiasis, in which the characteristic lesion of thrush is also more likely to be associated with erythema, patchy mucosal atrophy, and other forms of oral *Candida* infection that are discussed below.

The typical lesions in infants are described as soft, white, or bluish white, adherent patches on the oral mucosa, at times extending to the circumoral tissues (see Fig. 6-10). These bluish white intraoral lesions are generally painless and noted by the mother or nurse only if the mouth is carefully examined. They can be removed with little difficulty, but may leave a raw, bleeding surface. In the adult, inflammation, erythema, and painful eroded areas are more often associated with this disease, and at times the typical, pearly white or bluish white, plaquelike lesions are relatively inconspicuous. The lesions of thrush are by no means restricted to infants, however. Any mucosal area of the mouth may be involved: erythematous or white areas may develop beneath partial or complete dentures; alternatively, the white plaques may be found only in well-protected

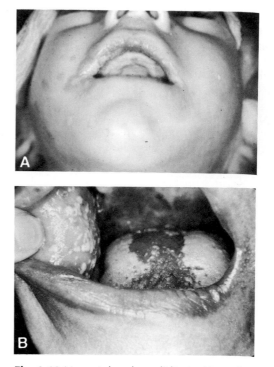

Fig. 6-10 Neonatal oral candidiasis. Note circumoral lesions (*A*) in addition to intraoral thrush (*B*).

areas. The lesions may involve the entire oral mucosa or relatively localized areas, where normal cleansing mechanisms are poor: the roof of the mouth, the mucobuccal fold, or the retromolar region. It is not unusual for the patient, and at times the dentist, to consider that the painful, inflamed areas are secondary to a bacterial infection and to continue the administration of a causative antibacterial antibiotic in increased dosages. As a rule, constitutional symptoms in thrush are nonexistent or mild in degree in comparison with other forms of stomatitis and pharyngitis such as Vincent's gingivostomatitis, primary herpes simplex infection, and stomatitis medicamentosa (contact stomatitis). In debilitated patients, the lesions of thrush may be discovered only on routine oral examination, both the patient and physician being unaware of the stomatitis.

A prodromal symptom of rapid onset of a bad taste and loss of taste discrimination is described by some adults. Burning of the mouth and throat may also precede the appearance of the white pseudomembranous lesions. Symptoms of this type in a patient receiving broad-spectrum antibiotics are strongly suggestive of thrush or other forms of oral candidiasis.

Differential diagnosis of thrush includes flecks of milk, other food debris or antacids remaining attached to the oral mucosa, particularly in a nursing infant or debilitated elderly patient. (This phenomenon has been referred to as *intern's thrush.*) Analogous pseudomembranous white lesions are caused by *Klebsiella* or other usually unspecified microbial agents, habitual cheek-biting, and rarely, a genetically determined epithelial abnormality such as white sponge nevus (see following section).

Causative Organism and Frequency

The yeastlike fungus that causes thrush and the other manifestations of candidiasis occurs in both yeast and mycelial forms in the oral cavity and infected tissues. Growth of the organism occurs by budding of the yeast cells to form germ tubes and individual hyphal elements, which undergo limited peripheral branching (to form a pseudomycelium; *see Fig. 3-21, 3-22, and 3-23*). These phenomena can be demonstrated in smears and tissue sections from the oral cavity or other involved tissues, as well as *in vitro,* and form the basis for confirmatory laboratory diagnostic tests for candidiasis (see Chap. 3).

Candida species are normal inhabitants of the oral flora of many individuals, but are present in the mouth of the healthy carrier in low concentration (fewer than 200 cells per milliliter of saliva). At this concentration, the organism cannot be demonstrated by direct microscopic examination of smears from the oral mucosa of the healthy carrier, and its presence can be demonstrated only by inoculation of a mouth swab onto a selective medium such as Sabouraud's agar, on which the bulk of the oral bacterial flora fail to grow. The frequency with which the organism can be demonstrated by this method varies with different populations studied and the sampling method used. Saliva samples, impression cultures, and imprint cultures have all been used for this purpose, although imprint cultures (using 2.5 cm × 2.5 cm plastic foam pads soaked in Sabouraud medium to obtain samples from different areas of the oral cav-

ity) reveal higher overall prevalence rates, as well as differential rates of colonization of various oral mucosal surfaces. Saliva samples give a carrier rate of 20% to 30% for healthy young adults, whereas imprint cultures, which sample colonized sites rather than detached cells and organisms in the mixed saliva, give a figure as high as 44%. Impression cultures are relatively insensitive and detect only a 13% healthy carrier rate. Imprint cultures also indicate that the papillae of the posterior oral surface of the tongue are the primary colonization site in the oral cavity, other areas being contaminated or secondarily colonized from this site.

The asymptomatic carrier state is affected by a number of known factors including contact with a hospital environment as a patient or health worker, smoking, prior use of antibiotics, and general health status. The carrier state is more prevalent in diabetics, and the density of *Candida* at various oral sites is also increased in this disease, although correlations with severity of diabetes, salivary or serum glucose levels or diabetic treatment have not been established. The wearing of removable prosthetic appliances has also been traditionally associated with higher asymptomatic carrier prevalence rates, based on the results of studies using saliva samples; however, imprint culture techniques suggest that removable appliances only increase the density of *Candida* in the mouth and hence the ease with which they can be detected by swabbing, but do not initiate the carrier state. Examples of carrier rates based on saliva samples are healthy young adults, 20%; hospital workers, 36%; hospital patients, 55% and higher; otherwise unselected adults, 50%; adults with removable dentures, 80% to 90%. Because *Candida* species are normal oral inhabitants, thrush and other forms of oral candidiasis may be classified as specific endogenous infections. A variety of species of *Candida* (*C. albicans, stellatoidea, tropicalis, parapsilopsis, pseudotropicalis, guilliermondi, krusei, famata, glabrata, rugosa,* and *pintolopesii*) have been isolated from carriers and from patients with candidiasis. The particular species involved with a given oral infection is not known to be of any significance, but *C. albicans* (a species that produces heavy-walled spores called chlamydospores on artificial media and rapidly buds in the presence of serum or special media such as rabbit coagulase plasma EDTA) is most commonly found in thrush. This species, together with *C. tropicalis* and *C. parapsilopsis,* is thought to be more highly pathogenic than the other species in regard to systemic infections. Severity and refractoriness of *Candida* infection to treatment depend more on site and predisposing factors than on properties of the infecting species, and the decreasing order of pathogenicity that has been described for *C. albicans* and the other species listed above has little clinical significance except for systemic human infections. Like other microorganisms involved in endogenous infections, *Candida* are of low virulence, are not usually considered contagious, and are involved in mucosal infection only where there is definite local or systemic predisposition to their enhanced reproduction and invasion (see also discussion below concerning candidiasis as a sexually transmitted disease).

Predisposing Factors

Currently there is no clear understanding of the mechanisms in oral candidiasis by which this organism colonizes broad areas of the oral epithelium rather than an isolated area of tongue papillae, but a variety of predisposing factors have been defined by clinical observation.

1. Marked changes in the oral microbial flora owing to administration of antibiotics (especially broad-spectrum) excessive use of antibacterial mouthrinses and xerostomia secondary to anticholinergic agents or secondary to salivary gland disease
2. Chronic local irritants (dentures and orthodontic appliances; heavy smoking)
3. Administration of corticosteroids (topical, oral and aerosolized inhalant; systemic)
4. Radiation to head and neck
5. Age (infancy, pregnancy, old age)
6. Hospitalization (age, debilitating disease, antibiotics)
7. Oral epithelial dysplasia
   congenital
   acquired (keratotic oral lesions)
8. Immunologic deficiency
   congenital (endocrine candidiasis syndrome, chronic familial mucocutaneous candidiasis, DiGeorge's and Nezelof's syndromes, thymoma, Swiss and Bruton type agammaglobulinemias)
   acquired (diabetes; leukemia and lymphomas; iatrogenic from cancer chemotherapy, bone marrow transplantation; acquired immune deficiency syndrome or AIDS)

So important are these predisposing factors in the etiology of this infection that it is extremely rare to find a case of oral candidiasis in which one or more of these factors cannot be identified. One study found, for example, that 78% of patients with thrush had an associated systemic disorder or recent antibiotic or corticosteroid administration. Topical, systemic, and aerosolized inhalant administration of corticosteroids are all important in this regard (see discussion in section dealing with treatment of lichen planus). A diagnosis of thrush should always be followed by a search for a possible hidden systemic problem, a review of the patient's medications, and a search for some locally acting predisposing factor such as an appliance, smoking habit, or mucosal abnormality (see Fig. 6-11).

Xerostomia and chronic local irritants presumably act by alteration of the oral mucous membranes, predisposing them to invasion by this organism. There have been only limited studies of the effects of these conditions on the oral flora, but shifts in the bacterial flora probably also accompany these situations and provide an opportunity for *Candida* species to increase. Radiation to the head and neck also affects the oral mucous membranes and produces xerostomia by causing obliterative changes in major and minor salivary glands. In Sjögren's syndrome, sarcoidosis, and other fibrosing diseases of the salivary glands, the onset of xerostomia is often gradual and tolerated by the patient until superinfection of the oral mucosa with *Candida* develops and the mucosal lesions, pain, and associated symptoms of thrush cause the patient to seek medical or dental care.

Several workers have followed the changes that occur in the oral flora of adults following topical treatment with an antibiotic, such as chlortetracycline (see Figs. 6-12 and 6-13). Brightman and associates found that from a

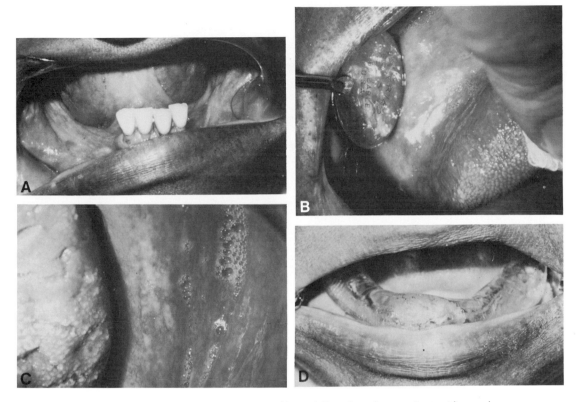

Fig. 6-11 Persistent oral candidiasis in a 58-year-old partially edentulous patient with poorly controlled diabetes mellitus and ill-fitting partial lower denture. *A, B,* and *C,* Lesions of pseudomembranous candidiasis are visible on the mandibular gingiva, lingual sulcus, and tongue dorsum. *D,* Lesions were controlled by application of nystatin cream under a plastic stent prior to construction of new denture.

normal value of approximately 10^9 organisms per 15 ml mouth-rinsing sample, the bacterial count dropped by a factor of 10^5 after 3 days of treatment with the broad-spectrum antibiotic. Counts of most bacteria remained at this low level throughout antibiotic treatment, although some species became resistant. The yeast count showed the reverse of the changes in bacterial counts. Yeasts appeared at countable levels on the fifth day of antibiotic treatment and gradually increased to an average of 10^5 organisms per sample after 14 days of treatment. This level was also maintained for at least 7 days after discontinuation of topical chlortetracycline. Three levels of yeast count, each with characteristic symptomatology and laboratory findings, were distinguished. Below a level of 10^5 yeast per 15 ml mouth-rinsing sample, all patients were asymptomatic, and 94% of mouth smears were free of yeasts and mycelia. Above 10^5, the frequency of symptoms increased, ranging in severity from bad taste, through soreness and burning of the mouth and throat, to clinically evident thrush and angular cheilitis. In this range, 72% of smears contained yeasts, and 33% of the patients had symptoms. Thrush was not evident unless counts rose above 10^6 yeasts per sample.

Similar results have been obtained by others, who suggest a concentration of fewer than 400 colony-forming units of *Candida* per milliliter of expectorated, unstimulated whole-mouth saliva as distinguishing asymptomatic carriers from those with candidiasis. These studies indicate that symptomatic oral candidiasis is largely a function of overgrowth of yeasts, with symptoms related to

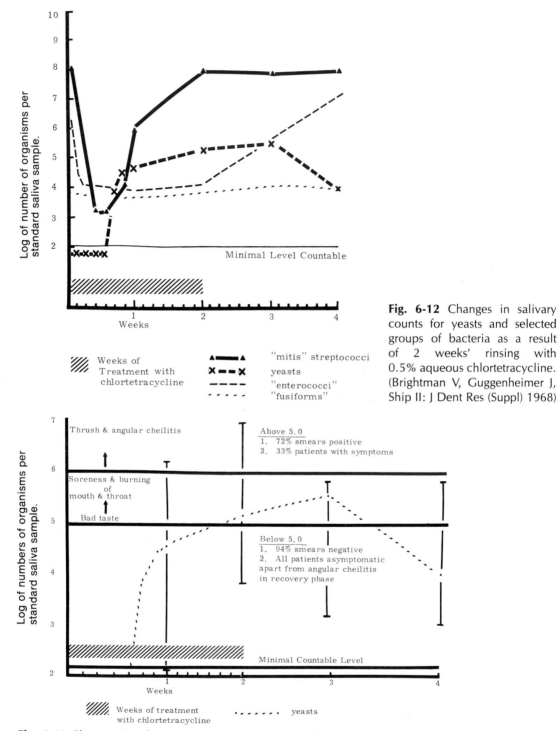

Fig. 6-12 Changes in salivary counts for yeasts and selected groups of bacteria as a result of 2 weeks' rinsing with 0.5% aqueous chlortetracycline. (Brightman V, Guggenheimer J, Ship II: J Dent Res (Suppl) 1968)

Fig. 6-13 Changes in salivary yeast count, laboratory findings, and symptomatology as a result of 2 weeks' rinsing with 0.5% aqueous chlortetracycline. (Brightman V, Guggenheimer J, Ship II: J Dent Res (Suppl), 1968)

the yeast concentration. The persistence of the high yeast counts after discontinuation of the antibiotic therapy also explains the persistence of lesions and symptoms into this period as is often noted clinically.

Histologic Features

Microscopic examination of the lesions of thrush reveals a localized superficial inflammatory reaction with ulceration of the surface. The ulcer is covered with a thick layer of cellular debris, fibrin, and inflammatory exudate, in which are found large numbers of yeasts and short mycelial filaments showing rudimentary branching. The fungi rarely penetrate below this superficial layer (see Fig. 10-14). This pseudomembrane imparts the characteristic white-flecked appearance to the mucosal lesions, and where it is removed by scraping or mastication of food, the underlying inflamed mucosa remains as an erythematous patch. On the basis of the rapidity of development of the lesions of thrush and their histologic appearance, thrush is correctly described as acute pseudomembranous candidiasis. Scanning electron microscopic examination of the lesions of thrush and the more adherent white scales that are seen in chronic mucocutaneous candidiasis reveal actual colonization of keratinized cells by pseudohyphae and small and large spores (blastospores and occasionally chlamydospores). These fungal elements appear to enter epithelial cells through holes in the keratinized cells. The origin of these holes is not known, whether for example they are produced by the organism or other cellular damage that provides an opportunity for the fungus to enter.

The adherence of *C. albicans* to both oral and vaginal epithelium is believed to be caused by a surface component of *germinated* yeast cells, possibly a surface protein of the yeast cell that binds to an epithelial glycoprotein receptor.

Diagnostic Features

Oral candidiasis may occur in a number of forms in addition to thrush. Because of this variability in appearance and the fact that oral lesions owing to other causes may be clinically indistinguishable from candidiasis, it is usually only by microscopic examination of scrapings or by histologic examination that a diagnosis of candidiasis can be confirmed.

In thrush, large numbers of yeasts and mycelia will be seen; in the chronic forms of oral candidiasis (see below) fewer organisms are present, but enough are usually present to allow a diagnosis to be made. In chronic atrophic candidiasis (denture sore mouth), scrapings of the palate may reveal few organisms, although the seating surface of the denture often is covered with a mat of mycelium mixed with food and cellular debris, and scrapings of the lesions of angular cheilitis often show mycelia. In chronic hyperplastic candidiasis, the organisms may disappear during topical antifungal therapy only to reappear from the depths of the epithelium as soon as therapy is stopped. It is always important to review what medications, mouthrinses, and denture cleansers the patient has used just before obtaining the specimen. Because of the high salivary carrier rate for this organism, salivary cultures using Sabouraud or other selective medium clinically are of little help, except to confirm the nature of the organisms demonstrated by examination of scrapings. Imprint cultures, however, provide information on the differential localization of *Candida* in various areas of the oral mucosa.

The high salivary carrier rate also prevents use of the presence or absence of serum or salivary antibody as a diagnostic test; however, the titers of serum and salivary antibody detected by fluorescence-labeling techniques are related to the presence of infection, and determination of these titers is a useful procedure in the diagnosis of the chronic forms of candidiasis (see Chap. 3).

Other Forms of Oral Candidiasis

Oral candidiasis is divided into four distinct categories based on the clinical appearance and natural history of the infection:*

* Lehner, T: Classification and clinico-pathological features of *Candida* infections in the mouth. In Winner HI, Hurley R (eds): Symposium on *Candida* Infections, p 119. Edinburgh, E & S Livingstone, 1966

Acute

Acute pseudomembranous candidiasis (thrush)

Acute atrophic candidiasis (antibiotic sore-mouth)

Chronic

Chronic atropic candidiasis (denture sore-mouth, angular cheilitis, and possibly median rhomboid glossitis), and chronic hyperplastic candidiasis.

Acute Atrophic Candidiasis

Acute atrophic candidiasis includes antibiotic sore-mouth and other instances in which a red patch of atrophic, raw, painful mucosa persists for some time with minimal evidence of pseudomembranous (white) lesions. Antibody levels against *C. albicans* are present in patients with this type of candidiasis, but they are usually not significant in thrush. Lehner reported one case in which the titer rose from 1:4 to 1:64 within 5 days of the use of oral tetracycline, although such a rise is certainly not characteristic in all patients who develop antibiotic sore-mouth. Antibiotic sore-mouth should be suspected in a patient who develops symptoms of oral burning, bad taste or sore throat during the convalesent period of an illness that has been treated with broad-spectrum antibiotics. Additional features of *Candida* infection may be present, such as angular cheilitis and thrush, and smears of the reddened painful mucosa are usually positive for yeasts and mycelia. The diagnosis of oral candidiasis may be obscured by a patient's vigorous use of mouthrinses or toothbrushing just before examination. The white flecks of thrush can be temporarily removed leaving only patchy red excoriation of the mucosa, a lesion that can still be described as candidiasis.

Chronic Atrophic Candidiasis

Chronic atrophic candidiasis (CAC) includes denture sore-mouth and angular cheilitis. Denture sore-mouth (DSM) is a diffuse inflammation of the maxillary denture-bearing area, with or without cracking and inflammation of the oral commissures (angular cheilitis; see Fig. 6-14). If both CAC and palatal papillary hyperplasia (PPH)* are present under a poorly fitting denture, the palatal lesions will be velvety or they may resemble the surface of an overripe berry and bleed on slight pressure. Pain and burning are usually reported during periods of exacerbation, but the red raw area will persist for years as long as the denture is worn. Significantly raised antibody titers against *C. albicans* are found in both serum and saliva in chronic atrophic candidiasis, a fact of considerable diagnostic importance, because the number of yeasts and mycelia present in the palatal and angular lesions is much fewer than in acute candidiasis.

The etiology of denture sore mouth remains a controversial topic, although the concept that it represents one form of chronic oral mucosal candidiasis has gained more support in recent years. The more traditional explanations for this lesion (trauma from a poorly fitting denture, loss of vertical dimension, and vitamin B deficiency) may all play a role in both the palatal mucosal and angular lesions; however, the resolution of the redness and soreness of the palate and of the angular fissures following antifungal treatment suggests that in this case, *Candida* species probably act as endogenous infecting agents on tissue predisposed to microbial invasion by chronic trauma. In over 80% of patients with angular cheilitis there is a coexistent denture stomatitis. Angular cheilitis is also rare in patients with a natural dentition. The term *perlèche*, originally used to describe cases of angular cheilitis as a result of vitamin B deficiency, is now used synonymously with angular cheilitis.

Denture sore mouth and palatal papillary hyperplasia (see Chap. 8) often coexist in one patient. There is no evidence that *Candida* is an etiologic agent in palatal papillary hyperplasia (smears may be positive, but biopsy and special staining fail to reveal the organism in the tissue), and while antifungal treatment will modify the bright red, "overripe strawberry" appearance of this combined DSM-PPH lesion, it will not resolve the basic

---

* Also referred to in the literature as IPH (inflammatory papillary hyperplasia).

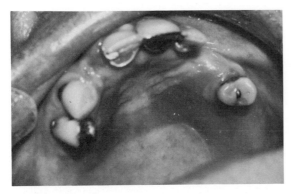

Fig. 6-14 Chronic atrophic candidiasis (denture sore mouth) affecting the mucosa in contact with a partial upper denture. The affected mucosa was bright red, had a velvety texture, and bled with mild trauma.

papillomatous lesion. Antifungal therapy in addition to removal of the denture is advisable before surgical excision of palatal papillary hyperplasia because elimination of the mucosal inflammation leaves a firmer tissue for surgery and often reduces the amount of tissue that needs to be excised.

The increased incidence of oral candidiasis among patients wearing dentures and other removable appliances is associated with a great increase in the number of *Candida* that can be cultivated from the mouth. Increased numbers are found not only in the lesions themselves but also on the tongue, palatal mucosa, in saliva, and attached to the tissue surface of the upper denture.

The presence of yeasts attached to the denture is considered an important etiologic factor in CAC, and this may be the only site where yeasts can be demonstrated by a stained smear. The extent of the attachment of yeast to the patient's appliances (and the severity of CAC) is increased by mucus and serum and decreased by the presence of salivary pellicle, suggesting an explanation for the severity of candidiasis in xerostomic patients. The contribution of other oral bacteria to yeast attachment is less clear, but rinsing of the appliance with 2% chlorhexidine solution *or* Mycostatin suspension will eliminate yeasts. Disinfection of the appliance is therefore considered an important part of treatment of CAC. Soft liners in dentures provide a porous surface and opportunity for additional mechanical locking of plaque and yeasts to the appliance. A small number of silicone rubber lining materials have been shown to contain inhibitory compounds for *C. albicans in vitro,* but the significance of this *in vivo* is not clear because of as yet unknown solubility and absorption factors. Most case reports of *Candida* colonization of soft liners have described liners of the silicone rubber type; in general, soft liners are considered to be an additional hazard for patients susceptible to oral candidiasis.

Denture sore mouth is rarely found under the mandibular denture. A possible explanation for this is that the negative pressure under the maxillary denture excludes salivary antibody from this region, and yeasts may reproduce undisturbed in the space between denture and mucosa. The closer adaptation of the maxillary denture and palate may also bring the large number of yeasts adhering to the denture surface in contact with the mucosa.

Median Rhomboid Glossitis. There is continuing debate over the identity of the lesion referred to as *median rhomboid glossitis* (see also Chap. 10) and whether it and other patches of atrophic papillae on the dorsum of the tongue are forms of chronic atrophic candidiasis. There is no doubt that the area of the anterior two thirds of the tongue affected by median rhomboid glossitis is commonly colonized by *Candida*. Imprint cultures demonstrate that the posterior half of the tongue in front of the row of vallate papillae has the highest density of *Candida* and is the primary oral reservoir of this organism; 36% of clinically normal tongues show fungal hyphae on smears of this area, over 40% of cadaver tongues contain fungal hyphae in the superficial epithelium, and smears from atrophic areas on the tongue dorsum also appear to have a higher density of hyphae. To date, however, a clear distinction is not possible among the various theories that propose that the lesions are caused by secondary *Candida* infection in areas of decreased vascular supply associated with diabetic arteriosclerosis, that the lesions represent a developmental anomaly, possibly with secondary *Candida* infection, or that the lesions are the result of the density of *Candida* infection in this area.

Chronic Hyperplastic Candidiasis

Chronic hyperplastic candidiasis includes a variety of clinically recognized conditions in which mycelial invasion of the deeper layers of the mucosa and skin occurs, and the host response is characterized by parakeratosis, acanthosis, pseudoepitheliomatous hyperplasia, microabscess formation, and an intense chronic inflammatory cell infiltration in the corium. Histologically, the lesions are quite different from those of thrush and atrophic candidiasis, and may be identified as leukoplakia unless special stains are used to demonstrate the invading mycelia. Lesions of the skin as well as the oral mucosa also characterize this group. *Candida leukoplakia* is an extremely chronic form of oral candidiasis in which firm, white, leathery plaques are found on the cheeks, lips, and tongue. Differentation of *Candida* leukoplakia from other forms of leukoplakia is difficult without special stains and antibody studies.

Chronic hyperplastic candidiasis (see Fig. 6-15) may occur as part of chronic mucocutaneous candidiasis (see following section), often with identifiable immunologic or endocrine abnormality as a major factor predisposing the patient to development of similar lesions around the nails and other skin sites or alternatively as isolated oral lesions. It is difficult to distinguish between chronic hyperplastic candidiasis of the oral mucosa that is not accompanied by other evidence of chronic mucocutaneous candidiasis and secondary opportunistic infection of keratotic white lesions caused by other etiologic agents.

A moderate degree of epithelial dysplasia is often seen in lesions of chronic hyperplastic candidiasis, but there are usually reversible changes that disappear with elimination of the *Candida* infection; however, the risk of malignant change in leukoplakia associated with chronic *Candida* infection has been estimated as greater than the 4% rate of malignant transformation usually seen with leukoplakia. *Candida* infection occurs in other chronic oral white lesions, but without any apparent increase in the tendency of these to malignant transformation. *Candida* infection

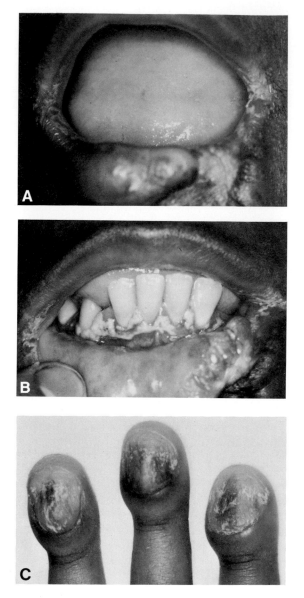

Fig. 6-15 Angular cheilitis and chronic hyperplastic candidiasis in 12-year-old with a congenital immunodeficiency. *A* and *B*, Note excoriation of labial commissure, thick leathery white membrane on lips and gingiva, and nodular lesion of lower lip. Defect of lower lip is the result of an earlier bacterial abscess of the lip. *C*, Chronic paronychial infection with *Candida* in same patient has led to destructive changes in the nail bed and clubbing of terminal phalanges of fingers caused by hypertrophic osteoarthropathy secondary to chronic pulmonary disease.

of the chorioallantoic egg membrane leads to epithelial hyperplasia and plaque formation, but similar lesions are produced by a variety of irritants and infectious agents in this system. Squamous cell carcinoma has been described as a complication of chronic oral hyperplastic candidiasis in relatively young patients with the chronic mucocutaneous candidiasis syndrome, but the incidence of squamous cell carcinoma in patients with this syndrome is not usually considered to be excessive.

The clinician who routinely treats chronic oral white lesions with topical antifungal agents before biopsy will often be surprised by the change that occurs in the appearance of many lesions with as little as 1 to 2 weeks of topical therapy. Many lesions become less extensive and less leathery, satellite plaques disappear, and on occasion white lesions are converted to red patches, which themselves also disappear with lengthier treatment. It seems likely therefore, that many if not all chronic oral mucosal lesions can become secondarily infected with *Candida,* in some cases to an extent where inflammatory changes, pseudomembrane formation, and even hyperplastic epithelial responses become the predominant feature of the lesion. On these grounds, long-term treatment of chronic oral white lesions with antifungal agents is justified, even though interrelationships between *Candida* infection, epithelial dysplasia, and the risk of future malignancy remain unsolved.

Id Reactions

Some persons with chronic *Candida* infections develop a secondary skin response characterized by a localized or generalized sterile vesiculopapular rash that is believed to be an allergic response to *Candida* antigens. These lesions, which are referred to as *monilids* or *id reaction,* usually resolve with treatment of the *Candida* infection. Lesions of this type as well as patches of erythema sometimes affect the perioral tissues of patients with oral candidiasis.

Extraoral Candidiasis

Disorders with evidence of more widespread *Candida* infection may be divided into those in which the mucosa of other body orifices (most often anogenital) or the skin is colonized and those in which other organs are involved. When organs are involved, *Candida* can also often be isolated from the bloodstream as well as the infected organs. Included here are diseases in which lesions analogous to oral thrush affect a number of skin and mucosal sites, as well as those in which immunologic deficiency or other systemic abnormality predisposes the patient to disseminated infection. Oral candidiasis in its various forms is often associated with a history or current evidence of extraoral candidiasis, although any single site or combination of sites may be affected.

Orificial and Intertriginous Sites

Candida species show preference for moist surfaces in contact with nutrients and tissue debris, especially where surface cleansing is inadequate. The mouth, vagina, colon, and rectum are therefore favored sites as are the variety of moist folds of skin (intertriginous areas) around the body orifices, waist, groin, armpits, knees, elbows and nails. Under special conditions, the mucosa of the glans penis, external ear canal, nares, and fistulas and surgically produced artificial bowel-openings can also be involved. Areas around indwelling catheters and lines inserted for intravenous solutions and parenteral hyperalimentation are particularly susceptible to local colonization with *Candida,* with the added risk of embolization and disseminated candidiasis. Tight and close-fitting garments encourage growth of *Candida* in many of these areas and often determine the site at which intertriginous candidiasis appears.

Candidal vulvovaginitis is an extremely common form of candidiasis, and many women with oral candidiasis have histories of vaginal candidiasis. Its frequency increases with pregnancy, diabetes, use of antibiotics and oral contraceptive agents, and local trauma. Candidal inflammation of the glans penis (*balanitis*) may occur in the sexual partner, leading to consideration of candidiasis in the adult in some instances as a sexually transmitted disease. Candidiasis of the *perineum, groin*, and *anorectal area* may develop as an extension of a vulvovaginitis, but is more often the result of colonization of the alimentary canal with contamination of the perineum, particularly in a child wearing diapers. *Candida* has a characteristic way of causing a dry pustulation with dissection at the lower levels of the stratum corneum of the skin. The lesion spreads from the affected orifice as an area of glazed, red skin with an easily detached overlying epidermis that is often denuded, leaving paperlike fringes along the margins. Satellite lesions often develop around these red, denuded areas.

Intertriginous candidiasis is usually accompanied by either oral or anogenital candidiasis and is considered to be caused by colonization from one of these sites. In general, the lesions are similar to those described as spreading peripherally for orificial candidiasis, with some modification imposed by the character of the particular skinfold involved. The axilla and submammary folds are most commonly affected, as are the ponderal creases secondary to obesity. Less extensive lesions usually affect the minor folds (retroauricular area, nail folds, interdigital folds, umbilicus, and prepuce).

Gastrointestinal Candidiasis

Gastrointestinal candidiasis is usually a complication of long-term broad-spectrum antibiotic and corticosteroid therapy. Leukemics and other immunosuppressed patients are particularly susceptible. This infection may present as an acute enterocolitis, diarrhea, or often simply as a proctitis with anal pruritis and perianal eczematization. Diagnosis is usually made on the basis of persistent culture of *Candida* in feces. *Esophageal candidiasis* with or with gastric ulceration is now described as the most common form of gastrointestinal candidiasis and is diagnosed by the characteristic appearance of the edematous and ulcerated mucosa on barium-swallow radiographic examination. Dysphagia, chest pain, and gastrointestinal bleeding may be presenting symptoms. Histologically, gastrointestinal candidiasis appears as a pseudomembranous inflammation, usually with localized ulcers that exhibit tuberculoid granulomas enclosing yeasts and hyphae. Oral candidiasis may or may not be evident in patients with gastrointestinal candidiasis.

Chronic Mucocutaneus Candidiasis (CMC)

Chronic infection with *Candida* usually occurs as a result of a defect in cellular immunity or structure of the epidermis. Both pseudomembranous and hyperplastic types of tissues response to the organism are seen in chronically infected patients, though hyperplastic mucocutaneous lesions, localized granulomas, and somewhat more adherent white plaques on affected mucous membranes are the prominent lesions that identify this syndrome. In many cases, persistent and significant predisposing factors can be identified. Four categories of CMC have been described: (1) *chronic familial mucocutaneous candidiasis*—a familial disorder affecting both sexes with a possible autosomal recessive inheritance and characterized by onset of chronic oral candidiasis and hyperplastic infection of the nail folds in infancy; (2) randomly occurring cases of severe mucocutaneous candidiasis with widespread skin involvement and development of *Candida* granulomas, often associated with other oportunistic fungal and bacterial infections; (3) *endocrine candidiasis syndrome*—an autosomal recessive disorder with early onset of chronic mucocutaneous candidiasis with subsequent appearance of hypoparathyroidism, hypoadrenocorticism, and other endocrine anomalies (see Fig. 6-16); and (4) *CMC of late onset* (>35 years); without any family history or other major clinical abnormality.

Resistance of the organism to antifungal agents is rarely a major factor in CMC, and in most patients the lesions can be maintained essentially free of detectable yeasts and hyphae with one or more of the available topical or systemic antifungal agents. Once treatment is discontinued, however, the organisms rapidly reappear, suggesting reinfection from other sites or that organisms that have penetrated deep into the tissues are protected from the antifungal agents. Histologic studies of the lesions of CMC confirm that

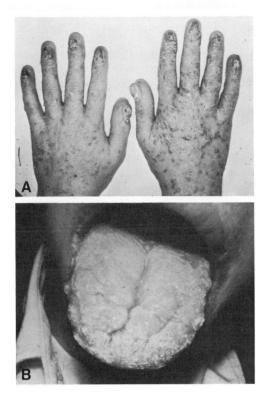

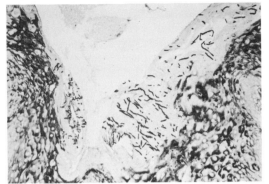

Fig. 6-17 Histologic section from gingiva of patient illustrated in Figure 6-16, stained to show depth of penetration of fungal mycelia.

Fig. 6-16 Clinical appearance of patient with endocrine candidiasis syndrome. *A,* The hands are covered with raised, dry, red lesions. Note fingernail deformities and paronychial inflammation. *B,* The tongue is atrophic, deeply fissured, and covered with an adherent white slough. (From Greenberg MS, Brightman VJ, Lynch MA, Ship II: Oral Surg 28:42, 1969)

the organism often penetrates to the corium of these patients (see Fig. 6-17). At this level it evokes both hyperplastic and inflammatory responses that lead to multiple areas of tissue thickening and granulomatous reaction affecting skin, mucous membranes, and nail folds. Involvement of other organs is rare. Mucocutaneous abnormalities that predispose to CMC are still rather poorly characterized, but some familial cases of CMC and cases in other patients for whom no endocrine problems or immune defect can be identified may be caused by genetically or metabolically determined epithelial abnormality. Iron and vitamin deficiencies probably act as predisposing factors at this level.

Diabetes, pregnancy, and steroid administration are recognized endocrine factors in almost all varieties of candidiasis. In addition, some patients with CMC present with multiple endocrine dysfunctions, justifying the description of one category of patients with CMC as the *endocrine candidiasis syndrome.* These patients usually have idiopathic hypoparathyroidism and/or Addison's disease, sometimes with accompanying thyroid, pituitary, and gonadal problems. A variety of organ-specific antibodies have been detected that account not only for the multiple endocrine hypofunction but also for the loss of hair, thin skin, keratitis, and intestinal malabsorption noted in this group of patients. Dental hypoplasia and severe caries are common, possibly as a result of the hypoparathyroidism, but probably also because of a generalized epithelial defect affecting tooth formation. Because in many cases chronic oral candidiasis and dental defects appear to predate the development of hypocalcemia or other endocrine anomalies in this syndrome, thorough evaluation of recurrent or chronic oral candidiasis in a child is important.

Defects in T-cell immunity have been detected in many patients with CMC, although no one type of defect is consistently found, and some patients also have B-cell and B- and T-cell interaction deficiencies. A number of tests of T-cell function are often abnormal in these patients (*e.g.*, cutaneous anergy, resistance to DNCB sensitization, lack of lymphokine formation and lymphocyte transformation, and decreased E-rosette formation). T-cell subset ratios may also be abnormal.

Both inherited and acquired immunodeficiency states are involved (DiGeorge's and Nezelof's syndromes, thymoma, Swiss and Bruton type agammaglobulinemias). Various efforts to restore immune competence have been used in the treatment of these patients (see following section), and when successful, persistent elimination of the chronic hyperplastic lesions is possible.

Oral lesions and severe dental defects are prominent features of many patients with CMC. Many of them become edentulous early in life, but are able to wear dentures without any particular increase in severity of their oral lesions. Isolated case reports of oral carcinoma developing in the chronic hyperplastic oral lesions in these patients suggest that continuous use of antifungal treatment together with long-term follow-up is advisable.

Systemic Candidiasis

This term is reserved for those situations in which there is evidence of focal necrotizing inflammation and *Candida* granuloma formation in one or more visceral organs, usually as a result of hematogenous dissemination of the organism. In almost all cases, the patient is immunocompromised as a result of leukemia, lymphoma, or steroid and cytotoxic therapy or debilitated from extensive surgery, especially open-heart surgery. Damaged heart valves, contaminated intravenous instruments, or indwelling catheters are the usual foci for dissemination of *Candida*. Use of contaminated drug paraphernalia by "mainlining" drug abusers accounts for a relatively high frequency of *Candida* fungemia, endocarditis, and systemic candidiasis in young adults. Systemic and gastrointestinal candidiasis are also common features of the recently described acquired immune deficiency syndrome (AIDS), a number of cases having occurred in drug abusers (see also Chap. 28).

Mucocutaneous candidiasis rarely leads to systemic candidiasis, usually only where granulomatous lesions develop around indwelling catheters or intravenous lines and provide intravenous seeding of *Candida*-infected emboli. Mycotic endocarditis and mycotic infection with *Candida* around artificial heart valves have been described following dental extractions, although attempts at demonstrating *Candida* fungemia followed dental extraction have not been successful, possibly because of the same factors that make demonstration of *Candida* fungemia accompanying systemic candidiasis or *Candida* endocarditis less efficient than techniques for demonstrating bacteremia. No clear associations have been found between thrush, denture stomatitis, or chronic oral hyperplastic candidiasis and systemic candidiasis. Oropharyngeal candidiasis associated with use of inhaled aerosolized corticosteroids does not involve the trachea or lower respiratory tract. In severely debilitated, terminally ill patients, saliva contaminated with *Candida* and loose pieces of a *Candida* pseudomembrane can be aspirated and contribute to the mixed microbial flora found in some aspiration pneumonias (see Figs. 10-15 and 10-16B and C). Pulmonary candidiasis with evidence of necrotizing inflammation around foci of yeasts and hyphae is relatively rare, indicating that *Candida* is a true opportunistic infectious agent as far as the visceral organs are concerned, despite the apparent ease with which it colonizes and produces superficial infections of skin and mucous membranes. Brain, heart, and kidney are the organs most often involved in systemic candidiasis, although hematogenous spread of infected emboli may produce foci in a variety of organs, including the skin.

It should be apparent from this description of extraoral candidiasis that there is no consistent relationship between oral candidiasis and extraoral infection, the exact pattern of lesions depending on the particular predisposing factors and situations that promote dissemination of the organism. Despite the frequency with which oral candidiasis occurs in hospitalized patients (thrush occurs in at least 10% of all hospital patients and one third of all hospital patients coming to autopsy), it is often neglected and considered a minor problem. There is no doubt, however, that treatment of this condition in desirable, and in immunocompromised patients and those predisposed to opportunistic infections, it is mandatory. Regular oral examinations of immunocompromised and debilitated patients with oral or nasal catheters or oral appliances should also be carried out to detect any localized *Candida* infections that could serve as foci of hematogenous spread.

Treatment of Oral Candidiasis

A variety of topical and systemically administered medications are now available to supplement the older antifungal antibiotics, mycostatin and amphotericin B. Several imidazole derivatives are available for topical use (clotrimazole and miconazole), and the most recently released, ketoconazole is administered as a tablet once daily. A number of new systematically administered drugs (miconazole, 5-fluorocytosine) in addition to amphotericin B are also available for treatment of the resistant lesions of CMC and for systemic candidiasis. The dye, gentian violet, is now rarely used even for superficial skin and mucous membrane infections.

The majority of acute oral *Candida* infections respond rapidly to topical mycostatin and will not recur provided the predisposing factors have also been eliminated. Seven to 10 days use of a mycostatin rinse,* three to four times daily is usually adequate, although some resistant cases may need a second course of treatment. Alternatively, mycostatin may be applied as a cream,† or by release from a lactose-containing vaginal tablet‡ allowed to dissolve slowly under the tongue. The location of the lesions and patient acceptance (of the three formulations, the lactose-containing tablets are the least distasteful) will usually determine the mode of application. Patients in whom predisposing factors such as xerostomia, immunodeficiency, or a loose denture cannot be eliminated will need either continuous or repeated treatment to prevent recurrences. Clotrimazole§ and miconazole‖ creams can also be used for treatment of oral lesions.

Owing to problems with patient compliance and the cost of mycostatin, a once daily dose of 200 mg ketoconazole# for 2 weeks is also now often used for acute oral candidiasis. When used for this short period, side-effects such as increased liver enzymes, abdominal pain, and pruritis are rare. Ketoconazole may also be more effective in some cases than topical mycostatin and imidazole compounds because it reaches the lesions by way of the bloodstream. Vaginal candidiasis responds to ketoconazole even more rapidly than does oral candidiasis, and the likelihood of reinfection is reduced by control of *Candida* at various sites. Both topical antifungal agents and ketoconazole can be used together, although the combination is rarely necessary. Ketoconazole, however, requires acid in the stomach for dissolution and absorption, and patients using antacids, anticholinergic agents, and histamine H_2 blockers should allow at least 2 hours between any of these medications and the dose of ketoconazole. Patients with achlorhydia need to use an acidified solution of ketoconazole.

The response of chronic oral candidiasis to either topical antifungal agents or ketoconazole may be less dramatic, usually because of the persistance of predisposing factors such as a loose denture, habit pattern, or underlying keratotic lesion. For the most part, however, mycostatin applied as a cream under a denture or to the lesions of angular cheilitis will eliminate redness and promote shrinkage of mucosa and healing of fissures. Two to four weeks of treatment with ketoconazole is equally effective. Treatment of denture sore-mouth and angular cheilitis must include elimination of *Candida* from the denture surface either by making a new denture or by re-lining an existing denture and maintaining it free of *Candida* by adding a few drops of mycostatin suspension before it is inserted in the mouth. Studies in Scandinavia have also shown that 0.2% chlorhexidine solution* and use of 1% chlorhexidine gel will eliminate denture sore-mouth and angular cheilitis. The addition of an absorbable corticosteroid (triamcinalone acetonide) and antibacterial agents to mycostatin creams and

---

* Mycostatin oral suspension, ER Squibb & Co. Inc, PO Box 4000, Princeton, NJ 08540
Nilstat oral suspension, Lederle Laboratories, Division American Cyanamid Co, Wayne, NJ 07470
† Mycostatin Cream or Nilstat Topical Cream
‡ Mycostatin or Nilstat vaginal tablets
§ Lotrimin Cream 1%, Schering Corp, Galloping Hill Rd, Kenilworth, NY 07033
§ Mycelex 1% cream, Miles Pharmaceuticals, Division Miles Labs, Inc., 400 Morgan Lane, West Haven, CT 06516
‖ Monistat-Derm Cream, Ortho Pharmaceuticals, 375 Mount Pleasant Ave, West Orange, NJ 07052

Nizoral Tablets, Janssen Pharmaceutica Inc, 501 George St, New Brunswick, NJ 08903
* Hibitane Mouthrinse, Stuart Pharmaceuticals, Division of ICI Americas Inc, DE 19897 (available in Europe and Canada, but not USA)

ointments accelerates symptomatic relief, and these preparations[†] are useful adjuncts for the treatment of angular cheilitis and perioral candidiasis. Treatment of angular cheilitis must also always involve treatment of denture stomatitis or other intraoral *Candida* lesions. Allergic reactions to chlorhexidine and to some of the ingredients in water-miscible creams used commercially as a vehicle for mycostatin have been described and should be watched for, particularly in the patient whose *Candida*-positive, patchy, red oral lesions or cheilitis seem to worsen with mycostatin cream.

Extraoral candidiasis requires treatment that is customized to the site and predisposing factors involved. In general, ketoconazole has been found to be more effective and cheaper than amphotericin B, which usually requires hospitalization of the patient if intravenous administration is needed. Resistant lesions of chronic mucocutaneous candidiasis are often eliminated by ketoconazole and it is also an effective means of controlling gastrointestinal candidiasis in patients with leukemia, lymphoma, or other immunocompromised state. Systemic candidiasis requires systemic administration of high doses of amphotericin B,[*] miconazole,[†] or 5-fluorocytosine,[‡] and increased doses of ketoconazole. Transfusions of transfer factor and transplantation of cultured thymic fragments have been used to correct the T-cell deficiencies associated with chronic mucocutaneous candidiasis. In some cases, resolution of the chronic skin and mucous membrane lesions occured along with improvement of *in vitro* T-cell functions.

Oral candidiasis that does not respond to topical or systemic antifungal treatment despite elimination of suspected predisposing factors or that recurs after adequate treatment

is an indication for a more thorough evaluation of the patient and a search for other predisposing factors including diabetes, hematologic abnormality, or other immunosuppressed state.

KERATOTIC WHITE LESIONS WITH NO INCREASED POTENTIAL FOR THE DEVELOPMENT OF ORAL CANCER

Stomatitis Nicotina

Stomatitis nicotina is a specific lesion that develops on the palate in heavy cigarette, pipe, and cigar smokers. These lesions have a characteristic appearance and are rarely missed because of their prominent location on the palate (Fig. 6-18A). Lesions of stomatitis nicotina are restricted to those areas exposed to a relatively concentrated jet of tobacco smoke; areas covered by an upper denture while smoking are not affected. The lesions are usually more prominent and well developed on the keratinized hard palate.

In the early stages the mucosa is reddened, but it subsequently becomes grayish white, thickened, and fissured. Focal thickening occurs around the orifices of the palatal minor salivary glands, which appear as white, umbilicated nodules with red centers that may be stained brown by deposits of tar. Histologically, the epithelium shows acanthosis and hyperkeratosis. The epithelium lining the ducts of the minor salivary glands often shows squamous metaplasia, and obstruction of ducts may lead to formation of small retention cysts. There is usually a moderate degree of chronic inflammation in the subepithelial connective tissue and around the gland acini (Fig. 6-18B).

Stomatitis nicotina represents one part of the spectrum of oral mucosal changes that follow heavy smoking. Unlike some other areas of leukoplakia and erythroplakia commonly found in the mouths of smokers, stomatitis nicotina is a reversible change that eventually disappears once smoking is stopped. Because squamous cell carcinoma of the hard palate and carcinoma of the palatal minor salivary glands are rare, it is generally believed that stomatitis nicotina has no pre-

---

[†] Mycolog Cream and Mycolog Ointment, ER Squibb & Co. Inc, PO Box 4000, Princeton, NJ 08540; Nystolone Cream and Nystolone Ointment, Henry Schein Inc, 8 Harbor Park Drive, Ft. Washington, NY 11050

[*] Fungizone Intravenous, ER Squibb & Co. Inc, PO box 4000, Princeton, NJ 08540

[†] Monistat IV, Janssen Pharmaceutica Inc, 501 George St, New Brunswick, NJ 08903

[‡] Ancobon Capsules, Roche Laboratories, Division Hoffman–LaRoche Inc, Nutley, NJ 07110

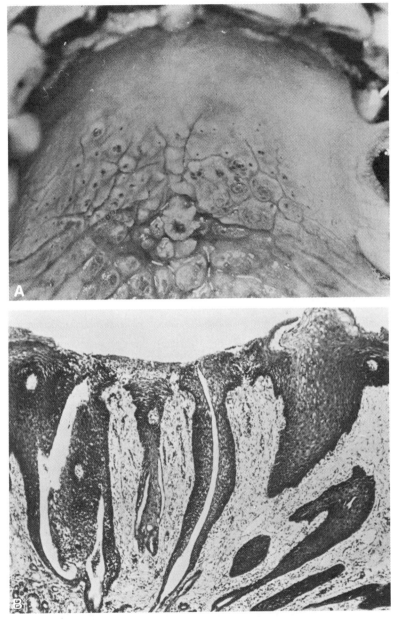

Fig. 6-18 Clinical and histologic appearances of stomatitis nicotina. *A,* The mucosa of the hard palate shows white, umbilicated nodules with red centers. *B,* Acanthosis and hyperparakeratosis of the surface epithelium with squamous metaplasia of the minor salivary gland ductal epithelium. (From WHO Collaborating Centre for Oral Precancerous Lesions: Definition of leukoplakia and related lesions: An aid to studies of oral precancer. Oral Surg 46:518, 1978; courtesy CV Mosby Co., St. Louis, MO 63141)

cancerous potential. Despite this fact, identification of areas of stomatitis nicotina can serve a useful purpose in educating patients about the hazards of smoking because the lesions are dramatic and easily seen. The lesions also serve the purpose of drawing the clinician's attention to localized erythematous areas of the soft palate and fauces, often with marginal tags of epithelium attached, that can represent more significant effects of smoking on the more susceptible nonkeratinized mucosa. Biopsy of stomatitis nicotina is rarely indicated except for assurance of a patient; biopsy or cytologic examination of related erythematous lesions of the soft palate is important however, particularly for lesions that do not rapidly disappear with cessation of smoking.

Reverse cigarette smoking as practiced in parts of Southeast Asia, the Caribbean, and

South America also produces a leukoplakic lesion of the palate. Unlike stomatitis nicotina seen in western countries, however, this lesion is often associated with epithelial dyskeratosis and an increased incidence of carcinoma (see following section on Oral Lesions Associated with Use of Tobacco and Alcohol).

Traumatic Keratoses

Traumatic keratosis refers to an isolated area of thickened whitish oral mucosa that is clearly related to an identifiable local irritant and that resolves following elimination of the irritant. Included in this definition are lesions that present in a similar manner but when promptly excised are demonstrated to be free of dysplastic changes. Histologically, lesions of this type show varying degrees of hyperkeratosis, parakeratosis, and acanthosis. Traumatic keratoses are particularly common and usually found in association with denture clasps, rough edges on dentures and broken teeth, on the lips of heavy cigarette smokers, and on the buccal mucosa opposite the molar teeth (see Fig. 6-19). When localized lesions of this type are found in association with identifiable, locally acting irritants, it is customary to try and remove the irritant and re-evaluate the lesion in 1 to 2 weeks. The majority of lesions will be reduced in size or completely gone (see Fig. 6-20). Use of a topical antifungal agent during this period of observation will also often hasten resolution of the keratotic area. On the return visit, any lesion that remains should be biopsied.

This policy of removing a suspected irritant and re-evaluating the area in 1 to 2 weeks should *not* be used in the following situations: where there is any doubt that the patient will return for re-evaluation; where the appearance of the lesion or other changes in the oral mucosa suggest that a more generalized leukoplakia or other mucosal disorder is present and may be contributing to the keratotic area in question; in patients who are otherwise predisposed to development of oral cancer (*e.g.*, heavy smokers and abusers of alcohol, diabetics, and patients with previous dysplastic oral lesions or susceptibility to multiple tumors); where there is any doubt about the association between the suspected irritant and the lesion; and where the keratotic tissue is located on the floor of the mouth or ventral surface of the tongue (or tongue dorsum in a patient with a history of syphilis), these being areas of increased frequency of oral carcinoma. In any of these circumstances, biopsy with histologic examination should be recommended and even carried out at the initial visit.

Provided the term *leukoplakia* is used simply as a clinical designation for a white lesion as was done for many years, clinical differentiation of leukoplakias exhibiting epithelial dysplasia from those that did not show this precancerous change was not possible—this distinction could only be made histologically. Based on this approach, biopsy of all white lesions is mandatory, but the practice led to the realization that few of the very large number of leukoplakic lesions biopsied showed dysplastic changes. (In surveys of leuko-

Fig. 6-19 Traumatic keratosis of cheek.

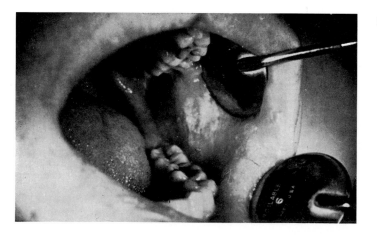

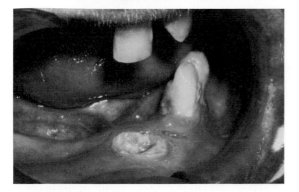

Fig. 6-20 Discrete white lesion of mandibular alveolus with rolled margins and ulcerated center located at the point of contact of solitary upper central incisor with mandibular mucosa. Following extraction of upper central incisor, lesion disappeared completely in 3 to 4 weeks confirming the clinical impression of traumatic keratosis.

plakic lesions submitted for biopsy, reported by Shafer and Waldron in 1961 and 1975, 80% to 82% of the lesions showed only varying degrees of hyperkeratosis, parakeratosis, and acanthosis and were without evidence of cellular atypia.) As redefined by the WHO Collaborating Reference Center for Oral Precancerous Lesions, leukoplakia is now used only for white lesions that remain after known diagnostic entities have been separated out.

Traumatic keratosis as defined above, "a white lesion that disappears following removal of a suspected irritant," is therefore no longer included within the definition of leukoplakia, although formerly such a lesion might have been referred to as a localized area of leukoplakia. As so defined and with the caveats listed above regarding delays in biopsy, traumatic keratosis represents a reversible and nonprecancerous lesion. Lesions of this type have also been referred to in terms of their histologic features: focal (or diffuse) keratosis, hyperkeratosis, hyperkeratosis simplex, or pachyderma oralis.

Intraoral Skin Grafts

Pieces of skin grafted into the oral mucosa, usually to line a surgically deepened buccal sulcus or to repair an antro-oral fistula or other extensive traumatic oral wound, retain many of the features of the donor site, such as thickness of the stratum corneum and a pigment layer. Such grafted tissue has occasionally been mistakenly identified as a white lesion, biopsied, and submitted for examination. The nature of the "lesion" will usually be apparent from its shape and location or the patient's dental history. The grayish white appearance of skin grafted into the oral cavity depends on imbibition of fluid by the thick stratum corneum and is analogous to the whitish wrinkled appearance that the skin of the fingertips develops following prolonged immersion. Normal keratinized oral mucosa does not exhibit this phenomenon.

Focal Epithelial Hyperplasia

Focal epithelial hyperplasia, or Heck's disease (also see discussion in Chap. 8), is a viral-induced oral mucosal change that has now been described in a wide range of population samples, including North American and Latin American Indians, Eskimos, Cape coloreds in South Africa and isolated whites in the United States and northern Europe. The lesions occur primarily on the lips and cheeks, and occasionally on the tongue and gingivae, as flat, slightly raised, whitish plaques with a roughened surface. Histologically, the lesions show localized acanthosis corresponding to the verrucous surface of the lesion and a lymphocytic infiltration. Dyskeratosis and epithelial atypia are not present, and the lesions have no precancerous potential. These lesions may regress and spontaneously disappear. They are less readily apparent when the mucosa is stretched.

Psoriasiform Lesions

Under this heading are grouped a number of lesions with clinical and histologic similarity to those seen in the oral cavity of patients with psoriatic dermatitis (psoriasis). Geographic tongue and ectopic geographic tongue, or erythema circinate migrans, and the oral lesions of Reiter's syndrome are included under this heading. There is no evidence to show that these various lesions are related in any way, and their clinical and histologic similarity may reflect a nonspecific mucosal response to a number of different etiologic agents.

Psoriasis

Psoriasis is a common dermatologic disease characterized by white, scaly papules and plaques on an erythematous base that preferentially affect the extremities and scalp. The disorder is usually chronic with periods of acute exacerbation; it is occasionally associated with a nonrheumatoid arthritis, which can affect many joints, the temporomandibular joint included. "Classical" skin lesions of psoriasis show parakeratosis, acanthosis, spongiosis, budding of the tips of rete processes, and thinning of the epithelium above the dermal papillae. Intra-epithelial microabscesses (Monro's abscesses) are formed by migration of polymorphonuclear leukocytes within the epithelium; the dermis shows a mixed inflammatory cell exudate.

Despite the prevalence of psoriasis, there appears to be no accurate data on the frequency of intra-oral lesions, and only some of the cases reported in the literature are accepted as oral psoriasis; others are thought to represent coexistent lichen planus or other keratotic changes. Mucous membrane involvement in psoriasis is generally considered to be rare, oral and anal lesions being somewhat more frequent than genital and conjunctival lesions. Two types of lesions have been observed on the oral mucous membranes of patients with psoriatic dermatitis and are accepted as psoriatic on the basis of their histologic appearance and clinical correlation with exacerbations and remissions of the skin lesions: white, scaly lesions that affect the palate and buccal mucosa and well-demarcated, flat, erythematous lesions with a slightly raised white annular or serpiginous border. Because of the clinical and histologic similarity of this latter type to the lesions of geographic tongue, erythema circinate migrans, and Reiter's syndrome, a diagnosis of intraoral psoriasis should not be made in the absence of histologically established skin psoriasis.

Reiter's Syndrome

Featuring a triad of urethritis, conjunctivitis, and arthritis, Reiter's syndrome is a disease of unknown origin that is considered an important cause of nongonococcal urethritis and is often acquired venereally (see also Chapter 28). A variety of infectious agents (*Mycoplasma*, *Bedsonia*, viruses, and trachoma-related agents) have been implicated with no firm etiologic relationship being established. Skin and mucous membrane lesions are common and are little different from those seen in psoriasis, either clinically or histologically. Annular lesions that are very similar to those seen in the mouth also occur on the glans penis and are referred to as circinate balanitis. Gray or red papules, which ulcerate leaving erythematous macules, shallow ulcers, and circinate lesions, are described in the oral mucosa of patients with this syndrome. Keratotic lesions may occur in the palms and soles (keratitis blenorrhagica) but are not a feature of the oral lesions. The disorder may be acute or run a chronic course with slow evolution of the different lesions over many months.

Geographic Tongue

Geographic tongue and ectopic geographic tongue, which also feature annular, circinate, or serpiginous lesions of the oral mucosa with a slightly depressed red atrophic center and a raised white border, are described in Chapter 10, Diseases of the Tongue. Because these conditions are relatively common and are indistinguishable from some of the oral lesions of psoriasis and Reiter's syndrome, it is very difficult to determine whether a patient with psoriatic dermatitis who has oral mucosal lesions of this type has oral psoriasis or psoriatic dermatitis with a geographic tongue. Where the oral lesions wax and wane in synchrony with the psoriatic dermatitis, the likelihood of the oral lesions being psoriatic is greater.

Areas of psoriatic dermatitis have a greatly increased epithelial cell turnover time of 2 to 4 days (normal 28 to 30 days) that approximates the normal oral turnover time of 4 to 8 days. This difference has been cited as a possible explanation for the rarity of oral lesions in psoriasis, and local variations in cell turnover time on the tongue surface might explain the appearance and migration of the lesions of geographic tongue. Studies of labeling indices for the buccal mucosa from psoriatic and nonpsoriatic individuals have not provided consistent evidence to support this hypothesis; however, and the concentration of the 70K protein characteristically found to be increased in areas of psoriatic dermatitis does not correlate with the psoriatic-versus-nonpsoriatic status of buccal mucosal epithelium.

Oral Genodermatoses

The term *oral genodermatoses* (an inherited disease affecting the oral mucosa) is most often used with reference to white sponge nevus and a number of less common genetically determined abnormalities of the oral mucosa. There are actually a large number of inherited and congenital syndromes associated with red and white lesions of the oral mucosa that need to be considered in the evaluation of both children and adults with chronic oral mucosal lesions. Brief descriptions of the salient features of the following syndromes are included in this section.*

- *Oral mucosal thickenings with or without secondary candidiasis*
  White sponge nevus
  Hereditary benign intraepithelial dyskeratosis
  Pachyonychia congenita
  Dyskeratosis congenita[†]
  Hyperkeratosis palmoplantaris with attached gingival hyperkeratosis
  Hyperkeratosis palmoplantaris with esophageal carcinoma and oral leukoplakia[†]
  Porokeratosis (Mibelli type)
  Tyrosinemia II (Richner–Hanhart syndrome)
- *Lesions primarily resulting from chronic candidiasis on basis of inherited immunodeficiency or epithelial dysplasia*
  Chronic familial mucocutaneous candidiasis; endocrine candidiasis syndrome; chronic mucocutaneous candidiasis associated with inherited immunodeficiency
  Acrodermatitis enteropathica
  Ectodermal dysplasia syndrome
  Juvenile diabetes mellitus
- *Lesions characterized by defective adhesion between epithelial cells[‡]*
  Dystrophic epidermolysis bullosa
  Keratosis follicularis (Darier's disease)
  Hereditary mucoepithelial dysplasia
- *Lesions caused by abnormal deposits in the oral submucosa*
  Pseudoxanthoma elasticum
  Hyalinosis cutis et mucosa oris

Candidiasis is an important factor in determining the appearance of some of the oral genodermatoses. In some, such as the endocrine candidiasis syndrome and acrodermatitis enteropathica, opportunistic infection by *Candida,* on the basis of immunodeficiency or epithelial dysplasia, largely determines the character of the lesions. In others (e.g., white sponge nevus and hereditary benign intraepithelial dyskeratosis) *Candida* appears to be a minor though fairly consistent component of the lesions, with an unspecified role in the genesis of the lesions.

Oral Genodermatoses Characterized by Thickened Patches of Oral Mucosa With or Without Secondary Candidiasis

White Sponge Nevus. Also referred to as Cannon's disease, white folded gingivostomatitis, and leukoedema exfoliativa, white sponge nevus is an autosomal dominant, inherited condition that usually affects only the oral mucosa; however, similar lesions have occasionally been described on the vaginal, penile, and anal mucosae. In the mouth, the buccal mucosa is the predominant area involved with the labial mucosa, alveolar ridges, and floor of mouth (decreasing order) as secondary sites (see Fig. 6-21). There is no sex predilection, and the majority of cases

---

* A number of syndromes in which the lesions of the oral mucosa are papillomatous or papular are described in Chapter 8 (*e.g.,* multiple mucosal neuroma syndrome, neurofibromatosis, tuberous sclerosis, acanthosis nigricans, Cowden's and Peutz–Jeghers syndromes, and the various syndromes involving generalized gingival fibromatosis).

† Associated with a tendency to malignant transformation—see section on Red and White Lesions with Defined or Uncertain Precancerous Potential

‡ Other diseases in this category such as pemphigus and pemphigoid, which are acquired rather than inherited or congenital, are described under Vesiculobullous Lesions in Chapter 5.

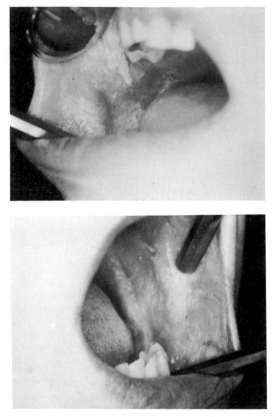

Fig. 6-21 White sponge nevus (white folded gingivostomatitis; Cannon's disease).

have been reported in whites. The abnormality may be detected in infancy but is often not recognized until adolescence or even adulthood. The lesions are asymptomatic and often first detected by a dentist or other person observing the unusual appearance of the individual's cheek lining in good illumination. The affected mucosa is white or gray, thickened, folded, and spongy. Friction from mastication may strip the superficial keratotic layers leaving zones of either apparently normal-looking epithelium or a raw area.

Histologically, the oral epithelium is hyperplastic with an irregular surface that becomes colonized by microorganisms, as does the papillary surface of the tongue. In the superficial epithelial layers, the cells become large and irregular with pyknotic nuclei and poorly stained, "washed out" or "empty" cytoplasm. The pyknotic nuclei are not displaced, however, in comparison with the changes seen in hydropic degeneration. The dermis is normal or has a small number of

chronic inflammatory cells. The histologic appearance is relatively characteristic and cytologic study will often reveal empty epithelial cells with centrally placed pyknotic nuclei.

Numerous pedigrees of families exhibiting this anomaly have been reported, including third and fourth generation offspring. It is relatively common, and a history of extensive leukoplakia or candidiasis in children or several members of a family should raise the possibility of this disorder. There is no evidence that these lesions undergo dysplastic change or predispose to oral cancer. The lesions in children are often first diagnosed as candidiasis, their true nature becoming apparent only after they fail to respond to antifungal therapy.

Hereditary Benign Intraepithelial Dyskeratosis. Also called Witkop—Von Sallman syndrome, this rare disorder was identified as an autosomal dominant trait with a high degree of penetrance in an isolated community in North Carolina with mixed white, black, and Indian ancestory. It was described in some detail 25 years ago by the oral pathologist and ophthalmologist whose names are recorded in the eponym for the syndrome. Affected individuals show oral mucosal thickenings that are clinically similar to but somewhat milder than those of white sponge nevus; in addition, superficial gelatinous-looking plaques occur on a hyperemic bulbar conjunctiva. Histologically and cytologically, the lesions differ from those of white sponge nevus and are characterized by a peculiar intraepithelial dyskeratosis in addition to ancanthosis and vacuolization of the stratum spinosum. The dyskeratotic cells are demonstrated well in Papanicolaou- or Giemsa-stained sections or cytologic scrapings as "tobacco cells" and "cells-within-cells." These abnormal cells are similar to those that occur in another genodermatosis, keratosis follicularis (Darier's disease), where they are referred to as *grains* and *corps ronds*, respectively (see following section). Photophobia and blindness caused by involvement of the cornea by plaque formation and scarring are common in the community studied. Consistent with the histologic similarity of these lesions to those of keratosis follicularis, there does not appear to be any tendency for the oral lesions of hereditary benign intraepithelial dyskeratosis to undergo malignant transformation.

The cell-within-a-cell phenomenon occurs more extensively in lesions of hereditary benign intraepithelial dyskeratosis than in lesions of keratosis follicularis. The same phenomenon has been described in cytologic smears of exfoliated buccal cells in patients under treatment with the cytotoxic drugs methotrexate and 5-fluorouracil.

Pachyonychia Congenita. The name, "pachyonychia congenita" (Jadassohn–Lewandowsky syndrome), which refers to congenital gross thickening of finger nails and toe nails, is used to describe another rare syndrome that includes palmoplantar keratosis and hyperhidrosis, follicular keratosis and oral leukokeratosis, as well as the striking nail changes. It also has an autosomal dominant inheritance pattern but with low penetrance. The nail lesions appear soon after birth and are characterized by thickened, hard, tubular nails filled with a horny brownish material that project upward from the nail bed at their free edges. Paronychial inflammation is common. The keratotic thickening of the palms and soles is quite apparent, as is the increased sweatiness of these areas in contrast with dry keratotic skin elsewhere. Bullae formation occurs on the feet, and secondary infection of these may lead to crippling deformity. Corneal dystrophy, thickening of the laryngeal commissures, tympanic membrane, and nasal mucosa, and mental retardation are also reported.

The oral leukokeratosis primarily affects the tongue dorsum, which becomes thickened and grayish white; the cheeks may also be involved at the interdental line. Histologically, these lesions are similar to those of white sponge nevus and show a uniform acanthotic thickening with marked intracellular vacuolization, parakeratosis, and absence of intercellular bridges in the stratum spinosum. Frequent oral aphthous ulceration and the occurrence of natal teeth are also features of this syndrome.

Hyperkeratosis Palmoplantaris with Attached Gingival Hyperkeratosis and Hyperkeratosis Palmoplantaris with Esophageal Carcinoma and Oral Leukoplakia. Keratotic thickening of the palms and soles (hyperkeratosis palmoplantaris or tylosis) occurs in a number of congenital syndromes* and is inherited as a autosomal dominant disorder. Two syndromes feature tylosis in association with hyperkeratotic and mucosal thickenings; of these, the syndrome in which *focal palmoplantar hyperkeratosis is associated with hyperkertosis of the normally keratinized oral mucosal areas* (attached gingivae, hard palate, tongue dorsum, retromolar pad, and buccal mucosa along the occlusal line) is a benign condition; the other, *palmoplantar hyperkeratosis with esophageal carcinoma and oral leukoplakia*, is also described here for comparison, although oral carcinoma often develops in the oral leukoplakia areas in this latter condition.

The syndrome with attached gingival hyperkeratosis is further characterized by the later onset of lesions (usually at puberty) and the presence of paranuclear bodies in the keratinocytes of the stratum spinosum and the stratum granulosum of the hyperkeratotic oral lesions. These bodies are visible as eosinophilic granules in both Papanicolaou-stained smears and hematoxylin-and-eosin stained sections and on electron microscopic examination appear to be condensed tonofilaments.

These granules are not seen in smears and tissue sections from the oral lesions in the syndrome with esophageal carcinoma and oral leukoplakia, suggesting an additional diagnostic aid for recognizing the benign and malignant form of leukoplakia associated with tylosis. In the "malignant" syndrome, oral lesions also begin much earlier, even during the preschool period, and involve the buccal mucosa and sulci with leukoplakia and preleukoplakia. Esophageal carcinoma and oral carcinoma are reported in these patients as early as 20 years of age.

Porokeratosis. Literally, keratosis of the pores, porokeratosis is a well-described though fairly rare genodermatosis, characterized by one or more isolated keratotic plaques on various skin surfaces. The plaques are surrounded by a distinct raised border of epi-

---

* Hyperkeratosis palmoplantaris is also a component of the Papillon–Lefèvre syndrome (see Chap. 8), isolated cases of dentinogenesis imperfecta, and a number of other disorders.

dermal proliferation with characteristic histology, referred to as the *cornoid lamella*. The plaques may or may not show a relationship with the pores of the skin and dermal appendages, and the name given to the disorder is a misnomer. The most likely explanation is that the plaques are produced by mutant clones of epidermal cells. Various clinical forms of the disorder have been described in addition to the type originally described by Mibelli in 1893, which is sometimes associated with mucosal lesions. Palatal lesions have been observed in a proportion of patients with the Mibelli type of porokeratosis and are described as "numerous small slightly depressed, opalescent rings and serpiginous lesions with hyperemic borders studded over the palate." On section, the oral lesions show the characteristic cornoid lamella and are unrelated to the openings of the palatal salivary glands.

Tyrosinemia II (also called the Richner–Hanhart syndrome). Tyrosinemia II is an autosomal recessive condition characterized by a genetically determined deficiency of hepatic tyrosine aminotransferase. Tyrosine and its metabolites accumulate in the blood and urine in the absence of this enzyme and may be detected there. Otherwise, renal and hepatic function in these individuals is normal, distinguishing them from those with the syndrome referred to as tyrosinemia I (or tyrosinosis), in which there is a more complicated pathophysiologic abnormality affecting a variety of metabolic pathways. Tryosinemia II features corneal erosion and plaques, palmoplantar erosions and hyperkeratosis in the neonatal period, and a variety of other lesions caused by an inflammatory response to local tissue deposits of tyrosine. Treatment with a diet low in tyrosine and phenylalanine is curative. Hyperkeratosis of the tongue is described in some children with these syndromes.

Lesions Primarily Resulting from Chronic Candidiasis on the Basis of Inherited Immune Deficiency or Epithelial Dysplasia

This category of oral genodermatosis includes various forms of chronic mucocutaneous candidiasis in which a familial pattern or congenital lesions suggest an inherited basis for chronic opportunistic infection with *Candida*. Several of these disorders (chronic familial mucocutaneous candidiasis, endocrine candidiasis syndrome, and chronic mucocutaneous candidiasis associated with inherited immune deficiency) have been described in a preceding section of this chapter. Other related disorders, in which the role of chronic mucocutaneous candidiasis was recognized long after description of the syndrome should be mentioned because the role of *Candida* in determining the characteristic appearance of these lesions is not always appreciated.

Acrodermatitis Enteropathica. A rare disease of infancy and childhood transmitted as an autosomal recessive character, acrodermatitis enteropathica is now recognized as a manifestation of zinc deficiency, probably on the basis of an inherited tendency to altered zinc absorption and metabolism. Zinc supplements appear to be curative, even though the pathogenesis of the characteristic lesions involves a number of etiologic factors.

The primary signs of the disorder are skin lesions, hair loss, nail changes and diarrhea. Erythematous, pustular, moist erosions of the orificial areas occur as an early manifestation, the perioral area usually being affected by weeping erosions, angular fissuring, and spreading dermatitis reminiscent of the orificial lesions of candidiasis on moist skin surfaces. *Candida* can be demonstrated in the lesions in a majority of patients with this disorder, and some cases have been mistakenly diagnosed as systemic thrush or candidiasis. In the fully developed condition, the buttocks, elbows, knees, fingers, and toes are affected by a vesiculobullous rash similar to that affecting the orificial areas. Loss of hair, retarded body growth, and mental changes also occur with some frequency. In addition to perioral lesions, the buccal mucosa, palate, gingivae, and tonsils present red and white spots, erosions, ulcers, and desquamation; lesions on the tongue are sometimes papillated; halitosis is often severe. To a large extent, these intraoral lesions can be explained on the basis of chronic candidiasis.

Inherited Anomalies That Involve Absence Or Defective Function of the Salivary

Glands. Defective salivary gland function is often associated with erythematous and white, plaquelike lesions secondary to xerostomia. *Candida* is a prominent feature of this type of stomatitis and probably contributes to the characteristic dry, red appearance of the oral mucosa described in *ectodermal dysplasia* and *juvenile diabetes.* Juvenile diabetes is also associated with defective neutrophil function, and this immune deficiency also contributes to the frequency of both acute and chronic hyperplastic forms of oral candidiasis observed in many juvenile diabetics.

Lesions Characterized by Defective Adhesion Between Epithelial Cells

The usual tissue response to separation of epithelial cells or separation of epithelium from the dermis is formation of a vesicle or bulla as a result of fluid accumulation in the intercellular clefts. Where the disorder is associated with a particularly fragile mucous membrane, frequent bulla formation with subsequent epithelial desquamation and infection will often lead to extensive scarring of the involved mucosa. Desquamating sheets of epithelium and plaquelike areas of scarring contribute to an overall effect of a white mucosa that may even obscure the basic bullous and ulcerative nature of the disorder. In yet another recently described "dyshesive disorder," the affected oral mucous membranes appear fiery red, similar to the change observed in desquamative gingivitis (see Chap. 5).

Dystrophic Epidermolysis Bullosa. Probably the best known of the inherited oral genodermatoses that feature a dyshesive process, the recessive, dystrophic form of epidermolysis bullosa involves separation of the epithelium from the dermis below the periodic acid-Schiff (PAS)-positive basement membrane of the dermo-epidermal junction. Trauma produces extensive bulla formation and desquamation, affecting the hands, feet, esophagus, and oral cavity. Within the oral cavity, the mucosa appears thick, gray, smooth, and bound down. The buccal and lingual sulci become obliterated with scarring; there is immobility of the lips and microstomia. Bulla formation with secondary scarring of the hands, feet, and other skin areas may interfere with growth and result in a dwarfed stature. Likewise, extensive lesions of the hands lead to an eventual claw-hand deformity with the distal part of the limb enclosed in a scarred, glovelike, epithelial sack. Conjunctival scarring, hoarseness, and laryngeal stenosis are associated problems. The older German literature includes a description of oral carcinoma secondary to epidermolysis bullosa; however, this is an extremely rare and uncertain phenomenon in epidermolysis bullosa, particularly because many severely affected patients die in childhood or adolescence from other causes.

Keratosis follicularis. Also called Darier's disease, keratosis follicularis is a rare, but well-described dermatosis inherited as an autosomal dominant condition. Clinically, the lesions are described as hyperkeratotic papules; histologically, there is hyperkeratosis, acanthosis, dyskeratosis, and formation of suprabasilar clefts caused by poor adhesion between cells. The dyskeratotic cells can be examined in section or in a cytologic smear and are described as "grains" (intensely basophilic-staining small elongated cells) and "corps ronds" (cells with homogeneous, eosinophilic material surrounding a basophilic, pyknotic nucleus, although corps ronds are said to be relatively rare in the oral lesions of these disorders. A dermal inflammatory exudate and a tendency to papillomatous changes (cobblestone lesions) also characterize the oral lesions in the more severely affected cases. In less severely affected cases, the intraoral lesions are keratotic and papular. The disorder is often misdiagnosed: clinically, it can be similar to stomatitis nicotina, and cytologic smears are sometimes misread as being premalignant on the basis of the unusual (but apparently benign) cells.

The skin lesions can become quite disfiguring as well as foul smelling and can cause the sufferer considerable social disability. An association with mental retardation and psychiatric disturbance is also reported by some authors. Similarity between the dyskeratotic cells in Darier's disease and those in hereditary benign intraepithelial dyskeratosis has been previously commented on.

Hereditary Mucoepithelial Dysplasia. The most recently recognized disorder in this group, hereditary mucoepithelial dysplasia was described by Witkop and associates in 1978. It is an autosomal dominant, inherited disorder affecting all the orificial mucosa and is characterized by cataracts, follicular keratosis of the skin, nonscarring alopecia, repeated episodes of pneumonia, spontaneous pneumothorax, and cor pulmonale. The oral lesion is a fiery red, flat or micropapillary-appearing mucosa most frequently involving the gingivae and hard palate. All oral and pharyngeal surfaces may be involved, and red, enlarged and fissured (scrotal) tongue is a common feature. Histologically, the oral lesions show a lack of cornified and keratinized cells, thinning of the epithelium, dyshesion, and dyskeratosis. Ultrastructural features include a paucity of desmosomes, intercellular accumulations of amorphous material and paranuclear lesions with strands of material resembling gap junctions and desmosomes. The condition is considered to be a basic defect in gap junction and desmosome formation. *Candida* infection does not appear to be a feature of this disorder. In one family described, well-developed changes affecting the oral mucosa were noted as early as 18 months of age.

Lesions Caused by Abnormal Deposits in the Oral Submucosa

Plaquelike (as distinct from generalized) deposits in the oral mucous membrane occur in a variety of conditions including amyloidosis, xanthomatosis, and a number of inherited conditions. In this last category, the disorders known as pseudoxanthoma elasticum and hyalinosis cutis et mucosa oris are worthy of mention because of confusion with Fordyce granules and leukoplakia.

Pseudoxanthoma Elasticum. In pseudoxanthoma elasticum, the basic defect involves the structure of elastin, making it susceptible to calcification. Raised, yellowish papules develop on areas of thickened, coarsely grained skin especially about the mouth, neck, axillae, elbows, and groin. The skin about the mouth may become redundant, producing a "hound dog" appearance. The mucosal surface of the lips, especially the lower lip, exhibits yellowish intramucosal nodules in

about 10% of cases. Other oral surfaces and the vaginal and rectal mucosae may be similarly affected. In addition to the dermatologic and oral changes, the syndrome includes brownish gray streaks of the optic fundus (angioid streaks), recurrent gastrointestinal hemorrhage, weak pulse, and failing vision. Histologically, the intramucosal nodules show large numbers of thickened and twisted elastic and collagen fibers.

Hyalinosis Cutis et Mucosa Oris. Also described as a cause of macroglossia (see Chap. 10), hyalinosis cutis et mucosa oris is an autosomal recessive trait, characterized by subdermal and submucosal infiltration of a hyaline glycoprotein material. Oral lesions are a prominent feature: elevated, pea-sized plaques affect all areas of the oral mucosa with eventual coalescence and cobblestone changes, leading to inelastic tissues and restriction of oral functions such as saliva flow, tooth eruption, and swallowing. In both this condition and pseudoxanthoma elasticum, the submucosal location of the deposits and the associated and characteristic skin changes serve to distinguish these lesions from leukoplakia.

RED AND WHITE LESIONS WITH DEFINED OR UNCERTAIN PRECANCEROUS POTENTIAL

Leukoplakia and Erythroplakia— Definitions

This section is concerned with keratotic white lesions of the oral mucosa that cannot be characterized clinically or histopathologically as any other disease *(leukoplakia)*, and bright red, velvety lesions that likewise cannot be characterized by similar criteria as any other disease *(erythroplakia)*. A large number of white and red lesions that can be assigned a definite diagnosis have already been discussed in this chapter, and additional specifically diagnosable white and red lesions that like leukoplakia and erythroplakia may be precursors of oral cancer will be discussed in subsequent pages. Leukoplakia and erythroplakia, however, are the two major lesions that have been implicated in the development of oral cancer. The relative importance given to leukoplakia versus erythroplakia in this regard has varied from time to time. Currently, erythroplakia is considered to have a far greater precancerous potential than does leukoplakia and has been identified by some authors (see Chap. 9) as the most common precursor lesion for oral cancer.

The background for the recommended current usage of the terms *leukoplakia* and *erythroplakia* is discussed at the beginning of this chapter; where possible, this usage has been followed in this chapter. It must be stressed, however, that the term *leukoplakia* is still used in different ways by many authors and that changing concepts and definitions of leukoplakia have produced a literature with many contradictions and undoubtedly, many statements that need to be re-examined in light of the current definition. It also seems clear that the epidemiology and natural history of leukoplakia have changed over the years with virtual elimination of some previously important etiologic factors (*e.g.,* tertiary syphilis and leukoplakia of the tongue dorsum) and more widespread influence of others (*e.g.,* more equal distribution of smoking habits among men and women in western countries). Revision of many of the statements from the literature that are reproduced in this section in particular should be expected. With the availability of new means of identifying and categorizing oral mucosal disorders, it is also to be expected that some lesions now included within the categories of leukoplakia and erythroplakia will be identified as specifically diagnosable disorders and excluded from these categories.

As currently defined, leukoplakia is almost synonymous with *idiopathic leukokeratosis,* a term that has been used by some authors to avoid confusion with earlier usages. Within the general category of leukoplakia, however, three etiologic subcategories are already developing: lesions caused by smoking, those associated with intraoral electrogalvanic reactions, and those associated with chronic candidiasis. For each subcategory, there are identifiable clinical and histopathologic features, although critical epidemiologic studies that might allow each to become a specifically diagnosable disorder are still lacking. In this sense, therefore, leukoplakia is not always an

idiopathic leukokeratosis, and the important etiologic roles of tobacco use, electrogalvanic reaction, and *Candida* infection can often be recognized in particular patients. In other patients, etiologic factors are very difficult to specify, and the leukoplakic lesion is truly idiopathic. The characteristics of leukoplakia associated with smoking habits and electrogalvanic reactions are described separately later in this section (and those of *Candida* leukoplakia in an earlier section) with this potential subcategorization in mind.

Erythroplakia, probably because of its much more recent appearance in the dental literature, remains a single category. Etiologic factors for erythroplakia are largely unrecognized, and its epidemiology and natural history are unsettled except for growing acceptance of the frequency with which carcinomatous changes occur in areas of erythroplakia.

Leukoplakia

Clinical Features

In addition to its occurring as either a localized lesion or diffuse change affecting a large area of the oral mucosa, leukoplakia is described as having three main clinical forms (Fig. 6-22): homogeneous (or leukoplakia simplex), nodular (or speckled), and verrucous. *Homogeneous leukoplakia* refers to a localized lesion or extensive white patch that presents a relatively consistent pattern throughout, even though the surface of the lesion may be described variously as corrugated ("like a beach at ebbing tide"), with a pattern of fine lines ("cristae"), wrinkled ("like dry, cracked mud"), or papillomatous. *Nodular (speckled) leukoplakia** refers to a mixed red and white lesion in which small keratotic nodules are scattered over an atrophic (or erythroplakic) patch of mucosa. This clinical variant is of a special importance because of its extremely high rate of malignant transformation, two thirds of cases in some series showing evidence of epithelial dysplasia or carcinoma on histopathologic examination.

Verrucous leukoplakia as a term is less well

---

* Also referred to as leukoplakia erosiva (Bánóczy) and as speckled erythroplakia.

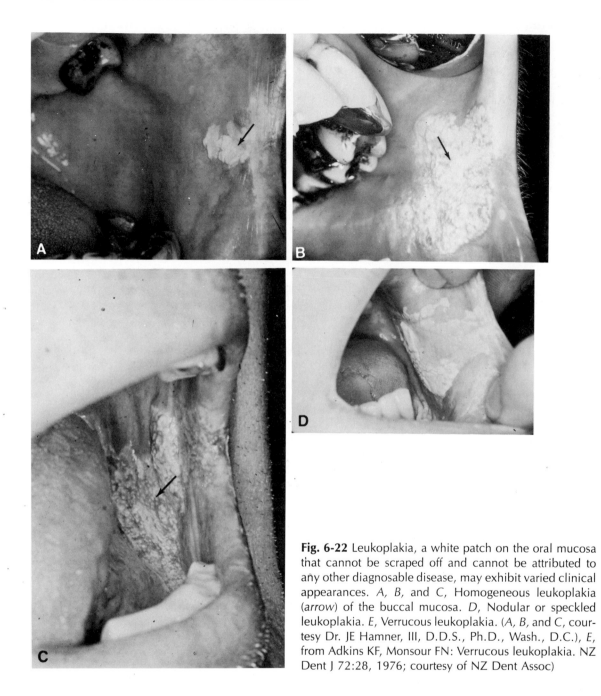

Fig. 6-22 Leukoplakia, a white patch on the oral mucosa that cannot be scraped off and cannot be attributed to any other diagnosable disease, may exhibit varied clinical appearances. *A, B,* and *C,* Homogeneous leukoplakia (*arrow*) of the buccal mucosa. *D,* Nodular or speckled leukoplakia. *E,* Verrucous leukoplakia. (*A, B,* and *C,* courtesy Dr. JE Hamner, III, D.D.S., Ph.D., Wash., D.C.), *E,* from Adkins KF, Monsour FN: Verrucous leukoplakia. NZ Dent J 72:28, 1976; courtesy of NZ Dent Assoc)

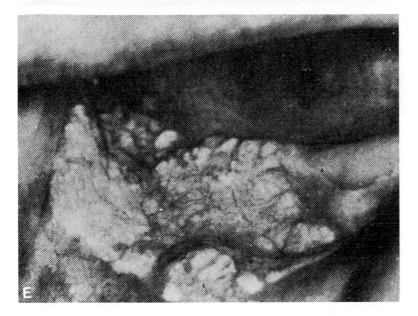

established in the literature, although a number of workers have used it to describe oral white lesions in which the surface is broken up by multiple papillary projections that may also be heavily keratinized, producing a lesion that bears some resemblance to the dorsum of the tongue. Some authors have used the term *verrucous hyperplasia* to describe similar lesions that are seen most often in the sixth to eighth decades of life on the alveolar mucosa and cheek, usually accompanied by homogeneous leukoplakia on the other oral surfaces. Extensive lesions of this type have also been described under the heading of *oral florid papillomatosis.*

Others prefer to avoid the term *verrucous leukoplakia* altogether to prevent confusion with verrucous carcinoma (see Fig. 6-23 and Chap. 9), a well-defined category of indolent oral carcinoma that rarely metastasizes and is frequently associated with use of snuff intraorally. Such lesions often arise on an area of leukoplakia and are said to be frequently underdiagnosed because of their degree of cellular differentiation, lack of cellular atypia, and slow progression from leukoplakia through pseudoepitheliomatous hyperplasia to carcinoma.

Descriptive terminology of this type is necessary for the clinician to characterize particular lesions. It is clear, however, that with the exception of nodular (speckled) leukoplakia, the clinical appearance of a given area of leukoplakia is in general a poor predictor of its behavior or histologic characteristics. Clinical grading of the severity of leukoplakia that was proposed nearly 50 years ago has been shown to be unreliable, and the necessity of examining a persistent white lesion histologically to determine the extent of dysplastic change is well established both in the literature and in the minds of most dentists. Controversy over the use of the term *verrucous leukoplakia* also reflects the concept that any patch of leukoplakia, if not established clinically as caused by some other disorder, should be considered potentially a carcinoma until another diagnosis is established by adequate histologic examination. Waldron and Shafer's 1975 study of over 3,000 cases of oral leukoplakia, covering the period of the 1960s and early 1970s when all "leukoplakias" were considered potentially carcinomatous and fairly aggressively biopsied, clearly demonstrated that lesions considered clinically to be possible squamous cell carcinomas often showed only extensive keratosis on microscopic examination, while conversely, a clinically innocuous leukoplakia occasionally proved to be an early infiltrating squamous cell carcinoma. The majority of leukoplakias are asymptomatic and probably are present

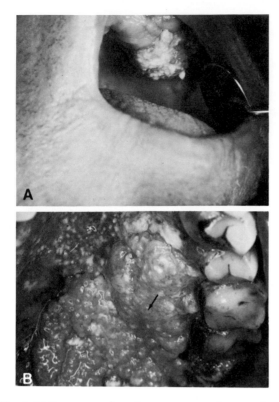

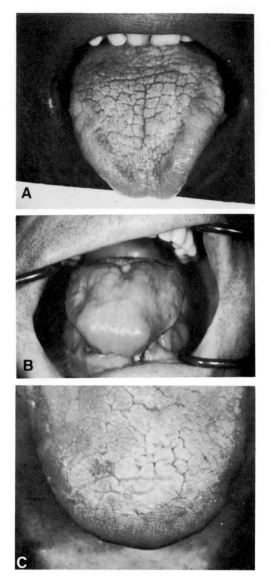

Fig. 6-23 Two examples of verrucous carcinoma. *A,* Verrucous form of leukoplakia associated with a squamous cell carcinoma of the alveolar ridge. *B,* Verrucous carcinoma of the palate in a 62-year-old black female. (*B,* Courtesy Dr. Soli K. Choksi)

Fig. 6-24 *A, B,* and *C,* Several examples of leukoplakia of the tongue reproduced from earlier editions of this text. Extensive lesions of this type are now fairly uncommon. (A) Leukoplakia of the tongue in a patient with positive serologic test for syphilis, (B) syphilitic atrophic glossitis with leukoplakia, (C) leukoplakia of the tongue in a 21-year-old male, heavy cigarette smoker.

for some time before they are recognized, reinforcing the need for prompt biopsy once other clinically identifiable disorders have been ruled out.

While leukoplakia may be found in almost any location in the oral cavity, it is more prevalent in some areas. Surveys of lesions submitted for biopsy published during the last decade list the buccal mucosa and the mandibular mucosa as the sites most often affected, with the lips and palate, maxillary mucosa, retromolar area, floor of the mouth, and tongue as less likely sites. Approximately 50% of lesions affect the cheeks, mandibular mucosa, and sulcus; leukoplakia of the floor of the mouth and tongue is only one quarter as prevalent as buccal leukoplakia. As mentioned earlier, the tongue has changed from being the most prevalent site in series published during the 1940s, to the least prevalent site since the 1960s (see Fig. 6-24).

The age of occurrence of leukoplakia has moved toward the older age group in more recent series, over 60% of cases in 1975 being over 50 years of age, possibly reflecting shifts in the mean age of the population. It is by no means only a disease of older age, however, and cases have been documented in patients under 20 years. The sex ratio has changed quite noticeably from a male–female ratio of 95:5 in the 1940s to approximately 3:2 in recent years, probably as a result of changes in the sex distribution of smoking habits. Because smoking habits vary from community to community, comparisons between sex ratios in different studies must include an investigation of smoking habits and other factors that are considered to be important in the etiology of oral leukoplakia.

Etiology

Local Factors. A number of locally acting etiologic agents (tobacco, alcohol, candidiasis, electrogalvanic reactions, mechanical and chemical irritants, and possibly herpes simplex virus) have been implicated in the etiology of leukoplakia. Of these, tobacco is identified as the major causative factor, based on both clinical observation and studies of experimentally induced leukoplakia in laboratory animals. The data relating to the role of various forms of tobacco use (and frequently associated use of alcohol) in producing leukoplakia are reviewed in the following section dealing with tobacco-induced leukoplakia. *Candida* is frequently present in sections of leukoplakia and is quite consistently associated with nodular (speckled) leukoplakias, as many as 60% of which show candidal infection compared with only 3% of homogeneous leukoplakias. *Candida* also produces hyperplastic reactions in the chorioallantoic membrane of the embryonated hen's egg and has been associated with dysplastic changes in oral leukoplakia by a number of authors. It is also claimed that on occasion treatment with antimycotic agents will eliminate dysplasia, and such treatment dramatically reduces the size and degree of hyperkeratinization of many leukoplakias. Critical experiments in laboratory animals are lacking, however.

The presence of measurable electrogalvanic currents has also been associated with oral leukoplakia in some patients, the majority of these lesions disappearing or spontaneously regressing with elimination of the electric cell produced by adjacent dissimilar metallic restorations (see also following section on Electrogalvanically Induced White Lesions). Lo-

cal mechanical irritants and a variety of chemical irritants produce hyperkeratosis with or without some dysplastic change. These lesions usually resolve with elimination of the irritant. Lehner and associates investigated cell-mediated immunologic reactions to herpes simplex type I in groups of patients with epithelial atypia and carcinoma. Patients with oral carcinoma had nonspecific depression of cell-mediated immunity. A specific increase in cell-mediated immunity to herpes simplex virus was demonstrated in leukoplakia with epithelial atypia, and sequential studies revealed fluctuations in the lymphocyte stimulation index to the virus with a fall associated with malignant transformation. Again, however, critical experiments in laboratory models are lacking, and the high frequency of herpes simplex virus infection in the community has prevented useful epidemiologic investigation of this topic.

Regional and Systemic Factors. In addition to these locally acting factors, the general condition of the oral mucous membrane as influenced by both regional and systemic disorders is important in enhancing the effectiveness of the locally acting factors. Tertiary syphilis, vitamin B_{12} and folic acid deficiency, sideropenic anemia (as seen most dramatically in the Plummer–Vinson syndrome; see Chap. 8), and possibly other nutritional deficiences are all associated with an atrophic glossitis and atrophic changes elsewhere in the oral mucous membrane that predispose these patients to both leukoplakia and oral carcinoma. More common, however, are patients with xerostomia caused by salivary gland disease, anticholinergic medications, or radiation, in whom the protective coating of saliva is reduced or absent. Both red and white lesions of the oral mucosa are increased in frequency, and the effects of even limited smoking are often quite noticeable. In animals rendered artificially xerostomic, the development of oral leukoplakia in response to a variety of carcinogens is greatly enhanced. Systemically administered alcohol, antimetabolite drugs, and specific antilymphocyte serum also enhanced the development of leukoplakia and carcinoma in experimental models, and agents like bacille Calmette Guérin (BCG) vaccine and levamisole, which stimulate immune mechanisms, retard the effect of locally acting factors. Certain nutritional supplements (*e.g.*, synthetic retinoids [13-cis-retinoic acid]) retard experimental leukoplakia development, a fact of some importance in justifying the use of topical vitamin A preparations in the treatment of leukoplakia.

Site and Malignant Transformation

The appearance of leukoplakia to some extent reflects the character of the particular area of mucosa involved, but more important, site determines the rate of malignant transformation. Factors concerned with the thickness and degree of keratinization of different areas of the oral mucosa, as well as those concerned with the more concentrated effect of particular irritants and predisposing factors at certain sites are probably involved. Table 6-1 illustrates the distribution and relative risk of malignant transformation by site for Waldron and Shafer's 1975 series of more than 3000 leukoplakias. As can be seen, the floor of the mouth is the site with the highest risk for leukoplakia: 43% of leukoplakias at this site showed some degree of epithelial dysplasia, carcinoma *in situ*, or invasive carcinoma in the biopsied tissue. Both lips and tongue (24% each) also showed a fair frequency of similar change, with palate, cheek, maxillary and mandibular mucosa, and sulci

having a relatively low risk (12% to 15%). It should be noted that in general, the intraoral sites less frequently involved (floor of mouth and ventral surface of the tongue) had the highest rate of transformation, indicating the clinical importance of leukoplakia at these unusual sites. The etiology of leukoplakia and carcinoma of the lips probably involves actinic radiation, as well as local application of heat from cigarettes and pipes, and is discussed in a subsequent section dealing with actinic keratoses.

The rate of transformation of oral leukoplakia to carcinoma is related to the number of years of follow-up as well as the original composition of the study population: regression of oral leukoplakias has also been documented and reported to occur in as many as 20% to 40% of cases followed over 10 years. This rate of regression is actually higher than the rate of 2% to 30% quoted for malignant transformation. The rate of malignant transformation in more recently published series has also been noted to be far lower than the rates quoted 30 to 40 years ago. This difference (an average of 30% quoted in 1961 versus 1% to 6% for current studies) may reflect changing patterns of disease, changing definitions of leukoplakia, better treatment and elimination of causative factors ("the majority of leukoplakias are reversible lesions that disappear with the elimination of smoking, alcohol and other local

Table 6-1. Oral Leukoplakia—Site and Relative Risk for Epithelial Dysplasia, Carcinoma *in situ*, and Invasive Carcinoma at Each Site

Site	% of Cases	Dysplasia/Cancer No. of Cases	Percent
Mandibular mucosa and sulcus	25	123/845	15
Buccal mucosa	22	121/736	17
Maxillary mucosa and sulcus	11	53/359	15
Palate	11	68/361	19
Lips	10	83/346	24
Floor of mouth*	9*	124/289	43*
Tongue	7	55/227	24
Retromolar	6	23/197	12
Total		650/3360	20

Data from Shafer WG: Basic clinical features of oral premalignant lesions. In Mackenzie IC et al (eds): *Oral Premalignancy.* Proceedings First Dows Symposium, 1980, Iowa City, University of Iowa Press.

*The relative infrequency but high malignant potential of leukoplakia of the floor of the mouth should be noted.

irritants"), and more precise criteria for definition of epithelial dysplasia.

Without minimizing previously stated cautions regarding the difficulty of predicting the likelihood of malignant change in a leukoplakia based on its clinical appearance, nodular (speckled) leukoplakias and verrucous leukoplakias do seem to have a more sinister prognosis than does homogeneous leukoplakia (leukoplakia simplex). In one series, 74% of cases of leukoplakia that subsequently underwent malignant transformation presented initially as nodular (speckled) lesions.

The question of what percentage of carcinomas arises from leukoplakia is less accurately documented. Current speculation tends to the belief that very few carcinomas start this way and that far more carcinomas arise in erythroplakic lesions. Without minimizing the importance of erythroplakia as a precancerous lesion, it must be recognized that a number of papers describe the frequency with which carcinoma and leukoplakia occur together and estimate the frequency of this association at somewhere from 16% to 32%. Studies of experimentally induced leukoplakia and oral carcinoma also show a progression of lesions over time with continuous application of carcinogens: in the case of hamster buccal pouch tumors (tongue lesions develop somewhat more slowly), hyperkeratosis and inflammation occur at 4 to 6 weeks, leukoplakia with microscopic hyperkeratosis and dysplasia at 6 to 8 weeks, carcinoma *in situ* at 8 to 10 weeks, and frankly invasive carcinoma at 10 to 12 weeks. Malignant transformation is inevitable once dysplasia has occurred, even if application of the carcinogen is stopped. The practice of classifying leukoplakias, according to their histopathologic structure, into dysplastic and nondysplastic and treating them conservatively or radically accordingly, thus has a sound scientific basis. Human oral lesions progress more slowly and are produced by lower concentrations of carcinogens acting over longer periods of time, but the same relationship probably holds.

Diagnosis

The most important issue in the diagnosis of oral leukoplakia is the determination of cellular dysplasia by microscopy. In general, the absence of dysplasia in the biopsy safely indicates a benign form, and treatment is usually determined by the results of the biopsy examination. Sampling errors no doubt do occur but will be mininized if the patient is followed over succeeding months and an attempt is made to obtain a biopsy that is representative of the various surface patterns exhibited by the lesion. For example, lesions that are without evidence of dysplasia can at a later date show such changes, but adequate follow-up and repeated biopsy help avoid this problem. Different areas of a very extensive leukoplakia can also show dysplasia, while others do not; in this case, multiple sites may need to be biopsied.

Benign forms of leukoplakia are characterized histologically by variable patterns of hyperkeratosis and chronic inflammatory cell infiltration in the corium. Dysplasia (see Fig. 6-25) is characterized by abnormal orientation of epithelial cells, cellular pleomorphism, and cellular atypia suggestive of early malignancy (irregular epithelial stratification, hyperplasia of the basal layer, drop-shaped rete pegs, increased number of mitotic figures, loss of polarity of basal cells, increased nuclear-cytoplasmic ratio, nuclear polymorphism and hyperchromatism, enlarged nucleoli, keratinization of single cells or cells in groups in the stratum spinosum, and loss of cellular adherence). Any degree of dysplasia and cellular atypia is probably significant of premalignant change; lesions showing severe grades of dysplasia merge with lesions diagnosable as carcinoma *in situ*. To some extent *dyskeratosis* has been used interchangeably with *dysplasia* in the literature on leukoplakia but has been replaced in recent years by the latter term. Dyskeratosis of some degree almost always accompanies the dysplastic changes and thus is not incorrect terminology, but *dysplasia* with its emphasis on cellular changes rather than abnormal patterns of differentiation is considered the more basic phenomenon.

Cytologic examination is usually of little assistance and cannot be relied on for the diagnosis of keratotic white lesions. Scraping of the surface of these lesions provides little else than superficial keratinized squames, and many studies have shown that there is poor correlation between cytologic findings in these lesions and the presence of atypia

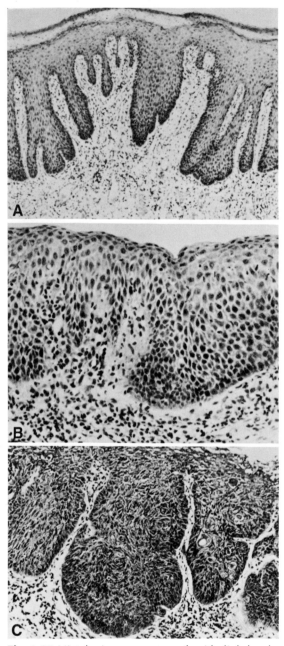

Fig. 6-25 Histologic appearance of epithelial dysplasia of varying degrees of severity. *A,* Slight epithelial dysplasia; elongated and drop-shaped rete processes; hyperparakeratosis (×65). *B,* Moderate epithelial dysplasia; increased nuclear-cytoplasmic ratio; disturbance of maturational sequence with cellular pleomorphism and nuclear hyperchromatism (×220). *C,* Severe epithelial dysplasia verging on carcinoma *in situ.* (From WHO Collaborating Centre for Oral Precancerous Lesions: Definition of leukoplakia and related lesions: An aid to studies of oral precancer. Oral Surg 46:518, 1978; courtesy CV Mosby Co, St. Louis, MO 63141)

detected on histopathologic section. By contrast, scanning electron microscopic examination of the surface cells from both erosive and verrucous leukoplakias has revealed the presence of surface irregularities to these cells that are associated with premalignant and malignant changes as detected by conventional light microscopic examination of tissue sections. Similar surface irregularities have been noted on cells exfoliated from dysplastic lesions at other sites (uterine cervix, larynx). In the scanning electron microscope, the surface cells of leukoplakia of the buccal mucosa were found to be different from those of normal buccal mucosa: in leukoplakia erosiva, the epithelial cells were dissociated; in verrucous leukoplakia, these cells were keratinized; dysplastic erosive leukoplakia was characterized by an atypical arrangement of superficial cytoplasmic projections (microrugae) of the epithelial cells that is not seen in normal tissue.

Differential Diagnosis

Differential diagnosis of oral leukoplakia involves consideration of the numerous other keratotic lesions described in this chapter. A diagnosis of leukoplakia is made when adequate clinical and histologic examination fails to provide evidence for an alternate diagnosis, and characteristic histopathological findings for leukoplakia are present. Important clinical criteria are the location; appearance, and texture of the lesion; known irritant factors, and clinical course. Candidiasis should always be considered as either a primary etiologic factor or opportunistic infectious agent and the lesion reevaluated after 1 to 2 weeks of continuous topical antifungal therapy and attempts at eliminating other suspected local irritants. A serologic test for syphilis should always be obtained in the case of leukoplakia of the tongue dorsum, and a complete blood count or other measure of iron deficiency manifesting in erythrocyte structure should be obtained to rule out sideropenia. In patients with borderline values or mild anemia, circulating iron stores should be measured more specifically. Extensive white lesions occurring in children suggest the possibility of candidiasis; when other children and members of the same family have similar white lesions, one of the genodermatoses is a consideration. In this latter case, additional search for associated anomalies (*e.g.*, palmo-plantar hyperkeratoses, other dermatologic lesions, and congenital abnormalities) is made.

Topically applied toluidine blue has been used with large leukoplakic lesions to identify areas that are more likely to show carcinomatous change and hence should be biopsied. In nodular (speckled) leukoplakia, topical application of toluidine blue is especially helpful in the evaluation of the erythroplakic areas. This technique is discussed more fully in the following section dealing with erythroplakia and also in Chapter 9.

The greatest area of uncertainty lies in differentiating leukoplakia from lichen planus of the oral mucosa. Although both are hyperkeratotic in nature, the more diffuse outline of the lesion in lichen planus, the frequent lack of change in the pliability of the involved tissue, the general distribution of the lesion, and existence of at least one area of lacelike appearance will permit a diagnosis of lichen planus. In a number of patients with chronic keratotic lesions a clear distinction between leukoplakia and lichen planus cannot be made based on clinical features and despite repeated biopsy over many years. The existence of this problem is perhaps not surprising, considering recent reports of both leukoplakia and lichen planus developing in association with at least two of the recognized etiologic agents for leukoplakia (*i.e.*, electrogalvanic currents and tobacco-betel nut-lime "quids").

Treatment

Initial treatment of suspected leukoplakia should include attempts at eliminating all possible local irritants and any identified systemic predisposing factors. Topical antifungal treatment should then be administered continuously for 1 to 2 weeks (antifungal rinses supplemented with vaginal tablets allowed to dissolve under the tongue). A specific appointment should be made for the patient to return for follow-up evaluation, with biopsy planned for that visit if significant resolution of the lesion has not occurred at that time. If the patient has habitually abused tobacco and alcohol, attempts should be made to eliminate these at least temporarily; if sig-

nificant withdrawal problems are expected, counselling and medical treatment should be arranged. No other treatment should be provided for the lesion before biopsy.

Because of the acknowledged difficulty in eliminating all suspected irritants, biopsy will often need to be carried out with something less than the complete elimination of likely irritant factors. Patients are often unconvinced of the role that tobacco and alcohol play in these lesions or are otherwise unwilling or unable to alter long-established habits. Elimination of electrogalvanic currents often cannot be achieved rapidly or without considerable expense. (Where a solitary area of leukoplakia or lichen planus is noted in direct apposition to a large metallic restoration, replacement with a temporary composite or other resin crown is certainly justified.)

Subsequent treatment of the lesions depends on the outcome of the biopsy. *If no evidence of dysplasia is found and the biopsy site is felt to be representative of the entire lesion, conservative treatment is acceptable.* Small lesions are often completely removed by the biopsy, and no additional treatment is needed apart from reassurance of the patient and instructions to report any apparent recurrences; this latter advice can be reinforced by means of a specific annual or biannual follow-up appointment. For larger lesions with no evidence of dysplasia on biopsy, there is a choice between removal of the remainder of the lesion and follow-up evaluation, with or without local medication. Given the evidence from experimental animal models that leukoplakia, dysplasia, and malignant change are related to the intensity of an irritant and the length of time it acts, repeated follow-up visits and repeat biopsy are essential particularly where complete elimination of irritants is not likely to be achieved. In such cases, removal of the entire lesion should also be strongly advised.

Administration of vitamin A has long been recommended for the treatment of leukoplakia that cannot be easily removed by surgery. More recently, a number of natural and artificial analogs of vitamin A, which are commonly referred to as *retinoids* (*e.g.*, 13-cis-retinoic acid; RO-7539; tretinoin*) and as a

---

* Retin A Brand Tretinoin, Ortho Pharmaceutical Corporation Dermatological Division, Raritan, NJ 08869 (see section on Treatment of Lichen Planus for details).

group are less toxic than vitamin A, have been tested for their effect on leukoplakia and a number of other chronic oral lesions such as lichen planus and geographic tongue. Vitamin A and its analogs cause metaplastic changes in squamous epithelium and reduce its tendency to keratinize. Topical administration of these agents reduces the size of leukoplakia lesions clinically, therapy for 2 to 3 weeks usually resulting in distinct changes. Various retinoids have been used for the chemoprevention of neoplastic and preneoplastic changes in a number of organs and are stated to be effective both clinically and in experimental animal models of gastric, esophageal, tracheobronchial, and bladder cancers. Studies on the effect of 13-cis-retinoic acid in DMBA-induced hamster chick pouch cancer remain controversial; however, one study at least showed that the metaplastic effect of the retinoid was independent of the carcinogenic effect of the DMBA and that neoplasia continued irrespective of administration of the retinoid.

At this time, there appear to be no clinical data available on the effectiveness of *systemically administered* vitamin A or retinoic acid on leukoplakia and no adequate experimental animal data to justify use of these compounds clinically for oral lesions without further controlled clinical trials. Overdosage with vitamin A can follow excessive systemic use and is characterized by irritability, fretfulness, itching, angular fissuring, and bleeding of the lips. Two or three weeks' use of topical vitamin A orally is stated not to cause toxicity, and similar treatment with vitamin A analogs is less likely to do so.

Treatment of the dysplastic forms of leukoplakia must take into consideration that the lesion has a greater potential for undergoing malignant change. In general, the greater the degree of cellular atypia observed in the biopsy, the greater the potential for malignant change; however, even moderate degrees of atypia indicate an increased potential for malignant change, with a greater chance of this being realized when recognized irritants cannot be eliminated. At the extreme are lesions in which the extent of dysplastic change is indistinguishable from what must be identified as carcinoma *in situ*. The closer the lesion appears to this extreme, the more it should be treated as carcinoma (see Chap. 9). Local excision of the entire lesion is indicated for all dysplastic leukoplakias of lesser degree than carcinoma *in situ*.

Surgical removal of extensive lesions (see Fig. 6-26) involves "stripping" of large areas of affected mucosa, and skin grafting may be necessary. Cryosurgery (localized application of freezing temperatures to vital tissues with formation of extra- and intracellular ice crystals, leading to a rapid build-up of toxic electrolyte concentrations, altered pH, protein denaturation, and destruction of cell membranes) is now available as an alternative to "stripping" and has been reported to produce good results in the treatment of extensive leukoplakias. Both "open-spray" and "closed probe" methods are used and following necrosis and sloughing of the treated tissue, will result in an area of normal appearing mucosa. Long-term follow-up of this treatment, however, is not available, and the question must be raised as to whether the replacement of a leukoplakic patch by normal appearing mucosa also ensures elimination of dysplastic tissue.

The effectiveness of surgical treatment for leukoplakia is also not entirely clear. Removal of etiologic factors has been shown to be the most important factor in treatment, and surgical treatment provides a better outcome when it is combined with elimination of etiologic factors. Leukoplakia can certainly redevelop on a healed surgical site or a graft when etiologic factors persist. Others have claimed that the incidence of carcinoma in leukoplakia is not altered by surgical treatment. While as many as 20% to 40% of leukoplakias, depending on severity, can be expected to regress with time, another 40% to 50% remain unchanged, and a small percentage (3% to 10%) can be expected to increase in size with persistence of etiologic factors. Evaluation of the effectiveness of particular treatments, therefore, must involve a relatively homogeneous sample of lesions, elimination or stability of etiologic factors, and statistical corrections for spontaneous regression and malignant transformation rates.

Important guidelines for the management of leukoplakia are as follows:

1. Clinical observation of suspected leukoplakia without biopsy is dangerous.

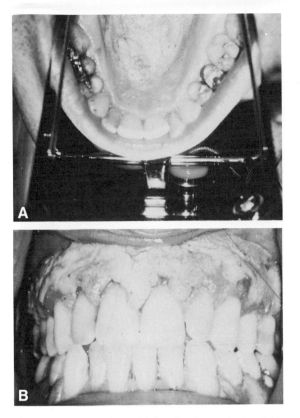

Fig. 6-26 Extensive thick, leathery leukoplakic plaques involving the palate (*A*), gingivae (*B*), and the tongue. Management of lesions of this extent requires use of all available diagnostic approaches to select the best areas for biopsy, as well as the use of antifungal agents, surgery, and possibly vitamin A analogs where the extent of the lesion or prompt recurrences limit the effectiveness of surgery.

2. The clinical response of hyperkeratotic areas of oral mucosa is unpredictable, and rebiopsy at 6- to 12-month intervals is indicated, particularly if the lesion changes in size or physical characteristics.

3. Somewhere between 6% and 10% of leukoplakias with evidence of dysplasia progress to malignancy. Except for a limited number of lesions and locations mentioned in item 4, the clinical features of leukoplakic lesions *in general* are a poor predictor of which will become malignant.

4. Because of the higher risk that nodular (speckled) and verrucous leukoplakia and leukoplakia of the floor of the mouth and tongue dorsum will become malignant, excision of these lesions with adequate follow-up is essential.

5. Recurrence will often follow removal of the lesion if recognized irritants and predisposing factors are not eliminated.

Erythroplakia

The term erythroplakia is applied to any area of reddened, velvety-textured mucosa that cannot be identified on the basis of clinical and histopathologic examination as being caused by inflammation or any other disease process. A number of workers have shown that the majority of oral lesions of this type, particularly those found under the tongue, on the floor of the mouth, and on the soft palate and anterior faucial pillars, exhibit a high frequency of cellular atypia and premalignant and malignant changes (see Fig. 6-27). The word is an adaptation of the French *erythroplasie de Queyrat*, which describes a similar appearing lesion of the glans penis having comparable premalignant tendency. While red lesions of the oral mucosa have been noted for many years, the use of the term *erythroplakia* in this context has been common for only about 25 years. Erythroplakic lesions are easily overlooked, and the true prevalence of the condition is not known. Red lesions of this type are far less common than leukoplakia in histopathologic series, but this probably reflects the fact that leukoplakias are more likely to be biopsied and emphasizes the lack of appreciation of the significance of erythroplakia clinically. Most authors have been impressed by the seriousness of the lesions submitted as red lesions or erythroplakia, and it has been proposed that these lesions are the most likely precursors of oral squamous cell carcinoma (see Chap. 9).

Several clinical variants of erythroplakia have been described by different investigators, but there is no generally agreed on classification. Shear in 1972 described "homogeneous erythroplakia, erythroplakia interspersed with patches of leukoplakia, and granular or speckled erythroplakia"; most authors consider this last category identical to speckled leukoplakia. (The suggestion has also been made that the term *speckled leukoplakia* be changed to *speckled erythroplakia*, to emphasize the frequency with which this particular lesion is associated with cellular atypia.) Mashberg in 1977 referred to "a gran-

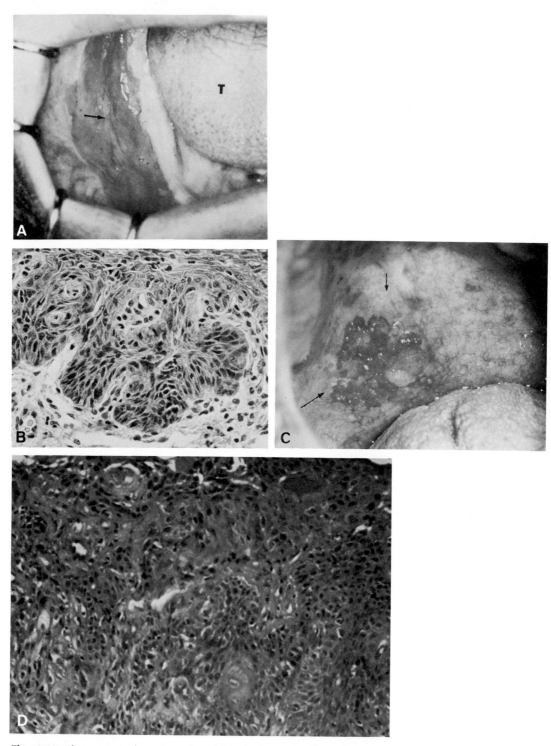

Fig. 6-27 Three examples of erythroplakic lesions. *A,* Clinical appearance of an area of erythroplakia on the buccal mucosa in a 49-year-old white female. (Courtesy Dr. JE Hamner, III, D.D.S., Ph.D., Wash., D.C.), *B,* Histologic appearence of an erythroplakic area adjacent to a squamous cell carcinoma of the floor of the mouth, showing marked epithelial hyperplasia with minimal atypia. *C,* Extensive erythroplakic area of the soft palate, which on biopsy *D* revealed invasive squamous cell carcinoma.

ular red, velvety lesion with either stippled or patchy areas of white keratin within or peripheral to the lesion," and "a smooth, non-granular lesion with minimal or no keratosis." Many of these lesions are irregular in outline, and some contain islands of normal mucosa within areas of erythroplakia, a phenomenon that has been attributed to coalescence of a number of precancerous foci. The high rate of premalignant and malignant changes previously referred to as a feature of erythroplakia is true for all clinical varieties of this lesion and not solely a feature of speckled erythroplakias. Different studies have demonstrated that 80% to 90% of erythroplakias are histopathologically either severe epithelial dysplasia, carcinoma *in situ*, or invasive carcinoma.

In view of the clinical significance of erythroplakias, their differentiation from other red, inflammatory lesions of the oral mucosa is critical. Similar appearing lesions are associated with candidiasis (vigorous oral hygiene just before examination of the mouth will remove a *Candida* pseudomembrane, leaving a red patch), and denture stomatitis is a red, patchy lesion. Tuberculosis (lupus vulgaris), histoplasmosis, areas of mechanical irritation, and a variety of nonspecific lesions may have an identical appearance. Confusion between erythroplakia and inflammatory lesions, however, is of less significance than is failure to notice a red patch or to disregard the patch as a transient, minor inflammatory lesion in the search for leukoplakia. The importance of drying the oral mucosa well when carrying out an oral cancer screening examination cannot be overemphasized, along with the need for careful examination of the floor of the mouth, ventral surface of the tongue and soft palate, and anterior faucial pillars, all prime areas for development of erythroplakia and carcinoma. In addition to their lack of dramatic clinical appearance, almost all erythroplakias are asymptomatic and unlikely to be drawn to the dentist's attention by the patient's complaint.

Because localized areas of redness are not uncommon in many mouths, areas of erythroplakia are likely to be disregarded by the examiner; they are often considered to be a transient inflammatory response to local irritation and not indicated for biopsy. Differentiation of erythroplakia with malignant change and other early squamous cell carcinomas (*e.g.*, erythroplastic carcinoma *in situ*, early small invasive carcinomas, patchy leukoplakic malignant tumors, and persistent postirradiation carcinomas) from benign inflammatory lesions of the oral mucosa can be enhanced by use of 1% toluidine blue (tolonium chloride) solution applied topically with a swab or as an oral rinse.* While this technique was previously found to have limited usefulness in the evaluation of many keratotic oral lesions, more recent prospective studies of the specificity of toluidine blue staining of areas of early carcinoma contained in erythroplakic and mixed leukoplakic and erythroplakic lesions report excellent results with false-negative (underdiagnosis) and false-positive (over-diagnosis) rates of well below 10%.

Early oral squamous cell carcinomas retain the stain owing to the increased DNA content of the malignant cells (*see Fig. 9-7*). Dysplastic areas stain less intensely than does carcinoma. False-positive reactions occur with traumatic ulcers and localized areas of inflammation, but the majority of such inflammatory lesions disappear and no longer stain after a 2-week period during which an attempt is made to free the mouth of identifiable local irritants. Small areas of intense staining sometimes occur from mechanical retention of the stain, but the 1% acetic acid rinse used after the toluidine blue solution usually eliminates these nonspecific reactions. Additional gentle local swabbing of a suspicious area with acetic acid after staining also helps differentiate those areas that easily decolorize under these circumstances from areas of carcinoma, which retain the stain more firmly. The papillae and crevices of the dorsum of the tongue usually retain stain that

---

* 1% toluidine blue (tolonium chloride) solution, composed of toluidine blue O powder (Fisher Scientific Co, Biological stain 56%) 1 g; acetic acid 10 ml, absolute alcohol 4.19 ml, distilled water to 100 ml, and *p*H adjusted with acetic acid to 4.5 or less. In the rinsing technique, the patient rinses with 1% acetic acid for 20 seconds, followed by two 20-second water rinses; 5 to 10 ml of the 1% toluidine blue solution is then used as a rinse and gargle, followed by a 1% acetic acid rinse for 1 minute and a final water rinse. No untoward effects have been noted as a result of topical use of this rinse.

may be transferred to the soft palate as a diffuse, amorphous coloration. Small asymptomatic early carcinomas stain dark blue; necrotic lesions and submucosal extensions of larger and symptomatic cancers usually do not stain. Keratin does not allow the stain to penetrate.

Unlike leukoplakia, erythroplakia has no apparent sex predilection; most cases reported have occurred in the sixth and seventh decades (similar to the current age distribution for leukoplakia). The etiology of erythroplakia is unknown, although it seems likely that smoking and alcohol abuse are important because they have been identified as prime etiologic factors for oral cancer.

Treatment of erythroplakia should follow the same principles outlined above for leukoplakia. Observation for 1 to 2 weeks following elimination of suspected irritants is acceptable, but prompt biopsy at that time is mandatory for lesions that persist. Because of confusion between areas of inflammation and dysplastic areas when the toluidine blue staining procedure is used, the toluidine blue solution should be reapplied following the period of elimination of suspected irritants. Lesions that stain on this second application very frequently show extensive dysplasia or early carcinoma. Where the epithelial dysplasia is severe and extensive or where actual carcinoma *in situ* has intervened, removal of the entire lesion is required. Actual invasive carcinoma must be treated promptly (see Chap. 9), despite the small size of most of the malignant erythroplakic lesions. Mashberg reports that 84% of these asymptomatic cancers that are identified as erythroplakia are 2 cm or less, 42% are 1 cm or less in diameter, and local excision with minimal soft tissue and bone loss is possible at this stage and produces excellent results and a recurrence rate of less than 5%.

Oral Lesions Associated with Use of Tobacco and Alcohol

There is extensive evidence establishing tobacco as a major etiologic factor in leukoplakia and squamous cell carcinoma of the oral cavity. This evidence includes epidemiologic study of risk factors for these lesions,

induction of leukoplakia and oral cancer in experimental animal models, regression of leukoplakia and milder degrees of epithelial dysplasia on elimination of smoking, and comparative studies of the effects of different forms of tobacco use on the oral mucosa. Publications by Pindborg and associates, Shklar, Graham, Wynder, and Banoczy, among others, should be consulted for detailed documentation of this evidence.

The relationship is undoubtedly more direct between smoking and leukoplakia than it is between smoking and oral cancer, and it appears that as many as 60% to 75% of leukoplakias, including a proportion with dysplastic changes, will either regress or disappear completely if smoking is eliminated for 1 year. The large number of active constituents that can be derived from tobacco include some that are considered to be initiators of the malignant process and others that promote it. The variability of effects that are associated with different forms of tobacco and the different uses to which it is put (see below) may possibly be explained on this basis in addition to certain inconsistencies in regard to tobacco as a carcinogen for oral cancer. For example, not all leukoplakias regress on cessation of smoking: malignant transformation of leukoplakias in patients without tobacco habits or who only smoke occasionally occurs five times more frequently than in those with daily smoking habits; among the inhabitants of Kerala state in India who have an exceptionally high rate of leukoplakia (2.1 and 1.5 per thousand for males and females, respectively), cigarette ("Bidi") smokers had an increased rate of leukoplakia but not malignant transformation, while those who chewed "pan" (a mixture of tobacco, betel nut, and sea-shell lime) had the highest rate of malignant transformation.

Mashberg and co-workers have recently drawn attention to the greater potential that alcohol abusers have for developing oral cancer when groups of subjects are compared after adjustment for smoking habits. The risk of developing oral cancer was found to be three to five times greater in those who consume more than the equivalent of 6 whiskeys daily, compared to those who consume fewer. Comparison of risk rates for alcohol versus smoking in this study also indicated that consumption of more than 6 whiskey equivalents daily is more harmful than smoking more than 40 cigarettes. Other workers have considered alcohol a co-carcinogen along with tobacco, chronic mouth irritation, diabetes, and syphilis but believe that it is a significant factor only where the patient also uses tobacco.

The variety of ways in which tobacco is used leads to considerable variation in the prevalence, site, and clinical presentation of lesions associated with tobacco. Cigarettes, cigars, and pipes are the major ways in which tobacco is used in western countries, but chewing tobacco and snuff dipping are other traditional usages that have increased somewhat in the United States in recent years as a result of warnings concerning the hazards of cigarette smoking. In some eastern countries and in a variety of indigenous cultures studied around the world, other methods such as chewing tobacco mixed with betel nut and lime and reverse cigarette and cigar smoking are prevalent.

Cigarette, Cigar, and Pipe Smoking. A comparison of cigarette, cigar, and pipe smoking indicates that cigar smoking is associated with fewer oral lesions than is either cigarette or pipe smoking, possibly because of the increased temperature of the combustion of the tobacco with the latter two methods. The highest prevalence of all oral lesions (stomatitis nicotina, leukoplakia, and carcinoma) is associated with pipe, or pipe and cigar smoking; cigarette smoking is associated with an increased prevalence of stomatitis nicotina over cigar and pipe smoking. Age is an important co-factor, oral lesions associated with smoking being more frequent in the over-50 age group. In defining tobacco usage, the dividing line between light to moderate and heavy usages is considered to be 30 cigarettes, or 4 cigars, or 6 pipes daily. Among high-risk groups (*e.g.*, armed services veterans), rates for leukoplakia were 3.8% for nonsmokers and 22.8% for smokers; there was an excess of lesions on the cheek, palate, and tongue in the smokers compared with nonsmokers, in whom leukoplakia was almost confined to the cheeks. At the moment, oral lesions associated with smoking are more common in males, but based on the increased smoking habits of young females in the last two decades, a change in this sex ratio is predicted in the next 20 to 25 years (see Fig. 6-28).

Snuff Dipping. Snuff dipping (placement or retention of finely ground or powdered tobacco in the oral vestibule) by comparison, has been recognized as associated with an exceptionally high rate of oral and pharyngeal cancer mortality among white women in the United States. In the southeastern states where the snuff dipping habit is popular in rural communities, a prevalence rate of 26 cases of cancer caused by this habit per 100,000 population has been calculated, making oropharyngeal cancer in this region next

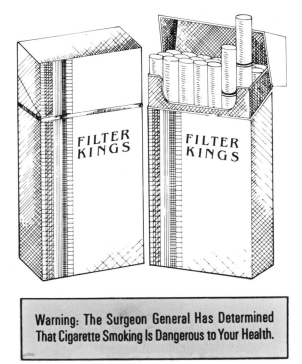

Fig. 6-28 A federal law requiring that all cigarette packages sold in the United States carry a warning about deleterious effects of cigarette smoking illustrates a trend believed to have had an influence on changing patterns of oral leukoplakia over the last two years.

in prevalence after cancers of the breast, uterus, ovary, colon, lung, and pancreas. Snuff dipping and cigarette smoking are often combined, and the effect of the latter obscures the carcinogenic effect of the snuff; in nonsmokers, snuff dippers have four times the risk of developing oral cancer than those who do not use snuff. Localized leukoplakia of the vestibule and gingiva are almost universal as a consequence of chronic snuff dipping, and the risk of cancer in these tissues (vestibule and gingiva otherwise have a low frequency of cancer) is about 50 times the rate in those who do not use snuff. Clinically, leukoplakia associated with snuff dipping is localized to the favored vestibular sulcus and adjacent gingiva, is often well circumscribed, and histologically exhibits a subepithelial band of hyalinization (see Fig. 6-29). Two thirds of the carcinomas that develop in these lesions are verrucous in type; additional leukoplakic zones may be found away from the snuff associated lesion, malignant transformation in these accounting for the increased general risk of cancer throughout the oral mucosa in snuff dippers.

The habit of snuff dipping is not consistently associated with increased rates of oral cancer, and in Scandinavia and South Africa, for example, leukoplakias associated with snuff dipping are said to rarely exhibit premalignant changes. These differences are attributed to variations in the composition of snuff, in particular to the amount of fermented or cured tobacco included in the mixture. The compound N^1-nitroso-nor-nicotine (NNN), which is derived partly from bacterial action on nicotine during the curing process and is contributed to by the action of salivary nitrites when the tobacco is held in the mouth, occurs in greater concentration in snuff tobacco and some pipe and cigar tobaccos than in cigarettes and has been implicated in the higher prevalence of leukoplakia and oral carcinoma in U.S. snuff dippers.

Tobacco and Betel-Nut Chewing. Similar local mucosal changes are produced by *other methods of chewing or holding tobacco in the mouth,* such as "pan" and "kharni" in India and southeastern Asia and New Guinea, and "nass" in some of the Soviet republics. In

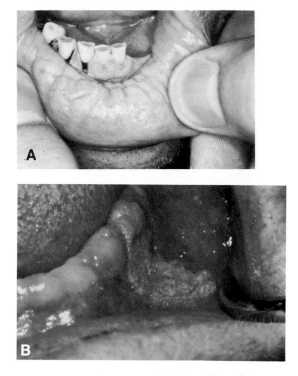

Fig. 6-29 *A,* Diffuse area of leukoplakia of the mucobuccal fold owing to the habit of holding snuff in this area. *B,* More localized area of leukoplakia in the mucobuccal fold and lateral aspect of the edentulous alveolus associated wiht habitual use of a quid of chewing tobacco and snuff.

each of these cases, varieties of cured and uncured tobacco are mixed with lime, oil, flavorings, and in India and southeast Asia, with the ground kernel of the betel nut, which contributes an intense brownish red color to the user's saliva, oral mucosa, and lips. In rural and industrial communities in the United States and the United Kingdom where *plug tobacco* is chewed, excess oral cancer rates are found in those who chew and smoke tobacco over those who only smoke. Extracts of betel nut produce both leukoplakia and carcinoma in the experimental hamster cheek pouch model; cured tobacco produces leukoplakia and increases the carcinogenic potential of betel nut extracts but alone, produces only leukoplakia. Like snuff dipping, these various forms of tobacco chewing are associated with increased rates of verrucous carcinoma at the site where the

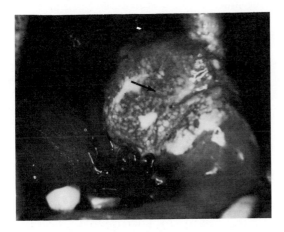

Fig. 6-30 Buccal carcinoma (*arrow*) in a 50-year-old Indian male who chewed betel quid. (Courtesy Dr. Fali S. Mehta)

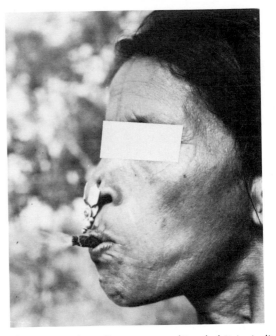

Fig. 6-31 "Chutta" reverse smoking habit in India. (Courtesy Dr. Fali S. Mehta)

"quid" or "pan" is held habitually (see Fig. 6-30).

Reverse Smoking. Considerable attention has also been given in the literature to an unusual practice of reverse cigarette or cigar smoking (*chutta*) that has been observed in indigenous isolated coastal communities of India, the Caribbean, and South America (see Fig. 6-31). This habit, which is said to allow smoking in localities or occupations exposed to high winds and water spray, is associated with an increased frequency of oral lesions, possibly caused by the higher intraoral temperatures and different combustion products. In an extensive study of 10,000 villagers in Andhra Pradesh in India, almost half of whom habitually reverse smoked, Pindborg and his associates recorded prevalences of 4.9% for leukoplakia (most of which occurred on the palate) and 9.5% for stomatitis nicotina, with rates for epithelial atypia in each case being 15.3% and 9.1%, respectively. Eighty percent of the palates biopsied showed hyperorthrokeratosis, and 73% showed epithelial hyperplasia. Unlike the palatal lesions seen in western smokers, both leukoplakia and stomatitis nicotina on the palate associated with reverse smoking (see Fig. 6-32) show high frequency of atypia that proceeds in many cases to carcinoma of the palate (see lack of premalignant potential of

stomatitis nicotina, described in preceding section). The epithelial atypia occurred mostly in the basal cell layer and were associated with delicately pointed rete pegs, kionoblastlike cells in the basal layer, migration of pigmented cells from the basal layer to the lamina propria, but only minimal inflammation of this zone.

Despite the attention that has been given to leukoplakia and carcinoma, tobacco usage in its various forms is also associated with other lesions of the oral mucosa. Increased thickness of the oral epithelium and increased keratinization of normally keratinized areas are common in chronic smokers, as is injection and generalized redness of the soft palate and fauces. Irregular red areas are also seen in this latter region and should be carefully examined and biopsied as possible erythroplakia. Burns and keratotic patches are common on the lips at the site of habitual cigarette smoking, particularly where the cigarette or cigar is retained as a stub for lengthy periods. Lichen planus-like lesions have also been described in association with betel-nut habits. Less significant but also associated

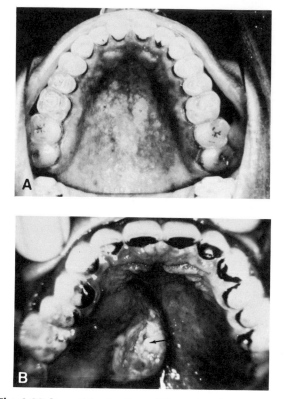

Fig. 6-32 Stomatitis nicotina of the palate in reverse cigarette smokers has a greatly increased potential for development of carcinoma than the same lesion observed in western "conventional" cigarette smokers. *A,* Stomatitis nicotina of the palate of a 50-year-old Indian female. *B,* Carcinoma of the palate *(arrow)* of a 42-year-old Indian female who practiced reverse smoking. (Courtesy Dr. Soli K. Choksi)

with smoking are discoloration of teeth from tarry deposits, increased oral mucosal pigmentation, increased rates of periodontal disease, and decreases in smell and taste acuity.

Oral Changes with Cessation of Smoking. The habitual smoker derives not only social standing and general physiological stimulation from the smoking habit, but also a considerable degree of oral sensory gratification. Sudden cessation of smoking frequently leads to withdrawal symptoms manifested by increased nervousness and desire for increased oral sensory stimulation. This leads many times to increased rates of cheek and lip biting, tongue thrusting, and other oral habits that may cause considerable mucosal

damage and symptomatology (burning tongue, tingling lips, etc). Other patients describe a constant awareness of their mouth and an inability to relax their jaws or free themselves from a sense of oral discomfort. Some patients complain of sensory changes at this time, such as increased roughness or sliminess of the lining of their mouths, sore throat, taste disorders, and others. Recurrent aphthae may recur, caused either by increased susceptibility of a thinner oral mucosa, increased tongue and cheek movement, or even psychosomatic causes associated with cessation of smoking. Often no physical cause can be found for these varied complaints, but their association with attempts at stopping smoking are often very clear. Small doses of muscle relaxants on a temporary basis may be needed to control these symptoms. The prevalence of these problems in consultative practice has increased in recent decades and can be expected to increase further, if warnings concerning the association of smoking with lung and oral cancer are taken realistically by more and more smokers.

Electrogalvanically Induced Oral White Lesions

Several workers have drawn attention to the possibility that electrogalvanic currents generated by dissimilar metallic restorations and prostheses in the oral cavity may be an important etiologic factor in oral lichen planus as well as leukoplakia. In one series, roughly half the lesions observed were lichen planus, the others leukoplakia. Many of these lesions resolved with elimination of the electrogalvanic stimulus. An electrogalvanic lesion is defined as one in close contact with a metallic restoration, and where different metals are present in the mouth (see Fig. 6-33). Additional evidences are signs of corrosion of metallic restorations and where equipment is available, measurement of an electric potential difference greater than 50 millivolts between two dissimilar metallic restorations in the mouth that are considered to be related to the lesion. Disappearance of the lesion following replacement of the restoration adjacent to the lesion with a nonmetallic substitute is also important information. Malignant

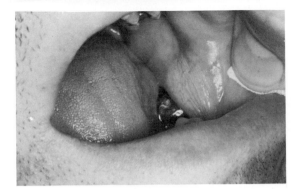

Fig. 6-33 Localized area of leukoplakia in contact with a large corroded amalgam restoration and with both gold and amalgam restorations present in each dental arch suggests the possibility of an electrogalvanically induced keratosis.

transformation was described in one third of the lesions reported in this particular series. Otherwise, no special histopathologic characteristics were noted to identify these electrogalvanic oral white lesions. Histologic and clinical similarities have been described between the lichen planus-like lesions seen in association with habitual betel-nut chewing and the electrogalvanically associated lichen planus lesions. Because of the high rate of malignant transformation noted in these white lesions, long-term follow-up is recommended even for lesions that regress clinically with elimination of the electrogalvanic stimulus.

Carcinoma *in Situ*

Severe dysplastic changes in a white lesion indicate considerable risk for the development of cancer. The more severe grades of dysplasia merge with the condition referred to as carcinoma *in situ* (see Fig. 6-25), which implies that the intraepithelial changes are the same as those seen in invasive cancers, even though there is no histologic evidence in the specimen submitted that malignant cells have left the confines of the epithelium. While various schemes have been devised for the grading of dysplasia in histologic sections, it is clear that there is no consensus among pathologists as to the relative value of different epithelial atypia (see Fig. 6-34). The WHO Collaborating Reference Center for

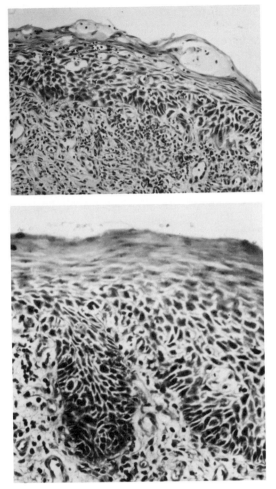

Fig. 6-34 Microscopically, carcinoma *in situ* demonstrates complete disorientation of cells throughout all epithelial layers yet the basement membrane remains intact. The change from normal to atypical epithelium is abrupt with variations in cellular shape and size, loss of rete pegs, hyperchromatic bizarre nuclei, and loss of cellular cohesion. As an alternative, other workers who have considered this definition too restrictive have defined carcinoma *in situ* as the presence of significant cellular abnormalities distributed vertically throughout the epithelial profile. Thus the presence of a surface flattening of squamous cells in a hyperkeratotic or hyperparakeratotic lesion would not impede this diagnosis. (Courtesy J.E. Hamner III, D.D.S., Ph.D., Washington, DC)

Oral Precancerous Lesions supports the convention of using the term carcinoma *in situ* only when the dysplastic change affects the whole or almost the whole thickness of the epithelium involved. This practice conforms to that used for evaluation of dysplasia in other mucosal sites (*e.g.,* cervix uteri, skin, larynx, esophagus and gastrointestinal tract); however, no adequate longitudinal data support the validity of this practice for the oral mucosa.

The use of the category of carcinoma *in situ* has been criticized on a variety of grounds in addition to the disagreements over its definition. For extensive leukoplakia, the tissue selected for biopsy may not be representative of all areas of the lesion, and the absence of invasion of the dermis in the sampled tissue may or may not reflect the situation elsewhere in the lesion. This problem is not unique to the diagnosis of carcinoma *in situ,* but it becomes very important when a decision is being made between dysplasia somewhere short of invasive carcinoma and invasive carcinoma. The discovery in recent years that a high percentage of erythroplakic lesions exhibit severe dysplasia and that many are in fact carcinoma *in situ* or invasive carcinoma has raised the question of the need for both categories, erythroplakia and carcinoma *in situ.* Textbook descriptions of carcinoma *in situ* usually describe it as varying from ''shiny atrophic patches, to leukoplakia, to erythroplakia.'' It is very possible, however, that the majority of carcinoma *in situ* presents as an erythroplakic lesion.

In many cases, lesions of carcinoma *in situ* are treated aggressively with local excision with a wide border of normal tissue. Exploration of regional nodes and dissection of nodes would not usually be included, unless there was clinical evidence of their involvement. Some surgeons, however, make no distinction between histologic diagnosis of carcinoma and one of carcinoma *in situ* as far as oral mucosal lesions are concerned.

Bowen's Disease

Bowen's disease is a localized, intraepidermal squamous cell carcinoma that may progress to invasive carcinoma over many years. It occurs most commonly on the skin, either on sun-exposed areas or on nonexposed skin as a result of arsenic ingestion. Clinically, it appears as a slowly enlarging erythematous patch with little to suggest a malignant process; histologically, the epithelial cells of the lesion lie in complete disarray, many with highly atypical, hyperchromatic nuclei and multiple nuclear forms. Individual cells located at any level of the epithelium may undergo keratinization, producing a characteristic histologic appearance. Lesions of this type caused by arsenic poisoning are often associated with visceral cancer, and Bowen's disease is therefore sometimes listed as a phakomatosis (see Chap. 8 for other examples of phakomatoses).

Bowen's disease also occurs on the male and female genital mucosae and in the oral mucosa as an erythroplakic, leukoplakic, or papillomatous lesion. Because of the superficial similarity between Bowen's disease and erythroplakia, both of which can be characterized as red patches of the mucous membrane that histologically contain severely dysplastic epithelium or intraepithelial carcinoma, the question has been raised as to whether they are the same disorder. Current opinion based on comparison of oral erythroplakias with the oral lesions of patients with well-documented Bowen's disease suggests that they are separate disorders.

Oral Submucous Fibrosis

Oral submucous fibrosis is a slowly progressive disease in which fibrous bands form in the oral mucosa, ultimately leading to severe restriction of movement of the mouth, including the tongue, (see Fig. 6-35). It occurs almost exclusively in India and its neighboring countries and Indian communities in Africa and Fiji. It is always associated with a juxtaepithelial inflammatory reaction followed by a fibroelastic change of the lamina propria with subsequent epithelial atrophy (see Fig. 6-36). These changes are associated with burning sensations in the mouth and occasionally with vesiculation of the mucosa. In the fully developed form, the outstanding clinical feature is the blanched atrophic epithelium. Leukoplakia often develops as a secondary change on areas of the affected epithelium; epithelial dysplasia is found in about 10% to 15% of cases and oral cancer in 6% to

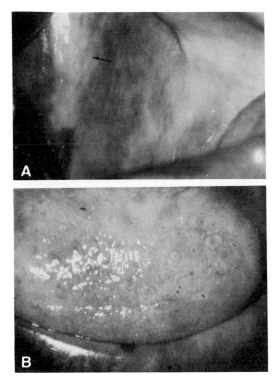

Fig. 6-35 Clinical appearance of oral submucous fibrosis. *A*, Fibrous bands (*arrow*) and marblelike clinical appearance of lesion involving the buccal mucosa. *B*, Atrophy of the filiform papillae of the tongue. (Courtesy J.E. Hamner III, D.D.S., Ph.D., Washington, DC)

30% of cases, depending on the population sampled. Based on these data, oral submucous fibrosis has been identified as an important premalignant condition in Indians. The etiology of the condition is unknown, hypersensitivity to spices and betel nut having been suggested but not established. There is no experimental animal model. This condition was also present in many of the Indian villagers in whom lichen planus-like lesions as well as leukoplakia were described in association with the betel-nut-and-tobacco chewing habit.

Actinic Keratosis, Elastosis, and Cheilitis

Actinic keratosis is a premalignant squamous cell lesion resulting from long-term exposure to solar radiation and may be found on the vermilion border of the lip as well as other

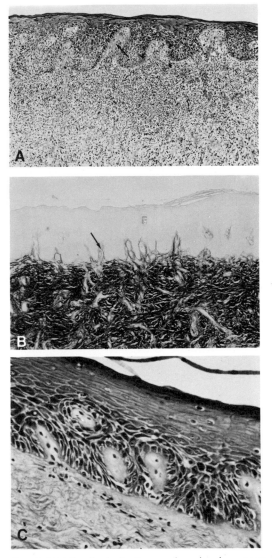

Fig. 6-36 Histologic features of oral submucous fibrosis include (*A*) epithelial atrophy, chronic inflammation, and juxtaepithelial band of amorphous nonbundular collagen (*arrow*), which is nonbirefringent under polarized light and stains in an atypical fashion with Rinehart stain (*B*). Many cases of oral submucous fibrosis demonstrate marked epithelial atypia that later progress to frank malignancy (*C*). (Courtesy J.E. Hamner III, D.D.S., Ph.D., Washington, DC)

sun-exposed skin surfaces. While on skin surfaces and the vermilion border of the lip, the lesion is crusted and keratotic; on the labial mucosa exposed to the sun, a white area of atrophic epithelium develops with underlying scarring of the lamina propria (referred to as *elastosis*). Where this atrophic tissue abrades or ulcerates, the term *actinic cheilitis* is appropriate. Neither of these lesions is, strictly speaking, leukoplakia, although true leukoplakia of the lip can occur in association with a heavy smoking habit. Both types of lesions may of course be combined.

At one time, a distinction was made between senile keratosis and elastosis and similar appearing actinic lesions in regard to supposed etiology and premalignant potential. Currently, little distinction is made between senile lesions found on the skin of elderly people with fair complexions and lesions associated with actinic radiation in a younger age group. As with leukoplakia, the clinical appearance of the lip lesion is a poor guide to the presence of dysplastic changes, and biopsy is indicated for lesions that do not regress with reduction in sun exposure or use of sun screens. Over 10% of these lesions are considered to undergo malignant transformation, and there is good evidence that actinic elastosis of the lip is a forerunner of lip carcinoma. Detailed examination of the lip and documentation of the extent of sun exposure are important components of an oral cancer screening examination in fair-skinned persons.

Early in the use of 5-fluorouracil as a systemic antimetabolite in the treatment of breast and gastric carcinomas, improvement of lip lesions was noted in patients with incidental actinic keratosis. Intentional use of this agent topically* for treatment of actinic keratosis and elastosis has therefore been recommended by a number of authors. Follow-up biopsy studies of a number of patients with actinic lip lesions who were treated in this fashion showed that while the clinical lesion could be reduced or eliminated in this way, dysplastic changes persisted in the apparently healthy lip mucosa that remained. Adequate follow-up and subsequent rebiopsy is therefore advised for patients who are treated in this fashion, rather than by surgical excision or lip "shaving" procedures. Application of 5-fluorouracil to the lip produces erythema followed by vesiculation, erosion, ulceration, necrosis, and re-epithelization. A topical corticosteroid (*e.g.*, betamethasone valerate†) is usually applied between treatments to control lip swelling.

Discoid Lupus Erythematosus

The range of oral lesions associated with the various clinical forms of lupus erythematosus is described in Chapter 24. Disagreements in the literature as to the relative frequency of oral lesions in discoid (DLE) and systemic (SLE) forms of lupus erythematosus appear to be related to the type of intraoral manifestation scored, as well as poor immunologic separation of DLE and SLE in earlier series of cases. Keratotic or mixed red and white lesions are possibly more common in DLE than in SLE; based on data collected in the 1960s, the frequency of oral lesions in all forms of lupus combined varies from 5% to 50%. The WHO Collaborating Reference Center for Oral Precancerous Lesions defines the oral lesions of DLE as "circumscribed, slightly elevated, white patches that may be surrounded by a (red) telangiectatic halo. A radiating pattern of very delicate white lines is usually observed." The classical discoid lesions are also described by others as a central atrophic area with white dots surrounded by a border with parallel white striae. The alternating red (atrophic), white (keratotic), and red (telangiectatic) zones provide a characteristic appearance (see Fig. 6-37). Early lesions may appear as irregular red patches without keratosis. The oral lesions may or may not be accompanied by skin lesions in both discoid and systemic forms (see Fig. 6-38). Clinically, differentiation from leukoplakia and lichen planus is difficult, and the older literature refers to the uncertainty of trying

---

* Efudex Topical Cream (2%), Roche Laboratories, Division Hoffman–LaRoche Inc, Nutley, NJ 07110; Fluoroplex Topical Cream (1%), Herbert Laboratories, Dermatology Division of Allergan Pharmaceuticals Inc, 2525 Dupont Drive, Irvine, CA 92713

† Valisone Cream (0.1%), Schering Corp, Galloping Hill Rd, Kenilworth, NJ 07033

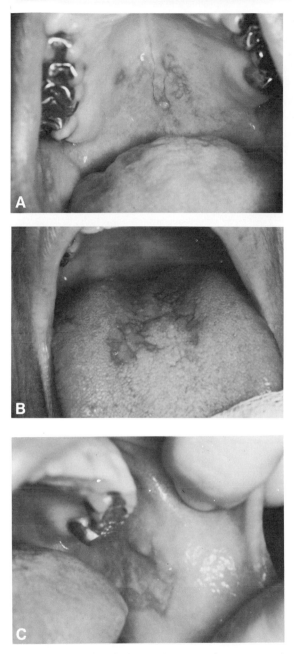

Fig. 6-37 Lesions of discoid lupus erythematosus affecting palate, tongue dorsum, and cheek. The alternating red (atrophic), white (keratotic), and red (telangiectatic) zones and location of lesions are characteristic.

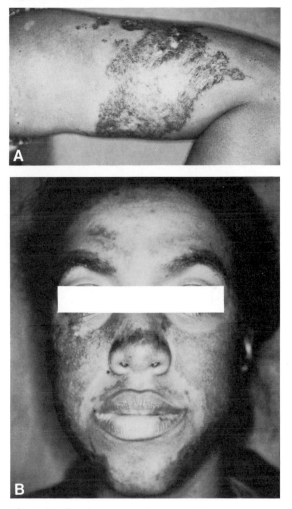

Fig. 6-38 Skin lesions on the arm (*A*) and malar and frontal skin of the face (*B*) in a patient with systemic lupus erythematosus.

to diagnose lupus erythematosus on the basis of the oral lesions. More recent studies using immunofluorescent techniques have shown a good correlation between the clinical appearance of the oral lesions and their histologic specificity. Lesions with features of both lichen planus and lupus erythematosus have also been described.

The histopathologic changes of oral DLE consist of hyperorthokeratosis with keratotic plugs, atrophy of the rete processes, "liquefaction degeneration" of the basal layer, and a bandlike infiltration of lymphocytes in the lamina propria. Immediately subadjacent to the epithelium is a band of slightly acido-

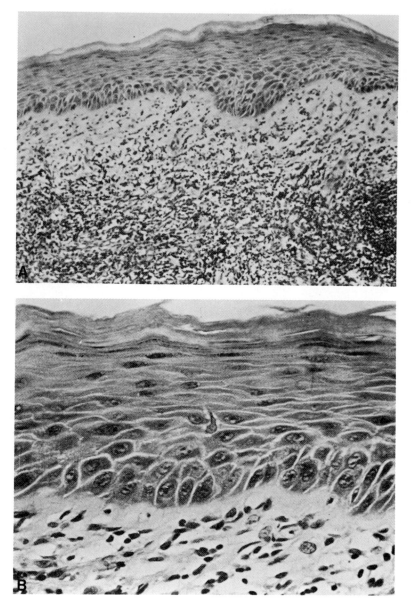

Fig. 6-39 Histologic appearance of discoid lupus erythematosus. *A,* Keratinized and atrophic epithelium with dense chronic inflammatory cell infiltrate, consisting mainly of lymphocytes in the superficial part of the lamina propria. Note that the infiltration is less dense in a zone close to the epithelium (×100). *B,* The band of eosinophilic material immediately subjacent to the basal cell layer also gives positive reactions with PAS and with labeled anti-immunoglobulin antisera by the immunofluorescent technique. (From WHO Collaborating Centre for Oral Precancerous Lesions: Definition of leukoplakia and related lesions: An aid to studies of oral precancer. Oral Surg 46:518, 1978; courtesy CV Mosby Co, St. Louis, MO)

philic, PAS-positive, diastase-resistant material that gives a positive reaction for immunoglobulin by the immunofluorescent technique. Positive cultures for *Candida* have been obtained in over 50% of patients with oral discoid lupus.

The majority of intraoral lesions in DLE occur on the cheeks, with the gingival tissues, labial mucosa, and vermilion border of the lip following in decreasing order of frequency. The lesions are frequently reported as symptomatic, with hot and spicy foods producing a burning sensation. Response to both topically and systemically applied corticosteroids is good.

The precancerous potential of intraoral discoid lupus has not been clearly defined. The older literature described occasional epithelioma formation in the healed scars of DLE on the skin, but such malignant change has also been attributed to the use of x-rays, radium, and ultraviolet light in the treatment of discoid lupus in the first half of this century. Development of squamous cell carcinoma has been described in lesions of discoid lupus involving the vermilion border of the lip, and an additional effect of actinic radiation acting on photosensitized tissues may play a role here. The literature on oral carcinoma supervening in chronic lupus appears to be limited to a number of isolated case reports, however.

A number of drugs (particularly hydralazine and procainamide) can precipitate a lupus-like disease with lesions of both the skin and the oral mucous membrane. Drugs that have been described as producing such lupoid lesions are as follows:*

- Gold (antiarthritic)[†]
- Griseofulvin (antifungal; Grifulvin, Grisactin)
- Hydralazine (antihypertensive; HHR Tablets)
- Isoniazid (antituberculosis; INH, Isoniazid tablets)
- Methyldopa (antihypertensive; Aldomet)
- Para-aminosalicylate (antituberculosis)[†]
- Penicillin (antibacterial; multiple formulations and products)
- Phenytoin (anticonvulsant; Dilantin, phenytoin sodium)
- Procainamide (antiarrhythmic; Pronestyl, Procan, Procainamide)
- Streptomycin (antibacterial; Streptomycin USP)
- Sulfonamides (antibacterial; multiple formulations and products)
- Tetracyclines (antibacterial; multiple formulations and products)

Dyskeratosis Congenita

This recessively inherited genodermatosis (also referred to as the Zinssner–Engman–Cole syndrome) is unusual in the high incidence of oral cancer that develops in young affected adults. It is a rare disorder, almost always seen in males, and is characterized by a series of oral changes that lead eventually to an atrophic, leukoplakic, oral mucosa with tongue and cheek most severely affected. The oral changes occur in association with severely dystrophic nails and a prominent reticulated hyperpigmentation of the skin of

* Modified from Scully C, Cawson RA: Medical Problems in Dentistry, Boston, PSG Wright, 1982. Fixed drug combinations are not included.
† See list of drugs associated with lichenoid lesions for formulations and products.

the face, neck, and chest. Many cases also exhibit hematologic changes including pancytopenia, hypersplenism, and an aplastic or Fanconi-type anemia (*i.e.*, an anemia associated with an inherited inability to repair DNA defects, leading to a high frequency of leukemia and lymphoma).

The oral lesions commence before age 10 as crops of vesicles with patches of white necrotic mucosa infected with *Candida;* ulcerations and erythroplakic changes and the nail dystrophy follow, with leukoplakic lesions and carcinoma supervening on these oral lesions in early adulthood.

Lichen Planus

Lichen planus is a relatively common dermatosis that occurs on the skin and oral mucous membrane. Lesions may be restricted to either location or may occur on both locations in one patient. About 50% of patients who have oral lichen planus also have skin lesions. The skin lesions are relatively constant, flat violaceous papules with a fine scaling on the surface (see Fig. 6-40); they may manifest in as many as six different forms, often with more than one form of the lesion evident in one patient. Because some lesions of oral lichen planus are erosive and others bullous, this disorder is also discussed in Chapter 5. The emphasis in this chapter is on the nonerosive, nonbullous forms of lichen planus, although the same basic pathologic process is probably involved in all forms.

The name *lichen planus* refers to the super-

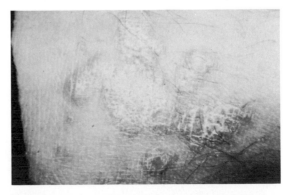

Fig. 6-40 Clinical appearance of skin lesions of lichen planus—flat, violaceous papules with a fine scaling of the surface.

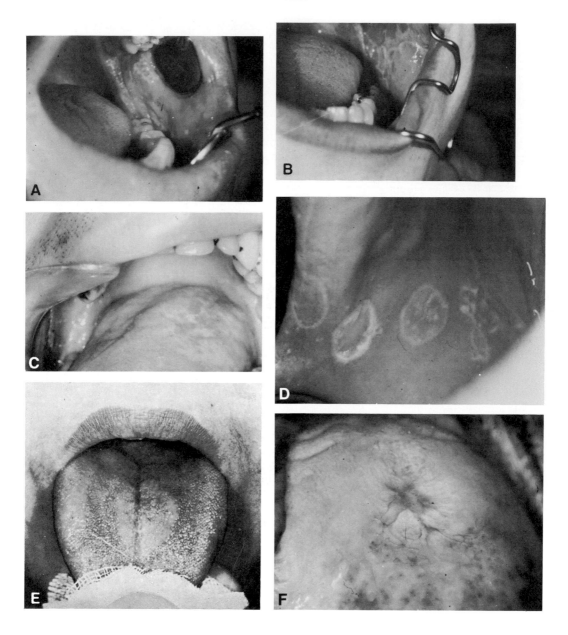

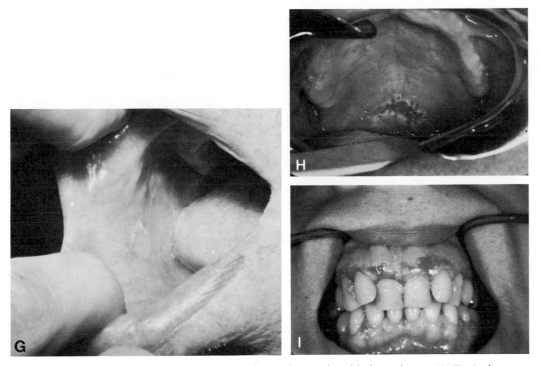

Fig. 6-41 Varied clinical appearance of the different forms of oral lichen planus: (A) Typical radiating linear lesions of reticular lichen planus, (B and C) lacelike pattern of the reticular form on cheek and tongue, (D) annular pattern of the reticular form, (E and F) extensive plaquelike lesions of the dorsum of the tongue that are difficult to distinguish from leukoplakia, (G) small asymptomatic erosive lichen planus of the buccal mucosa, (H) more extensive erosive lesion of the palate, and (I) papular lichen planus affecting attached gingiva with confluent plaquelike lesions of the nonkeratinized alveolar mucosa.

ficial similarity of the lesions of reticular lichen planus (see below) to the lacelike pattern produced by symbiotic algal and fungal colonies on the surfaces of rocks in nature (lichens). The name is unfortunate because no etiologic relationship exists between lichen planus and saphrophytic microorganisms, and the name only serves to increase patients' anxieties about the disorder.

The etiology of lichen planus has not been fully elucidated but probably involves an immunologically induced degeneration of the basal cell layer of the epithelium. Lichen planus is probably only one variety of a broader range of disorders in which an immunologically induced lichenoid lesion is the common denominator. Thus there are many clinical and histologic similarities between lichen planus and lichenoid dermatoses and

stomatitides associated with drugs, some immunologic disorders, graft-versus-host reactions, and some forms of lymphoma. While lichen planus may manifest as a particularly well-defined and characteristic lesion, the differential diagnosis for these lesions is quite extensive.

Clinical Features

Apart from the erosive and bullous forms of the disorder, lichen planus is quite frequently an indolent, painless lesion that many times has been present in a patient's mouth long before it is recognized during a routine dental examination or by the patient noticing that the cheek or lip mucosa is rougher than usual (see Fig. 6-41). The clinical features of the lesions in a given patient often vary with time, both in terms of the morphology of the clinical lesion and its extent and the area of erosion of the atrophic mucosa.

The *reticular* form (see Fig. 6-41 A-D) consists of slightly elevated, fine, whitish lines (Wickham's striae) that produce either a lace-like lesion, a pattern of fine radiating lines, or annular lesions. This is the most common and most readily recognized form of lichen planus, and the form for which the lesion is named. Most patients with lichen planus at some time exhibit some areas of the reticular form. The cheeks and tongue are preferentially affected in many patients with lichen planus; the lips, gingivae, floor of the mouth, and palate are less frequently involved. Because reticular lesions are the most common form, they are seen most often on the cheek and tongue, in many cases as bilateral lesions. *Papules,* (0.5 mm to 1 mm) whitish elevated lesions, are usually seen on the well-keratinized areas of the oral mucosa, but large *plaquelike lesions* that are often difficult to distinguish from leukoplakia may occur on the cheek, tongue, and gingivae (see Fig. 6-41 E,F + I).

Atrophic lichen planus describes inflamed areas of the oral mucosa covered by thinned, red epithelium. *Erosive* lesions probably develop as a complication of the atrophic process when the thin epithelium is abraded or ulcerated (see Fig. 6-41 G & H). Papular, placquelike atrophic, and erosive lesions are very frequently accompanied by reticular lesions. A search for these is an essential part of the clinical evaluation of a patient with suspected lichen planus, and when biopsy provides only a nonspecific diagnosis (*e.g.,* acute and chronic inflammation), the diagnosis of lichen planus is often confirmed by identifying an area of reticular pattern, even though at times only a small flamelike patch of striae or radially arranged white lines is found. Characteristically, the affected areas of the oral mucosa are not bound down or rendered inelastic by lichen planus, and the keratotic white lines cannot be eliminated either by stretching the mucosa or rubbing its surface.

The literature on oral lichen planus frequently refers to the personality of patients with this disorder as neurotic and overly concerned about health, work, and other problems and to the lesions as being psychosomatic in origin and developing or worsening in association with periods of heavy emotional stress, unresolved conflicts, and even physical stress. While many of these characteristics may be found in patients who seek consultation regarding lichen planus, this type of personality is common among patients with other chronic oral lesions and by no means characterizes the range of patients with lichen planus.

An association has been described between oral lichen planus, diabetes mellitus, and hypertension. This triad is referred to as *Grinspan's syndrome* and has been suggested as predisposing to the development of squamous cell carcinoma. Subsequent investigation of other series of patients with lichen planus have not confirmed Grinspan's findings, other than that a proportion of patients with chronic oral problems (especially those attending hospital clinics) will be found to have diabetes and hypertension (see also discussion regarding association of diabetes and lipid abnormalities with atypical facial pain, in Chap. 17). The naming of this syndrome has drawn attention to the need for quantitative measurement of blood sugars (oral glucose tolerance test) in all patients with lichen planus and the correction of any significant hyperglycemia as part of the treatment of the mucosal lesions. Prospective studies to justify this effort do not exist.

Histopathologic Features

Three features are usually considered essential for the histopathologic diagnosis of lichen planus: areas of hyperparakeratosis or hyperorthokeratosis, often with the thickening of the granular cell layer and a saw-tooth appearance to the retepegs; "liquefaction degeneration" or necrosis of the basal cell layer, which is often replaced by an eosinophilic band; and a dense subepithelial band of lymphocytes (see Figs. 6-42 and 6-43).

The main diagnostic feature that lichen planus shares with other lichenoid reactions is damage to the basal cell layer, including both vacuolar changes and cell death. Vacuolar change (liquefaction degeneration) is characterized by intracellular vacuoles, edema, separation of basal cells, and detachment of the lamina propria from the basal

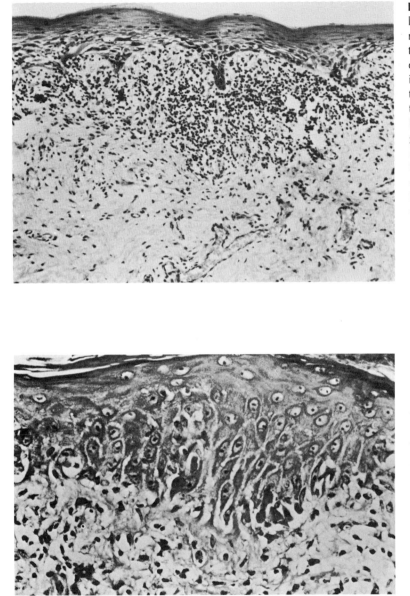

Fig. 6-42 Histologic features of lichen planus seen at low magnification (×90): atrophic epithelium, saw-tooth rete processes, bandlike lymphocytic infiltrate in the superficial part of the lamina propria and close to the epithelium. Civatte and colloid bodies, "liquefaction degeneration" of the basal cell layer, and a narrow band of eosinophilic material in the position of the basement membrane may be apparent on higher magnification. (From WHO Collaborating Centre for Oral Precancerous Lesions: Definition of leukoplakia and related lesions: An aid to studies of oral precancer. Oral Surg 46:518, 1978; courtesy CV Mosby Co, St. Louis, MO)

Fig. 6-43 Lichenoid tissue reaction in a fixed-drug eruption. There are shrunken Civatte bodies and some vacuolar change in the basal layer (H & E, ×400). (From Weedon D: The lichenoid tissue reaction. Int J Dermatol 21:203, 1982)

cells. Artifactual tears at this level are often seen in specimens mounted for light microscopy, raising the possibility of a vesiculobullous lesion, and bullae develop at this level in bullous lichen planus. The epidermal cell death noted in this disorder usually involves single basal cells, which are shrunken with eosinophilic cytoplasm and one or more pyknotic nuclear fragments. These dead cells are referred to as *Civatte bodies*, and there is ultrastructural evidence that they develop by a unique process referred to as *apoptosis*, in which cells are converted to filamentous bodies that are phagocytosed by macrophages or adjacent basal cells. Apoptosis evokes little inflammatory reaction, compared with cell death by necrosis, and the cells undergoing apoptosis in the basal layers of lichenoid epithelium are elsewhere often referred to as *dyskeratotic cells*. Some of the dead basal cells are incapable of being phagocytosed and are extruded into the underlying dermis where they become coated with immunoglobulins, particularly IgM, and are referred to as *colloid bodies* (see Figs. 6-43 and 6-44).

The lymphocytic infiltration is composed largely of T cells, most of which are small resting cells rather than lymphoblasts, suggesting that there is inadequate antigenic stimulus associated with the lesion to induce lymphocyte transformation. *Reactive follicle* formation is occasionally seen when the band of lymphocytes is unusually extensive or dense, and consideration must then be given to the possibility that the lesion represents a lymphomatous infiltration rather than lichen planus. In lichen planus, there is evidence that the activated T cells attach to the basal epidermal cells and produce death of these cells by apoptosis, and there is little evidence to interpret the bandlike layer of lymphocytes as an inflammatory response to cell death, rather than the agent of cell death.

Immunofluorescent Studies

Immunofluorescent studies of biopsy specimens from lesions of lichen planus reveal a number of features not seen in routine hematoxylin-and-eosin-stained sections that reflect the mode of development of these lesions (as described above) and also aid in distinguishing lichen planus from a number of other dermatoses. These studies have been carried out on both skin and oral mucous membrane lesions of lichen planus; in general, some of the staining patterns are noted more consistently in skin lesions, though more recent studies of oral lesions suggest that immunofluorescent staining reactions in many cases can also be helpful in separating oral lesions.

Lesions of lichen planus rarely give positive direct immunofluorescent staining reactions with anti-IgA, IgM, and IgG antisera at the level of the basement membrane and somewhat inconsistent reactions with anti-complement (C^1) antisera. By comparison, positive reactions at this level are common in mucous membrane pemphigoid. Positive immunofluorescent staining of aggregates of globular structures in the superficial layers of the dermis and the deeper part of the epithelium are a prominent feature of skin lichen planus (positive in 87% of cases) but also occur in 14% to 27% of oral lichen planus.

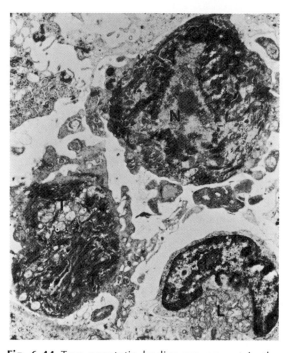

Fig. 6-44 Two apoptotic bodies are present in the basal layer in this case of lichen planus: one contains a large nuclear fragment (N), while the other is composed largely of tonofilaments (T) and cytoplasmic vacuoles. These two bodies probably have been produced during the apoptosis of a single basal cell. A lymphocyte (L) is nearby (× 3500). (From Weedon D: The lichenoid tissue reaction. Int J Dermatol 21:203, 1982)

This reaction is more often positive with anti-IgM than with anti-IgA and anti-IgG or anti-C^1 antisera. Similar globular staining reactions have also been described in lupus erythematosus, erythema multiforme, and mucous membrane pemphigoid. This finding alone therefore fails to specify lichen planus, although the extrusion of dead cells into the dermis and their subsequent coating with immunoglobulin is an important feature of the lichen planus lesion. The most consistent feature with direct immunofluorescent staining in both oral and skin lichen planus is the presence of subepithelial deposits of fibrinogen and antigenically related substances that are stainable by antifibrinogen antisera. Positive reactions with antifibrinogen antisera also occur in lupus erythematosus but are absent in pemphigus, mucous membrane pemphigoid, and erythema multiforme.

While there are discrepancies between different investigators regarding the proportion of cases of oral lichen planus and other oral lesions that give these reactions, there is sufficient consistency among the reports to indicate that a pattern of subepithelial fibrin deposit in the absence of positive immunofluorescence with anti-immunoglobulin and anti-C[1] antisera is sufficiently unique to be used as a diagnostic criterion for oral lichen planus. This finding is sufficiently specific to distinguish lichen planus from leukoplakia, mucous membrane pemphigoid, and erythema multiforme, and absence of staining with anti-immunoglobulin antisera allows separation of lichen planus from lupus erythematosus.

Successful immunofluorescent staining in lichen planus depends on sampling normal-appearing or erythematous perilesional mucosa. Tissue that has lost its epithelial covering is unsatisfactory, and a gentle biopsy technique and minimal handling of the tissue are essential. Mucosa at some distance from the attached gingiva is preferable because nonspecific immunofluorescent reactions are common in inflamed tissues. Similar nonspecific faint, finely granular immunofluorescence is occasionally noted in the basement membrane zone of lichen planus and erythema multiforme owing to the presence of a chronic subepithelial inflammatory exudate. The immunofluorescent staining reactions of lesions of lichen planus, mucous membrane pemphigoid, erythema multiforme, lupus erythematosus, pemphigus, and a number of other disorders in which the oral mucosa is the site of vesiculobullous lesions are summarized in Table 6-2 and illustrated in Figure 6-45.

Serum IgA, IgG, and IgM, and C[1] levels are occasionally elevated in lichen planus, but no consistent relationship has been noted. Dermal skin tests fail to show evidence of defective cellular immune responses, and the lack of B cells among the band of subepithelial lymphocytes indicates minimal local production of immunoglobulins.

Etiology

The etiology of lichen planus remains unknown; speculations about the nature of the general lichenoid reaction, of which lichen planus is one manifestation, are discussed in the next section on Lichenoid Reactions.

Differential Diagnosis

Differential diagnosis of lichen planus must consider the range of other lichenoid lesions (drug induced lesions, erythema multiforme, lupus erythematosus, graft-versus-host reaction, or secondary syphilis) as well as leukoplakia, squamous cell carcinoma, pemphigus, mucous membrane pemphigoid, and candidiasis. A detailed history and the clinical appearance and distribution of the lesions will often be very helpful.

While biopsy will not always provide an unequivocal diagnosis, it should always be carried out before treatment of the lesions because of the tendency for corticosteroids and chemical and surgical treatments to confuse the diagnosis even further if biopsy is delayed. Milder forms of reticular and annular lichen planus are often left untreated and are not biopsied over long periods of time; no doubt many such lesions occur without the patient's knowledge and never come to examination. Papular and plaquelike lesions should be biopsied to rule out dysplastic changes and leukoplakia, and erosive and bullous forms are usually biopsied, partly because they are symptomatic and more often brought to the clinician's attention and partly in order to differentiate them from other vesiculobullous disorders.

As a result of the diffuse distribution of some lichen planus lesions, care is needed in selecting a biopsy site and in processing the tissue so that sections contain the abnormal area and not just adjacent normal tissue. In the reticular, linear, and annular forms an attempt should be made to excise a single, distinct hyperkeratotic band or line (Wickham's stria) by means of two elliptical incisions at right angles to the hyperkeratotic line. Following 24 hours' fixation, the block is sectioned at right angles to ensure that serial sections cut from the surface of the block intersect the zone of hyperkeratosis and lymphocytic infiltration. The tissue is often friable and care must be taken to avoid artifactual tears in the subepithelial zone. Histologically, the presence of focal and deep lymphocytic infiltrates should be distinguished from the bandlike infiltrates of lichen

Table 6-2 Patterns* of Direct Immunofluorescence Staining in Tissue Sections of Lichen Planus, Pemphigus, Mucous Membrane Pemphigoid, Erthema Multiforme and Lupus Erythematosus

LESION	PATTERN OF STAINING[†]	ANTISERA				
		IgG	IgA	IgM	C[1]	FIBRINOGEN
Lichen Planus	Globular	+/−[‡]	+/−	+	−	+[§]
	SLP/BMZ	−	−	−	+	+ +
	ICS	−	−	−	−	−
Pemphigus	Globular	−	−	−	−	−
	BMZ linear	−	−	−	+/−	−
	ICS	+ +	+/−	+/−	+ +	−
Mucous Membrane Pemphigoid	Globular	−	−	−	+/−	−
	BMZ linear	+ +	+/−	+/−	+	+/−
	ICS	−	−	−	−	−
Erythema Multiforme	Globular	−	−	+/−	−	−
	BMZ	−	−	−	+[‖]	+/−
	ICS	−	−	−	−	−
Lupus Erythematosus	Globular	+	+/−	+	+ +	+ +
	BMZ linear	−	−	−	−	+ +
	ICS	+	+/−	+	+ +	−

*Based on data from Daniels TE and Quadra-White C: Direct immunofluorescence in oral mucosal disease: A diagnostic analysis of 130 cases. Oral Surg 51:38, 1981; Laskaris G, Sklavounou A and Angelopoulos A: Direct immunofluorescence in oral lichen planus. Oral Surg 53:483, 1982; Laskaris G and Angelopoulos A. Cicatrical pemphigoid: Direct and indirect immunofluorescent studies Oral Surg. 51:48, 1981; Schiødt M, Holmstrup P, Dabelsteen E and Ullman S: Deposits of immunoglobulins, complement and fibrinogen in oral lupus erythematous, lichen planus and leukoplakia. Oral Surg 51:603, 1981

Normal tissue and tissue from lesions of leukoplakia very rarely give positive reactions with these reagents

[†] Globular = Globular fluorescent staining in basement membrane zone and adjacent subepithelial connective tissue. In the case of lichen planus and lupus erythematosus, these structures correspond with colloid, cytoid, or Civatte bodies described in routine hematoxylin and eosin preparations.

SLP-BMZ (and BMZ linear) = Linear fluorescent staining of superficial lamina propria (SLP) and basement membrane zone (BMZ), unless specified otherwise

ICS = Intercellular spaces of epithelium.

[‡]Data roughly quantitated as:

Reaction positive in <10% of lesions   −

Reaction positive in 10-24% of lesions   +/−

Reaction positive in 25-50% of lesions   +

Reaction positive in 51-100% of lesions + +

§ Reaction more prominent in skin lichen planus (+ +) than in oral lichen planus (+/− to +)

‖ Nonspecific faint fine-granular fluorescence resulting from chronic subepithelial inflammation.

planus; the presence of eosinophils, neutrophils, or plasma cells in quantity in the infiltrate should also give concern that a process other than lichen planus is involved, particularly if the specimen has come from perilesional tissue. Germinal centers may indicate a lymphoma; marked dyskeratosis is unusual in lichen planus and suggests leukoplakia.

As discussed earlier, immunofluorescent studies can be of help in differential diagnosis of lichen planus (see Table 6-2), particularly in regard to separation of lichen planus from leukoplakia in chronic lesions. Because of the additional cost of immunofluorescent studies and the need for special specimen handling procedures, the majority of biopsies of lichen planus are submitted for routine hematoxylin and eosin sections only. Where previous biopsy has failed to provide specific diagnostic information on hematoxylin and eosin stain-

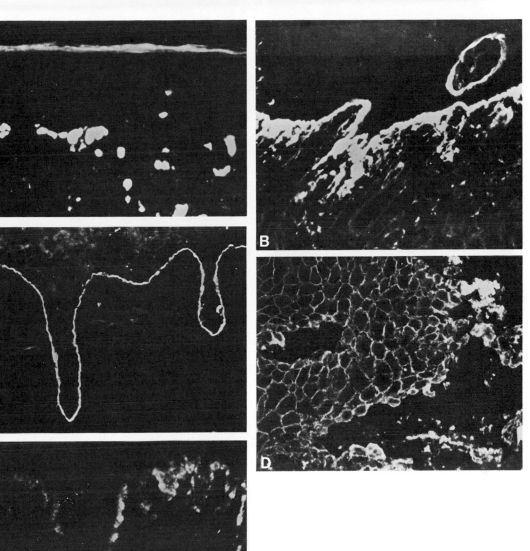

Fig. 6-45 Patterns of direct immunofluorescence in oral lichen planus, mucous membrane pemphigoid, pemphigus vulgaris, and lupus erythematosus. *A* and *B,* Oral lichen planus specimen showing aggregates of fluorescent globules in the superficial connective tissue and deep epithelium with anti-IgM. *C,* Oral mucous membrane pemphigoid specimen showing continuous linear fluorescence in the basement membrane zone with anti-C'3. *D,* Oral pemphigus vulgaris specimen showing intercellular space fluorescence throughout the epithelium with anti-IgG. *E,* Oral lupus erythematosus specimen showing coarse granular fluorescence in the basement membrane zone with anti-IgM (all figures ×156). (From Daniels TE, Quadra–White C: Oral Surg 51:38, 1981; courtesy CV Mosby Co, St. Louis, MO)

ing, repeat biopsy should always include submission of material for both immunofluorescence and routine staining. In a number of cases, clear histopathologic identification of lichen planus is not possible, and many authors describe cases with features of both lupus erythematosus and lichen planus or lichen planus and leukoplakia.

Clinical Course and Treatment

The lesions of oral lichen planus appear, regress, and reappear in a somewhat unpredictable fashion, and pending identification of the etiology of lichen planus, it is reasonable to assume that a heterogeneous group of conditions is included under this diagnostic category. The existence of the lichenoid reaction as a common denominator for disorders that are apparently as diverse as graft-versus-host reactions, drug reactions, and lupus erythematosus, for example, suggests that similar appearing lesions may develop and respond to a variety of circumstances. Figures are quoted for the rate of spontaneous healing of the various forms of oral lichen planus, but the course of an individual patient's lesions is often uncertain. Andreasen in his classical description of this disorder calculated that 41% of reticular lesions healed spontaneously and that 12% of the atrophic, 7% of the plaquelike lesions, and none of the erosive group healed without treatment. Silverman and Griffith reported that approximately 10% of a group of patients with predominantly erosive lesions had remissions, when followed longer than a year.

Treatment is usually initiated only if the lesions are symptomatic, and most of the information about the effects of treatment appears to be based on individual investigators' clinical experiences. Controlled trials of particular treatments, and comparisons of the effects of different treatments for oral rather than skin lichen planus are rare.

Lesions are usually too diffuse for surgical removal, although cryotherapy and cauterization have been used. Surgical excision also has a place in the treatment of long-standing erosive lesions. Symptomatic treatment of oral lesions can be provided by topical analgesics or antihistamine rinses or more specifically by use of topical corticosteroids to en-

courage healing of ulcerated areas and diminish inflammatory and hypersensitivity reactions around the lesion. Triamcinolone acetonide in a gel (e.g. Kenalog in Orabase*) or cream base (e.g., Kenalog Cream,* Aristocort Cream[†]) and betamethasone syrup or cream (Celestone[‡]), betamethasone dipropionate (Diprosone[‡]) or valerate (Valisone[‡]) creams are usually used for this purpose; beclomethasone dipropionate (Vanceril[‡]) and betamethasome valerate§ aerosol sprays are also reported as well tolerated and effective for oral lichen planus, provided the spray used is approved for oral use.§

Like many other oral white lesions, partial resolution of the lesion can often be obtained with 1 to 2 weeks' topical application of an antifungal agent, indicating a secondary role for *Candida* as an opportunistic agent in this disorder as well. Topical treatment with corticosteroids will also increase the extent of opportunistic *Candida* infection of the lesions, and during prolonged topical corticosteroid therapy, topical or systemic antifungal agents should be administered throughout, at least 1 week out of every four.

Weekly intralesional injections of triamcinolone acetonide (Kenalog-10 or Kenalog-40)* or triamcinolone diacetate (Aristocort Intralesional)[†] are useful in healing nonresponsive and extensively eroded areas of mucosa; the pain of the injection may be controlled by injecting the steroid in a 50% mixture with lidocaine. No more than two to three injections are usually required and healing of the previously ulcerated site occurs in 5 to 7 days, if the injections are well spaced and encompass the entire lesion.

---

* ER Squibb and Sons, Inc, PO Box 4000, Princeton, NJ 08540

[†] Lederle Laboratories, Division of American Cyanamid Co, Wayne, NJ 07470

[‡] Schering Corp, Galloping Hill Road, Kenilworth, NJ 07033

§ Bethamethasome valerate aerosol marketed in the United States by the Schering Corp (Valisone Aerosol), is stated to have potentially harmful or fatal consequences if used in concentrated form on mucous membranes and should not be prescribed for treatment of oral lesions. Bextasol marketed in Europe does not have these harmful effects and is recommended in a number of texts for the treatment of lichen planus and oral lesions responding to topical corticosteroids.

Topically applied tretinoin* (retinoic acid; vitamin A acid), though not without potential side-effects if applied to sun exposed areas like the lips, is reported to be quite effective in eliminating oral lichen planus. If mixed with Orabase to make an 0.9% gel, tretinoin can be applied directly to the lesions three to four times daily, with treatment extended as long as 1 to 2 months. Treatment with tretinoin and related retinoids (*e.g.*, RO10-7359) is less likely to produce toxic side-effects than is treatment with vitamin A, and fewer recurrences are reported.

Malignant Transformation

Malignant transformation has been reported in a small percentage (less than 5%) of patients with lichen planus followed over 5 to 10 years. Most authors report isolated examples of malignant transformation as having occurred in patients they have observed over a lengthy period, but usually there has been a longer period of observation of the patient than is common in most series of cases of lichen planus. A review of some 223 cases of malignant transformation in lichen planus described in the literature as of 1978, however, failed to find data to prove that the malignancies were clearly caused by transformation of lichen planus lesions. The rate of malignant transformation of less than 5%, quoted above is similar to that given for transformation of leukoplakia. In both cases, the figure is too low to be of help in elucidating etiologic relationships with oral cancer, but does justify follow-up observation and repeat biopsy as indicated by the clinical course of the lesion. In a number of reported cases of squamous cell carcinoma developing in lesions of lichen planus, other factors known to contribute to malignant change in oral lesions were present, and follow-up consequently needs to be more rigorous in the presence of sideropenic anemia, xerostomia, smoking, and alcohol abuse.

The results of a number of experimental studies are consistent with the concept that lichen planus is a preneoplastic condition. Hyman and colleagues have recently shown that lesions of lichen planus possess a "preneoplastic," ^{3}H cytidine autoradiographic labeling pattern when studied *in vitro*, based on the percentage of labeled cells, the concentration of label in the cells, and their intracellular distribution. Hakin and associates have described *in vivo* malignant transformation of cells derived from human lichen planus lesions.

Lichenoid Reactions

The inconstant association of oral and skin lesions of lichen planus (only 10% to 44% of patients *presenting* with oral lichen planus are reported to have skin lesions, whereas 70% or more of those presenting with skin lesions also have oral lesions) is sometimes cited as evidence that oral and skin lichen planus are separate disorders. There is little reason to assume this, however, and the results of electron microscopic and immunofluorescence studies provide considerable evidence for an identical pathogenesis for oral and skin lichen planus. It is therefore very likely that some of the disorders that mimic lichen planus on the skin and are referred to as *lichenoid dermatoses* or *lichenoid reactions* also have an oral counterpart.

The unifying feature of lichenoid reactions and lichen planus was originally the similar clinical and light microscopic appearance of the skin (and mucous membrane) lesions in the two conditions. Lichenoid reactions were differentiated from lichen planus on the basis of the associaton of lichenoid reactions with administration of a drug or a systemic disease and their resolution when the drug was discontinued or the disease treated. In recent years, however, the concept of lichenoid reactions has been extended to include a group of disorders characterized by a definite series of histopathologic changes that also probably relate to the etiology of these reactions. Lichenoid reactions thus are characterized by degeneration of basal epidermal cells as a primary event, with death of these cells manifested in a morphologically distinct process referred to as *apoptosis*. As a result of

---

* Retin-A Cream or Gel (Dermatologic Division Ortho Pharmaceutical Corp, Raritan, NJ 08869) is marketed for dermatologic use, but is used by many clinicians for treatment of oral lesions. Caution should be exercised in its use.

apoptosis, Civatte bodies develop in the lower layer of the epidermis and subepidermal tissues, with subsequent extrusion of filamentous rich apoptotic fragments into the dermis as colloid bodies. The cause of the cell death that initiates this process is postulated as a cell-mediated immune process in which the target cell is the basal cell layer of the epidermis. Clinically, lichenoid lesions may exhibit the classical appearance of lichen planus, but atypical presentations are seen, and some of the dermatologic lesions included show little clinical lichenification.

Table 6-3 lists some of the disorders that are currently proposed as constituting the group of lichenoid reactions. In addition to lichen planus, the group includes erythema multiforme; lupus erythematosus and dermatomyositis (the skin lesions of these two autoimmune disorders are often indistinguishable); lichenoid and fixed drug eruptions; graft-verus-host reaction; late secondary syphilis; and a number of dermatoses, consideration of which is beyond the scope of this text, except for stating that they are occasionally identified following dermatologic consultation for skin lesions noted in a patient presenting with oral "lichen planus." With the exception of these dermatoses and some of the lichenoid drug reactions, all of these lichenoid disorders may be represented by oral lesions as well.

In *erythema multiforme* (see also Chap. 5, for clinical features), severe liquefaction degeneration occurs in the upper layers of the epithelium with intraepithelial vesicle formation and loss of the basement membrane. The dermoepidermal interface is obscured by the predominantly lymphocytic cellular infiltrate, which also may contain neutrophils and eosinophils. Positive immunofluorescence reactions with anti-Ig and anti-C[1] antisera do not occur in the epithelium, but the majority of lesions show either globular or finely granular fluorescence in the basal membrane zone with anti-IgM, C[13] and antifibrinogen antisera. With *lupus erythematosus* and *dermatomyositis*, basal damage is focal and restricted to the points where the lymphocytic infiltration approaches the epidermis from perivascular regions in the dermis. Extension of perivascular lymphocytic infiltration deeper into

Table 6-3. Diseases Exhibiting the Lichenoid Tissue Reaction

SITE OF REACTION	DISEASE
Skin and Oral Mucosa	Lichen planus, lupus erythematosus, erythema multiforme, lichenoid and fixed drug eruptions, secondary syphilis, graft-versus-host disease
Skin	Lichen nitidus, lichenoid actinic keratosis, lichen striatus, lichenoid melanodermatitis, keratosis lichenoides chronica, poikilodermas, pityriasis lichenoides, lichenoid photodermatitis, morbilliform and other drug eruptions, lichen amyloidosis, disseminated superficial actinic porokeratosis, regressing seborrheic keratoses, plantar warts

Adapted from Weedon D: The lichenoid tissue reaction. Int J Dermatol 21:203, 1982, with permission of the International Society of Tropical Dermatology, Inc.

the skin, and alterations in the staining of the PAS-positive basement membrane are also characteristic. The basement membrane zone also fluoresces brightly as a continuous, coarsely granular band with anti-C[13] and anti-immunoglobin antisera. The presence of globular fluorescence in a definite percentage (10% to 20%) of lichen planus, erythema multiforme, lupus, and dermatomyositis, which was commented on earlier as a bar to this feature being accepted as diagnostic of lichen planus, is an integral feature of the lichenoid reaction.

Secondary syphilis should always be considered in the differential diagnosis of oral lichen planus because lichenoid lesions of both skin and mucous membranes can occur from this cause. Histologically, the lymphocytic infiltrate is usually deep as well as superficial, and small blood vessels in the dermis may show evidence of vasculitis as well as perivascular lymphocytic cuffing. Screening and specific tests for syphilis will be positive, and lesions will resolve following adequate antibiotic therapy.

Drug-Induced Lichenoid Reactions.

The following drugs and chemicals are reported to be associated with lichenoid dermatoses and intraoral lichenoid lesions:*

- *Antimicrobials*
    dapsone (leprosy, dermatitis herpetiformis)-Dapsone
    †para-aminosalicylate, PAS (tuberculosis)—Pamisyl Sodium, Parasal Sodium, Teebacin
    streptomycin—Streptomycin USP
    †tetracycline—Achromycin, Sumycin, tetracycline
- *Antiparasitics*
    antimony compounds (helminth infections)—stibophen (Fuadin); stibocaptate (Astiban)
    organic arsenicals (trypanosomiasis)—Arsobal, Melarsoprol
    chloroquine (malaria and amebiasis)—Aralen, Chloroquin
    †quinacrine (giardiasis; outmoded antimalarial)—Atabrine
- *Antihypertensives*
    chlorothiazide (thiazide diuretic)—Diuril
    hydrochlorothiazide (thiazide diuretic)—Esidrix, Hydrochlorothiazide, Hydrodiuril, Oretic
    labetalol (alpha- and beta-adrenergic blocker)
    mercurial diuretics (largely outmoded)
    methyldopa—Aldomet
    practotol (beta-adrenergic blocker; largely outmoded owing to side-effects)
- *Antiarthritics*
    aurothioglucose—Solganal
    colloidal gold (Europe only)
    †gold sodium thiomalate—Myochrysin

†gold sodium thiosulfate—Sanochrysin
- *Oral Hypoglycemic Agent of the Sulfonylurea Type*
    †chlorpropamide—Diabinese
    †tobutamide—Orinase
- *Miscellaneous Drugs, Chemicals, and Dental Restorative Materials*
    †iodides (expectorants, thyroid disease, radiographic contrast media)—Organidin, potassium iodide, Renografin
    penicillamine (chelating agent)—Cuprimine, Depen
    †quinidine sulfate (cardiac arrhythmias)—Quinidex, quinidine
    †substituted paraphenylenediamines used in color film developers
    †copper in dental casting alloys

For a number of these drugs, confirmed reports of intraoral lesions are lacking, but it is clear that a drug history can be one of the most important aspects of the evaluation of a patient with an oral, or oral and skin lichenoid reaction. Clinically, there is often little to distinguish drug-induced lichenoid reactions from lichen planus, and even authors who emphasize the uniqueness of lichen planus comment on the similarity of drug-induced lichenoid reactions to lichen planus. Histopathologically, lichenoid drug eruptions may show deep as well as superficial dermal lymphocytic infiltrates rather than the classical bandlike infiltrate of lichen planus, and eosinophils, plasma cells, and neutrophils may also be present in the infiltrate. The majority of drug-induced lichenoid reactions resolve promptly when the offending drug is eliminated, although a slow resolution of the lesion was a feature of one of the classical examples of drug-induced lichenoid reaction, the so-called New Guinea reaction caused by widespread use of quinacrine hydrochloride (Atabrine) as an antimalarial by Allied troops in southeast Asia during World War II. Gold therapy, diuretics, and oral hypoglycemic agents of the sulfonylurea type are all important causes of lichenoid reactions. It is also likely that the lichen planus-like lesions described in about a half of the patients who have oral mucosal white lesions associated with electrogalvanic currents may be caused by copper dental alloys.

* A number of drugs that were associated with lichenoid reactions in the past have been replaced with newer compounds. A listing of one or more trade names beside a drug indicates that it is currently available in the United States. A number of these drugs are also available in fixed combination with other drugs (*e.g.,* methyldopa and chlorothiazide—Aldochlor).
† Drugs associated with both oral *and* skin lichenoid reactions; for the remainder, only skin lesions have been documented.

Penicillamine, a chelating agent used to remove excess copper in Wilson's disease or other accumulations of toxic heavy metals and in the treatment of rheumatoid arthritis, primary biliary cirrhosis, and active liver disease is associated with many adverse reactions. As far as the oral cavity is concerned, these include lichenoid reactions, pemphiguslike lesions, lupoid reactions and stomatitis, and altered taste and smell functions.

A number of the drugs that have been associated with lichenoid reactions may also produce lesions of discoid lupus erythematous (*lupoid reactions*).

Lichenoid Lesions and the Graft-Versus Host Reaction

The *graft-versus-host reaction* is a complex, multisystem immunologic phenomenon characterized by engraftment of immunocompetent cells from one individual to a host, who is not only immunodeficient but who possesses transplantation isoantigens foreign to the graft and capable of stimulating it. Reactions of this type occur in up to 70% of patients who undergo bone marrow transplantation, usually for treatment of refractory acute leukemia. Both acute (under 100 days after bone marrow transplantation) and chronic (after day 100 post-transplantation) forms of the conditions are described. The pathogenesis is probably related to an antigen-dependent proliferation of thymus-dependent donor lymphocytes, which give rise to a generation of effector cells that react with

and destroy host tissues. Manifestations of the disorder are largely restricted to lymphocytic, hematopoietic, reticuloendothelial, and epithelial tissues. Of these, the epidermal (skin and mucous membrane) lesions are often most helpful clinically in establishing a diagnosis (see Table 6-4).

The epidermal lesions of *acute graft-versus-host reaction* are described under the heading of *toxic epidermal necrolysis* (Lyell's disease), a variety of erythema multiforme in which large flaccid bullae develop with detachment of the epidermis in large sheets leaving a scalded skin appearance. Oral mucosal lesions are only a minor component of this problem. Chronic graft-versus-host reactions are associated with lichenoid lesions that affect both skin and mucous membranes, exhibiting both clinical and histologic similarity with those of lichen planus (see Fig. 6-46) or scleroderma-like lesions. Salivary and lacrimal gland epithelium may also be involved by the graft-induced epithelial cell damage, and ocular and major and minor salivary gland changes analogous to the lesions of Sjögren's syndrome also occur. In some cases, the intraoral lichenoid lesions are extensive and involve cheeks, tongue, lips, and gingivae.

The mouth is a singularly sensitive reflector of a variety of reactions associated with bone marrow transplantation, and infectious and hemopoietic (neutropenic) complications of this form of therapy need to be distinguished from the specifically cytotoxic reactions that produce the lichenoid lesion. Over

Table 6-4. Major Mucocutaneous and Laboratory Manifestations of Chronic Graft-Versus-Host Reaction

SKIN AND MUCOUS MEMBRANES	LABORATORY TESTS
Erythematous rash	Elevated liver function values
Papulosquamous plaques	Eosinophilia
Reticular pigmentation	Autoantibodies
Lichenoid lesions	Hypergammaglobulinemia
Poikiloderma	
Atrophy and loss of elasticity	
Alopecia	
Xerophthalmia	
Xerostomia	

(Modified from Radu B, Gockerman JP: Oral manifestations of the chronic graft-versus-host reaction. JAMA 249:504, 1983)

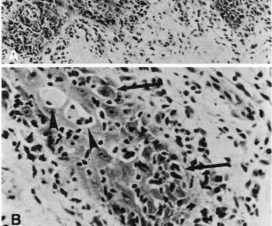

Fig. 6-46 Histologic appearance of lichenoid lesions associated with chronic graft-versus-host reaction. *A,* Sawtooth epithelial morphologic appearance with extensive lymphocytic infiltrate. Necrotic keratinocytes are circled (H&E, ×160). *B,* Basal vacuolar degeneration (*arrows*) and necrotic keratinocytes (*arrow heads*; H&E, ×400). (From Rodu B, Gockerman JP: Oral manifestations of the chronic graft-v-host reaction. JAMA 249:504, 1983; courtesy American Medical Association)

three quarters of patients who have bone marrow transplants develop oral infections. The majority are opportunistic *Candida* infections, although other unusual agents (*e.g., Aspergillus*), have also been described, and the supragingival dental plaque of immunosuppressed patients contains an increased population of *Candida* and catalase-negative diphtheroids. The differential diagnosis of oral lesions that develop in patients some months after bone marrow transplantation thus includes candidiasis and other opportunistic infections, toxic reactions to chemotherapeutic drugs that are often used concomitantly, unusual viral infections (chronic herpes), and lichenoid and other drug eruptions, in addition to lichenoid lesions of graft-versus-host etiology.

The specific etiology of the various disorders grouped together as lichenoid reactions remains unknown, despite the identification of a common pathogenesis and similar histologic features and the recognition that histocompatibility antigen HL-A3 is common to many patients with lichen planus. In graft-versus-host reactions the cause of the epithelial cell death is most likely a donor T-lymphocyte-mediated immune reaction (apoptosis has also been identified as the major mechanism of cell death in graft rejection phenomena). Similar immunologic reactions involving cell-associated drug molecules are possibly the basis for the reaction in lichenoid drug eruptions and some cases of erythema multiforme. The etiology of lichen planus remains completely unknown.

The consequence of this broad concept of lichenoid reactions (*c.f.* psoriasiform lesions and eczematous lesions as examples of other broad categories of epithelial disturbance, each with its own common underlying pathogenesis) is that considerably more attention needs to be given to a search for other causes of the lichenoid reaction in addition to lichen planus, when oral lichenoid reactions are being evaluated. Lichenoid drug reactions manifesting in the oral cavity have received some attention, and oral lichenoid graft-versus-host reactions have recently been well described, but it is likely that oral lichen planus as currently diagnosed represents a heterogeneous group of lesions that require more specific identification if their etiology and treatment is to be better understood.

BIBLIOGRAPHY

Variations in Structure and Appearance of Normal Oral Mucosa

Axell T and Henricsson: Leukoedema—An epidemiologic study with special reference to the influence of tobacco habits. Community Dent Oral Epidemiol 9:142, 1981

Axell TA: A prevalence study of oral mucosal lesions in an adult Swedish population. Odont Rev 27:1, 1979

Dolby AE (ed): Oral Mucosa in Health and Disease. Oxford, Blackwell Scientific Publications, 1975

Gorlin RJ, Pindborg JJ, Cohen MM, Jr: Syndromes

of the Head & Neck, 2nd ed. New York, Mc-Graw-Hill, 1976

Hamner JE et al: An epidemiologic and histologic study of leukoedema among 50,915 rural Indian villagers. Oral Surg 32:58, 1971

Hedin CA, Larsson Å: Physiology and pathology of melanin pigmentation with special reference to the oral mucosa. Swed Dent J 2:113, 1978

Kramer IR: Oral leukoplakia. Proc R Soc Med 73:765, 1980

Lever WF, Schaumberg–Lever G: Histopathology of the Skin, 5th ed. Philadelphia, JB Lippincott, 1975

Löning T and Burkhardt A: Dyskeratosis in human and experimental precancer and oral cancer. An immunohistochemical and ultrastructural study in man, mice and rats. Arch Oral Biol 27:361, 1982

McCarthy PL, Shklar G: Diseases of the Oral Mucosa, 2nd ed. Philadelphia, Lea & Febiger, 1980

Mackenzie IC et al: Oral Premalignancy. Proc First Dows Symposium, Iowa City, University of Iowa Press, 1980

Mashberg A, Garfinkel L: Early diagnosis of oral cancer: The erythroplastic lesion in high risk sites. Cancer 28:297, 1978

Mescon H, Grots IA, Gorlin RJ: Mucocutaneous disorders. In Gorlin RJ, Goldman HM (eds): Thoma's Oral Pathology, 6th ed. St Louis, CV Mosby, 1970

Monteil RA: Le grains de Fordyce: Maladie, hétérotopie ou adenome? Étude histologique et ultrastructurale. J Biol Buccale 9:109, 1981

Payne TF: Why are white lesions white? Observations on keratin. Oral Surg 40:652, 1975

Pindborg JJ: Atlas of Diseases of the Oral Mucosa, 3rd ed. Philadelphia, WB Saunders, 1980

Pindborg JJ: Oral Cancer and Precancer. Bristol, J Wright & Sons, 1980

Pindborg JJ, Mehta FS, Daftary DK: Incidence of oral cancer among 30,000 villagers in India in a 7-year follow-up study of oral precancerous lesions. Community Dent Oral Epidemiol 3:86, 1975

Robinson HC and Miller AS: Colby, Kerr and Robinson's Color Atlas of Oral Pathology, 4th ed, Philadelphia, J.B. Lippincott, 1983

Roed–Petersen B, Renstrup B: A topographical classification of the oral mucosa suitable for electronic data processing. Its application to 560 leukoplakias. Acta Odontol Scand 27:681, 1969

Rogers RS III, Jordan RE: Immunopathology of oral mucosal inflammatory diseases. Clin Exp Dermatol 2:97, 1977

Scragg MA and Johnson NW: Epithelial cell kinetics—(A) Review of methods of study and their application to oral mucosa in health and disease (B) Comparison of cell kinetics in normal and abnormal epithelia. J Oral Pathol 9:309, 1980; 11:102, 1982

Sedano H, Sauk JJ, Gorlin RJ: The Oral Manifestations of Genetic Diseases. Woburn MA, Butterworths, 1977

Sewerin I: The sebaceous glands in the vermilion border of the lips and in the oral mucosa of man. Thesis, Acta Odontol Scand 33:1, 1975, supp 68

Sewerin I and Praetorius F: Keratin-filled pseudocysts of ducts of sebaceous glands in the vermilion border of the lip. J Oral Path 3:279, 1974

Waldron CA: Oral epithelial tumors. In Gorlin RJ, Goldman HM (eds): Thoma's Oral Pathology, 6th ed, St Louis, CV Mosby, 1970

WHO Collaborating Centre for Oral Precancerous Lesions: Definitions of leukoplakia and related lesions: An aid to studies on oral precancer. Oral Surg 46:518, 1978

Nonkeratotic White Lesions

Ackerman A, Golfaden GL: Electrical burns of the mouth in children. Arch Dermatol 104:308, 1971

Bernstein ML: Oral mucosal lesions associated with excessive use of Listerine mouthwash. Oral Surg 46:781, 1978

Blanton PL, Hurt WC, Largeut MD: Oral factitious injuries. J Periodontol 48:33, 1977

Colby RA: Radiation effects on structure of the oral cavity. J Am Dent Assoc 29:1446, 1942

Halazonetis J, Harley A: Uremic stomatitis. Report of a case. Oral Surg 23:573, 1967

Hjørting–Hansen E, Holst E: Morsicato mucosae oris and suctio mucosae oris. An analysis of oral mucosal changes due to biting and sucking habits. Scand J Dent Res 78:492, 1970

Hovinga J, Roodvoets AP, Gaillard J: Some findings in patients with uraemic stomatitis. J Maxillofac Surg 3:125, 1975

Lauttamus A, Kasanen A, Oksala E, Tammisalo E: Oral manifestations in uremia. Proc Finn Dent Soc 70:50, 1974

Najjar TA: Harmful effects of "aspirin compounds." Oral Surg 44:64, 1977

Pitts W, Pickrell K, Quinn G, Massengill R: Electrical burns of lips and mouth in infants and children. Plast Reconstr Surg 44:471, 1969

Robinson JE: Dental management of the oral effects of radiotherapy. J Prosthet Dent 14:582, 1964

Candidiasis

Addy M et al: The effect of orthodontic appliances on the distribution of *Candida* and plaque in adolescents. Br J Orthod 9:158, 1982

Arendorf TM, Walker DM: The prevalence and intraoral distribution of *Candida albicans* in man. Arch Oral Biol 25:1, 1980

Aronson K, Soltani K: Chronic mucocutaneous candidosis: A review. Mycopathologia 60:17, 1976

Berdicevsky I et al: Oral *Candida* of asymptomatic denture wearers. Int J Oral Surg 9:113, 1980

Brightman V, Guggenheimer J, Ship II: Changes in the oral microbial flora during treatment of recurrent aphthous ulcers Program and Abstract of Papers, International Association for Dental Research, 46th General Meeting San Francisco, Calif., March 21 to 24, 1968. Abstract 353, p 126. Suppl., J Dent Res 1968

Brown LR et al: Comparison of plaque microflora in immunodeficient and immunocompetent dental patients. J Dent Res 58:2344, 1979

Budtz–Jörgensen E: The significance of *Candida albicans* in denture stomatitis. Scand J Dent Res 82:151, 1974

Cawson RA: Symposium on denture sore mouth. II. The Role of *Candida*. Dent Pract 16:138, 1965

Cawson RA: Chronic oral candidiasis and leukoplakia. Oral Surg 22:582, 1966

Cawson RA: Leukoplakia and oral cancer. Proc R Soc Med 62:610, 1969

Chervinsky P et al: Incidence of oral candidiasis during therapy with triamcinalone acetonide, Ann Allergy 43:80, 1979

Cohen J et al: Infection and immunosuppression. A study of the infective complications of 75 patients with immunologically mediated disease. Q J Med 51:1, 1982

Cooke BED: Median rhomboid glossitis. Candidiasis and not a developmental anomaly. Br J Dermatol 93:399, 1975

de Vries–Hospers HG et al: The effect of amphotericin B lozenges on the presence and number of *Candida* cells in the oropharynx of neutropenic-leukemic patients. Infection 10:71, 1982

DeWilde T et al: Prevalence of *Candida albicans* in patients receiving total parenteral nutrition. Sabouraudia 20:169, 1982

Dreizen S et al: Unusual mucocutaneous infections in immunosuppressed patients with leukemia. Postgrad Med 66:131, 1979

Drutz DT: Newer antifungal agents. In Remington JS and Schwartz MN (eds): Current Clinical Topics in Infectious Diseases 3 New York, McGraw-Hill, 1982

Eelkema H H et al: Thrush complicating radiotherapy of the mouth and neck. Radiology 72:26, 1959

Eidelman D et al: Dental sepsis due to *Candida albicans* urticaria: case report, Ann Allergy 41:179, 1978

Epstein JB et al: Quantitative relationships between *Candida albicans* in saliva and the clinical status of human subjects. J Clin Microbiol 12:475, 1980

Farman AG et al: Central papillary atrophy of the tongue. Oral Surg 43:48, 1977

Farman AG et al: Central papillary atrophy of the tongue and denture stomatitis. J Prosthet Dent 40:253, 1978

Feigin RD et al: Treatment of mucocutaneous candidiasis with transfer factor. Pediatrics 53:63, 1974

Freedman CR: Infective endocarditis and other intravascular infections: In Current Topics in Infectious Diseases, Greenough WB and Meigan TC (eds) Plenum Med Bk Co, NY, 1982

Greenberg MS et al: Idiopathic hypoparathyroidism, chronic candidiasis, and dental hypoplasia. Oral Surg 28:42, 1969

Guggenheimer J, Brightman VJ, Ship II: Effect of chlortetracycline mouthrinses on the healing of recurrent aphthous ulcers: a double-blind controlled trial. J Oral Ther 4:406, 1968

Higgs, Wells: Chronic mucocutaneous candidiasis: new approaches to treatment. Br J Dermatol 89:179, 1973

Hill HR: Immunodeficiency disease. Prog Clin Pathol 8:205, 1981

Holbrook WP et al: Candidal infections: Experience in a British dental hospital. Oral Surg 49:122, 1980

Holmberg K: Oral mycoses and antifungal agents. Swed Dent J 4:53, 1980

Hong R, Dibbell DG: Cultured thymus fragment transplant in chronic candidiasis complicated by oral carcinoma. Lancet 1:773, 1981

Hory R et al: Thymic transplantation for relief of immunodeficiency disease. Surg Clin North Am 59:299, 1979

Hory R et al: Cultured thymus fragment transplant in chronic candidiasis complicated by oral carcinoma. Lancet 1:773, 1981

Jennison RF: Thrush in infancy. Arch Dis Child 52:747, 1977

Jones HE: Therapy of superficial fungal infection. Med Clin North Am 66:873, 1982

Kessel LJ et al: Chronic mucocutaneous candidiasis—Treatment of the oral lesions with miconazole: Two case reports. Br J Oral Surg 18:51, 1980

Lehner T: Candidal fungaemia following extraction of teeth and its relationship to systemic candidiasis. Br Dent J 117:253, 1964

Lehner T: Classification and clinico-pathological features of *Candida* infections in the mouth. In Winner HI, Hurley R (eds): Symposium on *Candida* Infections, pp 138–153. Edinburgh, E. and S. Livingstone, 1966

Lehner T: Immunofluorescent investigation of

Candida albicans antibodies in human saliva. Arch Oral Biol 10:975, 1965

Lerner PI, Weinstein L: Infective endocarditis in the antibiotic era. N Engl J Med 274:199, 1966

Lighterman L: Oral moniliasis, a complication of aureomycin therapy. Oral Surg 4:1420, 1951

Monaco JD: The role of *Candida* in inflammatory papillary hyperplasia. J Prosthet Dent 45:470, 1981

Myllarniemi S, Perheentupa J: Oral findings in the autoimmune polyendocrinopathy-candidosis syndrome (CAPECS) and other forms of hypoparathyroidism. Oral Surg 45:721, 1978

Neill DJ: Symposium on denture sore mouth. I. An aetiological review. Dent Pract 16:135, 1965

Renstrup G: Occurrence of *Candida* in oral leukoplakias. Acta Pathol Microbiol Scand 78:241, 1970

Rockoff AS: Chronic mucocutaneous candidiasis. Arch Dermatol 115:322, 1979

Rose HD, Sheth NK: Pulmonary candidiasis. A clinical and pathological correlation. Arch Intern Med 138:964, 1978

Sadeghi EM et al: The presence of *Candida albicans* in hereditary benign intraepithelial dyskeratosis. An ultrastructural observation. Oral Surg 48:342, 1979

Sahay JN: Inhaled corticosteroid aerosols and candidiasis. Br J Dis Chest 73:164, 1979

Sams WM, Jr et al: Chronic mucocutaneous candidiasis. Immunologic studies of 3 generations of a single family. Am J Med 67:948, 1979

Sauaranayak LP et al: Factors affecting the *in vitro* adherence of *Candida albicans* to acrylic surfaces. Arch Oral Biol 25:611, 1980

Scherr SA et al: Chronic candidiasis of the oral cavity and esophagus. Laryngoscope 90:769, 1980

Silva–Hutner M, Cooper BH: Yeasts of medical importance. In Lennette EH, Balows A, Hausler WJ, Jr, Truant JP (eds): Manual of Clinical Microbiology, 3rd ed. Washington DC, American Society of Microbiologists, 1980

Sjoberg KH: Moniliasis–An internal disease? Three cases of idiopathic hypoparathyroidism with moniliasis, steatorrhea, primary amenorrhea and pernicious anemia. Acta Med Scand 179:157, 1966

Sobel JD et al: Adherence of *Candida albicans* to human vaginal and and buccal epithelial cells, J Infect Dis 143:76, 1981

Symoens J et al: An evaluation of two years of clinical experience with ketoconazole. Rev Infect Dis 2:674, 1980

Tapper–Jones LM et al: Candidal infections and populations of *Candida albicans* in mouths of diabetics. J Clin Pathol 34:706, 1981

Tkach JR et al: Severe hepatitis associated with ketoconazole treatment for chronic mucocutaneous candidiasis. Cutis 29:482, 1982

Toogood JH et al: Candidiasis and dysphonia complicating beclomethasone treatment of asthma. J Allergy Clin Immunol 65:145, 1980

Turrell AJ: Aetiology of inflamed upper denture-bearing tissues. Br Dent J 120:542, 1966

Tyldesley WR et al: Oral lesions in renal transplant patients. J Oral Pathol 8:53, 1979

Vogt FC: The incidence of oral candidiasis with use of inhaled corticosteroids. Ann Allergy 43:205, 1979

Wells RS, Higgs JM and McDonald A: Familial chronic muco-cutaneous candidiasis. J Med Genetics 9:302, 1972

Wilborn WH et al: Scanning electron microscopy of oral lesions in chronic mucocutaneous candidiasis. JAMA 244:2294, 1980

Woodruff PW, Hesseltine HC: Relationship of oral thrush to vaginal mycosis and incidence of each. Am J Obstet Gynecol 36:467, 1938

Wright BA et al: Candidiasis and atrophic tongue lesions. Oral Surg 51:55, 1981

Wright BS: The effect of soft lining materials on the growth of *Candida albicans*. J Dent 8:144, 1980

Keratotic White Lesions with No Increased Potential for the Development of Oral Cancer

Anneroth G, Isacsson G, Langerholm B, Lindvall AM, Thyresson N: Pachyonychia congenital. A clinical histological and microradiographic study with special reference to oral manifestations. Acta Derm Venereal 55:387, 1975

Archard HO, Heck JW, Stanley HR: Focal epithelial hyperplasia: An unusual oral mucosal lesion found in Indian children. Oral Surg 20:201, 1965

Banóczy J et al: White sponge nevus: Leukoedema exfoliativum mucosae oris. A report of 45 cases. Swed Dent J 66:481, 1973

Banóczy J, Szabo L, and Csiba A: Migratory glossitis. A clinical-histologic review of seventy cases. Oral Surg 39:113, 1975

Basu MK, Moss N: Warty dyskeratoma, a note concerning its occurrence on the oral mucosa and its possible pathogenesis. Br J Oral Surg 17:57, 1979–1980

Bauer EA et al: Recessive dystrophic epidermolysis bullosa. Evidence for increased collagenase as a genetic characteristic in cell culture. J Exp Med 148:1378, 1978

Buchner A, Ramon Y: Focal epithelial hyperplasia: Report of two cases from Israel and review of literature. Arch Dermatol 107:97, 1973

Cataldo E et al: Psoriasis with oral manifestations. Cutis 20:705, 1977

Chernovsky MF: Porokeratosis. In Fitzpatrick et al

(eds): Dermatology in General Medicine, 2nd ed. New York, McGraw Hill, 1979

Clausen FP: Histopathology of focal epithelial hyperplasia: Evidence of viral infection. Tandlaegebladet 73:1013, 1969

Danbolt N: Acrodermatitis enteropathica. Br J Dermatol 100:37, 1979

Danielsen L, Kobaysai T: Pseudoxanthoma elasticum: An ultrastructural study of oral lesions. Acta Dermatovenerol 54:173, 1974

Dawson TAJ: Microscopic appearance of geographic tongue. Br J Dermatol 81:827, 1969

Geist ET et al: Third and fourth generation white sponge nevus: Report of a case. J Oral Surg 39:457, 1981

Goldsmith LA: Tyrosinemia and related disorders. In Stanbury JB et al (eds): The Metabolic Basis of Inherited Disease, 5th ed, p 287. New York, McGraw-Hill, 1983

Gorlin RJ, Chaudhry AP: The oral manifestations of keratosis follicularis . Oral Surg 12:1468, 1959

Gorlin RJ: Genetic disorders affecting mucous membranes. Oral Surg 28:512, 1969

Gorlin RJ: Heritable mucosal disorders. In Stewart RE, Prescott GH (eds): Oral Facial Genetics, p. 360. CV Mosby, St Louis, 1971

Harrison PV et al: A comparative study of psoriatic and non-psoriatic buccal mucosa. Br J Dermatol 106:637, 1982

Jorgenson RJ, Levin S: White sponge nevus. Arch Dermatol 117:73, 1981

Kousa M: Clinical observations on Reiter's disease with special reference to the venereal and nonvenereal aetiology. Acta Dermatovenerol 58:1, 1978

Larregue M et al: Syndrome de Richner-Hanhart ou tryrosinase oculocutanée. Ann Dermatol Venerol 106:53, 1979

Maser ED: Oral manifestations of pachyonychia congenita: Report of a case. Oral Surg 43:373, 1977

Mawhinney H et al: Pachyonychia congenita with candidiasis. Clin Exp Dermatol 6:145, 1981

Miller RL et al: Darier's disease of the oral mucosa: clinical case report with ultra-structural evaluation. J Oral Pathol 11:79, 1982

Milhail and Wertheimer FW: Clinical variants of porokeratosis (Mibelli). Arch Dermatol 98:124, 1968

Ritter SB, Petersen G: Esophageal carcinoma, hyperkeratosis and oral leukoplakia: Occurrence in a 25 year old woman. JAMA 235:1723, 1976

Sadeghi EM, Witkop CJ: The presence of Candida albicans in hereditary benign intra-epithelial dyskeratosis. An ultrastructural observation. Oral Surg 48:342, 1979

Savolainen ER et al: Deficiency of galacto sylhydroxylysyl glucosyltransferase, an enzyme of collagen synthesis, in a family with dominant epidermolysis bullosa simplex. N Engl J Med 304:197, 1981

Spouge JD et al: Darier-White's disease: a cause of white lesions of the mucosa. Oral Surg 21:441, 1966

Steiner GA: Successful treatment of acrodermatitis enteropathica with zinc sulfate. Am J Hosp Pharm 35:1535, 1978

Svendsen IB, Albrechtsen B: The prevalence of dyskeratosis follicularis (Darier's disease) in Denmark. Acta Dermatovenerol 39:256, 1959

Tyldesley WR: Oral leukoplakia associated with tylosis and oesophageal carcinoma. J Oral Pathol 3:62, 1974

Tyldesley WR, Kempson SA: Ultrastructure of the oral epithelium in leukoplakia associated with tylosis and esophageal carcinoma. J Oral Pathol 4:49, 1975

Weathers DR, Baker G, Archard HO, Burkes EJ, Jr: Psoriasiform lesions of the oral mucosa (with emphasis on "ectopic geographic tongue"). Oral Surg 37:872, 1974

Weathers DR, Driscoll RM: Darier's disease of the oral mucosa: Report of five cases. Oral Surg 37:711, 1974

White DK et al: Intraoral psoriasis associated with widespread dermal psoriasis. Oral Surg 41:174, 1976

Witkop CJ, Jr: Disorders affecting cellular communications in oral tissues: Gap junctions. In Daws BS (ed): In Vitro Epithelia and Birth Defects. Birth Defects 16:197, 1980

Witkop CJ, Jr, Gorlin RJ: Four hereditary mucosal syndromes. Arch Dermatol 84:762, 1961

Young WG: Familial white folded dysplasia of the oral mucous membrane. Br J Oral Surg 5:93, 1967

Young WG et al: Focal palmoplantar and gingival hyperkeratosis syndrome: Report of a family, with cytologic, ultrastructural and histochemical findings. Oral Surg 53:473, 1982

Red and White Lesions with Defined or Ulcerative Precancerous Potential

Adkins KF, Monsour FN: Verrucous leukoplakia. N Z Dent J 72:28, 1976

Anderson DL: Cause and prevention of lip cancer. J Can Dent Assoc 37:138, 1971

Andreasen JO: Oral lichen planus. I A clinical evaluation of 115 cases, II A histologic evaluation of 97 cases. Oral Surg 25:31, 158, 1968

Banóczy J: Oral leukoplakia Dev Oncol 8, Martinus Nijhoff Pubs, Hingham, Mass. 1982

Bánóczy J: Occurrence of epithelial dysplasia in

oral leukoplakia. Analysis and follow-up study of 12 cases. Oral Surg 42:766, 1976

Bánóczy J et al: Clinical and histologic studies on electrogalvanically induced oral white lesions. Oral Surg 48:319, 1979

Bánóczy J et al: Scanning electron microscopic study of oral leukoplakia. J Oral Pathol 9:145, 1980

Baric JM, Alman JE, Feldman RS, Chauncey HH: Influence of cigarette, pipe and cigar smoking, removable partial denture and age on oral leukoplakia. Oral Surg 54:424, 1982

Bazemore J et al: Relation of quinacrine hydrochloride to lichenoid dermatitis (atypical lichen planus). Arch Dermatol 54:308, 1946

Beckman BI: Valisone aerosol spray contraindicated in mucous membranes. J Am Acad Dermatol 4:233, 1981

Berry HH, Landwerlen JR: Cigarette smoker's lip lesion in psychiatric patients. J Am Dent Assoc 86:657, 1973

Craig RM: Speckled leukoplakia of the floor of the mouth. J Am Dent Assoc 102:690, 1981

Daftary DK et al: An oral lichen planus-like lesion in Indian betel-tobacco chewers. Scand J Dent Res 88:244, 1980

Daniels TE et al: Direct immunofluorescence in oral mucosal disease: A diagnostic analysis of 130 cases. Oral Surg 51:38, 1981

Dreizen S et al: Oral complications of bone marrow transplantation in adults with acute leukemia. Postgrad Med 66:187, 1979

Dusek JJ, Frick WG: Lichen planus: Oral manifestations and suggested treatments. J Oral Maxillofac Surg 40:240, 1982

Ehrl PA: Clinical study of an aromatic retinoid (RO l0-9359) for the treatment of oral hyperkeratosis. Dtsch Zahnaerzl, 2 35:554, 1980

Eisenberg E et al: Pemphigus-like mucosal lesions: A side effect of penicillamine therapy. Oral Surg 51:409, 1981

Fellner MJ: Lichen planus. Int J Dermatol 19:71, 1980

Feuske NA, Greenberg SS: Solar-induced skin changes. Am Fam Physician 25:109,1982

Fiumara NJ, Grande DJ, Giunta JL: Papular secondary syphilis of the tongue. Oral Surg 45:540, 1978

Freedman A, Shklar G: Alcohol and hamster buccal pouch carcinogenesis. Oral Surg 46:794, 1978

Garb J, Rubin G: Dyskeratosis congenita with pigmentation, dystrophia ungium and leukoplakia oris. Arch Dermatol Syph 50:191, 1944

Gardner HL et al: The vulvar dystrophies, atypias and carcinoma in situ. An invitational symposium. J Reprod Med 17:131, 1976

Gilmore W et al: The effect of 13-cis-retinoic acid

on hamster buccal pouch carcinogenesis. Oral Surg 51:256, 1981

Gongloff RK, Gage AA: Cryosurgical treatment of oral lesions: Report of cases. J Am Dent Assoc 106:47, 1983

Gorlin RJ: Bowen's disease of the mucous membrane of the mouth; A review of the literature and a presentation of six cases. Oral Surg 3:35, 1950

Graham S: Dentition, diet, tobacco and alcoholism in the epidemiology of oral cancer. J Natl Canc Inst 59:1611, 1977

Gupta PC et al: Incidence rates of oral cancer and natural history of oral precancerous lesions in a 10-year follow-up study of Indian villagers. Community Dent Oral Epidemiol 8:283, 1980

Hakim AA et al: In vivo malignant transformation of cells from human oral lichen planus lesions. Neoplasma 29:189, 1982

Hay KD, Muller HK, Reade PC: D-penicilla-mine-induced mucocutaneous lesions with features of pemphigus. Oral Surg 45:385,1978

Hazel OG et al: Leukoplakia buccalis. AMA Arch Dermatol 61:781, 1950

Hellinger M I et al: Clinicopathologic correlation of oral white lesions. Oral Surg 16:1365, 1963

Hillman R: Hypervitaminosis A, experimental induction in a human subject. Am J Clin Nutr 4:603, 1956

Hobaek A: Leukoplakia oris. Acta Odontol Scand 7:61, 1946

Holmstrup P, Pindborg JJ: Erythroplakic lesions in relation to oral lichen planus. Acta Dermatovenerol 59:77, 1979

Hyman GA et al: Autoradiographic studies of oral lichen planus. Oral Surg 54:172, 1982

Keller AZ: Alcohol, tobacco and age factors in the relative frequency of cancer among males with and without liver cirrhosis. Am J Epidemiol 106:194, 1977

Kramer IRH, El–Labban N, Lee KW: The clinical features and risk of malignant transformation in sublingual keratosis. Br Dent J 144:1717, 1978

Krutchkoff DJ et al: Oral lichen planus. The evidence regarding potential malignant transformation. J Oral Pathol 7:1, 1978

Laskaris G et al: Direct immunofluorescence in oral lichen planus. Oral Surg 53:483, 1982

Lindquist C, Teppo L: Epidemiological evaluation of sunlight as a risk factor of lip cancer. Br J Cancer 37:983, 1978

Macdonald DG: Premalignant lesions of the oral epithelium. In Dolby AE (ed): Oral Mucosa in Health and Disease, p 335. Oxford, Blackwell Scientific Publications, 1975

Maidhof R et al: Cell proliferation in lichen planus of the buccal mucosa. Acta Dermatol Venerol

(Stockh) 61:17, 1981

Marefat P, Shklar G: Experimental production of lingual leukoplakia and carcinomas. Oral Surg 44:578, 1977

Mashberg A: Erythroplasia vs leukoplakia in the diagnosis of early asymptomatic oral squamous carcinoma. N Engl J Med 297:109, 1977

Mashberg A: Reevaluation of toludine blue application as a diagnostic adjunct in the detection of asymptomatic oral squamous carcinoma: A continuing prospective study of oral cancer III. Cancer 46:758, 1980

Mashberg A: Alcohol as a primary risk factor in oral squamous carcinoma. Cancer 31:146, 1981

Mashberg A: Final evaluation of tolonium chloride rinse for screening of high-risk patients with asymptomatic squamous carcinoma. J Am Dent Assoc 106:319, 1983

Mason C, Grisius R, McKean T: Stomatitis medicamentosa associated with gold therapy for rheumatoid arthritis. US Navy Med 69:23, 1978

Mehta FS et al: Chewing and smoking habits in relation to precancer and oral cancer. J Cancer Res Clin Oncol 99:35, 1981

Meyboom RHB: Metal antagonists. Side Effects Drugs 8:529, 1975

Neumann–Jensen B, Holmstrup P, Pindborg JJ: Smoking habits of 611 patients with oral lichen planus. Oral Surg 43:410, 1977

Nisengard RJ et al: Diagnostic importance of immunofluorescence in oral bullous diseases and lupus erythematosus. Oral Surg 40:365, 1975

Paissat DK: Oral submucous fibrosis. Int J Oral Surg 10:307, 1981

Peck GL et al: Toxic epidermal necrolysis in a patient with graft-vs-host reaction. Arch Dermatol 105:561, 1972

Pindborg JJ: Pathology of oral leukoplakia. Am J Dermatopathol 2:277, 1980

Pindborg JJ et al: Reverse smoking in Andhra Pradesh, India: A study of palatal lesions among 10,169 villages. Br J Cancer 25:10, 1971

Pinkus H: Lichenoid tissue reactions. Arch Dermatol 107:840, 1973

Quigley LF et al: Reverse cigarette smoking in Caribbeans: Clinical histologic, and cytologic observations. J Am Dent Assoc 72:867, 1966

Rodu B, Gockerman JP: Oral manifestations of the chronic graft-vs-host reaction. JAMA 249:504, 1983

Roed–Petersen B: Effect on oral leukoplakia of reducing or ceasing tobacco smoking. Acta Dermatol Venerol (Stockh) 62:164, 1982

Romero RW et al: Unusual variant of lupus erythematosus or lichen planus. Arch Dermatol 113:741, 1977

Sale GE et al: Oral and ophthalmic pathology of graft-versus-host disease in man. Predictive value of the lip biopsy. Hum Pathol 12:1022, 1981

Schiodt M et al: A clinical study of 32 patients with oral discoid lupus erythematosus. Int J Oral Surg 7:85, 1978

Schiødt M et al: Oral findings in glass blowers. Community Dent Oral Epidemiol 8:195, 1980

Schiødt M et al: Deposits of immunoglobulins, complement and fibrinogen in oral lupus erythematosus, lichen planus and leukoplakia. Oral Surg 51:603, 1981

Schottenfeld D: Editorial: Snuff dippers cancer. N Engl J Med 304:778, 1981

Seehafer JR et al: Lichen planus-like lesions caused by penicillinamine in primary biliary cirrhosis. Arch Dermatol 117:140, 1981

Shafer WG, Waldron CA: A clinical and histopathologic study of oral leukoplakia. Surg Gynecol Obstet 112:411, 1961

Shafer WG, Waldron CA: Erythroplakia of the oral mucosa. Cancer 36:1021, 1975

Shear M, Pindborg JJ: Verrucous hyperplasia of the oral mucosa. Cancer 46:1885, 1980

Shklar G: Modern studies and concepts of leukoplakia in the mouth. J Dermatol Surg Oncol 7:996, 1981

Shklar G, McCarthy PL: Histopathology of oral lesions of chronic discoid lupus erythematosus. Arch Dermatol 114:1031, 1978

Silverman S Jr. and Griffith M: Studies on oral lichen planus II. Follow-up on 200 patients, clinical characteristics, and associated malignancy. Oral Surg 37:705, 1974

Silverman S, Ware WH: Comparison of histologic cytologic and clinical findings in intraoral leukoplakia and associated carcinoma. Oral Surg 13:412, 1960

Sloberg K et al: Topical tretinoin therapy and oral lichen planus. Arch Dermatol 115:716, 1979

Sprague WG: A survey of the use of the term "leukoplakia" by oral pathologists. Oral Surg 16:1067, 1963

Sundström B, Mörnstad H, Axéll T: Oral carcinomas associated with snuff dipping. Some clinical and histological characteristics of 23 tumors in Swedish males. J Oral Pathol 11:245, 1982

Tyldesley WR, Harding SM: Betamethasone valerate aerosol in the treatment of oral lichen planus. Br J Dermatol 96:659, 1977

Waldron CA, Shafer WG: Current concepts of leukoplakia. Int Dent J 10:350, 1960

Waldron CA, Shafer WG: Leukoplakia revisited. A clinicopathologic study of 3256 oral leukoplakias. Cancer 36:1386, 1975

Walker DM: Identification of subpopulations of lymphocytes and macrophages in the infiltrate of lichen planus lesions of skin and oral mucosa. Br J Dermatol 94:529, 1976

Warnock GR, Fuller RP, Jr, Pelleu GB, Jr: Evaluation of 5-fluorouracil in the treatment of actinic keratosis of the lip. Oral Surg 52:501, 1981

Weedon D: Apoptosis in lichen planus. Clin Exp Dermatol 5:425, 1980

Weedon D: The lichenoid tissue reaction. Int J Dermatol 21:203, 1982

Winn DM et al: Snuff dipping and oral cancer among women in the southern United States. N Engl J Med 304:745, 1981

Zak FG et al: Toxic epidermal necrolysis (Lyell): The scalded-skin syndrome. Am J Med 37:140, 1964

Zegarelli DJ: Lichen planus: A simple and reliable biopsy technique. J Oral Med 36:18, 1981

7

Pigmentation of the Oral Tissues

LESTER W. BURKET

Pigmentation of the oral mucosa and skin may be of endogenous or exogenous origin. An example of the former is the pigmentation typical of black and some European peoples. Such pigmentation of endogenous origin serves as a protection against prolonged exposure to sun rays. Of particular interest to the dentist is the endogenous pigmentation of the oral mucosa and the circumoral tissues that are associated with a wide variety of systemic diseases, particularly those of endocrine origin. Some of these systemic diseases have osseous manifestations in the jaws and skull that may be seen on dental radiographs. Certain neoplasms, the melanomas, are characterized by abnormal production of melanin, and some medications may stimulate melanin production.

Many medicaments and foreign particulate substances are responsible for exogenous pigmentation. They are not the products of substances manufactured within the body and gain access to the human tissues coincident to the treatment of disease or by trauma when they may become imbedded in the tissues.

ENDOGENOUS PIGMENTATION

The exact nature of abnormal endogenous pigmentation varies with the disease but in most cases it is melanin. This is an insoluble polymer of high molecular weight. In mammals it is always bound to protein. It varies from brown, blue-black, to black depending on the vascularity of the overlying tissues and the epithelium.

In man, the development of melanin requires the precursor acid, tyrosine. In albinism, the complete absence of melanin on the skin represents an inhibited state of the tyrosine–tyrosinase system.

In malignant melanomas, and in blacks, the inhibitory factors of melanin production are absent. There are certain tissues in which melanin production is greatest, for instance the areola about the nipples, the genitalia, and the dorsal surfaces of the forearms. It is least on the palmar surfaces of the hands and the soles of the feet. Areas of the oral cavity where melanosis is more common include the gingiva, buccal mucosa, tongue, and hard palate. Pigmentation is less common on the floor of the mouth. The color variations may be uniform, symmetrical, or blotched.

Pigmented nevi occur frequently on the skin and much more rarely on the oral mucosa where they are usually located on the lower lip and less commonly, on the gingiva and palate. They are usually referred to as moles and contain melanin pigment varying in color from light brown to purplish brown-black. There have been reports of white, nonpigmented nevi, which are recognized from biopsy. Intraorally, nevi are flat or slightly raised well-demarcated lesions. It is this discrete demarcation that differentiates them from the typical patches of melanin pigmentation seen so often in people with increased melanin pigment in the skin, as is seen in blacks and others with dark skin. A review by Trodahl of 135 melanotic lesions of the oral mucosa over a 28-year period showed 42 of them to be malignant and 25% of the malignant ones appeared clinically innocuous as melanotic "spots." Malignancy was more likely to occur on gingival and palatal lesions than on those of the lip.

Abnormal melanosis is common about the skin of the oral commissures in a number of systemic diseases. The presence and distribution of melanosis in some systemic diseases may be diagnostic or at least cause the clinician to suspect a certain systemic alteration. Abnormal melanin deposition occurs in a number of the following medical conditions.

Addison's Disease

Abnormal pigmentation of the skin and mucous membranes (see Fig. 7-1) is one of the earliest signs of Addison's disease. This abnormal pigmentation has a tendency to develop in scars and folds of skin. It may also appear on the oral mucosa where it resembles blotches of bluish purple ink that appear to have been thrown on the oral mucosa. In the typical well-developed Addison's disease, the skin may be a bronze color.

Historically the most common cause of this disease was decreased adrenocortical hormone production caused by destruction of the adrenal cortex associated with tuberculosis, some chronic parasitic infection, or ma-

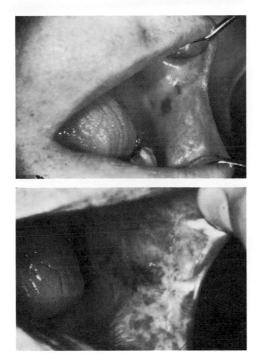

Fig. 7-1 Oral mucosal pigmentation in Addison's disease.

lignancy. Today most cases are of unknown cause.

The general systemic symptoms of Addison's disease are weakness, nausea, and vomiting with an associated low blood pressure. A series of sophisticated laboratory procedures permit the diagnosis of this disease by the physician, including 24-hour urinary determinations of 17-ketosteroids or 17-hydroxycorticosteroids. There is often an associated eosinophilia that may reach as high as 80% to 90%. This disease usually responds to appropriate hormone replacement therapy.

The alert dental clinician may be the first to suspect this disease because of the characteristic pigmentation of the oral mucosa and general symptoms of malaise with a lowered blood pressure.

Peutz–Jeghers Syndrome

This syndrome (Figs. 7-2 and 7-3), associated with pigmentation of the oral tissues and frequently both large and small intestinal polyposis, is an inherited condition found in equal frequency in both sexes. There is abnormal melanin pigmentation of the circumoral areas of the face, and the interdigital areas of the hands may be involved. Polyposis of the uterus and nasal fossa may be associated with similar abnormal pigmentation. These areas of pigmentation present no obvious features to distinguish them from the pigmented sites in Addison's disease.

There is no known physiological basis for the location of pigmented areas, which in themselves are harmless and require no therapy. The areas about the eyes, lips, and nostrils are 1 mm to 10 mm in size and usually have a clearly demarcated margin.

The intestinal polyps may produce symptoms such as bleeding and abdominal pains. The lesions rarely (less than 3%) undergo malignant degeneration. This should not be confused with *familial colonic polyposis,* which does *not* exhibit abnormal pigmentation and has a *very high* incidence of malignant transformation.

Hyperfunction of the Pituitary Gland

The pituitary gland plays an important role in melanin production, and the production of melanin is increased in some cases of hyperpituitarism.

Pregnancy and Female Sex Hormones

In the third trimester of pregnancy, abnormal pigmentation of the skin is not uncommon. This usually involves the circumoral tissues and it is extremely common about the nipples. This form of pigmentation is often spoken of as chloasma (see Fig. 7-4). The use of oral contraceptives may be associated with th3same form of pigmentation to a lesser degree. This was especially true when preparations contained larger dosages of the sex hormones.

Neurofibromatosis

This rare condition, also known as von Recklinghausen's disease, may be associated with discrete pigmented areas on the skin known as *café au lait* spots. These pigmented spots are associated with sessile tumors of the skin and the mucous membranes. The sessile tu-

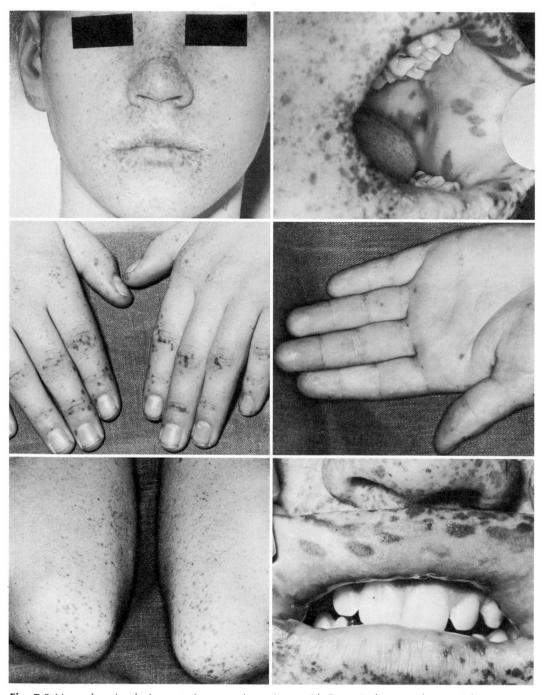

Fig. 7-2 Lip and perioral pigmentation seen in patients with Peutz-Jeghers syndrome. (Klostermann GF: Dtsch Med Wochenschr 81:631)

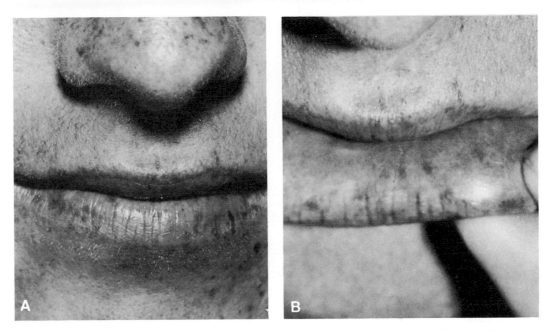

Fig. 7-3 *A,* Pigmented spots of the lips extend into the immediate perioral region. *B,* Pigmented spots are seen on labial mucous membrane of everted lower lip. (Rohrs LC: Intestinal polyposis and pigmented spots of lips. JAMA 165:209, 1957)

mor developments are overgrowths of the structures of the peripheral nerves. Oral manifestations of this disease may consist of multiple sessile appendages on the lips, tongue, and gingiva.

Hemochromatosis

This endogenous pigmentation results from the deposition of abnormal amounts of iron as well as melanin in the body tissues. It represents disordered iron metabolism and may result from increased dietary iron intake, excessive transfusions or other parenteral iron-containing medications, or increased intestinal iron absorption. The combination of the iron pigmentation with melanin results in a characteristic bronze color that is an important clinical feature of this disease. This skin pigmentation has been reported to occur in from 90% to 97% of cases and is more often due to melanin than to iron or a combination of the two. The skin pigmentation is similar to that found in Addison's disease. A classic tetrad of liver cirrhosis, diabetes, cardiac failure, and bronzed skin occurs in 82% of cases. It is uncommon in the young patient with

onset usually being between 40 and 60 years of age. This disease can be diagnosed by special staining techniques of biopsy specimens and in the laboratory by increased plasma iron concentration.

The intraoral findings consist of a bluish gray pigmentation of the hard palate with lesser involvement of the attached gingival tissues. Pigmented changes in these tissues may suggest this disease to the dentist or periodontist. At least 15% to 25% of the persons with this disease have oral pigmentation.

Pigmentation Due to Therapy with Quinacrine Hydrochloride and Related Antimalarial Drugs

Quinacrine hydrochloride and other antimalarial drugs have been shown on occasion to produce a blue-black mucocutaneous hyperpigmentation. Histologic studies of skin biopsy specimens from these patients show yellowish to dark brown granules that resemble melanin, although the exact composition is not known. The facial, subungual, and pretibial tissues are most often involved, and

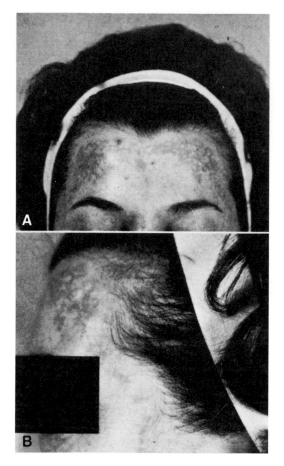

Fig. 7-4 Melasma of the forehead (*A*) and cheeks (*B*). (Resnick S: JAMA 199:602)

orally there is pigmentation of the hard palate with a sharp demarcation between the hard and soft palate. It has been found that the patient must take the drug for a minimum of 4 months for such pigmentation to occur. The pigmentation generally disappears on discontinuing the drug.

Carotenemia

Carotenemia is a condition that results from chronic excessive levels of carotin pigments in the tissues. This usually results from the long and continued consumption of foods containing large amounts of carotene such as carrots, sweet potatoes, and egg yolks. Disturbances in the metabolism of these foods in the production of vitamin A may also give rise to excessive amounts of carotene.

In carotenemia an orange-to-yellow pigmentation of the skin and oral mucosa occurs. This is comparable to the changes in these tissues that are observed with high circulating bile pigments but does not involve the sclera. This color change is most intense on the palms and soles and in the area of the soft palate. Diagnosis is made by the laboratory findings of normal serum bilirubin, which excludes jaundice, and elevated levels of serum carotene.

No specific therapy is indicated. Slow resolution usually occurs following decreased dietary intake.

Jaundice

Jaundice (icterus), which is due to increased levels of bilirubin in the blood, causes a yellowish discoloration of the skin and oral mucosa. It is evident earliest in the sclera because of that tissue's normal white color and high content of elastic tissue, which has an affinity for bile pigments. Causes of jaundice are discussed in Chapter 20. Diagnosis is made by measuring the serum bilirubin level.

EXOGENOUS PIGMENTATION

The most common intraoral forms of local or exogenous pigmentation are foreign substances imbedded in the gingival tissues. These often result from accidents during the childhood years. If one falls on a gravel or cindered road, small particles of the road surface material may become imbedded in the gingiva and the other exposed oral tissues. The common use of charcoal dentifrices traditionally caused an important type of oral pigmentation; however, charcoal-containing tooth powders are rarely used in the United States (they are still used in European countries). Pencil points are occasionally broken off in the gingival tissues; if the fragments are not completely removed, may cause permanent discoloration of the tissue.

A common cause of iatrogenic pigmentation is small particles of dental amalgam that may become imbedded in the gingiva or in the mucosa of the cheek when restorations are removed from the teeth or when the teeth are extracted. This form of pigmentation is infrequently observed today because of air-powered handpieces, which are less frequently associated with trauma to the soft tissues. Also, better techniques of tooth removal minimize tooth fracture. Pigmentation due to small particles of dental amalgam are purplish gray in color and fairly discrete. If the pigmentation is associated with the removal of a lower molar or bicuspid tooth, the particles, aided by the force of gravity, may lodge in the alveolus of the extracted tooth. Pigmentation of the alveolus is therefore more common in the mandible and fairly uncommon on the maxilla. At times, the small particles of amalgam can be recognized in the usual periapical films. No treatment is indicated.

Deposits of metallic sulfides in the marginal gingivae, the interdental papillae, or the oral mucosa are also causes of exogenous pigmentation. These metals may enter the body as the result of occupational exposure, habits, or therapeutic administration and are discussed in detail later in this chapter. Pigmentation of the oral tissues may be the first evidence of toxicity to the metal.

General Considerations in Metallic Stomatitides

The mechanism of production of lesions in bismuth, lead, and mercurial stomatitis is in part similar to that of acute necrotizing ulcerative gingivitis (ANUG). The absorption of these metals and the deposition of their salts in the gingival tissues interfere with the circulation and the nutrition of the marginal gingiva and the interdental papilla, permitting secondary invasion of mouth bacteria especially the fusospirochetal organisms. Metallic salts secreted in the saliva also are irritating.

Bismuthism

Considering the widespread medicinal use of bismuth, there are comparatively few toxic symptoms. Chronic manifestations consist of vague gastrointestinal disturbances, nausea, bloody diarrhea, "bismuth grippe," and jaundice. "Bismuth lines" can be demonstrated radiologically in the growing ends of bones. Bismuth pigmentation rarely appears either

in children or in women during pregnancy. The skeletal system of the developing fetus serves as a ready storage depot for the absorbed metal. The urine is the chief avenue of excretion, with only traces of this metal being found in the saliva.

Medicinal use of bismuth-containing preparations by the patient represents the most frequent cause of bismuthism. Occupational sources are unimportant. The incidence of stomatitis has decreased markedly with the replacement of bismuth salts by penicillin in the treatment of syphilis. A bismuth line or bismuth stomatitis usually develops as a result of ingestion or injection of bismuth salts for therapeutic purposes. The soluble subnitrate and subcarbonate salts are prescribed orally for nonspecific forms of diarrhea and colitis, and bismuth salts are frequently found in analgesia anal suppositories. These drugs may occasion rapid development of a bismuth line or bismuth stomatitis because of the more complete absorption from the inflamed gastrointestinal tract. Many proprietary drugs contain bismuth salts, and bismuth-containing salves or pastes may result in bismuth pigmentation if they are applied repeatedly to the granulating wound surfaces.

Symptoms. A bismuth line (see Fig. 7-5) may exist without symptoms, but there is often a metallic taste, and the patient often experiences a burning sensation of the oral tissues. In most instances the patient complains of an annoying gingivostomatitis with symptoms

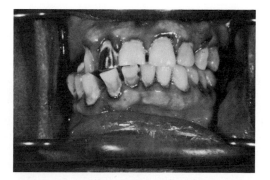

Fig. 7-5 Bismuth deposition in the marginal gingiva at the sites of local irritation. Note the localized distribution of the pigmentation in the tissues.

identical with those described for ANUG. The tongue is frequently sore and enlarged. Painful ulcerative lesions may develop where the oral tissues come in contact with calcareous or other irritants.

Signs. Large, extremely painful, shallow ulcerations are seen at times on the cheek mucosa in the molar region.

The bismuth salts in the bloodstream are believed to unite with hemoglobin or an acid radical of the blood. The blue-black bismuth sulfide granules are formed by the action of H_2S produced by the action of bacteria on the organic material remaining in areas of poor oral hygiene (see Fig. 7-6) or areas associated with dental plaque.

The blue-black bismuth line appears to be well demarcated to the eye, but if it is examined with a hand lens, the pigmentation is observed to be diffusely distributed (compared with lead). In mild cases there may be involvement of only the interdental papillae, the gingival tissues about erupting third molars (see Fig. 7-7), or the lingual gingiva of the mandibular incisors especially those with calcareous deposits or local areas of inflammation (see Fig. 7-8). The tongue, the lips, and the cheeks may have pigmented areas where these tissues contact ulcerative lesions of the gingiva as a result of increased capillary permeability. Regional adenopathy may be present.

Diagnosis. An ulcerative gingivostomatitis accompanied by a discrete blue-black pigmentation of the interdental papilla and the marginal gingiva in a patient chronically receiving oral or anal administration of bismuth compounds is sufficient for a tentative diagnosis.

Pigmentation resulting from other metals, usually lead, or other causes of gingival discoloration must be ruled out. The "paper test" will indicate whether the pigmentation is actually in the gingival tissues. If the discoloration is accentuated when the corner of a small piece of white paper (see Fig. 7-9) is inserted in the gingival sulcus, the presence of the pigmented area in the gingival tissues is verified; if the discoloration disappears, the suspected pigmentation is due to discoloration of the adjacent root surface, usually from calculus.

The absence of constitutional symptoms usually permits differentiation from lead intoxication. The hemogram, with changes characteristic of lead poisoning, may assist in doubtful cases. The urine can be tested for bismuth content, and urine and blood lead levels may be obtained.

Treatment. Special attention should be given to establishing and maintaining the best possible oral hygiene. Bismuth pigmentation of the oral mucosa and painful ulcerative lesions can be prevented in most instances if the physician administering bismuth-containing preparation would emphasize the necessity for maintaining scrupulous oral hygiene. The treatment of the painful ulcerative lesion follows the procedures described for ANUG.

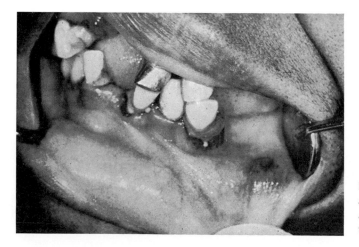

Fig. 7-6 Bismuth pigmentation localized to areas of poor oral hygiene and irritation. An area of contact pigmentation is present on the lip.

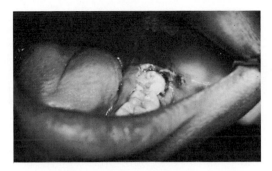

Fig. 7-7 Acute pericoronal infection with bismuth pigmentation and traumatic irritation.

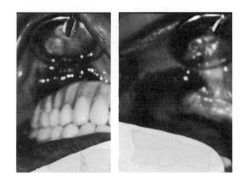

Fig. 7-8 Bismuth pigmentation persisting in an edentulous patient who had a severe decubital ulcer due to an ill-fitting denture.

The disappearance of the bismuth line following the institution of the above treatment is unpredictable.

Prognosis. The prognosis of acute bismuth stomatitis is good, but response to treatment will not be as prompt as in uncomplicated ANUG because of the persisting deposits of bismuth and the disturbance in the nutrition of the marginal gingiva.

Lead Poisoning

Few metals have had a more widespread detrimental effect on human health than lead. From the beginning of recorded history, there are anecdotal reports concerning the hazards associated with the use of this metal and its salts. In more recent times, plumbism has been shown to be caused by lead in pigments, paints, glazes, cooking vessels, containers, ointments, and batteries. Even "moonshine," an illicit alcoholic beverage

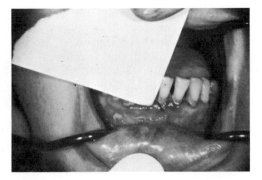

Fig. 7-9 The "paper test," which is used to differentiate between stain on the root surfaces and pigmentation in the marginal gingival tissues. The dark line on the gums persists after the paper is inserted above the tooth. Case of bismuth stomatitis.

distilled in car radiators, has been shown to cause acute lead poisoning. Efforts to curtail the unrestricted use of lead have met with some success; however, the use of tetraethyl lead as an antiknock compound in gasoline has introduced a new source of lead into the environment. Excessive absorption of lead from automobile exhausts and dust and dirt derived from house paint is known to affect a large number of poor children living in rundown urban centers. Diagnosis of this type of asymptomatic chronic exposure is difficult, and for most children, treatment is limited.

Children who live in old housing in city centers are considered to be at risk. While it is difficult to obtain reliable estimates of the number of children involved, the Surgeon General reports that as many as a quarter of a million may suffer the consequences of elevated lead exposure. As far as acute exposure is concerned, this is often work related and associated with employees in foundries, smelters, battery plants, munitions, and garages. A considerable number of reports describe lead poisoning in printers, welders, and painters.

The most common pathways for lead absorption are through the alimentary tract and the lungs, but only about 10% of ingested lead is absorbed in the gut; absorption is modulated by the vitamin D and calcium status of the individual. The lungs represent a more efficient pathway for lead absorption. The size of the inhaled particle is a major factor controlling absorption in the alveolus. As might be expected, lead in an aerosol form is absorbed with high efficiency. A minor pathway of lead absorption is through the skin. Plumbism caused by the dermal absorption of organic lead compounds has been described.

Irrespective of the absorption pathway, lead is taken up by circulating erythrocytes and bound to reactive sulfhydryl groups of proteins. From the circulation, lead is transferred to all the soft tissues, and in high concentrations it will inhibit a number of metabolic pathways. In the red cells, lead inhibits enzymes associated with hemoglobin synthesis; hence, abnormal activities of enzymes such as aminolevulinic acid dehydrogenase and intermediates such as aminolevulinic acid and protoporphyrins are frequently seen.

Systemic Aspects. Lead has a high affinity for cells in both the central and peripheral nervous system. The developing central nervous system of the child is particularly sensitive to lead. In acute poisoning, demyelination and axonal degeneration can occur. The most serious effect of lead is termed *lead encephalopathy;* mental retardation, cerebral palsy, and seizures are sequelae of survivors.

Over 90% of lead present in the body is contained within the calcified tissues. As an ion "sink," lead atoms can be adsorbed into the crystallite hydration shell or be incorporated into the crystal lattice. When incorporated into bone, lead can interfere with cellular metabolism and change the rates of bone resorption and aposition. Indeed, evidence of disturbed calcification is used as a diagnostic indicator of plumbism. Lead is also stored in the teeth, and high levels of lead are found in the outer enamel, cementum, and secondary dentine. Data from analyses of lead levels in shed primary teeth have been used to provide information on the prevalence and incidence of plumbism in children. Recent studies using dentine lead as an indicator of cumulative exposure indicate that deficits in school performance are related to the lead burden.

Oral Aspects. *Symptoms.* The oral tissues are exposed to lead through direct contact with the ingested lead and through secretion of absorbed lead into the saliva. The oral symptoms of plumbism are vague and always overshadowed by the systemic manifestations of the disease. Probably the most important symptom is metallic taste. There are reports in the literature to indicate that this may be accompanied by excessive salivation and dysphagia.

Signs. When lead exposure is high and acute and when there is poor oral hygiene, a "lead line" (see Fig. 7-10) can be seen. The line is grey-black in color and it is present along the gingival margin. The lead line is probably caused by the formation of a lead sulfide salt in the gingival crevice. Of course, if the periodontal condition is good, a lead line will not be present. Other manifestations of plumbism have also been described. These include pallor of the lips and poor muscle tone, and the face is often ashen in color because of an associated anemia. In children another type of lead line can be seen on radiographs of the skull. These radiographic densities were originally thought to be caused by the deposition of lead in the bone; however, more recent studies indicate that the lines are a lead-related interference in bone turnover and growth.

Diagnosis. Diagnosis of lead poisoning is based on clinical tests that include measurements of the whole blood lead (95% of lead in blood is found in association with red blood cells) and free erythroporphyrin levels. In the past, and still in common use are mea-

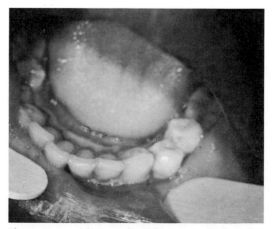

Fig. 7-10 Lead line on lingual marginal gingiva.

surements of aminolevulinic acid and aminolevulinic acid dehydratase and synthetase levels in the blood. A common indication of lead poisoning is the presence of basophilic stippling of red cells. The presence of lead in the intestinal tract and lead lines in the long bones and skull provide radiographic evidence of lead poisoning. These lead lines do not represent radiologically visible lead but rather represent deranged calcium metabolism that results from the activity of lead on osteoclastic activity and calcium resorption. Abnormal neurologic values for both the peripheral and central nervous system are also indicative of lead poisoning. When there is a question concerning the level of lead, a lead mobilization test can be used to provide an index of the lead burden. In children, additional information on the level of exposure can be gained by measurements of the tooth lead level. For adults, the hair lead concentration is commonly used as an indicator of exposure.

Treatment. As with most environmental diseases, the first step in treatment is to ascertain the source of the toxic element. The patient should then be moved away from the source; if the condition is acute and severe, lead can be removed from the body using a chelating agent such as calcium edetate (EDTA) or penicillamine. It should be emphasized that this form of treatment can have undesirable side-effects and should not be lightly undertaken.

Prognosis. The oral lesions are of secondary importance and can be eliminated once the disease has been diagnosed and treated.

Mercurialism

Mercury compounds are readily absorbed by inhalation, ingestion, injection and inunction. Mercurialism (ptyalism) develops as a result of occupational contact, drug overdosage, suicide attempts, or self-medication with mercurial compounds. With the reduction of industrial hazards, mercury intoxication has become a comparative rarity. Prolonged administration of mercurial diuretics are a potential cause of mercurialism as well as occasional agranulocytosis. The frequent use of night creams containing inorganic salts may produce a distinctive discoloration of the face, usually limited to folds of the skin and eyelids.

A mercury hazard exists in paints containing mercurial salts such as phenylmercuric propionate. These salts are incorporated in many water base paints to prevent the growth of mold.

The ingestion of mercurial compounds by children may result in a symptom complex called *acrodynia*. Cases of acrodynia have been reported from the inhalation of mercury vapors arising from paints containing mercurial salts. These paints should be appropriately labeled as being dangerous for use indoors or in poorly ventilated rooms.

The potential occupational hazard of dentists and members of the dental team from improper use of dental amalgam alloys is well known, and standards for the handling of mercury in the dental office have been developed and published in *The Journal of the American Dental Association*. The dermatitis and the stomatitis associated with amalgam fillings represent an allergic reaction to this element rather than a true intoxication.

Because of the costly damage and the danger that may result from the contact of mercury with the metal skin of an airplane, all airlines have placed an embargo on the commercial air shipment of mercury. Dentists attending postgraduate courses or clinicians should ship the mercury by other means or obtain the mercury in the city where it will be used.

The pathogenesis of the mercury line is similar to that described for bismuth, but the mercuric sulfide is more irritating to the oral tissues.

Systemic Aspects. The general symptoms of mercurialism include intestinal colic, diarrhea, headache, insomnia, tremor of the fingers, and at times, of the tongue. Renal symptoms indicate severe intoxication, and they are usually the cause of death. Long-continued exposure to mercury vapor can result in permanent neurologic changes.

Oral Aspects. *Symptoms.* A marked increase in flow of a ropy, viscid saliva is characteristic of mercurialism. The "hot mouth," the itching sensation, and the metallic taste are caused by the mercuric salts in the saliva.

The lips are dry, cracked, and swollen. A faint diffuse grayish pigmentation of the alveolar gingiva is a variable finding. Any or all of the symptoms of ANUG may be present. A marked periostitis with exfoliation of the teeth or fragments of the jaw occurs in severe cases.

Signs. Oral mucosal ulcerations are more prone to occur than in bismuth or lead intoxication, and the ulcerations are more likely to spread to the palate, the throat, and the pharynx. The tongue usually is enlarged and painful, and frequently it is ulcerated (see Figs. 7-11, 7-12, and 7-13). Along its borders are indentations produced by the teeth. The lymph and salivary glands are enlarged, and

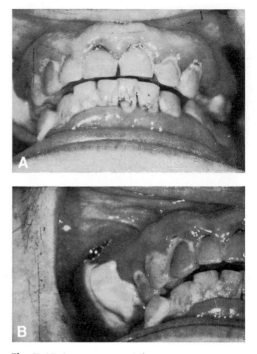

Fig. 7-12 Acute mercurial stomatitis in a 56-year-old woman resulted from therapy with this metal. *A,* Note the marked swelling and hyperemia of the gums with ulceration of the marginal gingivae. *B,* The large calcareous mass indicates the poor oral hygiene in this patient.

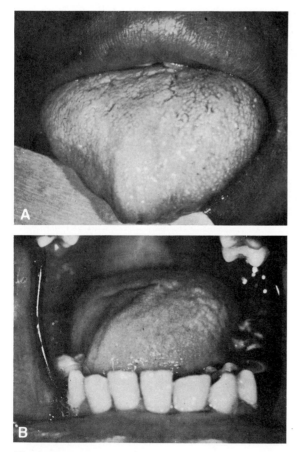

Fig. 7-11 *A,* Acute oral reaction to mercurial rubs. The marked swelling of the tongue caused it to protrude from the mouth. Also note swelling of upper lip. *B,* Same case 10 days later after the use of hot physiological saline irrigations and the cessation of mercurial rubs.

frequently the latter structures are very painful.

Rahimo and Shimasaki reported an interesting case of mercurial necrosis of the cheek in a patient receiving a mercurial diuretic. The initial differential diagnoses included diphtheria and a fungal infection.

Diagnosis. Usually, the oral symptoms overshadow the systemic complaints. In obscure cases, the saliva and the urine can be analyzed for this metal. The diagnosis is made usually on the basis of a history of occupational, therapeutic, accidental, or suicidal contact with this metal. Mucosal or gingival ulcerations in a patient who gives a history of taking a diuretic by injection should be suspected of having mercurialism. The patient's physician should be consulted, and if a mercurial diuretic is being prescribed, a nonmercurial diuretic should be substituted.

Treatment. Systemic treatment includes bedrest and a suitable dietary regimen adjusted

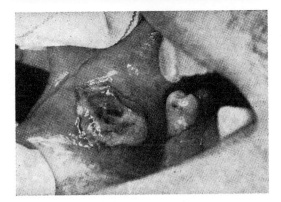

Fig. 7-13 Mercurial necrosis of the cheek. (Rahimo, Shimasaki: Oral Surg 13:55)

for the renal damage. The treatment of the oral lesions follows that described for ANUG. Extractions in the acute stage are contraindicated because extensive tissue necrosis and slough may result.

Atropine or belladonna can be prescribed to lessen the salivary flow and the corresponding mucosal irritation. Response to treatment is slow.

Prognosis. Death in acute mercurialism results usually from renal failure. In chronic intoxication the ultimate prognosis is good, although extensive destruction of the gingival tissue and even loss of the teeth may occur.

Argyria

Argyria is characterized by a permanent discoloration of the skin and the mucous membranes resulting from local or systemic absorption of silver compounds. It may result from the use of silver-containing nasal drops or sprays or formerly, silver-arsphenamine injections used to treat syphilis. Chewing pieces of photographic film over an extended period also will result in argyria of the exposed areas of the hands, the face, and the neck. In former years argyria was seen in patients with gastric ulcer who were treated with silver nitrate. This treatment is no longer used.

Signs and Symptoms. The exposed body surfaces, including the nail beds, are usually deeply discolored. Patients with argyria ap-

pear to be extremely ill, although they experience few if any subjective symptoms. The skin is slate gray, violet, or cyanotic, and in marked cases there is even a suggestion of a metallic luster. The skin discoloration may be mistaken for the cyanosis associated with heart disease. The pigmentation is distributed diffusely throughout the gingival and the mucosal tissues.

Buckley, using chemical solubility techniques and electron microscopy, demonstrated that silver-containing particles in localized argyria were silver sulfide, and that the particles were predominantly intracellular. The silver-containing compounds enter the skin through the sweat pores.

Localized argyrosis may develop following the long-continued use of topical silver-containing preparations. Pigmentation occurs early in the mouth, but it is rarely observed by the patient, since there are no systemic or local symptoms.

Diagnosis. The diagnosis of argyria is made on the objective findings and the history of occupational or therapeutic contacts with silver or its compounds. In doubtful cases biopsy studies will establish the diagnosis.

In the differential diagnosis there must be considered cyanosis of cardiac or pulmonary origin, pigmentation resulting from other metals, or disease and cyanosis due to the administration of drugs such as acetanilid. In cyanosis of cardiac or pulmonary origin or in cyanosis secondary to drug therapy, the tissues are more bluish purple in color, and there is a blanching of the tissue when the blood is forced out by pressure. This can also be determined readily by firm pressure on the fingernails.

Treatment. The source of contact with the silver compounds should be eliminated. Complicated, painful, and not too successful techniques have been described for removal of the pigmentation.

Auric Stomatitis

Gold salts are used primarily in the treatment of rheumatoid arthritis, but have also been used in lupus erythematosus, leprosy, and other dermatologic lesions that are resistant to the usual forms of treatment. Purpura and malignant neutropenia have been reported occasionally following gold therapy, but dermatitis and stomatitis are the most commonly observed toxic reactions. They occur in from 10% to 40% of the patients who receive intensive gold therapy. Vesiculation and ulceration of the oral mucosal and the gingival tissues occur in the more acute reactions.

The diagnosis of auric or gold stomatitis is made on the basis of the therapeutic administration of gold compounds and the exclusion of other diseases known to cause similar symptoms. The treatment of auric stomatitis consists of the discontinuance of the auric therapy and palliatively, a mildly alkaline mouthwash.

Arsenic

Most patients with arsenism have developed it from industrial exposure or accidental or intentional poisoning. Chronic gastritis and colitis are frequently the only symptoms. Keratosis of the palms of the hands and the soles of the feet is commonly observed. Dermatitis, pigmentation, or ulcerations of the skin may develop from long-continued arsenic therapy such as with Fowler's solution.

Oral Aspects. The symptoms of arsenic stomatitis are similar to those experienced in mercurial stomatitis. The oral tissues are extremely painful, and they are deep red in color. In contrast with mercurialism, the mouth in arsenic stomatitis is dry.

Treatment. The treatment of arsenic burns or periostitis is unsatisfactory. A surface anesthetic ointment or rinse such as lidocaine or dyclonine solution can be used for symptomatic treatment of soft-tissue lesions.

Stomatitis Due to Copper, Chromium, Cadmium, or Zinc

Exposure to copper compounds may result in the development of a bluish green line of the gingiva and the teeth. Frequently, the tooth discoloration is permanent because of the etching of the enamel. Chronic increased intake of copper salts may be associated with the development of anemia.

Chrome platers are exposed to a fine spray of chromic acid that is irritating and corrosive to the mucous membranes of the nose and the throat. Burning, soreness, and dryness of the mouth associated with swelling of the tongue have been reported by Lieberman and may precede painful ulcerations of the nasal septum, which frequently result in perforation. The oral lesions are usually confined to those portions of the mouth that come in contact with the chromic acid spray, but multiple ulcers may appear on the oral mucosa. The teeth may become etched and show a persistent deep orange stain. Similar symptoms and lesions have also been reported in cadmium platers.

Zinc intoxication is an occupational hazard in galvanizers, zinc oxide and molten brass workers, and at times, electric arc welders. The acute symptoms are similar to an anaphylactic response with chills, fever, sweating, a rapid pulse, nausea, vomiting, and dryness and burning of the upper respiratory tract. Chronic zinc stomatitis is characterized by congestion and suppuration of the gingival tissues with a bluish gray line and a metallic taste. The teeth may become loose due to destruction of the alveolar process, although little pain is experienced. Painful submaxillary lymph node and salivary gland involvement does occur however.

Phosphorus Poisoning

The outstanding symptom of phosphorus poisoning ("phossy jaw") is a periostitis and an osteomyelitis of the jaws—usually the mandible. A localized area of necrosis may develop at the site of an injury, a retained root, a decayed tooth, or a periodontal pocket. It is accompanied by pain and at times by a garliclike odor. The necrotic process may spread to involve a large portion of the jaw. Rapid disintegration of the teeth has also been noted.

The osteomyelitis is extremely resistant to treatment. Once this process heals, however, there appears to be no contraindication to placing tissue-bearing dentures on the healed tissues.

The oral hygiene of all phosphorus workers should be maintained in the best possible state. If surgical procedures are indicated on involved tissue, heavy prophylactic antibiotic therapy is indicated. Extreme care should be taken when the surgery is performed to prevent unnecessary trauma to the hard and the soft tissues.

BIBLIOGRAPHY

Aberder DN: Oral contraceptives and dental care. Br Med J 4:417, 1967

Buckley WR, et al: Localized argyria. Arch Dermatol 92:697, 1965

Cohen GJ, Ahrens WE: Chronic lead poisoning. J Pediatr 54:271, 1959

Egorin MJ, Trump DL, Wainwright CW: Quinacrine ochronosis and rheumatoid arthritis. JAMA 236:385, 1976

Frantzis TG et al: Oral manifestations of hemochromatosis. Oral Surg 33:186, 1972

Heinmann H: Chronic phosphorus poisoning. Indust Hygiene Toxicol 28:142, 1946

Hirschfeld I, Hirschfeld L: Oral pigmentation and a method of removing it. Oral Surg 4:1012, 1951

Hirschman SS et al: Mercury in house paint as a cause of acrodynia. JAMA 269:889, 1963

Kehoe RA: Lead absorption and lead poisoning. Med Clin North Am 26:1261, 1942

Kopito L et al: Chronic plumbism in children. JAMA 209:243, 1969

Levine SA, Smith JA: Argyria confused with heart disease. N Engl J Med 226:682, 1942

Lieberman H: Chrome ulcerations of the nose and throat. N Engl J Med 225:132, 1941

Lynn BD: "The pill" as an etiologic agent in hypertrophic gingivitis. J Oral Surg 24:333, 1967

Needleman HL (ed): Low Level Lead Exposure. New York, Raven Press, 1980

Needleman HL, Davidson I, Sewell EM, Shapiro IM: Subclinical lead exposure in Philadelphia school children. N Engl J Med 290:245–248, 1974

Patterson CC: Contamination and natural lead environments of man. Arch Environ Health 11:344, 1965

Plack W, Bellizzi R: Generalized argyria secondary to chewing photographic film. Oral Surg 49:504, 1980

Rahimo AA, Shimasaki WW: Mercurial necrosis of the cheek. Oral Surg 13:54, 1960

Resnik S: Melasma induced by oral contraceptive drugs. JAMA 199:601, 1967

Rohrs LC: Intestinal polyposis and pigmented spots of lips. JAMA 165:208, 1957

Ross EM: Argyria caused by chewing of photographic film. N Engl J Med 269:798, 1963

Ross E: First symposium on oral pigmentation. J Periodontol 31:345, 1960

Simpson TH: Mucocutaneous pigmentation: Peutz-Jeghers syndrome? Oral Surg 17:331, 1964

Spencer MC: Topical use of hydroquinone for depigmentation. JAMA 194:114, 1965

Spiegel L: Discoloration of skin and mucous membrane resembling argyria, following use of bismuth and silver arsphenamine. Arch Dermatol Syph 23:266, 1931

Toto PD: Neurofibromatosis. Oral Surg 7:423, 1954

Trodahl JN, Sprague WG: Benign and malignant melanocytic lesions of oral mucosa. Cancer 25:812, 1970

Tuffanelli D, Abraham RK, Dubois EI: Pigmentation from antimalarial therapy. Arch Dermatol 88:419, 1963

Waldron HA, Stofen D: Subclinical Lead Poisoning. New York, Academic Press, 1974

Zegarelli EV: Melanin spots of the oral mucosa and skin associated with polyps. Oral Surg 7:972, 1954

Zegarelli EV et al: An atlas of oral lesions observed in the syndrome of oral melanosis with associated intestinal polyposis. Oral Surg 15:411, 1962

8

Benign Tumors of the Oral Cavity, Including Gingival Enlargements

VERNON J. BRIGHTMAN

This chapter is concerned with the clinical features, diagnostic characteristics, and management of localized, nonmalignant growths of the oral cavity and adjacent tissues. A variety of lesions of miscellaneous etiologies are discussed, only some of which are properly classified as true neoplasms. Malignant tumors are discussed in Chapter 9 (Oral Cancer); normal structures, sometimes mistakenly identified as tumors, in this chapter and in Chapters 10 and 17; and leukoplakia and some other persistent epithelial lesions that are only slightly raised above the mucosal surface, in Chapter 6 (Red and White Lesions). This chapter is organized into sections dealing with the following:

1. Normal structural variants
2. Inflammatory hyperplasias
3. Hamartomas
4. Cysts of the jaws and benign odontogenic tumors
5. Salivary cysts and benign tumors of the salivary glands
6. Benign viral-induced oral tumors
7. Syndromes with benign oral neoplastic or hamartomatous components
8. Gingival enlargements
9. Cervicofacial actinomycosis

IMPORTANCE OF BIOPSY

Although some of the lesions discussed in this chapter, if untreated, will lead to extensive tissue destruction and deformity and others interfere with mastication and become secondarily infected following masticatory trauma, the major clinical consideration in the management of these tumors is to identify their benign nature and to distinguish them from potentially life-threatening malignant lesions. Since this decision usually can be made with certainty only by microscopic examination of excised tissue, biopsy (see Chaps. 3 and 9) is an important and even essential step in the treatment of many of the lesions discussed in this chapter.

Only if excisional biopsy (removal of the entire lesion) will itself lead to mutilation and deformity should consideration be given to retaining these lesions. In such cases, incisional biopsy (removal of a representative sample of the lesion with a scalpel or electro-cautery) is mandatory. For example, excisional biopsy is rarely carried out in the case of fibrous dysplasia of the jaws and hemangioma, because of the extent of the lesion, and in the case of hemangioma, because of the possibility of severe hemorrhage. Large cysts in the body and ramus of the mandible are also often marsupialized rather than curetted, due to the likelihood of fracture of thinned bony plates. However, in both cases a small sample of tissue should be excised for histologic examination. A small minority of the growths described in this chapter will undergo shrinkage and regression with time, as occurs with some inflammatory hyperplasias (clinical fibroma, pyogenic granuloma, pregnancy epulis) when inflammatory or hormonal stimuli contributing to the lesion subside. However, the majority either remain static or increase in size (expand), if they are untreated or incompletely removed.

Excisional biopsy has the additional advantage that in most circumstances the lesion is removed permanently and does not remain as a constant source of anxiety to both patient and dentist. When a lesion is only partially excised, even after microscopic examination of an incisional biopsy specimen has failed to reveal any evidence of malignancy, the problem of whether the biopsy specimen was a representative sample remains. Further biopsy may be necessary, particularly if the lesion alters in appearance and character after biopsy. Paradoxically, management of extensive benign lesions of the oral cavity that cannot be thoroughly removed by excision, electrocoagulation, or cryotherapy, is often more difficult than management of localized lesions of more aggressive nature that can be "cured" by surgery. This problem is caused by the anxiety regarding oral cancer that often develops when a visible lesion is left in a patient's mouth. Attempts at reassuring a patient that a lesion is benign are often futile as long as it remains as a daily reminder whenever he examines his mouth or explores (and magnifies the size of) the lesion with his tongue. Symptoms associated with the lesion and changes in its appearance as a result of trauma further reinforce the patient's belief that he has a progressively enlarging and perhaps invasive lesion.

On the other hand, anxiety that a chronic

oral lesion may be cancerous is not unreasonable. Epidemiologic studies of oral cancer support the belief that early diagnosis and treatment reduce the high death rate from this cause and also emphasize the nonspecific appearance of many early oral cancers. Over 7,000 deaths from oral cancer occur annually in the United States, and one of every three persons with intraoral cancer dies within 5 years. It has been predicted that as many as 80% of all oral cancer deaths could be prevented by early recognition of the disease. Among the reasons for the delay in recognizing oral cancer is the fact that it may present as a benign-appearing lesion, and receive either conservative (nonsurgical) treatment or no treatment for a considerable time before its true nature is recognized. All surgeons are aware of patients in whom an oral lesion was considered to be the result of chronic irritation for many months, during which it enlarged, invaded neighboring tissue, and revealed its true cancerous nature. Such unfortunate occurrences emphasize the need for all oral growths to be considered cancer until proven otherwise by microscopic examination of a representative biopsy. Lesions that have been classified as benign by histopathologic study should also be rebiopsied if they change in character, increase rapidly in size, or if in the opinion of the responsible dentist or physician, their appearance and behavior appear to contradict their histologically benign structure. For the majority of benign oral growths, exfoliative cytology is of little help in determining whether the benign appearance of the lesion may hide malignant cells, and it is no substitute for biopsy in these circumstances.

Given the desirability of biopsy (and if possible, complete excision) of all benign tumors of the oral cavity (as has been argued in the preceding paragraphs), the question remains of how soon the biopsy should be done. When done immediately after the lesion is observed, any risk of the patient's not returning for the biopsy is eliminated; but this advantage should be weighed against the possibility that such aggressive treatment may frighten the patient and reduce the chance of his returning for essential follow-up studies. Likewise, when a patient is referred to a surgeon for diagnosis and treatment of an oral tumor or cyst, the dentist should follow the referral with a telephone call to determine that the patient appeared for the consultation. When the lesion is very likely the result of chronic irritation (e.g., in the case of a suspected inflammatory hyperplasia or periapical cyst), the logical first step is removal of the irritant, delaying the biopsy for some time following complete removal of the suspected irritant (e.g., 1 to 2 weeks in the case of an inflammatory hyperplasia and 3 to 6 months in the case of a periapical cyst) to determine whether the lesion regresses.

Biopsy should not be delayed, if any of the following are noted: rapid increase in the size of the lesion (that cannot be convincingly explained by inflammation, edema, and opening of new vascular channels as with some hemangiomas and lymphangiomas, or by a generalized growth spurt, as with some hamartomas); absence of any recognized irritant, particularly where the lesion is chronically ulcerated or hemorrhages spontaneously; presence of firm regional lymph nodes, especially where they seem fixed to surrounding tissue; destruction of tooth roots and loosening of teeth; and evidence of rapid expansion of the jaw with lifting of the periosteum and production of a "sunray" effect radiographically. Further justifications for prompt biopsy are a history of cancer elsewhere in the body, previous history of oral cancer and radiation therapy to the oral cavity.

Many benign oral tumors can be identified with some degree of certainty from their clinical and radiographic appearances and their behavior, but it is hazardous to rely on these criteria alone. Microscopic examination of biopsied tissue not only convincingly confirms a lesion's benign nature but also provides for its accurate identification. All excised tissue should always be submitted for histopathologic examination, and in the case of oral lesions it is important that the examining pathologist be familiar with the characteristics of oral lesions. For instance, pseudoepitheliomatous hyperplasia (see below) that is found in association with several oral lesions is often mistakenly identified as carcinomatous infiltration, and the wide variety of odontogenic neoplasms frequently proves a puzzle even for experienced oral pathologists.

Benign oral tumors can also serve as a clue

to predisposition to various systemic malignancies, even when the oral lesion itself carries no premalignant potential. Accurate histologic identification of an oral lesion (*e.g.*, odontogenic keratocyst, multiple osteomas, a neurofibroma, or papillomatosis) may be the first step in the recognition of a syndrome that includes a high risk of carcinoma in another organ (see Syndromes with Benign Oral Neoplastic or Hamartomatous Components). If the findings of the oral biopsy are clear-cut and unequivocal, further diagnostic procedures and even exploratory surgery may be justified to eliminate the possibility of an associated malignancy elsewhere in the body. In a similar fashion, giant cell lesions of the jaw bone occasionally can lead to the discovery of parathyroid tumors or hyperplasia.

NORMAL STRUCTURAL VARIANTS

Structural variations of the jaw bones and overlying oral soft tissues are sometimes mistakenly identified as tumors. Overly anxious individuals with otherwise unexplained oral symptoms frequently make this error (see also Chap. 17), but in most cases, a dentist with some experience will recognize the suspected lesion as within the range of normal variation for the oral cavity and be able to reassure the patient. Biopsy in these cases is rarely indicated. Examples of such structural variants are ectopic lymphoid nodules (small, slightly reddish nodular elevations of a localized area of the oral mucosa as distinct from the pharyngeal mucosa); tori (see below); a pronounced retromolar pad remaining after extraction of the last molar teeth; localized nodular connective-tissue thickening of the attached gingiva; the papilla associated with the opening of Stensen's duct; vallate and other papillary projections of the tongue dorsum; and lingual varicosities in older individuals.

Localized nodular enlargements of the cortical bone of the palate (*torus palatinus*; see Figs. 8-1*A*, *B*, and *D*) and jaws (*torus mandibularis*; see Fig. 8-1*C*) occur frequently and are usually considered normal structural variants of these bones and analagous to the spurs that are frequently encountered on other bones (*e.g.*, on the malleoli of the tibia and fibula). The lack of obvious irritants for most tori and their negligible growth after an initial slow but steady period of development also suggest that tori are in most cases neither inflammatory hyperplasias nor neoplasms. Histologically, tori consist of layers of dense cortical bone covered by a thin epithelium with minimal rete-peg development. Clinically, they can be insignificant, or quite important lesions; however, patients are often concerned that such nodular growths represent a neoplasm.

Tori may pose a severe mechanical problem in the construction of dentures, and as a result of their prominent position and thin epithelial covering, they are frequently traumatized, and the resulting ulcers are slow to heal. Rarely, tori on the palate or lingual mandibular ridge may become sufficiently large to interfere with eating and speaking. Unless a torus is exceptionally large, its surgical removal when dictated by a patient's anxiety or mechanical concerns is not a major procedure provided splints or stents are fabricated beforehand to provide a protective dressing during healing.

Similar nodular growths may also be seen from time to time on the buccal aspect of the maxillary and mandibular alveolae and must be differentiated from bony hyperplasia secondary to a chronic periapical abscess. Nodular bony enlargements of the alveolus also can occur in fibrous dysplasia and Paget's disease, where they represent superficial evidence of a more generalized bony dysplasia.

INFLAMMATORY HYPERPLASIAS

The term *inflammatory hyperplasia* is frequently used to describe a large range of commonly occurring nodular growths of the oral mucosa that histologically resemble inflammatory granulation tissue. This resemblance may be greater or lesser depending on the degree to which one or more of the components of the inflammatory reaction and healing response are exaggerated in the particular lesion. Some appear to be predominantly epithelial overgrowths with only scanty connective tissue stroma; others are fibromatous with minimal epithelial covering and may exhibit either angiomatous, desmoid (collagenous), or fibroblastic features. In many lesions, different sections may reveal examples

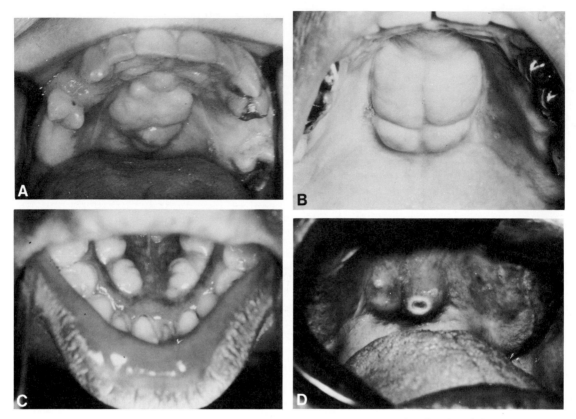

Fig. 8-1 Torus palatinus (*A* and *B*) and torus mandibularis (*C*) are common localized nodular enlargements of the cortical bone of the palate and jaws, usually considered to be normal structural variants of these bones. When traumatized, the resulting ulcers (*D*) are often slow to heal because of the dense relatively avascular bone in these lesions and their susceptibility to recurrent trauma.

of each of these histologic patterns. Like scar tissue, some inflammatory hyperplasias appear to mature and become less vascular (paler and less friable) and more collagenous (firmer and smaller) with time. Others appear to have almost unlimited ability for exophytic growth until they are excised.

This variability of histologic appearance is reflected in the wide range of clinical characteristics that inflammatory hyperplasias show and in the clinical names many of them have acquired, suggesting a specific etiology or natural history. Names such as (clinical) "fibroma" and "papilloma" are therefore often used to describe these lesions, even though there is no evidence to suggest that they have a neoplastic etiology. The major etiologic factor for these lesions is generally assumed to be chronic trauma (such as that produced by ill-fitting dentures, calculus,

overhanging dental restorations, and fractured teeth) and in many cases chronic irritants can be convincingly demonstrated (*e.g.*, palatal papillary hyperplasia). In some (*e.g.*, pregnancy epulis, and the central giant cell tumor associated with hyperparathyroidism), the level of circulating hormones also undoubtedly plays a role. The majority occur on the surface of the oral mucous membrane where irritants are quite frequent. Two deeper lesions (pseudosarcomatous fasciitis and giant cell reparative granuloma of bone) are also classified as inflammatory hyperplasias on the basis of their histologic structure and clinical behavior.

As surface outgrowths of the oral mucous membrane, most inflammatory hyperplasias are subject to continual masticatory trauma and frequently are ulcerated and hemorrhagic. Dilated blood vessels, acute and chronic inflammatory exudates, and localized abscesses are additional reasons for the swollen, distended, red to purple, "overripe," "inflamed" appearance of some inflammatory hyperplasias. Epithelial hyperplasia frequently produces a lesion with a textured surface or an area of mucosa resembling carpet pile. Erosion of the underlying cortical bone rarely occurs with inflammatory hyperplasia of the oral mucosa; and when it is noted, there should be a strong suspicion that a malignancy is involved, and a section of the affected bone should be included with the biopsy specimen.

Provided the chronic irritant is eliminated at the time the lesion is excised, the majority of inflammatory hyperplasias will not recur, thereby confirming the benign nature of these lesions as would be expected from their histologic structure. On the other hand, on rare occasions the oral surgeon and oral pathologist are confronted by recurrent lesions with an unusually aggressive growth rate that histologically show an abundance of young, proliferating, epithelial, fibroblastic, or endothelial cells. Differentiation of these lesions from carcinoma and sarcoma is not always easy on either clinical or histologic grounds, and the surgeon may be justified in excising a block of tissue surrounding the lesion rather than simply trimming the recurrent growth. In these situations, experience with the particular type of inflammatory hyperplasia involved is critical for both surgeon and pathologist, since some oral hyperplasias show neoplastic tendencies much more than others.

The following are all examples of inflammatory hyperplasias; fibrous inflammatory hyperplasias (clinical fibroma, papilloma, epulis fissuratum, and pulp polyp); palatal papillary hyperplasia; pyogenic granuloma; pregnancy epulis; giant cell reparative granuloma (giant cell epulis and central giant cell tumor of the jaw); pseudosarcomatous fasciitis; and pseudoepitheliomatous hyperplasia.

Fibrous Inflammatory Hyperplasia

Fibrous inflammatory hyperplasia may occur on any surface of the oral mucous membrane as either pedunculated or sessile (broadbased) growths (Fig. 8-2). They are more likely to be identified as papillomas if they are pedunculated and keratinized, and as fibromas if they are sessile, firm, and covered by thin squamous epithelium. On the gingiva, a similar lesion is often referred to as an epulis (plural, epulides), that is, a growth on the gum (Fig. 8-3). The majority remain small, and lesions more than 1 cm in diameter are rare on the cheeks, tongue, and floor of the mouth, possibly because masticatory trauma restricts their size through necrosis and ulceration. An exception to this rule occurs in the case of lesions associated with the periphery of ill-fitting dentures, the so-called *epulis fissuratum*, because the growth is often split by the edge of the denture, one part of the lesion lying under the denture and the other between the lip or cheek and the outer denture surface. This lesion may extend the full length of one side of the denture. Many such hyperplastic growths will become less edematous and inflamed following removal of the associated chronic irritant, but they rarely resolve entirely. In the preparation of the mouth to receive dentures, these lesions are excised to prevent further irritation and to ensure a soft-tissue seal for the denture periphery. *Pulp polyps* (chronic hyperplastic pulpitis) are an analogous condition involving the pulpal connective tissue, which proliferates through a large pulpal exposure and fills the cavity in the tooth with a mushroom-shaped polyp connected by a stalk to the pulp chamber. Masticatory pressure usually leads to keratinization of the epithelial covering of these lesions. Characteristically, pulp polyps (like granulation tissue) contain few sensory nerve fibers and are remarkably insensitive. This feature distinguishes them from hyperplastic overgrowths of the gingiva, which may also produce a polypoid mass filling a tooth cavity and are usually quite sensitive to pressure and curettage. The superstructure of teeth affected by pulp polyps is usually so badly destroyed by caries that endodontic treatment is not considered; however, when mechanical considerations do not preclude it, root canal therapy can be satisfactorily completed on these teeth following extirpation of the polyp and remaining pulp tissue.

Differential diagnosis of fibrous inflammatory hyperplasias should include consideration of the possibility that the lesion is a true papilloma (a cauliflowerlike mass made up of

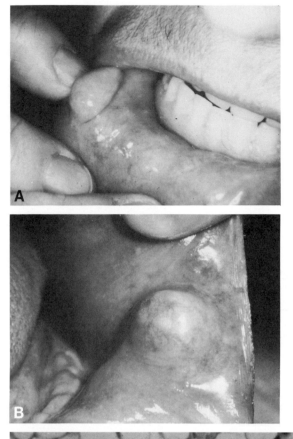

multiple fingerlike projections of stratified squamous epithelium with a central core of vascular connective tissue) or a small verrucous carcinoma. It should also be remembered that multiple oral papillomatous lesions may be viral induced (*i.e.*, warts) or one feature of a syndrome with more serious manifestations in other organs (*e.g.*, acanthosis nigricans or ichthyosis hystrix). On the dorsal surface of the tongue, nodular lesions may represent scars, neurofibroma, and myoblastoma, as well as fibrous inflammatory hyperplasias. Both pedunculated and broad-based nodules on the pharyngeal surface of the tongue are usually lymphoid nodules or cystic dilatations of mucous gland ducts (see Figure 10-3C).

Fibrous inflammatory hyperplasias probably have no malignant potential, and recurrences following excision are almost always a result of failure to eliminate the particular form of chronic irritation involved. The occasional report of squamous cell carcinoma arising in an area of chronic denture irritation, however, underlines the fact that no oral growth, even those associated with an obvious chronic irritant, can be assumed to be benign until proven so by histologic study.

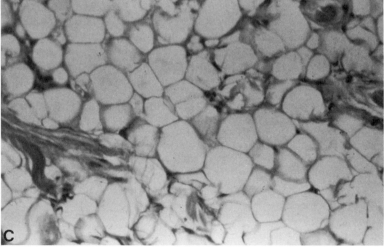

Fig. 8-2 *A*, Pedunculated fibrous inflammatory hyperplasia of the cheek possibly associated with dental trauma. *B* and *C*, A comparable soft nodular swelling of the lip, which on biopsy proved to be a small benign growth made up of mature fat cells (lipoma). (*B* and *C*, Courtesy of Gary Cohen, D.M.D., Philadelphia, PA)

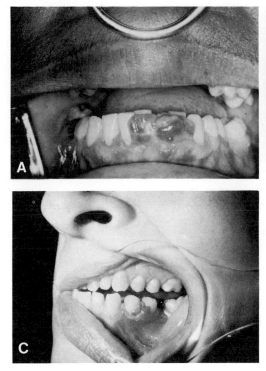

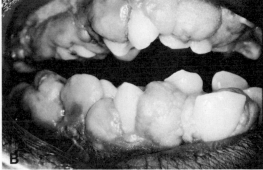

Fig. 8-3 Three examples of inflammatory hyperplasia affecting the gingiva. *A,* A fibrous epulis associated with calculus. *B,* Generalized hyperplasia of the gingivae as a result of local irritants in a brain-damaged child maintained on phenytoin (Dilantin). *C,* A pregnancy epulis in an otherwise healthy dental arch; oral hygiene was excellent and the epulis was associated with a "food-pack" area that developed after loss of the mandibular first molar. The lesion resolved after delivery.

In other words, where possible, all fibrous inflammatory hyperplasias of the oral cavity should be treated by local excision.

Palatal Papillary Hyperplasia

Palatal papillary hyperplasia (also known as palatal epithelial hyperplasia, or palatal papillomatosis) is a common lesion with a characteristic clinical appearance that develops on the hard palate in response to chronic denture irritation in approximately 3% to 4% of denture wearers. Full dentures in which relief areas or "suction chambers" are cut in the palatal seating surface appear to be the strongest stimuli for the lesion, but it is also seen under partial dentures, and occasional care reports have described the lesion in patients who have never worn dentures. A similar lesion is sometimes seen on the lingual alveolar mucosa under a lower denture.

The palatal lesion is usually associated with some degree of denture stomatitis due to chronic candidal infection, which influences the appearance of the papillary hyperplasia. When so complicated by candidal infection, the lesion may be red to scarlet in appear-

ance, and the swollen, tightly packed projections resemble the surface of an overripe berry. Such lesions are friable, often bleed with minimal trauma, and may be covered with a thin whitish exudate. When the candidal infection is eliminated, either by removing the denture or by topical administration of an antifungal agent, the papillary lesion becomes little different in color from the rest of the palate and consists of more or less tightly packed nodular projections. If tiny, the nodular projections simply give a feltlike texture to that portion of the palate, and the lesion may even pass unnoticed unless it is stroked with an instrument or disturbed by a jet of air. If larger, the polypoid projections are obvious, and the patient is usually aware of the condition.

The microscopic appearance of these lesions is little different from that of "papillomas" elsewhere in the mouth, although the degree of branching and polypoid proliferation that develops on the epithelial surface occluded by the denture is often quite surprising. Low-power examination of these lesions demonstrates their exophytic nature, and neither epithelial invasion of the submucosa nor resorption of the palatine bone occurs, even under large or long-standing lesions. Despite their sometimes bizarre clinical appearance, these lesions appear to have almost no neoplastic potential, a finding that is borne out by the absence of atypia and cellular dysplasia in biopsy specimens. Since squamous cell carcinoma is also extremely rare on the palate, surgical removal of palatal papillary hyperplasia would not appear to be mandatory.

Where surgical preparation of the alveolar ridges is carried out prior to making new dentures, papillary hyperplasia lesions are usually excised or cauterized, and the old denture or a palatal splint is used to maintain a surgical dressing over the denuded area postoperatively. Small lesions are often left intact and may disappear after a new denture has been worn for some time. There is no evidence that astringent or antibacterial mouthrinses or salves will control these lesions, but they may shrink considerably and become less inflamed with use of topical antifungal agents to eliminate the superimposed *Candida*-induced denture stomatitis.

When florid papillomatosis of the palate occurs or persists in the absence of dentures, consideration should also be given in the differential diagnosis to the several granulomatous or chronic infectious diseases that may manifest intraorally in this fashion (*e.g.*, sarcoid, leprosy, the Melkersson–Rosenthal syndrome, blastomycosis, and histoplasmosis, especially where both ulceration and papillary lesions occur together).

Pyogenic Granuloma

Pyogenic granuloma is a small, pedunculated, hemorrhagic nodule that occurs most frequently on the gingiva and has a strong tendency to recur following simple excision. Chronic irritation localized to these lesions may sometimes be hard to identify, but the fact that they are usually located close to the gingival margin suggests that calculus and overhanging margins of dental restorations are important irritants that should be eliminated when the lesion is excised. Their friable, hemorrhagic, and frequently ulcerated appearance results from their histologic structure; they are composed largely of proliferated endothelial tissue, much of which is canalized into a rich vascular network with minimal collagenous support. Polymorphs, as well as chronic inflammatory cells, are consistently present throughout the edematous stoma with microabscess formation. A frank discharge of pus is not present, however (despite the common name for the lesion), and where it occurs, one is probably dealing with a fistula from an underlying periodontal or periapical abscess the opening of which is often marked by a nodule of granulation tissue.

Identical lesions with the same histologic structure occur in association with the florid gingivitis and periodontitis that may complicate pregnancy. Under these circumstances, the lesions are referred to as *pregnancy epulis (or tumor)*; see Fig. 8-3C. The increased prevalence of pregnancy epulides toward the end of pregnancy when levels of circulating estrogens are highest, and the tendency for these lesions to shrink after delivery (when there is a precipitous drop in circulating estrogens) indicate a definite role for these hormones in the etiology of the lesion. Like pregnancy gingivitis, these lesions do not occur in mouths that are kept scrupulously free of even minor gingival irritation, and local irritation is clearly also an important etiologic factor. The relatively minor degree of chronic irritation that may be necessary to produce a pregnancy epulis is worth noting, however.

There is some evidence that both pyogenic granuloma and pregnancy epulis may mature and become less vascular and more collagenous, gradually converting to a fibrous epulis. Similar lesions also occur intraorally in extragingival locations. Histologically, differentiation from hemangioma (see below) is important.

The existence of these lesions always indicates the need for a periodontal consultation, and treatment should include elimination of subgingival irritants and gingival "pockets" throughout the mouth as well as excision of the gingival growth. Small isolated pregnancy tumors occurring in a mouth that is otherwise in excellent gingival health sometimes may be observed for resolution following delivery, but the size of the lesion, episodes of hemorrhage or superimposed acute necrotizing ulcerative gingivitis, and the presence of a generalized pregnancy gingivitis usually dictate treatment during pregnancy. When possible, surgical and periodontal treatment should be completed during the second trimester with continued surveillance of home care until after delivery.

Giant Cell Granuloma

Giant cell granuloma occurs either as a peripheral lesion on the gingiva (giant cell epulis, osteoclastoma, peripheral giant cell reparative granuloma) or as a centrally located lesion within the jaw bone that radiographically appears "cystlike" (see Figs. 8-4 and 8-5). Both types of lesions are histologically similar and are considered examples of benign inflammatory hyperplasia in which cells with fibroblastic, osteoblastic, and osteoclastic potentials predominate. The lesions are also highly vascular; hemorrhage is a prominent clinical and histologic feature and also contributes a brown stain to the rarer central lesions. These lesions may appear under the stimulus of increased circulating parathormone (primary and secondary hyperparathyroidism) or in the presence of normal levels of the hormone. True giant cell neoplasms, such as the giant cell tumor that occurs in the humerus and femur, rarely occur in the jaw and usually only as a complication of Paget's disease.

Peripheral giant cell granulomas are five times as common as central lesions. Central lesions occur preferentially in the mandible, anterior to the first molar, and often cross the midline. Several large series of both peripheral and central giant cell granulomas have been reported in the literature, and their histologic structure has been studied in detail (Figs. 8-4B, C, 8-6 and 8-8).

Since some degree of bony destruction usually accompanies even small peripheral giant cell granulomas, treatment of both peripheral and central lesions requires referral to an oral surgeon. Another important consideration in the management of these lesions is the necessity to search for evidence of hyperparathyroidism in all patients with histologically confirmed giant cell lesions of the jaw. There are documented examples of parathyroid lesions having been discovered as a result of blood and urine chemistry studies requested by a dentist following diagnosis of a giant cell lesion. The frequency with which this is likely to happen has not been

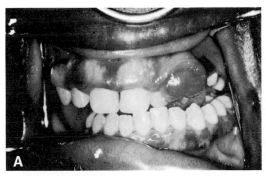

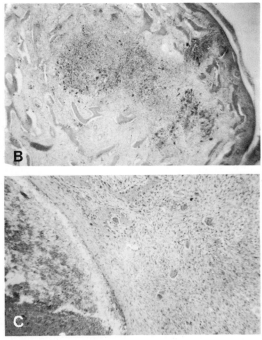

Fig. 8-4 Giant cell reparative granuloma (peripheral giant cell tumor); an example of an inflammatory hyperplasia featuring osteoblastic and osteoclastic proliferation with a vascular stroma. The lesion in this case was not associated with evidence of hyperparathyroidism. A, Clinical appearance of the lesion. B and C, Low- and higher-power views of stained sections from the lesion.

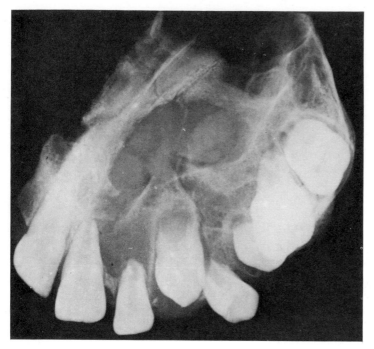

Fig. 8-5 An active giant cell tumor; roentgenograph of a surgical specimen. (Courtesy of J.E. Hamner III, D.D.S., Ph.D., Washington, DC)

calculated, however, and is probably quite low since in most series of cases of hyperparathyroidism, lesions of the jaw have been among the last clinical manifestations of the disease to appear. Fewer than 10% of patients with hyperparathyroidism have radiographically visible cystic jaw lesions (Fig. 8-7) or even "loss of the lamina dura" (another effect of hyperparathyroidism often used clinically to screen for the disease). Since the cost of serum calcium, phosphorus, and alkaline phosphatase determinations is not great, they should be requested prior to surgical removal of a jaw bone lesion that radiographically is compatible with a giant cell granuloma and immediately following the histologic diagnosis of giant cell granuloma in either central or peripherally located lesions. Any abnormality in these determinations would justify further medical or endocrinologic consultation, at which time the need for specific measurement of parathormone levels could be determined (see also Chapter 3).

In large lesions of the jaw bone, the chance that a biopsy specimen is not representative of the entire lesion is quite high. Removal of a section of bone and tumor is technically difficult, and the pathologist is usually supplied with multiple small fragments curetted from the bony cavity rather than a solid specimen. In interpreting the results of the biopsy, therefore, consideration should be given to the possibility that the granulomatous, giant cell-containing tissue observed microscopically does not represent simply a normal reparative response to some other bone lesion rather than an inflammatory hyperplasia. Areas of osteoclastic activity are also found in many other bone lesions, and a firm diagnosis of a large centrally located jaw-bone lesion may not be obtained until the lesion has been removed and examined thoroughly by the pathologist.

Pseudosarcomatous Fasciitis

Pseudosarcomatous fasciitis, a nonneoplastic connective tissue proliferation, usually occurs on the trunk or extremities as a rapidly growing nodule that histologically imitates a malignant mesenchymal neoplasm but clinically behaves as benign. Many cases are originally diagnosed as sarcoma, although published series of cases suggest that certain histologic features may help to identify this entity and confirm its hyperplastic nature. Similar le-

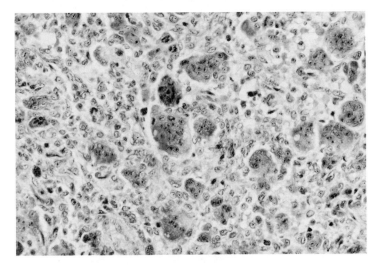

Fig. 8-6 A benign giant cell tumor. H&E stain ×250 (Courtesy of J.E. Hamner III, D.D.S., Ph.D., Washington, DC)

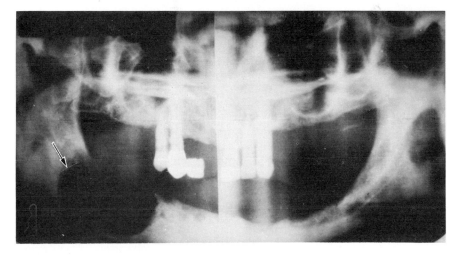

Fig. 8-7 Panorex roentgenograph of a hyperparathyroid tumor at the angle of the right mandible (*arrow*). (Courtesy of J.E. Hamner III, D.D.S., Ph.D., Washington, DC)

sions have been described in the head and neck regions but apparently not intraorally.

Pseudoepitheliomatous Hyperplasia

Pseudoepitheliomatous hyperplasia is a rather common exuberant response of oral epithelium to chronic irritation in which the rete pegs are extended in an irregular fashion deep into the underlying connective tissue. Keratin pearl formation may be prominent, but other signs of cellular atypia characteristic of carcinoma are absent. Neutrophilic infiltration about the elongated rete pegs is also prominent in contrast with carcinoma. Sections may show isolated clumps of epithelial cells in the depth of the lesion, but these are apparently due to the plane of sectioning cutting across long, narrow rete pegs, and true neoplastic invasion does not occur.

Clinically, lesions exhibiting pseudoepitheliomatous hyperplasia may be indistinguishable from epidermoid carcinoma, and if unnecessary surgery and radiation are to avoided, the pathologist diagnosing the biopsy must be familiar with the existence of this bizarre type of epithelial hyperplasia that is relatively common in the oral cavity. Even

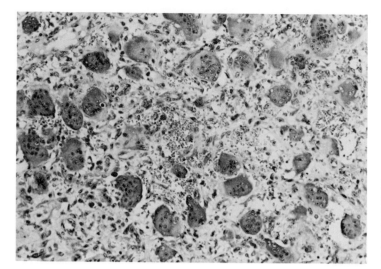

Fig. 8-8 Tumor seen with hyperparathyroidism. (Hematoxylin and eosin [H&E] ×160). Compare with Figures 8-4C and 8-6. (Courtesy of J. E. Hamner III, D.D.S., Ph.D., Washington, DC)

so, differentiation of this lesion is not always easy, and experienced oral pathologists may be hesitant in deciding whether a particular lesion features this change or is, in fact, a carcinoma.

Two oral lesions (the *granular cell myoblastoma of the tongue* and the *keratoacanthoma of the lip*), which are described later in this chapter, also characteristically exhibit pseudoepitheliomatous hyperplasia along the periphery of the lesion, and errors of diagnosis in which these lesions are wrongly identified as carcinoma are unfortunately not uncommon. Submission of a biopsy that includes the entire lesion and accurate documentation of the history and clinical appearance of the lesion can aid the pathologist significantly in recognizing pseudoepitheliomatous hyperplasia. This change is also commonly seen in epulis fissuratum. Like other inflammatory hyperplasias, pseudoepitheliomatous hyperplasia is cured by local excision, provided the chronic initiating irritant is also eliminated.

HAMARTOMAS

Hamartomas are tumorlike malformations characterized by the presence of particular histologic tissues in improper proportions or distribution, with a prominent excess of one type of tissue. On the one hand hamartomas are to be distinguished from malformations such as extra digits, supernumerary teeth, and ectopic salivary gland tissue in which excessive tissue is present in its usual histologic relationship; on the other hand, they are to be distinguished from true benign tumors with relatively unlimited capacity for expansive growth, which may continue after the exciting agent has ceased to operate.

Hamartomas are usually congenital and have their major period of growth at the time the rest of the body is growing. Once they have achieved their adult dimensions, they do not extend to involve more tissue and rarely increase in size unless trauma, thrombosis, or infection cause edema, inflammatory infiltration, and filling of new vascular channels. They are also to be distinguished from the excessive proliferation of reparative tissue described earlier in this chapter (Inflammatory Hyperplasias) and for the most part are easily separated histologically from such lesions. Hamartomas are found in many tissues of the body, and a tendency to such malformations is often hereditary. Individual oral hamartomas are therefore often found in association with other gross and microscopic developmental abnormalities that assist considerably in their clinical diagnosis.

Hemangioma (both solitary and when found in association with other developmental anomalies in the various angiomatosis syndromes), lymphangioma, glomus tumor, granular cell myoblastoma of the tongue and granular cell epulis, neurofibromatosis, fibrous dysplasia of bone (ossifying fibroma), various odontomas and some odontogenic tumors, and possibly the melanotic neuroectodermal tumor of infancy are all examples of hamartomatous development in the oral region. To a greater or lesser extent, these lesions all possess the characteristics of hamartomas, although "transitional forms" in which the lesion shows some characteristics of aggressive neoplastic growth certainly occur and cause serious management problems. These variants aside, the treatment of hamartomas is essentially a cosmetic problem, and complete removal of these lesions is often neither desirable nor possible.

Teratomas, which are often thought of as malformations, but are in fact neoplasms of developing tissues, are mentioned at the end of this section to allow their comparison with hamartomas.

Hemangioma

This tumorlike malformation is composed of seemingly disorganized masses of endothelial-lined vessels that are filled with blood and connected to the main blood vascular system. They have been described in almost all locations in and about the oral cavity and face and may involve deep structures such as the jaw bones, salivary glands, and temporomandibular joint as well as the surface mucosa and skin. They may occur as isolated lesions in the oral cavity (see Fig. 8-9), as multiple lesions affecting different parts of the body, and in association with other developmental anomalies in the various angiomatous syndromes described below. They range from simple red patches or birthmarks (port wine stains), which do not raise the mucosal or skin surface, to large fungating masses, which bury teeth and cause serious deformity and disfiguration. Small lesions may be clinically indistinguishable from pyogenic granulomas and superficial venous varicosities, but histologic examination often reveals other epithelial and neural abnormalities in the surrounding tissues that aid in separating them from highly vascular granulation tissue. Both cavernous and capillary types are described, the former consisting of relatively large blood-filled lakes, the latter of masses of proliferating vessels of capillary dimension. In both cases, there is a simple endothelial lining to the vascular channels and little connective tissue stroma. Such lesions characteristically bleed profusely when traumatized.

Many hemangiomas are evident at birth, and they frequently increase in size with general bodily growth. Filling of previously empty vascular channels also accounts for an increase in size of these lesions, such changes sometimes occurring very rapidly following trauma. While such growth is to be distinguished from neoplastic growth, this distinction may not be easy to make clinically, and the clinician quite reasonably will sometimes be concerned that what is assumed to be a hamartomatous lesion may be developing a neoplastic tendency.

When located on the surface of the skin or oral mucous membrane, hemangiomas are usually readily identified. Large lesions are warm and may even be pulsatile if associated with a large vessel. Hemangiomas of the tongue and gingiva are often covered by un-

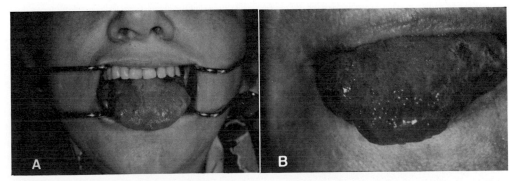

Fig. 8-9 Bilateral hemangiomas of the tongue.

usually rugose epithelium. Differentiation should be made from vascular inflammatory hyperplasias, from varicosities of the superficial veins on the ventral surface of the tongue that are common after 50 years of age, and from pigmented nevi, telangiectasias of various etiologies, and hematomas. Centrally located hemangiomas must be distinguished from the many osteolytic tumors and cystlike lesions that affect the jaws, as well as both congenital and acquired arteriovenous aneurysms of the jaw. Care should be taken in biopsying or excising hemangiomas, partly because of their tendency to uncontrolled hemorrhage and partly because of the difficulty of knowing the extent of the lesion, only a small part of which may be evident in the mouth. Gingival hemangiomas often connect with similar lesions in the jaw bone, and radiographic examination of the bone may not always reveal an abnormality of the trabecular architecture. Hemorrhage from centrally located hemangiomas of the jaw is especially difficult to control, and surgery should be attempted on hemangiomas only when provision has been made beforehand to control any untoward hemorrhage that may occur (typed and crossmatched blood, splints, and the means of tying off branches of the external carotid artery). In general, electrocoagulation causes less postoperative hemorrhage than does incision with a scalpel. Some assistance in defining the extent of bony hemangiomas may be given by scintigraphic bone scans, and radiographic examination of the affected tissues may reveal not only bony defects, but also *phleboliths* in the cheek and salivary glands that mark the location of abnormal vessels.

Treatment of hemangiomas continues to be a difficult problem fraught with the danger of uncontrollable hemorrhage. In addition to conventional surgical techniques and the injection of sclerosing solutions, methods involving cryosurgery, intravascular embolization with silicon spheres and other nonsurgical approaches have been described in recent years. Although radiation can be used successfully to sclerose these lesions, the risk of inducing neoplastic change later in life is very high and its use is contraindicated, particularly in children. Many of the reported cases of malignant change in hem-angiomas undoubtedly are the result of radiation treatment.

Hemangiomas of the skin and oral mucous membrane often coexist with similar lesions of the central nervous system and the meninges. A variety of such *angiomatous syndromes* have been described with eponyms applied to both complete and incomplete variants of each syndrome. Although the skin and oral lesions are at the most deforming and disfiguring, the central nervous system lesions are often associated with serious problems of epilepsy, hemiplegia, mental retardation, and retinal changes.

Sturge–Weber syndrome (encephalofacial or encephalotrigeminal angiomatosis) is probably the most common of these malformations (Fig. 8-10). It is characterized by angiomatosis of the face (nevus flammeus) with a variable distribution sometimes matching the dermatomes of one or more trigeminal nerve divisions, leptomeningeal angiomas particularly of the parietal and occipital lobes of the brain with associated characteristic intracranial calcifications, contralateral hemiplegia, and one or more of the neurologic symptoms just mentioned. Oral changes occur in about a third of the cases of this syndrome and may include massive growths of the gingiva and asymmetric jaw growth and tooth eruption sequence (due to differential blood flow to the affected area).

Since many patients with this syndrome are treated for many years with phenytoin (Dilantin) as an anticonvulsant, a distinction needs to be made in these patients between gingival hypertrophy due to phenytoin and that due to angiomatous changes, particularly if gingivectomy is planned. Classically, the intraoral lesions in this syndrome occur on the same side of the body as other angiomas in the patient, but the classical pattern is not always found either in the distribution or expression of the various components of the syndrome. Fortunately, this serious malformation is apparently not of hereditary origin (compare Osler–Weber–Rendu syndrome, Chap. 23).

Other, rarer, angiomatous syndromes are those of *Maffucci* (multiple angiomas of the skin and enchondromas of bone) and *von Hippel–Lindau* (a familial syndrome involving hemangioblastomas in retina and cerebellum,

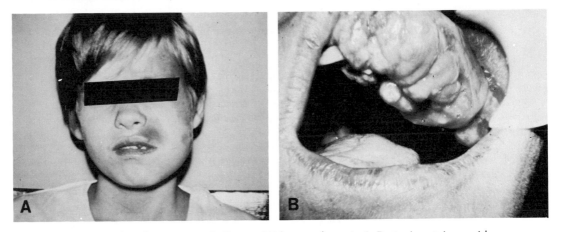

Fig. 8-10 Encephalofacial angiomatosis (Sturge–Weber syndrome). *A*, Port-wine stain on side of face. *B*, Massive intraoral hemangioma of maxilla. (Courtesy of E.P. Rossi, D.D.S., M.S., Cleveland, OH)

pancreatic and renal cysts, renal adenomas, and hepatic hemangiomas). Syndromes such as Sturge–Weber and von Hippel–Lindau, which involve a visible congenitally acquired external lesion (birth spot or "phakos") and other systemic anomalies, are sometimes referred to as the *phakomatoses*.

Many reviews and case reports of both isolated oral hemangiomas and the various angiomatous syndromes are available and attest to the problems associated with treatment of these nonneoplastic lesions.

Lymphangioma

Lymphangioma is histologically and etiologically similar to the hemangioma, except that the abnormal vessels are filled with a clear, protein-rich fluid containing few cells (lymph) rather than blood. Lymphangiomas may occur alone or more frequently, in association with hemangioma or other anomalous blood vessels with which the lymphangiomatous vessels are anastomosed. The tongue is the most common oral location for this lesion, and together with hemangioma it is an important cause of *congenital macroglossia*.

Lymphangiomas are frequently without clear anatomical outline, presenting on clinical examination as soft masses that dissect tissue planes and turn out to be more extensive than anticipated. Large lymphangiomas spreading into and distending the neck are referred to as *cystic hygromas*. Differential diagnoses for lymphangiomas include, in the tongue—hemangioma, congenital hypothyroidism, mongolism, amyloidosis, neurofibromatosis, various storage diseases (*e.g.*, Hurler's syndrome and glycogen storage disease), and primary muscular hypertrophy of the tongue, all of which may cause macroglossia (see also Chap. 10); and in the neck—various inclusion cysts, cellulitis, and ranula, as well as other causes of congenital wryneck (*torticollis*) that large angiomas of the neck may simulate. Abnormalities of the mucosa overlying a lymphangioma may give the appearance of a localized glossitis and draw attention to the presence of a small lesion buried in the tongue. The problems of management of lymphangioma are similar to those of hemangioma.

Glomus Tumor and Other Vascular Endothelial Growths

An unusual abnormality, glomus tumor develops as a small painful unencapsulated nodule as a result of hamartomatous proliferation of the cells found in the characteristic type of peripheral arteriovenous anastomosis known as the glomus. In addition to having a characteristic histology, these lesions also may secrete various catecholamines. The glomus tumor is rare or nonexistent in the mouth, but similar lesions arising in the carotid and aortic bodies and glomus jugulare may produce neck masses. Differentiation of the glomus tumor from other masses of proliferating vascular endothelial cells (*hemangioendothelioma* and *hemangiopericytoma*), which may represent hamartomas or benign neoplasms, requires special stains and considerable histopathologic diagnostic skills. Other important diagnostic features that characterize at least some glomus tumors are an autosomal dominant inheritance pattern and a tendency to be removed while still quite small because of the associated pain.

Granular Cell Myoblastoma and Granular Cell Epulis

The so-called granular cell myoblastoma or granular cell tumor is an important oral hamartomatous lesion because of its frequent occurrence as a nodule on the dorsum of the tongue, and in its variant form on the gingiva, as a congenital epulis (Fig. 8-11); controversy as to its nature and cytologic structure; and the overlying pseudoepitheliomatous hyperplasia that often leads to a misdiagnosis of squamous cell carcinoma and unnecessarily radical surgery. Histologically, these lesions are composed of masses of large eosinophilic, granular cells interspersed with a collagenous stroma and covered with hyperplastic lingual mucosa. The large granular cells have been variously identified as of muscle cell (*Abrikossoff myocytes*), histiocytic, Schwann cell, and fibroblastic origin; and electron microscopic studies have not conclusively solved the problem.

About a third of oral myoblastomas occur on the tongue; those occurring elsewhere in the mouth (palate, gum, floor of mouth and lips) and on the skin are similar in most of their clinical and histologic features. Important distinctions between lingual and extralingual myoblastomas are, in the latter, the absence of overlying pseudoepitheliomatous hyperplasia and the presence of female sex predilection. Quite innocent looking and often long-standing tongue nodules biopsied in adults may turn out to be granular cell tumors. Treatment of these oral lesions both on the tongue and in extralingual locations is by

local excision. Differential diagnosis for congenital epulis includes other hamartomatous and hyperplastic oral mucosal lesions, odontogenic tumors, and ectopic tooth germs. Multiple and familially occurring oral granular cell myoblastomas have been reported on several occasions. In contrast to the prevalence of the granular cell myoblastoma, true neoplasms of the muscle of the body of the tongue (*rhabdomyoma*) are exceedingly rare, and some examples probably represent hamartomatous lesions better classified as granular cell tumors. Histochemical and electron microscopic observations usually allow separation of these two distinct lesions.

Neurofibroma

These developmental abnormalities (*i.e.*, hamartomas and not neoplasms) arise from both nerve sheath (neurilemmal) cells as well as from perineural fibroblasts. Although solitary neurofibromas do occur, the main clinical feature of neurofibroma is its tendency to be multiple and to be associated with a variety of other familial abnormalities in the syndrome of *von Recklinghausen's neurofibromatosis,* which is inherited as an autosomal dominant condition and in which there is also a tendency to develop sarcoma (see following section on syndromes with benign oral neoplastic—in this case, hamartomatous—components). Since 5% of patients with neurofibromatosis develop sarcoma, recognition of an otherwise innocent-appearing nodule in the oral cavity as a neurofibroma can be an important diagnosis. Histologically, neurofibromas are to be distinguished from neurilemmomas (tumors of the nerve sheath; schwannomas). Both are encapsulated tumors that show patterns of whorled connective tissue elements interspersed with readily recognizable axons with or without a myelin sheath. Neurilemmomas also exhibit a characteristic palisading of nuclei and other suggestions of histologic organization referred to as an organoid structure; both features are usually absent from neurofibromas. Both neurofibromas and neurilemmomas may occur as isolated lesions or in patients with neurofibromatosis. Although neurofibromas are generally classified as

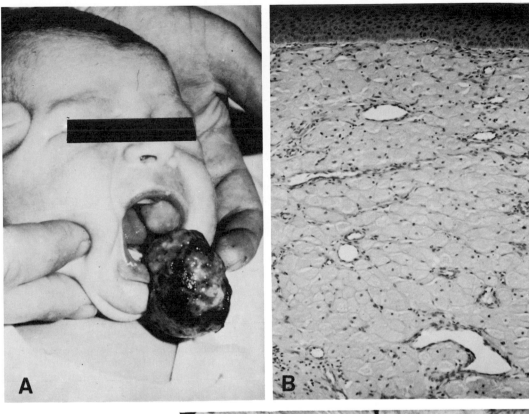

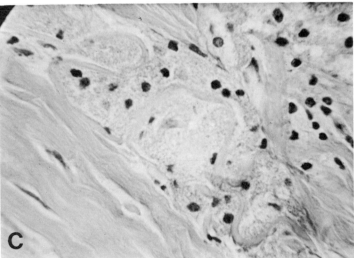

Fig. 8-11 *A*, Congenital epulides arising from upper and lower jaw of a 2-day-old infant. *B*, Section of one of these tumors; both showed identical histologic structure despite different clinical appearances. The lesion is composed of masses of granular eosinophilic cells characteristic of the granular cell-type of congenital epulis. (Blair A, Edwards DM: Congenital epulis of the newborn. Oral Surg 43, May, 1977) *C*, Similar cells from a granular cell myoblastoma presenting as a painless indurated mass in the anterior third of the tongue of a 49-year-old man. (Courtesy of E.P. Rossi, D.D.S., M.S., Cleveland, OH)

hamartomas, neurilemmomas are usually referred to as benign neoplasms. Oral lesions are usually asymptomatic and do not recur after local excision (Fig. 8-12).

Melanotic Neuroectodermal Tumor of Infancy

This tumor has been classified both as a hamartoma and as a benign neoplasm, with recent authors favoring the latter etiology. It is a rare tumor occurring both orally and extraorally, usually in children under 6 months of age, and showing a characteristic histologic picture of melanin-containing epithelial cells lining cuboidal or slitlike spaces. It is probably a tumor of neural crest origin (the embryonic layer which contributes greatly to cranial and oral development), although histologic similarities to the enamel organ have led some to consider it of odontogenic origin and to the use of such synonyms as *melanotic ameloblastoma* and *pigmented epulis*. Theories assigning its origin to ectopic retinal epithelium have produced the synonyms of *retinal anlage tumor* and *melanotic progonoma*. The lesion usually protrudes into the mouth and may also involve underlying bone. The lesions do not necessarily appear pigmented clinically. It is rarely an aggressive lesion, although recurrences after local excision have been described.

Pigmented Nodules and Macules in the Oral Mucosa

Pigmented nodules and macules are common adjacent to the teeth and usually can be shown by biopsy and electron probe analysis to be local accumulations of silver or gold particles, probably introduced as a result of soft-tissue trauma during placement or polishing of a dental restoration (*amalgam tattoo*). Intraoral moles (*pigmented nevi*) also occur and should be removed, partly for the same reasons outlined for the majority of benign oral tumors in the introduction to this chapter and partly because the relationship of intraoral moles to malignant melanoma remains uncertain.

Pigmented nevi, along with freckles (lentigo), are nonneoplastic, melanin-containing hamartomas, but on the skin at least, there

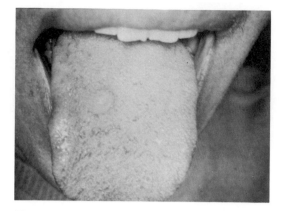

Fig. 8-12 Asymptomatic neurofibroma of the tongue. This lesion was not associated with other evidences of neurofibromatosis.

is evidence that some malignant melanomas arise by neoplastic changes in pigmented nevi. Skin cancer prevention thus rightly emphasizes changes in the appearance of a mole as a danger signal warranting surgical consultation and usually excision of the lesion for histologic examination. Perhaps because of the relative rarity of intraoral pigmented nevi, there is no good evidence indicating whether these oral lesions are predisposed to malignant change. Approximately 30% of oral melanomas are preceded for several months by a patch of pigmentation of the oral mucosa, but it is not known whether this patch is a nevus or simply slow development of the melanoma. On the skin, some melanomas arise from the specific histologic varieties of nevi described as junctional or combined, but others also seem to arise in normal skin and freckled (macular pigmented) areas. The majority of intraoral nevi are histologically classified as intradermal; junctional and combined lesions are unusual; blue nevi (Jadassohn–Tièche) are said to be the next most common type of intraoral nevus after the intradermal.

Since intraoral nevi are usually single, their removal is not a major undertaking and is strongly recommended. Unfortunately, fewer than two thirds of oral nevi are pigmented, this fact once again suggesting a good reason for excision of all oral mucosal nodules, since many oral nevi are undoubtedly clinically identified as fibrous hyperplasia or clinical fibroma and are not removed. Differentiation of amalgam tattoos from pigmented oral nevi may also be difficult, particularly when the lesion is located well away from the teeth and there is no clear history of accidental trauma to the area from dental instruments. Differential diagnosis of a pigmented nodule that has recently appeared in the oral mucosa should include accidental trauma and hematoma as well as primary or metastatic melanoma, although only a fraction of metastatic melanomas are pigmented.

Nevi are also discussed later in this chapter in reference to the multiple nevoid basal cell carcinoma syndrome.

Fibrous Dysplasia of Bone and Other Benign Fibro-Osseous Lesions

Fibrous dysplasia of bone results from an abnormality of development of bone-forming mesenchyme. This is manifested by replacement of spongy bone by a peculiar fibrous tissue within which trabeculae or spherules of poorly calcified fiber (nonlamellar) bone are formed by osseous metaplasia. Histologically, a given lesion may show a great variability of pattern with some fields predominantly collagenous, some osteoid, and others fully ossified and calcified. Radiographically, the lesion will usually present varying degrees of radiopacity and lucency, some areas resembling compact bone, others cystic areas. Surgical exploration of such "cystic areas" usually reveals either a soft fibrous tissue or more characteristically, a tissue that is gritty on section or curettage. Because these lesions often develop to quite a large size with few symptoms other than a slowly developing asymmetry of the bone, when examined radiographically they may exhibit quite dramatic deformity and apparent bony destruction. Patients may have a small, solitary focus (monostotic form) or may have many bones affected with multiple lesions (polyostotic form). Rare cases exist in which the lesions of fibrous dysplasia coexist with other developmental bony defects or with extraskeletal changes, notably a blotchy cutaneous hyperpigmentation and precocious puberty. The term *McCune–Albright's syndrome*, or simply *Albright's syndrome*, has been used to describe these more dramatic cases

occurring in children. Solitary foci are far more common than are multiple lesions, particularly in the jaw bone. Except that in the polyostotic form a greater variety of histologic pattern and size of lesion are seen, there is no essential difference between the two lesions. The cause of the endocrine manifestations in Albright's syndrome (thyrotoxicosis, precocious puberty, hypogonadotrophic hypogonadism, acromegaly, vitamin D-resistant rickets, etc.) is not known, but is thought to be related to hypothalamic secretion of releasing hormone.

The hamartomatous nature of the condition is exemplified by the existence of congenital forms of the disease, the association of fibrous dysplasia with other developmental bone problems in the same patient, the frequency with which increasing size of the lesion correlates with periods of increased skeletal growth rate, the association of endocrine abnormalities with bony lesions in Albright's syndrome, and the rarity of malignant transformation of these lesions, considering the frequency with which fibrous dysplasia is seen. Recent reviews have stressed that malignant transformation of these lesions probably occurs more frequently than is usually believed because small foci of fibrous dysplasia are often overlooked in evaluating a patient with a malignant bone lesion. Fibrous dysplasia in most cases can be safely handled as a benign developmental anomaly, and superficial recontouring of the lesion or curettage of a large "cystic" lesion remain appropriate management, provided an adequate and representative bone biopsy has been obtained. Radiotherapy is contraindicated in its treatment. The role that surgical intervention and radiotherapy administered in earlier decades of this century play in recurrences of fibrous dysplasia and in the rare cases of malignant transformation is not known.

The extensive size of some lesions in fibrous dysplasia and their nonuniform radiographic appearance pose a problem to the surgeon who needs to obtain representative biopsies with minimal disturbance of the lesion. Biopsies of these lesions, like other bone biopsies, only too frequently reveal nothing more than superficial layers of reactive normal bone formation. Curettage of one of the "cystic" cavities usually provides material of more diagnostic value. At times, the hypercellularity, pleomorphism, and aggressiveness of the fibrous tissue in these lesions will lead the pathologist to suspect that he is dealing with a fibrosarcoma or osteogenic sarcoma, and consideration of both the clinical behavior of the lesion and the histologic appearance are needed to arrive at a diagnosis. Fibrous dysplasia has been described in association with giant cell reparative granuloma of bone, aneurysmal bone cyst, and a number of other fibro-osseous lesions, and the coexistence of different histologic pictures in one lesion or in one patient can provide added diagnostic difficulties.

The clinical problems associated with fibrous dysplasia of bone are related to the site and extent of involvement. Many small foci probably remain unrecognized throughout life. In the long bones, deformity and fractures are common complications that often lead to initial diagnosis of the lesion. In the jaws and other parts of the craniofacial skeleton, involvement of adjacent structures such as the cranial sinuses, cranial nerves, ocular contents, and so on can lead to serious complications in addition to cosmetic and functional problems. Intracranial lesions arising from the cranial bones may produce seizures and changes in the electroencephalogram. Extension into and occlusion of the maxillary and ethmoid sinuses and mastoid air spaces is common; proptosis, diplopia, and interference with jaw function also often prompt surgical intervention.

Computerized tomography and ^{99m}Tc bone scans have proven of great help in diagnosing lesions of fibrous dysplasia. Trimming and surface contouring of the affected bone, curettage of bony cavities, and packing with bone chips remain the recommended treatments. Attempts at treating advanced cases of the polyostotic form with calcitonin have not been greatly successful even though the hormone is useful in other disorders characterized by increased bone resorption and formation, such as osteoporosis, Paget's disease, and metastatic bone carcinoma. Laboratory evidence of increased bone turnover, increased alkaline phosphatase, and high urinary hydroxyproline levels with normal serum calcium and phosphate levels oc-

cur in large monostotic lesions of fibrous dysplasia and in the polyostotic form. Opinions differ as to whether pain is a common feature of fibrous dysplasia. Small lesions are undoubtedly often asymptomatic. Larger lesions associated with cortical fractures are painful, incapacitating, and lead in many cases to extreme degrees of deformity. The extent of the deformity may be as great as that associated with untreated von Recklinghausen's disease of bone due to hyperparathyroidism, and in the early part of this century, fibrous dysplasia was often confused with this metabolic bone disorder.

Other Benign Fibro-Osseous Lesions

Before 1970, *fibrous dysplasia* was used as an all-inclusive term that encompassed both the monostotic and polyostotic forms of fibrous dysplasia as described above and a variety of other *fibro-osseous* lesions, notably ossifying fibroma, fibrous osteoma, and osteoblastoma. Histologic studies often failed to establish definitive differences between these lesions, particularly when the problems of maturation of the connective tissue elements with time, the inhomogeneity of large lesions and inadequate biopsy specimens were considered. The problem of separating these different lesions in the jaw bone is further compounded by the occurrence in the jaw of lesions with cemental as well as osseous dysplasia (Fig. 8-13), and the frequency of giant-cell type reparative granulomas in this region. A number of papers published by oral pathologists during the late 1960s and early 1970s emphasized the variety of histologic appearance in fibro-osseous lesions derived from the periodontal membrane and distinguished them from similar lesions arising from medullary bone origin. An example of such a classification is presented in Table 8-1 and includes a number of lesions considered elsewhere in this chapter. Ossifying fibroma, aneurysmal bone cysts, and cherubism are discussed below.

The difficulty of differentiating tumors of periodontal membrane origin from tumors of medullary bone origin—fibro-osteoma, osteoblastoma, cherubism, giant cell tumor, aneurysmal bone cyst, "brown tumor" of hyperparathyroidism, and Paget's disease—has

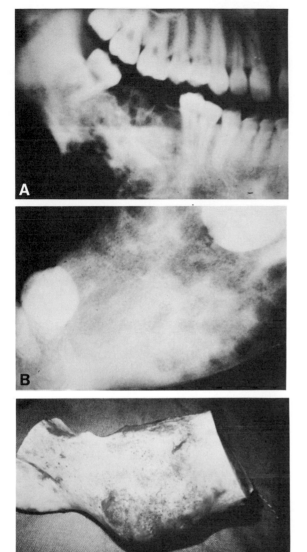

long been recognized. Differentiation between tumors of periodontal membrane origin and tumors of medullary bone origin is important because the latter tumors usually behave in a more aggressive fashion, even though they are benign. The absolute proof of medullary bone origin in this group of tumors is yet to be shown, however. Benign fibro-osseous lesions of periodontal membrane origin are much more prevalent in the jaws than are fibro-osseous lesions of medullary bone origin. These latter lesions may be differentiated using clinical, radiographic, hematologic, and histopathologic considerations. For additional information on this controversy, the reader should consult the reviews by Hamner, Waldron, and Eversole.

Ossifying Fibroma

Differentiation of solitary lesions of *ossifying fibroma* and fibrous dysplasia can be quite difficult on histologic grounds alone, but most current authors state that the lesions can be distinguished if radiographic and clinical criteria are used in addition to the appearance of a biopsy from the central part of the lesion. Fibrous dysplasia has a diffuse margin radiographically; ossifying fibroma is an expansile process with a clearly defined cortical margin and more closely resembles a benign tumor. Fibrous dysplasia tends to favor the maxilla whereas ossifying fibroma more often occurs in the mandible. Both are slow growing and originate early in life, but fibrous dysplasia grows endosteally and follows the general

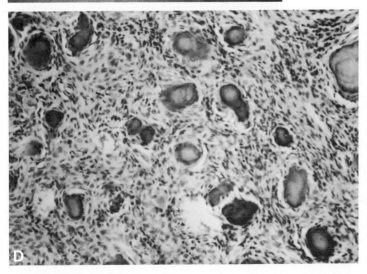

Fig. 8-13 Large cemento-ossifying fibroma of the mandibular molar region in a 21-year-old black female. The patient had a 2-year history of localized enlargement of the body of the mandible associated with a dull throbbing pain and loosening of the teeth in this region. Radiographic examination (*A* and *B*) revealed a large multilocular lesion extending from the third molar to the premolar area with expansion of the bone in all directions. Histologic examination of the excised lesion (*C* and *D*) revealed spherules of bone and cementum in a fibrous matrix. (Courtesy of Todd Beckerman, D.D.S., Baltimore, MD)

Table 8-1. Fibro-Osseous Lesions of the Jaw Bones

Origin	Lesion
Periodontal membrane	Cementifying fibroma (cementoma)
	Ossifying fibroma
	Cemento-ossifying fibroma
	Fibroma
Medullary bone	Fibro-osteoma
	Active juvenile ossifying fibroma
	Cherubism
	Fibrous dysplasia
	Giant cell tumor
	Aneurysmal bone cyst
	Hyperparathyroidism jaw lesion
	Paget's disease

structure of the affected bone, usually producing a thickening and irregular deformation of the bone. Ossifying fibroma, by contrast, grows into and fills cavities like the nasal cavity and accessory sinuses and destroys surrounding bone as it enlarges. Management of the two benign lesions is similar, although more aggressive behavior can be expected from the ossifying fibroma. Malignant transformation of ossifying fibroma is no more common than in fibrous dysplasia.

Aneurysmal Bone Cyst

Aneurysmal bone cyst, unlike ossifying fibroma and fibrous dysplasia, occurs less frequently in the jaw bones than in the long bones, usually involving the mandible rather than the maxilla. Microscopically, curetted material from the cavity resembles the giant cell reparative granuloma but has more prominent vascular spaces with evidence of old and recent hemorrhages and thrombosis and hyalinization of some of the vascular spaces. Like the giant cell reparative granuloma, it has no epithelial lining despite the common usage of "cyst" to describe it, and both lesions are believed to arise from an intraosseous hematoma. Aneurysmal bone cyst is to be differentiated from the so-called *traumatic bone cyst* (the name given to solitary and usually asymptomatic cavities found in the man-

dible, usually without any epithelial or other distinguishing lining and which contain only serum or are apparently empty), for which a traumatic etiology seems to be less convincingly established. In both cases, thorough curettage of the lesion and its walls and packing with bone chips results in healing of the defect.

Cherubism

Cherubism is a tumorous lesion of the jaws affecting children and is characterized by bilateral, painless mandibular (and often corresponding maxillary) swellings that cause fullness of the cheeks, firm protuberant intraoral alveolar masses, and missing or displaced teeth (Fig. 8-14). Submaxillary lymphadenopathy is described as an early, fairly constant feature that tends to subside after 5 years of age and usually has regressed by 12 years. Maxillary involvement can often produce a slightly upward turning of the child's eyes, revealing an abnormal amount of sclera beneath them. It was the upward, "looking toward heaven" cast of the eyes, combined with the characteristic facial chubbiness of these children that prompted the term *cherubism.*

In a review of the genetic pedigrees of 65 patients in 21 families, cherubism was related to a dominant gene with a penetrance of nearly 100% in males and between 50% and 75% in females; however, the exact cause of cherubism remains unknown, and total agreement on the genetic aspects of this malady does not exist.

Cherubism has a very early clinical onset, the youngest reported child by Hamner and Ketchum being 14 months old. Rapid progression of the disorder may occur during the next several years, encompassing all of the areas that will become affected and causing clinical features that vary according to the anatomy involved and the severity of the genetic disorder. The typical initial painless, bilateral, symmetrical enlargement of the posterior mandible and rami has been described in all of the reported cases; however, the maxillae are often affected simultaneously, giving rise to the upward cast of the eyes by tumor encroachment on the orbital floor and often causing partial obliteration of the palatal vault with a resulting "V"-shaped cleft.

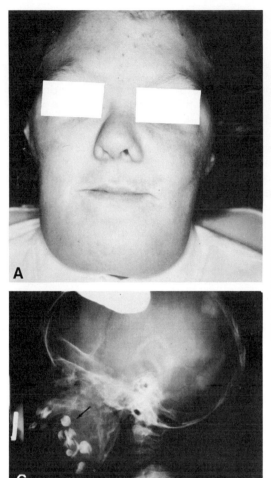

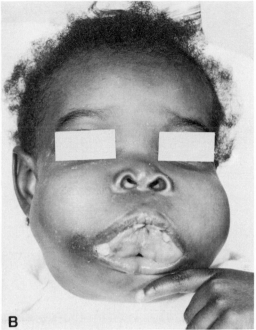

Fig. 8-14 Three examples of cherubism: (*A*) in a 23-year-old white female, and (*B*) a severe case in a 3-year-old black female. (*C*) Lateral head film depicting the radiographic features of cherubism. (*A*, Courtesy of Sheldon Rovin, D.D.S., Ph,D., Philadelphia, PA; *B & C*, Courtesy of J. E. Hamner III, D.D.S., Ph.D., Washington, DC)

The clinical appearance may vary from barely discernible posterior swellings of a single jaw to marked anterior and posterior grotesque expansion of both jaws with concomitant difficulties in mastication, speech, swallowing, and respiration.

The early rapid rate of size increase usually declines with advancing age. As the child reaches puberty, the facial appearance may begin to improve as the normal bony growth pattern evolves toward adulthood facial features. The maxillary lesions often tend to regress, although the mandibular lesions may continue to progress until 15 years of age. Reshaping of the bone has been described between 20 and 30 years of age with regression of the mandibular lesions, resulting in a mandible that is only a bit larger than normal.

Radiographically, the lesions of cherubism appear as multiple, well-defined, multilocular radiolucencies in the mandible and maxillae. These rarefactions begin in the posterior alveolar and rami regions and can spread anteriorly. They are irregular in size and usually cause marked destruction of the alveolar bone. Numerous displaced and unerupted teeth appear to be floating in radiolucent spaces.

Serum calcium and phosphorus are within normal limits for cherubism patients, whereas the serum alkaline phosphatase level may be elevated.

Histologically, the cherubism jaw lesion can bear a close resemblance to the benign giant cell reparative granuloma. Other specimens have been described as being more

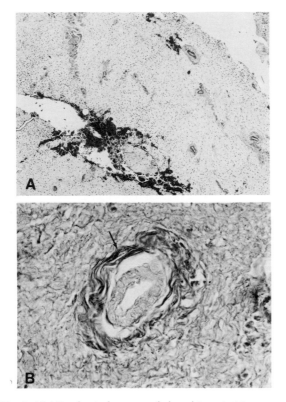

Fig. 8-15 Histologic features of cherubism *A,* Masson trichrome stain of tissue that bears a close resemblance to giant cell reparative granuloma. *B,* Perivascular cuffing of collagen that contributes the prominent eosinophilic cuffing noted around capillaries in these lesions. (Courtesy of J.E. Hamner III, D.D.S., Ph.D., Washington, DC)

mature with a greater amount of fibrous tissue and collagen and fewer giant cells. The prominent eosinophilic perivascular cuffing material noted around capillaries in these lesions has been proven to be collagen; and this finding is a distinctive histologic diagnostic feature (Fig. 8-15).

The problem of clinical management and surgical treatment is an arduous one, and each child must be evaluated individually according to the degree of tumor manifestation. The reported treatment of cherubism has varied considerably with advocates for each of the following methods: no active treatment, extraction of teeth in the involved areas, surgical contouring of expanded lesions, and complete curettage.

The statement has been repeated in the literature that many occurrences of cherubism have resolved spontaneously when there was no treatment instigated, yet no one has documented such a philosophy of "watch and wait" with any long-term follow-up of actual case results. The belief that a policy of nonsurgical interference will eventually result in an adult with a symmetrical facial appearance obviously has been based on casual familial histories of a parent having vague jaw swellings as a child that eventually did "regress," so that the typical manifestation of cherubism was not present in adulthood; however, no child with early typical cherubism has been carefully followed to adulthood without some form of treatment.

There has been considerable debate concerning the advantages of the proposed various treatments for this disorder. Based on the experience of cases treated at the National Institutes of Health, cherubism is a relentless process in the early stages, and if the jaws are extensively involved or even moderately so, thorough curettage of all possible tumor, taking pains to spare as many of the teeth as possible, is the treatment of choice. These cases exhibited steady progression of the tumor lesions whether the initial surgery was extensive or more conservative.

If the lesions are mild on initial manifestation with minimal bone involvement and are noticed only on radiographs, they can be observed and followed closely in relationship to the corresponding jaw growth. A surge in tumor growth can occur quickly. Lesions causing initial expansion of the rami appear to enlarge steadily if left untreated. Curettage and recontouring must usually be combined to obtain the best esthetic result. Merely trimming a large lesion is not satisfactory.

The prognosis is enhanced if cherubism occurs in only one jaw, preferably the mandible. Anterior as well as posterior lesions in both jaws present a grave situation. Cherubism lesions in the maxillae act in a more aggressive manner than do their mandibular counterparts and because of the anatomical considerations pose the more serious problem. The use of radiation in any form of therapy for cherubism is now universally condemned because of the dangers of sarcoma induction, osteoradionecrosis, and interference in bone growth and facial development in these children.

Teratomas and Dermoid Cysts

Teratomas are neoplasms composed of a mixture of tissues, more than one of which exhibits neoplastic proliferation. They are congenitally acquired and usually found in the ovary. Rare examples have been described in children, either arising from the oral cavity or protruding into the oral cavity from the base of the skull. The finding of various organlike structures (teeth, tissue, hair, skin) in these tumors and their common location in the ovary may give the misleading impression that they are fetal malformations rather than neoplastic growths of developing tissue. The latter currently accepted explanation clearly provides a more convincing explanation for oral teratomas than does the former. Those arising in the base of the skull often extend into the cranial cavity as well as into the oral cavity, and newborn infants with such lesions rarely survive. No single histological picture is characteristic, although the usual histological appearance of disorganized neoplastic tissues of various types readily identifies the lesion to the pathologist.

Teratomas of the ovary are often referred to as dermoid cysts (because they may include epidermal tissue and even hair follicles). Unfortunately the same term, *dermoid* or *epidermoid cyst*, is also used to describe inclusion cysts of the face, neck, and floor of the mouth (*i.e.*, cystic degeneration of epithelium trapped in these tissues at the time of closure of the embryonic fissures). These cysts also feature epidermal tissues and even hair follicles, sweat and sebaceous glands in the cyst wall, and keratin and sebum in the cyst cavity. Such lesions are *not* teratomas and *not* neoplastic. Unlike oral teratomas, which are usually apparent at birth or soon after, most dermoid cysts of the head and neck do not appear until after puberty, perhaps because of increased glandular secretory activity of the trapped epithelium.

CYSTS OF THE JAWS AND BENIGN ODONTOGENIC TUMORS

Cysts of the Jaw

Cysts (*i.e.*, fluid-filled, epithelial-lined cavities in the jaw bones and soft tissues of the face, floor of the mouth, and neck) may cause either intraoral or extraoral swellings that clinically resemble a benign tumor. Unilocular and multilocular radiolucencies discovered in the jaw bones by radiographic examination must also be differentiated from solid growths in the jaw, a distinction that cannot always be made by inspection of the radiograph. The majority of cysts, however, are small, do not distend surface tissues and are often first recognized in routine dental radiographic examinations. Others are discovered during investigation of a nonvital tooth or acute dental abscess due to secondary infection of the cyst, or by loosening of teeth, and (rarely) jaw fracture. Small isolated radiolucencies in the jaw bone that are not associated with loss of pulp vitality are usually observed over several months for increase in size before surgical exploration. Cysts that are large enough to be suspected of being benign tumors warrant surgical removal, since aspiration of the cyst alone will usually be followed by recurrence.

Radiographic examination rarely provides a conclusive diagnosis as to the nature of a radiolucency in the jaw, although it may be used to gauge the rate of growth of such lesions and to detect erosion of tooth roots and cortical destruction; both features are uncommon in cysts and benign tumors but characteristic of malignant lesions. Contrary to traditional lore, there is no size range that separates periapical cysts from dental granulomas, and microscopic examination of periapical lesions frequently reveals tiny cystic areas and areas of epithelial proliferation in what is clinically thought to be a granuloma. Similarly, caution must be used in diagnosing even large radiolucent jaw lesions as cysts simply because they appear "spherical" in the radiograph. The differential diagnosis of multiple radiolucencies in the jaw should include consideration of multiple myeloma, eosinophilic granuloma and other histiocytoses, metastatic carcinoma, hyperparathyroidism, multiple dental granulomas, periapical cysts, cemental dysplasia, ossifying fibroma, and fibrous dysplasia.

Unfortunately, even microscopic examination of the contents of cysts and material curetted from the cyst wall does not always produce a definitive diagnosis. Diagnosis of cysts, therefore, often has to be made on the basis of whatever historical, clinical, radiographic, and microscopic evidence can be collected and may still be equivocal. The classical example of this is the large asymptomatic, centrally located cyst of the mandible, which may involve both body and ramus and be unassociated with any teeth and which on surgical exploration proves to be an incompletely fluid-filled space with no epithelial lining and only a thin connective tissue membrane separating it from surrounding normal bone. Conversely, there are many occasions on which microscopic examination of the cyst wall provides a clear diagnosis of some importance in the management of the lesion, and submission of all excised tissue for histopathologic examination (including fragments scraped from the wall of the jaw cyst and periapical tissues curetted at the time of dental extraction or apicoectomy) is strongly urged.

The treatment of choice for a cyst is local excision with complete removal of the cyst lining. With larger lesions, the surgeon may decide to curette the lining through a relatively small window, and removal of the lining can be expected to be incomplete with recurrence a possibility. Alternatively, the lining of larger cysts may be sutured to the oral mucosa adjacent to the surgically created window and the cyst "marsupialized." If such lesions are kept patent by repeated irrigation, the lesion will cease to expand, will not become secondarily infected, and the defect in the jaw will gradually even out. Surgical management of large lesions by techniques involving closure of the defect left by excision of the cyst calls for the use of bone chips or other artificial means of stimulating fibrous and bony replacement of the defect and the use of splints to prevent pathologic fracture while the defect heals.

An extensive list of different types of cysts affecting the jaws and adjacent oral tissues has been accumulated, but it is beyond the scope of this chapter to include detailed discussion of the clinical, radiographic, and histologic features of each type. The reader is referred to more extensive coverage provided in most textbooks of oral pathology and oral radiology, as well as to articles that review particular classes of cysts. A useful classification separating them into those of nonodontogenic origin and those arising from cells associated with the dental lamina (odontogenic cysts) is provided in Table 8-2. The radiographic appearance of some odontogenic and nonodontogenic cysts is illustrated in Figure 8-16.

Carcinoma arising in the wall of dentigerous cysts provides further justification for histopathologic examination of all tissue curetted from jaw cysts. *Odontogenic keratocysts* (Fig. 8-17) are described in more detail in the following section on syndromes with benign oral neoplastic components. *Cysts of the maxillary sinus*, although not usually of oral origin, should be mentioned because of the frequency with which they have been recognized in panoramic dental radiographs that have come into almost universal use in dental practice in recent years. The discovery of such lesions (which are to be distinguished from normal bony lamellae common within the maxillary sinus) warrants otorhinologic consultation, even though the majority are asymptomatic, benign cystic hyperplasias of the sinus mucosa that require no treatment. Cysts arising in the maxilla, especially peri-

Table 8-2. A Classification of Cysts of the Jaw

NONODONTOGENIC	ODONTOGENIC*
Fissural cysts (including globulomaxillary, nasoalveolar, median mandibular, anterior lingual, dermoid, epidermoid, newborn palatal, and nasopalatine cysts)	Dentigerous
	Eruption
	Gingival and periodontal
Pseudocysts (aneurysmal, static, and solitary bone cysts)	Radicular (periapical)
Thyroglossal duct cysts	Cystic keratinizing tumor
Lymphoepithelial (branchial cleft) cysts	Odontogenic keratocysts

* Excluding odontogenic tumors, which also often exhibit cystic degeneration (Modified from Gorlin RJ, Goldman HM: Thoma's Oral Pathology, 6th ed. St. Louis, CV Mosby, 1970)

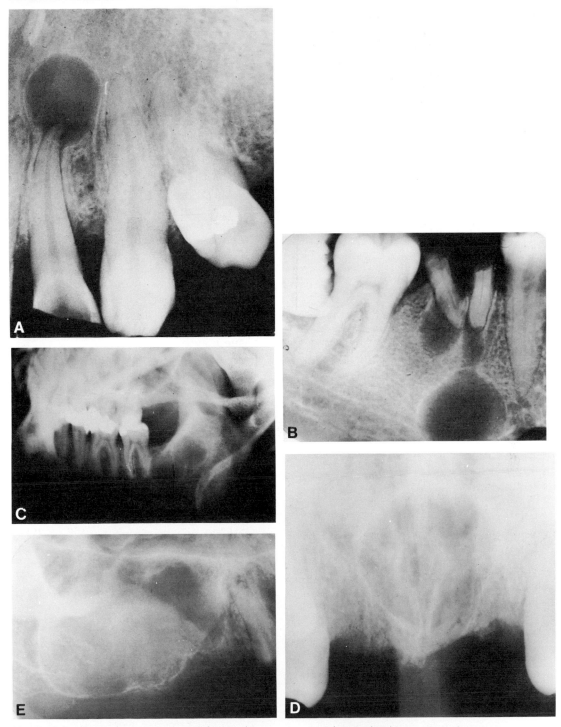

Fig. 8-16 Radiographic appearance of several jaw cysts. *A* and *B,* Radicular (periapical) cysts as a result of pulpal necrosis and infection. *C,* Two primordial cysts (dentigerous cysts derived from the odontogenic epithelium associated with unformed third and fourth molars). *D,* A nonodontogenic fissural cyst in the midline of the anterior maxilla (note intact nasopalatine canal). *E,* Mucus cyst of the maxillary sinus. (Radiographs courtesy of Robert Beideman, D.M.D., Philadelphia, PA)

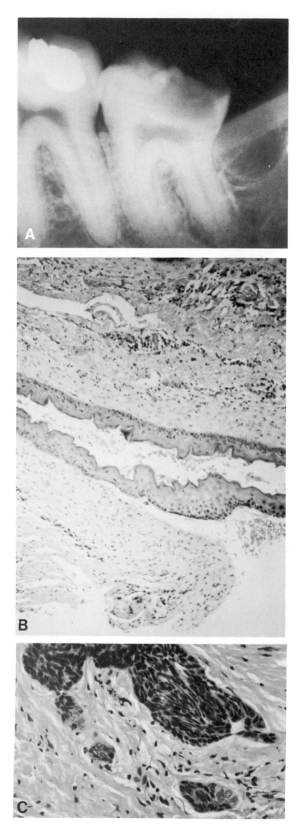

apical cysts of the molars and premolars, may extend into the maxillary sinus but usually do so by expanding the floor of the sinus ahead of them.

Cystic degeneration may also occur in *benign odontogenic tumors*, but the hamartomatous or neoplastic nature of the odontogenic tumors requires that they be given special consideration (see following section). The misleading, so-called cystic radiographic appearance of many odontogenic tumors, the majority of which develop within and expand the jaw (and which is perpetuated in the synonym of "multilocular cyst" for the ameloblastoma), also leads to clinical confusion between the two classes of lesions. Cystic degeneration is a common change in odontogenic tissue, and it is not surprising that odontogenic tumors frequently contain cystic areas. The importance of thorough histopathologic examination of all curetted material is once again underlined by the fact that tumor tissue may be recognized in only a small section of a lesion, the bulk of which is represented by a relatively nonspecific odontogenic cyst.

Benign Odontogenic Tumors

If fibro-osseous jaw lesions, nonodontogenic hamartomas of the jaw, and malformations such as enamel pearls (small globules of enamel lying free or attached to the roots near the bifurcation of multirooted teeth) are excluded, *odontogenic tumors* are quite rare, probably constituting fewer than 1% of all jaw cysts and tumors, and are an insignificant cause of oral cancer. Some, such as the ameloblastoma and the Pindborg tumor, are undoubtedly neoplastic; others, such as the

Fig. 8-17 *A,* Asymptomatic odontogenic keratocyst in the mandibular third molar region noted as an incidental finding in a periapical radiograph; histologically, the cyst has a well-keratinized epithelial lining (*B*) with nests of cells of presumed odontogenic origin (*C*) located in the surrounding connective tissue.

Table 8-3. Histopathologic Classification of Odontogenic Tumors

ECTODERMAL ORIGIN	MESODERMAL ORIGIN	MIXED ORIGIN
Ameloblastoma Adenomatoid odontogenic tumor (adenoameloblastoma) Calcifying epithelial odontogenic tumor (Pindborg tumor)	Odontogenic fibroma Odontogenic myxoma Ossifying fibroma Cementifying fibroma Cemento-ossifying fibroma	Ameloblastic fibroma Ameloblastic odontoma Odontoma (compound or complex)

Table 8-4. Comparison of Features of the Three Odontogenic Tumors of Ectodermal Origin

	AMELOBLASTOMA	ADENOMATOID ODONTOGENIC TUMOR	CALCIFYING EPITHELIAL ODONTOGENIC TUMOR
Incidence	1% of all oral tumors and cysts	100 reported cases	40 reported cases
Age of occurrence	20–49 years	11–19 years	13–78 years ($\bar{x}$ − 42)
Sex incidence	Male and female equal	Females > males	Male and female equal
Location	Mandible > maxilla (molar ramus area)	Maxilla > mandible (cuspid area)	Mandible > maxilla (premolar–molar area)
Radiographic appearance	Multilocular radiolucency	Radiolucency (1 2 cm diameter) with small masses of calcification	Radiolucency with radiopaque islands
Signs and symptoms	Destructively invasive "locally malignant" swelling with few true metastases	Expands cortical bone but is not invasive	Swelling with local invasion and destruction
Treatment	Surgical resection with adequate margins (Block excision)	Curettement	Surgical resection with adequate margins

compound odontoma and some varieties of cementoma, are most likely hamartomas. Malignant variants of several odontogenic tumors also attest to the neoplastic nature of at least some odontogenic growths. Although there have been many attempts at classifying the odontogenic tumors, lack of knowledge concerning the cells of origin of many of these lesions, the bewildering array of histologic types of odontogenic tumors that result from inductive changes in the mesodermal component of these lesions and their relative rarity cause much confusion in their histopathologic diagnosis. A classification based on histopathologic appearance is illustrated in Table 8-3, and the features of the three odontogenic tumors of ectodermal origin are compared in Table 8-4.

Ameloblastoma

This is without doubt the best-known odontogenic tumor, and its behavior is often used as the norm by which other odontogenic tumors are judged.* Most tumor registeries also

* Discussion of ameloblastoma under the heading of Benign Tumors of the Oral Cavity may be questioned because the capacity for local invasion that this tumor can show certainly belies a "benign" character. Distant metastasis is, however, quite rare, and the local invasion shown by this tumor probably differs biologically from that shown by squamous cell carcinoma, for example. Provided the student fully recognizes the locally destructive tendency of this tumor and the need for block excision in its treatment, it is conveniently discussed at this point, because it provides a useful comparison with other, rarer odontogenic tumors.

list it as the most prevalent odontogenic tumor; but since these data are based on biopsied lesions and well-differentiated and calcified lesions such as compound odontomas are often never removed, the data may not reflect the true frequency. Bhaskar, on the basis of 429 odontogenic tumors in 20,575 oral biopsies submitted to the Armed Forces Institute of Pathology, found the ameloblastoma to occur about as frequently as the odontogenic fibroma (20%). However, the prevalence of ameloblastomas ensures that all pathologists have encountered them, and there is fairly good agreement among surgeons that ameloblastomas should be treated by block excision due to their tendency for local invasion, so that description of a given odontogenic tumor as "more aggressive" or "less aggressive" than an ameloblastoma can be a useful means of communication in this rather uncertain field. Undoubtedly, misdiagnosis and controversy over diagnosis are common with odontogenic tumors, and both unnecessary and inadequate surgical treatment are often seen. In this field, more than in any other in oral medicine and surgery, the need for competent oral pathologists experienced in the wide variety of tumors peculiar to the oral cavity is most obvious.

In defining the ameloblastoma as the norm for odontogenic tumors, care must be given to the range of lesions accepted as ameloblastoma, since several lesions of quite different nature have been included under this diagnosis in past years. In particular, it is important that the melanotic neuroectodermal tumor of infancy (sometimes referred to as a melanotic ameloblastoma), the adenomatoid odontogenic tumor (adenoameloblastoma) and ameloblastic odontoma (odontoameloblastoma) are excluded from the definition of ameloblastoma. Used in this restricted sense, ameloblastoma is a slowly growing, benign neoplasm with a strong tendency to local invasion (which may be a property of all odontogenic epithelium rather than evidence of neoplastic infiltration) and which can grow to be quite large without metastasizing (Fig. 8-18). Rare examples of distant metastasis of an ameloblastoma in lungs or regional lymph nodes do exist, but this should not be a concern, except perhaps in a very large lesion of many years' duration.

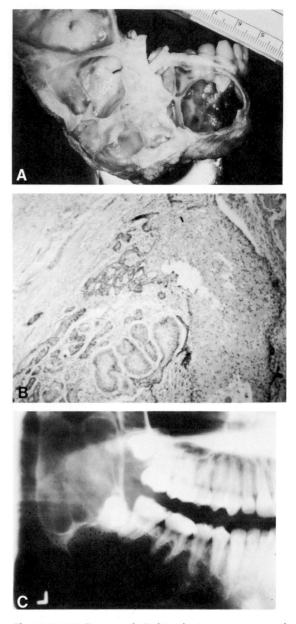

Fig. 8-18 (A) Gross and (B) histologic appearance of a very large multilocular ameloblastoma that occupied and distended the entire mandible. C, Radiograph of an ameloblastoma of similar dimension.

Ameloblastomas are rare in children, the greatest period of prevalence being in the 20-to-50 age range. The majority occur in the mandible and over two thirds in the molar-ramus area. Curettage of the unilocular or multilocular lesions (both radiographic appearances are characteristic) is often followed by local recurrence, and block excision of the lesion with a good margin of unaffected bone (or hemisection of the mandible for a large lesion) is the treatment of choice that is rarely followed by recurrence.

Microscopically, all ameloblastomas show a fibrous stoma with islands or masses of

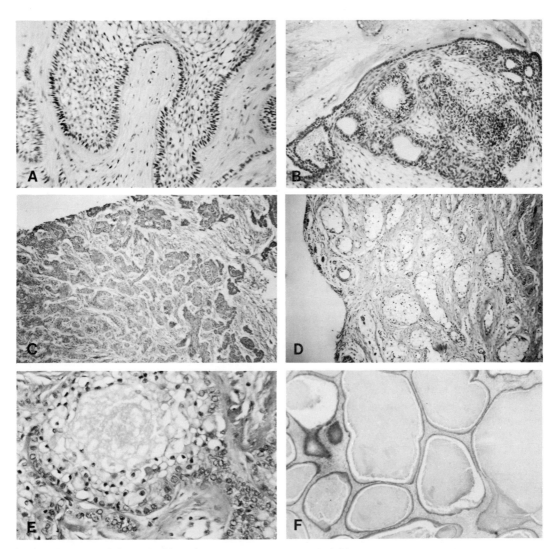

Fig. 8-19 Some of the varied histologic pictures seen in ameloblastoma. (H & E sections). *A,* Follicular pattern. *B,* Cystic degeneration in area of embryonal odontogenic epithelium. *C,* An area resembling basal cell carcinoma derived from odontogenic epithelium. *D,* Cystic degeneration of odontogenic follicles giving effect reminiscent of sebaceous cells (*sebaceous cell* variant). *E,* Detail of cystic degeneration of a follicle. *F,* Keratin-containing cysts lined by odontogenic epithelium sometimes referred to as a *kerato-ameloblastoma,* but more accurately as the keratinizing and calcifying odontogenic cyst (Gorlin cyst; see also Fig. 8-20*A* and 8-20*B*).

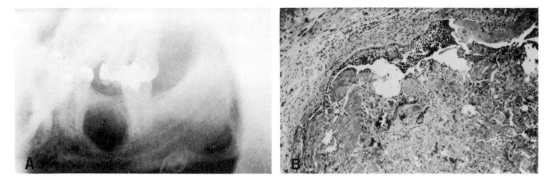

Fig. 8-20 *A* and *B,* Asymptomatic lesion of the mandible of a 55-year-old male; discovered on routine radiographic examination. Histologic examination revealed a cystic lesion lined by a double-layered epithelium and containing larger eosinophilic masses of keratin and a calcified product resembling osteoid or dentinoid. Diagnosed as a cyst of odontogenic origin of the keratinizing and calcifying type—a Gorlin cyst. (Gorlin RJ, Pindborg JJ, Clausen FJ, Vickers RA: The calcifying odontogenic cyst—A possible analogue of the cutaneous calcifying epithelioma of Malherbe. Oral Surg 15:1235, 1962; Courtesy of Charles E. Tomich, D.D.S., M.D., Indianapolis, IN)

proliferating epithelium that always resemble the odontogenic epithelium of the enamel organ to some degree. *Follicular, plexiform,* and *acanthomatous* histologic variants are described in which the appearances of basal cells, stellate reticulum (with varying degrees of cystic degeneration), and squamous metaplasia are reproduced. These histologic variants show no correlation with either the clinical appearance of the lesion or its behavior, and different sections of the same tumor may show one or the other histologic variation (Figs. 8-19 and 8-20).

The *follicular ameloblastoma* tends to resemble the enamel organ with the outer cells similar in appearance to the inner dental epithelium. The center portion of the epithelial island contains a loose, delicate network of cells, similar to the stellate reticulum. Squamous metaplasia of epithelial cells within the stellate reticulumlike central area has given rise to the term *acanthomatous ameloblastoma.* Cystic degeneration can occur within the follicle areas and the stroma *per se.*

The *plexiform-type ameloblastoma* exhibits irregular masses and strands of epithelial cells, which resemble ameloblasts or basal cells. Cystic degeneration of the central portion is common. Ameloblastomas occasionally contain large granular cells, giving rise to the term *granular cell ameloblastoma.*

Distinction between an area of proliferating odontogenic epithelium in the wall of a dentigerous cyst and early ameloblastoma may be difficult to make (Figs. 8-21 and 8-22). There is no clear origin for the ameloblastoma, and the dentigerous cyst is only one possibility, with remnants of the dental lamina and the basal layer of the oral mucosal epithelium also being strong contenders. However, there does seem to be good reason for repeated curettage or excision of the bony wall of a cyst in which such a change has been noted, especially in young patients.

There is no justification for the use of radiation therapy in the treatment of ameloblastomas; its use in past years has been associated with a considerable incidence of radiation-induced sarcoma.

The *adenomatoid odontogenic tumor* (also referred to as an *adenoameloblastoma*) differs considerably from the ameloblastic norm and is usually now excluded from that category. By contrast with ameloblastoma, it is a well-encapsulated lesion that rarely recurs even with conservative curettage, and recognition of its characteristic histology should prevent the need for block excision of the lesion. Clinically, it may be suspected because of its preference for the maxilla rather than the mandible and for anterior segments of the jaws rather than posterior. Often it presents as a

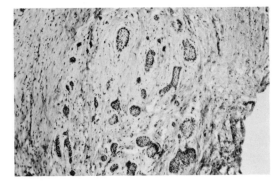

Fig. 8-21 Proliferation of odontogenic epithelium in a dental granuloma (H & E).

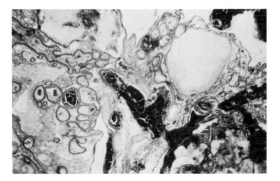

Fig. 8-22 Ameloblastoma developing in the wall of a dentigerous cyst (H & E).

cystic lesion that is not associated with a missing tooth and that on biopsy is found to have several masses of tumor tissue in its wall. These mural nodules are composed of characteristic masses of ductlike structures lined with basal or columnar cells with peripherally placed nuclei. The "lumen" of some of these "ducts" is nonexistent, that of others dilated with an eosinophilic or fibrillar material giving some suggestion of poorly formed stellate reticulum. Amorphous calcification may be apparent both microscopically and radiographically (Fig. 8-23).

Ameloblastic Odontoma

Calcification within an ameloblastoma is rare, and this feature can serve to distinguish it from both the adenomatoid odontogenic tumor and the ameloblastic odontoma (sometimes referred to as an odontoameloblastoma, the enamel-producing ameloblastoma of early authors). This latter lesion consists of ameloblastic tissue found in association with an abnormal mass of partially calcified dental tissues that histologically may contain enamel, dentin, osteodentin, bone, cementum, and pulp tissue as well as various developing stages of these tissues. Such mixtures of a complex odontoma (see below) with ameloblastomatous tissue apparently behave in much more benign fashion than does an ameloblastoma and may be treated safely by local excision or curettage.

Calcifying Epithelial Odontogenic Tumor

The *Pindborg tumor* (or *calcifying epithelial odontogenic tumor;* see Fig. 8-24) also shows

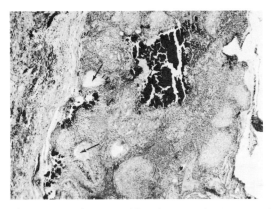

Fig. 8-23 Adenomatoid odontogenic tumor with ductlike structures (*arrows*) H & E, ×65; (Courtesy of J. E. Hamner III, D.D.S., Ph.D., Washington, DC)

considerable calcification but behaves like an ameloblastoma in that it is locally invasive even though histologically it does not resemble ameloblastoma. This odontogenic tumor is composed of masses of polyhedral epithelial cells with little stroma. The cells may be eosinophilic, exhibit intercellular bridges, and be quite pleomorphic with multiple giant nuclei. In many ways it appears microscopically like a potentially aggressive squamous cell carcinoma with a predominance of cells resembling those of the stratum spinosum of oral epithelium, and undoubtedly many cases have been wrongly diagnosed as squamous cell carcinoma. The central location of the tumor in the jaw, often with expansion of the cortex (rather than the destructive lesions characteristic of carcinoma), and the areas of spotty calcification radiographically

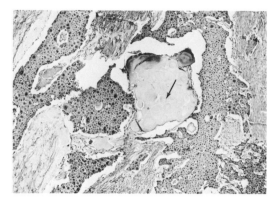

Fig. 8-24 Calcifying epithelial odontogenic tumor with Liesegang calcification (*arrow*) H & E, ×65; (Courtesy of J. E. Hamner III, D.D.S., Ph.D., Washington, DC)

should alert the clinician to the possibility of a Pindborg tumor. Sections of such a tumor should be examined for the characteristic hyaline, concentrically calcified globules of amyloid within the masses of epithelioid cells that confirm the lesion as of odontogenic origin. Larger areas of calcification and dentin formation may also be found. Treatment is by local block excision, but exploration of regional nodes and follow-up radiation (as might be used for squamous cell carcinoma) are quite unjustified for this odontogenic lesion.

Other Epithelial Odontogenic Tumors

Other epithelial odontogenic tumors in which varying degrees of dentin and enamel matrix (with or without calcification) occur are the *ameloblastic fibroma* (a tumor of children which resembles an ameloblastoma radiologically and histologically except that the stroma consists of pulp tissue rather than undifferentiated connective tissue and which behaves less aggressively than ameloblastoma; see Fig. 8-25), *dentinoma* (a similar lesion in which the pulp tissue also shows evidence of dentin and predentin formation), and various *odontomas* such as ameloblastic odontoma (described above) and complex and compound varieties (see following text).

Complex and compound odontomas are nonaggressive lesions that are more likely hamartomatous than neoplastic. They are often small and may remain undiscovered for many years until they are revealed by routine

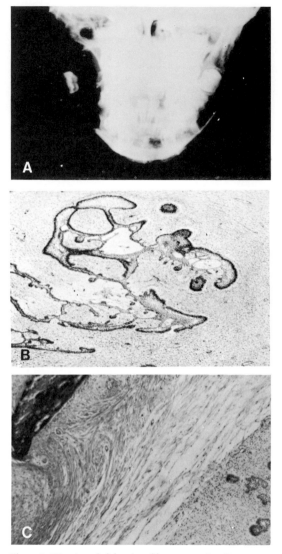

Fig. 8-25 Ameloblastic fibroma. *A*, Roentgenographic appearance (Charles Halstead, D.D.S., M.S.D., Atlanta, GA). *B*, Histologic structure showing pulplike stoma enclosing proliferating odontogenic epithelium. *C*, Erosion of bone adjacent to tumor.

panoramic radiography or a search for a missing permanent tooth. Their radiographic appearance is often characteristic, and if their presence does not interfere with orderly tooth eruption, they may be safely left undisturbed. Dentigerous cysts may form in association with these lesions and this possibility may justify their removal and certainly justifies repeated radiographic examination for new cyst development every 2 to 3 years. The term *complex odontoma* is used for lesions that contain mature calcified dental tissue that is poorly differentiated as to its exact identity as enamel, dentin, or cementum. Such lesions characteristically appear as dense radiopaque objects sometimes lying in a "clear space" or associated with a "cyst," but more often are enclosed by a well-defined "lamina dura." *Compound odontomas* contain calcified structures that grossly and radiographically resemble poorly formed and often small teeth in which enamel and dentin and cementum can be distinguished. Remembering the common meanings of complex (complicated, hard to separate or analyze) and compound (a joining together of parts so as to form a whole) may help the student distinguish these two types of odontoma which are, in fact, quite aptly described by these terms.

Myxomas (tumors composed of very loose cellular connective tissue containing little collagen and large amounts of intercellular substance that is rich in hyaluronic acid) occur with some frequency in the jaw bones. Since similar lesions are rare in other bones and since some oral myxomas contain tiny epithelial remnants resembling inactive odontogenic epithelium, this tumor is assumed to be of odontogenic origin and to be composed of hyperplastic connective tissue resembling dental pulp. It is a slowly growing but invasive tumor of jaw bone that sometimes reaches quite large dimensions and distends the jaw. It produces a radiographic appearance that may be indistinguishable from ameloblastoma, fibrous dysplasia, giant cell reparative granuloma, cherubism (an inherited condition that is usually seen only in children and is characterized by familial occurrence of multilocular radiolucencies of the jaw bone that contain mature fibroblastic tissue with multinucleate giant cells; see discussion earlier in this chapter under Fibrous Dysplasia and Other Fibro-Osseous Lesions), and the jaw lesions of hyperparathyroidism (osteitis fibrosa cystica). Treatment is similar to that recommended for ameloblastoma, although tooth root resorption in an area affected by a myxoma and recurrence after simple curettage may give the impression of a more aggressive lesion.

The *odontogenic fibroma* (which is composed of mature fibroblastic tissue with rare nests and strands of odontogenic epithelium) is a slowly growing and nonaggressive lesion that may be the mature end-result of the odontogenic myxoma. Unlike the myxoma it does not recur after curettage.

Cementoma

This term is commonly used to describe the localized masses of radiopaque, condensed areas of the alveolus adjacent to the roots of the teeth. On the one hand, this lesion merges with *hypercementosis* (excessive but evenly spread layers of cementum around the apical third of a tooth root, often causing considerable difficulty in extraction) and on the other with fibrous dysplasia of bone, in which both bone and cemental matrix formation are often observed (see Fig. 8-13).

Periapical cementomas are often multiple and are distinguished from chronic periapical abscesses by their being associated with vital teeth. There is good evidence that periapical cementomas pass through an osteolytic phase in which they can be distinguished from periapical cysts and granulomas only by the retention of vitality in the tooth, through a stage in which one or more radiopaque zones appear within the radiolucent area, to a final stage of uniform radiopacity. The term *periapical cemental dysplasia* is often used for such lesions to emphasize their relationship to fibrous dysplasia and to distinguish them from hypercementosis (Fig. 8-26). Provided such lesions do not increase in size or otherwise exhibit atypical behavior, there seems to be no reason to remove them. Should caries or other pulpal disease warrant endodontic treatment of a tooth with a cementoma, apicoectomy with removal of the dense periapical lesion is desirable, if only to prevent complication in the postoperative evaluation of the success of the endodontic therapy.

Middle-aged females appear to be preferentially susceptible to a widespread form of cementoma formation in which both maxilla and mandible may be occupied by large globular masses of cementum. Differentiation of this condition (*familial multiple gigantiform cementoma*) from *chronic sclerosing osteomyelitis of the jaws* (Fig. 8-27) and *ossifying fibroma* is of-

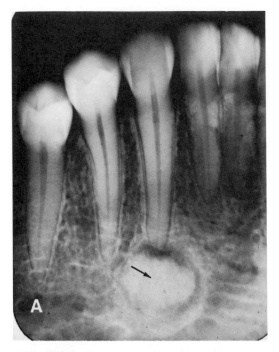

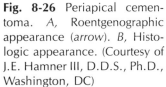

Fig. 8-26 Periapical cementoma. *A,* Roentgenographic appearance (*arrow*). *B,* Histologic appearance. (Courtesy of J.E. Hamner III, D.D.S., Ph.D., Washington, DC)

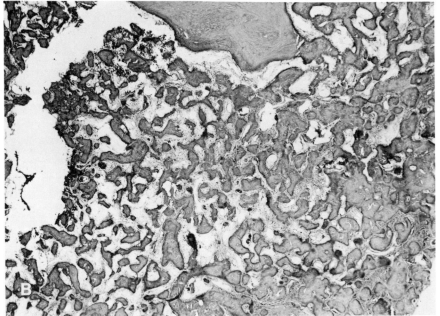

ten difficult. Biopsies may not clearly show the identity of the sclerotic substance, and since unnecessary surgical treatment is contraindicated in this avascular tissue, representative biopsies are often not available.

Extraction of teeth frequently leads to chronic osteomyelitis in areas of the jaw bone

affected by this lesion, adding to the difficulty of accurate diagnosis. Treatment should be conservative, and surgical intervention kept to a minimum. Chronic sequestrum and sinus formation are common and should be managed by irrigation and gentle debridement of exposed sequestra rather than by

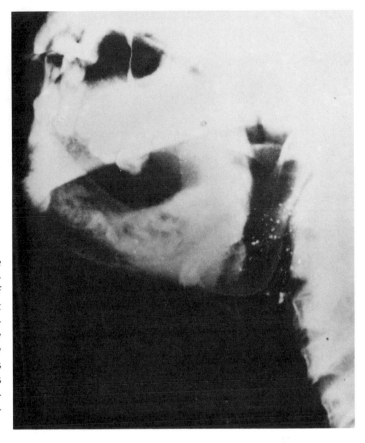

Fig. 8-27 Roentgenograph. Appearance of chronic sclerosing osteomyelitis affecting the major portion of the body of the mandible. Clinical and histologic differentiation of this lesion from ossifying fibroma may be difficult, particularly if teeth have been extracted or surgery carried out adjacent to the area. (Nichols C, Brightman, VJ: Parotid calcifications and cementoma in a patient with Sjögren's syndrome and idiopathic thrombocytopenia. J Oral Pathol 6:51, 1977)

surgical excision. Exploration of these lesions rarely leads to the finding of a distinct sequestrum and usually causes even more extensive bony necrosis. It is also doubtful whether long-term antibiotic therapy is helpful, and antibiotics should be used only when acute inflammatory exacerbation associated with pain, soft-tissue swelling, and marked production of pus occur. Such episodes are in fact unusual, and an antibiotic chosen on the basis of its efficacy against microorganisms contained in freely flowing pus can be used to treat them on these occasions.

SALIVARY CYSTS AND BENIGN TUMORS OF THE SALIVARY GLANDS

Nodules and swellings may affect both the major salivary glands and the extensive areas of minor salivary gland tissue distributed throughout the mucosal surface of the lips, cheeks, palate, floor of the mouth, and posterior third of the dorsum of the tongue. Because of their location, swellings of the major glands are almost always much larger than those affecting the more superficially placed minor glands at the time they are observed. Tumors of the major salivary glands are relatively rare yet frequently poorly localized in the gland and subject to recurrence and spread, a fact that may be related to their relatively larger size at the time of discovery. It follows that prompt removal of nodules from the major salivary glands is desirable as soon as they are noted, despite the risk of damage to the 5th and 7th cranial nerves and the risk of salivary fistula that accompanies surgery on the parotid and submandibular glands.

Salivary Cysts

The *mucocele*, a common lesion on the inner aspect of the lips and the cheeks, resembles

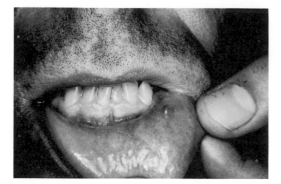

Fig. 8-28 Small mucocele of the lower lip.

a small cyst but is in reality a small mucus-filled mucosal bleb caused by extravasation and pooling of the secretion of a minor salivary gland in the periductal tissue (Fig. 8-28). These lesions are thought to be traumatic in origin (they may be produced experimentally by cutting but not by ligating the gland duct), the extravasated secretion producing an intense inflammatory response in the periductal tissue. The majority of these lesions rupture during mastication and heal spontaneously. Occasionally, recurrent lesions suggest the need for surgical excision of the affected tissue. Such an approach may result in damage to adjacent gland ducts, however, and is recommended as a last resort when multiple recurrences and scar formation have led to formation of a nodule, rather than as a routine method of treatment.

Mucous retention cysts of the minor salivary glands also occur and clinically are difficult to distinguish from mucoceles, except that they rarely occur on the lower lip, the site of predilection for the mucocele. Mucous retention cysts also may be found as pea-sized swellings of the ducts of mucous glands on the pharyngeal surface of the tongue.

Retention cysts of the submandibular and sublingual glands may achieve a large size and burrow into the tissue planes of the neck before becoming apparent in the floor of the mouth as a pale, bluish-green fluid-filled swelling. These cysts are traditionally referred to as *ranula* because of the supposed resemblance of the sublingual swelling to the skin of a frog's belly (*Rana* is the generic name for one variety of frog) and may recur if inadequately removed, a common consequence of their location and dissecting tendency.

Similar cystic lesions do not apparently affect the parotid gland, and the major cyst in that gland (excluding cystic degeneration of tumors) is the *branchial cleft cyst*. This is characterized by a lining composed of stratified squamous epithelium surrounded by a layer of lymphoid nodules. Branchial cleft cysts, as the name implies, are traditionally thought to be inclusion cysts formed from remnants of the cervical sinus (the branchial cleft separating the hyoid and first cervical embryonic arches). A more current hypothesis with some experimental confirmation is that this lesion in the parotid gland arises by cystic degeneration of salivary gland epithelium trapped within lymphoid nodules during development. Lesions histologically similar to branchial cleft cysts also occur in the floor of the mouth and in the tongue where a similar etiology is likely.

Nodular swellings affecting the orifices of the minor salivary glands of the posterior palate are common lesions in smokers and are referred to as *stomatitis nicotina*. The lesion is characterized by swelling and blockage of the orifice of these glands with an easily visible brownish plug of tar-stained salivary debris. The nodules usually occur on an area of leukoplakic or hyperkeratotic palatal mucosa. The nodular lesion contains elements of hyperkeratosis and acanthosis as well as squamous metaplasia of the gland duct and some degree of chronic sialadenitis. The lesion usually regresses with cessation of smoking. Leukoplakia occurring elsewhere in the oral cavity as a result of heavy smoking is usually considered a precancerous condition, but some authors have questioned whether stomatitis nicotina is a precancerous lesion even though it results from smoking, since carcinoma of the palate is a very rare condition. However, stomatitis nicotina can serve as a useful indicator of excessive smoking, and attempts to eliminate the lesion are desirable since they draw the patient's attention to the need to reduce, or preferably eliminate, smoking (see also Chapter 6).

Necrotizing sialometaplasia, another nodular lesion of the palate, is not specifically related to smoking, but may be mistaken for mucoepidermoid or squamous cell carcinoma if the pathologist is not familiar with this benign hyperplastic lesion in this location. It is a benign, ulcerative, inflammatory process of the minor salivary glands, primarily found in the hard palate. The lesion develops rapidly and heals spontaneously in 6 to 12 weeks. It occurs primarily in persons between the ages of 40 and 60 and has been reported more frequently in men than in women. In necrotizing sialometaplasia, the squamous metaplasia and tissue necrosis are confined to the existing ductal and lobular pattern of the salivary glands, a unique characteristic that aids in diagnosis (Fig. 8-29). No specific treatment is required, although healing that occurs by secondary intention is usually slow.

Sjögren's syndrome is discussed in Chapter 11. Rapid increase in size of the parotid or other major salivary glands affected by this autoimmune process may simulate a tumor and may even be the cause for the biopsy that establishes the nature of this disease. In view of the recognized incidence of malignant lymphomatous change in the salivary glands in Sjögren's syndrome, repeated biopsy may be necessary in the parotid gland that is irregularly enlarged or nodular in this condition.

Benign Tumors of the Salivary Glands

The benign and malignant forms of salivary gland tumors are compared in Table 8-5 according to their proportionate percentage of occurrence. Many classifications exist, chiefly because there is not universal agreement among pathologists as to the cell of origin for many of these lesions. These neoplasms are rare, also, comprising 1% to 4% of all head and neck tumors; the benign varieties account for 65% of the total number.

Diagnosis of salivary gland tumors is based upon patient history, palpation, clinical signs and symptoms, sialography, radioisotope scans, and surgical biopsy.

In comparison with benign salivary tumors, the malignant tumors exhibit no sex predominance and tend to be more prevalent after 50 years of age. Clinical signs and symptoms typically include pain, sudden growth, facial nerve paralysis, a firm consistency, poor demarcation with infiltration into the surrounding tissues, and metastatic spread by either lymphatic or hematogenous routes for malignant tumors.

In terms of anatomic site, 80% of salivary gland tumors occur in the parotid gland, 10%

in the submandibular gland, 1% in the sublingual gland, and 9% in minor salivary glands.

Treatment is most often surgical resection or surgery in conjunction with radiation therapy. Salivary gland tumors tend to recur because of the difficulty of complete surgical eradication without damage to the branches of the facial nerve in the case of parotid tumors.

Pleomorphic Adenomas

The most common salivary gland tumor is the *pleomorphic adenoma* also known as a *mixed salivary tumor.* This latter term is possibly a misnomer since the hyaline cartilagelike areas seen in these epithelial tumors appear to be the result of inductive change in the connective tissue stroma produced by the neoplastic myoepithelial cells of the tumor. The term *pleomorphic adenoma* is also misleading, since carcinomatous change is quite common in these lesions, and it is probably wise to assume that all pleomorphic adenomas irrespective of their histologic type are, in fact, adenocarcinomas and to treat them accordingly. Most pleomorphic adenomas are encapsulated, but they frequently recur if simply "shelled-out" of the gland.

The histologic criteria for diagnosing a malignant mixed tumor are not thoroughly established, and reliance is usually placed on the nuclear changes of malignancy (such as nuclear hyperchromatism and pleomorphism, increased or abnormal mitoses, and increased nuclear/cytoplasmic ratio), in addition to evidences of hematogenous, lymphatic, or neural invasion, focal necrosis and peripheral infiltration. Removal of the affected salivary gland lobule, or preferably the entire gland, results in fewer recurrences and usually prevents the local infiltrative growth and lymphatic spread that occur in about 25% of cases.

Both major and minor salivary gland tissues are affected by this lesion, but there are differences in incidence and behavior of the tumor in the two locations. The sites of predilection in order of importance are the palate, lip, buccal mucosa, and tongue. Palatal and submandibular lesions, though rare, are considered to be more malignant than those in other regions.

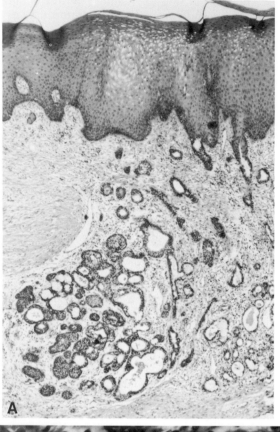

Fig. 8-29 *A,* Minor salivary gland shows distinctive signs of necrotizing sialometaplasia with squamous cell metaplasia of salivary acini and ducts. Note maintenance of salivary gland architecture, hyperplasia of pseudoepitheliomatous surface epithelium, acinar degeneration, and mucus inspissation. Upper right corner falsely appears as ingrowth of squamous cell from surface epithelium, mimicking squamous cell carcinoma, which actually represents squamous metaplasia of ductal elements as they approach surface epithelum (× 40). *B,* Squamous metaplasia of salivary gland ducts showing thickening of walls of some ducts and total obliteration of lumens of other salivary ducts. Normal salivary ducts are only one or two cell layers thick. Note bland nuclear morphology and lack of cellular atypia (× 125).

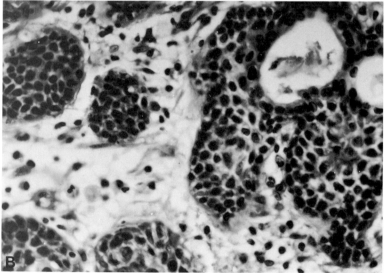

Fig. 8-29, cont., C, Squamous metaplasia of salivary ducts and acini showing acinar degeneration and mucus pooling. Note maintenance of acinar architecture (×125). (Grillon GL, Lally ET: Necrotizing sialometaplasia: Literature review and presentation of five cases. J Oral Surg 39:747, 1981)

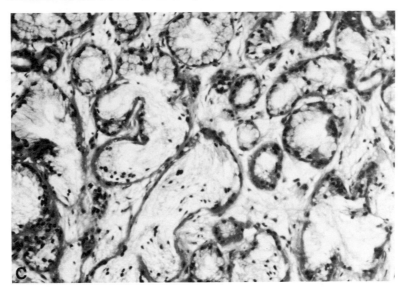

Salivary gland tumors are usually first noticed because of a swelling in the major gland or the oral cavity (Fig. 8-30A). Some are discovered by routine palpation of the glands, and oral examination should include palpation of the major salivary glands as well as the entire oral mucosa to detect nodules that may not be visible on inspection; others cause pain, and a small number encroach on the facial nerve in the parotid gland and cause facial paralysis. Pain is traditionally considered a sign of poor prognosis, and facial paralysis due to this cause usually occurs only with large tumors infiltrating beyond the gland capsule. A small number are first detected as nodular areas of poor "filling" in a sialogram. Because of the unpredictable nature of salivary gland tumors, oral mucosal nodules and unidentified nodules in the major glands that are discovered by palpation or sialography should be biopsied (Fig. 8-30B).

The salivary gland tumor is sometimes referred to as a *cylindroma,* and is characterized histologically by groups or rosettes of epithelial cells of reasonably benign appearance that enclose a cylinderlike space containing hyaline or mucinous material. This type of tumor is well known as a particularly malignant lesion, and the term has been properly replaced by that of *adenoid-cystic carcinoma* (Fig. 8-31).

Monomorphic Adenomas

Epithelial neoplasms of the salivary glands that do not exhibit inductive changes in the stroma and are made up of a single type of cell (compare pleomorphic adenoma) are sometimes referred to as *monomorphic adenomas*. Unlike pleomorphic adenomas, these lesions are usually benign. The most common of these lesions is *Warthin's tumor (papillary cystadenolymphomatosum),* a histologically exotic growth made up of a triple-layer epithelial proliferation *within* a cyst wall (*i.e.,* a cystadenoma). The villous structure within the cyst consists of two layers of epithelium and a layer of lymphocytic tissue with germinal centers. Because of its encapsulated cystic nature, it can often be easily diagnosed by needle aspiration (a controversial technique that may be of little help with other major salivary gland tumors) and by its characteristic appearance in scintigrams of the parotid using the isotope ^{99m}Tc-pertechnetate. It is also one of the few growths of the parotid gland that occurs bilaterally (compare sialoadenitis), and this fact can have diagnostic value at times (7.5% of cases are bilateral and 2% recurrences).

Warthin's tumor and onkocytomas (see Fig. 8-32 and below) originate in the onkocytes, which are derived from ductal epithelium. Onkocytes are relatively large, polyg-

Table 8-5. Salivary Gland Tumors

	Type of tumor	Percentage of Occurrence*
Benign	Mixed tumor (pleomorphic adenoma)	58
	Papillary cystadenoma lymphomatosum (Warthin's tumor)	6
	Oncocytoma (oxyphilic adenoma)	1
Malignant	Mixed tumor	7
	Mucoepidermoid carcinoma	12
	Adenocarcinoma	11
	Adenoid cystic carcinoma (cylindroma)	
	Acinic cell adenocarcinoma	
	Epidermoid carcinoma	5

* Major salivary gland tumors

onal, eosinophilic cells with a granular cytoplasm that contain a large number of mitochondria and are actively secreting cells similar to the striated duct cells in the normal gland. These cells, like ductal epithelium, can extract large anions from blood, such as pertechnetate and iodides, and secrete them into a central lumen lying within clumps of cells. Because Warthin's tumors and onkocytomas do not connect with an organized duct system as in normal gland tissue, the anions accumulate in cystic spaces in the tissue without being discharged and account for the characteristic scintigraphic appearance.

Onkocytoma (oxyphil adenoma) and other cystadenomas composed of onkocytic or sebaceous cells also occur as benign growths of salivary tissue. Onkocytes and sebaceous cells are also found in normal salivary gland tissue and other salivary gland neoplasms. *Onkocytic hyperplasia* is a common age-change in both the parotid and small serous glands of von Ebner and mucous glands associated

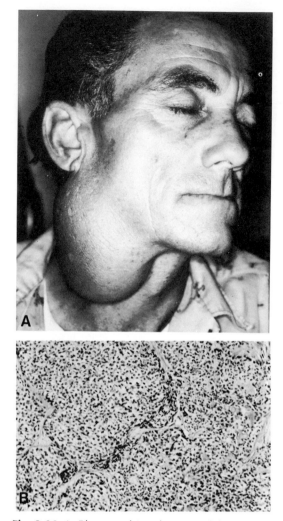

Fig. 8-30 *A*, Pleomorphic adenoma of the parotid in a 49-year-old male; a mass slowly enlarging over the previous 5 years. (Courtesy of Robert M. Howell, D.D.S., M.S.D., Lincoln, NB) *B*, Histologic appearance of a characteristic area of malignant mixed tumor. (Courtesy of J. E. Hamner III, D.D.S., Ph.D., Washington, DC)

with the vallate and foliate papillae of the tongue.

Familial cases of Warthin's tumor in association with onkocytic metaplasia of the pharynx and larynx have been reported. This observation, and the frequent multiple occurrence of Warthin's tumor in the one patient suggest that Warthin's tumor is also a metaplastic rather than a neoplastic process,

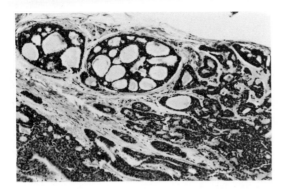

Fig. 8-31 Adenoid cystic carcinoma, a particularly malignant salivary gland tumor despite the term *cylindroma* often used to describe it. It is composed of small, darkly staining uniform cells closely arranged in anastomosing cords or ductlike patterns, the central portion of which may contain mucoid or hyaline material. The end result is a honeycomb or Swiss cheese appearance. The stromal tissue often becomes hyalinized, and because it surrounds the tumor cells, a cylindromatous pattern evolves. This tumor is extremely malignant, yet the histologic appearance is deceptively benign. (Courtesy of J.E. Hamner III, D.D.S., Ph.D., Washington, DC)

with the associated lymphoid reaction being in the nature of a delayed hypersensitivity response.

Malignant change is apparently rare in most monomorphic adenomas, and conservative local excision or shelling-out of the lesion is considered adequate treatment.

BENIGN VIRAL-INDUCED ORAL TUMORS

Several benign oral epithelial growths are thought to be examples of virus-induced neoplasms. Papilloma, warts, keratoacanthoma, and focal epithelial hyperplasia probably belong in this category, although conclusive evidence on this point and diagnostic techniques for isolation and identification of the causative viruses are not available. Wart virus has been isolated from similar skin lesions, and the virus of molluscum contagiosum can also be demonstrated in the inclusion bodies of that lesion on both oral and skin surface and can be transmitted to tissue culture cells.

(The likelihood of Paget's disease being a multicentric, viral-induced tumor of osteoclasts is discussed later in this chapter, under Syndromes with Benign Oral Neoplastic or Hamartomatous Components; nasopharyngeal carcinoma, a malignant tumor associated with a persistent infection with Epstein–Barr virus, is described in Chapter 10.)

Molluscum contagiosum, a dermatologic infection acquired by direct skin contact and characterized by clusters of tiny firm nodules that can be curetted from the skin, is histologically composed of clumps of proliferating epithelial cells with prominent eosinophilic inclusion bodies. It is not a neoplasm but is included here as one of the spectrum of oral epithelial proliferations that result from viral infection. Both intraoral and labial lesions of molluscum contagiosum have been reported (see also Chapter 28).

Oral papillomas and *warts (verruca vulgaris)* share many similarities. The latter term usually is applied when a crop of lesions develops, sometimes in association with similar skin lesions. When they occur on the keratinized surface of the lips, alveolar gingivae, or palate, these lesions are well keratinized and wartlike, often with a definite narrow pedicle (Figs. 8-33 and 8-34). On the nonkeratinized mucosal surface they may appear soft and redder and be hard to differentiate from the lesions of fibrous hyperplasia described earlier in this chapter. A rugose, cauliflowerlike, exophytic lesion is more likely to be a papilloma than fibrous hyperplasia. Local excision of these lesions is desirable, electrocoagulation being the treatment of choice on the lips where they cause a cosmetic problem.

Although these lesions are probably infectious, a history of direct contact with another infected person is unusual except in the case of multiple and often recurrent oral warts associated with sexual contact, which are referred to as *condyloma acuminatum* (see also Chap. 28). Intraoral papillomatosis may be inherited in such rare conditions as ichthyosis hystrix, but other manifestations of this syndrome (a congenitally acquired deforming skin papillomatosis) serve to differentiate these lesions from other congenital conditions, such as Down's syndrome in which florid papillomatosis may also occur.

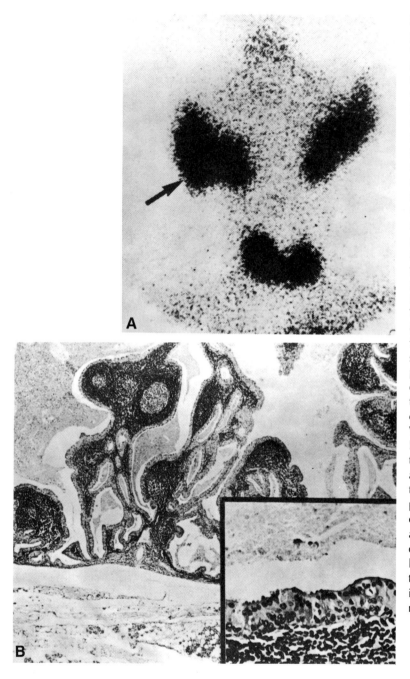

Fig. 8-32 *A,* Scintigraphic appearance of Warthin's tumor located in right tail of the parotid gland. In this anterior view of a sodium pertechnetate radionuclide scan 20 minutes postinjection (see Chap. 11 for description of technique), the radioisotope concentration at this location (*arrow*) is increased. The upper central accumulation of the radionuclide at the level of the midfacial structures represents early oral salivary excretion of the sodium pertechnetate. This scintigraphic appearance is virtually diagnostic of Warthin's tumor. *B,* Low-power (×6) and higher-power (×100) photomicrographs of the Warthin's tumor demonstrated in (*A*) following excision by superficial parotid lobectomy. The sections show typical papillary projections into a cystic, protein-containing lesion. Inset shows the characteristic double-layered oncocytic epithelial lining of Warthin's tumor with abundant lymphocytes immediately below the epithelium. *A* and *B* are from an unusual case of familial Warthin's tumor. Oncocytic metaplasia, the basic histopathologic change in Warthin's tumor may also occur elsewhere in the oropharyngeal mucosa as an isolated finding or sometimes as in the case illustrated by *A* and *B* in association with Warthin's tumor.

Fig. 8-32, cont., *C* and *D*, On-kocytic hyperplasia of the glands of the tongue dorsum noted at autopsy in a 61-year-old female with advanced arteriosclerosis. Two cystic areas lined by onko-cytes (*arrow*) lie adjacent to a deep midline fissure in the re-gion of the foramen cecum that probably represents the remains of the thyroglossal duct. (*A* and *B*, Courtesy of A.M. Noyek, M.D., Toronto, Ont; J Otolar-yngol 9:90, 1980)

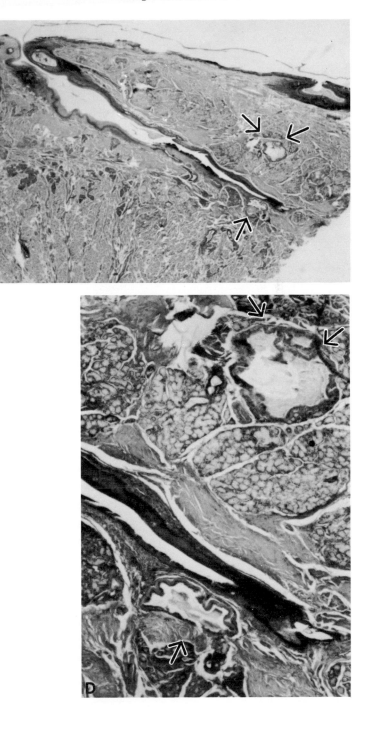

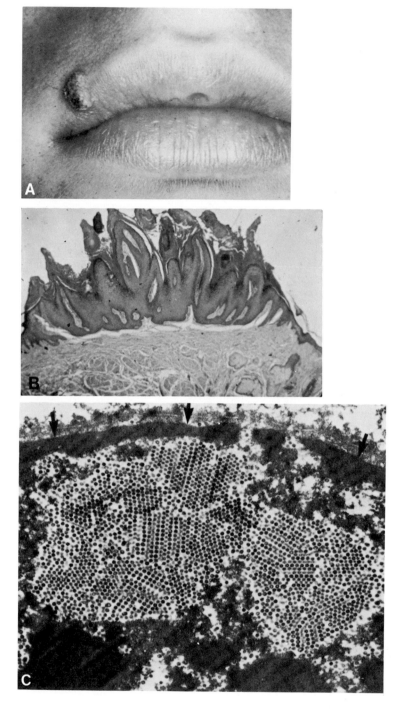

Fig. 8-33 *A,* A crop of viral warts (verruca vulgaris) on the keratinized skin surface of the upper lip of a 16-year-old male; lesions were removed by electrocautery. *B,* Histologic section of a wart on the upper lip showing the exophytic epithelial hyperplasia and keratin-capped papillae. (H & E). *C,* Portion of a superficial cell nucleus from an intraoral lesion diagnosed histopathologically as verruca vulgaris. Note the presence of numerous paracrystalline viral particles within the nucleus. Nuclear membrane is indicated by arrows; × 16,000 (Wysocki, GC, Hardie J: Ultrastructural studies of intraoral verruca vulgaris. Oral Surg 47:58, 1979)

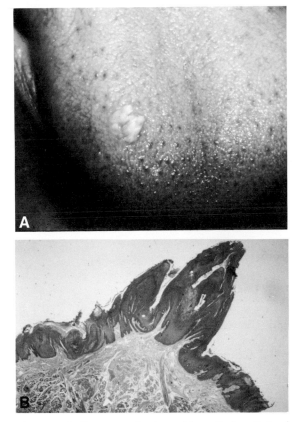

Fig. 8-34 Solitary exophytic and heavily keratinized wart on the dorsum of the tongue of a 22-year-old female. Before infiltration anesthetic, wart was inverted below surface of tongue.

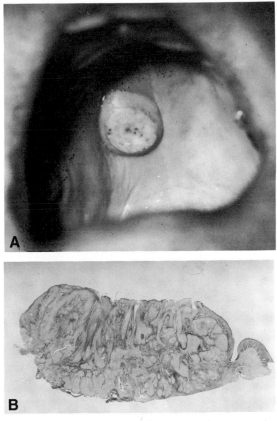

Fig. 8-35 Solitary intraoral keratoacanthoma on the hard palate of a 28-year-old white male cigarette smoker who also had a mild stomatitis nicotina. Lesion noted three weeks previously; no associated bony or regional lymph node involvement; no recurrence following local soft tissue excision. *A*, Clinical view of the lesion, which is well circumscribed, abruptly elevated above the mucosal surface, and presenting a roughened, whitish surface. *B*, Overall microscopic morphology of the lesion. Note the cup-shaped configuration, the sharply circumscribed margin, and the thinned surface epithelium that tends to "lip" the central cell mass. Epithelium at the margins of the lesion was well differentiated with minimal pleomorphism and hyperchromatism. (From Scofield HH, Weining JT, Shukes RC: Solitary intraoral keracanthoma. Oral Surg 37:889, 1974; courtesy CV Mosby Co., St Louis, MO).

Focal epithelial hyperplasia (Heck's disease), a condition that is characterized by numerous soft papules distributed throughout the oral mucosa, is endemic in some Eskimo and American Indian communities but quite rare in Caucasians. Examples in Puerto Ricans and more recently in Negroes suggest that further search for this lesion may show it to be more widespread. Histologically, it is characterized by nondyskeratotic, nodular acanthosis, which forms the basis of the papules, and a subepithelial lymphocytic infiltration. A viral etiology is likely, based on the consistency of electron microscopic demonstration of viral particles in these lesions. Once identified, the lesions require no treatment; malignant transformation is unknown.

If the preceding lesions in this section seem difficult for the reader to accept as neoplasms (and indeed there is no certainty that they are), such is not the case with *keratoacanthoma*, a lesion whose rapid growth may be quite frightening and is often mistakenly diagnosed as squamous or basal cell carcinoma (Fig. 8-35). Like some carcinomas, these lesions appear fixed to the surrounding tissue,

Table 8-6. Syndromes in Which Benign Tumors of the Oral Cavity Are Associated with a Predisposition to Internal Malignancy

SYNDROME	ORAL LESIONS	OTHER SKIN LESIONS	ASSOCIATED ABNORMALITIES	ASSOCIATED MALIGNANCY
von Recklinghausen's Neurofibromatosis	Intraoral neurofibromas (especially of tongue) leading to macroglossia; Rarely, intrabony neurofibromas of jaws	Multiple neurofibromas (especially trunk and extremities); Café-au-lait spots (especially trunk, axilla, pelvis); Axillary freckles; Giant nevi	CNS tumors; acoustic neuromas; meningioma and glioma; plexiform neuromas; Bone cysts and hyperplasia associated with neuromas; Mental retardation	Malignant neurilemmoma (5% of cases); Pheochromocytoma; Astrocytoma and glioma
Gardner's Syndrome	Multiple osteomas of cranial and facial skeleton (especially frontal bone, mandible, and maxilla); Compound odontomas and hypercementosis	Epidermoid and sebaceous cysts; Desmoid tumors, lipomas, fibromas, and leiomyomas	Polyposis of the colon	Adenocarcinoma of colon (very high incidence)
Nevoid Basal Cell Carcinoma Syndrome	Multiple jaw cysts (simple, primordial, and odontogenic keratocysts); Dilaceration of teeth adjacent to cysts; Facial abnormalities (frontal bossing, sunken eyes, and wide nasal bridge; mild mandibular prognathism)	Epidermoid cysts; Milia and calcium deposits	Rib and vertebral anomalies; Short metacarpals; Ovarian fibromas; Calcification of ovarian fibromas and dura	Basal cell carcinoma of skin (often without sunlight exposure); Medulloblastoma; Ameloblastoma and fibrosarcoma of jaws (low incidence)
Multiple Mucosal Neuroma Syndrome (Multiple Endocrine Neoplasia Type III)	Neuromas of lips, tongue and buccal mucosa (oral cavity most common site); Thick or "bumpy" lips; Prognathism (infrequent)	Neuromas of eyelids and nasal laryngeal mucosa; Abnormal triple response to intradermal histamine injections (no flare)	Parathyroid adenomas; Hypertension	Medullary carcinoma of thyroid; Pheochromocytoma

Condition	Oral manifestations	Associated skin/other lesions	Other features	Neoplasms
Tuberous Sclerosis	Adenoma sebaceum Gingival lesions and enamel hypoplasia Cranial defects	Adenoma sebaceum	Epilepsy Mental retardation Hamartomas of brain, heart, and kidney	Astrocytoma and glioblastoma
Acanthosis Nigricans	Perioral and oral mucosal papillomatosis with areas of black pigmentation	Similar lesions on neck, axilla, and groin	*Absence* of endocrine abnormalities, obesity, and family history	Gastric adenocarcinoma
Peutz-Jeghers Syndrome*	Pigmented macules* of lips and oral mucosa	Similar lesions on fingers and toes	Intestinal polyposis (small intestine)	Gastric, duodenal, and colonic adenocarcinoma (low incidence)
Albright's Syndrome	Solitary or multiple foci of fibrous dysplasia of jaw bones Oral pigmentation (rarely)	Café-au-lait spots	Polyostotic fibrous dysplasia and bony deformities (1% of cases) Precocious sexual development	Fibrosarcoma and osteogenic sarcoma developing in areas of fibrous dysplasia
Paget's Disease† (Osteitis Deformans)	Localized or generalized bony jaw growths Hypercementosis	—	Large head, curved back, and bowed legs deformity Raised serum alkaline phosphatase with normal calcium and phosphorus levels	Osteogenic, chondro-, and fibrosarcoma, and giant cell tumor of bone developing in affected areas
Cowden's Syndrome (Multiple Hamartoma and Neoplasia Syndrome)	Papillomatosis of lips, gingivae, palate, pharynx, and fauces Pebbly, fissured tongue	Lichenoid and papillomatous lesions of perioral, perinasal, and periorbital areas, ear, and neck	Hamartomas of skin, gastrointestinal tract, breasts, and thyroid	A variety of neoplasms affecting principally the ovaries, colon, ear canal, and various soft and hard tissues

* Peutz-Jeghers syndrome is included because it represents another oral lesion associated with intestinal polyposis. The oral lesions are usually flat, pigmented macules and unlikely to be mistaken for a tumor.

† Oral lesions are only one part of a generalized neoplastic bone disease, any part of which, including the oral lesions, can undergo malignant change.

357

often grow rapidly, and are usually capped by thick keratin. Occasionally the lesion matures, exfoliates, and heals spontaneously, but more frequently, block excision is carried out and the diagnosis becomes apparent when the entire lesion is examined microscopically. Incisional biopsy specimens are almost always diagnosed as carcinoma, since they lack the panoramic view of the entire lesion which is of greatest help in its differentiation from carcinoma.

Epithelial tissue adjacent to the lesion is sharply demarcated from that of the lesion, which thus appears to lie in a cup-shaped depression. The proliferating epithelium constituting this amazing lesion consists of masses of reasonably well-differentiated squamous cells that often produce keratin pearls and show little cellular atypia. Clumps of cells that appear to be separated along the base of the lesion and the accompanying chronic inflammatory exudate in this region presumably are the cause for the mistaken diagnosis of carcinoma that seems, at the time, to be confirmed by the aggressive clinical appearance of the lesion. This latter fact, namely the rapid growth of this lesion, as well as its usual location on the upper lip (where squamous cell carcinoma of actinic etiology is rare compared with the lower lip) should remind the clinician to consider keratoacanthoma in his differential diagnosis. Intraoral lesions are quite rare. Treatment of this lesion remains controversial; some authors, who believe it is not clearly separable from squamous cell carcinoma, advocate wide excision to prevent recurrence.

SYNDROMES WITH BENIGN ORAL NEOPLASTIC OR HAMARTOMATOUS COMPONENTS

The main emphasis in this chapter has been on the accurate identification of benign oral tumors by means of histopathologic examination so that they may be clearly separated from malignant lesions and treated accordingly. Although only a small minority of the lesions in this chapter can be considered precancerous, the clinician must always bear in mind the possibility that he is dealing with a malignant lesion until he has accurately iden-

tified the nature of the oral swelling or bony defect under consideration; in many cases this assurance can only be provided by biopsy and microscopic examination of the excised tissue. Continuous awareness concerning oral and facial malignancy is a creditable attitude for all clinicians even though the frequency with which an individual practitioner may actually be confronted with a malignant oral lesion is fortunately low.

The oral cavity and face can also provide evidence of malignancy elsewhere in the body, and clinicians need to be aware of a variety of oral signs that can serve as an index of internal malignancy. Carcinoma is discussed in Chapter 9 and amyloidosis secondary to multiple myeloma is described in Chapter 22, and also as a differential diagnosis for macroglossia in an earlier section of this chapter and in Chapter 10. Addison's disease due to adrenal carcinoma and carcinoid syndrome as the result of pheochromocytoma may also be revealed by changes in the pigmentation and color of the oral mucosa (see Chap. 7). Recurrent herpes zoster and erythema multiforme (Chap. 5) may signal the presence of an otherwise undetected lymphoma or carcinoma.

In addition to these signs and of particular pertinence to this chapter are a group of conditions in which quite benign oral growths, which are themselves quite without any precancerous potential, are associated with a predisposition to a malignancy in another organ system. Such conditions, which are usually familial (often with autosomal dominant inheritance), are uncommon, but the very frequent association of a particular oral lesion with the internal malignancy in such families makes the recognition of these oral lesions very important.

Several authors have reviewed cancer syndromes associated with characteristic skin lesions. Table 8-6 summarizes those syndromes that are associated with benign oral tumors. A brief discussion of these syndromes follows.

Von Recklinghausen's Neurofibromatosis

This condition is inherited as an autosomal dominant condition, but only half the cases exhibit a familial history. The syndrome is characterized by the simultaneous occurrence of areas of light brown pigmentation usually on the trunk, axilla, and pelvic areas (café-au-lait spots, light brown macules with a smooth outline "like the coast of California"; the finding of six or more macules with a diameter of 1.5 cm or greater is diagnostic of neurofibromatosis*) and a wide variety of nerve and nerve sheath tumors, in both central and peripheral nervous systems. The peripheral lesions are often indistinguishable from those described earlier in this chapter (Hamartomas–Neurofibroma); the central lesions, because of their location within a bony cavity often in association with various nerve roots, lead to neurologic symptoms, mental retardation, and vertebral anomalies. Large infiltrating lesions that occur both peripherally and centrally and lead to severe deformity are referred to as *plexiform neuromas* (Fig. 8-36).

Malignant transformation of one or more neurofibromas occurs in about 5% of patients with this syndrome. Pheochromocytomas (tumors of the adrenal medulla and paraganglia) also may occur and produce hypertension by secretion of excess catecholamines. Approximately 5% of patients with neurofibromatosis have well-developed oral lesions with macroglossia (the tongue being the most common oral location for neurofibroma both in this syndrome and in solitary oral neurofibroma; see Fig. 8-12). This condition and the associated oral lesions are said to be more prevalent in patients in mental institutions. The lesions may be asymptomatic, about a third being recognized on routine physical examination.

Gardner's Syndrome

Although it is rare, Gardner's syndrome is of importance because of the high frequency with which carcinomatous transformation occurs in the polypoid intestinal lesions characteristic of this condition. Recognition of the multiple osteomas of the face and jaws and accompanying skin cysts and tumors fully justifies radiographic examination of the bowel and the resection of all polypoid tissue

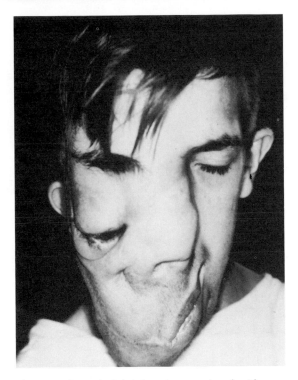

Fig. 8-36 Gross facial deformity associated with neurofibromatosis in a 25-year-old male. (Courtesy of Robert M. Howell, D.D.S., M.S.D., Lincoln, NB)

even in young adults (Fig. 8-37). Approximately 15 years may elapse between development of the polyps and adenocarcinomatous change, but since this is a condition with autosomal dominant inheritance with marked penetrance, examination of all family members beyond puberty, often by elective laparotomy, is usual.

Nevoid Basal Cell Carcinoma Syndrome

This is inherited in a similar fashion to the preceding syndrome, and thorough examination of all family members is justified when individuals with the characteristic jaw cysts, facial and other bony abnormalities, and skin lesions are detected. Although basal cell carcinoma is frequently a treatable lesion, in this condition the multiple nature of the carcinomas, their appearance at an early age, and their tendency to occur anywhere on the skin surface, often on areas covered by clothing, make early recognition and treatment difficult.

---

* Café-au-lait spots are also found in 10% of the normal population, especially in fair-skinned persons. Similar skin lesions with the same name occur in Albright's syndrome.

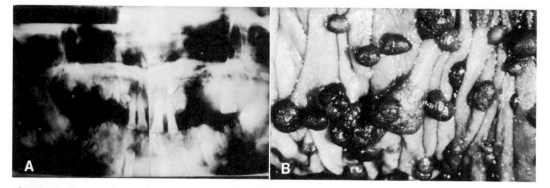

Fig. 8-37 Gardner's syndrome in a 43-year-old black female with a history of multiple osteomas and odontomas of the jaws and multiple colonic polyps, one of which showed adenocarcinomatous change. Death occurred following surgical removal of a larger desmoid tumor of the abdominal wall. Additional findings at autopsy included an adrenal cortical adenoma, fibroadenoma of the breast, multiple leiomyomata of the uterus, multiple hamartomas of the kidney, and an exostosis above left eyebrow. *A,* Panoramic roentgenograph of jaws showing osteomas, odontomas, and multiple unerupted teeth. *B,* Multiple adenomatous polyps of the colonic mucosa. (Archard HO: In Fitzpatrick TB [ed]: Dermatology in General Medicine, p 927. New York, McGraw-Hill, 1971)

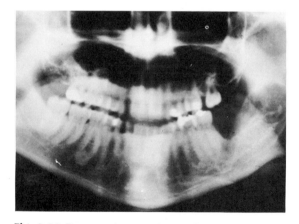

Fig. 8-38 Bony cavity remaining after curettage of a large odontogenic keratocyst lying close to but distinct from the crypt of an unerupted mandibular third molar. (Courtesy of Louis Guernsey, D.D.S., Philadelphia, PA)

Many of the jaw cysts in affected individuals have a keratinized epithelial lining and may be filled with layers of desquamated squames. Such cysts are referred to as *primordial* or *odontogenic keratocysts.* Considerable interest has been shown in cysts of this type in recent years because they frequently "bud" and produce daughter cysts, which may lead to incomplete removal and recurrence of the cyst, and because a keratinizing cyst lining is more common in "dentigerous" cysts that have undergone carcinomatous change. Such cysts also occur without other evidence of this syndrome (Fig. 8-38), and in the older literature they were often referred to as *epidermal inclusion cysts of the jaws* (compare epidermoid or dermoid cysts, described under hamartomas, which also contain various epidermal appendages). The finding of multiple odontogenic keratocysts, however, should always suggest the possibility of the syndrome and a search for its other features.

Pitting of the soles and palms (milia, local areas of undermaturation of the epithelial basal cells) is an obvious additional finding in about half of the individuals affected by the syndrome, and the facies with ocular hypertelorism may be prominent. There is no evidence that development of squamous cell carcinoma is a hazard associated with the odontogenic keratocysts in this syndrome, but occasional ameloblastoma and fibrosarcoma of the jaws have been reported.

All odontogenic keratocysts (both solitary and multiple) should be followed indefinitely postoperatively because of their capacity for recurrence and infiltration. A poor phosphate diuresis in response to parathormone is apparently not a feature of this syndrome (earlier reports to the contrary). The word "nevus" used in the name of this syndrome and in certain other connotations (*e.g.*, nevus flammeus in Sturge–Weber syndrome; nevus unius lateris for ichthyosis hystrix) refers to a genetically determined hamartoma or birthmark, not to a melanocytic nevus or mole.

Multiple Mucosal Neuroma Syndrome

More recently identified as *multiple endocrine neoplasia Type III* (MEN), the multiple mucosal neuroma syndrome is one of a group of familial syndromes in which neoplastic change occurs in several endocrine glands in one individual. MEN Type I involves lesions in some combination of pancreatic islets, adrenal cortex, parathyroid, and pituitary glands and includes the Zollinger–Ellison syndrome (multiple pancreatic islet cell adenomas secreting gastrin or secretin and leading to gastric hypersecretion and peptic ulceration). MEN Type II involves the thyroid gland (medullary carcinoma: a rather nonaggressive and clinically firm malignant tumor of the thyroid gland with a fibrous stroma with prominent amyloid deposits), adrenal medulla (pheochromocytoma), and parathyroid gland (chief cell hyperplasia or adenoma). Neither Type I nor II is associated with any oral findings, but a group of patients (Type III) in whom medullary carcinoma of the thyroid and pheochromocytoma (with hypertension) are found in association with parathyroid adenomas also exhibit neuromas of the lips, tongue, buccal mucosa, eyelids, and nasal and laryngeal mucosa.

Almost all individuals with MEN Type III have oral mucosal neuromas, which may be extensive enough to thicken the lip and produce a characteristic "bumpy lip" appearance. Although there are complex interactions between the various involved endocrine organs in each of these three variant syndromes, the finding of multiple neoplastic endocrine involvement is thought to be due to a widespread predisposition to cancer in many tissues derived from neuroectoderm, rather than to endocrine interactions. Endocrine interaction is also evident in the occurrence of Cushing's syndrome, hyperinsulinism, hypertension, and hyperparathyroidism in some affected individuals. Various combi-

nations of abnormalities are found in the relatives of affected individuals. The finding of oral mucosal neuromas in association with a family history of carcinoma of the thyroid or pheochromocytoma indicates a need to search for other evidences of this syndrome.

Tuberous Sclerosis

This inherited disorder is characterized by fits and mental retardation in association with hamartomatous glial proliferations and neuronal deformity in the central nervous system. Fine, wartlike lesions (adenoma sebaceum) occur in a butterfly distribution over the cheeks and forehead, and histologically similar lesions (vascular fibromas) have been described intraorally. Characteristic hypoplastic enamel defects may also be seen. Rhabdomyoma of the heart and other hamartomas of kidney, liver, adrenal, and pancreas are described. Neoplastic transformation of the glial proliferations constitutes the "internal malignancy" of this syndrome.

Acanthosis Nigricans

The finding of the typical velvety areas of papillomatosis on a background of melanin-pigmented skin (*acanthosis nigricans*) is associated in some cases with a predisposition to gastric adenocarcinoma. Unfortunately, acanthosis nigricans is not a specific entity and is also found in association with endocrine abnormalities and obesity and in an inherited form. In the presence of these abnormalities, acanthosis nigricans is not indicative of a predisposition to gastric adenocarcinoma. Intraoral papillomatosis has also been described in this condition.

Albright's Syndrome

Polyostotic fibrous dysplasia with café-au-lait spots* on the skin, bony deformities, and precocious sexual development is referred to as (*McCune-*) *Albright's syndrome* (see also discussion under Fibrous Dysplasia and Other

---

* These lesions (compare those of neurofibromatosis) are usually fewer than six in number though they are sometimes quite large and characteristically have an irregular border ("coast of Maine"). They are usually on the same side as bony lesions and may overlie them.

Fibro-Osseous Lesions, earlier in this chapter), and is an inherited form of fibrous dysplasia, usually with multiple bone involvement. Osteosarcoma develops in about 1% of patients with the syndrome. Since osteosarcoma also occasionally develops in patients with long-standing monostotic fibrous dysplasia (in some cases as the result of radiation therapy, but in others even without such treatment) and in view of the greater volume of dysplastic bony tissue in which sarcoma can develop in polyostotic fibrous dysplasia, it is not known whether the lesion of Albright's syndrome is more predisposed to malignant transformation than that of monostotic fibrous dysplasia. Polyostotic fibrous dysplasia may occur in the absence of the other components of the syndrome, namely, café-au-lait spots and precocious sexual development, and bone scans are indicated in patients with large lesions of fibrous dysplasia of the jaws as well as in those with multiple jaw lesions, even in the absence of skin pigmentation.

Paget's Disease (Osteitis Deformans)

This is by far the most common disease among those listed in Table 8-6, affecting about 3% of the population over 45 years of age and about 6% to 7% of hospitalized patients; it is rare in patients under 40 years. The nature of this bone disease is unknown, although evidence to suggest that it is a multicentric benign tumor of osteoclasts has been presented. No endocrine basis for the disease has been found, and the frequency with which malignant transformation occurs (1% to 2% of patients, especially those with multiple foci) and the heterogeneity of the osteoclasts in biopsies of patients with Paget's disease suggest that the disease itself is a benign (hormone-sensitive) neoplasm of bone cells.

The possibility of an infective, viral etiology for Paget's disease is suggested by the ultrastructural demonstration of intranuclear inclusions in the abnormal osteoclasts found in these patients, as well as in osteosarcoma cells in Paget's lesions that have undergone malignant transformation. Similar inclusions have not been demonstrated in other human sarcomas or in osteoclasts in normal bone, fibrous dysplasia, and metabolic bone disorders such as hyperparathyroidism and rickets; however, similar inclusions have been reported in a giant cell tumor of bone. These inclusions consist of bundles of microfilaments with an electron-lucent core and usually show evidence of paracrystalline array. Similar inclusions are seen in measles and subacute sclerosing panencephalitis virus infections. Measles virus and respiratory syncytial (RS) virus antigens have also been reported in osteoclasts from Paget's lesions, and it is possible that paramyxovirus infections modified by genetic or environmental factors are involved in the etiology of this multifocal neoplasm.

The bony lesions of Paget's disease produce characteristic deformities of the skull, jaw, back, pelvis, and legs and are readily recognized both clinically and radiologically. Irregular overgrowth of the jaw bones, especially the maxilla, may occur leading to the facial appearance described as "leontiasis ossea." A "ground-glass" change in the alveolar bones, often associated with loss of the lamina dura and root resorption, is described in dental radiographs in the early (osteolytic) phase of the disease. Subsequently, the jaws and other affected bones are occupied by dense sclerotic bony deposition that fixes the deformed skeleton in its characteristic shape and provides diagnostic features to the calvarium ("cotton wool" appearance between widened bony tables of the skull), maxilla, and maxillary sinuses and elsewhere. Healing of dental extraction wounds in affected areas is poor. The narrowing of skull foramina can cause ill-defined neuralgic pains (see discussion of Atypical Facial Pain, Chap. 17). There is an increased incidence of both salivary and pulpal calculi. Jaw fractures do not usually occur (c.f., Paget's disease of the long bones), but benign giant cell tumors and malignant sarcomatous transformation affect both the jaw bones and the long bones of these patients with some frequency; multicentric sarcomas are not uncommon.

Although a few patients with Paget's disease are without symptoms, many suffer considerable pain and deformity. These problems, associated medical problems such as cardiac failure and hypercalcemia, and the high incidence of malignant transformation have encouraged the use of a variety of new treatments for this disease, many of which are still being tested. The majority of these agents are designed to suppress some of the metabolic events by which bone cells remodel the calcified tissue and influence exchange of mineral ions between bone and the circulating fluids. They include antibiotics (mithramycin and actinomycin D), hormones of human and animal origin (calcitonin and glucagon), and salts (fluoride and diphosphonates). Marked reduction in pain and some slowing in the progression of the disease have been obtained with many of these agents. Radiotherapy is still also used. Urinary levels of hydroxyproline (as a measure of collagen metabolism) and serum alkaline phosphatase levels (as a measure of osteoblastic activity) are also used as indices of improvement in this disease in addition to bone scans with radiofluoride and radiostrontium.

Usually not manifest until the fifth decade, Paget's disease has a definite familial distribution, susceptibility to this disease probably being inherited, like the majority of the syndromes in Table 8-6, as an autosomal dominant condition. It is clearly not the same category of disease as are the other syndromes listed, in which benign oral lesions may signal the presence of internal malignancy. The oral lesions in Paget's disease are simply the jaw bone manifestation of a widespread bone disease; however, it is well for the dentist to realize that the patient with oral Paget's changes has an increased chance of developing sarcoma both orally and wherever else his disease is manifested. In view of the rarity of a giant cell tumor in the jaws except as a complication of Paget's disease, the finding of this lesion in a patient over 40 should also raise the possibility of previously undiagnosed Paget's disease.

Cowden's Syndrome

Cowden's syndrome (multiple hamartoma and neoplasia syndrome) is characterized by hamartomatous involvement of many organs with a potential for neoplastic transformation. It is inherited as an autosomal dominant character. Multiple papules on the lips and gingivae are often present, as are papillomatosis of the buccal, palatal, faucial, and oropharyngeal mucosae. The tongue is pebbly, fissured, or scrotal. Multiple papillomatous nodules (histologically inverted follicular keratoses) are often present on the perioral, perinasal, and periorbital skin and also on the pinnae of the ears and neck. A variety of neoplastic changes occur in the organs exhibiting hamartomatous lesions.

Xanthomas

Mention should be made of benign growths made up of lipid-containing histiocytes (*xanthomas*) that may occur intraorally and on the face of individuals with a variety of disorders (lipidoses) characterized by abnormal concentration of lipids in tissues or extracellular fluids. Many of these conditions are inherited, and some are secondary to diseases such as hypothyroidism, diabetes mellitus, obstructive liver diseases, and dysproteinemia, such as multiple myeloma. Isolated xanthomas sometimes occur in the absence of recognizable systemic abnormality, but when multiple lesions are found and when they are associated with similar lipid deposits elsewhere on the skin, in the eyelids (xanthelasma), and the cornea and with nodules on the tendons, they are almost certain to be a manifestation of a lipidosis. It is important that these lesions are recognized and the patient referred for plasma triglyceride, cholesterol, and lipoprotein measurement and medical consultation, since several of the inherited lipidoses are associated with early onset of severe coronary atherosclerosis and diabetes mellitus, which are likely to be fatal if not treated. A thorough description of the occurrence of oral and facial xanthomatosis in association with the various lipidoses does not appear to have been published, although there are case reports of oral lesions of this type. Many of the lipidoses are characterized in terms of the associated plasma lipoprotein abnormality (see Chap. 3). Xanthomatosis is manifest in Types I to III and V hyperlipoproteinemias, and mucous membrane eruptions are frequent in Types I and V (both of which exhibit hyperchylomicronemia). Xanthomas of the tendons, skin, and eyes and atheromatosis of the vascular endothelium are prominent features of Types II and III (carbohydrate-induced hyperlipoproteinemia), both of which carry a high risk of lethal ischemic heart disease.

In *Tangier disease*, a familial high-density lipoprotein deficiency (a rare autosomal recessive condition), affected children and adults exhibit startling orange or yellowish gray discolorations and swelling of the tonsils and pharyngeal mucosa in association with hypocholesterolemia and enlargement of other organs of the reticuloendothelial system (spleen, liver, lymph nodes).

Osteolytic jaw lesions, xanthomas, and other oral soft-tissue swellings also occur in a variety of granulomatous diseases associated with lipid storage. These diseases (usually referred to under the generic name of *Histiocytosis X*) include such variants as eosinophilic granuloma, Letterer–Siwe disease, and Hand–Schuller–Christian disease. Widespread proliferation of reticuloendothelial cells characterizes these diseases, which are often not benign and therefore beyond the scope of this chapter.

GINGIVAL ENLARGEMENTS

Gingival enlargement is usually caused by local conditions such as poor oral hygiene, food impaction, or mouth breathing; systemic conditions such as hormonal changes, drug therapy, or tumor infiltrates may complicate the process or even set the stage for the development of unfavorable local conditions leading to food impaction and difficulty with oral hygiene.

Traditionally a distinction was made between hypertrophy of the gingiva (an increase in the size of the cellular elements making up the gingiva) and hyperplasia (an actual increase in the number of the cellular elements). Both of these elements are usually present in inflammatory disease of the gingiva. In this section, the word "hyperplasia" is used simply to describe clinically evident gingival enlargement without reference to a particular histologic process underlying the change.

Gingival enlargement has been associated with a wide variety of local and systemic factors (see Tables 8-7 and 8-8). Enlargement is seen more consistently with some of these, for example administration of the anticonvulsant drug phenytoin (Dilantin) and its derivatives, pregnancy and other hyperestrogenic states characterized by increased blood levels of estrogens, monocytic leukemia, and clinical scurvy. A number of these conditions are discussed elsewhere in this and other

Table 8-7. Causes of Gingival Enlargement (Inflammatory and Fibrotic)

LOCAL INFLAMMATORY AND TRAUMATIC FACTORS	SYSTEMIC PREDISPOSING FACTORS
Poor oral hygiene	Endocrine
Accumulations of calculus	Puberty
Malposed teeth	Menstruation and pregnancy
Inadequate contact areas	Hypothyroidism and pituitary dysfunction
Incorrect toothbrush habits	Diabetes
Occlusal interferences	Gonadal disturbances
Irritation from ill-fitting crowns, clasps, prosthetic or orthodontic appliances	Contraceptive medications
Mouth breathing	Nutritional
	Scurvy
	Subclinical nutritional deficiencies of mixed types, including B complex
	Blood dyscrasias
	The leukemias—particularly monocytic and myelogenous
	Polycythemia vera
	Drugs
	Phenytoin
	Congenital and Inherited (see Table 8-8)

chapters (*e.g.*, congenital epulis and pregnancy epulis, phenytoin-induced hyperplasia, pyogenic granuloma, leukemic gingival hyperplasia enlargement, diabetic gingivitis, scurvy, and some of the congenital and inherited gingival enlargements).

Inflammatory Gingival Enlargement

Inflammatory enlargement of the gingivae (Fig. 8-39) is encountered more commonly than fibrotic enlargement (Fig. 8-40). In most instances it begins at an area of poor oral hygiene, food impaction, or other local irritation that can be readily eliminated or controlled by the dentist. The interproximal gingivae are usually involved first. They bulge from between the teeth, producing favorable sites for food impaction and secondary infec-

Table 8-8. Syndromes Commonly Associated with Diffuse Gingival Enlargement

SYNDROMES WITH GINGIVAL HYPERPLASIA	SYNDROMES WITH GINGIVAL FIBROMATOSIS
Congenital enlargement of the gingivae, altered eruption of teeth, and corneal dystrophy (*Rutherford syndrome*)	Gingival fibromatosis with ear, nose, bone, and nail defects and hepatosplenomegaly (*Zimmerman–laband syndrome*)
Mucolipidosis II (*I-cell disease*)	Gingival fibromatosis with hypertrichosis, epilepsy, and mental retardation
Gingival enlargement, hypopigmentation, micro-ophthalmos, oligophrenia, and athetosis (*Cross syndrome*)	Gingival fibromatosis with multiple hyaline fibromas (*Murray–Puretic–Drescher syndrome*)
Fetal face syndrome (*Robinow syndrome*)	
Hyperkeratosis palmoplantaris and periodontoclasia in childhood (*Papillon–Lefevre syndrome*)	
Encephalofacial hemangiomatosis (*Sturge–Weber syndrome*)	
Multiple hamartoma and neoplasia syndrome (*Cowden's syndrome*); gingival papillomas as part of widespread oral, pharyngeal, and facial papillomatosis (see Table 8-6)	

tion. The tissues are glossy, smooth, and edematous, often pitting on pressure. They bleed readily. The inflammatory enlargement tends to spread and gradually involves the labial and buccal gingivae.

The pseudopockets formed by the gingival enlargements make the maintenance of good oral hygiene difficult, perpetuating a cycle of inflammation and fibrosis. These tissues are susceptible to secondary infection. A fetid odor may result from the decomposition of food debris and accumulation of bacteria in these inaccessible areas.

Loss of interseptal bone and drifting of the teeth occur in long-standing cases of inflammatory enlargement. Chronic inflammation of the gingival tissues predisposes to the formation of new connective tissue fibers and the development of a fibrotic type of enlargement. These changes are commonly referred to as *gingivitis,* or *periodontal disease* where the process involves loss of interproximal bone.

Gingival inflammation affecting primarily the maxillary anterior region is observed in mouth breathers. Some of the patients have a severe class II malocclusion. Several theories have been offered to account for the gingival enlargement in mouth breathers. It is believed that the alternate moistening and dehydration of the gingivae result in mild inflammatory changes that lead to a hypertrophic reaction. In some patients abnormal facial development or malocclusion leads to a continued opening of the mouth and lips predisposing these patients to this form of gingivitis.

Varying degrees of gingival hypertrophy, probably due to hormonal changes, have been observed in association with the use of contraceptive pills.

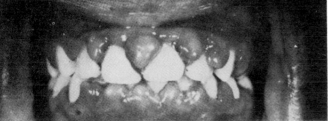

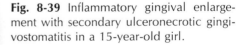

Fig. 8-39 Inflammatory gingival enlargement with secondary ulceronecrotic gingivostomatitis in a 15-year-old girl.

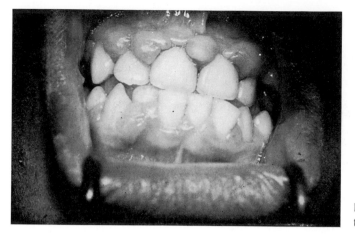

Fig. 8-40 Fibrosis of the gingiva secondary to long-standing inflammatory disease.

The periodontal status of 89 women taking oral contraceptives was compared with that of 72 women matched for age but not taking the pill. The study showed no significant difference in gingivitis between the two groups when all women in both groups were compared; however, women receiving oral contraceptives for longer than 1½ years had significantly more periodontal destruction than did the control group. The effects of contraceptive drugs on gingiva and alveolar bone of rats have also been studied, but again with equivocal results.

The diagnosis of inflammatory gingival enlargement should present no difficulty. The edema of the tissues, their bright red or purplish red color, and their tendency to hemorrhage should permit differentiation from fibrotic gingival enlargement. Gingival enlargement associated with local factors is usually limited to the buccal and labial gingival tissues. It is important for the clinician to remember that although most gingival enlargements are inflammatory in nature, benign and malignant neoplasms of the gingivae also occur, and a biopsy should be obtained whenever the cause is unclear or the lesion does not respond to local therapy (see Figs. 8-41, 8-42, and 8-43).

Treatment of the inflammatory type of gingival enlargement consists of the establishment of excellent oral hygiene, the elimination of all local predisposing factors if possible, the elimination of any recognized systemic predisposing causes, and proper home care by the patient.

The treatment of hyperplastic gingivitis usually is difficult, and many times it is not entirely successful, possibly because of the failure to discover all the causative factors or to eliminate them. Much of the success of the treatment of hyperplastic gingivitis rests with the patient who because of his age or indifference to the condition may not always be impressed with his important role in treatment.

When the diagnosis of gingival hyperplasia has been established and the more important systemic predisposing factors have been ruled out, the first step in treatment is careful removal of all hard and soft deposits about the teeth. Special attention should be given to instructing the patient in the proper method of toothbrushing and gingival massage. Other local predisposing factors such as poor dentistry should be corrected. All local irritative factors such as calculus, the margins of cervical cavities, or areas of food impaction should be corrected. Local treatment is often of value, even when the gingival hyperplasia is associated with systemic disease. Although systemic factors should be removed whenever possible, the elimination of local irritative factors may be all that is necessary to obtain a reasonably satisfactory clinical result.

In patients with extensive gingival hyperplasia, the affected tissues must be removed surgically. When this is done, it is very important that the remaining tissues have the proper architecture and contour.

The gingival changes associated with pu-

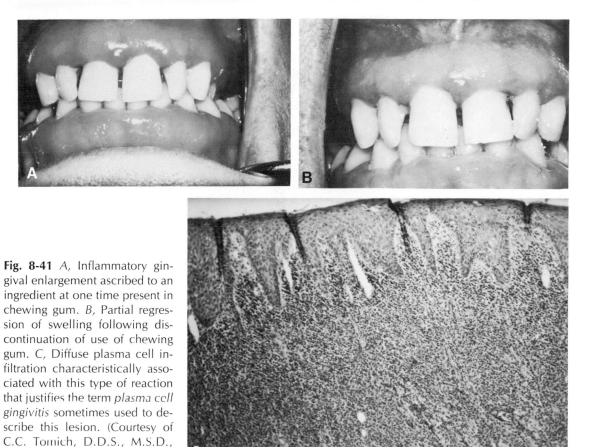

Fig. 8-41 *A,* Inflammatory gingival enlargement ascribed to an ingredient at one time present in chewing gum. *B,* Partial regression of swelling following discontinuation of use of chewing gum. *C,* Diffuse plasma cell infiltration characteristically associated with this type of reaction that justifies the term *plasma cell gingivitis* sometimes used to describe this lesion. (Courtesy of C.C. Tomich, D.D.S., M.S.D., Indianapolis, IN)

berty, menstruation, and pregnancy may resist all forms of local treatment other than surgery. At times the gingival enlargement during adolescence will regress spontaneously between 15 and 17 years of age. If the gingival enlargements are removed surgically, a satisfactory and permanent result is usually obtained.

The successful treatment of gingival enlargement in mouth breathers depends mainly on the elimination of the habit. The patient should be referred to an otolaryngologist to determine whether there is some obstruction of the upper air passages, such as enlarged adenoids. Orthodontic treatment may be required to correct any malocclusion and to permit the normal closure of the lips during sleep. Some clinicians advocate the use of a protective ointment on the gums at night.

The oral changes associated with the blood dyscrasias are described in the sections devoted to this subject. A generalized gingival enlargement (Fig. 8-43) is occasionally one of the earlier symptoms of these diseases. A complete history should be taken in these patients, including a careful review of systems to see if other symptoms of systemic disease exist.

Fibrotic Gingival Enlargement

Proliferative types of gingival lesions have the normal pink color or they may be slightly paler than normal. The tissue is firm, hard, and fibrous in consistency, due to the increase in fibrous tissue; it does not bleed readily or pit on pressure. Typical examples of gingival fibrosis are found in the gingival enlargements associated with the administra-

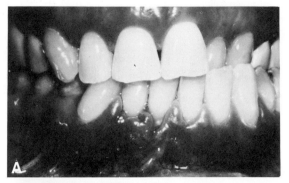

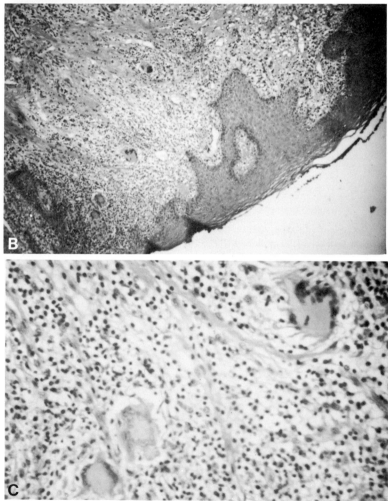

tion of phenytoin (Dilantin) and its derivatives and in diffuse fibromatosis of the gingiva. A fibrotic gingival enlargement may develop in any patient with long-standing gingival hyperplasia. Phenytoin-induced hyperplasia is also discussed in Chapter 27.

Phenytoin-induced gingival hyperplasia affects at least 40% to 50% of patients who use the drug beyond 3 months. More severe effects may not develop until after several years of continued use. Evidence from animal studies, individual case reports, and clinical trials

Fig. 8-42 Inflammatory gingival enlargement associated with a noncaseating granulomatous tissue response. Lesions such as this have been described in patients with a diagnosis of Melkersson–Rosenthal syndrome and Crohn's disease and are often seen in association with granulomatous cheilitis and nodular enlargements of the tongue and other areas of the oral mucosa.

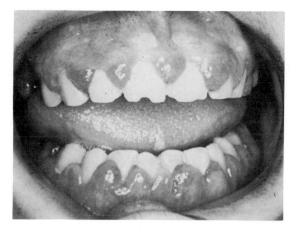

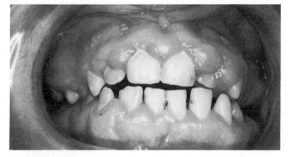

Fig. 8-44 Fibrotic gingival enlargement associated with administration of phenytoin (Dilantin) in a 17-year-old female.

Fig. 8-43 Generalized gingival enlargement associated with a leukemic infiltrate in a patient with untreated monocytic leukemia.

indicates that both the drug and local irritation from plaque and calculus or restorations and appliances are etiologic factors. If gingival irritation can be eliminated, gingival hyperplasia will at the most be only minimal. Continuous and obvious irritation such as that associated with banded orthodontic appliances is often associated with very severe hyperplasia. The pathogenesis of the gingival changes caused by phenytoin is still unsettled; earlier suggestions that the gingival collagen is modified or that reduced serum and salivary IgA associated with chronic use of phenytoin are the cause of the hyperplasia have not been confirmed. In fact, the available data indicate that the mature fibrous-type phenytoin-induced gingival lesion represents neither hypertrophy, hyperplasia, nor fibrosis but is an example of uncontrolled growth of a connective tissue of apparently normal cell and fiber composition. The term *phenytoin (or DPH)-induced hyperplasia* is still commonly used, however.

The clinical appearance of phenytoin-induced gingival hyperplasia is usually characteristic (Fig. 8-44), although numerous variants are seen depending on the location of the lesion, the particular irritant involved, and the extent of secondary inflammatory changes. The diagnosis is made from the history of chronic phenytoin use and the clinical appearance of the lesions; biopsy and measurement of the serum levels of phenytoin offer no additional diagnostic information.

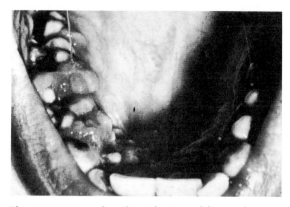

Fig. 8-45 Unusual unilateral gingival hyperplasia in a 35-year-old female is associated with administration of phenytoin (Dilantin) for treatment of post-infarct focal motor epileptic seizures. The patient had not brushed her teeth on the left side for 2 years because of the strange feeling there (dysesthesia secondary to stroke) and had actually carried out a controlled trial proving that despite low serum IgA levels she could almost prevent the hyperplasia on the right side by careful brushing. (Kristensen CB: One-sided gingival hyperplasia after treatment with diphenylhydantoin. Acta Neurol Scand 56:353–356, 1977. Copyright © 1977 by Munksgaard International Publishers, Ltd., Copenhagen, Denmark.)

With very rare exceptions, the hyperplasia is restricted to the gingivae, and following extraction of teeth and excision of the hyperplastic tissue, there is no recurrence.

Treatment of phenytoin-induced gingival hyperplasia should emphasize elimination of local gingival irritants, scrupulous oral hygiene, and interdental massage (Fig. 8-45). In a number of patients, seizures can be controlled by other nonhydantoin derivatives,

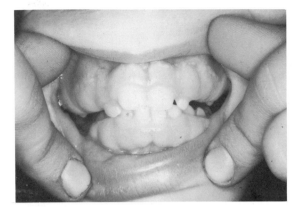

Fig. 8-46 Familial gingival hyperplasia.

and the physician, the patient, and the family may be willing to experiment with supervised alteration of the patient's anticonvulsive medications in order to reduce the hyperplasia.

The menarche frequently beings a period of difficult management, partly because of the increased frequency of seizures that may occur at this time, partly because orthodontic treatment is usually begun about this time, and partly because of the patient's increased awareness of any orofacial cosmetic defects as adolescence progresses. Some authors advocate that phenytoin be routinely avoided in treating female adolescents to exclude the possibility of both gingival hyperplasia and hirsutism. The epileptic patient's medication should at least always be reviewed before orthodontic treatment is begun.

Topically applied medications including antiplaque agents such as chlorhexidine have no effect on the gingival changes once hyperplasia is established. Hyperplasia of any degree will not resolve simply by removing local gingival irritants, and excision of hyperplastic gingivae, root planing, and elimination of rough margins on restorations are usually necessary before adequate gingival hygiene and plaque control can be established. If gingivectomy is not followed by institution of adequate home care and use of interdental massage, the hyperplasia will recur. A customized splint may be constructed to retain the periodontal dressing needed after gingivectomy, ligating it to anterior and posterior teeth to prevent the pack being dis-

lodged and aspirated during a convulsive seizure. The brain-damaged and retarded epileptic patient often presents a difficult management problem, particularly if neither parents nor nurses can provide adequate tooth brushing and gingival hygiene. In such cases, the value of gingivectomy must be carefully considered, and resorted to only when the overgrowth interferes with closure of the teeth or lips or is a source of severe halitosis or hemorrhage.

Phenytoin taken during pregnancy, with or without barbiturates produces a two- to threefold increase in congenital anomalies. Affected offspring exhibit a variety of musculoskeletal growth defects, psychomotor retardation, and facial deformities including ocular hypertelorism, depressed nasal bridge, hypertrichosis, and wide mouth. While broad alveolar ridges have been reported in 30% of cases, gingival fibromatosis apparently does not occur with this route of administration.

Diffuse fibromatosis of the gingiva is a less common form of gingival hyperplasia, and in many cases it is a congenital or inherited disorder (Fig. 8-46), although diffuse enlargement of the gingivae can also be a response to widespread local irritants with or without a systemic factor. The enlargement may be present at birth or only become apparent with the eruption of the deciduous or permanent dentitions. A variety of pathogenetic mechanisms are involved: hemangiomatous enlargement, infiltration of the gingival tissues with histiocytes and other cells containing abnormal metabolic products, fibrotic reaction in gingivae overlying multiple impacted or grossly carious or hypoplastic teeth, or idiopathic fibrosis, possibly on a genetic basis. In many cases, affected individuals have received phenytoin therapy to control the effects of associated central nervous system abnormalities and seizures. Here it may be difficult to separate the basic gingival abnormality from a secondary phenytoin-induced hyperplasia.

If well developed, the dense, firm gingival tissue results in varying spacing of the teeth and changes in the profile and general facial appearance (Fig. 8-47). The hyperplasia may be so excessive as to crowd the tongue, interfere with speech, cause difficulty in chewing food, and prevent normal closure of the lips.

The surface of the hyperplastic tissue usually has a nodular appearance because of the thickened, hyperkeratinized epithelium. There is usually little difficulty in differentiating simple hyperplasia of the gingivae from diffuse fibromatosis. The medical history will enable the physician to rule out phenytoin-induced hyperplasia, and physical examination will often reveal other oral or systemic physical anomalies to suggest the likelihood of an inherited problem, even if no specific syndrome can be identified. Pedigree analysis based on the family history may also provide evidence for a genetically determined factor. One fairly common form of familial gingival fibromatosis is inherited as an autosomal dominant trait. The treatment of gingival fibromatosis is often unsatisfactory. Gingivectomy is usually necessary, although the tissue may regrow.

A listing of the syndromes that are most consistently associated with diffuse gingival enlargement is provided in Table 8-8: (See also Fig. 8-48.)

CERVICOFACIAL ACTINOMYCOSIS

Actinomycosis is an infectious disease caused by a slender, gram-positive, rod-shaped bacterium, *Actinomyces israelii,* that exhibits a number of simple fungal-like characteristics, such as a tendency to grow as a mass of rounded bodies (clubs) and filaments in tissue (hence the term "ray fungus"), low virulence, and the property of eliciting suppuration, necrosis, and a chronic granulomatous tissue response. Based on the shared feature of a granulomatous tissue response, actinomycosis, tuberculosis, and syphilis were once grouped as the "specific granulomatous diseases." However, there is little else in common among these three infections as far as their natural history, clinical features or treatment are concerned, even though chronic pulmonary infection with *Actinomyces* on occasion can be confused clinically and radiographically with tuberculosis. Since *Actinomyces israelii* is an anaerobic or microaerophilic species, isolation of the organism in pure culture is difficult and iden-

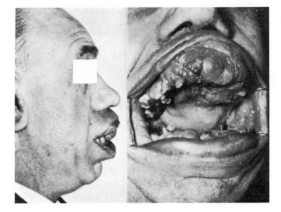

Fig. 8-47 Profile view and intraoral appearance of a 49-year-old male patient before all visible and easily accessible teeth were removed, after which he was able for the first time in his life to appose his lips. Gingivae had been resected several times before. The father, son, and daughter all suffered from hereditary gingivofibromatosis. (Winstock D: Hereditary gingivofibromatosis. Br J Oral Surg 2:61, 1964)

tification is often based on demonstration of the organisms stained in tissue sections, or as microcolonies ("sulphur granules") in pus (see Chapter 3). When special efforts are made to isolate the organism, it can be shown to be part of the normal oral bacterial flora, especially concentrated in dental plaque, calculus, carious lesions, and the tonsillar crypts. It is probable that almost all cervicofacial actinomycotic infections are endogenous in origin and occur when dental plaque, calculus, or gingival debris contaminates relatively deep wounds around the mouth. While the classical lesions of cervicofacial actinomycosis are chronic, low-grade, persistent infections that may be difficult to eradicate, careful bacteriologic study of acute jaw and soft tissue abscesses following surgical or other trauma has demonstrated that *Actinomyces iraelii* may also be involved in acute and rapidly resolving suppurative lesions. Microscopic examination of periapical tissues of non-vital and endodontically treated teeth may also, on occasions, reveal an isolated periapical actinomycotic granuloma, suggesting that this otherwise noninvasive organism can also be walled off and tolerated in the oral tissues for long periods of time without evidence of active disease.

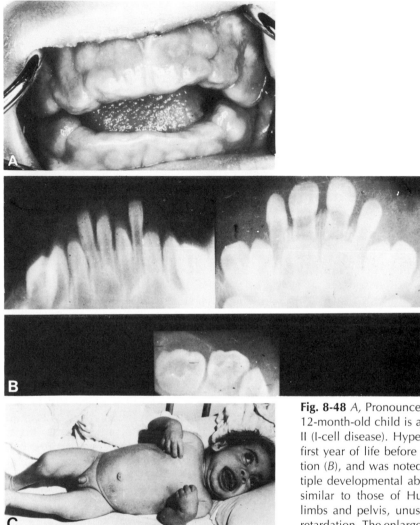

Fig. 8-48 *A,* Pronounced gingival hyperplasia in this 12-month-old child is associated with mucolipidosis II (I-cell disease). Hyperplasia developed during the first year of life before eruption of deciduous dentition (*B*), and was noted in association with (*C*) multiple developmental abnormalities, skeletal changes similar to those of Hurler syndrome in the lower limbs and pelvis, unusual facies, and psychomotor retardation. The enlarged gingival tissue was firm and hard and obstructed mastication and closure of the mouth.

Pulmonary actinomycosis is generally believed to result from aspiration of oral or tonsillar debris, with areas of localized atelectasis secondary to obstruction of small air passages providing the necessary anaerobic conditions for growth of the *Actinomyces.* It is also possible that pulmonary actinomycosis may arise hematogenously from an infected oral or cervicofacial focus. *Ileocecal* (intestinal) *actinomycosis* is the commonest other form of actinomycosis, and usually arises following rupture of an inflamed appendix with development of a mass in the right iliac fossa. In recent years, *pelvic actinomycosis* has been

recognized as an important complication of some intrauterine contraceptive devices (IUD's). Bloodstream spread in immunocompromised individuals may occur from any of these primary foci of infection.

Approximately 60% of all actinomycotic infections occur in the cervicofacial area and there is a history of tooth extraction or jaw fracture in about 15% to 20% of cases. It was once believed that the organism was implanted in the oral tissues by chewing wood splinters, blades, or stalks of grass, and that the infection was more common in agricultural workers. More recent data fail to sup-

Fig. 8-48, cont. *D,* Fibroblasts cultured from the skin biopsy showed numerous granular inclusions and complete absence of lysosomal beta-galactosidase activity. *E,* Electron microscopic examination of gingival fibroblasts showed numerous membrane-limited empty vacuoles distending these cells. (Courtesy of Daniel Galili, D.M.D., Jerusalem, Israel; *A* through *C,* Galili D et al: Oral Surg 37:533, 1974; *D,* Terashima Y et al: Am J Dis Child 129:1083, 1975; *E,* Mart JJ et al: Acta Neuropathol 33:285, 1975)

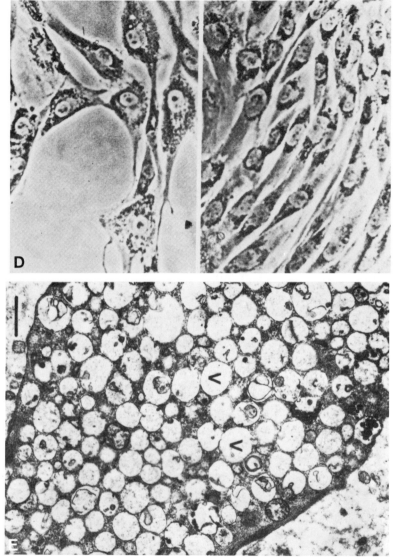

port this idea and have also cast doubt on *Actinomyces* as the universal etiologic agent for a cattle disease referred to as "lumpy jaw," which was believed to be analogous to cervicofacial actinomycosis in man.

The submandibular region is the most frequent site of involvement in human cervicofacial actinomycosis, the disease usually spreading by direcct tissue extension. There may be associated changes detectable at the portal of entry such as a nonhealing tooth socket, exuberant granulation tissue, or periosteal thickening of the alveolus. On many occasions, however, the chronic infection spreads from the periapical region with minimal clinical signs until it is well established. Then, soft-tissue swelling or development of a fistula causes the patient to seek treatment. The cheeks, the masseter region, and the parotid gland may also be involved. Extension to the skull and the meninges has occured on rare occasions.

One of the characteristics of actinomycosis is the lack of immediate tissue reaction following implantation of the infection. An actinomycotic infection and an abscessed or a pulpless tooth will produce similar submandibular swellings. If the swelling and the trismus persist after the removal of the tooth, actinomycosis should be suspected. Several

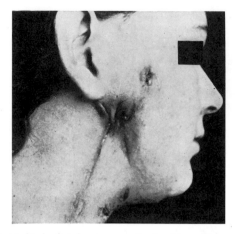

Fig. 8-49. Multiple fistulas in a patient with actinomycosis of the cervicaofacial region. (Courtesy the late Dr. Robert H. Ivy, Philadelphia PA).

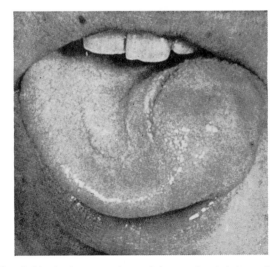

Fig. 8-50. Actinomycotic nodule on the left lateral aspect of the dorsum of the tongue in a 27-year-old man. (From Dorph–Peterson L, Pindborg JJ: Actinomycosis of the tongue: Report of a case. Oral Surg 7:1178, 1954; Courtesy CV Mosby Co St Louis MO 63141)

hard, circumscribed, tumor-like swellings may develop and break down, discharging a yellowish fluid containing the characteristic macroscopic "sulfur granules." It usually requires 6 weeks or longer for an actinomycotic swelling to break down and discharge pus. The multiple discharging sinuses that subsequently develop (see Fig. 8-49) are almost pathognomonic of the disease. The adjacent tissues usually have a hard, doughy consistency. The skin surrounding the discharging fistulae is purplish, and there may be small areas of hypertrophic granulation tissue. Acute pain is uncommon.

Primary actinomycosis of the tongue (see Fig. 8-50) must be differentiated from neoplasms, tuberculous ulcerations, syphilitic gumma, and other chronic infectious granulomatous diseases such as histoplasmosis. In actinomycosis of the tongue, there is usually found a small, deep-seated nodule, which is painless at first and causes little discomfort. The lesion gradually increases in size, and the overlying tissues soften and rupture. There may be temporary healing, after which the process is repeated with the development of a more extensive lesion. Dysphagia is a prominent symptom in cases of extensive involvement.

Diagnosis

Any indolent inflammatory process in the submandibular area with induration and persistently draining multiple fistulae is suggestive of actinomycosis. A purplish or dark-red discoloration of the skin surrounding the sinuses is additional evidence. The discharge should be examined grossly for the "sulfur granules" and cultured anaerobically for the causative organism.

Actinomycosis of the cervicofacial region may be confused with osteomyelitis. In osteomyelitis, pain is more severe with greater destruction of bone and more rapidly developing suppuration. Radiological studies aid in the diagnosis. Tuberculous adenitis and other causes of submandibular and cervical lymphadenopathy, such as cat-scratch disease, lymphogranuloma venereum, and Hodgkin's disease should be considered. The board-like induration found in actinomycosis, and the examination of the exudate for acid-fast organisms help in making a diagnosis.

Presumptive diagnosis can be made if "sulfur granules" are present and gram-positive mycelia can be demonstrated. Positive diagnosis can be made only from anaerobic culture and isolation of actinomyces from infected tissue or pus; as previously discussed, the opportunity for positive diagnosis in this disease is limited, and will occur only when the clinician and microbiologist collaborate to confirm a suspected actinomycotic infection or when the organism is demonstrated in tissue section.

Chronic cervicofacial actinomycosis is traditionally considered a difficult infection to eradicate, but more recent texts suggest that penicillin and tetracyclines are quite effective, particularly if high doses are used and continued for several weeks of treatment. The optimal dose of penicillin is not known, but at least 4 million units should be given daily intramuscularly. Tetracyclines are administered 500 mg every 6 hours. Preference is usually given to use of tetracyclines for treatment of this infection to avoid the repeated intramuscular injections of penicillin. Iodides, sulphonamides, and radiation were all used at one time but no longer have any place in the treatment of these infections. Antifungal antibiotics do not effect the growth of actinomycetes. Surgical drainage of definable foci of infection may be needed and, on occasion, alone may be curative. The major problem associated with treatment of actinomycosis is the development of allergic reactions to the prolonged high doses of antibiotics.

Otherwise, asymptomatic periapical actinomycotic foci that are demonstrated in association with necrotic dental pulp tissue or endodontic treatment rarely result in progressive actinomycotic infection. The apicoectomy procedure is that by which such foci are demonstrated, alone being adequate treatment in most cases. The finding of the "ray fungus" in a periapical granuloma always raises the question of whether additional antibiotic treatment is needed. If antibiotics are given in this circumstance, a somewhat shorter period of administration (*e.g.*, 1 to 2 weeks) is probably adequate.

Acute alveolar abscesses that are shown to be associated with *Actinomyces* infection have likewise usually resolved with the initial antibiotic treatment prior to recognition of *Actinomyces* as a possible causative agent. Once again, increased doses of penicillin or tetracyclines may be given for an additional 1 to 2 weeks, but the need for this is not well established. The widespread use of penicillin and other antibiotics prophylactically after dental extractions, jaw fractures, and other orofacial trauma is considered to be responsible for a decreasing prevalence of cervicofacial actinomycosis over recent decades.

BIBLIOGRAPHY

Bhaskar SN: Oral pathology in the dental office: Survey of 20,575 biopsy specimens. J Am Dent Assoc 76:761, 1968

Early detection of oral cancer. [Editorial]. J Am Dent Assoc 76:700, 1968

Gorlin RJ, Goldman HM: Thoma's Oral Pathology, 6th ed. St. Louis, CV Mosby, 1970

Gorlin RJ, Pindborg JJ, Cohen MM: Syndromes of the Head and Neck, 2nd ed. New York, Blakiston, McGraw-Hill, 1976

Mescon H, Grots IA, Gorlin RJ; Mucocutaneous disorders. In Gorlin RJ, Goldman HM (eds): Thoma's Oral Pathology, 6th ed. St. Louis, CV Mosby, 1970

Sedano HO et al: Oral Manifestations of Inherited Disorders. Boston, Butterworth, 1977

Shafer WG et al: A Textbook of Oral Pathology, 3rd ed. Philadelphia, WB Saunders, 1974

Shklar G, McCarthy PL: The Oral Manifestations of Systemic Disease. Boston, Butterworth, 1976

Stafne EC, Gibilisco JA: Oral Roentgenographic Diagnosis, 4th ed. Philadelphia, WB Saunders, 1975

Vickers RA: Mesenchymal (soft tissue) tumors of the oral region. In Gorlin RJ, Goldman HM (eds): Thoma's Oral Pathology, 6th ed. St. Louis, CV Mosby, 1970

Waldron CA: Oral epithelial tumors. In Gorlin RJ, Goldman HM (eds): Thoma's Oral Pathology, 6th ed. St. Louis, CV Mosby, 1970

Inflammatory Hyperplasias

Ackerman LV, McGavran MH: Proliferating benign and malignant epithelial lesions of the oral cavity. J Oral Surg 16:400, 1958

Adkins KF, Martinez MG, Hartley MW: Ultrastructure of giant-cell lesions. A peripheral giant-cell reparative granuloma. Oral Surg 28:713, 1969

Adkins KF, Martinez MG, Robinson LH: Cellular morphology and relationships in giant-cell lesions of the jaws. Oral Surg 28:216, 1969

Avioli LV: The diagnosis of primary hyperparathyroidism. Med Clin North Am 52:451, 1968

Chapnick P: A review of hyperparathyroidism, and an interesting case presenting with a giant cell lesion. Trans Cong Int Assoc Oral Surg 4:44, 1973

Dehner LP: Tumors of the mandible and maxilla in children. I. Clinicopathologic study of 46 histologically benign lesions. Cancer 31:364, 1973

Giansanti JS, Waldron CA: Peripheral giant cell

granuloma: Review of 720 cases. J Oral Surg 27:787, 1969

Guernsey LH: Reactive inflammatory papillary hyperplasia of the palate. Oral Surg 20:814, 1965

Hobaek A: Dental prosthesis and intraoral epidermoid carcinoma. Acta Radiol 32:259, 1949

Kerr DA: Granuloma pyogenicum. Oral Surg 4:158, 1951

Macchia AF, Cassalia PT: Primary hyperparathyroidism: Report of a case. J Am Dent Assoc 81:1153, 1970

Price EB, Jr, Silliphant WM, Shuman R: Nodular fasciitis: A clinicopathologic analysis of 65 cases. Am J Clin Pathol 35:122, 1961

Rose HP: Papillomas of the oral cavity. Oral Surg 20:542, 1965

Silverman S, Jr, Ware WH, Gillooly C, Jr: Dental aspects of hyperparathyroidism. Oral Surg 26:184, 1968

Waldron CA, Shafer WG: The central giant cell reparative granuloma of the jaws: An analysis of 38 cases. Am J Clin Pathol 45:437, 1966

Hamartomas

Adams RD, DeLong GR: Developmental and other congenital abnormalities of the nervous system. In Wintrobe MM et al (eds): Harrison's Textbook of Internal Medicine, 7th ed. New York, McGraw-Hill, 1974

Baden E, Pierce HE, Jackson WF: Multiple neurofibromatosis with oral lesions: Review of the literature and report of a case. Oral Surg 8:263, 1955

Bell RH: The non-surgical treatment of benign vascular lesions of soft tissue. Trans Cong Int Assoc Oral Surg 4:53, 1973

Boysen ME: Fibro-osseous lesions of the craniofacial bones. J Laryngol Otol 93:793, 1979

Chaudhry AP, Hampel A, Gorlin RJ: Primary malignant melanoma of the oral cavity: A review of 105 cases. Cancer 11:923, 1958

Czernobilsky B et al: Rhabdomyoma. Report of a case with ultrastructural and histochemical studies. Am J Clin Pathol 49:782, 1968

El Deeb M et al: Congenital monostotic fibrous dysplasia—A new possibly autosomal recessive disorder. J Oral Surg 37:520, 1979

El Deeb M et al: Aneurysmal bone cyst of the jaws. Report of a case associated with fibrous dysplasia and review of the literature. Int J Oral Surg 9:301, 1980

Erich WE: Teratoid parasites of the mouth (episphenoids, epipalati [epurani] epignathi). Am J Orthod Oral Surg 31:650, 1945

Eversole LR et al: Fibrous dysplasia: A nosologic problem in the diagnosis of fibro-osseous lesions of the jaws. J Oral Pathol 1:189, 1972

Friedman JM et al: Cavernous hemangioma of the oral cavity: Review of the literature and report of a case J Oral Surg 31:617, 1973

Gorlin RJ, Chaudhry AP: Oral melanotic pigmentation in polyostotic fibrous dysplasia, Albright's syndrome. Oral Surg 10:857, 1957

Grabias SL et al: Fibrous dysplasia. Orthop Clin North Am 8:771, 1977

Hamner JE III, Ketcham AS, Swerdlow H: Cemento-ossifying fibroma of the maxilla. Oral Surg 26:579, 1968

Hamner JE III, Scofield HH, Cornyn J: Benign fibro-osseous jaw lesions of periodontal membrane origin. Cancer 22:861, 1968

Hamner JE III: The demonstration of perivascular collagen deposition in cherubism. Oral Surg 27:129, 1969

Hamner JE III, Ketcham AS: Cherubism: An analysis of treatment. Cancer 23:1133, 1969

Hidano A, Nakajima S: Earliest features of the strawberry mark in the newborn. Br J Dermatol 87:138, 1972

Higashi T et al: Computed tomograhy and bone scintigraphy in polyostotic fibrous dysplasia: Report of a case. Oral Surg 50:580, 1980

Hjelmstedt A et al: A case of Albright's syndrome treated with calcitonin. Acta Orthop Scand 50:251, 1979

Huang T et al: The use of cryotherapy in the management of intra-oral hemangiomas. South Med J 65:1123, 1972

Johnston MC, Bhakdinaronk A, Reid YC: An expanded role of the neural crest in oral and pharyngeal development. In Bosma JF: Fourth Symposium on Oral Senses and Perception, Development in Fetus and Infant. Chap. 3. U.S. Dept. HEW, NIH. Bethesda, MD, 1973

Kerr DA, Pullon PS: Study of the pigmented tumors of the jaws of infants (melanotic ameloblastoma, retinal anlage tumor, progonoma), Oral Surg 18:759 1964

Kohout E, Stout AP: The glomus tumor in children. Cancer 14:555, 1961

Koop CE, Moschakis EA: Capillary lymphangioma of the tongue complicated by glossitis. Pediatrics 27:800, 1961

Lichenstein L: Diseases of Bone and Joints. St. Louis, CV Mosby, 1975

Longacre JJ, Benton C, Unterthiner RA: Treatment of facial hemangioma by intravascular embolization with silicone spheres. Case report. Plast Reconstr Surg 50:618, 1972

Lund BA, Dahlin DC: Hemangiomas of the mandible and maxilla. J Oral Surg 22:234, 1964

Lustmann J et al: Central giant cell granuloma and periapical fibrous dysplasia occurring in the same jaw. Int J Oral Surg 7:11, 1978

Mahour GH et al: Teratomas in infancy and childhood; experience with 81 cases. Surgery 76:309, 1974

Moscovic EA, Azar HA: Multiple granular cell tumors ("myoblastomas"). Case report with electron microscopic observations and review of the literature. Cancer 20:2032, 1967

Nance FL et al: Technetium bone imaging as an adjunct in the management of fibrous dysplasia. Oral Surg 50:199, 1980

New EB, Erich JB: Dermoid cysts of the head and neck. Surg Gynecol Obstet 65:48, 1937

Obisesan AA et al: The radiologic features of fibrous dysplasia of the craniofacial bones. Oral Surg 44:949, 1977

Palladino VS, Rose SA, Curran T: Salivary gland tissue in the mandible and Stafne's mandibular "cysts." J Am Dent Assoc 70:388, 1965

Rao AA: Ehlers–Danlos syndrome with monostotic fibrous dysplasia. Postgrad Med 25:186, 1979

Rintala A, Ranta R: Separate epignathi of the mandible and the nasopharynx with cleft palate: case report. Br J Plast Surg 27:103, 1974

Romaniuk K, Becker R: Two cases of aneurysmal bone cysts of the jaw. Int J Oral Surg 1:48, 1972

Shafer AD: Primary macroglossia. Clin Pediat 7:357, 1968

Shklar C, Meyer I: Vascular tumors of the mouth and jaws. Oral Surg 19:335, 1965

Shuster HL et al: Radionuclide bone imaging as an aid in the diagnosis of fibrous dysplasia: Report of a case. J Oral Surg 37:267, 1979

Strong EW, McDivitt RW, Brasfield RD: Granular cell myoblastoma. Cancer 25:415, 1970

Stuhler T et al: Fibrous dysplasia in the light of new diagnostic methods. Arch Orthop Trauma Surg 94:255, 1979

Waldron CA: Fibro-osseous lesions of the jaws. J Oral Surg 28:58, 1970

Waldron CA, Giansanti JS: Benign fibro-osseous lesions of the jaws: A clinical–radiologic–histologic review of sixty-five cases. Oral Surg 35:190, 1973

Warrick CK: Some aspects of polyostotic fibrous dysplasia. Possible hypothalamic to account for an associated endocrine change. Clin Radiol 24:125, 1973

Weathers DR, Waldron CA: Intraoral cellular nevi. Review of the literature and report of five cases. Oral Surg 20:467, 1965

Willis RA: Hamartomas and hamartomatous syndromes. In The Borderland of Embryology and Pathology. London, Butterworth, 1962

Woods JE et al: The challenge of large facial hamartomas and other benign conditions of the head and neck. Am J Surg 138:521, 1979

Odontogenic Tumors

Baden E: Odontogenic tumors. Pathol Annu 6:475, 1971

Barros RE, Dominguez FV, Cabrini RL: Myxoma of the jaws. Oral Surg 27:225, 1969

Becker R, Pertl A: Zur Therapie des Ameloblastoms. Deutsch Zahn Mund Kieferheilk 49:423, 1967

Bhaskar, SN, Cutright DE: Multiple enostosis: report of 16 cases. J Oral Surg 26:321, 1968

Chaudhry AP, Spink JH, Gorlin RJ: Periapical fibrous dysplasia (cementoma). J Oral Surg 16:483, 1958

Gardner DG, Michaels L, Liepa E: Calcifying epithelial odontogenic tumor: An amyloid-producing neoplasm. Oral Surg 26:812, 1968

Giansanti JS, Someren A, Waldron CA: Odontogenic adenomatoid tumor (adenoameloblastoma). Survey of 3 cases. Oral Surg 30:69, 1970

Gorlin RJ et al: The calicifying odontogenic cyst–a possible analogue of the cutaneous calcifying epithelioma of Malherbe–an analysis of fifteen cases. Oral Surg 15:1235, 1962

Gorlin RJ, Meskin LH, Brodey R: Odontogenic tumors in man and animals: pathologic classification and clinical behavior–A review. Ann NY Acad Sci 108:722, 1963

Hamner JE III, Pizer ME: Ameloblastic odontoma. Report of two cases. Am J Dis Child 115:332, 1968

Hamner JE III, Scofield HH, Cornyn J: Benign fibro-osseous jaw lesions of periodontal membrane origin. An analysis of 249 cases. Cancer 22:861, 1968

Hooker SP: Ameloblastic odontomas. An analysis of twenty-six cases. Abstracts of papers presented at 21st annual meeting. Am Acad Oral Pathol Miami Beach, April, 1967

Krolls SO, Pindborg JJ: Calcifying epithelial odontogenic tumor. A survey of 23 cases and discussion of histomorphologic variations. Arch Pathol 98:206, 1974

Lucas RB: Pathology of Tumors of the Oral Tissues, 3rd ed. New York, Longman, 1974.

Nichols C, Brightman VJ: Parotid calcifications and cementomas in a patient with Sjögren's syndrome and idiopathic thrombocytopenic purpura. J Oral Pathol 6:51, 1977

Pindborg JJ, Kramer IRH: International histological classification of tumors No. 5, Histological typing of odontogenic tumors, jaw cysts and allied lesions. Geneva, World Health Organization, 1971

Pizer ME, Hamner JE III: Odontogenic tumors: A survey of their manifestations in childhood. Clin Pediatr 6:593, 1967

Sehdev MK et al: Ameloblastoma of maxilla and mandible. Cancer 33:324, 1974

Small IA, Waldron CA: Ameloblastomas of the jaws. Oral Surg 8:281, 1955

Stanley HR, Diehl DL: Ameloblastoma potential of follicular cysts. Oral Surg 20:260, 1965

Salivary Cysts and Tumors

Arguelles MT et al: Necrotizing sialometaplasia. Oral Surg 42:86, 1976

Batsakis JG et al: Monomorphic adenomas of major salivary glands: A histologic study of 96 tumors. Clin Otolaryngol 6:129, 19-1

Bhaskar SN: Lymphoepithelial cysts of the oral cavity. Report of twenty-four cases. Oral Surg 21:120, 1966

Caldwell EH: Malignant transformation of a Warthin's tumor: Case report, review of the literature and discussion of pathology. Ann Plast Surg 3:177, 1979

Cummings NA et al: Sjögren's syndrome. Newer aspects of research, diagnosis and therapy. Ann Intern Med 75:937, 1971

Eneroth CM, Frazén S, Zajicek J: Aspiration biopsy of salivary gland tumors. A critical review of 910 biopsies. Acta Cytol 11:470, 1967

Grillon GL et al: Necrotizing sialometaplasia: literature review and presentation of five cases. J Oral Surg 39:747, 1981

Noyek AM et al: Familial Warthin's tumor, 1. Its synchronous occurrence in mother and son; 2. Its association with cystic oncocytic metaplasia of the larynx. J Otolaryngol 9:90, 1980

Seifert G et al: Histologic subclassification of cystadenolymphoma of the parotid gland—Analysis of 275 cases. Virchow's Arch (Pathol Anat) 388:13, 1980

Siddiqui AR et al: Possible explanation for the appearance of Warthin's tumor on I-123, and Tc-99M-pertechnetate scans. Clin Nuc Med 6:258, 1981

Other Benign Oral Neoplasias

Archard HO, Heck JW, Stanley HR: Focal epithelial hyperplasia: An unusual oral mucosal lesion found in Indian children. Oral Surg 20:201, 1965

Eisinger M et al: Propagation of human warts virus in tissue culture. Nature 256:432, 1975

Iverson RE, Vistnes LM: Keratoacanthoma is frequently a dangerous diagnosis. Am J Surg 126:359, 1973

Morris AL, Eversole LR, Sorenson HW: Oral florid papillomatosis in Down's syndrome. Oral Surg 37:202, 1974

Schiff BL: Molluscum contagiosum of the buccal mucosa. Arch Dermatol 78:90, 1958

Scofield HH, Werning JT, Shukes RC: Solitary intraoral keratoacanthoma. Oral Surg 37:889, 1974

van Wyck CW, Staz J, Farman AG: Focal epithelial hyperplasia in a group of South Africans: Its clinical and microscopic features, and its ultrastructural features. J Oral Pathol 6:1, 14, 1977

Wallace JR: Focal epithelial hyperplasia (Heck's disease): Report of a case. J Am Dent Assoc 93:118, 1976

Benign Oral Tumors and Internal Malignancy

Ayres WW, Delaney AJ, Backer MH: Congenital neurofibromatous macroglossia associated in some cases with von Recklinghausen's disease; A case report and review of the literature. Cancer 5:721, 1952

Bowerman JE: Polyostotic fibrous dysplasia with oral melanotic pigmentation. Br J Oral Surg 6:188, 1969

Brannon RB: The odontogenic keratocyst. A clinicopathologic study of 312 cases. Part I. Clinical features. Oral Surg 42:54, 1976

Browne RM: The odontogenic keratocyst. Histological features and their correlation with clinical behaviour. Br Dent J 131:249, 1971

Casino AJ, Ohm GL, Winston J, Wolk D: Oral facial manifestations of the multiple endocrine neoplasia syndromes. Oral Surg 51:516, 1981

Curth HO: How and why the skin reacts. In Conference on Paraneoplastic syndromes. Part VIII. A spectrum of organ systems that respond to the presence of cancer. Ann NY Acad Sci 230:435, 1974

Donoff RB, Guralnick WC, Clayman L: Keratocysts of the jaws. J Oral Surg 30:880, 1972

Erbe RW: Current concepts in genetics: inherited gastrointestinal-polyposis syndromes. N Engl J Med 294:1101, 1976

Gorlin RJ, Chaudhry AP: Multiple osteomatosis, fibromas, lipomas and fibrosarcomas of the skin and mesentery, epidermoid inclusion cysts of the skin, leiomyomas and multiple intestinal polyposis: A heritable disorder of connective tissue. N Engl J Med 263:1151, 1960

Gorlin RJ et al: Multiple basal-cell nevi syndrome. An analysis of a syndrome consisting of multiple nevoid basal-cell carcinoma, jaw cysts, skeletal anomalies, medulloblastoma and hyporesponsiveness to parathormone. Cancer 18:89, 1965

Gorlin RJ et al: Multiple mucosal neuromas, pheochromocytoma and medullary carcinoma of the thyroid—a syndrome. Cancer 22:293, 1968

Gray TK, Ontjes DA: Clinical aspects of thyrocalcitonin. Clin Orthop 111:238, 1975

Haynes HA, Fitzpatrick TB: Cutaneous manifestations of internal malignancy. In Wintrobe MM et al (eds): Harrison's Principles of Internal Medicine, 7th ed, Chap. 367, New York, McGraw-Hill, 1974

Holmes LB et al: Mental Retardation. An Atlas of Diseases Associated with Physical Abnormalities. New York, Macmillan, 1972

Kaufman RL, Chase LR: Basal cell nevus syndrome: normal responsiveness to parathyroid hormone. Birth Defects 7:149, 1971

Khairi MRA et al: Mucosal neuroma, pheochromocytoma and medullary thyroid carcinoma: multiple endocrine neoplasia type 3. Medicine 54:89, 1975

Lowe NJ: Peutz-Jeghers syndrome with pigmented oral papillomas. Arch Dermatol 111:503, 1975

Neal CJ, JR: Multiple osteomas of the mandible associated with polyposis of the colon (Gardner's syndrome). Oral Surg 28:628, 1969

Papanayotou P, Vezirtzi E: Tuberous sclerosis with gingival lesions. Report of a case. Oral Surg 39:578, 1975

Robbins SL: Pathologic Basis of Disease, Chap. 23, pp 1074–1075. Philadelphia, WB Saunders, 1974

Schwartz DT, Alpert M: The malignant transformation of fibrous dysplasia. Am J Med Sci 247:1, 1964

Scully RE, Galdabini JJ, McNeely BU: Case records of the Massachusetts General Hospital. Weekly clinicopathological exercises. Case 14-1976. N Eng J Med 294:772, 1976

Steiner AL, Goodman AD, Powers SR: Study of a kindred with pheochromocytoma, medullary thyroid carcinoma, hyperparathyroidism and Cushing's disease: multiple endocrine neoplasia, type 2. Medicine 47:371, 1968

Zeligman I, Houston FM: Tuberous sclerosis with adenoma sebaceum of face and hypopigmented macular lesions of the trunk. Birth Defects 7:311, 1971

Paget's Disease

Avioli LV, Berman M: Role of magnesium metabolism and the effects of fluoride therapy in Paget's disease of bone. J Clin Endocrinol Metab 28:700, 1968

Barry HC: Paget's Disease of Bone. Edinburgh, ES Livingstone, 1969

Goldfield EB: Newer agents in treating Paget's disease of bone. Geriatrics 29:61, 1974

Hutter RVP, et al: Giant cell tumors complicating Paget's disease of bone. Cancer 16:1044, 1963

Levison V: The treatment of Paget's disease of bone by radiotherapy. Ann Phys Med 10:230, 1970

McGowan DA: Clinical problems in Paget's disease affecting the jaws. Br J Oral Surg 11:230, 1974

Mills BG: Comparison of the ultrastructure of a malignant tumor of the mandible containing giant cells with Paget's disease of bone. J Oral Pathol 10:203, 1981

Mills BG et al: Immunohistological demonstration of respiratory syncytial virus antigens in Paget's disease of bone. Proc Natl Acad Sci 78:1209, 1981

Rasmussen H, Bordier P: The cellular basis of metabolic bone disease. N Engl J Med 289:25, 1973

Rosenmertz SK, Schare HJ: Osteogenic sarcoma arising in Paget's disease of the mandible. Review of the literature and report of a case. Oral Surg 28:304, 1969

Seldin HM et al: Giant cell tumor of the jaws. J Am Dent Assoc 55:210, 1957

Sherman RS, Wilner D: Roentgen diagnosis of Paget's disease (Osteitis deformans): The usual, the unusual and the complications. D Radiog Photog 43:51, 1970

Singer FR: Paget's disease of bone: A slow virus infection (Edit). Calcif. Tissue Int 31:185, 1980

Smith BJ, Everson JW: Paget's disease of bone with particular reference to dentistry. J Oral Pathol 10:233, 1981

Spilka CJ, Callahan KR: Review of the differential diagnosis of oral manifestations in early osteitis deformans. Oral Surg 11:809, 1958

Viola MV et al: Virus-like inclusions in osteosarcoma cells arising in Paget's disease. Lancet 1:848, 1982

Xanthoma

Fleischmajer R, Dowlati Y, Reeves, JR: Familial hyperlipidemias. Diagnosis and treatment. Arch Dermatol 110:43, 1974

Fredrickson DS et al: Tangier disease: Combined staff conference at the National Institutes of Health. Ann Intern Med 55:1016, 1961

Fredrickson DS, Lees RS: Familial hyperlipoproteinemia. In Stanbury JB, Wyngaarden JB, Fredrickson DS (eds): Metabolic Basis of Inherited Disease. 3rd ed. New York, McGraw-Hill, 1972

Miller AS, Elzay RP: Verruciform xanthoma of the gingiva: report of six cases. J Periodontol 44:103, 1973

Raffle EJ, Hall DC: Xanthomatosis presenting with oral lesions. Br Dent J 125:62, 1968

Gingival Enlargement

Araiche M, Brode H: A case of fibromatosis gingivae. Oral Surg 12:1307, 1959

Darling AI, Fletcher JP: Familial white folded gingivostomatosis. Oral Surg 11:296, 1958

Emerson TG: Hereditary gingival hyperplasia: A family pedigree of four generations. Oral Surg 19:1, 1965

Emslie RD et al: Mouth breathing: Etiology and effects. J Am Dent Assoc 44:506, 1952

Englert RJ, Levin IS: Diffuse osteofibromatosis; a symptom complex. Oral Surg 7:837, 1954

Giles WS, Agnew RG: Idiopathic fibrous hyperplasia of the edentulous maxillary ridges. J Periodontol 31:210, 1960

Hassel TM et al: Summary of an international symposium on phenytoin-induced teratology and gingival pathology. J Am Dent Assoc 99:652, 1979

Krohn S: Effect of the administration of steroid hormones on the gingival tissues. J Periodontol 29:300, 1958

Laband PF et al: Hereditary gingival fibromatosis. Oral Surg 17:339, 1964

Lewis AB: Effects of smoking on oral mucosa. Oral Surg 8:1026, 1955

Nally FF: Gingival hyperplasia due to primidone "mysoline." J Irish Dent Assoc 13:113, 1967

Ramfjord S: The histopathology of inflammatory gingival enlargement. Oral Surg 6:516, 1953

Savara BS et al: Hereditary gingival fibrosis: study of a family. J Periodontol 25:12, 1954

Smith QT: Gingival fibrosis during phenytoin ingestion. Northwest Dent 57:23, 1978

Tamagna JA: Familial white folded dysplasia of the oral mucous membranes. Clin Stomatol Conf 6:56, 1965

Witkop CJ: Heterogeneity in gingival fibromatosis. Birth Defects 7:215, 1971

Zegarelli E, Kutscher A: Familial white folded hypertrophy of the mucous membranes. Oral Surg 10:262, 1957

Cervicofacial Actinomycosis

Barclay JK: Actinomycosis of the mandible. Case report. Aust Dent J 23:477, 1978

Bazhanov NN et al: Use of hyperbaric oxygenation in the therapy of maxillofacial actinomycosis. Stomatologiia 59:28, 1980

Blair GS: An unusual dental abscess. Br Dent J 147:17, 1979

Blake GH et al: Cervicofacial actinomycosis associated with Eikenella corrodens: case report. Milit Med 147:414, 1982

Borssén E et al: Actinomyces of infected dental root canals. Oral Surg 51:643, 1981

Bronner M, and Bronner M: Actinomycosis, 2nd Ed. Bristol, England, John Wright and Sons. 1971

Choukas NC: Actinomycosis of the mandible. Oral Surg 11:14, 1958

Davis MIJ: Analysis of 46 cases of actinomycosis with reference to its etiology. Am J Surg 52:447, 1941

Fergus HS: Actinomycosis involving a periapical cyst in the anterior maxilla. Report of a case. Oral Surg 49:390, 1980

Fitzgerald JE et al: Systemic immune response to oral colonization. J Periodont. Res 17:237, 1982

Freeman LR et al: Conservative treatment of periapical actinomycosis. Oral Surg 51:205, 1981

Gold L and Doyne EE: Actinomycosis with osteomyelitis of the alveolar process. Oral Surg 5:1056, 1952

Gondor S et al: Appendicovesical fistula caused by ileocecal actinomycosis. Can J Surg 25:23, 1982

Happonen RP, Viander M, Pelliniemi L and Aitsalo K: Actinomyces israelii in osteoradionecrosis of the jaws; Histopathologic and immunocytochemical study of five cases. Oral Surg 55:580, 1983

Holst E et al: Cervicofacial actinomycosis. A retrospective study. Int J Oral Surg 8: 194, 1979

Hunter GC and Westrick CM: Cervicofacial abscess by actinomyces. Oral Surg 10:793, 1957

Hurt DF et al: Clinicopathologic conferences Case 39, Part III Cervicofacial actinomycosis. J Oral Maxillofac Surg 40:367, 1982

Johnson S, et al: Actinomycosis of mandible, U.S. Armed Forces Med J 8:1214, 1957

Kirsch SA: Cervicofacial actinomycosis following surgical trauma in rats. Oral Surg 46:827, 1978

Kubo M et al: A histological and ultrastructural comparison of the sulfur granule of actinomycosis and actinobacillosis. Nat Inst Anim Health 20:53, 1980

Kuepper RC et al: Actinomycosis of the tongue: Report of a case. J Oral Surg 37:123, 1979

Laforgia P et al: Nodular isolated actinomycosis of the tongue—a case report. Dent Surv 55:48, 1979

Lane SL, et al.: Oxytetracycline in the treatment of oro-cervical facial actinomycosis. JAMA 151:986, 1953

Lopez-Majano V et al: Cervico-facial actinomycosis. Eur J Nucl Med 7:143, 1982

Mitchell RH: Actinomycosis and the dental abscess. Br D J 120:423, 1966

Musser LB et al: Actinomycosis of the anterior maxilla. Oral Surg 44:21, 1977

Perna E et al: Actinomycotic granuloma of the Gasserian ganglion with primary site in a dental root. J Neurosurg 54:553, 1981

Robbins TS et al: Actinomycosis: the disease and its treatment. Drug Intell Clin Pharm 15:99, 1981

Seyfert H: Cervico-facial actinomycosis—Frequence and change in a period of 29 years. Zahn Mund Kieferheilkd 66:699, 1978

Sundqvist G et al: Isolation of Actinomyces israelii from periapical lesion. J Endod 6:602, 1980

Sykes GS et al: Actinomyces-like structures and their association with intrauterine contraceptive devices, pelvic infection and abnormal cervical cytology. Br J Obstet Gynecol 88:934, 1981

Valicenti JF Jr et al: Detection and prevalence of IUD-associated Actinomyces colonization and related morbidity. A prospective study of 69,925 cervical smears. JAMA 247:1149, 1982

Villa VG: Pulp abscess associated with actinomyces. Oral Surg 10:207, 1957

Walker S et al: Mandibular osteomyelitis caused by Actinomyces israelli. Oral Surg 51:243, 1981

Wesley RK et al: Periapical actinomycosis: Clinical considerations. J Endod 3:352, 1977

9

Oral Cancer

KENNETH KENT, ALAN SAMIT

Figures 9-18, 9-20 through 9-24, 9-27 A–E, 9-30, 9-31 A–E, 9-32, and 9-35 A and D are used by courtesy of the Department of Dental Oncology, M.D. Anderson Cancer and Tumor Hospital, Houston, Texas.

This year at least 12,000 Americans will die as a result of oral cancer and more than 26,000 new cases will be diagnosed. Oral cancer represents approximately 5% of all malignancies in men and 2% in women. Although the oral cavity is examined routinely and relatively frequently, the majority of new cases of intraoral cancer will be discovered only after the patient becomes symptomatic and seeks professional care (Fig. 9-1). More than 60% of these tumors will be well advanced when first detected, and the treatment results will be generally disappointing.

Advanced cancer, which mandates aggressively applied combined treatment modalities, results in significant disability and deformity. The long-term prognosis for patients with oral cancer is discouraging, with overall survival following definitive treatment approaching only 30% at 5 years. Death usually results from failure to control the primary lesion, cervical lymph node metastases, or both. Common terminal events in oral cancer patients include exsanguination, aspiration pneumonia, or airway obstruction. Malnutrition is nearly always a major contributing factor.

The detection of oral cancer at its earliest clinical manifestation is essential because there is a direct correlation between survival and the stage of the disease at the time of diagnosis.

SURVIVAL (IN MONTHS) FOR ORAL CANCER PATIENTS

- Stage I—47.4 months
- Stage II—27.5 months
- Stage III—13.8 months

Early detection provides the patient with the best opportunity for successful management and possible cure. The orderly, predictable nature of oral cancer permits lesions to be clinically detected before the patient becomes symptomatic. Not only are the chances for survival increased, but deformity and dysfunction after treatment are minimized.

Head and neck cancers with the best prognosis, such as the vocal cord or lower lip, tend to become clinically obvious or symptomatic at an early stage; conversely, lesions that are inaccessible for direct examination or become symptomatic very late, such as the base of the tongue or tonsillar pillar, usually have a less favorable prognosis. The capacity of the tumor to involve the lymphatic system also significantly affects the therapeutic prognosis. Cancers of the base of the tongue or the soft palate, which frequently metastasize to the neck early or bilaterally, are more difficult to manage successfully than are tumors of the anterior floor of the mouth, which tend to metastasize unilaterally and somewhat later during the course of the disease.

An understanding of the nature and behavior of aerodigestive cancer is essential to

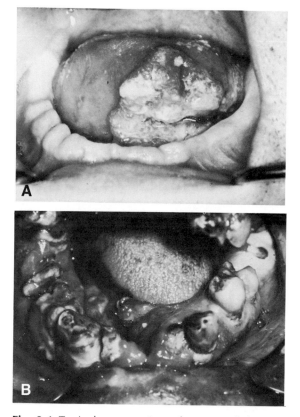

Fig. 9-1 Typical presentation of cancer of the oral cavity when detected by the patient. The disease is well advanced and was detected only when the patient became symptomatic and sought treatment. Treatment of such advanced disease usually results in deformity and disfigurement; unfortunately, the prognosis is also unfavorable. *A,* Squamous cell carcinoma of the anterolateral tongue. *B,* Extensive squamous cell carcinoma of the anterior floor of mouth that has invaded the tongue and anterior mandible.

adequate evaluation of oral pathosis or management of patients with oral cancer. The predominant role of squamous cell carcinoma in head and neck malignancy must be recognized. An awareness of the most common sites, a knowledge of the appearance of early lesions, and a high index of suspicion are required for the dentist or physician to discover asymptomatic oral cancer. An understanding of the pathophysiology of the disease and awareness of current modalities of therapy, treatment sequelae, and morbidity are necessary for successful management of the cancer patient.

TRADITIONAL CONCEPTS

Unfortunately, several of the traditional concepts of oral cancer create potential impediments to comprehensive patient evaluation and often frustrate early diagnosis. These classical concepts, which are concerned primarily with the appearance of oral cancer and the specific intraoral sites in which cancers are found, are outmoded and convey erroneous and misleading information. Only by setting aside these antiquated concepts and adopting new currently recognized criteria for the detection of early cancer can the best interests of the patients be served.

Oral cancer is classically described as an indurated, ulcerated lump or sore that may or may not be painful and is often associated with cervical adenopathy. Unfortunately, this is a description of advanced disease, which has usually been present for many months or longer. When these classical criteria for the detection of oral cancer are applied, only well-established, late, symptomatic lesions are discovered. *Recent studies have demonstrated that early lesions have a characteristic appearance and can be predictably recognized.* It is inexcusable to continue to overlook asymptomatic lesions now that their clinical appearance has been well documented.

The oral cavity has traditionally been divided into anatomic regions for purposes of cancer site reporting, for example, the tongue, buccal mucosa, lips, alveolar processes, floor of the mouth, and hard and soft palates. Although these classical divisions are certainly convenient, the actual clinical distribution of oral cancer does not follow this arbitrary arrangement. Instead, localization of cancer within the oral cavity is essentially confined to three distinct areas. Geographic and national variations in cancer localization are fairly well recognized and can be readily explained on the basis of regional and environmental factors or local customs.

Historically, oral cancers have been arbitrarily segregated from other cancers of the

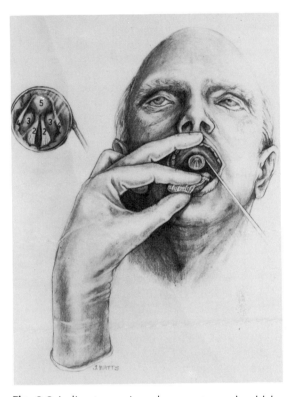

Fig. 9-2 Indirect or mirror laryngoscopy should be used to evaluate the hypopharyngeal and laryngeal regions. The patient is comfortably seated in an upright position in the dental chair. The mouth is opened and the protruded tongue is grasped with a sponge between the thumb and index finger while the middle finger retracts the upper lip. A warm mirror is used to displace the uvula superiorly and posteriorly. Indirect examination of (1) the glottic chink, (2) true vocal chords, (3) vestibular folds (false vocal chords), (4) aryepiglottic folds, and (5) epiglottis is performed. Illumination with a headlamp is necessary. Phonation is required to completely visualize the vocal chords and assess their mobility; for the dentist a prolonged "eee" sound is optimal. Topical anesthetic or nitrous oxide—oxygen analgesia—may be necessary to control a hyperactive gag reflex.

aerodigestive tract. Consideration of oral, pharyngeal, laryngeal, or esophageal cancers as distinctly unrelated lesions creates artificial boundaries that can frustrate the early diagnosis of nonoral mucosal malignancies. Because many patients visit the dentist more often than the physician, the dentist should be encouraged to extend his examination procedures to include the entire upper aerodigestive tract. Palpation of the base of the tongue and hypopharynx, and indirect mirror examination of the vallecula, hypopharynx, epiglottis, and supraglottic larynx should be routine procedures in the dental office (Fig. 9-2). By this means, the number of early asymptomatic lesions detected deep to the oral cavity might be increased with a subsequent reduction in morbidity and mortality.

ETIOLOGIC FACTORS IN AERODIGESTIVE CANCER

A definitive etiology for cancer of the aerodigestive mucosa has not yet been established. Evidence indicates that the induction of malignant changes within tissues is probably a multifactorial process dependent on several as yet undefined variables. It has even been suggested that malignant transformation may be a frequent occurrence and that clinical tumors develop only when the immune system fails to recognize or overcome the abnormal cells. Although no definite etiology has been determined, several risk factors are apparently associated with an increased incidence of oral cancer. Some of these risk factors are well established and generally acknowledged; others are relatively controversial.

Patient factors, especially age, sex, and family history appear to be extremely significant determinants in the development of oral cancer. Most oral cancers occur in males older than 40 years. The incidence is further increased in patients with a family history positive for cancer. Although other factors are also significant, it is probable that a hereditary predisposition to develop cancer can be genetically transmitted.

Alcohol and tobacco abuse are implicated as local factors in nearly all cases of oral cancer. The evidence is inconclusive as to whether alcohol or tobacco abuse is more significant, although many investigators have tentatively assigned a predominant role to alcohol. The specific mechanism, either direct local tissue injury or indirect systemic effects, has not been identified. Malnutrition and metabolic abnormalities secondary to alcohol abuse may also be contributory. The frequency, chronicity, and type of alcohol consumed appear to be significant. Tobacco abuse measured in pack-years (the number of packs of cigarettes smoked per day times the number of years the patient has been smoking) is also associated with an increased incidence of aerodigestive cancer. As with alcohol, specific mechanisms have not yet been identified.

Patients with a history of a previous oral cancer are often encouraged to modify or desist from their use of alcohol and tobacco; however, some studies indicate that the incidence of subsequent primary cancers may not depend on continued exposure to alcohol or tobacco once the initial disease has developed. The implication is that the pathophysiologic changes necessary for cancer development have already become operational and are no longer affected by continuing or abstaining from the noxious habits; however, efforts to discourage alcohol and tobacco abuse can be justified on the basis that progressive heart, lung, or liver damage is associated with sustained indulgence.

Environmental factors such as exposure to the sun, natural carcinogens, or industrial pollutants affect not only the incidence of oral cancer but may also explain regional variations in the intraoral distribution of cancer. Greater actinic exposure results in an increased incidence of lip cancer in the southwestern United States. Reverse smoking (the lighted end of the cigarette held within the mouth) explains an increased incidence of hard palate cancers in the rain forests of South America. Betel nut chewing accounts for the disproportionate number of cancers of the buccal mucosa in India.

Correlation of the patient and local and environmental factors in any particular geographic locale determines the high-risk patient. In the industrialized northeastern United States, males over 40 years of age who abuse alcohol and tobacco are apparently at the highest risk; a previous oral cancer or a

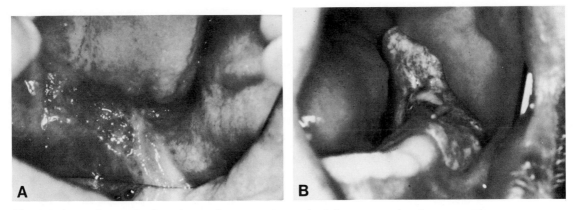

Fig. 9-3 According to both patients, these tumors resulted from recent local trauma. The large size of the lesions is not consistent with the short history of trauma described by the patient. The traumatic event probably caused the patient to become aware of an asymptomatic lesion that was present for many months. *A,* Described by the patient as irritation secondary to a 2-week-old fracture of the distobuccal flange of an old denture. *B,* Described by the patient as irritation resulting from trapping a peanut under the denture only 3 weeks ago.

family history of cancer additionally increases the risk. These patients should be given the highest priority for regular, systematic, and comprehensive head and neck cancer evaluations. Although no sex or age group is without cancer incidence, the highest yield of early asymptomatic lesions will be found when the patients at high risk are identified and carefully screened.

Some authorities and many patients attribute a significant role to trauma in the development of oral cancer. Patients often relate the initiation of a lesion to a specific, memorable traumatic event, such as biting the tongue, breaking a denture, or injury from hot or coarse food. Recognizing that oral cancer usually develops in a relatively slow, predictable fashion, it is often difficult to correlate the tumor size at presentation, which may be rather large, with the recent traumatic incident (Fig. 9-3). More likely, the traumatic event marked the time that the patient first became aware of a previously asymptomatic lesion, rather than the start of the lesion. The role of acute trauma in the initiation of oral cancer is probably negligible.

Lichen planus has also been implicated in the etiology of oral cancer. Although a direct cause and effect relationship has not yet been established, occasional reports demonstrate an apparent association between lichen planus and subsequent oral carcinoma. Patients with a history of lichen planus, especially the erosive form, should be considered at high risk until additional longitudinal studies are completed.

EVALUATION

Identification of Early Asymptomatic Lesions

When the classical criteria for the detection of oral cancers are applied, the number of asymptomatic early lesions discovered is disappointingly small, despite frequent localization to areas that are readily accessible for examination. Most cancer screening programs fail to detect a significant number of early lesions; however, use of recently established criteria for the clinical identification of asymptomatic carcinoma can dramatically increase the number of early lesions that are diagnosed.

Early oral cancers are asymptomatic, usually less than 2.0 cm in diameter, predominantly red, with or without a white component, and smooth or minimally elevated. Nearly 95% of early lesions have an erythroplastic (red) component, whereas fewer than 5% are exclusively white. Leukoplakia, traditionally considered a premalignant lesion,

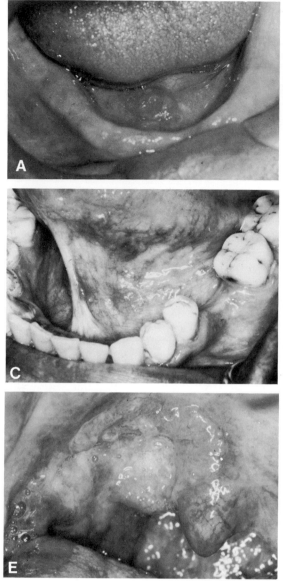

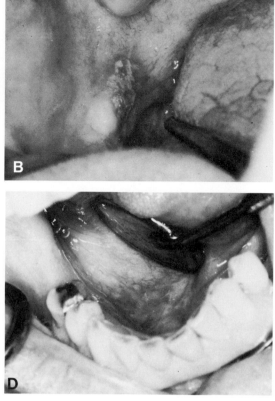

Fig. 9-4 The clinical appearance of early, asymptomatic oral cancer is far different from that of advanced disease. The lesions, which often appear to be insignificant, are predominantly red, may or may not have a white component, and are usually less than 2 cm in diameter. Textural changes may be minimal, but roughness, granularity, ulceration, or induration increase the probability of invasion. *A,* Anterior floor of mouth, squamous cell carcinoma. *B,* Retromolar trigone, squamous cell carcinoma. *C,* Anterior floor of mouth, squamous cell carcinoma. *D,* Anterior floor of mouth, squamous cell carcinoma. *E,* Soft palate, clear cell carcinoma. (Courtesy of Keith Kent, D.M.D.)

has been shown to undergo malignant transformation only rarely. Textural changes associated with areas of erythroplasia, such as roughness, granularity, ulceration, or induration, greatly increase the probability that the lesion is malignant. It is apparent that oral cancer can be reliably detected earlier than was previously believed (Fig. 9-4).

Additional studies have established that these early, asymptomatic cancers are essentially localized to three specific areas within the oral cavity (Fig. 9-5). The floor of the mouth accounts for more than 45% of all early oral carcinomas. The soft palate complex, consisting of the soft palate and uvula, the anterior tonsillar pillars, and the lingual aspect of the retromolar trigones, accounts for nearly 30% of the lesions. The ventral aspect of the tongue and the middle and posterior thirds of the lateral aspect of the tongue account for about 15% of the lesions. Only 10% of early cancers are located outside these three areas in various sites within the oral cavity. It must be appreciated that the distribution of oral cancers just described is based on data obtained in the industrial northeastern United States and that regional and geographic variations must be anticipated.

Meticulous examination of patients at high risk, with particular attention to areas of erythroplasia in high-risk sites, facilitates the diagnosis of asymptomatic cancer. Early lesions are often amenable to aggressive local treatment with minimal deformity, negligible loss of function, and optimal survival.

Initial Evaluation of Suspected Lesions

When a suspected lesion is detected, especially in a high-risk site in a patient at high risk, a standardized protocol should be used to ensure adequate assessment and minimize inappropriate intervention.

Initially, detailed medical and social histories and a history of the lesion, if available, should be recorded. The entire oral cavity, pharynx, and larynx should be evaluated by palpation, direct inspection, and indirect mirror visualization. Additional areas of mucosal abnormality that are detected should be documented. All lesions should be described in detail, with attention to location, size, color, texture, and other significant physical characteristics. Photographs, especially color transparencies, often prove invaluable for subsequent comparison. Diagrams are occasionally useful if completed accurately. Careful examination of the neck for adenopathy should be performed with specific attention to the size, location, texture, mobility, and the absence or presence of tenderness in any palpable nodes. Enlarged nodes that are soft, freely mobile, and tender suggest inflammatory reaction; palpable nodes that are firm or hard, not freely mobile, or nontender are strongly suggestive of metastatic involvement.

Indulgence in potentially noxious habits should be ascertained. Probable sources of irritation should be reduced or eliminated when possible. An observation appointment for re-evaluation of the lesion should be scheduled 10 to 14 days later. The waiting

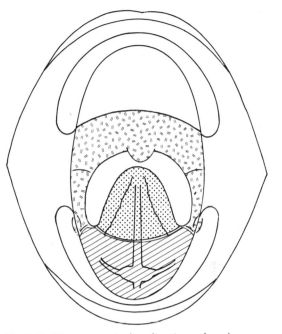

Fig. 9-5 Diagrammatic localization of oral cancers depicting high-risk sites. The anterior floor of mouth accounts for 45% of all early, asymptomatic cancers. The soft palate complex accounts for 30% of the lesions, and the ventral and posterolateral tongue, 15%. The remainder of the oral cavity accounts for only about 10% of all oral cancers.

period permits resolution of purely inflammatory lesions resulting from acute trauma or irritation. *Lesions persisting beyond the observation period without apparent cause should be considered malignant until proven otherwise by biopsy and microscopic evaluation.*

When the diagnosis of oral cancer appears to be obvious on the basis of clinical appearance but the cervical examination is not grossly positive, the biopsy should be deferred until an examination can be completed by the practitioner or oncology team who will definitively treat the patient. This courtesy minimizes confusion that can arise when a small primary lesion is distorted by the biopsy or when cervical adenopathy not found by the initial examiner before biopsy is discovered after biopsy by the second examiner. It is then uncertain whether the newly detected nodes are merely reactive to the biopsy or were present before biopsy, but not appreciated by the initial examiner. Once an evaluation has been performed by the individual or team who will ultimately assume responsibility for the treatment of the patient, the biopsy may be obtained without risk of introducing confusion.

Grossly positive lesions with obvious cervical node involvement can probably be biopsied immediately by the initial examiner without introducing confusion. The diagnosis can thereby be established more quickly, and entry into a formal evaluation and treatment system can be facilitated. Specific protocols for the biopsy of suspected oral lesions will generally be established by the individual cancer treatment teams in each community.

Toluidine Blue Vital Staining

In the evaluation of early asymptomatic oral cancers, areas of redness that persist beyond the observation period must be biopsied. Because the erythroplastic region is generally composed of an area of inflammatory reaction as well as possible foci of tumor cells, it is essential to obtain a tissue specimen that represents the true nature of the lesion. Obtaining multiple random samples from the entire area is not a reliable diagnostic procedure because small foci of tumor cells can still be missed.

Toluidine blue, a basophilic vital nuclear dye, can guide biopsy by localizing small foci of tumor cells within the larger area of inflammation. Topical application of the staining medium to the oral mucosa is followed by a rinse of 1.0% acetic acid. The dye, retained predominantly in the abnormal nuclei of tumor cells, produces areas of uptake seen as discretely blue-stained tissue (Fig. 9-6). Rinsing is performed to remove dye retained by debris or within irregularities of the mucosal surface. Positive areas of uptake do not represent ulceration or disruption of the mucosa; they represent retention of dye by the increased nuclear DNA content of tumor cells in the intact mucosa. Biopsy of dye retention areas is most likely to demonstrate foci of invasive cancer on microscopy.

It is readily apparent that toluidine blue could be used as a general intraoral rinse for gross screening purposes. Routine use of this technique without due consideration of all other factors essential to diagnosis should be discouraged. Casual overreliance on an apparently effective, yet simple, screening modality encourages the examiner to become complacent regarding the comprehensive integration of history and clinical examination, which are essential to the reliable detection of early cancer.

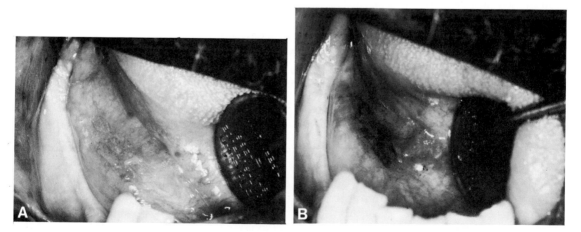

Fig. 9-6 Discrete foci of invasive cancer can be localized within the generalized area of inflammatory reaction by use of toluidine blue. The dye is taken up in the nuclei of abnormal (DNA-rich) cells and serves as a guide to selection of the most productive biopsy site. Two early, asymptomatic, erythroplastic lesions of the anterior floor of mouth are shown before and after staining. The erythroplastic areas that have not stained in a positive fashion represent inflammatory changes; stained areas revealed squamous cell carcinoma upon histologic examination.

Toluidine blue staining is remarkably reliable. False-negative and false-positive rates are low. Although highly suggestive of malignancy, a positive toluidine blue reaction is not conclusive in establishing the diagnosis of cancer. Biopsy and histologic evaluation are required for a definitive diagnosis.

Biopsy Techniques

Biopsy diagnosis of malignant lesions is an absolute requirement before ablative cancer therapy can be initiated. To provide an adequate biopsy specimen, certain criteria must be met. The specimen obtained should be representative of the lesion under investigation. Adequate depth (through the epithelium into connective tissue) is necessary to determine the integrity of the basement membrane and to search for nests of invasive tumor cells. Most pathologists do not require or request that the specimen include a zone of adjacent, clinically normal tissue in order to recognize malignant changes; however, when ulceration is present, specimens obtained from the ulcerated areas may reveal only nondiagnostic necrosis. Central necrosis occurs in tumors because rapidly enlarging lesions often outgrow their blood supply. In such instances, viable tumor is usually present at the periphery of the lesion, adjacent to normal tissue. Inclusion of some clinically uninvolved tissue in the specimen when ulceration is present, usually ensures a representative sample of active nonnecrotic tumor.

Intentional excisional biopsy (total removal of all abnormal tissue for diagnostic purposes) has absolutely no role in the diagnosis of oral cancer. Planned excisional biopsy of a lesion clinically suspected to be malignant cannot be justified by any rationale and should be condemned. Adequate excision of a malignant lesion usually requires at least a 1.5-cm margin of clinically uninvolved tissue along each periphery (Fig. 9-7); if the diagnosis is benign, it is impossible to justify removal of

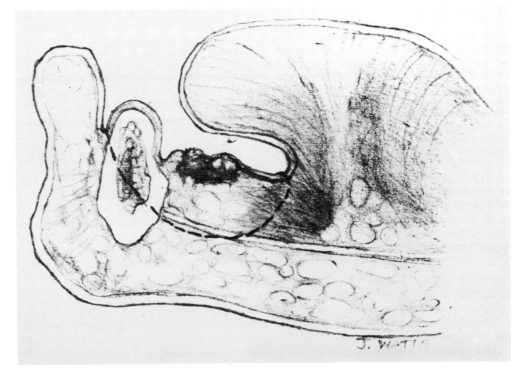

Fig. 9-7 Adequate excision of a malignant lesion requires a margin of at least 1.5 cm of clinically uninvolved tissue in all directions. This precludes intentional excisional biopsy of clinically suspected lesions. (The dimensions of adequate margins may vary depending on the specific histopathology of the lesion.) Margins of 1.5 cm are demonstrated for a small lesion.

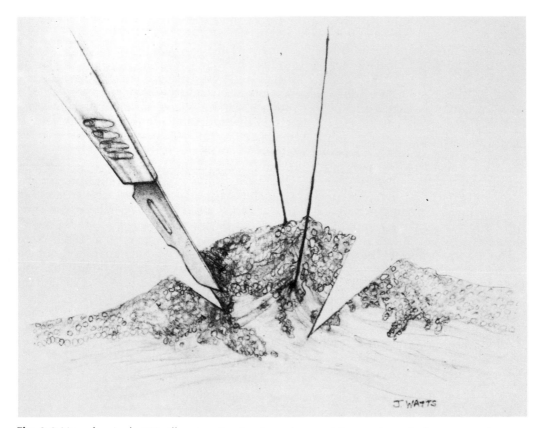

Fig. 9-8 Use of a single 3/0 silk suture to elevate and control the specimen is demonstrated. Incision must be extended to include the submucosa to evaluate the integrity of the basement membrane and determine the degree of invasion. Maceration of the specimen or implantation of surface cells into deeper layers can result if a tissue forceps is used to control the specimen.

such a large block of tissue (a specimen 3.1 cm × 3.1 cm × 1.6 cm for a 1.0-mm lesion). If the diagnosis is malignant, any specimen with less than 1.5 cm of clinically normal tissue along each margin is inadequate, and retreatment of the lesion would be mandated. Excision of a lesion for diagnosis is justifiable only when the lesion is almost certainly benign or when the lesion is so minute that total removal is required to ensure an adequate volume of tissue for microscopic evaluation. In most cases, every reasonable attempt should be made to obtain an incisional specimen (removal of a small representative portion of the lesion).

Anesthetic requirements for incisional biopsy of the oral mucosa are minimal. Block or remote infiltration anesthesia using lidocaine with epinephrine is adequate in all ac-

cessible regions of the oral cavity. Specimens can occasionally be obtained with topical anesthetic or without anesthetic, but patient comfort and the adequacy of the specimen are often better assured by profound local anesthesia. Postoperative analgesic requirements are usually minimal.

Local anesthetics should not be infiltrated directly into or through clinically involved tissue. Malignant cells can be inadvertently implanted into deeper tissues, and microscopic artifacts can be created that will interfere with diagnosis. Artifacts can also occur when sharp tissue forceps are used to grasp or manipulate the specimen or when the lesion is biopsied with electrosurgical instrumentation.

After adequate local anesthesia is obtained, a 000 silk suture is introduced into the tissue to be biopsied. The suture is used to gently elevate and manipulate the specimen (Fig. 9-8). A small elliptical incision is created with a scalpel. The ellipse should be oriented parallel to the suture. The incisions are carried into the underlying connective tissue, and the specimen is removed on the suture. The tissue is suspended over the specimen bottle and the suture is cut, allowing the specimen to fall into the preservative. It is not necessary to remove the suture because it does not interfere with processing and can be readily identified by the pathologist on microscopic sections. Unintentional introduction of artifacts or distortion of the specimen are minimized by this technique.

The use of a biopsy forceps rather than a scalpel may offer certain advantages, especially in the oral cavity posteriorly or in relatively inaccessible areas such as the uvula or retromolar trigone. The functional portion of the instrument consists of a cupped beak and a cutting beak. After anesthesia is obtained, a small portion of the lesion to be biopsied is grasped in the beaks, which are then closed tightly. The specimen is excised with a rapid twisting and pulling movement (Fig. 9-9) and is then gently teased from the cupped beak into the specimen bottle with a needle or other suitable instrument. Care must be exercised when biopsy forceps are used on movable tissue such as the soft palate, uvula, or the floor of the mouth to ensure that the specimen obtained includes the underlying connective tissue. A dull or damaged forceps or improper technique can result in significant tearing or partial deepithelialization of a large area of adjacent tissue.

Regardless of the biopsy technique used, the elastic components of the mucosa cause the excised specimen to contract. A specimen that initially seemed adequate may appear inadequate. Similarly, contraction of the elastic tissues in the biopsy site produces a defect that is often larger than anticipated. The clinician should not be disconcerted by these findings. Expectation of this phenomenon should preclude unnecessary harvesting of additional specimens or closure of biopsy sites.

The routine use of sutures to close biopsy sites should be discouraged unless required

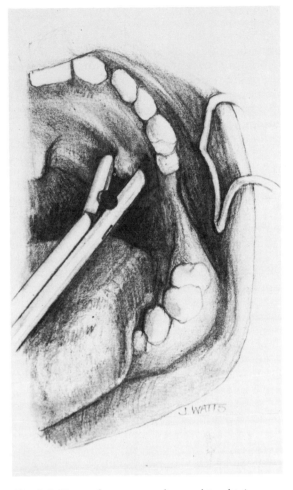

Fig. 9-9 Biopsy forceps may be used to obtain specimens from relatively inaccessible areas. The tissue is grasped firmly and removed with a rapid twisting and pulling movement. Care must be exercised to ensure an adequate depth of tissue and to prevent stripping of large areas of the mucosa.

to ensure adequate hemostasis. The risk of introducing malignant cells into adjacent or deep tissues during suture placement outweighs the benefits of obtaining primary closure of a small surgical site.

Microscopy specimens should immediately be placed into an amount of 10% formalin that is at least ten times the volume of the tissue mass. This ratio of formalin to tissue ensures proper fixation and negates autolysis that might render the specimen nondiagnostic. The tissue is then transported to the pathologist in the sealed formalin bottle along with a detailed report. The report should include the patient's age; the history, location and description of the lesion; and a clinical differential diagnosis. When indicated, radiographs or additional pertinent clinical information should also be provided. Following processing and microscopic review, the pathologist will return a report containing a gross description of the specimen, the microscopic findings, and the diagnosis.

Microscopic interpretation is subjective, and occasionally pathologists will disagree on the diagnosis, especially in terms of degree or extent. When the biopsy report is negative but clinical suspicion is high or toluidine blue uptake is strongly positive, several options are available. Review of the slide material with the pathologist, reorientation and resectioning of the specimen, or obtaining additional opinions from other pathologists are all appropriate. Serial sections (*i.e.*, sections obtained at regular intervals from the entire specimen) may clarify the diagnosis. Repeat biopsy should also be considered when the clinical suspicion remains high, despite negative microscopic findings.

Occasionally, patients are seen with obvious cervical node involvement without evidence of a primary lesion. After an exhaustive search for the "occult" or "unknown" primary lesion remains negative, random biopsy specimens are harvested from areas that are difficult to visualize and those apparently normal tissue sites which are most frequently involved with cancer of the head and neck.

(These sites include the nasopharynx, the soft palate complex, the base of the tongue, and the pyriform sinus.) If negative, these "blind" biopsies should be repeated. Occult primaries are frequently located within the nasopharynx, an area that is difficult to examine. In addition, nasopharyngeal lesions have the propensity to be responsible for node involvement disproportionate to the apparently insignificant size of the primary lesion. Distant primary lesions (such as lung or kidney) may also manifest as cervical lymph nodes or other head and neck metastases.

Diagnoses established on the basis of exfoliative cytology (examination of cells scraped from the surface of a lesion) *must* be confirmed by biopsy. False-negative cytology results are not uncommon. Cytology, if selectively used and properly applied in conjunction with other techniques, can serve as a valuable initial screening modality, but is not an alternative to definitive diagnosis by histologic examination of biopsy specimens.

Histopathology

Microscopic evaluation of clinically abnormal areas of aerodigestive mucosa can reveal a wide range of histopathologic diagnoses (Fig. 9-10). Benign findings include parakeratosis, orthokeratosis, hyperkeratosis, acanthosis, pseudoepitheliomatous hyperplasia, and acute and chronic inflammation. These entities are usually reactive in nature and are characterized by cellular normalcy with some variation in tissue architecture (Fig. 9-11).

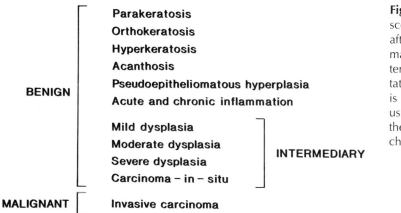

BENIGN
Parakeratosis
Orthokeratosis
Hyperkeratosis
Acanthosis
Pseudoepitheliomatous hyperplasia
Acute and chronic inflammation

INTERMEDIARY
Mild dysplasia
Moderate dysplasia
Severe dysplasia
Carcinoma – in – situ

MALIGNANT
Invasive carcinoma

Fig. 9-10 The range of microscopic diagnosis likely to be seen after biopsy is extensive. Findings may be benign, malignant, or intermediary. Although the interpretation of histopathologic changes is subjective, most pathologists usually concur on the nature of the changes, if not the degree of changes.

Fig. 9-11 Microscopic sections demonstrating (*A*) hyperkeratosis, (*B*) acanthosis, and (*C*) pseudoepitheliomatous hyperplasia. These benign changes are characterized by cellular normality with variation in tissue architecture.

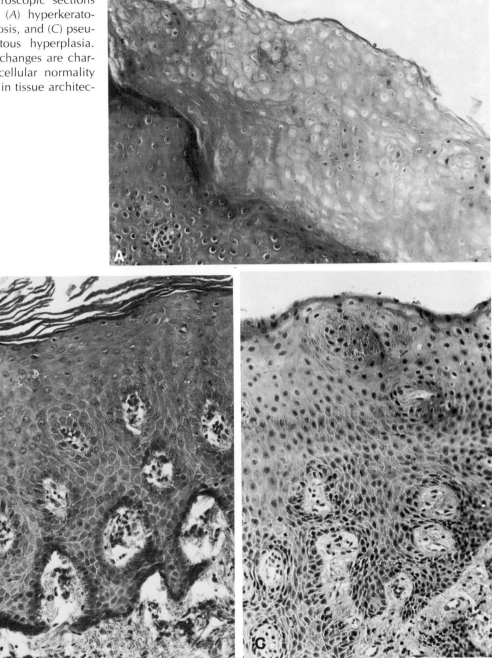

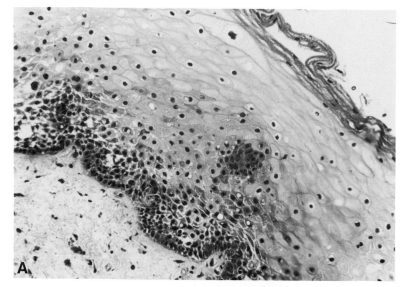

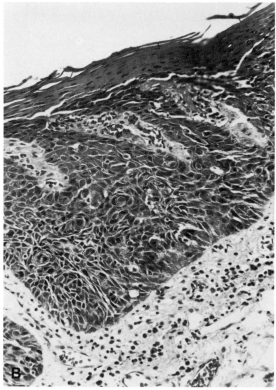

Fig. 9-12 Dysplasia is characterized by abnormalities in cell size and orientation, altered maturation, and bizarre, pleomorphic, hyperchromatic nuclei. Atypia may be (A) mild to (B) severe depending on what percentage of epithelium is abnormal.

Elimination of the responsible etiologic factors often permits resolution of the lesion. Benign lesions that do not resolve should be regularly re-evaluated or conservatively excised.

Dysplasia (atypia) is characterized by cellular abnormality involving only a portion of the epithelium. Changes seen in cellular atypia include variations in cell size, morphology, orientation, and alteration in the normal maturation sequence (Fig. 9-12). Dysplasia may be mild, moderate, or severe depending on the extent of the epithelium involved. Although a diagnosis of atypia is benign, increasing degrees of involvement indicate a greater probability of malignant progression.

When the cellular dysplasia involves the entire thickness of the epithelium, but is confined to the epithelium by an intact basement membrane, the diagnosis is carcinoma *in situ* (Fig. 9-13). Carcinoma *in situ* (Ca *in situ*) demonstrates all of the microscopic cellular changes seen in malignancy except invasion. Ca *in situ* usually does not have the capacity to metastasize. This diagnosis implies an increased potential for malignant transformation in the future or that the specimen may have been obtained immediately adjacent to an area of frank malignancy. When the diagnosis is severe atypia or Ca *in situ*, total excision of the lesion is indicated, and frequent repeated biopsy and microscopic evaluation are advisable.

Squamous cell carcinoma is characterized by cellular abnormality, the presence of abnormal cells throughout the entire thickness of the epithelium, and disruption of the basement membrane by nests or sheets of abnormal cells extending into the underlying connective tissue. Microscopic cellular changes consistent with carcinoma include variable cell size and orientation, disturbances in maturation, increased mitotic figures, altered nuclear size and shape, and hyperchromatism. The significance of squamous cell carcinoma in head and neck cancer cannot be overstated because more than 90% of all aerodigestive malignancies above the clavicles are squamous cell carcinomas.

The degree of differentiation, determined by how closely the lesion resembles normal

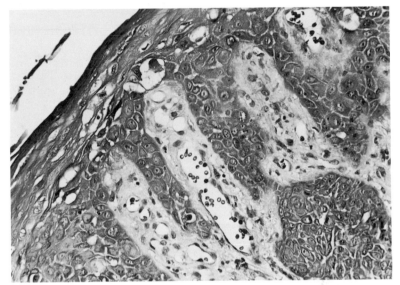

Fig. 9-13 Carcinoma *in situ* is characterized by cellular atypia involving the entire thickness of the epithelium; the basement membrane remains intact. Carcinoma *in situ* represents the most extreme tissue changes that can occur short of frank invasion. All areas of the specimen must be examined to detect small, local areas of invasion of the underlying mucosa that would change the diagnosis to invasive squamous cell carcinoma.

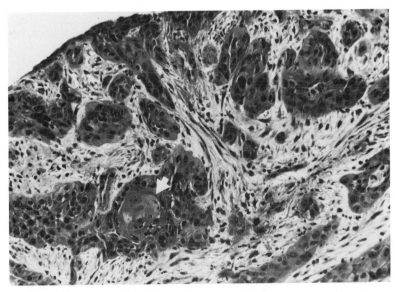

Fig. 9-14 Squamous cell carcinoma, which accounts for 90% of all head and neck cancers, is characterized by cellular abnormality, involvement of the entire thickness of the epithelium, and disruption of the basement membrane with invasion of abnormal cells into the connective tissue. The degree of differentiation depends on how closely the tumor resembles normal epithelium microscopically. Well-differentiated squamous cell carcinoma may form keratin localized in keratin pearls (*arrow*).

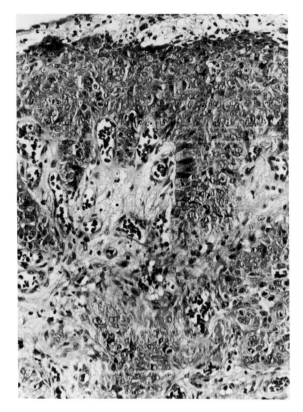

Fig. 9-15 Poorly differentiated squamous cell carcinoma is characterized by a lack of order or organization. Little resemblance to normal epithelium is apparent.

epithelium microscopically, is generally reported by the pathologist. Well-differentiated squamous cell carcinomas, like normal squamous epithelium, can form keratin. This occurs in characteristic nests of cells called keratin pearls (Fig. 9-14). Well-differentiated lesions approach normal tissue in their response to radiotherapy and are generally considered somewhat less aggressive, although the clinical behavior of individual lesions may not be distinguishable from less well-differentiated lesions. Poorly differentiated squamous cell carcinoma is seen microscopically as a totally disorganized mass of bizarre, frankly abnormal cells with little order or uniformity (Fig. 9-15). Although these tumors are generally more aggressive, they are also considered to be relatively more radioresponsive. To some extent, the degree of differentiation correlates with the aggressiveness and probable relative radiosensitivity of the tumor.

Evidence shows that the degree of inflammatory reaction seen microscopically in response to the tumor may have prognostic significance. The implication is that the host immune mechanisms are partially capable of recognizing malignant cellular differences and can participate to some degree in control of the tumor.

OTHER AERODIGESTIVE CANCERS

Occasionally, squamous cell carcinoma assumes a papillary configuration in which the lesion is mostly exophytic. This entity is termed *verrucous carcinoma* (Fig. 9-16). Ulceration is relatively uncommon, and extensive invasion usually does not occur until late in the course of the disease. Verrucous carcinoma has an apparent predilection for the buccal mucosa and a reported tendency to become more aggressive in response to radiotherapy.

Basal cell carcinoma, an insidious, locally destructive cutaneous cancer that usually does not metastasize, is also encountered in the head and neck region with moderate frequency. The exposed areas of the scalp and face are most frequently involved, and sensitivity to actinic radiation is considered the major etiologic factor. Typically, these lesions are detected late and appear as persistent indurated skin ulcers with rolled margins (Fig. 9-17). Early lesions may present as pearly gray nodules with flaking and fine surface telangectasis. These lesions may be easily detected by the dentist examining exposed susceptible areas of the skin of the head and neck. Small lesions can be treated successfully by surgery, irradiation, topical chemotherapy, or cryosurgery; large lesions may be extremely disfiguring and resistant to treatment. Basal cell carcinomas have a tendency to recur or manifest second primaries; therefore, frequent re-examination of patients with a history of basal cell carcinoma is mandatory.

Melanoma, an extremely aggressive cutaneous pigmented cancer may be detected in the skin of the head and neck region, intra-

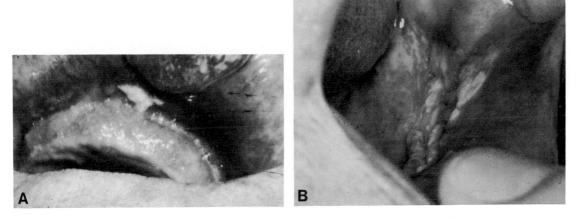

Fig. 9-16 Verrucous carcinoma tends to be slower growing and less aggressive. Lesions are most common on the buccal mucosa. Verrucous carcinoma has a predilection for becoming more aggressive in response to radiation therapy. *A,* Verrucous carcinoma of the maxillary labial frenum. *B,* Verrucous carcinoma of the buccal mucosa. (Photos courtesy of Keith Kent, D.M.D.)

orally as a primary lesion, or as distant metastases from another part of the body (Fig. 9-18). Primary skin lesions initially present with variations in the color, outline, and height of pigmented skin lesions. Induration may occasionally be present. Satellite lesions (local cutaneous metastases) are common. Melanoma is disseminated by both hematogenous (blood-borne) and lymphatic routes. The prognosis of patients with malignant melanoma is usually extremely unfavorable, unless the diagnosis is made early when the lesion is less than 0.76 mm in depth and aggressive treatment is initiated immediately. Intraoral melanoma is very rare and has a much worse prognosis than melanoma of the skin. It is usually detected as a pigmented mucosal lesion that has recently undergone a change in character. Intraoral melanoma is most frequently reported as occurring in the maxilla. Treatment usually consists of radical resection.

DISSEMINATION OF SQUAMOUS CELL CARCINOMA

Dissemination of squamous cell carcinoma occurs by direct extension of the primary tumor into adjacent tissues and by lymphatic metastases in the early and middle stages of the disease. Involvement of the cervical lymph nodes generally follows an orderly and predictable course dependent on the location of the primary tumor (Fig. 9-19). The ipsilateral submandibular, jugulodigastric, and deep cervical nodes usually become involved first with eventual spread to other nodes. Occasionally, contralateral or bilateral nodal involvement may be seen earlier than expected, especially with lesions of midline structures (*e.g.,* the base of the tongue or soft palate). Rarely, metastatic spread will skip expected node groups, and the disease may initially become evident in noncontiguous cervical nodes. In such cases, it is imperative to re-evaluate for the existence of a second primary lesion.

Oral cancers that have advanced through adjacent tissues to involve the overlying skin have a poor prognosis. Skin involvement is usually associated with insidious, diffuse metastases through the dermal lymphatics. The extent of dermal lymphatic spread is often difficult to assess and impossible to control, even when the primary lesion is successfully managed.

Generalized dissemination of head and neck cancer to bone and other organs is the result of hematogenous spread. This typically occurs with sarcomas or only in the later stages of aerodigestive cancer after the re-

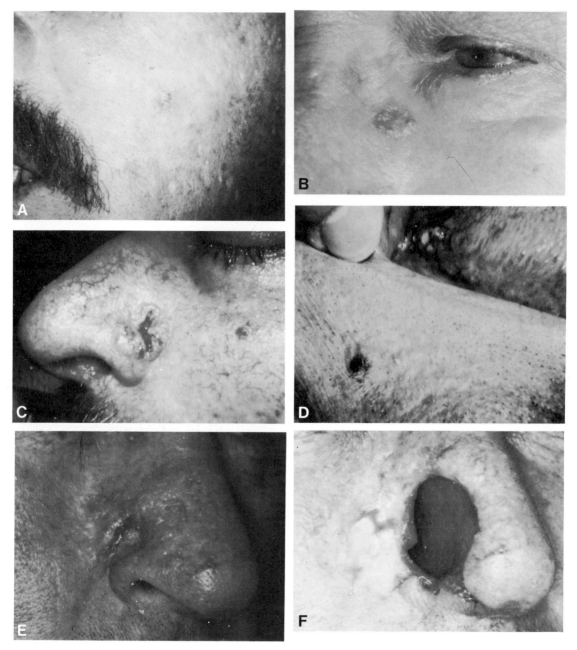

Fig. 9-17 (continued)

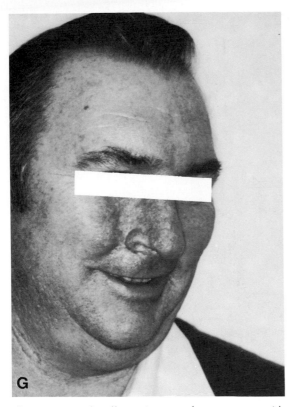

Fig. 9-17 Basal cell carcinoma often presents with rolled margins; exposed areas of the face and scalp are most frequently involved. Basal cell carcinomas of the skin of (A) the cheek, (B) the lateral aspect of the nose, (C) ala of the nose, (D) the lower lip with a synchronous squamous cell carcinoma of the lateral border of the tongue, (E) the nasolabial fold (large, recurrent lesion) before treatment, (F) following surgical resection, and (G) following prosthetic reconstruction. (Photos A, C, and D courtesy of Keith Kent, D.M.D.)

gional lymph nodes are already involved. The documentation of the presence of widely disseminated disease is most frequently a postmortem finding because most oral cancer patients die as a result of failure to control the primary lesion or cervical node disease, before distant metastases appear. The occurrence of an early oral primary lesion with evidence of bone or organ metastases implies that the oral lesion is probably not the only primary tumor. The likelihood of a synchronous second primary cancer site such as the

esophagus or lung is great (approximately 15%). The evaluation of all cancer patients before and after therapy should include an aggressive search for additional primary lesions.

Lesions of the soft palate prove particularly difficult to control and require inclusion of wide margins in the treatment specimen because of a tendency for submucosal involvement of apparently normal adjacent tissues. Microscopic examination of specimens obtained from the soft palate at some distance from a known primary palatal lesion are often positive for microscopic disease. The terms *field cancerization* or *condemned mucosa* have been applied to describe this phenomenon or cases in which multiple aerodigestive primary lesions occur synchronously.

EVALUATION OF THE PATIENT WITH BIOPSY-PROVEN DISEASE

Once the diagnosis of oral cancer is established by biopsy, a comprehensive evaluation of the patient is indicated to assure that appropriate and adequate therapeutic measures are applied. These procedures are generally well standardized, although individual institutions or practitioners may vary the format.

The patient is admitted to the hospital, and a complete history and physical examination are performed. Routine radiographic and laboratory studies are obtained. Additional studies such as renal or pulmonary function tests are completed to evaluate the patient's ability to withstand organ toxicity associated with some therapies, especially if chemotherapy protocols are anticipated.

Depending on the nature and extent of the disease, radionuclide scans may be obtained. Technetium-99 phosphonates taken up in areas of active bone metabolism can indicate bone involvement before lytic lesions become evident on routine radiographs. Complete skeletal scans may be obtained to rule out generalized metastases, although these would be unexpected in cases without established cervical involvement. On positive scans, "hot spots" define areas of increased

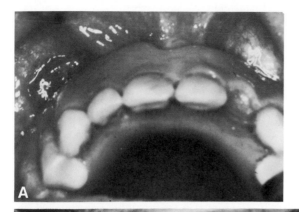

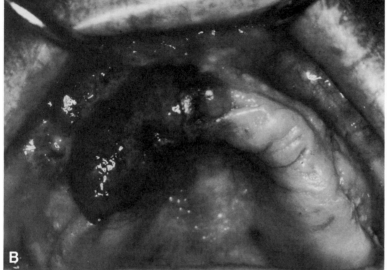

Fig. 9-18 Melanoma is an extremely aggressive pigmented epithelial cancer that may arise intraorally. The prognosis of cases of intraoral melanoma is very poor. Dental prostheses must always be removed during examination to detect the existence and extent of oral lesions.

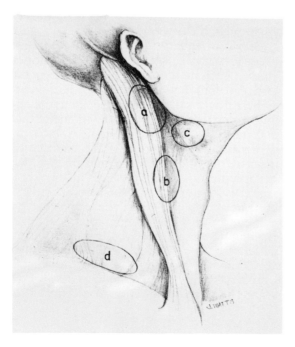

Fig. 9-19 Squamous cell carcinomas in particular primary sites frequently metastasize to specific node groups. Tumors of the base of the tongue and tonsillar pillar usually involve the jugulodigastric nodes(a). Tumors of the tonsillar pillar, tongue, larynx, hypopharynx, and sinus often involve the deep cervical nodes(b). Tumors of the floor of the mouth, posterolateral tongue, and soft palate frequently involve the submandibular nodes(c). Supraclavicular or lower deep cervical nodes may be involved in carcinoma originating below the clavicles(d). Knowledge of typical metastatic patterns can often indicate the most likely sites for the primary tumor.

bone deposition that may be the result of reaction to tumor invasion. Routine radiographs are obtained to evaluate areas of increased activity. False-positive scans can result from chronic sinusitis, acute and chronic dental disease, degenerative joint disease, and recent or old trauma, rather than tumor.

A liver-spleen scan may be obtained to evaluate the presence of metastatic organ involvement, especially if liver function tests are abnormal. Metastatic organ involvement, like generalized bone metastases, would be unlikely in the absence of obvious cervical nodes. Positive skeletal findings or organ involvement without established neck disease are suggestive of a primary cancer not of the head and neck region in addition to the known oral lesion.

Patients with carcinoma of the hypopharynx, supraglottic or subglottic regions, or esophagus are generally evaluated by barium swallow radiographs and laryngotomography or computerized axial tomography (CT scan). Patients with accessible oral lesions would probably not undergo these special studies unless the physical examination or symptoms suggested a second primary lesion. CT scan can be used to accurately determine the extent of deep tumor invasion into adjacent tissues.

The most important diagnostic procedure performed for all patients with head and neck cancer is panendoscopy. Panendoscopic evaluation includes deep hypopharyngeal palpation and direct visualization of the hypopharynx, larynx, trachea, mainstem bronchi, and esophagus. Both rigid and flexible instrumentation is available to facilitate examination of these areas. Indirect mirror examination or fibroscopic examination of the nasopharynx should be included. Panendoscopy can be performed under general anesthesia or topical anesthesia and sedation. The procedure is not without risks, and morbidity can be significant. The objectives of panendoscopy, however, are critical to proper patient evaluation and include accurate staging of the tumor; evaluation and biopsy of mucosal lesions in areas not accessible for direct examination or instrumentation; search for additional, synchronous (present at the same time) primary tumors; and evaluation of the

response to treatment and assessment of the status of residual, recurrent, or new metachronous (separated in time) primary disease. Accurate staging is defined by the following hierarchy.

TNM CLASSIFICATION—ORAL CAVITY

T—Size of primary tumor
- T0—No evidence of primary tumor
- Tis—Carcinoma *in situ*
- T1—Primary tumor $\leq$ 2 cm
- T2—Primary tumor > 2 cm and $\leq$ 4 cm
- T3—Primary tumor > 4 cm
- T4—Primary tumor > 4 cm with invasion of deep structures or skin

N—Node (cervical) metastases
- N0—No clinically positive nodes
- N1—Single homolateral node $\leq$ 3 cm
- N2a—Single homolateral node $\geq$ 3 cm but > 6 cm
- N2b—Multiple homolateral nodes all < 6 cm
- N3a—Homolateral node(s), at least one > 6 cm
- N3b—Bilateral nodes
- N3c—Contralateral nodes only

M—Distant metastases
- M0—No known metastases
- M1—Distant metastases present

STAGING

- Stage I—T1 N0 M0
- Stage II—T2 N0 M0
- Stage III—T3 N0 M0; any T1, 2 or 3, N1, M0
- Stage IV— T4, any N, M0;
  any T, N2 or N3, M0;
  any T, any N, M1

Consultations are obtained from all of the various services that may contribute to the patient's care, including surgery, radiation therapy, chemotherapy, dental service, dietetics, psychiatry, speech therapy, social services, rehabilitation medicine, and a member of the clergy. The active participation of these specialists results in a coordinated, comprehensive, orderly treatment sequence for the individual patient and his particular needs.

The Team Approach

One of the most important factors in the successful management of cancer patients is the use of a team approach to diagnosis, treatment planning, control of the disease, rehabilitation, and follow-up. The concept of a single professional without support treating the cancer patient should be relegated to history. The optimal cancer treatment team should be composed of a variety of health care specialists, including professional, paraprofessional, and lay representatives. The specific composition of each team will vary at different treatment centers and will often be determined by the specific disease under treatment.

MEMBERS OF THE ONCOLOGY TEAM

- Surgeons
- Radiation therapists
- Physicists
- Hematology oncologists
- Dentists
- Speech pathologists
- Social workers
- Nurses
- Psychologists
- Psychiatrists
- Physical therapists
- Physiatrists
- Occupational therapists
- Enterostomal therapists
- Pharmacists
- Clergy
- Patients
- Patients' family

Excellent communication between members of the treatment team is absolutely essential to all phases of successful cancer patient management. Iatrogenic treatment failures can often be attributed to lack of early recognition or diagnosis, inadequate treatment coordination, poor follow-up mechanisms, and most unfortunately, communications breakdown.

The Role of Dentist on the Treatment Team

The dentist should be an active member of every oncology team, especially teams responsible for managing patients with oral cancer. The dentist can play an integral role in all phases of treatment from detection to follow-up. Without the active participation of a dentist, an oral cancer team is limited in its ability to deliver comprehensive care to its patients.

Dentists are often the first professionals consulted for oral complaints, so they frequently have the earliest opportunity to discover malignant lesions when the chances for successful management are best. Because his professional interest and expertise focus around the oral cavity, the dentist can often detect asymptomatic or innocuous lesions, easily overlooked by other professionals, that may prove to be early cancers. The dentist may also provide a reliable clinical diagnosis for many oral lesions, distinguishing normal anatomy from benign or malignant pathosis (Fig. 9-20). Evaluation of suspected lesions can be accomplished after the dentist has eradicated all extraneous sources of irritation, trauma, and inflammation.

Dental pretreatment planning recommendations can contribute to successful cancer management by decreasing or controlling associated morbidity. Intraoral complications related to the tumor, unfavorable oral treatment sequelae, and symptomatic oral conditions are usually best managed by the dentist, who is the team member most familiar with oral physiology and pathophysiology. Definitive management of the tumor and reduced morbidity can frequently be facilitated by individually designed and fabricated dental prostheses (Fig. 9-21). Dental intervention and support can often be critical to the control of associated treatment morbidity and rehabilitation of the patient following cancer treatment therapy (Fig. 9-22).

The prime objective of every cancer treatment team should be the total eradication of the disease and the restoration of the patient to a viable position in society. Treatment of head and neck cancer may lead to severe cosmetic and functional deformities or may be associated with significant morbidity secondary to unfavorable sequelae. A cure is not achieved until adequate restoration of dysfunction and deformity are established and adverse treatment sequelae are controlled (Fig. 9-23). The specially trained dentist is

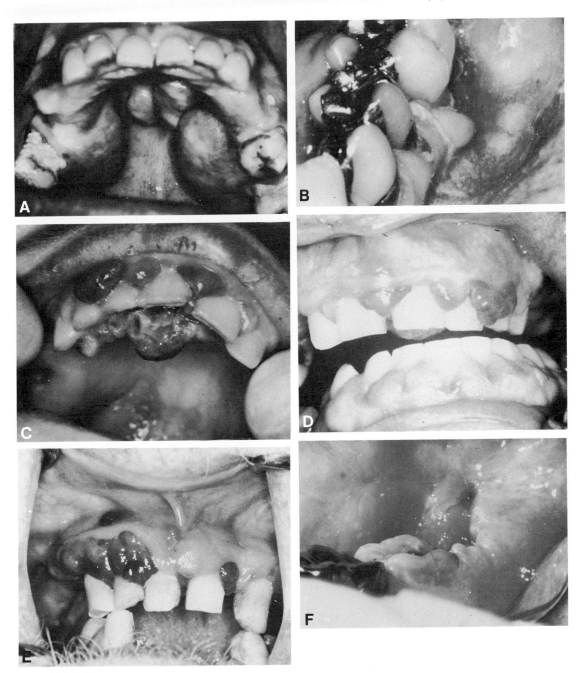

Fig. 9-20 The dentist may often be consulted to provide differential diagnoses of lesions such as (A) palatal tori and exostoses, (B) invasive squamous cell carcinoma misdiagnosed originally as trauma from a toothbrush, (C) focal necrosis superimposed on leukemic infiltrate, (D) leukemic infiltrate occurring synchronously with Dilantin hyperplasia, (E) leukemic infiltrate misdiagnosed as periodontal disease, and (F) an extraction site failing to heal because of the presence of invasive squamous cell carcinoma.

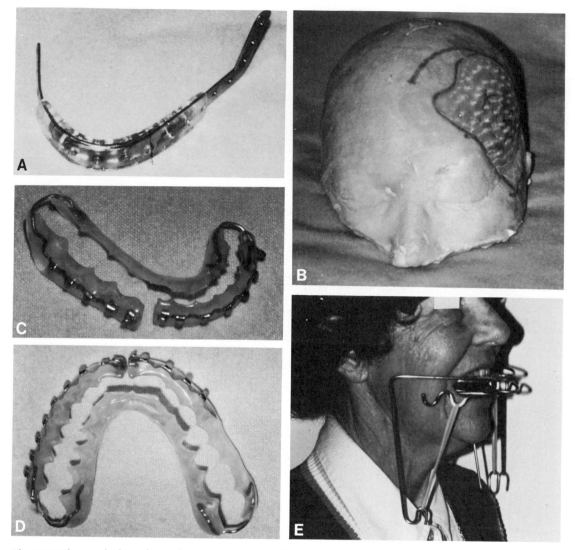

Fig. 9-21 The morbidity of oncologic treatment may be reduced by cooperative participation on the treatment team. Special prostheses may be fabricated to facilitate reconstruction following ablative surgery such as (*A*) mandibular implant to restore discontinuity secondary to a segmental mandibulectomy and (*B*) cranial implant for use following a craniotomy. Stents such as (*C*) maxillary and (*D*) mandibular labiolingual removable arch bars may facilitate intermaxillary fixation to minimize the severity of the medial and inferior rotation of the mandible secondary to scar contracture and fibrosis following mandibular resection. A dynamic bite opener (*E*) facilitates exercise and physiotherapy to overcome trismus.

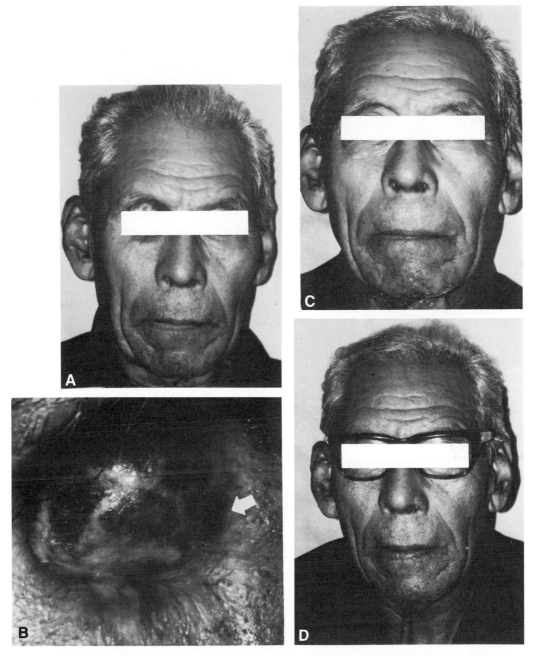

Fig. 9-22 Surgical resection often results in both cosmetic and functional deformity. Orbital exenteration (*A*) may compromise the ethmoid sinuses. (*B*) (*arrow*) Facial reconstruction (*C*) provides adequate cosmesis as well as sealing the perforation of the sinuses. Eyeglasses (*D*) are often useful to mask margins of the prosthesis as well as to correct vision.

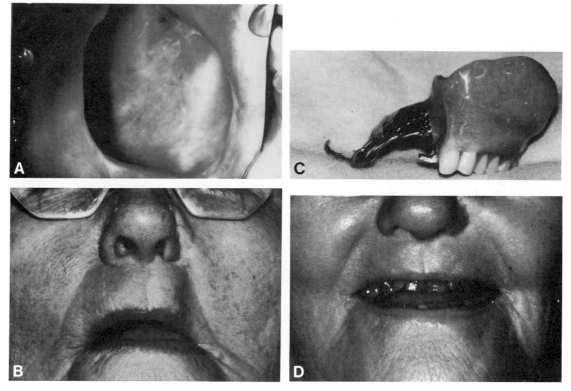

Fig. 9-23 A total maxillectomy (*A*) often results in an oroantral communication causing residual hypernasality of speech, nasal reflux, compromised occlusion, and facial deformity (*B*). A prosthetic obturator (*C*) may be designed to replace missing anatomic structures and restore adequate cosmesis by restoring facial contours (*D*).

often the team member most qualified to supervise the nonsurgical management and restoration of orofacial defects. Correction of cosmetic deformity, communication disorders, inadequate nutrition, sensory impairments, altered responses to infection or irritation, as well as protection of oral tissues can be provided. With proper training, orientation, and cooperation, the dentist should be an indispensable member of the cancer treatment team and can contribute significantly to the successful management of the patient.

Dental Evaluation

A thorough pretreatment dental evaluation is indicated for every patient with head and neck cancer. This evaluation should be initiated and com- *pleted as soon as possible after the diagnosis of cancer is established but before presentation to the hospital's tumor board.*

The dental evaluation should be comprehensive and systematic. A review of the medical, social, and dental histories should be documented and an assessment of the medical risk for dental treatment established. A thorough review and interpretation of records of previous surgery or radiation therapy is essential. The results of ongoing medical evaluations, special tests, and laboratory studies should be assessed and recorded. Special precautions necessary for elective or emergency dental care should be determined.

A leisurely initial evaluation of the patient's adaptability and capacity for maintenance of meticulous oral hygiene is often im-

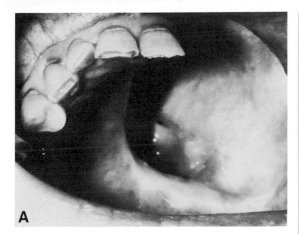

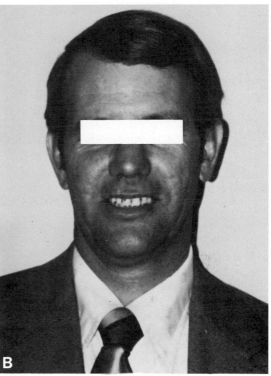

Fig. 9-24 Preservation of key abutment structures, adequate preparation of the surgical defect including control of the location of the cicatrix resulting from placement of skin grafts, and careful technique to minimize scarring and deformity can result in return of the patient to a viable role in society. *A,* Retentive scar on lateral border of maxillectomy defect. *B,* Minimal facial scar at columella.

possible because of time constraints. Frequently, definitive cancer therapy and dental treatment must be initiated as soon as possible, often before extensive preventive dental education or hygiene instruction can be completed; therefore, patient compliance and tolerance must be determined on the basis of the presenting dental condition and the prior dental and social histories. A comprehensive initial patient interview can often provide a reliable psychological assessment of the patient and can aid in the formulation of a prediction of the patient's tolerance for and probable response to dental treatment.

The preservation of sound, healthy teeth should be encouraged. The traditional premise that all teeth must be removed before definitive treatment of oral cancer by radiotherapy is no longer tenable. In certain cases, aggressive application of oral hygiene maintenance techniques and control of dental decay can minimize the incidence and severity of associated complications. Coordination of surgical and prosthodontic efforts can result in the retention of abutment and bearing

structures that may eventually be essential to successful reconstructive and rehabilitative efforts. The preservation of abutment teeth provides improved masticatory efficiency, facilitates nutritional support, and can be a positive factor in the patient's self-image.

Dental records should include articulated intraoral study casts. Extraoral diagnostic study casts, or moulages, are often very useful. Intraoral and extraoral photographs or color transparencies should be obtained. Pretreatment dental and facial color shades, patterns, and profiles should also be recorded. Dental charting and diagrams should be completed as indicated.

Appropriate dental radiographs, including a panoramic dental radiograph, must be obtained. Periapical radiographs of all clinically or radiographically suspected areas of dental pathosis and potential abutment teeth should be evaluated. Specific attention should be directed to areas of osteolysis, periodontal or periapical pathoses, retained roots, irregular osseous contours, temporomandibular joint abnormalities, antral defects or inclusions, and sialoliths. Additional radiographs, such as occlusal views (for anterior floor of mouth lesions) and sialograms (for salivary gland tumors), may be indicated to accurately assess tumor extent and possible osseous involvement. The dental examination should include a thorough intraoral and extraoral inspection using direct and indirect visualization of all hard and soft tissues of the oral cavity, perioral structures, the oropharynx, and the hypopharynx. Bimanual palpation of accessible regions including the neck should be performed to detect tissue masses and irregularities.

Periodontal evaluation should include a determination of the tissue color and consistency, bleeding score index, plaque index, periodontal pocket depth, zones of attached tissue, tooth mobility, amounts of calculus, furcation involvements, and other defects. The patient's current level of oral hygiene maintenance, a key factor in determining dental treatment recommendations, must be assessed. Tissue changes as a result of previous treatment should be recorded. Evidence of prior periodontal or endodontic surgery therapy may be indicative of a high level of dental awareness or suggestive of a history of chronic neglect with periods of intermittent aggressive intervention. Areas of gingival recession require close scrutiny. Large amounts of exposed root surfaces or cementum, particularly in areas of the dental furcations, may also indicate overly aggressive attempts at hygiene, but are difficult for the patient to maintain and are especially susceptible to decay. Unfavorable dental architecture and periodontal defects that are inaccessible and difficult or impossible to cleanse must be eliminated.

Endodontic evaluation should not be overlooked. Tenderness to percussion, thermal sensitivity, and abnormal electrical pulpal responses should be noted. Existing or incipient pulpal and periapical pathosis should be treated. These areas have been shown to serve as a source of infection or reservoir for bacteria in the immunosuppressed patient. Endodontic emergencies during treatment, which can usually be easily avoided, may cause unnecessary distress or life-threatening danger to the patient and may compromise successful cancer therapy.

The restorative evaluation must be thorough. The patient's caries, plaque, periodontal bleeding score, and DMF (decayed, missing, filled) indices can serve as reasonably effective indicators of dental awareness and compliance. All incipient and existing carious lesions must be detected and treated as rapidly as possible. Existing dental restorations must be closely scrutinized for adequacy and integrity. All restorations should be carefully evaluated to detect marginal leakage and contours unfavorable to adequate hygiene maintenance.

Examination of the temporomandibular joint complex can be informative. Treatment procedures such as hemimandibulectomy or radiation therapy may exacerbate existing subclinical, pathologic conditions (including crepitus, clicking, and deviation on movement). Existing or potential speech abnormalities should be assessed by the dentist in cooperation with the speech pathologist. Existing or anticipated abnormalities in mastication, deglutition, or oral function that may result from treatment must be considered and corrective measures planned. Rehabilitative treatment may include physiotherapy or fabrication of special stents and speech and swallowing aids.

Prosthodontic examination should include an assessment of all potential prosthetic-bearing and retentive regions. Areas of tissue undercuts, alveolar irregularities, bony prominences, unfavorable muscle attachments, and hypermobile tissues should be noted and corrected, when possible, at an appropriate time in the treatment sequence. Existing removable prostheses must be stable, retentive, nonirritating, atraumatic, and cleansible. Poorly fitting prostheses should be revised or removed. Oral surgical intervention and preprosthetic tissue preparation, which may facilitate subsequent reconstruction and rehabilitation, must be closely correlated with the comprehensive cancer treatment program. Uncoordinated scheduling of oral surgical procedures may cause significant treatment delays or complications in treatment of the tumor.

Teeth with a limited or unfavorable prognosis should be extracted. Simultaneous alveolectomy to allow primary wound closure and eliminate sharp, irregular osseous contours should be performed. Necessary pre-prosthetic surgery should be expeditiously performed. Efforts must be directed to prevent the need for subsequent surgical intervention in regions that are to be irradiated. Extractions and indicated preprosthetic surgical procedures should be performed in advance of radiotherapy if a slight delay will not adversely affect the prognosis. Radiation treatment can begin once mucosal integrity is re-established (usually within 2 to 4 weeks). If a delay in the start of radiotherapy is not feasible, the indicated surgery should be deferred until after the completion of the radiotherapy when the severe phase of radiation-induced mucositis has resolved. The 6-week period following radiation therapy, which is characterized by mucosal inflammatory and reparative processes, has been termed the *golden period*. Surgical intervention usually can be safely completed before the end of this interval, before significant tissue fibrosis, endarteritis, and periosteal degeneration are manifested.

Osteoradionecrosis, discussed more fully in Chapter 13, is a progressive refractory infection and necrosis of the bone secondary to radiation-induced vascular changes that can follow minor trauma and elective or emergency surgical procedures completed more than 6 weeks after radiotherapy. Osteoradionecrosis may also result if radiotherapy is initiated prior to adequate soft tissue repair after surgery or if surgery is performed within the treatment fields during the course of radiation. Tissues undergoing rapid initial reparative processes are especially susceptible to the lethal effects of irradiation. Once the golden period has transpired, endodontic therapy or conservative symptomatic management of dental pathoses are preferable to surgical management. One of the primary objectives of the initial dental evaluation is to eliminate the need for oral surgery, and to reduce the likelihood of mucosal trauma, which may occur during and after radiotherapy.

The definitive dental treatment plan should be reviewed by the entire cancer treatment team. Alternative dental treatment plans should be formulated to correlate with the requirements of all possible alternative cancer treatment modalities. Immediate den-

tal intervention should be instituted unless it will cause intolerable delays or jeopardize the overall success of the cancer therapy. If possible, the dentition and oral structures should be restored to optimal states in order to negate the potential risks of unexpected surgical intervention or posttreatment dental complications.

Tumor Board

Once the preceding evaluations have been completed and the findings correlated, the patient is presented at the tumor board, or its equivalent. The tumor board generally consists of representatives from each of the major specialties involved in the management of head and neck cancer patients. The functions of the tumor board are as follows:

1. To ensure the most accurate assessment of each patient's disease and to determine the therapeutic options
2. To provide a forum for discussion of the available treatment options and their particular applicability to the specific patient
3. To provide a forum for the correlation of treatment results
4. To provide a mechanism for the selection of patients for assignment to approved experimental treatment protocols
5. To provide instruction in the principles of management of head and neck cancer patients for students, interns, and residents

The recommendations of the tumor board are formulated after the patient is re-examined by each of the members of the diagnostic, treatment, and rehabilitative teams and the available treatment options are discussed. The recommendations are then presented to the patient, who should participate actively in the final decision on the type and extent of treatment he will receive. While the findings of the tumor board are not binding, the recommendations, which are based on the combined expertise of the members, are usually followed closely. Appropriate treatment can then be administered.

The development and acceptance of a comprehensive treatment plan before initiation of definitive therapy is a requisite to successful treatment. Unilateral alterations in treatment delivery, modality, sequence, or extent, especially after treatment has been initiated, should be discouraged, except in the most unusual emergency situations.

TREATMENT MODALITIES

General Considerations

The treatment of head and neck cancer is continuously undergoing change and modification; new advances are being made daily at cancer treatment centers throughout the world. As a result of aggressive research endeavors and rapid technologic advances, many new treatment modalities have evolved and are under investigation. During the past 10 years, dramatic improvements in treatment capabilities have lead to greater success, enhanced survival and life expectancy, and decreased morbidity in the management of head and neck cancer.

Cancer treatment modalities are of four basic types: surgery, radiation therapy, chemotherapy, and combined therapy. Early stages of disease can often be successfully treated with single modes of therapy. The complete eradication of more advanced disease often depends on combinations of surgery and radiotherapy. The use of aggressive chemotherapy for the treatment of oral cancer is still in experimental stages. Adjunctive chemotherapy is often used for late, extensive lesions where the prognosis is severely limited, regardless of treatment.

Surgery

The surgical treatment of oral cancer as a primary modality is ablative in nature. All clinical disease must be excised with an adequate margin of adjacent normal tissue. The excision of a wide margin of uninvolved tissue in all dimensions about the tumor is necessary to ensure that residual elements of microscopic disease do not remain within the surgical field. When clinical metastases to cervical nodes have occurred or microscopic metastases are probable or suspected, the management of the cervical lymphatic system must be included to ensure adequate therapy.

The extent of surgery performed depends on the extent of disease determined to be present. Localized lesions without apparent or suspected cervical lymphatic involvement can generally be managed by wide local excision. The technique preferred for tumor removal is "en bloc" resection, which involves removal of the entire surgical specimen consisting of the tumor and an adequate margin of surrounding tissue in continuity as one intact specimen, without incision through involved tissues.

Localized lesions with suspected or proven cervical lymphatic involvement require wide resection of the primary tumor in continuity with dissection of the involved neck. The standard radical neck dissection involves excision of the cervical lymphatic system and removal of the sternocleidomastoid and omohyoid muscles, the internal and external jugular veins, the accessory nerve (causing shoulder drop), the submandibular gland, and the inferior pole of the parotid gland. More conservative and accepted variations of the radical neck dissection include preservation of the accessory nerve, sternocleidomastoid muscle, and the internal jugular vein. These modified procedures are usually performed when only microscopic cervical involvement is suspected or when the cervical lymphatics are clinically negative and are treated prophylactically in high-risk cases. From a physiologic standpoint, radical neck dissection is a relatively benign procedure and although extensive, is generally well tolerated by most patients.

Large, deeply infiltrating primary lesions with neck involvement mandate a composite resection or "commando" procedure, which includes en bloc resection of the primary tumor with the involved adjacent osseous structures (usually a portion of the mandible) and a total radical neck dissection.

Debulking procedures, or the deliberate, subtotal removal of nonresectable cancers provides palliation of acute symptoms and can be justified on the basis of relief of pain, control of infection, or alleviation of airway obstruction. Although the benefits of palliative surgery are only temporary, these procedures can improve the quality of life for the terminal patient.

Surgical resection of even the smallest malignant intraoral lesion must be relatively extensive because of the need for adequate margins and can result in moderate deformity and debility. The need to acquire surgical access and achieve adequate excision of advanced lesions can result in extreme deformity and severe disability, often involving structures that are critical for communication, nutrition, or social interaction. Acceptable cosmetic and functional reconstruction of anticipated surgical defects can be facilitated by coordinated pretreatment planning and can be achieved postoperatively by combined surgical, prosthetic, and rehabilitative efforts (Fig. 9-24).

Surgical intervention, although apparently destructive, offers certain advantages over other treatment modalities. Immediate microscopic examination of the surgical margins can be performed during surgery by means of frozen section techniques to ensure the adequacy of the excision. Comprehensive postoperative review of permanent sections of the surgical specimens allows additional evaluation of the adequacy of treatment procedures. Surgical defects can often be simply and satisfactorily revised using primary or secondary reconstructive procedures.

The surgical management of cancer permits additional therapeutic intervention if necessitated by the discovery of residual, recurrent, or new primary disease. Adjunctive surgery can also be used in combination with other principal treatment modalities. Bulky tumors, often poorly vascularized, can be surgically reduced prior to primary radiotherapy, which is more effective on well-oxygenated tissue. Surgery can also be used in the management of many of the unfavorable sequelae that frequently accompany other treatment modalities, such as reconstruction of mandibular discontinuity following composite therapy or debridement of osteoradionecrosis following radiotherapy.

Radiation Therapy

Radiation therapy is being used with increasing frequency as a primary treatment modality in the management of oral malignancies. Generally used in the treatment of early,

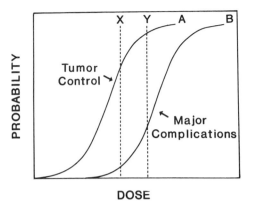

Fig. 9-25 Radiation therapy dosage is determined as that amount that will have a maximal tumoricidal effect while minimizing major complications. Sigmoid curves representing tumoricidal effect (A) and major injury to normal tissues (B). At a given dose (X) tumor control may be achieved with a high probability and minimal major complications. At a given dose (Y), a higher probability of tumor control is achieved with a more significant incidence of major complications.

well-vascularized lesions, radiotherapy is also effective in eradicating small foci of malignant cells present in very early lesions, peripheral to a large lesion, or associated with early cervical lymphatic metastases. Tumor regression is usually complete, often with negligible residual deformity, following the use of properly administered radiotherapy.

Although radiotherapy has been used successfully in the treatment of malignancies for many years, rapid developments in medical radiotherapy instrumentation and technology have resulted from recent research in military and civilian applications for nuclear energy. Advanced equipment and new therapeutic techniques are finding application in the treatment of oral cancer.

Radiotherapy uses either high-energy electromagnetic radiation (x-rays and gamma rays) or high-energy particulate matter to disrupt the reproductive ability of malignant cells. Ionizing radiation causes cell death (absence of clonogenic viability) by disrupting intracellular DNA configuration and function by cleaving the double-strand DNA molecule. Radiation sensitivity is cell-cycle depen-

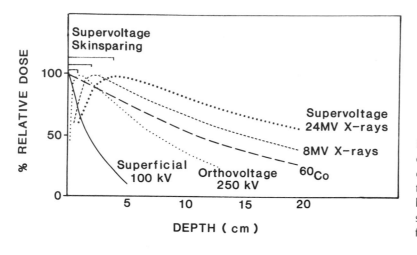

Fig. 9-26 Dose curves for different types of ionizing radiation at comparative depths demonstrate that greater depth of penetration by higher energy radiation results in a greater skin-sparing effect.

dent and oxygen dependent. Cells have the capacity to repair sublethal injury. Cells in reproductive phases or tissues composed of cells with rapid life cycles are likely to be more radiosensitive; however, clinical response may differ from tissue culture sensitivity. Normal tissue and tumor respond to radiation in varying degree. The normal tissue response accounts for the associated treatment morbidity (Fig. 9-25).

Radiation-induced abnormalities of DNA structure can lead to cell injury or death or disruption of reproductive capabilities or have no discernible effect at all. Normal cells, which are susceptible to the same radiation changes, can, in addition, undergo malignant transformation. An increased incidence of malignancies has been documented in populations following occupational, military, or therapeutic exposure to varying levels of radiation. Protective precautions should be observed wherever ionizing radiation is used.

Radiotherapy can be administered in different forms. External beam (radiation originating from a source outside the body) techniques are most frequently used in the treatment of oral cancer. Gamma rays are a product of the decay of a radioactive material such as ^{60}Co. Radiation can also be generated by accelerating particulate matter across a high-energy differential (voltage) and directing the particles against a heavy-metal target to produce x-rays. The diagnostic dental x-ray machine uses a peak, variable kilovoltage potential (Kev), while current radiotherapy

devices, such as linear accelerators, use a variable megavoltage potential (Mev). Other particulate matter, such as neutrons and *pi* mesons accelerated in a cyclotron, can be used for therapeutic irradiation of tissues. The higher the energy of the radiation used, the greater will be the penetration of the tissue, with less damage to the overlying structures (skin-sparing effect) (Fig. 9-26).

A course of therapeutic radiation is fractionated into multiple, small daily doses called *fractions*. Total dose, fraction size, and elapsed time from initiation to completion of therapy are prescribed to induce a maximal tumoricidal effect while minimizing normal cellular and tissue response. Repair of sublethal injury in normal cells usually occurs within 4 hours of each daily fraction. Fractionated radiotherapy is administered over the course of many treatment sessions and requires significant patient cooperation. Interruptions in therapy either from patient noncompliance or because of the severity of radiation side effects can compromise the result.

External beam radiotherapy is often delivered in daily divided doses of 180 rad to 250 rad, five times per week. The total treatment dose administered for oral cancer generally ranges from 4,500 rad to 7,500 rad (45 Gy to 75 Gy) depending on the purpose and nature of the irradiation, the location and type of tumor, and the technique used. The use of multiple portals (irradiation of the tumor from different directions) and fractionated doses is calculated to maximize tumor damage while minimizing adverse effects on normal tissues.

Adjuncts to external beam radiotherapy include brachytherapy and the use of radioactive implants. Brachytherapy, or intracavitary radiation therapy, involves the application of the radioactive source, contained in a custom-fabricated carrier device, directly to the surface of the tumor. Brachytherapy is most effective in treating small tumors on or close to the surface. The radioactive material can also be implanted directly within the tumor and adjacent tissues. Intracavitary and direct implantation radiotherapy are often used in conjunction with external beam irradiation to boost or increase the dose of radiation delivered to a localized area of tumor involvement beyond that which could be safely delivered by a single modality. The dentist is frequently requested to fabricate special positioners and locators used to accurately and rapidly position the radioactive material in a stable and immobile, predetermined position (Fig. 9-27).

Radiation therapy can be used to treat cancer patients who are poor risks for anesthesia or surgery or where the tumor is surgically inaccessible. Judicious application of radiation delivered to a large volume of tissue to eradicate microscopic foci of disease can result in minimal effect on normal tissue. While radiation generally produces a smaller defect than does ablative surgery, the effects can cause normal tissue damage. The damage to both tumor and normal tissue is dose related: the higher the dose, the greater the tissue response. Radiotherapy is generally most effective when the tumor is well vascularized and well oxygenated.

The oral mucosa is particularly responsive to radiation injury because the cell life cycle and turnover rate are relatively rapid. This susceptibility is manifested as mucositis, tissue fragility, and fibrosis. Injury to serous salivary acini results in qualitative and quantitative changes in saliva characterized by increased pH, increased viscosity, and diminished flow. The superimposition of xerostomia on damaged mucosa can produce severe symptomatology.

The unfavorable effects of radiation on healthy tissue account for the major complications and morbidity associated with therapy. Unlike surgical complications, which are immediately evident, permanent, and nonprogressive, the complications associated with radiotherapy can be immediate and temporary or gradual in onset and relentlessly progressive in nature. The list of radiotherapeutic complications associated with the treatment of oral cancer is extensive.

RADIATION-INDUCED CHANGES IN THE ORAL CAVITY

- Fibrosis of the musculature
- Fibrosis of connective tissues
- Trismus
- Capillary fragility and friability
- Decreased vascular elasticity
- Decreased vascular permeability
- Telangiectasia
- Tissue fragility and friability
- Decreased repair potential
- Susceptibility to soft tissue necrosis
- Susceptibility to osteoradionecrosis
- Increased susceptibility to caries
- Mucositis
- Susceptibility to infection
- Salivary changes (increased acidity; increased immunoproteins; increased lysozymes; increased numbers of *Streptococcus mutans*, lactobacilli, actinomycoses, and fungi; decreased quantity; increased proportion of mucoid component; decreased proportion of serous component (increase in thickness and ropiness)

Radiotherapy is also associated with an extremely poor retreatment potential. Tissues irradiated with tumoricidal doses often cannot tolerate additional treatment with therapeutic radiation. The healing of irradiated tissues following surgery for the management of residual recurrent or new primary disease is variable, depends on dose and host response to prior radiation, and is generally unfavorable.

Radiation therapy is often used as an adjunctive treatment modality. Preoperative radiation delivered before definitive surgical treatment can be used to decrease tumor bulk and facilitate subsequent surgery; however,

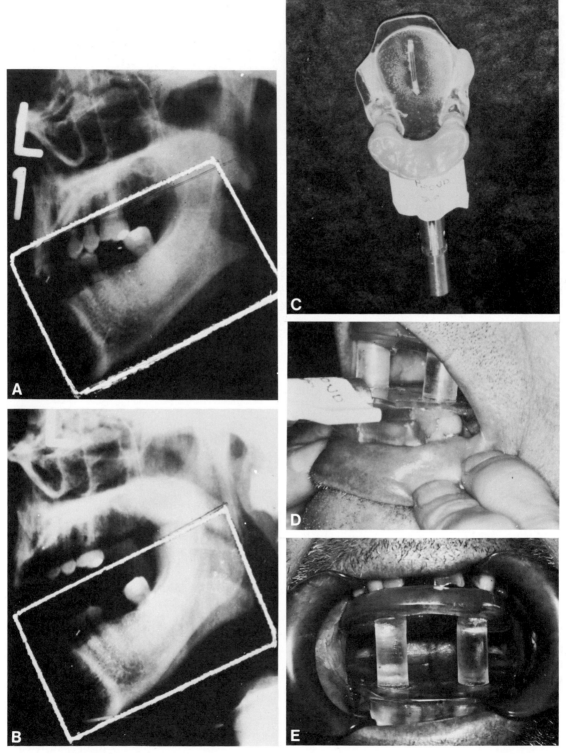

Fig. 9-27 (continued)

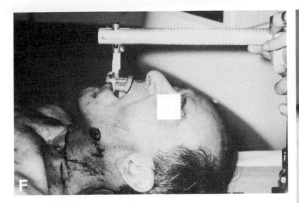

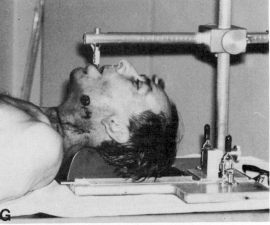

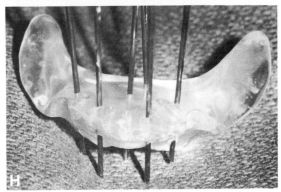

Fig. 9-27 Specially fabricated dental prostheses may be used to displace adjacent structures out of the treatment field. *A,* Treatment field includes the inferior aspect of the maxilla when the teeth are in maximal intercuspation. *B,* The same treatment field does not include the maxilla if the mandible is positioned properly. *C, D, E,* The intraoral component of a specially fabricated positioner. *F* and *G,* The extraoral component of the positioner is adaptable, rigid, indexed to allow accurate and rapid repositioning of the patient, and comfortable. Special prostheses (*H*) are also used to position radioactive implants.

a favorable clinical response to preoperative radiotherapy does not allow the extent of the surgical resection to be decreased. Tumors that were initially nonresectable do not become resectable when response to radiotherapy is favorable. Preoperative radiotherapy can also be used to sterilize islands of microscopic cancer that may be present in tissues adjacent to the tumor. This minimizes the risk of inadvertent implantation or seeding of tumor cells into healthy tissues during surgery.

Alternatively, postoperative radiotherapy can be used to ensure that microscopic disease is not left at the margins of the surgical resection. Postoperative radiotherapy can also be used prophylactically when gross clinical metastases to the regional lymph nodes are absent but subclinical or micro-

Fig. 9-28 Most squamous cell carcinomas of the lower lip occur halfway between the midline and the commissure. Patients often attribute lesions of the lip to chronic irritation or cold sores. Lip lesions should be detectable in their early stages because of their prominent, visible location.

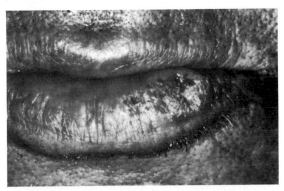

scopic metastases are suspected or likely. Radiation therapy has been demonstrated to prevent neck node recurrence when the primary is controlled.

Chemotherapy

Chemotherapy has demonstrated only minimal effectiveness in the management of oral squamous cell carcinoma. Current chemotherapy regimens produce only temporary or partial tumor regression and are rarely used as the primary treatment modality for oral cancer. Substantial progress is being achieved using adjunctive chemotherapy on an experimental basis in combination with primary radiotherapy and surgery. In addition, chemotherapy can be used for palliation when treatment for cure is not possible. Chemotherapeutic debulking of the tumor can result in greater patient comfort and improved function, at least temporarily.

Chemotherapeutic effect depends on selective cellular toxicity with tumor cells having greater susceptibility than normal cells. Most agents affect an enzyme or substrate related to DNA synthesis or function, resulting in disruption of the DNA strand configuration or strand cross-linking. Cells undergoing active DNA synthesis or replication are selectively inhibited or adversely altered. Chemotherapeutic agents currently used in the treatment of oral cancer include methotrexate, adriamycin, bleomycin, cis-platinum, vincristine, and hydroxyurea.

The morbidity associated with chemotherapy is high. Adverse effects include bone marrow suppression, immunosuppression, stomatitis, gastrointestinal toxicity, alopecia, renal failure, hepatic dysfunction, and pulmonary fibrosis. Most chemotherapeutic agents are metabolized by the liver and excreted by the kidney. Renal or hepatic dysfunction drastically decreases the patient's tolerance for aggressive therapy, and morbidity and mortality are increased. High levels of chemotherapeutic agents may also be concentrated and secreted by the salivary glands, resulting in excessive intraoral levels. This can compound an existing oral mucositis and further impair the patient's ability to maintain adequate nutritional intake and oral hygiene.

Alternate Therapies

Cryosurgery and hyperthermia are infrequently used as primary treatment measures in the management of oral cancer. Cryosurgery, which involves the removal of heat from the tissues by application of a cryogen (liquid nitrogen), produces cell death from protein denaturation, disruption of cell membranes and organelles, and enzyme release as a result of multiple freeze–thaw cycles. Although cell and tissue death are controllable and certain, cryosurgery offers little advantage over surgery or radiotherapy in the management of most lesions. Cryosurgery is most frequently used for the control of early lesions in debilitated patients or for palliation of nonresectable lesions in patients unsuitable for surgical or radiotherapeutic debulking procedures. Hyperthermia may be used in conjunction with chemotherapy or radiotherapy to increase the tumoricidal effect. Great care must be exercised when selecting patients for alternative treatment modalities to ensure that conventional management would not be more effective or appropriate.

SITE-SPECIFIC BEHAVIOR OF HEAD AND NECK CANCER

Squamous cell carcinoma of the aerodigestive mucosa is essentially a unified disease process that can develop in any number of diverse primary sites within the head and neck region. The incidence of clinical tumors in each of these sites depends on a host of multiple factors, as yet poorly understood. Most primary head and neck cancers demonstrate relatively consistent site-specific behavior patterns that reflect tumor size, symtoms, frequency of metastases, and probable responses to treatment. A knowledge of the site-specific characteristics of the more common head and neck lesions can contribute significantly to improved patient management.

The floor of the mouth is the most common site for intraoral squamous cell carcinoma. The degree of infiltration apparent at the initial presentation of lesions of the floor of the mouth may be deceptive because invasion of the tongue and mandibular periosteum occur frequently but may be difficult to assess clinically. Metastases generally appear in the middle stages of the disease and tend to be ipsilateral. The treatment of early lesions can often be accomplished by surgery or radiotherapy with comparable results. Late lesions require radical combinations of surgery and radiotherapy.

Lesions of the soft palate complex frequently develop contralateral or bilateral node metastases. "Clean" (disease-free) surgical margins are often difficult to achieve because the malignant changes usually extend well beyond the clinical lesion. Radiotherapy is often indicated as the primary treatment modality for soft palate tumors because of the difficulty of achieving disease-free surgical margins and because surgery may often produce a greater degree of functional deformity.

Cancers of the anterolateral and posterolateral tongue, when symptomatic, present with localized pain as the initial clinical symptom. Ipsilateral node metastases are more likely with anterior lesions, but the tendency for bilateral node metastases is increased as the lesions occur more posteriorly. In a similar fashion, the prognosis becomes more grave as more posteriorly located lesions are detected because of the tendency for later detection and greater access to regional lymphatics.

Squamous cell carcinoma of the lips is rare in black patients. Most lesions of the lower lip occur halfway between the midline and the commissure (Fig. 9-28), usually metastasize late, and can be managed by radiotherapy or surgery with essentially equal results. An increase in the incidence of metastases and a more unfavorable prognosis are seen with lesions at or near the commissure. Lesions of the maxillary lip occur nearer the midline, tend to be more aggressive, and metastasize earlier and bilaterally. A history of primary herpes simplex may be a predisposing factor in the etiology of cancers of the lip (Fig. 9-29).

Lesions at the base of the tongue are generally advanced when detected. Voice changes secondary to immobility of the tongue and referred ipsilateral ear pain are common but occur late in the disease. Involvement of the vallecula and epiglottis are

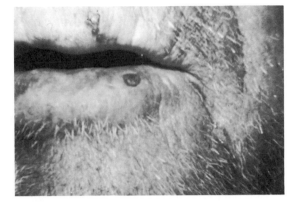

Fig. 9-29 A history of herpes simplex may be a predisposing factor in the etiology of cancers of the lip. Squamous cell carcinomas of the lip are demonstrated at sites of prior herpetic lesions. (Photo courtesy of Keith Kent, D.M.D.)

frequent and may result in aspiration and severe swallowing problems. Node metastases are often bilateral or contralateral. Treatment usually consists of major ablative surgery, radiotherapy, or both, and the prognosis is generally unfavorable.

Lesions of the pyriform sinus are particularly insidious because this area is essentially "silent"; diagnostically significant symptoms are infrequent. A sore throat and pain on swallowing may result when adjacent structures are invaded, but the diagnosis is usually established only after cervical nodes are apparent. The prognosis and response to treatment are not encouraging.

Squamous cell carcinoma of the intrinsic larynx has a relatively favorable prognosis because small lesions produce voice changes and persistent hoarseness, which facilitate earlier detection. Neck node metastasis is rare in early vocal cord lesions because the true vocal cord has no lymphatic drainage. Radiotherapy is often preferred for early lesions because the voice can be preserved. Late lesions can be managed reasonably well in many cases by a combination of radiotherapy and total laryngectomy, but the voice is permanently lost, and some means of artifical speech must be adopted.

Tumors of the esophagus have a very poor prognosis. These lesions tend to be detected only very late in the course of the disease

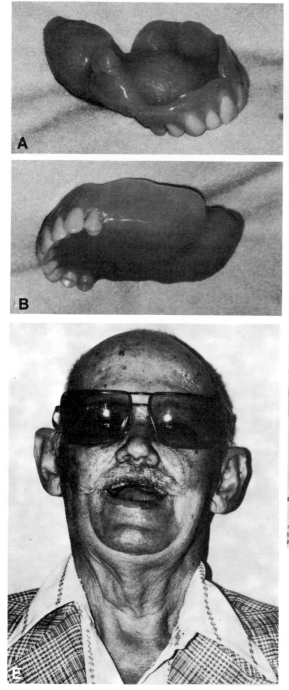

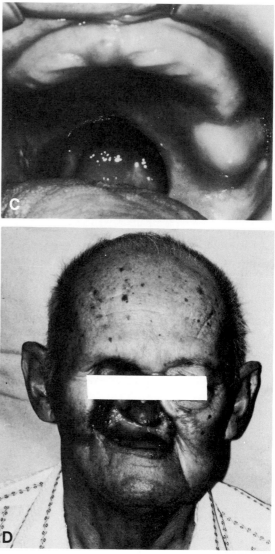

Fig. 9-30 The dentist often provides a significant contribution to the rehabilitation of the cancer patient, including intraoral reconstruction with a combined obturator (*A*), and palatal drop (*B*) to restore hard and soft palate defects (*C*) and compensate for limited tongue motion secondary to neurologic deficit. Combined intraoral–extraoral prostheses can adequately restore a patient with a large defect (*D*) to a functional role in society (*E*).

because the tumor must become sizable before symptoms are evident. "Sticking" of solid foods, then difficulty with liquids, and finally, total blockage of oral intake are common. Weight loss may be extensive. The proximity and early involvement of the mediastinal nodes adversely affect the prognosis. Survival rates are extremely poor despite the most aggressive treatment regimens.

DENTAL MANAGEMENT OF UNFAVORABLE TREATMENT SEQUELAE

All of the therapeutic modalities currently applied in the management of head and neck cancer produce adverse treatment sequelae that are often manifested in the oral cavity.

ORAL MANIFESTATIONS OF ADVERSE TREATMENT SEQUELAE

- Abnormal speech
- Masticatory inadequacy
- Impaired deglutition
- Dysphagia
- Altered salivary flow
- Altered appearance—disfigurement
- Altered response to normal flora
- Altered response to irritation
- Altered response to infection
- Restriction of normal movement
- Mandibular deviation
- Velopharyngeal incompetence (hypernasality; nasal reflux)
- Oroantral communication
- Alteration in sensory perception
- Anesthesia, paresthesia, or sensitivity
- Inability to care for self
- Fear
- Depression
- Edema
- Impaired lymphatic drainage
- Fibrosis
- Trismus
- Necrosis
- Mucositis
- Vascular stenosis
- Vascular fragility
- Petechiae
- Hemorrhage
- Caries susceptibility
- Oral incompetence
- Microstomia
- Desquamation

Many of these symptomatic and debilitating conditions can occur during the course of therapy and can compromise successful treatment by causing delays or interruptions. Unfavorable treatment sequelae can also occur following therapy and can be as debilitating or destructive as the original tumor. Most of these complications can be predicted or anticipated; many can be prevented, controlled, or minimized. Aggressive dental support facilitates the completion of therapy without compromise or interruption and can significantly reduce patient discomfort and disability following therapy.

Ablative surgery can produce anatomic deformitites or sensory deficiencies that may severely impair the patient's ability to function normally. In all cases, patients should be realistically advised preoperatively regarding the nature and extent of the complications that are anticipated following surgery. The patient should be reassured and informed of successful methods of overcoming the anticipated deformity. Oral hygiene instruction and dental education should be supplemented when indicated by instruction in modified patterns of eating and swallowing, as well as alternative methods of communication. Speech therapy may include the technique of substitution for difficult-to-form sounds or electrolaryngeal and esophageal speech. Immediate surgical and postsurgical prostheses designed by the specially trained dentist can be used to restore surgically created anatomic or neurologic deficiencies. Improvements in speech, mastication, swallowing, and cosmetic rehabilitation can be accomplished through the coordinated efforts of the dentist and other members of the oncologic treatment team (Fig. 9-30).

The oral mucosa can be adversely affected by both radiotherapy and chemotherapy. Mucositis and an increased susceptibility to infection and injury are common mucosal reactions (Fig. 9-31). Severe oral discomfort can lead to inadequate nutritional intake and weight loss. In many treatment centers, tumoricidal therapy is usually interrupted if the

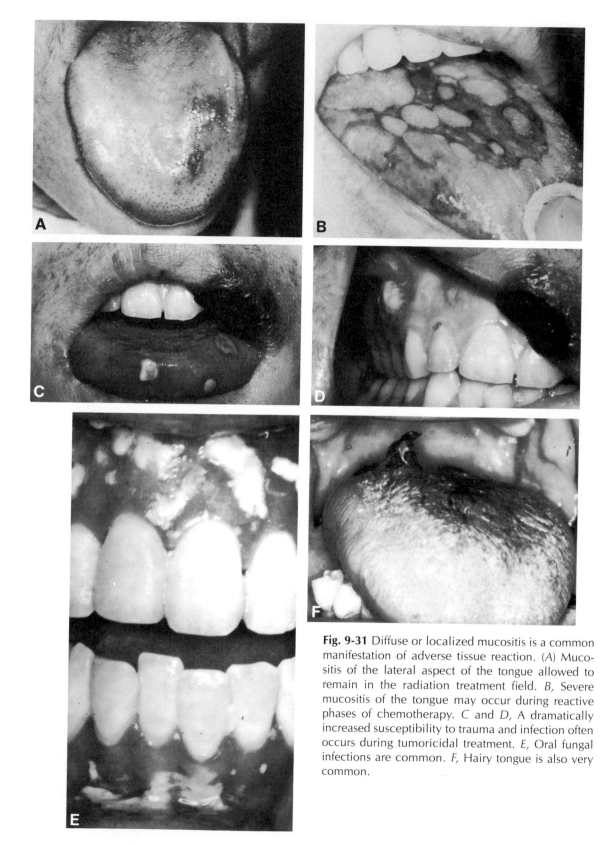

Fig. 9-31 Diffuse or localized mucositis is a common manifestation of adverse tissue reaction. (*A*) Mucositis of the lateral aspect of the tongue allowed to remain in the radiation treatment field. *B*, Severe mucositis of the tongue may occur during reactive phases of chemotherapy. *C* and *D*, A dramatically increased susceptibility to trauma and infection often occurs during tumoricidal treatment. *E*, Oral fungal infections are common. *F*, Hairy tongue is also very common.

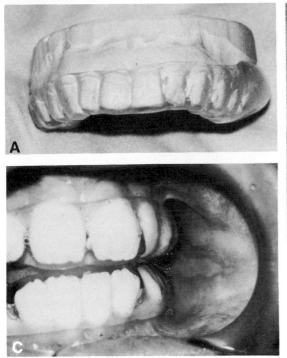

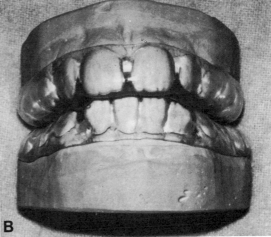

Fig. 9-32 Soft mouthguards may be used to protect or displace friable mucosa from chronic irritation.

patient's normal body weight is decreased by more than 10%. Delays imposed to allow the mucositis to abate and to permit recovery of body weight critically diminish the effectiveness of the tumor treatments. Dental support in the form of oral hygiene instruction and symtomatic relief of acute conditions can significantly reduce the severity of the mucositis and increase the patient's tolerance for the indicated tumoricidal therapy.

Some degree of mucositis in response to cancer therapy is unavoidable and should be controlled by maintaining tissue hydration systemically and topically. Adequate fluid intake, frequent intraoral rinses, and the use of a room humidifier should be encouraged. Because the inflamed mucosa is more susceptible to bacterial and fungal infections, improved oral hygiene and the use of topical and systemic antimicrobial agents guided by frequent culture and sensitivity testing of the infective organisms can reduce the incidence and severity of secondary infections. Patient comfort can also be improved by judicious use of topical anesthetics, steroids, and protective coating agents.

TOPICAL AGENTS FOR ORAL USE

- Artificial saliva
- Water
- Normal saline (buffered)
- Nystatin oral suspension
- Nystatin suppositories
- Hydrogen peroxide (0.25% to 3%)
- Viscous xylocaine
- Kaopectate and Benadryl
- Cellulose base topical dressings
- Hemostatic agents
- Topical fluorides and others

Oral rinses and frequent irrigations with buffered normal saline (one teaspoonful of baking soda per quart of saline solution) should be encouraged. The use of artificial saliva may temporarily relieve xerostomia. Intraoral rinses with effervescent hydrogen peroxide can be used to debride inaccessible areas and provide topical oxygenation to injured or irritated soft tissues. Concentrations should range from 0.25% to 1.5% as determined by individual patient needs and tolerance. Special oral hygiene aids are readily available to assist the patient who is unable to tolerate or adequately manipulate a tooth-brush or dental floss.

Emphasis should be placed on minimizing trauma to the teeth, supporting structures, and oral mucosa. Patients should be encour-aged to discontinue or significantly reduce noxious habits. Tobacco and alcohol abuse, ingestion of spicy or hot foods, continued use of poorly fitting prostheses, and other sources of irritation should be eliminated. Special prostheses may be individually de-signed and fabricated to protect the soft tis-sues, such as the tongue and buccal mucosa, from habitual trauma (Fig. 9-32).

Commercial mouthwashes and breath fresheners are frequently self-administered by cancer patients to cleanse the oral cavity, mask fetor oris, and temporarily provide a sense of fresh taste. Unfortunately, most commercial products contain alcohol, pre-servatives, fixatives (phenol), and caustic fla-voring agents (citric acid or citrates). Patients should be cautioned against the use of these irritants, which can severely aggravate an ex-isting oral mucositis.

The serous acinar cells of the major and minor salivary glands are especially suscep-tible to radiation-induced injury. Radiother-apy produces quantitative and qualitative changes in saliva. Salivary flow is dimin-ished, the consistency becomes thick and ro-pey, and the pH is significantly decreased. The lubricating and cleansing capacity of the saliva is severely affected. An existing mu-cositis can be further aggravated, and masti-cation and swallowing are often severely im-paired. Salivary changes drastically increase the patient's susceptibility to dental decay be-cause acidic salivary pH provides an excellent environment for the proliferation of cari-ogenic bacteria and contributes to gradual de-mineralization of the teeth. A dramatic in-crease in cervical, incisal, and line-angle caries is often noted (Fig. 9-33). Restorative materials should be selected with considera-tion for the altered intraoral environment. Impression materials containing eugenol should be avoided because of the increased propensity to cause mucosal chemical burns. The use of acid-soluble restorative materials such as silicates and many composites is con-traindicated. Amalgam is the material of

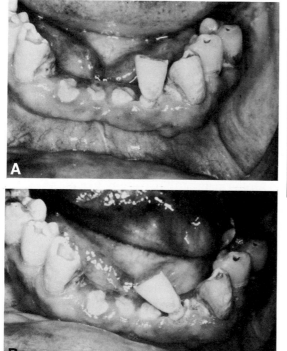

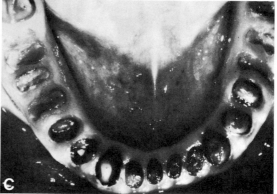

Fig. 9-33 Alteration in salivary quality and quantity leads to an increased susceptibility to caries, espe-cially of cervical areas, incisal edges, and line an-gles. Amputation of clinical crowns often results. Residual roots within the boundaries of prior radia-tion treatment fields must be avoided.

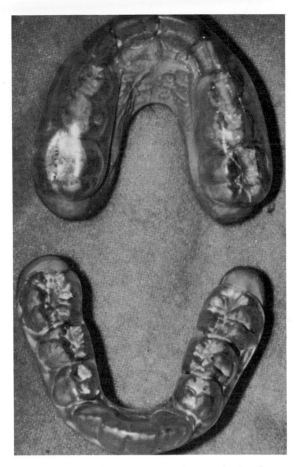

Fig. 9-34 Fluoride carriers or other methods of providing daily topical application of fluoride are necessary for all patients with increased caries susceptibility.

choice for most intracoronal restorations. Meticulous oral hygiene, control of plaque and calculus formation, and the avoidance of a cariogenic diet must be reinforced.

Topical fluorides should be applied to the remaining tooth surfaces on a daily basis for the rest of the irradiated patient's life. Sodium fluoride is available in neutral pH preparations and is most effective when applied in a custom-fabricated carrier (Fig. 9-34). A nonaqueous 0.4% stannous fluoride, which has an acid pH, can be effectively self-applied with a toothbrush. Attention to meticulous daily home care and topical fluoride application should never be discontinued because the changes in the oral flora, salivary consis-

tency, and pH are usually progressive and permanent. Fluorides should be applied after debridement of plaque and debris to ensure maximum contact with susceptible surfaces. Accidental or intentional ingestion of the fluorides should be avoided. Nausea and vomiting may indicate systemic fluoride toxicity, which can be fatal. Milk is a specific antidote to toxic levels of fluoride.

Necrosis of oral structures can follow all forms of cancer therapy and can result in as much deformity and disability as the original tumor. Necrosis of tissue occurs secondary to a loss or deficiency of the blood supply to a localized area and may be difficult to control. The vascular impairment can be attributed to generalized tissue fibrosis and scaring, fibrosis of the intimal layer of the blood vessels with a loss of vascular elasticity and permeability, tissue tension producing anoxia of distal areas, or an altered autoimmune response. Following radiotherapy, efforts to preserve teeth, avoid acute and chronic mucosal injury, and maintain oral hygiene are directed to prevent or minimize the need for elective or emergent surgical intervention so that the risk of osteoradionecrosis may be avoided (Fig. 9-35)

FOLLOW-UP EVALUATION

The management of patients with head and neck cancer does not end when the patient is discharged from the hospital. Many patients will require additional surgical and prosthodontic reconstructive procedures, physical therapy, rehabilitation training including speech and swallowing instructions, occupational therapy, and psychiatric and social counselling. Following definitive cancer treatment, the use of these services is often essential to the restoration of the patient to a viable role in society.

The single most important function of subsequent follow-up care is the continual, periodic re-evaluation of the patient's status relative to cancer. The detection of residual, recurrent, metastatic, or new primary disease at an early stage requires regular, intensive re-examination. Each clinical manifestation of subsequent malignant disease is an unfavorable occurrence, and retreatment success rates are much lower than are initial treatment rates. Early discovery and appropriate treatment offer the patient the best opportunity for successful management.

Residual disease represents original tumor that persists following the initial cancer treatment and is usually manifested clinically within 1 to 6 months after definitive therapy. Residual lesions occur at the original tumor site or in adjacent regions and are likely the result of inadequate or incomplete tumor ablation.

Recurrent disease is cancer that develops at or adjacent to the original primary tumor site, but only after an interval of time sufficient to indicate that it is probably a regrowth rather than persistence of the tumor. Recurrent cancer generally becomes clinically evident 6 months or more following completion of definitive therapy. In some cases, the distinction between residual and recurrent tumors is difficult to establish, essentially academic, and of little clinical significance.

The appearance of cervical or generalized metastases following treatment represents failure of the initial therapeutic efforts to adequately control the disease process. Subsequent metastatic involvement may also reflect either an inadequate initial evaluation or the clinical appearance of previously undetected disseminated microscopic disease. Definitive treatment of metastatic disease should be initiated when the metatases become clinically evident.

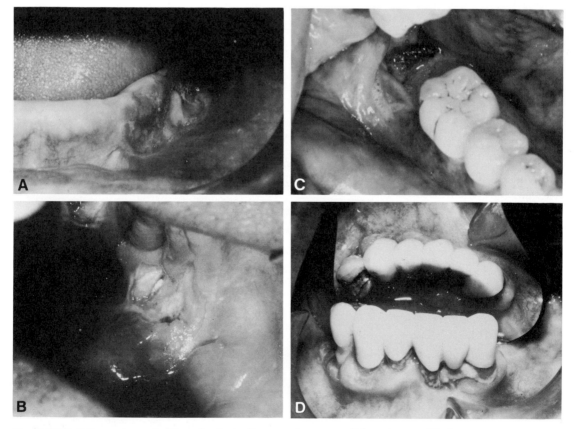

Fig. 9-35 Soft tissue necrosis (A) and osteoradionecrosis can result from trauma (B), inappropriate extraction of teeth (mandibular third molar) that were in a previously irradiated area (C), or traumatic manipulation of tissues during routine dental procedures (D).

Patients with a previous head and neck primary cancer are at significantly increased risk of developing additional, distinctly separate primary tumors, and therefore should be thoroughly and frequently re-evaluated. The interval of time between the occurrence of two or more primary cancers has significant prognostic value. When the lesions occur simultaneously or within a short time, the prognosis is severely limited. As the interval between the development of separate primary lesions increases, patient survival following treatment of the second primary appears to increase. Greater host participation in tumor resistance on an immunologic basis may contribute to improved patient survival.

Intensive initial follow-up is indicated for treated patients because residual, recurrent, cervical, or new primary diseases is most likely to become clinically apparent during the early posttreatment period. All head and neck cancer patients should be re-examined monthly for the first year following initial therapy. Evaluations should be completed every 2 months during the second year, then quarterly for the next year. Patients who remain free of disease are then seen every 6 months for 1 year and thereafter are re-examined annually. Patients who remain free of disease at 5 years are less likely to develop additional lesions but are still regularly evaluated for the remainder of their lives. Patients should be advised to contact the clinic for the next earliest appointment whenever significant problems arise between appointments.

The clinical manifestations of residual, recurrent, or metastatic disease are not unlike those that accompanied the original tumor. The detection of these lesions, however, may be more difficult because of alterations in anatomy and physiology that have resulted from the original cancer and previous treatment. Although a large number of diverse problems may follow treatment of the original lesion, mucosal abnormalities, progressive dysphagia, persistent cough, hoarseness or voice changes, and weight loss are significant. Weight loss is perhaps the most ominous. Inability to maintain body weight is an extremely reliable prognosticator of tumor regrowth or new aerodigestive cancer. Failure to thrive in the presence of adequate nutritional intake is strongly suggestive of tumor development and also indicates that the response to therapy is not likely to be very favorable.

At each follow-up visit, the patient's history, especially regarding the previous tumor and its treatment, should be ascertained. Careful inspection and palpation of all accessible mucosal surfaces are performed with attention to areas of abnormality, especially in high-risk sites or in previous primary tumor sites. Erythema, roughness, granularity, friability, and induration characterize high-risk lesions. Biopsy is indicated for areas of mucosal change that persists 2 weeks without obvious etiology. Additional testing such as barium swallow radiography or endoscopy is indicated to evaluate dysphagia, voice changes, hoarseness, or weight loss that persists without apparent cause.

Pain is generally not a prominent feature of residual, associated metastatic, or new primary cancer and is most commonly associated with surgical or radiotherapeutic complications. Assessment of these unfavorable treatment sequelae and corrective measures can be accomplished synchronously with the cancer re-evaluations.

Secondary surgical reconstructive procedures should be deferred for a minimum of 1 to 2 years following the initial cancer treatment if the patient is stable and adequate function and cosmesis can be obtained with a prosthesis. Evaluation for residual or recurrent disease is facilitated by maintaining the original tumor site inviolate and accessible for direct observation.

•　　　　　•　　　　　•

The dentist should be active in all phases of the treatment of patients with cancer. Aggressively applied combined modalities used in the management of carcinomas of the head and neck region often dramatically affect a patient's oral cavity with resulting severe functional and cosmetic deformity. The costs of current therapeutic techniques, including medical care provider time, patient disfigurement and dysfunction, financial expense, and treatment failures are prohibitive. The best currently available method of controlling treatment costs and morbidity is to treat the lesion at the earliest possible time.

Efforts to establish the cause of cancer of the aerodigestive tract are continuing. Only when a distinct cause is defined will cancer be preventable or curable. Until the specific etiology of cancer is clarified, research should emphasize early detection and patient education. The treatment of advanced lesions only offers most patients false hopes. The discovery and aggressive management of early lesions offers patients with oral cancer their only real chance for successful treatment.

BIBLIOGRAPHY

Ackerman LV, delRegato JA: Cancer Diagnosis, Treatment and Prognosis, 4th Ed. St Louis, CV Mosby, 1970

American Joint Committee for Cancer Staging and End-Results Reporting (AJC): Manual for Staging of Cancer 1978, pp 27–52. Chicago, AJC, 1978

Ansfield FJ, Ramirez G, Davis HL Jr et al: Treatment of advanced cancer of the head and neck. Cancer 25:78–82, 1970

Anderson R, Hoopes JE (eds): Symposium on Malignancies of the Head and Neck. Third Symposium on Cancer of the Head and Neck. St Louis, CV Mosby, 1975.

Aramany M, Drane JB: Radiation displacement prostheses for dentulous patients. J Prosthet Dent 27:212–216, 1972

Aramany M, Drane JB: Radiation protection prosthesis for edentulous patients. J Prosthet Dent 27:292–296, 1972

Ash CL: Oral cancer: A twenty-five year study. AJR 87:417–430, 1962

Baker HW: Staging of cancer of the head and neck: oral cavity, pharynx, larynx, and paranasal sinuses. Cancer 33:131, 1983

Bascom PW: Oral cancer and prosthodontics. J Prosthet Dent 19:164–173, 1968

Batsakis, JG: Tumors of the Head and Neck: Clinical and Pathologic Considerations. Baltimore, Williams & Wilkins, 1979

Berger DS, Fletcher GH, Lindberg RD et al: Elective irradiation of the neck lymphatics for squamous cell carcinomas of the nasopharynx and oropharynx. AJR 111:66–72, 1971

Bertino JR, Boston B, Capizzi RL: The role of chemotherapy in the management of cancer of the head and neck: A review. Cancer 36:752–758, 1975

Bertino JR, Mosher MB, DeConti RC: Chemotherapy of cancer of the head and neck. Cancer 31:1141–1149, 1973

Beumer J et al: Radiation complications in edentulous patients. J Prosthet Dent 36:193, 1976

Beumer J, Curtis TA, Firtell DN: Maxillofacial Rehabilitation, Prosthodontic and Surgical Considerations. St. Louis, CV Mosby, 1979

Beumer J, Silverman S, Benak S: Hard and soft tissue necrosis following radiation therapy for oral cancer. J Prosthet Dent 27:640–644, 1972

Bhaskar SN: Synopsis of oral pathology, 2nd Ed. St. Louis, CV Mosby, 1981

Bocca E, Pignataro O: A conservative technique in radical neck dissection. Ann Otol Rhinol Laryngol 76:975–987, 1967

Bodey GP, Buckley M, Sathe YS, Freireich EJ: Quantitative relationships between circulating leukocytes and infection in patients with acute leukemia. Ann Intern Med, 64:328, 1966

Borgelt BB, Davis LW: Combination chemotherapy and irradiation for head and neck cancer: A review. Cancer Clin Trials 1:49–59, 1978

Bosl GJ: Adjuvant chemotherapy in management of Stage III and Stage IV tumors of the head and neck. Cancer 33:139, 1983

Brooks JM, Fielding AF: Newest techniques, concepts and responsibilities of the dentist in treating diagnosed oral cancer patients. J DC Dent Soc pp 39–44, Summer, 1978

Bulbudian AH: Maxillofacial prosthetic: Evolution and practical application in patient rehabilitation. J Prosthet Dent 15:554, 1965

Burns HP, van Nostrand AWP, Bryce DP: Verrucous carcinoma of the larynx: Management by radiotherapy and surgery. Ann Otol Rhinol Laryngol 85:538–543, 1976

Byars LT, Lampe I: Radiation vs. radical surgical resection of tumors of the mouth, lips and tongue. Postgrad Med 22:591–602, 1957

Byers RM et al: Squamous carcinoma of the oral cavity: Choice of therapy. Curr Probl Cancer 65:27, 1981

Cancer, A Manual for Practioners. Boston, American Cancer Society, Massachusetts, 1978

Carl W: Oral and dental care for the irradiated patient. Quintessence Int 10, 1974

Carl W et al: Oral care of patients irradiated for cancer of head and neck. Cancer 30:448, 1972

Carl W et al: Radiotherapy and the dentist. Am J Roentgenol, Radiat Ther Nucl Med 120:1: 188, 1974

Carl W, Drinnan AJ: Dental management of cancer patients: Curricular implications. J Dent Educ 38:11: 642, 1974

Carl W, Schaaf NG: Dental care for the cancer patient. J Surg Oncol 6:293, 1974

Carter SK: The chemotherapy of head and neck cancer. Semin Oncol 4:413–424 1977

Castigliano SG et al: Master metal cast for swaging lead masks in treatment on carcinoma of the skin. Am J Orthodont (Oral Surg Sect) 33:319–325, 1947

Castigliano SG: A master facial cast for rigid portal delineation in roentgen therapy of carcinoma about the face. Am J Roentgenol Radium Ther 59:19, 1948

Chalian VA, Drane JB, Standish SM: Maxillofacial Prosthetics Multidisciplinary Practice. Baltimore, Williams & Wilkins, 1971

Clark RL, Howe CD: Cancer Patient Care at M.D. Anderson Hospital and Tumor Institute. Chicago, Year Book Medical Publishers, 1976

Clark WH, Jr, In Bernardino EA, Mihm, MC: The histogenesis and biologic behavior of primary human malignant melanomas of the skin. Cancer Res 29:705–727, 1969

Clark WH, Jr, Mihm MC, Jr: Moles and malignant melanoma. In Dermatology in General Medicine, pp 491–511. New York, McGraw Hill, 1971

Curtis TA et al: Complete denture prosthodontics for the radiation patient. J Prosthet Dent 36:66, 1976

Daly TE et al: Management of dental problems in irradiated patients. Presented before The Radiological Society of North America, Chicago, Ill, December 2, 1970

Daly TE: Radiation complications in head and neck cancer. Cancer Bull 20:90–91, 1968

Daly TE, Drane JB: Management of dental problems in irradiated patients. Annual meeting of the Radiological Society of North America. Chicago, November 26–29, 1972

Davis NC et al: Primary cutaneous melanoma: A report from the Queensland Melanoma Project. American Cancer Society Professional Education Publication

David DJ and Barritt JA: Psychosocial implications of surgery for head and neck cancer. Clin Plast Surg 9:327, 1982

Davis NC, Herron JJ, McLeod GR: The macroscopic appearance of malignant melanoma of the skin. Med J Aust 2:883–886, 1966

Delclos L: Radiotherapy for head and neck cancer (Teamwork: Problems common to physicians and dentists). J Prosthet Dent 15:157–167, 1965

Delclos L, Lindberg, RD, Fletcher GH: Squamous cell carcinoma of the oral tongue and floor of the mouth. Am J Roentgenol 126:223–228, 1976

del Regato JA, Spjut HJ: Ackerman and del Regato's Cancer: Diagnosis, Treatment and Prognosis, 5th ed, pp 264, 281, 341–342, 345. St. Louis, CV Mosby, 1977

del Regato JA, Sala JM: The treatment of carcinoma of the lower lip. Radiology 73:839–844, 1959

Department of Head and Neck Surgery and Oncology: Cancer of the Head and Neck, A Collection of Papers. Buffalo, NY, Rozwell Park Memorial Institute, 1981

Dowell KE, Armstrong DM, Aust JB, Cruz AB, Jr: Systemic chemotherapy of advanced head and neck malignancies. Cancer 35:1116–1120, 1975

Drane JB: Development plan for the department of dental oncology. M. D. Anderson Hospital and Tumor Institute, February, 1976

Einhorn J, Wersall J: Incidence of oral carcinoma in patients with leukoplakia of the oral mucosa. Cancer 20:2189–2193, 1967

Engelmeier RL and King GE: Complications of head and neck radiation therapy and their management. J Prosthet Dent 49:514, 1983

Facts and Figures. New York, American Cancer Society, 1982

Feldman JG, Hazan M, Nagarajan M, Kissin B: A case-control investigation of alcohol, tobacco, and diet in head and neck cancer. Prev Med 4:444, 1975

Fleming TJ: Osteoradionecrosis associated with definitive radiation therapy for head and neck malignancies. J Prosthet Dent 49:675, 1983

Fletcher GH: Basic principles of the combination of irradiation and surgery. Int J Radiat Oncol Biol Phys 5:2091–2096, 1979

Fletcher GH: Elective irradiation of subclinical disease in cancers of the head and neck. Cancer 29:1450–1454, 1972

Fletcher GH: Textbook of Radiology. Philadelphia, Lea & Febiger, 1980

Fletcher GH, Jesse RH, Healey JE, Jr et al: Oropharynx. In MacComb WS, Fletcher GH (eds): Cancer of the Head and Neck, pp 179–212. Baltimore, Williams & Wilkins, 1967

Fletcher GH, Jing BS: The Head and Neck, p 168. Chicago, Year Book Medical Publishers, 1968

Fletcher GH, MacComb WS, Braun EJ: Analysis of sites and causes of treatment failures in squamous cell carcinomas of the oral cavity. AJR 83:405–411, 1960

Fletcher GH, MacComb WS, Chau PM, Farnsley WG: Orthovoltage and higher-energy irradiation in the treatment of Oropharyngeal cancers: Cobalt 60 teletherapy and betatron X-irradiation. In Pack GT, Ariel IM (eds): Treatment of Cancer and Allied Diseases, 2nd Ed, Vol. 3, pp 192–219. New York: Hoeber, 1962

Fraument JF, Jr: Geographic distribution of head and neck cancers in the United States. Laryngoscope (Supp 8) 88:40–44, 1978

Fretwell DL: The head and neck irradiated patient: Dental considerations. VA Dent J 54:8–15, 1977

Fried MP et al: Cervical metastases from unknown primary. Ann Otolaryngol Rhinol Laryngol 84:152–157, 1975

Fries R et al: Carcinoma of the oral cavity: On the prognostic significance of the primary tumor site (by organs) in the oral cavity. J Millofacial Surg 8:25–37, 1980

Frisch J: Dental treatment after irradiation. J Prosthet Dent 12:182–189, 1962

Gage AA: The role of the dentist in the therapy of oral cancer by radium. NY Univ J Dent 9:178–182, 1951

Gaisford JC (ed): Symposium on cancer of the head and neck. Pittsburgh, 1968. In Total Therapy and Reconstructive Rehabilitation, Vol. 2. St. Louis, CV Mosby, 1969

Gehrig JD: Should teeth be removed prior to radiation therapy? Dent Clin North Am 13:4:929–938, 1969

Gilbert HA, Kagen AR: Modern Radiation Oncology, Classic Literature and Current Management. Hagerstown, MD, Harper & Row, 1978

Goffinet DR, Bagshaw MA: Clinical use of radiation sensitizing agents. Cancer Treat Rev 1:15–26, 1974

Goldsmith MA, Carter SK: The integration of chemotherapy into a combined modality approach to cancer therapy, V. Squamous cell cancer of the head and neck. Cancer Treat Rev 2:137–158, 1975

Gottlieb JA, Burgess MA, Bodey GP, Livingston RB: Recent developments in chemotherapy for head and neck cancer. In Neoplasia of Head and Neck. M.D. Anderson Hospital, pp 121–133. Chicago, Year Book Med, 1974

Griem ML, Barnhart GW: Use of a resilient material for intraoral radium mold featuring an after loading technic. Radiology 79:856–859, 1962

Hamberger AD, Fletcher GH, Guillamondegui DM, Byers RM: Advanced squamous cell carcinoma of the oral cavity and oropharynx treated with irradiation and surgery. Radiology 119:433–438, 1976

Hardingham M, Dalley VM, Shaw HJ: Cancer of the floor of the mouth: Clinical features and results of treatment. Clin Oncol 3:227–246, 1977

Hickey AJ, Drane JB: Prosthetic treatment and rehabilitation: Use in patients with cancer of the head and neck. Current Problems in Cancer. Chicago, Yearbook Medical Publishers, 1978

Holoye PY, Byers RM, Gard DA et al: Combination chemotherapy of head and neck cancer. Cancer 42:1661–1669, 1978

Hulbert M et al: A flexible plastic material for use in the construction of radium applicators. Br J Radiol 27:413–414, 1954

Jesse RH, Barkley HT, Lindberg RD et al: Cancer of the oral cavity: Is elective neck dissection beneficial? Am J Surg 120:505–508, 1970

Jesse RH, Fletcher GH: Metastases in cervical lymph nodes from oropharyngeal carcinoma: Treatment and results. AJR 90:990–996, 1963

Jesse RH, Lindberg RD: Efficacy of combined radiation therapy with a surgical procedure in patients with cervical metastases from squamous cancer of the oropharynx. Cancer 35:1163–1166, 1965

Keys HM, McCasland JP: Techniques and results of a comprehensive dental care program in head and neck cancer patients. Int J Radiat Oncol Biol Phys 1:859–866, 1976

Kogelnik HD, Fletcher GH, Jesse RH: Clinical course of patients with squamous cell carcinoma of the upper respiratory and digestive tracts with no evidence of disease 5 years after initial treatment. Radiology 115:423–427, 1975

Kramer S: Radiation therapy and chemotherapy combination. JAMA 217:946–947, 1971

Lampe I: The place of radiation therapy in treatment of carcinoma of the lower lip. Plast Reconstr Surg 24:34–44, 1959

Lattes R: Precancerous lesions of the oral cavity and larynx. Presented at the International Workshop on Cancer of the Head and Neck, New York, 1965

Lederman M: Cancer of the Nasopharynx: Its Natural History and Treatment. American Lecture Series #432. Springfield, Charles C Thomas, 1961

Lindberg RD: Distribution of cervical lymph node metastases from squamous cell carcinoma of the upper respiratory and digestive tracts. Cancer 29:1446–1449, 1972

Lindberg RD, Fletcher GH: The role of irradiation in the management of head and neck cancer: Analysis of results and causes of failure. Tumori 64:313–325, 1978

Lindberg RD, Jesse RH: Treatment of cervical lyumph node metastases from primary lesions of the oropharynx, supraglottic larynx and hypopharynx. AJR 102:132–137, 1968

Loré JM: Head and Neck Surgery, 2nd ed. Philadelphia, WB Saunders, 1973

MacComb WS: Leukoplakia of the intraoral cavity. Postgrad Med 27:349–355, 1960

MacComb WS, Fletcher GH: Cancer of the Head and Neck. Baltimore, Williams & Wilkins, 1968

Malanoma AM et al: Oral cancer in 57,518 industrial workers of Gujarat, India: A prevalence and follow-up study. Cancer 37:1882–1886, 1976

Maldonado O, Dreizen S, Matalon V et al: Dental oncology. Cancer Bull 29:57, 1977

Mancuso AA, Hanafee WN, Juillard GJF et al: The role of computed tomography in the management of cancer of the larynx. Radiology 124:243–244, 1977

Manual for Staging of Cancer, 1977, American Joint Committee for Cancer Staging and End-Results Reporting. Chicago, AJCCS, 1977

Markwell BD, Whittle RJM: Displacement appliances in radiography. Br Dent J 124:564–568, 1968

Mashberg A: Erythroplasia: The earliest sign of asymptomatic oral cancer. J Am Dent Assoc 96:615–620, 1978

Mashberg A: Erythroplasia vs leukoplakia in the diagnosis of early asymptomatic oral squamous carcinoma. N Engl J Med 297:109–110, 1977

Mashberg A: Final evaluation of tolonium chloride rinse for screening of high-risk patients with asymptomatic squamous carcinoma. J Am Dent Assoc 106:319, 1983

Mashberg A: Reevaluation of toluidine blue application as a diagnostic adjunct in the detection of asymptomatic oral carcinoma. Cancer 46:758–763, 1980

Mashberg A, Garfinkle L: Early diagnosis of oral cancer: The erythroplastic lesion in high risk sites. CA 28:5, 1978

Mashberg A, Meyers H: Anatomical site and size of 222 early asymptomatic oral squamous cell carcinomas: A continuing prospective study of oral cancer. II Cancer 37:2149–2157, 1976

Mashberg A, Meyers H, Garfinkel L: Criteria for the diagnosis of asymptomatic oral squamous cell carcinoma. Presented at Third International Symposium on Detection and Prevention of Cancer, New York, 1976

Mashberg A, Morrissey JB, Garfinkel L: A study of the appearance of early asymptomatic squamous cell carcinoma. Cancer 32:1436–1445, 1973

McGovern VJ et al: The Classification of malignant melanoma and its histological reporting. Cancer 32:1446–1457, 1973

Mihm MC, Fitzpatrick TB, Lane–Brown MM et al: Primary detection of primary cutaneous malignant melanoma—Early clinical signs: A color atlas. N Eng J Med 289:989–996, 1973

Million RR: Cancer in the head and neck. In DeVita VT, Hellman S, Rosenberg SA (eds): Cancer: Principles and Practice in Oncology, Chap 13. Philadelphia, JB Lippincott, 1981

Moertel CG, Dockerty MB, Baggenstoss AH: Multiple primary malignant neoplasms. Cancer 14:221, 1961

Moore C: Anatomic origins and location of oral cancer. Am J Surg 114:510, 1967

Moore C: Cancer control. Presidential address given before the Annual Meeting of The Society of Head and Neck Surgeons (April 1976)

Moore C: Smoking and cancer of the mouth, pharynx, and larynx. JAMA 191:107–110, 1965

Moss WT, Brand WN, Battifora H: Radiation Oncology, Rationale, Technique, Results, 5th ed. St. Louis, CV Mosby, 1979

Muggia FM, Cortes–Funes H, Wasserman TH: Radiotherapy and chemotherapy in combined clinical trials: Problems and promise. Int J Radiat Oncol Biol Phys 4:161–171, 1978

Neel HB: Cryosurgery for the treatment of cancer. Laryngoscope 90:1, 1980

Neoplasia of the Head and Neck. 17th Annual Clinical Conference on Cancer. MD Anderson Hospital & Tumor Institute. Chicago: Year Book Medical Publishers, 1974

Nethery WJ, Delclos L: Prosthetic stent for gold grain implant to the floor of the mouth. J Prosthet Dent 27:81–87, 1970

Niebel HH, Chomet B: In vivo staining test for delineation of oral intra-epithelial neoplastic change. Preliminary report. J Am Dent Assoc 68:801, 1964

Parel SM, Drane JB, Williams EO: Mandibular replacements: Review of the literature. J Am Dent Assoc 94:120, 1977

Peterson DE and Overholster CD: Increased morbidity associated with oral infection in patients with acute nonlymphocytic leukemia. Oral Surg 51:390, 1981

Phillips, Benak: Radiation modalities in treatment of cancer of the oral cavity. J Prosthet Dent 27:413–418, 1972

Pindborg JJ: Current concepts of oral precancerous lesions. Presented at the Greater New York Dental Meeting, New York, 1976

Pindborg JJ et al: Studies in oral leukoplakia. Acta Odontol Scand 21:407, 1963

Price LA, Hill BT, Calvert AH et al: Improved results in combination chemotherapy of head and neck cancer using a kinetically-based approach: A randomized study with and without adriamycin. Oncology 35:26–28, 1978

Rahn AO, Boucher LJ: Maxillofacial Prosthetics, Principles and Concepts. Philadelphia, WB Saunders, 1970

Rahn AO, Drane B: Dental aspects of the problems, care, and treatment of the irradiated oral cancer patient. J Am Dent Assoc 74:957–966, 1967

Rahn AO, Drane JB: Prosthetic evaluation of patients who have received irradiation to the head and neck region. J Prosthet Dent 19:174–179, 1968

Richman SP, Livingston RB, Gutterman JU et al: Chemotherapy vs. chemoimmunotherapy of head and neck cancer. Report of a randomized study. Cancer Treat Rep 60:535–539, 1976

Robinson JE: Dental management of the oral effects of radiotherapy. J Prosthet Dent 14:582–587, 1964

Rosenthal LE, Wilkie B: The effects of radiotherapy on oral tissue. J Prosthet Dent 15:153–156, 1965

Rothman K, Keller A: The effect of joint exposure to alcohol and tobacco on risk of cancer of the mouth and pharynx. J Chronic Dis 25:711, 1972

Rouviere H: Anatomy of the Human Lymphatic System, p 53. Ann Arbor, Mich, Edwards Brothers, 1938

Rubin P (ed): Current Concepts in Cancer, pp 1–116. Parts I–VIII. Chicago: American Medical Association, 1974

Rudd KD et al: Maxillary appliance for controlled radium needle placement. J Prosthet Dent 16:782–787, 1966

Rudd KD et al: Radium source appliance for treatment of nasopharyngeal cancer. J Am Dent Assoc 72:852–866, 1966

Santiago R: Use of intraoral prostheses in radiotherapy. Med Rec Ann 58:3–11, 1965

Scannel JB: Practical considerations in the dental treatment of patients with head and neck cancer. J Prosthet Dent 15:764–769, 1965

Schuller DE et al: Preoperative reductive chemotherapy for locally advanced carcinoma of the oral cavity, oropharynx and hypopharynx. Cancer 51:15, 1983

Scully C: The immunology of cancer of the head and neck with particular reference to oral cancer. Oral Surg 53:157, 1982

Shafer WG, Waldron CA: Erythroplakia of the oral cavity. Cancer 36:1021–1028, 1975

Shannon IL: A saliva substitute for dry mouth relief. Presented at the Harvard University–Veterans Administration Geriatric Symposium, Boston, MA, 1977

Shannon IL, Edmonds EJ: Effect of fluoride concentration on rehardening of enamel by a saliva substitute. Int Dent J (in press)

Shannon IL, McCrary BR, Starcke EN: A saliva substitute for use by xerostomic patients undergoing radiotherapy to the head and neck. Oral Surg 44:656–661, 1977

Shannon IL, Starcke EN, Wescott WB: Effect of radiotherapy on whole saliva flow. J Dent Res 56:693, 1977

Shannon IL, Trodahl JN, Starcke EN: Radiosensitivity of the human parotid gland. Proc Soc Exp Biol Med 157:50–53, 1978

Shannon IL, Trodahl JN, Starcke EN: Remineralization of enamel by a saliva substitute designed for use by irradiated patients. Cancer 41:1746–1750, 1978

Shannon IL, Wescott WB, Starcke EN, Mira J: Laboratory study of cobalt-60 irradiated human dental enamel. J Oral Med 33:23–27, 1978

Shedd DP: Clinical characteristics of early oral cancer. JAMA 215:955, 1971

Shedd DP et al: Further appraisal of in vivo staining properties of oral cancer. Arch Surg 95:16–22, 1967

Shedd DP, Hukill P, Bahn S: In vivo staining properties of oral cancer. Am J Surg 110:631, 1965

Silverberg E and Lubera JA: Cancer statistics 1983. Cancer Vol 33 No 1, 1983

Starcke EN, Shannon IL: How critical is the interval between extractions and irradiation in patients with head and neck malignancy? Oral Surg 43:333–337, 1977

Strauss, Spatz: Irradiated dentition: Dentist's responsibilities. J Prosthet Dent 27:209, 1972

Strong EW: Preoperative radiation and radical neck dissection. Surg Clin North Am 49:271–276, 1969

Strong MS, Vaughn CW, Ineze JS: Toluidine blue in the management of carcinoma of the oral cavity. Arch Otolaryngol 87:527, 1968

Tapley N: Clinical Applications of the Electron Beam, pp 125–129. New York, John Wiley & Sons, 1976

Totten RS: Tumors of the Oral Cavity, Larynx, and Pharynx. In Rubin P (ed): Current Concepts in Cancer, pp 4–6. Chicago: American Medical Association, 1974

Trowbridge J, Carl W: Oral care of the patient having head and neck irradiation. Am J Nurs 75:12:2146, 1975

University of Rochester, School of Medicine and Dentistry Clinical Oncology for Medical Students and Physicians: A Multidisciplinary Approach. Rochester, NY, American Cancer Society, 1978

Van Aken J, Verhoeven JW: Factors influencing the design of aiming devices for intraoral radiography and their practical application. Oral Surg 47:378–388, 1979

Vincent RG, Marchetta F: The relationship of the use of tobacco and alcohol to cancer of the oral cavity, pharnyx or larynx. Am J Surg 105:501–505, 1963

Waldron CA, Shafer WG: Leukoplakia revisited. A clinicopathologic study of 3,256 oral leukoplakias. Cancer 36:1386–1392, 1975

Wescott WB, Mira JG, Starcke EN et al: Alterations in whole saliva flow rate induced by fractionated radiotherapy. Am J Roentgenol 130:145–149, 1978

Wescott WB, Starcke EN, Shannon IL: Chemical protection against postirradiation dental caries. Oral Surg 40:709–719, 1975

Wynder EL, Bross IJ, Feldman RM: A study of the etiological factors in cancer of the mouth. Cancer 10:1300, 1957

Zach GA: Planning dental treatment for the preradiation patient. J Hosp Dent Pract 9:17, 20–21, 1975

10

Diseases of the Tongue

VERNON J. BRIGHTMAN

ANATOMY OF THE TONGUE

Muscles and Nerve Supply

The tongue is essentially a complex muscular organ that is anchored to the hyoid bone, styloid process, and genial tubercles of the mandible at the points of insertion of three extrinsic tongue muscles (hyoglossus, styloglossus, and geniohyoglossus). It is loosely attached to neighboring structures by two other extrinsic muscles (palatoglossus and glossopharyngeus) and by extensions of the oral and pharyngeal mucous membranes covering the tongue. The bulk of the tongue is composed of four groups of intrinsic muscles that are attached to a well-developed median fibrous raphe and a similar dorsal submucous fibrous raphe. The tongue is divided into a small anterior oral portion and a larger posterior portion* *(base of the tongue)* situated below the angles of the mandible and more or less inaccessible to physical examination. The superior (oral) and posterior (pharyngeal) surfaces of the tongue are invested with specialized mucous membranes from which a variety of different papillary projections are developed, some of which carry special receptors for taste as well as fine nerve endings essential to the highly developed perceptual function of the tongue. The inferior (oral) surface is covered with a poorly keratinized mucous membrane that merges with and is indistinguishable from that of the floor of the mouth. The extrinsic and intrinsic muscles are innervated by the hypoglossal (12th cranial) nerve, with the exception of the palatoglossus and glossopharyngeus (see Table 10-1). The lingual branch of the trigeminal (5th cranial) nerve transmits general sensation from the anterior two thirds of the tongue, also bearing within its sheath fibers of the chorda tympani branch of the facial (7th cranial) nerve which carry special taste

sensations from the anterior two thirds of the tongue. The glossopharyngeal (9th cranial) nerve carries general sensation and special taste sensation from the pharyngeal surface. Proprioceptive sensation from the tongue muscles is transmitted by the hypoglossal nerves to the nodose ganglia, where branches of the vagus (10th cranial) nerve carry it to the brain.

Dissection in a vertical direction from the dorsal surface of the tongue reveals four or five alternating layers of intrinsic and extrinsic muscles lying below the dorsal submucous raphe (see Table 10-1; Fig. 10-1). A portion of the geniohyoglossus lies directly below the anterior portion of the ventral surface of the tongue, some of its fibers forming the very prominent anterior lingual frenum. Further distally, the ventral mucous membrane covers the hyoglossus, which is intermingled with the horizontal portion of the styloglossus along the lateral margin of the tongue. Diagnostic biopsies from the dorsal surface of the tongue rarely penetrate deeper than the submucous raphe, although some fibers of the superior lingualis intrinsic muscle may be found attached to its deeper surface. Biopsies from the margins of the tongue usually include at least the more superficial fibers of some of the extrinsic muscles. The mucous membrane of the pharyngeal surface is thicker, and biopsies in this area only occasionally include hyoglossal fibers and a few from the glossopharyngeus.

Deeper fibers of the geniohyoglossus, hyoglossus, and styloglossus also run vertically and horizontally through the body of the tongue to attach to the midline and dorsal submucous raphes. Protrusion and retrusion of the tip of the tongue are controlled by fibers of the geniohyoglossus, which also depresses the midline of the tongue to form an anteroposteriorly directed channel along which fluids pass as in sucking. The hyoglossus depresses the side of the tongue, rendering it convex. The styloglossus draws the tongue upward and backward, and activation of the palatoglossus raises the base of the tongue. The intrinsic muscles control a variety of complex movements that modify the size of the tongue in three dimensions.

At autopsy, the tongue is easily removed

---

* When viewed through the lips or when extended, the oral portion of the tongue is prominent and is commonly referred to as the *anterior two thirds,* with the *posterior third* less well visualized. When the tongue is removed *in toto* and is not extended, the oral portion may appear no larger than the posterior pharyngeal portion.

Table 10-1. Extrinsic and Intrinsic Muscles of the Tongue

MUSCLE	ATTACHMENTS AND INSERTIONS	NERVE SUPPLY	ACTIONS
Extrinsic Group			
Geniohyoglossus	Genial tubercles of the mandible; hyoid bone; median raphe of the tongue	Hypoglossal	Retracts, depresses, and protrudes the tongue
Hyoglossus	Body and greater horn of the hyoid bone; side of the tongue	Hypoglossal	Depresses tongue and draws down its sides
Styloglossus	Styloid process and stylomandibular ligament; side of the tongue	Hypoglossal	Raises and retracts the tongue
Palatoglossus (anterior palatine pillar)	Soft palate; side of the tongue	Spinal accessory via pharyngeal plexus	Contracts anterior faucial pillars and raises base of the tongue
Glossopharyngeus (lingual fibers of superior constrictor of pharynx)	Side of the tongue; midline pharyngeal raphe	Pharyngeal plexus	Contracts oropharynx
Intrinsic Group			
Superior lingualis	Submucous dorsal raphe and median raphe of the tongue; tip and sides of the tongue	Hypoglossal	Shortens tongue and raises its edges and tip
Transverse lingualis	Median raphe of the tongue; sides of the tongue	Hypoglossal	Narrows and stretches tongue and lifts its edges
Vertical lingualis	Upper and lower surfaces of the tip and sides of the tongue	Hypoglossal	Flattens tip of tongue
Inferior lingualis	Hyoid bone and undersurface of the tongue at its base; tip of the tongue	Hypoglossal	Shortens tongue

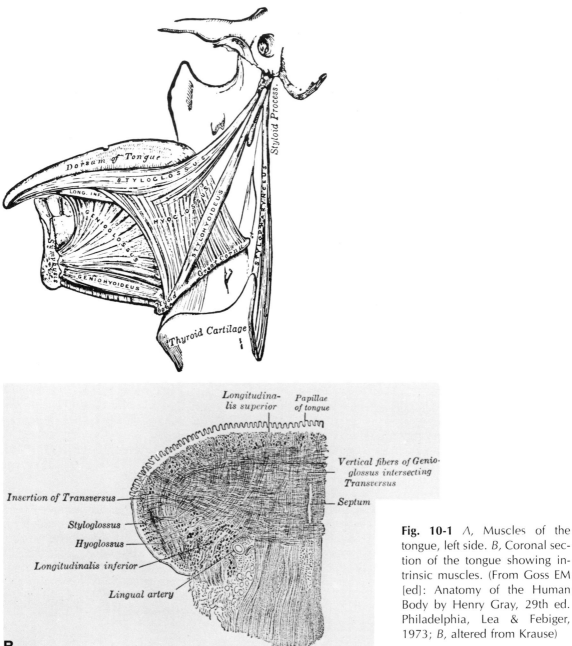

Fig. 10-1 Λ, Muscles of the tongue, left side. B, Coronal section of the tongue showing intrinsic muscles. (From Goss EM [ed]: Anatomy of the Human Body by Henry Gray, 29th ed. Philadelphia, Lea & Febiger, 1973; B, altered from Krause)

along with the larynx, trachea, and other prevertebral structures, once its muscle and mucous membrane attachments to the inside of the mandible and soft palate have been severed. While the tongue is no longer routinely removed at autopsy, the fact that this can be accomplished via the standard Y-shaped chest incision and without risk of facial disfigurement means that considerably more can be learned about the histopathology of the human tongue than of the parotid gland or other oral adnexal structures.

Superficial Features of the Anterior Two Thirds

The mucosa of the anterior dorsal surface of the tongue is characterized by two types of papillae with defined functions (*filiform* and *fungiform*) and a number of other elevations without any clear function (see Fig. 10-2). *Filiform papillae* are slender connective tissue papillae, each with several secondary papillae with heavily keratinized caps, that are found in rows radiating anteroposteriorly over the anterior dorsal surface. The concentration of these papillae in man has been calculated at about 500/cm^2; none are found on the pharyngeal surface. They are most heavily concentrated in the center of the dorsum and function primarily in licking and to convey food distally; they also probably have an important role in modulating textural and pressure sensations on the tongue and are supplied with numerous nerve endings and an arterial and venous blood supply, the latter equipped with contractile elements to control blood flow.

The *fungiform papillae,* likewise, are found only on the anterior two thirds of the tongue and number about 100/cm^2 on the tip and 50/cm^2 in the middle of the tongue. These mushroom-shaped structures have a rich capillary network that along with their larger size makes them easily identifiable as reddish dots against a carpet of filiform papillae. Fungiform papillae carry taste buds varying in number from 0 to as many as 20 to 30 per papilla. In most individuals, fewer than one half of the fungiform papillae bear taste buds and function as taste receptors at any one time. Of the remainder, more than three quarters have one to three taste buds. It is not known whether there is a turnover and regeneration of taste buds among different fungiform papillae. When the chorda tympani is sectioned, taste buds on the anterior two thirds of the same side of the tongue disappear rapidly; the fungiform papillae may also disappear slowly over subsequent years. Taste buds on the fungiforms also depend on capillary blood flow, taste function rapidly declining with occlusion of blood flow in the capillary bed.

Taste-bud bearing papillae can be readily identified with low-power magnification of blocks of biopsied tissue following topical application of protein stains or Alcian blue, which stain the pore of the taste bud intensely. *In vivo* fungiform papillae are also often easily recognized by tiny particles of melanin pigment; unlike the keratinized filiform papillae, they do not elongate when normal wear decreases, and do not pick up secondary staining from food, tobacco, and bacteria.

The anterior two thirds of the tongue is relatively free of mucous or serous glands except directly under the tip where the small mucous glands of Blandin and Nuhn are found.

Superficial Features of the Posterior Third

At the junction of the anterior two thirds and posterior third of the tongue is found the V- or Y-shaped row of vallate (also referred to as circumvallate) papillae that terminates on the lateral margins of the tongue with a cluster of leaflets known as the foliate papillae (see Fig. 10-3). Posteriorly, the pharyngeal surface of the tongue is thrown into a number of rounded elevations by subepithelial aggregations of lymphoid tissue (lingual tonsils). Each vallate papilla is surrounded by a moat and cuff, and foliate leaflets are separated by similar grooves. Vallate* and foliate papillae contain large numbers of taste buds on their walls, a nonkeratinized epithelium, specialized connective tissue cores with a complex of vascular loops, numerous fine endings of the 9th cranial nerve, clusters of very prominent serous glands (glands of von Ebner) that drain into the moat, and a parasympathetic ganglion probably associated with glandular secretion (see Fig. 10-4).

Recently, the secretion of the glands of von Ebner has been shown to contain a lipoprotein lipase (or pregastric esterase) that is important for the digestion of fat in the neonate

---

* Based on limited data, figures of approximately 200 to 250 taste buds per vallate papilla are quoted for individuals below age 20, with numbers decreasing to 200 or less during maturity and to fewer than 100 beyond age 75.

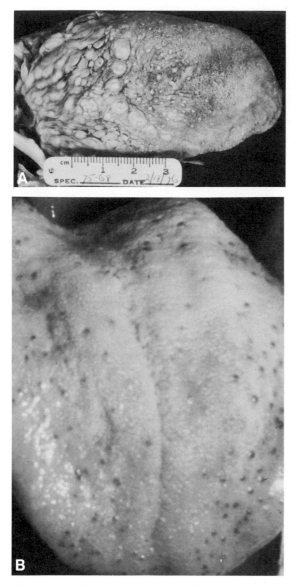

Fig. 10-2 *A,* View of entire upper (dorsal) and posterior (pharyngeal) surfaces of tongue removed at autopsy from a 61-year-old male with coronary atherosclerosis and myocardial infarction. A row of vallate papillae separates anterior two thirds from the pharyngeal portion. Some relatively larger fungiform papillae are apparent on the anterior two thirds. *B,* Clinical photograph of anterior third of dorsum of the tongue. Numerous fungiform papillae are evident in this illustration because of localized aggregations of melanin on the top of these papillae. Other fungiform papillae can usually be easily distinguished if the carpet of filiform papillae is disturbed with dental air spray or stroked with an instrument.

before the full development of the exocrine pancreas and secretion of intestinal lipase. The strategic location of these lipase-rich glands of von Ebner, close to the point at which milk is discharged from the nipple, and the absence of vallate and foliate papillae in nonmammalian species and those mammals that lack true suckling mechanisms suggest that the vallate and foliate papillae function biologically in suckling and have only a secondary function as organs of taste in adult mammals. Lipoprotein lipase development in von Ebner's glands is first noted *in utero* at about the time taste buds appear; suckling stimulates formation of lipoprotein lipase; the role of taste and other stimuli in stimulating secretion from these glands is still unknown. The glands of von Ebner are found clustered in a definite zone below the row of vallate papillae and adjacent to the foliate papillae. The remainder of the pharyngeal surface is packed with numerous mucus-secreting acini.

Vascular Supply

The tongue is supplied by right and left lingual arteries that arise from the external carotid artery soon after it branches from the common carotid. Near the base of the tongue, the lingual artery divides into three branches: a dorsal branch, a deep lingual artery that flows through the body of the tongue giving off numerous vertical branches towards the dorsal surface, and a sublingual artery that supplies the ventral surface of the tongue and the floor of the mouth. The vertical branches of the deep lingual artery and the dorsal branch anastomose to form two capillary plexuses that lie above and below the dorsal raphe. The extensive capillary networks of the lingual papillae are derived from the more superficial of these two plexuses. It is commonly stated that there are few connections between vessels on the right and left sides of the tongue except at the tip and posteriorly; however, bleeding often continues even though the ipsilateral lingual artery is occluded, and occlusion of either the lingual artery or external carotid artery on one side does not produce ischemic changes in the tongue muscles. Infarcts of the tongue usually develop on the basis of lingual arteritis

and not from carotid or lingual arteriosclerosis.

Microbial Flora of the Dorsum

The extensively papillated anterior dorsal
surface of the tongue provides an ideal hab-
itat for a variety of bacterial and fungal species depending on the state of the oral environment.

Facultative streptococci are the predominant cultivable bacteria isolated from this region, and they constitute about 38% of the

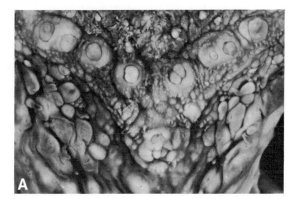

Papillae vallatae accessoriae laterales
Papillae vallatae medianae anteriores
Papilla vallata lateralis
Papilla vallata centralis
Papillae vallatae medianae posteriores

Fig. 10-3 Structures on the posterior (pharyngeal) surface of the tongue. *A,* Close-
up view of tongue illustrated in Fig. 10-2A to show array of vallate papillae and
submucosal aggregates of lymphoid cells that distend the posterior surface and
constitute the lingual tonsils. *B,* Nomenclature for describing vallate papillae. In *A,*
one central, and two lateral and three lateral accessory papillae can be distinguished
on each side. *C,* Anteroposterior section through pharyngeal mucosa of the tongue
to show lingual tonsils with inspissated secretions, lymphoid follicles, and submucosal mucous glands. (*B,* Oppel A: Lehrbuch der Verg Mikroskopischen Anatomie
der Wirbeltiere. Jena, Fischer, 1900)

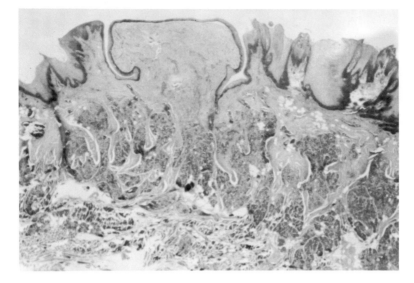

Fig. 10-4 Anteroposterior section showing histology of the vallate papillae of the human tongue: keratinized papillae of anterior two thirds of the tongue dorsum, vallate papilla; specialized gustatory epithelium containing taste buds on both the papillary and lateral walls of moat, epithelium of pharyngeal surface of the tongue, acini of von Ebner's glands draining through ducts to base of moat, acini of mucous glands, parasympathetic ganglion, and specialized connective tissue and nerve and vascular plexus making up core of papilla.

tongue flora. *Veillonella* (12% to 15%), facultative and anaerobic diphtheroids (approximately 20%), micrococci–staphylococci, and *Bacteroides* (approximately 5% each) are the next most prevalent groups. Twenty to fifty-five percent of the facultative streptococci are identified as *Streptococcus salivarius* with *Streptococcus mitis* constituting another 18%. Comparisons between the predominant cultivable flora of dental plaque, gingival crevice, cheek, tongue, and salivary specimens indicate that the tongue and not the dental plaque or gingival crevice is the major source of salivary bacteria (see Table 10-2). *Bacteroides melaninogenicus, Fusobacterium* species, and spirochetes, which are prominent members of the gingival crevice flora, make up less than 1% of the tongue flora. Likewise, *Streptococcus sanguis* and *Streptococcus mutans,* the predominant organisms in dental plaque, are the least prevalent type of streptococci on the tongue.

It is uncertain whether dental plaque is recolonized by *S. sanguis* and *S. mutans* from the tongue following tooth cleaning and flossing because these organisms are a minor component of the tongue flora. Because these dextran- and levan-synthesizing streptococcal species largely disappear from the oral cavity once all teeth are removed, an equally good case can be made that streptococci of this type normally found on the tongue are derived from dental plaque. Tongue hygiene (brushing and scraping the dorsum) is often recommended as an essential part of oral hygiene directed to caries prevention, even though the scientific basis for this practice is not clear. The association of *S. salivarius* with the tongue is related to the preferential affinity of this species for epithelial surfaces in contrast to the affinity of *S. sanguis, S. mutans,* and *Actinomyces* for adhering to and colonizing tooth surfaces.

Development of the Tongue

The anterior two thirds of the tongue develops *in utero* by the fusion of two lateral lingual swellings and a midline swelling referred to as the *tuberculum impar;* all of these structures arise from the first branchial arch. The lateral lingual swellings subsequently merge with and grow over the tuberculum impar, and retention of this structure in some individuals is hypothesized as the origin of the anomaly known as *median rhomboid glossitis.* The posterior portion of the tongue develops from the second and third branchial arches. The point of fusion between the tuberculum impar of the anterior two thirds and the rudimentary posterior portion of the tongue (referred to as the *copula*) corresponds

Table 10-2. Approximate Proportional Distribution of Bacteria on Various Oral Surfaces and in Saliva*

BACTERIA	GINGIVAL CREVICE	CORONAL PLAQUE	TONGUE DORSUM	BUCCAL MUCOSA	SALIVA
Streptococcus salivarius	< 0.5	< 0.5	20	11	20
Streptococcus mitis	8	15	8	60	20
Streptococcus sanguis	8	15	4	11	8
Streptococcus mutans	?	0–50	< 1	< 1	< 1
Enterococci	0–10	< 0.1	< 0.01	< 0.1	< 0.1
Gram-positive filaments	35	42	20	?	15
Lactobacilli	< 1	< 0.005	< 0.1	< 0.1	< 1
Veillonella species	10	2	12	1	10
Neisseria species	< 0.5	< 0.5	< 0.5	< 0.5	< 1
Bacteroides oralis	5	5	4	?	?
Bacteroides melaninogenicus	6	< 1	< 1	< 1	< 1
Vibrio sputorum	5	1	< 0.5	< 0.5	?
Spirochetes	2	< 0.1	< 0.1	< 0.1	< 0.1
Fusobacterium	3	4	1	?	< 1

* Data calculated as a percentage of total flora cultivable on anaerobically incubated blood agar. Estimates derived from the data of several authors (Reproduced with permission from Gibbons RJ, van Houte J: Bacterial adherence in oral microbial ecology. Annu Rev Microbiol 29:19–44, 1975. Copyright © 1975 by Annual Reviews Inc.)

to the site of invagination of the epithelial cells that subsequently migrate inferiorly to form the thyroid gland. In the adult, this point is marked by the foramen caecum, which may or may not still lead into an epithelial-lined tract called the *thyroglossal duct*. The foramen caecum and the arms of the V-shaped row of vallate papillae that extends anteriorly and laterally from it mark the separation of the oral and pharyngeal portions of the tongue.

FUNCTIONS OF THE TONGUE

The tongue serves numerous functions in all animal species including man. An awareness of these functions is of considerable assistance in diagnosing and managing local and systemic disorders affecting the tongue and provides some understanding of the distress that usually accompanies limitation of function of this organ.

Prehension and Ingestion. Because the tongue can be extended beyond the mouth and can be molded by muscular action to serve as a scoop, a brush, or other sampling device, it functions prominently in many species as a means of collecting both liquid and solid food and propelling the food to the pharynx. Licking, sucking, and chewing movements all involve coordinated muscular activity of the tongue as well as the jaws, lips, and cheeks. Compared to the tongues of other species, the human tongue is less extensible and has a relatively poorly developed coating of filiform papillae on the dorsum; however, it can be used very effectively to lick icecream and stamps, for example, and to sample food before ingestion. *Suckling* is a highly specialized form of ingestion characteristic of the infant mammal: in the human, the mother's nipple and surrounding areola are drawn deep into the open mouth, the everted lips form a seal, and the dorsum of the tongue is applied to the nipple and areola, which are rhythmically compressed by the jaw and tongue, discharging milk onto the dorsum of the tongue at about the level of the row of vallate papillae.

Swallowing. Swallowing is a coordinated muscular activity involving the tongue and constrictor muscles of the pharynx to close the palatal velum and the epiglottis allowing passage of the bolus into the esophagus without regurgitation into the nose or lower respiratory tract. Hypoglossal paralysis or even less significant problems such as localized but painful tongue lesions or topical anesthesia of the base of the tongue and pharynx (particularly in the elderly) are often associated with aspiration or choking because of a lack of coordinated control of swallowing function.

Perception. The specialized mucosa and general and special sensory nerve supply of the tongue dorsum provide sensitive assessment of temperature, texture, taste, pain, and general sensation. Proprioceptors in the lingual muscles, periodontal membrane, and masticatory muscles modulate spatial (stereotactic) sensation. The closeness of different receptors on the dorsum of the tongue and the fact that branches of the same cranial nerve carry a variety of sensory information make diagnosis of sensory complaints difficult; in the absence of specific therapies for modifying pain, taste, or tactile sensation, attempts at controlling a given symptom (*e.g.*, use of a topical analgesic) usually result in other equally unpleasant sensory side-effects.

Phonation. Adequate muscle strength and control as well as an intact lingual sensory system are needed for accurate enunciation; partial glossectomy can limit communication as effectively as can laryngectomy.

Respiration. Recent electromyographic studies of the tongue muscles (genioglossus, in particular) suggest that the position of the jaw and tongue, by contributing to lingual muscular tonus, influences respiratory control. These studies have led to a better understanding of the various sleep apnea syndromes and the role of severe malocclusion and hypotonicity of the tongue in some of these problems.

Jaw Development. Muscular pressures from the tongue are an important factor in developing the shape of the mandibular arch and the position of anterior and posterior tooth segments. Both hypoglossia and macroglossia significantly affect jaw development, and increasing tongue size in the adult as a result of acromegaly or tumors will cause spacing of teeth and other deformities. Tongue thrusting is considered to be an important etiologic factor in anterior open bite problems.

Symbolic Functions. Functions that are traditionally associated with the tongue but that have no anatomic or physiologic basis should be mentioned because images of this type are well established by cultural and literary tradition and must frequently influence a patient's perception of a lingual abnormality. The human tongue is not used for stroking and grooming (although this is common in carnivore and nonhuman primates), but soft speech and ululatory sounds and conversational "stroking" serve the same function. Expressions such as "speaking with a forked tongue," "poisonous speech," and "speaking in a different tongue" all ascribe mental attitudes and behaviors to the visible organ by which they are expressed; conversely, disease, deformity, and pain in the tongue can "imply" the same personality traits. The tongue may figure prominently in sexual encounters, playing both a physical and symbolic phallic function (see also discussion in Chap. 17).

EXAMINATION OF THE TONGUE

Procedures for routine examination of the tongue are described in Chapter 2, and examination of 5th, 7th, and 9th cranial nerve functions is discussed in Chapter 16 with reference to evaluation of the patient with chronic oral pain or taste abnormalities. This section briefly describes a number of specialized examination procedures that have been developed in recent years and that have already proved useful in the evaluation of some tongue disorders. It is expected that further development of these and other new diagnostic approaches will help considerably in improving our understanding and management of many problems such as glossodynia, tongue thrusting, hypotonicity, taste disorders, and depapillation that are now only poorly understood.

Cineradiographic studies of the oral cavity and pharynx during drinking, chewing, suckling, phonation, and other activities have added immeasurably to our understanding of the position and shape of the tongue in motion and help diagnose abnormalities of swallowing, phonation, and other functions associated with congenital and surgically induced defects. *Computer-assisted tomography* (CT scan) has been used in a number of instances to identify space-occupying lesions and muscular atrophy secondary to hypoglossal nerve damage, where the lesion was deep in the base of the tongue and not detectable by other approaches (see Fig. 10-5). *Pulsed (Doppler) ultrasound* has been used to study the characteristics of arterial blood flow in the tongue, and abnormal pulse waves have been noted in the lingual arteries of individuals with evidence of compromised flow in other branches of the carotid arterial tree (see Fig. 10-6). *Real-time (gray scale, B mode) ultrasound* is also adaptable for the study of the tongue provided probes of sufficiently small cross-sectional diameter are available for exploring the ventral surface of the tongue. This approach can be used to produce an image of a cyst or other lesion

within the tongue and also to estimate tongue size (Fig. 10-7).

Isotopic scanning techniques are also useful in cases where a mass in the tongue is composed of specialized secretory tissue or other tissue such as thyroid, which selectively concentrates intravenously administered radioactive ^{131}I or ^{99m}Tc-pertechnetate. *Electromyography* has been used for many years to study action potentials in actively contracting muscles and has contributed to an understanding of lingual and masticatory muscular function. Recently, noninvasive techniques using surface electrodes (earlier techniques that required a thin-needle electrode inserted in the muscle to be studied) have been introduced with considerable success.

The *scanning electron microscope* (SEM) is well established as a tool for studying the surface topography of the tongue dosrum, the character and morphology of the different types of tongue papillae, and the distribution and morphology of bacteria on the papillated areas of the dorsum (Fig. 10-8). *Transmission electron microscopy* (TEM) has been used successfully in the study of pathologic changes affecting the taste buds of animals with xerostomia, lesions of the 7th and 9th cranial

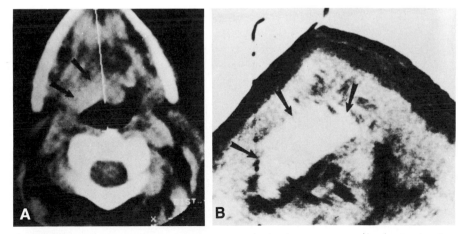

Fig. 10-5 Visualization of a mass in the tongue by both computer-assisted tomography (CT) and real-time ultrasound. *A* demonstrates a well-defined mass in the posterior right tongue (*arrows*). In this case, it is a verrucous carcinoma. *B,* Transverse sonogram of the same lesion (*arrows*) has excellent definition. (Mettler FA et al: Gray-scale ultrasonography in the evaluation of neoplastic invasion of the base of the tongue. Radiology 133:781, 1979)

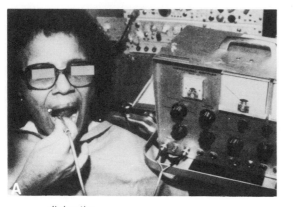

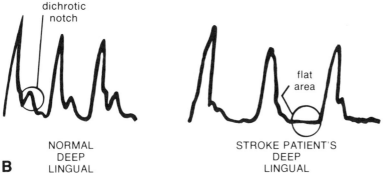

dichrotic notch

NORMAL
DEEP
LINGUAL

B

flat area

STROKE PATIENT'S
DEEP
LINGUAL

Fig. 10-6 Characteristics of arterial blood flow in the tongue as detected by pulsed (Doppler) ultrasound. *A,* Demonstration of clinical use of Doppler flowmeter, including probe placement on ventral surface of the tongue. *B,* Comparison of velocity pulse curves in deep lingual arteries of normal and stroke patients. Notice especially the deep dicrotic notch in the normal curve and its virtual absence in the stroke patient's curve. Notice also the flat area between pulses in the stroke curve. (Myers DE et al: Evaluation of lingual artery hemodynamics in stroke patients using Doppler ultrasound. Oral Surg 51:252, 1981)

nerves, and those resulting from a variety of toxins and DNA inhibitors; the application of TEM to the study of tongue biopsies of patients with various taste complaints is also being explored. TEM has also helped establish the nature of the granular cells found in a lesion referred to as granular cell myoblastoma, which is frequently found in the tongue. *Direct microscopic examination of the tongue papillae,* and the capillary blood flow in the fungiform papillae in particular, is possible with intravenously administered fluorescein dye. This basic technique has been used in ophthalmology for some years to study changes in retinal vessels, and the ophthalmologic microscope is easily adapted to study of capillary blood flow on the tongue dorsum. While there is a small risk of anaphylactic or other untoward allergic reaction to the dye, the technique is clinically acceptable and has been used to demonstrate changes in the taste papillae, as well as localized areas of decreased blood flow on the tongue secondary to diabetic angiopathy. *Psychophysical evaluation* of lingual sensory

function includes various methods for evaluating taste function (taste testing with a series of concentrations of sweet, sour, bitter, and salty solutions; electrogustometry; and regional "tongue mapping" for localized taste dysfunction); tactile sensation testing by means of von Frey fibers, a single or two-point esthesiometer, or a series of objects of graded texture; and testing for stereotactic sensitivity by means of a set of National Institute of Health shapes or other three-dimensional objects. This latter approach has been particularly helpful in evaluating speech disorders.

INHERITED, CONGENITAL, AND DEVELOPMENTAL ANOMALIES

A number of conditions are included under this heading: some that occur sufficiently frequently to be considered normal variants (these probably have multifactorial etiologies); significant deformities of the tongue that occur along with other orofacial and systemic defects, and in many cases help define

Fig. 10-7 Real-time ultrasonographic imaging of the base of the tongue. *A,* Patient positioning for scanning the base of the tongue with a small hand-held ultrasonic probe. *B,* Anatomical diagram of main structures involved. *C,* Normal longitudinal real-time ultrasonographic image of the base of the tongue with identification of the soft palate (S), tongue (T), geniohyoid (G), mylohyoid (M), and acoustical shadowing caused by the hyoid (H). (Mettler FA et al: Gray-scale ultrasonography in the evaluation of neoplastic invasion of the base of the tongue. Radiology 133:781, 1979)

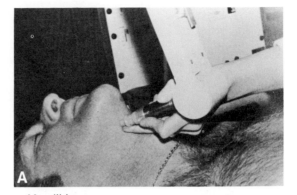

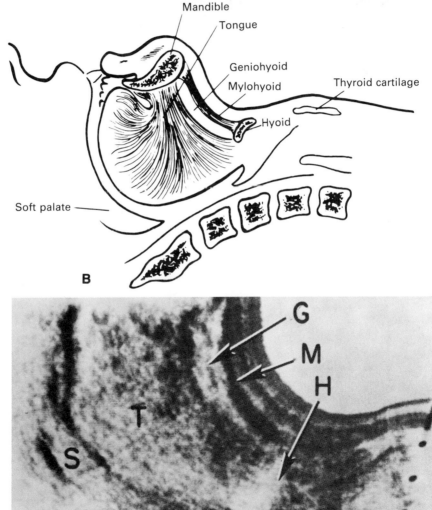

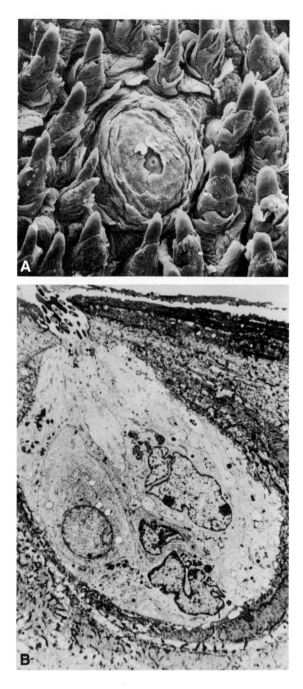

Fig. 10-8 Scanning (SEM) and transmission (TEM) electron microscopy of the dorsum of the tongue. *A,* SEM view (×355) of a fungiform papilla with a taste pore *(arrow)* indicating the location of a taste bud; the fungiform papilla is surrounded by numerous filiform papillae, each with a keratinized cap. *B,* TEM view (×3000) of a section of a human vallate papillae taste bud showing pore and taste bud cells in longitudinal section and anastomosing nerve cells around the base of the bud. The pore of this taste bud contains an aggregation of bacteria. Such aggregates have been described as being common in the taste buds of xerostomic rats, but their significance in the human is not known. (*A,* Kessel RG, Kardon RH (eds): Tissue and Organs: A Text-Atlas of Scanning Electron Microscopy. San Francisco, WH Freeman, 1979. Copyright © 1979; *B,* Courtesy of Dr. Max Listgarten, Philadelphia, PA)

of inheritance clearly established or evident in every example of the disorder.

Normal Variations in Tongue Morphology and Function

Partial Ankyloglossia

Partial ankyloglossia (tongue-tie, see Fig. 10-9) refers to congenital shortness of the lingual frenum or a frenal attachment that extends nearly to the tip of the tongue, binding the tongue to the floor of the mouth and restricting its extension. Because of the imprecise functional definition of this condition, estimates of its prevalence vary from 1 in 250 to 1 in 2500 newborns. Severe degrees of ankyloglossia are easily recognized, and often exhibit a midline mandibular diastema; but milder forms of the condition probably do not represent a pathologic condition and do not influence jaw development, tooth position, or phonation. Requests for treatment of alleged ankyloglossia should be viewed with caution—in many instances, requests for treatment of partial ankyloglossia come from families in which there is evidence of behavioral problems in the parents or child, and the relatively minor but psychologically frightening operation (clipping or snipping the frenum with scissors) may be seen as a

a number of inherited syndromes; and a group of miscellaneous conditions that show evidence of developmental etiology, even though the disorder may not become apparent until late infancy or adolescence. In only a few of these conditions is the exact mode

punitive measure. Reports of partial ankyloglossia affecting several generations suggest a possible genetic basis for this minor variation in the attachment of the geniohyoglossus.

The clinician is better able to make a judgment concerning the need for treatment of a patient with suspected ankyloglossia if he considers the following items: history of poor sucking or inability to chew some foods; recurrent tongue biting; demonstrated inability to clean the teeth and lick the lips with the tongue; speech defects, especially the sounds t, d, n, l in words such as ta, te, time, water, cat; as well as the general intelligibility of the speech. In some instances, speech defects of this type can be handled satisfactorily by a speech therapist without need for cutting the frenum.

Extreme degrees of ankyloglossia occur more rarely and include complete attachment of the tongue to the floor of the mouth or alveolar gingiva, attachment of the tip of the tongue to the hard palate (*glossopalatine ankylosis* or *ankyloglossum superius syndrome,* which is often seen in association with cleft palate), and cases in which the lingual frenum is only one of several grossly hyperplastic frenums present (*e.g.,* orofacial digital syndrome I; also discussed below with tongue clefting syndromes). Ankyloglossia also occurs as a minor finding in the cleft lip–palate–congenital lip pit, cryptophthalmos, trisomy 13, and Pierre Robin syndromes.

Variations in Tongue Movements

The ability to fold and curl or deform the margins of the tongue is apparently under partial genetic control. Ability to curl up the lateral borders of the tongue into a tube is noted in 65% of Caucasians and is inherited as an autosomal dominant trait; less frequent is the ability to fold back the tip of the extended tongue without the aid of the teeth. Other individuals can voluntarily deform the tip of the tongue into a clover-leaf pattern (trefoil tongue), although no clear inheritance pattern has been identified here. Unusual extensibility of the tongue, both forward to touch the tip of the nose (Gorlin sign) and backward into the pharynx, occurs in other-

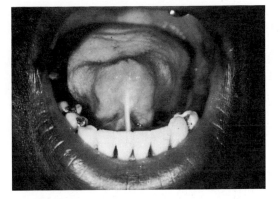

Fig. 10-9 Partial ankyloglossia.

wise normal individuals, as well as in the *Ehlers–Danlos syndrome.* The extreme degrees of extensibility noted in this syndrome are caused by inherited defects in collagen metabolism that affect all tissues and are responsible for the hyperelastic skin, loose jointedness, and more severe cardiovascular and gastrointestinal complications that are also characteristic of the syndrome. The tongue in *tuberous sclerosis* has been described as "long and narrow" as a consequence of hyperostosis and thickening of the mandible but is not abnormally extensible. The mobility of the tongue in *epidermolysis bullosa* may also be severely restricted as a result of fibrous scars secondary to blister formation.

Tongue Thrusting

Tongue thrusting is the positioning of the tongue between the anterior teeth during swallowing, speaking, or at rest. Almost all newborns exhibit this phenomenon, which is therefore referred to as the *infantile swallowing pattern,* to distinguish it from the adult pattern characteristic of the larger adult mandible with a more posteriorly located tongue. The prevalence of tongue thrusting declines to about 3% by 12 years of age, but there are no data to define at what age retention of the infantile swallowing pattern should be considered abnormal. There is considerable controversy regarding the role that persistent tongue thrusting plays in the etiology of anterior open bite, whether the treatment of both the tongue thrusting and the orthodontic anomaly are both necessary to correct the open bite, and whether myofunctional therapy is effective in controlling tongue thrusting. Anterior open bite associated with macroglossia or cerebral palsy should be distinguished from simple tongue thrusting. There is little evidence to suggest that the tongue thrusting habit represents an inherited anomaly or syndrome or that it is other than a variant of the normal developmental process. Anterior open bite secondary to tongue thrusting is a common clinical diagnosis, however, and myofunctional therapy directed to controlling the habit is customarily provided by speech therapists.

Fissured Tongue

Fissured tongue (see Fig. 10-10) occurs as a normal variant affecting less than 10% of the population. Twin studies suggest that it is probably genetically determined, although the frequency of individuals with well-marked fissuring increases with age, as does the number, width, and depth of the fissures in affected individuals. The frequency of fissured tongue has been found to be four to five times greater in institutionalized, mentally retarded and psychotic individuals, a fact at least partly explained by the frequency of fissured tongue in trisomy 21 mongolism. Fissured tongue is also a feature of several

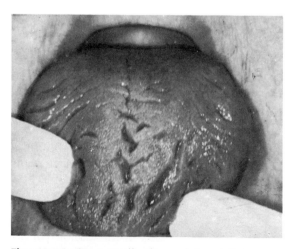

Fig. 10-10 Congenitally fissured (scrotal) tongue. Other members of the same family were similarly affected.

inherited syndromes (see Table 10-3) as well as the Melkersson–Rosenthal syndrome (see Chap. 8). Various terms are used to describe well-accentuated and distinct patterns of fissuring (e.g., plicated, scrotal, or cerebriform tongue), but no good evidence shows that fissuring itself or any one pattern of fissuring is diagnostic of a particular anomaly or disease, various case reports to the contrary.

Increased efforts at tongue hygiene are often prescribed for individuals with fissured tongue who complain of burning or other symptoms (see Chap. 17), on the assumption that bacteria and debris retained in the fissures contribute to the symptoms. While fissured tongues frequently lack the "clean" appearance of nonfissured tongues and are usually redder, no evidence suggests that this represents inflammation or a pathologic condition or that it is the cause of the tongue symptoms. It is customary to separate the walls of deep tongue fissures and examine the base of each fissure for ulcers, nodules, and other lesions when carrying out an oral examination.

Patent Thyroglossal Ducts, Thyroglossal Duct Cyst, and Lingual Thyroid

The thyroid gland develops from an anlage of endothelial cells in the midline of the floor of the pharynx between the first and second branchial arches, just posterior to the future tuberculum impar. These cells sink into the base of the developing tongue, descend into the neck, and proliferate below the larynx to form the thyroid gland. Remnants of epithelium along this path are referred to as the thyroglossal duct. The oropharyngeal opening of this duct is located immediately *behind* the apex of the V-shaped row of vallate papillae and is referred to as the foramen caecum. In the adult, this foramen may or may not be patent as determined by probing. In autopsy specimens, most tongues have a sinuslike defect at this point, but it rarely penetrates beyond the superior longitudinal muscle band. On histologic examination (see Fig. 10-11) it is usually a stratified squamous epithelial-lined tract with or without adjacent lymphoid aggregates and mucous acini. Vallate papillae, taste buds bearing epithelium,

Table 10-3. Inherited and Congenital Syndromes Associated With Particular Tongue Deformities*

DEFORMITY	SYNDROME
Ankyloglossia	Cleft palate–congenital lip pit syndrome Cryptophthalmos syndrome Orofacial digital syndromes I and II
Macroglossia	Lipoid proteinosis† (hyalinosis cutis et mucosa; glycoprotein) Mucolipidosis II† (I cell disease; abnormal lysozymes; see Fig. 8-48) Mucopolysaccharidosis I-H† (Hurler's syndrome; acid mucopolysaccharides, heparan, and dermatan sulfate) Mucopolysaccharidosis II† (Hunter's syndrome; sulfoiduronate sulfatase deficiency) Mucopolysaccharidosis III† (Sanfilippo syndrome; heparin sulfate or n-acetyl D α-D glucosamine) Mucopolysaccharidosis VI† (dermatan sulfate) Gm$_1$ gangliosidosis† (Gm$_1$ ganglioside and keratan sulfate) Fetal face syndrome Macroglossia—omphalocele–visceromegaly (Beckwith's syndrome) Glycogen storage† (Pompe's disease; glycogen) Congenital lymphangioma Trisomy 21 mongolism (Down's syndrome) Cretinism Hemangiomatosis (Sturge-Weber syndrome)
Bald and Depapillated Tongue	Dyskeratosis congenita Epidermolysis bullosa Hyalinosis cutis et mucosa syndrome Endocrine candidosis Familial dysautonomia
Fissured Tongue	Multiple hamartoma and neoplasia syndrome (Cowden's syndrome) Ectrodactyly; ectodermal dysplasia; clefting syndrome Deep midline fissure (Coffee–Lowry syndrome)
Cleft, Bifurcated, and Tetrafurcated Tongue	Fetal face syndrome Meckel's syndrome Orofacial digital syndromes I and II
Long, Narrow, or Hyperextensile Tongue	Tuberous sclerosis Ehlers–Danlos syndrome
Papillomatous Tongue	Meckel's syndrome Congenital lymphangioma Neurofibromatosis Anderson–Fabry syndrome

* The appearance of the tongue alone is usually not diagnostic; however, it may be helpful in determining a range of possible diagnostic categories. The same type of tongue abnormality may also occur as a normal variant or as a result of trauma, infection, or other postdevelopmental event (see text).

† Defined on the nature of the metabolite (listed after the name of the syndrome) accumulating in the affected tissues.

inflammatory cell infiltrates, and oncocytic cells are also occasionally noted in these defects. On rare occasions, sebaceous and apocrine glands and even rudimentary hair follicles have been found on histologic examination of specimens from this region, justifying the term choristoma of the thyroglossal duct. Fungal (*Candida*) colonization of this developmental defect is present in about one half of autopsy specimens.

In about 10% of autopsy specimens, typical colloid-containing, epithelial-lined follicles representing microscopic heterotopic lingual thyroid tissue are found associated with the

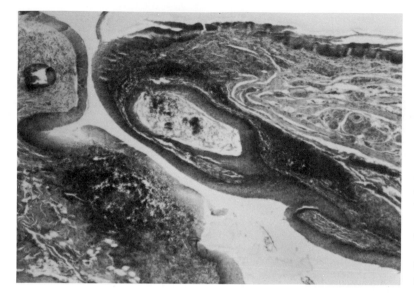

Fig. 10-11 Histologic appearance of the opening of the thyroglossal duct in the region of the foramen cecum of the tongue. Higher power magnification of case illustrated in Fig. 8-31 *C* and *D*. Note squamous epithelium-lined tract with accessory sinuses appearing as cysts in cross-section, and subepithelial lymphoid aggregates. Considerable variation is seen in the histologic appearance of this region; fewer than 10% of autopsy specimens exhibit the typical colloid-containing epithelial rests commonly associated with the term *thyroglossal duct.*

thyroglossal duct. Isotopic studies indicate that approximately 30% of individuals have functioning thyroid tissue along the path of the thyroglossal duct; in 70% of those with heterotopic thyroid, the thyroid gland is contained entirely within the tongue. Enlargement of the lingual thyroid, cystic changes, or malignancy may be first recognized due to symptoms of an enlarging tongue, dysphagia, or less commonly, hypoglossal palsy. Thorough removal of lingual thyroid tissue in such cases will often result in hypothyroidism requiring hormonal supplementation.

Newer diagnostic tools, gray-scale ultrasound, CT scan, and specific localization of functional thyroid tissue with ^{131}I and ^{99m}Tc-pertechnetate scans have greatly improved presurgical evaluation of these problems. The opening of the thyroglossal duct on the surface of the tongue is quite difficult to identify clinically owing to its location. In the absence of cystic degeneration (which may occur anywhere along the length of the thyroglossal duct), the thyroglossal duct usually remains unrecognized.

Median Rhomboid Glossitis

Median rhomboid glossitis describes a rounded or roughly lozenge-shaped, raised area that occurs in the midline of the tongue dorsum just *anterior* to the vallate papillae (see Fig. 10-12). The area is devoid of filiform or other papillae although it may be fissured or lobulated. Histologically, it is characterized by hypoplastic, acanthotic epithelium with elongated rete pegs, a subepithelial chronic inflammatory infiltrate, vascular dilatation and fibrosis, and hyalinization of the underlying muscle. Clinically, it should be differentiated from areas of traumatic depapillation and tumors; concern about the latter often leads to excisional biopsy of the area.

For many years, median rhomboid glossitis was accepted as a developmental anomaly resulting from persistence of the tuberculum impar. Such an explanation is consistent with the common location of these areas, as well as the rare cases that occur somewhat anteriorly but usually still in the midline. The histologic resemblance of these areas to naturally occurring and experimentally induced chronic hyperplastic candidiasis (see Chap. 6) and the demonstration that *Candida* can often be identified in the keratin layer of this area on section or by microbial culture have led to the developmental etiology being discarded by some authors in favor of an infectious origin; however, there appears to be inadequate information available to distinguish between these two proposed etiologies and both developmental and infectious phenomena could be involved. The paucity of

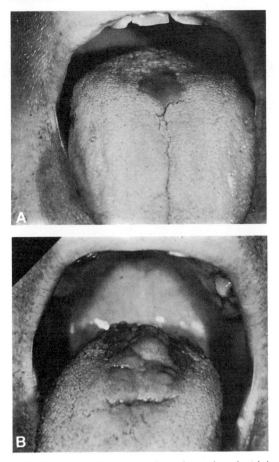

Fig. 10-12 *A,* Small lesion of median rhomboidal glossitis. *B,* Raised and fissured lesion of median rhomboidal glossitis. These are frequently considered to be malignant lesions.

reported cases in neonates and children argues against a solely developmental etiology.

Carcinomatous change in this region is very rare, although the possibility is a prominent concern of patients who have these areas pointed out to them but inadequately explained and those who discover the "lesion" themselves while searching for a cause of burning tongue or other symptoms. Like the other common variants of tongue structure described in this chapter (fissured tongue and geographic tongue), there is no evidence to associate median rhomboid glossitis with symptomatology. The underlying muscular fibrosis and hyalinization described in biopsies of this condition possibly repre-

sent sections of the dorsal submucosal raphe rather than any degenerative change. The traditionally reported male predominance of median rhomboid glossitis is not confirmed by all reported series. A figure of 2% to 3% is usually given for the prevalence of this anomaly.

Major Inherited, Congenital and Developmental Abnormalities

Cleft, Lobed, Bifurcated, and Tetrafurcated Tongues

Separation of the anterior two thirds of the tongue by deep midline or accessory clefts is an unusual though a very distinct malformation, frequently associated with defined congenital syndromes. This type of malformation is characteristic of the *orofacial digital syndromes I and II;* here it occurs in association with ankyloglossia and multiple frenums, and in some cases with small hamartomas in the midline of the ventral surface of the tongue that are composed of fibrous and salivary gland tissues, muscle fibers, and cartilage. Deformities of the eyes, nose, upper lip, palate, and digits are also present. Midline clefting is also a feature of the *fetal face syndrome* and *Meckel's syndrome* (in which the surface of the cleft tongue is also thrown into multiple papilomatous projections). Deep midline fissuring without actual clefting may be seen in other syndromes.

Aglossia, Hypoglossia, and Macroglossia

Aglossia (more accurately, *hypoglossia*) is a rare congenital anomaly usually associated with severe deformation of the limbs and digits (*hypoglossia–hypodactylia syndrome*), in which only a tiny nodule of tongue tissue develops from the copula. Despite the lack of a functional tongue and associated multiple oral anomalies, the speech of these patients is usually said to be not severely impaired.

Macroglossia is a component of numerous syndromes, most of them associated with inborn metabolic anomalies in which the increase in tongue size is caused by deposit of unusual lipid or carbohydrate intermediates in the tongue. In all cases, other abnormalities accompany the macroglossia. Eight syndromes of this type are listed in Table 10-3. Other inherited syndromes with macroglossia that do not have a specified genetically determined metabolic basis include the *fetal face syndrome* (which is associated with tongue clefting) and the *macroglossia–omphalocele–visceromegaly syndrome (Beckwith's syndrome)* in which high birth-weight, umbilical hernia, enlargement of the viscera, and linear indentations in the earlobe are associated with macroglossia.

Because the tongue is a mobile muscular organ of variable size, it has been difficult in many cases to distinguish between macroglossia caused by increase in tongue muscle bulk and apparent macroglossia, or the basis of poor muscular control. Tongue size may be accurately estimated now with ultrasound techniques, and the question whether the protruding tongue characteristically associated with trisomy 21 mongolism (Down's syndrome), cretinism, and the storage diseases just mentioned is caused by increased tongue bulk can be answered.

By far, the most common cause of congenital macroglossia is a *lymphangioma* (or *hemangio–lymphangioma*) restricted to the tongue or in continuity with a *cystic hygroma* of the neck (see Chap. 8). The surface of tongues so affected is usually nodular and very irregular. Persistent enlargement of the tongue results in pressure deformities of the dentition and dental arches. This secondary abnormality is seen commonly in Down's syndrome and where larger tongue masses are left untreated for some time, as is often the case with hemangiomas or other tongue anomalies associated with mental retardation. Macroglossia is also a feature of *acromegaly* (caused by excessive production of growth hormone in the fully mature adult) and commonly leads to distortion of the mandibular arch even though the space between the two bodies of the mandible is also increasing by deposition of new bone at the condylar growth centers.

Hamartomas and Dermoids

The tongue may be enlarged or distorted by the presence of a variety of tumorlike growths of developmental origin (hamarto-mas—*neurofibromas, hemangiomas*) or by epithelial inclusion cysts (*dermoids and branchial cleft cysts*). While the origin of these is developmental, they may not become apparent until adolescence or later because of increased secretory activity of glandular tissue or to cystic degeneration of the epithelial remnants. Dermoids are rarely found in the tongue (where they are described as *median lingual cysts*), although they may extend into or distort the tongue by extension from their usual location in the floor of the mouth or neck (see Chap. 8 for additional description).

Bald or Depapillated Tongues

Atrophy of the filiform papillae as a result of iron or vitamin deficiency is discussed in the following section under the heading of glossitis. Depapillation or absence of papillae may also be caused by a congenital anomaly, or develop as a secondary feature. In *familial dysautonomia* (Riley–Day syndrome), there is congenital absence of both fungiform and vallate papillae as well as a variety of neurologic abnormalities resulting in vasomotor problems, absent reflexes, feeding difficulties, and diminished pain and taste sensation. The filiform papillae that are not dependent on the 7th and 9th cranial nerve innervation for their development are unaffected. Loss of papillae secondary to congenital anomalies that result in scarring of the tongue dorsum occurs in *epidermolysis bullosa, dyskeratosis congenita, endocrine candidosis,* and *hyalinosis cutis et mucosa* syndromes.

Papillomatous Changes

In several congenital disorders the surface of the tongue is covered with multiple papillomas. When extensive, this abnormality is referred to as a *pebbly tongue*. Lesions of this type are associated with congenital, lingual *lymphangiomas, neurofibromatosis,* and the *Anderson–Fabry* syndrome and *Meckel's* syndrome. Similar appearances may develop in adults, but usually on a basis of a chronic granulomatous infection or allergic response (*e.g., Melkersson–Rosenthal* syndrome, *acanthosis nigricans, leprosy*) or a familial predisposition (*e.g., multiple mucosal neuroma* syndrome; see Chap. 8). In some cases, the multiple tongue nodules are irregular in size, and the terms *cobblestoned* or *lumpy* are used.

DISORDERS OF THE LINGUAL MUCOSA

Despite its heavily keratinized dorsal surface, the mucosa of the tongue is affected by the same inflammatory and degenerative processes that occur elsewhere in the oral cavity. In addition, the filiform papillae respond to a number of systemic and local physical factors that have less dramatic effect on the nonkeratinized oral mucosa. The term *glossitis* is frequently used to describe tongue changes, particularly those in which portions of the tongue appear denuded or redder than usual. Use of the term does not necessarily imply a primary inflammatory process in all cases. Changes in the surface of the tongue are usually associated with alteration of the microbial flora of the tongue dorsum. Not uncommonly, secondary inflammatory changes occur as a consequence of this changed microbial flora and superficial bacterial or fungal invasion of the mucosal barrier rather than as part of the primary disorder.

Disorders of the lingual mucosa will be discussed under the following headings: Changes in the Tongue Papillae, including keratotic and nonkeratotic white lesions; Depapillation and Atrophic Lesions; Pigmentations; Ulcers and Infectious Disease; Superficial Vascular Changes; and Disorders of the Lingual Mucosal Glands. Where the tongue lesion differs only slightly from similar lesions that commonly occur elsewhere in the mouth, discussion will be brief and the reader should refer to appropriate sections of Chapters 5, 6, and 7.

Changes in the Tongue Papillae

Geographic Tongue

Geographic tongue (benign migratory glossitis; see Fig. 10-13) refers to irregularly shaped, reddish areas of depapillation and thinning of the dorsal tongue epithelium that are usually surrounded by a narrow zone of regenerating papillae that is whiter than the surrounding tongue surface. Spontaneous development and regeneration of affected areas accounts for the terms *wandering rash*, *migratory glossitis*, and *geographic tongue*. Figures of 1% to 2% or even higher are usually quoted for the prevalence of this condition. It is often accompanied by minor variations in tongue structure, such as fissured tongue, irregularities at the junction of dorsal and ventral epithelium along the tongue margins, and even isolated patches of keratinized epithelium below this junction. Histologically, sections that include both the white and red areas show papillae of variable height with some submucosal round cell infiltration, as well as areas of spongiotic epithelium with localized intraepithelial infiltrates of polymorphonuclear leukocytes, the so-called intraepithelial spongiotic pustules, or Monro's abscesses. Clinically and histologically similar lesions also occur in Reiter's syndrome, dermatitis herpetiformis, and pustular psoriatic dermatitis.

Lesions are not always restricted to the tongue, and similar irregular or circinate lesions occurring elsewhere in the oral cavity are referred to as *ectopic geographic tongue*, *erythema circinata migrans*, or *annulus migrans*. Because these also contain the characteristic spongiotic pustules, they are sometimes diagnosed as "compatible with" Reiter's syndrome or psoriatic stomatitis.

The etiology of geographic tongue remains obscure, and the existence of similar lesions in association with other dermatoses only confuses the issue. An immunologic reaction has been proposed on the basis of the associated inflammatory infiltrate that may on occasion be dominated by eosinophils. The same infiltrate is said to justify an allergic etiology when considered along with the results of surveys showing a higher incidence of atopic predisposition (increased serum IgE, associated hay fever, asthma, and eczematous dermatitis) in patients with geographic tongue and their families. No particular inheritance pattern has been established. Based on interviews and psychometric evaluation of college students with and without geographic tongue, a personality type character-

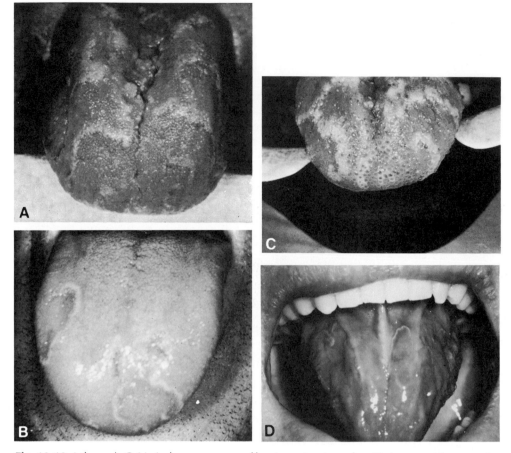

Fig. 10-13 *A* through *C*, Varied appearances of benign migratory glossitis (geographic tongue). Note irregularly shaped depapillated areas outlined by a zone of regenerating papillae. Fungiform papillae are readily distinguished in some of these atrophic areas as a result of atrophy of the surrounding carpet of filiform papillae. *D*, Lesions of erythema circinata migrans on the ventral surface of the tongue; patient had characteristic lesions of geographic tongue on the dorsum and lesions similar to these on both cheeks.

ized as "more prone to complain or verbalize discomfort" has been associated with the lesion of geographic tongue, independent of whether the lesion was associated with symptoms. On this basis and the exaggerated fear of oral cancer that is often expressed by patients with geographic tongue, a psychosomatic background has been cited. Specific interaction between emotional state and tongue papillation has not been identified, other than reports of more active-appearing lesions in patients with geographic tongue when they are exposed to psychological stress. Psychotropic medications do not affect

tongue papillation or eliminate the lesions, although they will reduce muscular tension in the tongue and any tendency to crenation of the margins against the dental arch.

Controversy exists as to whether the lesions of geographic tongue are ever symptomatic. Symptoms of burning, stinging and pain are often reported by patients who are noted to have geographic tongue lesions, but in many cases this is probably caused by chance association, in the same way that fissured tongue and median rhomboid glossitis are sometimes reported to be symptomatic (see also discussion of glossodynia in Chap.

17). Treatment of geographic tongue, where attempted for the control of chronic burning pain or other oral sensory abnormality, usually consists of the application of topical local anesthetic agents of the lidocaine variety or aqueous antihistamines such as 0.5% aqueous dyclonine hydrochloride or diphenhydramine, administered as a mouth rinse over crushed ice before meals. Transient anesthesia of the mucous membrane is obtained, which some patients find preferable to the burning sensations and other irritations reportedly caused by spicy or hot foods.

Cautious topical applications of salicylic acid and tretinoin (retinoic acid or vitamin A acid), which are sold in a variety of commercial preparations for the treatment of acne, have been recommended by some authors as an effective means of eliminating lesions (and symptoms) of geographic tongue. Because these preparations are usually specified for external use only, they should be applied to the tongue sparingly with a cotton applicator and only with informed patient consent. There is currently no justification for the use of systemic preparations of 13-cis-retinoic acid* (which have recently been approved as an acceptable systemic inhibitor of sebum formation in patients with severe cystic acne) in the treatment of geographic tongue. Side-effects of this systemic medication are common and do not warrant its use for the treatment of geographic tongue, until there is better understanding of the effect of topically applied tretinoin on geographic tongue.

Coated or Hairy Tongue

In health, the heavily keratinized surface layers of the filiform papillae are continuously desquamated through friction of the tongue with food, the palate, and the upper anterior teeth and are replaced by new epithelial cells from below. When tongue movements are limited by illness or painful oral conditions, the filiform papillae lengthen and become heavily coated with bacteria and fungi (see Fig. 10-14). The longer papillae give the

tongue a coated or hairy appearance and retain debris and pigments from substances such as food, tobacco smoke, and candy. These changes primarily affect the middorsum of the tongue, which often becomes discolored in a very startling way. Extreme degrees of this phenomenon occurring in dehydrated, debilitated, terminally ill patients can lead to very thick, leathery coatings on the tongue that are referred to as "earthy" or "encrusted" tongue (see Fig. 10-15).

Because such changes in the tongue coating are evident to any observer and are associated at times with systemic illness, they were once looked upon as a mirror of general health status. While depapillation may result from general metabolic abnormality, there appears to be no evidence that increase in the length of the filiform papillae or the halitosis that often accompanies it is anything other than the result of local oral environmental changes. The condition known as black hairy tongue that can be induced in dogs by nicotinamide deficiency is apparently not documented in man, even though both humans with pellagra (see discussion under Depapillation and Atrophic Lesions) and dogs develop stomatitis and glossitis as a result of this nutritional deficiency.

The likelihood of developing hairy tongue is increased with use of a number of local and systemic medications, probably as a result of secondary changes in the oral microbial flora. These include systemic antibiotics, topical hydrogen peroxide, perborate, and similar oxidizing agents used in some mouth rinses.

Thorough cleaning and scraping of the tongue, application of topical keratolytic agents, and prescription of yogurt or other *Lactobacillus acidophilus* cultures have been used in the treatment of this problem; however, the affected papillae usually rapidly return to normal when antibiotic treatment is discontinued and normal jaw and tongue activity is restored. The old distinction made between true hairy tongue and pseudo-hairy tongue (a stained coating on the tongue dorsum without extreme elongation of the filiform papillae; at one time thought to be produced by a change in the tongue microbial flora) appears to have disappeared from the

---

* Accutane brand of isotretinoin, Roche Laboratories, Nutley, NJ 07110

literature. Both lack of function and changes in the flora probably play a role in the etiology of this condition.

Nonkeratotic and Keratotic White Lesions

As discussed in Chapter 6, the diagnosis of white lesions of the oral cavity is commonly restricted to a small number of standard lesions (for example, candidiasis, lichen planus, leukoplakia, white sponge nevus, lupus), which are identified on a combination of clinical and histopathologic features, in some cases with the assistance of immunofluorescence techniques. These diagnoses are often equivocal and even inaccurate when they fail to consider the wide range of disorders in which white lesions of the oral cavity have been described. This situation is par-

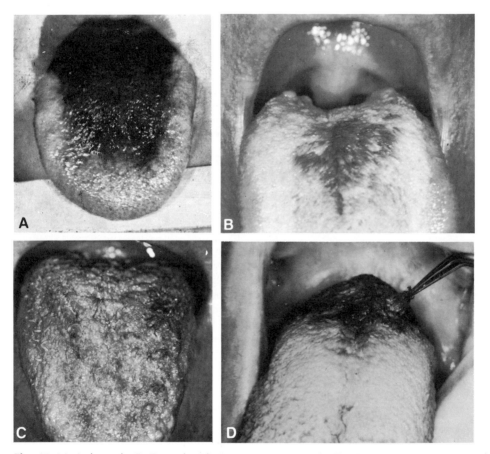

Fig. 10-14 *A* through *C,* Coated or hairy tongue. *A,* Markedly discolored tongue resulting from the use of hydrogen peroxide, chromic acid, and potassium permanganate during treatment of fusospirochetal gingivitis. *B,* Hypertrophy of the filiform papillae with secondary discoloration; note vallate papillae visible posteriorly near the lateral margins of the tongue. *C,* Brown, discolored, abnormally coated tongue developed following a course of penicillin therapy. *D,* Elongated and discolored filiform papillae well justifying the term *black hairy tongue.*

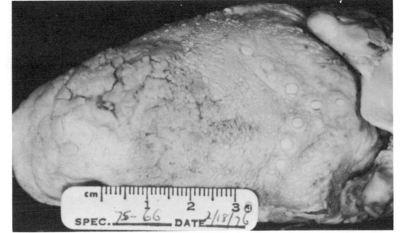

Fig. 10-15 An "encrusted" tongue with thick microbial deposits on its dorsal surface noted at autopsy in a 54-year-old woman dying with a multifocal necrotizing bronchopneumonia with cavitation. Demonstration of *Candida* sp. in this deposit and in the lung lesions suggests the possibility that the pneumonia resulted from aspiration of pieces of this membrane.

ticularly true of white lesions of the tongue, where the clinical and histopathologic appearances of the lesion are further compounded by the heavily keratinized papillary structure of the tongue dorsum and the effect of the adherent microbial flora. For many patients with chronic white lesions of the tongue, specific diagnoses are often not established despite multiple biopsies and studies, particularly if the tongue lesion is not accompanied by similar changes elsewhere on the oral mucosa. Superinfection with *Candida* species also commonly occurs with most keratotic lesions of the tongue, and an initial period of treatment with a topical antifungal agent often significantly alters the clinical and histopathologic picture of the lesion and may make specific diagnosis easier.

Nonkeratotic White Lesions

Thrush. Thrush (acute pseudomembranous candidiasis; see Fig. 10-16) often appears as the classical pearly white, pinhead-sized flecks scattered over the dorsal surface. Microscopic examination of smears prepared from these soft flecks should reveal large numbers of yeasts and pseudomycelia. Lesions of this type are often seen in immunosuppressed patients, in patients on corticosteroids or cholinergic medications, in patients with xerostomia from other causes, and in neonates.

Burns. The thick, keratinized dorsal surface of the tongue with an adherent coat of saliva is more resistant to chemical and thermal burns than are thinner, drier areas of the mucosa, such as the palate. Patients who scald or burn their tongues on hot foods may well experience some persistent pain and hypersensitivity of the tongue, but rarely exhibit any lesion except at the tip of the tongue, unless the burn is of sufficient intensity to necrose the surface tissues. Examples of the latter are the severe burns caused by electric contacts and ingestion of lye. Before sloughing of the dead tissue, the burned area often becomes white and leathery (see Fig. 10-17).

White Sponge Nevus and Pachyonychia Congenita. White sponge nevus and pachyonychia congenita (see Chap. 6) are inherited anomalies in which the surface of the tongue as well as other parts of the oral mucosa are involved by white spongy plaques without significant hyperkeratosis; the white appearance is probably caused by fluid absorption by the thickened spongiotic surface layers of the mucosa.

Vesiculobullous and Other Desquamating Disorders. While not usually considered under the heading of white lesions, desquamating disorders are often mistakenly identified as white lesions because of the coalescence of areas of whitish desquamating

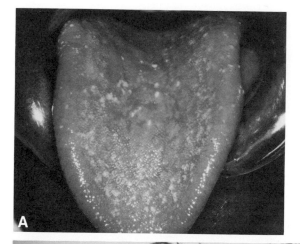

epithelium with areas of papillary atrophy and scarring. Patches of regenerating papillae may also be interspersed, giving the tongue an overall picture of alternating red and white areas in a marblelike pattern. Changes such as these are often observed in patients with well-established, *benign mucous membrane pemphigoid* and *bullous* and *erosive lichen planus* (see below), as well as those with congenital disorders associated with friable and desquamating mucosa (*e.g., epidermolysis bullosa* and *acrodermatitis enteropathica*). Secondary infection with *Candida* species is usual in these disorders and contributes to the appearance of the oral lesions.

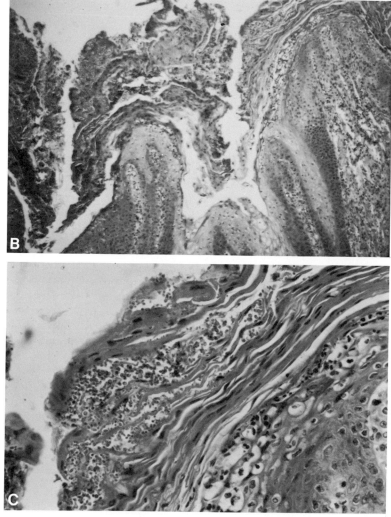

Fig. 10-16 *A,* Soft, pearly white, easily dislodged plaques constitute the lesions of thrush on the tongue of a woman maintained on long-term corticosteroid therapy for idiopathic thrombocytopenic purpura. *B* and *C,* Histologic examination of lesions of thrush reveals layers of keratin, fibrin, yeasts, and cellular exudate closely applied to the tongue papillae, with an underlying acute mucosal inflammatory response. Lesions illustrated in *B* and *C* were noted at autopsy in an 80-year-old woman dying with confluent bronchopneumonia consistent with aspiration of both *Candida* sp. and coliform bacteria.

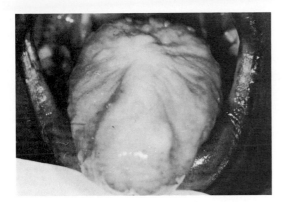

Fig. 10-17 Lye burn of tongue in 12-year-old boy.

Keratotic White Lesions

Lichen Planus. Lacelike, erosive and bullous varieties of this disorder may affect the tongue in addition to the cheeks, lips, and gingivae. Lesions on the tongue may exhibit characteristic clinical appearances and appear similar to those on the cheeks (see Fig. 6-41). On occasion, the lesions in only one location are characteristic, and the diagnosis is made on that basis, with the assumption that lesions in other areas are variants of the same disorder. Chronic lichen planus often leads to considerable atrophy and scarring of the tongue dorsum, making the lesions indistinguishable both clinically and histologically from a number of other atrophic lesions of the tongue (see below).

Leukoplakia. (See Fig. 6-26.) The problems associated with the varied usages of the term *leukoplakia* as a clinical and microscopic diagnosis are discussed in Chapter 6. For the reasons outlined at the beginning of this section, leukoplakia is often the diagnosis by exclusion used for many keratotic tongue lesions that have no other specific identity even after histologic examination. Irrespective of the term used to describe the lesion, it is important to know whether there is any evidence of dysplastic change in any of the tissue available for biopsy examination and whether these tissue samples are representative of the entire lesion; whether there is any laboratory evidence of syphilis or diabetes; the extent to which the patient consumes alcohol and smokes, and whether there is any evidence of cirrhosis. Depending on the answers to these questions, management of the lesion can be conservative, or total excision of the lesion may be advisable.

In the literature before about 1950, leukoplakia of the tongue appeared as a prevalent and important lesion (see earlier editions of this textbook). In at least two surveys based on material submitted for histopathologic diagnosis published since that time, the tongue is described as being relatively infrequently involved by leukoplakia in comparison with the buccal mucosa and alveolar ridges, for example. It is not clear whether this represents a change in prevalence or whether it simply reflects changing custom in the use of the term *leukoplakia* in describing keratotic tongue lesions. *Because of the greater frequency of oral carcinoma on the lateral margins and ventral surface of the tongue, leukoplakia in these regions should be evaluated very carefully and repeatedly on regular follow-up visits if the lesion cannot be excised completely.*

Depapillation and Atrophic Lesions

Localized or more extensive loss of the papillae from the anterior two thirds of the tongue may result from a number of causes: chronic trauma, nutritional deficiency and hematologic abnormalities, medications, and peripheral vascular disease. Diabetes and chronic candidiasis are associated with a condition referred to as *central papillary atrophy* or *atrophic glossitis*, although it is not clear whether the *Candida* infection is a primary or secondary etiologic factor. Long-standing lichen planus, tertiary syphilis, lupus and scleroderma, and a number of congenital anomalies (see previous section) are associated with extensive scarring of the submucosal tissues and atrophy of the underlying papillae. An unusual chronic sclerosing disorder affecting the oral mucosa, pharynx, and esophagus that is referred to as *oral submucous fibrosis* has been described as having a prevalence of 0.2% to 0.5% in some communities in India. The etiology of this disorder, which may predispose to extensive leukoplakia, is not known. Long-standing xerostomia (drug- or radiation-induced, or as a result of Sjögren's syndrome) is also associated with atrophy of tongue papillae.

Chronic Trauma. Localized areas of depapillation are often noted on the tongue in association with jagged teeth or rough margins of restorations, and there is usually evidence of papillary regeneration around these areas. In patients hypersensitive to eugenol, an area of depapillation matching the location of a temporary dressing may occur. Inadvertent contact of the tongue with dental medicaments such as phenol may be followed by temporary local depapillation.

Nutritional Deficiencies and Hematologic Abnormalities. Redness, loss of papillae, and painful swelling of the tongue are characteristically found in *deficiencies of several B vitamins*—niacin (pellagra), riboflavin (ariboflavinosis), pyridoxine, folic acid, and vitamin B_{12} (pernicious anemia, sprue; see Fig. 10-18). Similar changes are also associated with *iron deficiency.* Each of these factors is involved in the production of both epithelial cells and erythrocytes, and manifestations of the deficiency affect other mucosal surfaces, skin, circulating erythrocytes, and bone marrow, as well as the tongue papillae. Various changes occur in other organs also. Deficiencies of one of these factors alone rarely occurs on the basis of a dietary deficiency, although specific deficiencies may result from *malabsorption syndrome* (pernicious anemia, sprue) or from *drug-conditioned deficiencies* (*e.g.,* isoniazid and pyridoxine deficiency). Excessive loss of iron as well as deficient intake is usually involved in iron-deficiency states. The term *atrophic glossitis* is commonly used to describe the appearance of the tongue that results from these various nutritional deficiencies and hematologic abnormalities.

Various descriptive terms (*e.g.,* "raw," "beefy," "magenta," or "bright red" tongue; Hunter's glossitis) have been used to describe the tongue with atrophic glossitis, and at one time the appearance of the tongue was considered to be reasonably specific for particular vitamin deficiencies. The appearance of the tongue with atrophic glossitis is probably conditioned by other factors associated with these deficiency states (*e.g.,* secondary candidiasis) and by itself does not provide adequate information for an accurate diagnosis. Hematologic studies (CBC and differential, total iron-binding capacity, and serum iron level), as well as measurement of circulating levels of specific vitamins, where indicated by abnormal hematologic values, are needed. As discussed in Chapters 3 and 22, it is important to realize that iron deficiency (sideropenia) can exist in the face of normal hemoglobin and erythrocytic values because iron stores have to be drastically reduced before signs of anemia develop.

Sideropenic anemia shares the features of atrophic glossitis, angular cheilitis, generalized atrophic oral muscosa, oral ulcerations, and secondary candidiasis with the other classical deficiency states listed above; in addition, it may be accompanied by dysphagia and predisposition to oropharyngeal carcinoma. In this well-developed form, apparently more common in women of northern European descent, it is referred to as the *Plummer–Vinson syndrome* or *Paterson–Kelly syndrome.* Associated signs to be noted in this syndrome are thin, narrow lips with a narrow orifice; pale, dry atrophic skin; brittle and spoon-shaped fingernails (koilonychia); and possibly dryness and atrophic changes of the conjunctiva and vaginal and anal mucosae. Differential diagnosis from Sjögren's syndrome (which carries its own risk of predisposition to lymphoma rather than carcinoma) is important.

Prevalence rates for esophageal, pharyngeal, and oral carcinoma (in order of decreasing importance) are increased in individuals with the Plummer–Vinson syndrome. The majority of surveys of this disorder were carried out in Scandinavia before 1940; compulsory addition of iron to bread at that time was apparently responsible for a greatly decreased prevalence of this problem.

In many cases, depapillation of the tongue and atrophic glossitis resolve completely following administration of the appropriate factor or correction of a malabsorption problem. Pernicious anemia is classically associated with atrophic gastritis, folic acid and vitamin B_{12} deficiencies, ileitis, or surgical bypasses involving portions of the small intestine concerned with absorption of these factors. Recently, glossitis and other signs accompanying vitamin B_{12} deficiency anemia have also

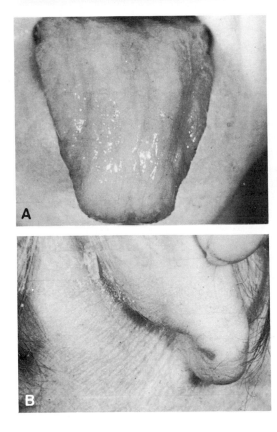

Fig. 10-18 The tongue and vitamin deficiencies. *A* and *B,* Smooth, red, painful tongue in patient with vitamin B-complex deficiency associated with a scaly dermatitis evident here behind the ear. *C,* Acute glossitis with ulceration in a patient with pellagra. *D,* Early tongue changes in niacin deficiency. *E,* Bald red tongue in patient with pernicious anemia. (*C,* Courtesy of J. H. Stine, D.D.S., Bryn Mawr, PA)

been noted as a complication in patients undergoing surgical stapling of the stomach for treatment of morbid obesity.

The frequency with which vitamin or iron deficiency underlies complaints of burning or painful tongue is low, at least from the perspective of the oral consultant. There is no doubt that atrophic glossitis associated with nutritional deficiency is associated with symptoms of this type, but the general availability of multivitamins and publicity given over the years to their association with tongue symptoms usually result in early treatment of the deficiency by the primary care physician or internist. Exceptions are those cases in which sideropenia has gone unnoticed because of normal hemoglobin levels or where an unusual malabsorption problem is involved. The main danger associated with indiscriminate administration of multivitamins and vitamin B_{12} for the treatment of glossodynia in the absence of atrophic glossitis or adequate hematologic evaluation is that accurate diagnosis of an anemia becomes impossible, and problems requiring specific therapy (*e.g.*, pernicious anemia with its neurologic complications) may be overlooked.

In vitamin B_{12} deficiency and other macrocytic anemias, changes analogous to those occurring in the erythrocyte series (see Chaps. 3 and 22) have been demonstrated in buccal mucosal cells by exfoliative cytology; presumably, similar changes affect the lingual mucosa and underlie atrophic glossitis. The literature states that the filiform papillae are most susceptible to nutritional deficiency and disappear first, followed by the fungiform papillae; regeneration occurring in the reverse order. Vallate and foliate papillae on the posterior third are stated not to be affected; however, these statements have apparently not been tested with detailed documentation or modern techniques using electron microscopy or psychophysical and other measures of lingual sensory function. In view of the increased susceptibility of the pharyngeal mucosa to dysplastic change with iron deficiency, it seems unlikely that mucosal changes are restricted to reduction in the height of the filiform papillae.

Medications. Depapillation of the tongue has been described as a side-effect of a number of medications, usually antibiotics, cancer chemotherapeutic agents, or anticholinergic agents. In these cases mechanisms similar to those described above (inhibition of epithelial reproduction, secondary candidiasis, and the effects of chronic xerostomia) are probably involved.

Peripheral Vascular Disease. Decreased nutritional status of the lingual papillae as a result of vascular changes affecting the subpapillary dorsal capillary plexus or lingual vessels supplying it presumably underlies the atrophic glossitis sometimes seen in diabetes. Fibrosis of the submucosal tissues secondary to obliteration of small vessels by an autoimmune process is responsible for the scarred, shrunken, and atrophic appearance of the tongue in scleroderma. In lupus erythematosus, isolated irregular areas of lingual mucosal atrophy and ulceration are caused by the arteritis that along with specific immunologic tests provides histologic confirmation of this disease when it affects the lingual mucosa.

With increasing use of newer microvascular diagnostic techniques, additional information about the role of blood flow in maintaining the normal dorsal lingual mucosa is expected. Studies to date using fluorescence-enhanced capillary microscopy in humans have documented variations in the fungiform papillae associated with age, sex, and the number and shape of terminal vessels in the papillae, as well as changes following section of the chorda tympani. Susceptibility of the superficial lingual capillary plexus and taste sensitivity to increased barometric pressure have also been described as well as alterations in the superficial capillaries of the fungiform papillae in diabetes. Scanning electron microscopic observation of the filiform papillae has also revealed changes associated with congenital heart disease.

Infarcts of the tongue (see also below under Diseases Affecting the Body of the Tongue) may be associated with shrinkage of the affected side of the tongue and atrophic changes in the overlying mucosa.

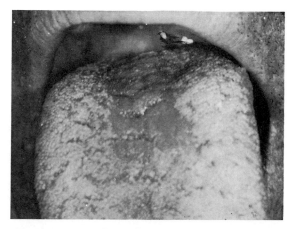

Fig. 10-19 Central papillary atrophy of the tongue. A condition that is poorly distinguished from median rhomboid glossitis and like it has been etiologically associated with chronic candidiasis.

Diabetes and Chronic Candidiasis. Considerable debate in recent years has centered about the role of chronic candidiasis and diabetes in central papillary atrophy of the dorsum, a condition in which a relatively large area of low, flat papillae or completely atrophic papillae is noted in the middorsum of the tongue anterior to the row of vallate papillae and often with minimal changes in the more marginal dorsal tongue mucosa (see Fig. 10-19). Both diabetes and chronic candidiasis have been identified as the cause of this lesion, based on the frequency of blood sugar abnormalities in affected individuals and demonstration of *Candida* in biopsy specimens and on culture of the lesion. Associated findings of denture stomatitis and angular cheilitis are also cited in support of a fungal etiology, together with the existence of similar lesions in patients with the endocrine candidiasis syndrome and demonstration of localized depapillation in rats with experimentally induced candidiasis as a result of tetracycline administration. Epidemiologic studies alone are unlikely to solve this debate, and the possibility of increased prevalence of oral *Candida* infections in diabetics (another unproven association) suggests that *Candida* play an important role as secondary invaders here, as they probably do in a large number of chronic oral mucosal disorders.

The dorsal submucosal raphe is also frequently more prominent and hyalinized in tongues exhibiting central papillary atrophy, and the role of this structure and changes in the vascular plexuses surrounding it in this condition should be more fully explored (see Fig. 10-20).

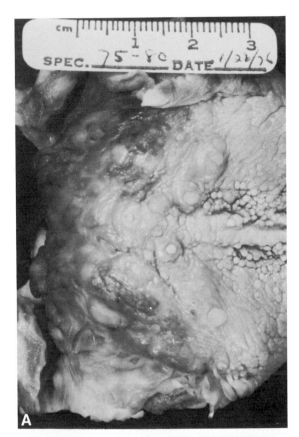

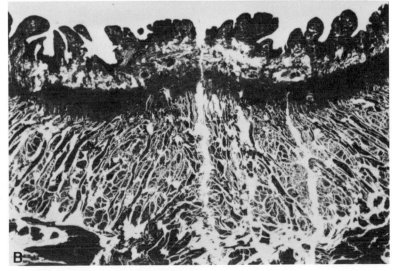

Fig. 10-20 *A,* Tongue of an 80-year-old male exhibiting an atrophic depressed area anterior to the row of vallate papillae. *B,* Thickened, hyalinized dorsal raphe and shrunken overlying papillae seen in vertical section through this area.

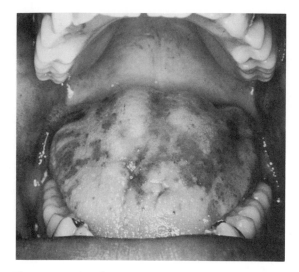

Fig. 10-21 An otherwise normal tongue showing an unusual pattern of melanin pigmentation with no diagnostic significance.

Tertiary Syphilis and Interstitial Glossitis. The tongue in tertiary syphilis may be affected by gumma formation or a more diffuse chronic granulomatous lesion referred to as *interstitial glossitis*. Tongues affected in this way are said to exhibit "nonulcerating, irregular indurations with an asymmetric pattern of grooves alternating with leukoplakia and smooth (atrophic) fields covering the entire dorsum." "Initially the tongue is often enlarged but later can undergo marked shrinkage" (see Fig. 28-15). Syphilitic interstitial glossitis occurs predominantly in males, and affected individuals have a one in three chance of developing squamous cell carcinoma. With the decreased prevalence of tertiary syphilis in many countries, this condition is now only rarely described. Routine laboratory testing for evidence of active syphilis is still indicated in patients (particularly males) with leukoplakia and atrophic glossitis, however, and special attention should be given to the regular follow-up examination of males with persistently positive serologic tests for syphilis and white or atrophic tongue lesions to check for possible carcinomatous change. Carcinoma developing on the dorsum of the tongue in a patient with interstitial glossitis appears to be an exception to the general finding that carcinoma of the tongue is rare on the dorsum.

Pigmentation

The tongue may exhibit various patterns of racial melanin pigmentation (see Fig. 10-21), although the deposits observed in man are minimal compared with the extensive, patchy melanin deposits occurring in other species, including nonhuman primates. Endogenous pigmentation is rarely identifiable on the dorsum because of the thickness of the epithelium, but jaundice may be apparent under the thinner ventral mucosa. Exogenous pigmentation of the filiform papillae of the normal and coated or hairy tongue is very common and results from microbial growth and metabolic products, food debris, and dyes from candy, beverages, and mouth rinses. Tattooing of the lateral margins and ventral surface of the tongue is not uncommon as a result of deposits of amalgam and other metals from lacerations during dental treatment.

Pigmentation of the tongue and other oral mucous membranes has been described with a commonly used cancer chemotherapeutic agent, doxorubicin hydrochloride,* which also discolors the patient's urine and sometimes the nail beds and skin folds. As it is not an antimicrobial agent, this discoloration is probably not caused by changes in the tongue flora and may represent absorption of a colored compound by keratin as occurs in carotinemia.

Extravasation of red cells around lingual varicosities may give a patchy, bluish red discoloration, usually to the anterior ventral surface of the tongue. The thin tissue overlying a ranula is said to have a greenish blue appearance.

Ulcers and Infectious Diseases

Ulceration of the tongue may result from an extremely wide variety of physical and infectious agents, acting on either the normal mucosa or the mucosa that has been already damaged by atrophic changes, vesiculobullous disease, or immunologic reactions. The mobility of the tongue and its close association with the dentition and dental prostheses

* Adriamycin, Adria Laboratories, Inc, 5000 Post Road, Dublin, Ohio 43017

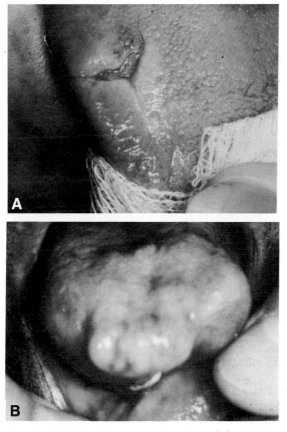

Fig. 10-22 *A,* Healing traumatic ulcer of the tongue in a 15-year-old epileptic caused by inadvertent biting of the tongue during a seizure. *B,* Badly scarred and deformed tongue in an older epileptic.

normal individuals, rough surfaces on restorations and jagged, broken cusps rapidly cause ulceration of the tongue if they are in a position that the tongue cannot avoid. As in the case of ulcers associated with chronic trauma elsewhere on the oral mucosa, adequate follow-up should be established following elimination of the suspected irritant whenever there is suspicion that a chronic ulcer may be a malignant lesion (Fig. 10-23). Inflammatory hyperplasias (fibromas) often develop on the dorsal or ventral surfaces of the tongue as a response to chronic irritation or biting trauma (Fig. 10-24).

The fimbriated folds on either side of the lingual frenum and the openings of the submandibular and sublingual glands are especially liable to be aspirated during dental procedures with resultant ulceration and ecchymosis (see Fig. 10-25); the lateral margins and ventral surface of the tongue are also frequently damaged by contact with rapidly revolving burs, discs, or other dental equipment. Ulcers of the lingual frenum in neonates with natal lower incisors are referred to as Riga's ulcers or Riga–Fede disease and are caused by abrasion of the tongue by

contribute to its susceptibility to physical trauma, which together with the mixed oral flora play important roles in the etiology of all tongue ulcers.

Quite severe ulcers, which are more in the nature of lacerations and contusions, are produced by sudden biting trauma, either during an epileptic seizure (see Fig. 10-22) or as a result of a sudden blow to the jaw while the tongue lies between the upper and lower teeth. More chronic ulcers of the same type are seen in patients with uncontrolled grinding and chewing movements as a result of ischemic or other brain damage. Special "tongue-depressing splints" that remove the tongue from the occlusal table are sometimes needed to prevent extensive tongue damage in these patients. Because of the more or less continuous activity of the tongue, even in

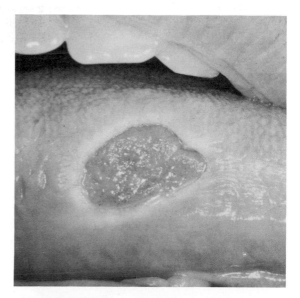

Fig. 10-23 Chronic, nonhealing ulcer resulting from treatment of a traumatic ulcer with aspirin-containing chewing gum. The clinical appearance of this ulcer would strongly suggest a malignant lesion, although in this case prompt healing occurred on discontinuing the aspirin-containing gum.

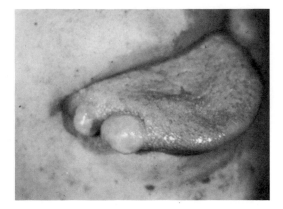

Fig. 10-24 Fibromas developing following tongue trauma.

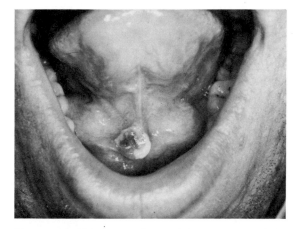

Fig. 10-25 Traumatic ulcer of the junction of the frenum and lingual folds caused by a saliva ejector.

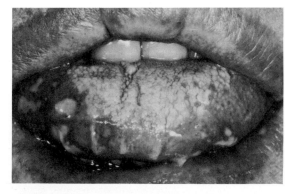

Fig. 10-26 Severe recurrent aphthous ulcers involving the tongue and other oral mucous membranes.

the teeth during suckling. The benefits of breast feeding are sufficiently important to justify extraction of natal teeth even though they are only rarely supernumeraries.

Shallow but persistent tongue ulcers, especially along the posterior ventral surfaces, are common in *patients with lichen planus, the various nutritional deficiencies* and *hematologic problems* described above under Depapillation and Atrophic Lesions, and in patients with *xerostomia*. In cases of xerostomia, lack of protective lubrication as well as the atrophic mucosa are important etiologic factors. The persistence of ulcers in these locations will often cause concern about the possibility of carcinomatous change, although as pointed out elsewhere, the frequency of carcinoma developing from lichen planus is quite low, and classical cases of Plummer–Vinson syndrome with an increased predisposition to oropharyngeal cancer are now rare.

The lateral margins and tip of the tongue are frequently involved in severe episodes of *recurrent aphthous ulcers* (see Fig. 10-26) and the related *Bechet's syndrome;* the well-keratinized dorsum is rarely ulcerated in these conditions. *Vesiculobullous disorders* (pemphigoid, pemphigus, erythema multiforme) also may involve the lingual mucosa, but often spare the dorsal surface.

Both ulcerative and proliferative lesions of the tongue occur in a number of *chronic granulomatous infections,* and special histologic studies and cultures are usually necessary for identification of the specific infectious agents and accurate diagnosis. *Tuberculosis* of the tongue usually manifests as a chronic ulcer most often located on the posterior ventral surface or pharyngeal surface. Similar chronic ulcers may also result from *histoplasmosis, blastomycosis, cryptococcosis, sporotrichosis,* and *mucormycosis* (phycomycete infections). The anterior third of the tongue may also be the site of an extragenital chancre in *primary syphilis* (see Fig. 28-11), and oral lesions of *lymphogranuloma venereum* likewise may be located on the tongue. The mucous patch of secondary syphilis may involve the tongue as well as other parts of the oral mucosa.

In *primary herpes simplex gingivostomatitis,* the dorsum, ventral surface, and lateral margins of the tongue may be ulcerated. While recurrent herpes simplex infection occurs intraorally much less frequently than it affects the external surfaces of the lips, the observable intraoral lesions are confined to localized areas of well-keratinized mucosa including palate, attached gingivae, and tongue dorsum. Because of the limited extent of each mucosal lesion in recurrent intraoral herpes simplex virus infection and the continuous movements of the tongue, intact vesicles are rarely, if ever, seen on the tongue. *Herpes zoster* may affect the lingual branch of the mandibular division of the 5th cranial nerve and produce a series of ulcers along the anterior third of the tongue on one side, often with similar lesions on the lips or intraorally following the distribution of the mental branch of the same nerve on the same side. The tongue as well as other regions of the oral cavity can be the location for a crop of ulcers accompanying a number of acute virus infections (*e.g.,* strains of coxsackie A and other enteroviruses).

Possibly as a result of the extensive normal oral bacterial flora, specific *bacterial stomatitides* are unusual, unless the normal flora has been eliminated by antibiotic therapy or xerostomia, for example. While unusual species may colonize the mouth and become the predominant oral flora under those conditions, these "infections" lack specificity of mucosal reaction or organism. In many cases, neither the tongue nor other areas of the oral mucosa exhibit any unusual appearance. The one clear exception to this rule is the classical pseudomembranous mucositis (and often glossitis) that results from superinfection with *Candida*. Acute inflammation of the oral mucous membrane, the tongue included, is described as a result of both *beta-hemolytic streptococcal* and *gonococcal infections.* Here also, data are lacking to establish whether these cases represent examples of acute inflammation of the oral mucosa as a result of these organisms or simply contamination of the tongue and saliva with organisms from localized specific pharyngitis. In infections with erythrogenic, toxin-producing *Streptococcus pyogenes* (scarlet fever), the classical sign of "strawberry tongue" is described because of prominent red fungiform papillae against a whitish pink coating. The specificity of this sign and a number of other classical

descriptions of the tongue in infectious disease (*e.g.,* "baked tongue," the dry, brown, coated tongue of typhoid fever; and "parrot tongue," the dry, horny, immobile tongue of chronic low-grade fevers) is questionable; as graphic as these descriptions are, it is likely that they reflect the effects of dehydration, lengthy illness, and secondary bacterial infection and methods of treating severe bacterial infections in the preantibiotic era.

Lesions of *acute necrotizing ulcerative gingivitis* (ANUG) may spread to adjacent marginal surfaces of the tongue producing characteristic irregular necrotic defects, especially if the tongue is traumatized by rough tooth margins, roots, and so on.

In recent years, a number of cases of acute glossitis and septicemia associated with positive oral and blood cultures for *Hemophilus influenzae* B have been described in children. While this organism has been previously associated with buccal cellulitis and septicemia, the unusual feature of a rapidly enlarging red tongue in association with fever may be an important diagnostic clue for investigating the possibility of infection with this organism, and for starting the IV ampicillin that is needed for adequate treatment. The glossitis rapidly resolves with no residual effects following this treatment. Multiple pseudomembranous ulcerations of the tongue and palate have also been noted with septicemia caused by *Capnocytophaga** species in granulocytopenic patients.

It is of considerable importance that *ulcers of the tongue due to carcinoma* be accurately identified, so that adequate surgical or radiation therapy can be instituted as early as possible. Because of the greater incidence of oral carcinoma on the ventral surface of the tongue, lesions in this region should be examined as carefully as possible and biopsied if there is the least suspicion that the lesion may be carcinomatous (see Fig. 10-27). A number of benign tumors that are sometimes mistakenly diagnosed as carcinoma are mentioned at the end of this chapter, and discussed more fully in Chapter 8. The so-called *solitary eosinophilic ulcer* or *traumatic granuloma*

---

* Carbon dioxide-preferring gram-negative oral bacteria, previously classified as *Bacteroides* and associated with production of lytic periodontal lesions.

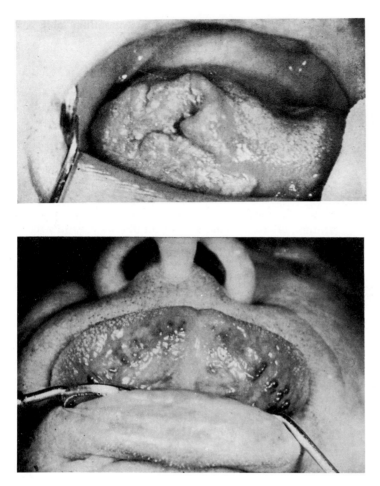

Fig. 10-27 Squamous cell carcinoma of the right side of the tongue producing marked induration and deformity.

Fig. 10-28 Superficial lingual varicosities.

of the tongue is also of importance in this regard. Eosinophils are common in many oral mucosal lesions and may at times be the most prominent type of granulocyte in a section of an oral ulcer. The term solitary eosinophilic ulcer, however, refers to a rapidly developing and often large (1 cm to 2 cm) ulcer of the tongue that histologically reveals no evidence of carcinoma or other malignant process and that contains numerous eosinophils. Such ulcers heal spontaneously in 2 to 3 weeks; they do not represent lesions of histiocytosis X (in that there are no associated bone lesions or rod-shaped "X-granules" demonstrable in the cytoplasm of the eosinophils or associated histiocytes on ultrastructural study); and they do not recur. Similar lesions have been described on the gingiva.

Because of the prominent position of the tongue when the mouth is open and the fact that it is often used to explore unfamiliar environments, it is subject to a variety of *unusual and sometimes bizarre injuries and infections*. Among these are insect stings, and even infestation by fly larvae (myiasis); animal bites including snakebite; human bites; electrical burns; frostbite; syphilitic chancres; and other sexually acquired infections.

Superficial Vascular Changes

Lingual varicosities are evident as prominent purplish blue spots, nodules, and ridges, usually on the anterior ventral surface of the tongue (see Fig. 10-28) and around the sub-mandibular-sublingual gland orifices; occasionally, they extend further posteriorly along the ventral surface and may also be seen on the posterior pharyngeal surface of the tongue. Thrombus formation, fibrosis, and even calcification may raise them above the mucosal surface as firm nodules and ridges, but they are rarely symptomatic. They usually increase in number with age and have no other known correlates. Their existence does not appear to be related to either jugular venous pressure or obstruction to the portal venous system, as is the case with esophageal varices and rectal hemorrhoids. The frequency with which lingual varices are found suggests that they represent a normal age change and prevents any clear information being obtained in regard to a number of alleged associations between abnormal superficial lingual vessels and other conditions. For example, the finding of angiomas of both the tongue and scrotum (referred to as the Fordyce lesion or Fordyce angiokeratoma) in younger individuals is stated to be a predictor of jejunal angiomas, which could be a potential source of occult gastrointestinal bleeding. A similar association of oral mucosal (but not lingual) and scrotal and penile angiomas occurs in the congenitally acquired *Anderson–Fabry syndrome* (angiokeratoma corporis diffusum). It has also been suggested that the relatively rare intracranial venous angioma, as distinct from the more usual cerebral arteriovenous aneurysm, may also be associated with sublingual venous angiomas; such lesions might be difficult to distinguish from the more common lingual varicosities.

Petechial hemorrhages and *telangiectases* also can usually be demonstrated on the ventral tongue surface as well as elsewhere on the oral mucosa in individuals with thrombocytopenia and hereditary hemorrhagic telangiectasia, respectively. *Hemangiomas* are relatively common on the tongue and may represent either a solitary localized lesion or one component of a more widespread hamartomatous syndrome such as Sturge–Weber syndrome (see Chap. 8).

Disorders Affecting Lingual Mucosal Glands

Very little is known about changes affecting the lingual mucosal glands (which occur predominantly on the pharyngeal surface or the anterior ventral surface) or the serous glands

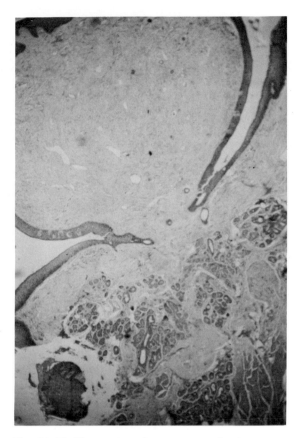

Fig. 10-29 Obstruction phenomena and acinar atrophy affecting von Ebner's glands in a biopsied vallate papilla from a patient with complaints of dry, sore mouth, persistent salty taste, and evidence of pansialadenitis, diabetes mellitus, and Type II hyperlipproteinemia (see also Fig. 11-11).

of von Ebner. Small cystic dilations of the pharyngeal mucosal glands are common, but of no apparent clinical significance. The lingual mucosal glands are affected in Sjögren's syndrome and other pansialadenites (see Fig. 10-29). The glands of von Ebner are apparently not affected in cystic fibrosis because they can produce the bulk of the lipoprotein lipase needed for fat digestion when pancreatic lipase production is decreased as a result of this inherited disorder; however, specific description of the histopathology of these glands in cystic fibrosis patients does not appear in the literature. Large cysts of the sublingual glands that often distend the overlying floor of the mouth and displace the tongue are referred to as *ranula* (see Chap. 8). Cysts of the anterior lingual glands of Blandin and Nuhn have been described.

DISEASES AFFECTING THE BODY OF THE TONGUE

The following diseases can be the cause of swelling of the body of the tongue or lingual neuromuscular dysfunction: amyloidosis; infections (lingual abscesses, Ludwig's angina, actinomycosis, cysticercosis, and trichinosis); neuromuscular disorders (*e.g.,* amyotrophic lateral sclerosis, muscular dystrophy, hypoglossal nerve damage, glossoptosis and sleep apnea syndrome, and temporomandibular joint myofascial dysfunction); vascular disorders (arteriosclerosis, cranial arteritis, and infarcts); angioneurotic edema; and a variety of tumors (see following section).

Amyloidosis

Involvement of the tongue is described in both the *primary* and *secondary* forms of amyloidosis; the characteristic fibrous glycoprotein of this disease is deposited in the submucosa as well as in the deeper muscular layers of the tongue. Generalized enlargement of the tongue (macroglossia) and fungating swelling may result, usually as a late manifestation of the disorder. Both oral and rectal biopsies (as well as appropriate biopsies of other affected organs, such as the kidney) are used for the diagnosis of suspected amyloidosis. Biopsy of the tongue is positive in 90% of cases in primary amyloidosis. Special stains (Congo red, crystal violet) and the use of polarizing microscopy and fluorescence microscopy following staining with thioflavine-T are needed to identify amyloid deposits in biopsies. Amyloidosis should be considered in the differential diagnosis of tongue enlargements and indurated swellings of the tongue in adults, particularly where there is a history of multiple myeloma or long-standing tuberculosis, rheumatoid arthritis, or severe anemia to provide the antigenic stimulus for amyloid formation. There seems to be no evidence to suggest that this disorder also leads to painful burning tongue.

Infections

Infections of the body of the tongue usually result from contaminated traumatic injuries that have been sutured superficially with inadequate debridement or drainage of the deeper parts of the wound. *Ludwig's angina* (acute phlegmonous bacterial infection of the tissue spaces above and below the mylohyoid muscle, usually from periapical abscesses of the mandibular molars and with spread into the submental and sublingual spaces) is not properly an infection of the tongue; however, it is characterized by an indurated swelling of the whole floor of the mouth and base of the tongue, which pushes the tongue upward and prevents the patient from closing the mouth. Dysphagia is a common complication of all enlargements of the base of the tongue.

Actinomyces species are not uncommonly isolated from tongue abscesses especially where deep lacerations of the tongue have been contaminated with calculus and tooth fragments. Such acute actinomycotic infections respond well to antibiotic treatment. Chronic actinomycosis of the tongue with induration and multiple draining sinuses (the so-called wooden tongue of cattle) is very rare.

Localization and encystment of cestode and nematode parasites in the tongue muscles have been described on a number of occasions with the larval stages of the pork tapeworm, *Taenia solium* (cysticerosis) and trichina worm, *Trichinella spiralis* (trichiniasis or trichinosis) most commonly involved. When demonstrated, such infections are simply representative of the general infestation of skeletal muscle that occurs in these diseases and are usually accompanied by muscle aches, fever, and marked eosinophilia. Tongue biopsies are not usually used for diagnosis of these parasitic infections; biopsies of deltoid and gastrocnemius muscles are preferred.

Neuromuscular Disorders

Neuromuscular disorders of central, peripheral, or muscular origin may produce symptoms of dysphagia and choking as well as disordered mastication and speech problems.

Dysphagia caused by weakness of the tongue muscles is referred to as *oropharyngeal dysphagia* to distinguish it from esophageal dysphagia. Symptoms of oropharyngeal dysphagia include aspiration while swallowing, regurgitation of fluid into the nose, pharyngeal pain on swallowing, and inability of the tongue to move the bolus of food into the pharynx. Dilation or atony of the pyriform sinuses and pharynx and retention of contrast media in the valleculae are characteristic radiographic findings. Aspiration of contrast medium into the trachea, regurgitation into the nose, and apparent obstruction of the upper esophageal sphincter may also be noted. Neuromuscular disorders are the most common cause of oropharyngeal dysphagia, although similar findings occur in patients with Sjögren's syndrome and sideropenic dysphagia (Plummer–Vinson syndrome). Acute pharyngitis, Vincent's angina, glossitis, and retropharyngeal abscesses will produce the same problem on a transient basis.

Speech problems caused by neuromuscular disorders involving the tongue are often severe but may also be the first symptom noted by the patient because fine coordination is needed for accurate articulation and phrasing. Problems of this type are referred to as *dysarthria* to distinguish them from cerebral disorders in which the ability to produce or comprehend spoken languages is limited (aphasia or dysphasia). The dysarthric patient understands what he hears, and if literate, has no difficulty writing. Depending on the location of the neuromuscular deficit causing the dysarthria, characteristic speech defects are discernible, and the pattern of speech at times may provide important diagnostic data about the nature of the neurologic abnormality involved. The reader is referred to texts on neurology and speech therapy for further details.

In those conditions characterized by *repetitive, uncontrolled movement of the tongue, head, and jaws,* depapillation, burning sensations, and traumatic ulcers of the tongue are common (*e.g.,* buccolingual-facial dyskinesia [BLFD] or senile tremor, parkinsonism, and the tardive dyskinesias. The tongue is frequently severely damaged by the *destructive ruminatory jaw movements* that occur in decerebrate patients, as a result of injuries to the

cerebral cortex, trigeminal nuclei, and hypothalamus. Levodopa (the most effective drug used to treat parkinsonism may also be responsible for hypermobility of the tongue. In the *tardive dyskinesias* (a broad group of extrapyramidal tract motor disorders that have been observed as long-term side-effects of neuroleptic drugs such as phenothiazines, butyrophenone tranquilizers, and reserpine derivatives), the tongue, lip, and jaw movements are often quite marked and have traditional descriptions. Fine tremors and fasciculation* of the tongue are described as "vermicular movements," rapid darting movements of the tongue as "fly-catcher's tongue" or "bon-bon" sign, and when associated with involuntary mouthing, chewing and smacking movements of the lips with constant lip tremor, as "rabbit syndrome."

Weakness of the tongue can occur in *polymyositis, multiple sclerosis,* and the various diseases described under the heading of *muscular dystrophy.* During the acute stage of polymyositis or in advanced muscular dystrophy, the flaccid small tongue that cannot be extended and that falls backward in the mouth blocking the airway is adequate evidence of this weakness. On recovery from polymyositis and in milder disorders, various forms of dynamometers that measure the force exerted when the tongue is pressed against the instrument are used to detect lingual muscle weakness. Because tongue and cheek muscle pressures are needed to retain a full lower denture, some evaluation of muscle strength in these patients prior to denture construction can provide information on the likelihood of problems with the prosthesis (see also Chap. 2 for methods of evaluating strength of muscles innervated by particular cranial nerves).

The tongue and perioral muscles are affected at different stages in the progression of various muscular dystrophies. For example, in *Duchenne's muscular dystrophy,* shoulder and pelvic girdle muscles are first affected, producing problems of posture and locomotion, and the tongue is involved only late in the disease. In *myotonic dystrophy,* on the other hand, oral, facial, neck, and tongue

---

* A series of visible contractions passing over a muscle while it is at rest.

muscles are commonly affected along with the muscles of the hands, forearms, and legs. Damage to the hypoglossal nerve, the main motor nerve supplying the tongue musculature, leads to *hypoglossal palsy.* If bilateral, the tongue cannot be extended; if unilateral, the tongue deviates to the unaffected side when extended.

Two other diseases, myasthenia gravis and amyotrophic lateral sclerosis, deserve comment because tongue dysfunction is prominent and because patients with these problems in an early stage may consult the dentist complaining of difficulty with chewing or swallowing that they mistakenly identify as of dental origin. With progression of the disease, the diagnosis usually becomes apparent, but routine use of a thorough oral examination procedure (as described in Chap. 2) can help tremendously in recognizing patients with potential problems of this type.

Myasthenia gravis is characterized by weakness and easy fatigability, which more frequently affects facial, oculomotor, laryngeal, pharyngeal, and respiratory muscles rather than lingual muscles. It is believed to be caused by a specific myoneural junction defect that is reversible by the administration of anticholinesterase drugs. Protrusive movements of the tongue may become weak, leading at times to posterior collapse of the organ with airway obstruction. Dysphagia and regurgitation of food into the mouth are common; and there is poor control of saliva, particularly following administration of anticholinesterase drugs, which stimulate additional salivary flow.

Amyotrophic lateral sclerosis (ALS, a steadily progressive disorder of motor neurons in the cerebral cortex, brainstem, and spinal cord, which is manifested clinically by muscular weakness, atrophy, and spasticity with exaggerated reflexes and is usually fatal in 2 to 5 years) sooner or later affects the muscles supplied by the brainstem, resulting in weakness, atrophy, and obvious fasciculations in the tongue and facial muscles, associated with dysarthria and impairment of chewing and swallowing. The sensory system and higher centers are unaffected. The aura of hopelessness that surrounds a diagnosis of ALS, at least in the early stages of the disease, also generates an attitude of denial in some patients, who may continue to seek medical and dental care from numerous consultants even though there is no doubt about the diagnosis. Such patients vainly hope that a new denture or a tooth extraction or treatment of a burning tongue will cure their symptoms. It is important that the dentist, through adequate history taking and communication with the various physicians the patient has consulted, becomes aware of the patient's diagnosis and undertakes dental treatment only with full understanding of the reality of the patient's condition. Once the oropharyngeal musculature is involved in ALS, fasciculations of the tongue and facial muscles are usually pronounced and recognizably pathologic. Occasionally, "benign" fasciculations unrelated to this or any other neuromuscular disorder also occur in normal patients.

The number of central nervous system and peripheral neuromuscular disorders that are associated with neuromuscular abnormality of the tongue is large, and the reader is referred to neurology texts for discussion of diseases such as cerebral palsy, stroke, and vascular accidents, ataxia, cerebellar atrophy, poliomyelitis, bulbar palsy, infantile muscular atrophy, chorea, brain tumors, and cranial trauma and their effects on the oropharyngeal region. (Additional material may be found in Chapters 15, 16 and 27.)

The Sleep Apnea Syndrome

In recent years, there has been increased interest in a miscellaneous group of disorders characterized by episodes of apnea (periodic cessation of respiration) associated with regular sleep or a pattern of hypersomnolence. All of these disorders are characterized by underventilation of the pulmonary alveoli with resultant alveolar hypoxemia and hypercapnia (hence they are also classified as the alveolar hypoventilation syndromes). While such problems can occur as a primary disorder (Ondine's curse), or secondary to barbiturate intoxication or respiratory center damage (*e.g.,* from bulbar poliomyelitis or brainstem infarcts), it has become apparent that a number of similar problems are caused by blockage of the pharyngeal airway by the tongue. The blockage occurs either as a result of congenital deformity (Pierre Robin syndrome or severe retrognathism from other causes), muscular weakness, or altered tonus of the genioglossus muscles (pickwickian syndrome; "Fat-boy" syndrome described very clearly in Charles Dickens' *The Pickwick Papers*, which includes morbid obesity, hypersomnolence, periodic breathing with hypoventilation, and cor pulmonale or hypertrophy of the right ventricle secondary to pulmonary disease), and possibly the sudden infant death syndrome.

Based on electromyographic recordings, it has been shown that the genioglossus muscles, which pull the tongue forward, function as muscles of respiration by opposing a tendency of the pharynx to collapse as a result of the negative pressure induced by inspiratory chest movements. Electrical activity has been demonstrated in the genioglossus muscles in phase with inspiratory activity, ensuring that a patent airway is maintained while the diaphragm and other inspiratory muscles enlarge the chest cavity and draw air into the lungs. Pharyngeal obstruction occurs whenever the force of the negative pressure in the pharynx exceeds the force exerted by the genioglossus muscles. Phasic activity in the genioglossus is maintained by cerebral carbon dioxide levels.

In the *Pierre Robin syndrome* (or more accurately, the Robin anomalad, because a number of different disorders are involved, all characterized by the combination of micrognathia, cleft palate, and posteroinferior positioning of the tongue, referred to as *glossoptosis*), the primary defect is hypoplasia of the mandible, which prevents the normal descent of the developing tongue between the medially growing palatal shelves. In addition to the strikingly receded mandible ("Andy Gump" facies) apparent at birth, these infants have difficulty during the inspiratory phase of respiration with periodic cyanotic attacks, labored breathing, and pectus excavatum; nursing or any form of feeding by mouth is almost impossible. Despite much debate on the subject, the basic problem in this syndrome appears to be the lack of support afforded to the tongue by the hypoplastic mandible, allowing it to fall downward and backward into the lower posterior pha-

ryngeal space and obstruct the epiglottis. The tongue acts as a ball valve preventing inhalation but allowing exhalation. Provided death does not occur in the first few months of life from aspiration pneumonia, unresolved apnea, or starvation and inanition, many affected individuals gradually improve with postnatal growth of the mandible providing more space for the tongue and better genioglossus development. A number of surgical procedures have been devised to aid the growth process. Ankyloglossia is a commonly associated complaint, and opinions vary as to whether the tongue is of normal size, small, or large. In many cases, this orofacial syndrome occurs in association with multiple skeletal deformities and mental retardation.

Temporomandibular Joint Myofascial Dysfunction

Evidence indicates that the muscles of mastication, the tongue muscles, and the strap muscles of the neck function as a unit and that dysfunction in one group of muscles is frequently associated with altered tonus and symptoms of "tension" in the other related groups. Tongue thrusting and inability to relax the tongue, which often follow sudden changes in occlusion such as placement of a new crown or bridge, presumably result from a mechanism of this type, and the therapeutic value of a "nonfunctional bite splint" in the management of many tongue dysfunctions may derive partly from the same mechanism. Reflex interactions within the central nervous system between proprioceptive signals from the tongue musculature carried by cranial nerves 10 and 12, from the periodontal membrane and masticatory muscles by cranial nerve 5, and motor output carried in the appropriate branches of the same nerves probably account for these phenomena.

Other more unusual syndromes involving interaction between cranial and cervical nerves have also been described; for example, the so-called *neck–tongue syndrome* characterized by unilateral upper nuchal or occipital pain with or without numbness in these areas and accompanied by simultaneous numbness of the tongue on the same side. This is explained by compression of the root of the second cervical nerve in the atlantoaxial (C1 to C2) space on sharp rotation of the neck. Afferent fibers from the lingual nerve travelling by the hypoglossal nerve to the second cervical root provide the explanation for the tongue numbness. The lingual nerve forms loops of communication with the hypoglossal nerve as the two course together over the hyoglossus muscle below the tongue.

Vascular Disease of the Body of the Tongue

The human lingual arteries are highly susceptible to the development of atherosclerotic changes. Microscopic evidence of plaques with intimal thickening, lipid infiltration, and fragmentation of the internal elastic lamina is found in the large and medium-sized arteries of the tongue in over 90% of individuals older than 10 years (see Fig. 10-30). Unlike the situation in the other branches of the carotid tree, atherosclerosis of the lingual vessels is rarely complicated by thrombotic, hemorrhagic, or ulcerative changes, which elsewhere contribute to the vascular occlusions that usually complicate atherosclerosis with advancing age. The extent of the lingual atherosclerosis increases with age, but age does not bring ischemic complications secondary to the atherosclerosis. Calcification may occur in the lingual atherosclerotic plaques and is more common in the lingual vessels of patients with arteriosclerotic heart disease or coronary arteriosclerosis.

Doppler ultrasound studies of the deep lingual arteries of stroke patients have revealed absence of a dicrotic notch to the pulse wave, indicating a period of negligible flow in the lingual artery during diastole (see Fig. 10-6). Presumably, these changes are the result of occlusion in the external carotid artery transmitted to the lingual artery and not caused by occlusion within the tongue. The significance of these disturbances of flow in producing symptoms in the tongue is not known, but they could conceivably contribute to some of the lingual sensory problems (pain, burning, loss of taste sensation) reported by convalescing stroke patients.

Infarcts of the tongue are fairly rare but do occur as an unusual complication of giant cell ("temporal") arteritis that normally affects the temporal, facial, vertebral, ophthalmic, and ciliary arteries but spares the internal and external carotid, cerebral, and central retinal arteries. Once again, the lesion that causes the sudden ischemia of the tongue lies either in the external carotid or the first part of the lingual artery. Considerable deformity of the tongue following fibrosis and shrinkage of the infarcted muscle occurs in patients surviving this event.

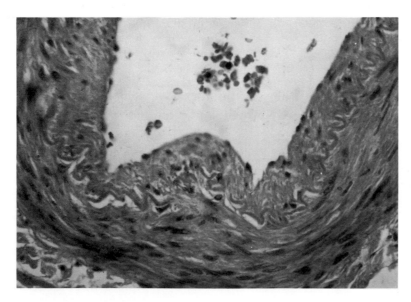

Fig. 10-30 Atherosclerotic changes involving lingual arteries within the body of the tongue. In the case of this 80-year-old woman, advanced atherosclerotic changes were found in many organs; however, changes such as these affect the lingual vessels at all ages, though they rarely occlude the vessels.

Angioneurotic Edema

Angioneurotic edema is one form of acute anaphylactic reaction representing an immediate hypersensitivity response allied to urticaria, allergic rhinitis, and asthma. The clinical response in this case is a relatively well-demarcated, localized edema involving the deeper layers of the skin and subcutaneous tissues. When this reaction is localized to the mucosa of the tongue, oropharynx, and larynx, considerable swelling of the tongue, glottis, and laryngeal structures occurs with rapid occlusion of the airway. It may also occur on a hereditary basis, when it is associated with deficiency in the function of an inhibitor of the first component of complement. Both acute and chronic forms of the disorder are described: recurrent episodes that become self-limited after 6 weeks are called acute; attacks persisting beyond this period are referred to as chronic. A variety of antigenic stimuli may be involved: seasonal respiratory allergens, animal danders, bacterial antigens, foods such as shellfish, chocolate, nuts, various drugs, and occasionally cold and physical trauma to the tongue. Other evidences of predisposition to the immediate type of hypersensitivity reactions may or may not be present. Antihistamine and sympathomimetic agents such as IM adrenalin provide symptomatic relief and are sometimes life saving. Recurrent episodes are sometimes controlled by consistent daily administration of antihistamines (*e.g.*, 50 mg to 75 mg diphenhydramine hydrochloride daily). In milder forms of the disorder, crenation of the tongue margins, a sensation of recurrent swelling of the tongue, and associated rhinitis and sinusitis may be the extent of the findings.

MALIGNANT TUMORS OF THE TONGUE*

Over 90% of malignant tumors of the tongue are epidermoid carcinomas occurring on either the anterior two thirds or the posterior third of the organ. The remainder include occasional verrucous carcinomas and adeno-

* Benign tumors are considered in Chapter 8.

carcinomas arising in the minor salivary glands of the tongue. Sarcomas are rare but include those arising from fibroblasts, skeletal muscle, nerve sheaths and vascular endothelium, as well as Hodgkin's and non-Hodgkin's lymphomas, representing the full spectrum of connective tissue, neuroectodermal elements, and lymphoid tissue from which the tongue is derived. A summary of case reports of tongue tumors published annually reveals a wide range of individual tumor types that reads somewhat like an encyclopedia of neoplasms, and attests in most cases to the rarity of the tumor. Metastatic tumors to the tongue likewise are rare and mainly derived from melanomas of the skin and carcinomas of the breast and lung.

The remainder of this section will be limited to a discussion of epidermoid carcinomas of the tongue and a small number of benign conditions that are sometimes confused with epidermoid carcinoma. The reader is referred to standard texts on head and neck tumors as well as the *Cumulative Index Medicus* for information on the less common carcinomas and sarcomas mentioned above.

Squamous Cell Carcinoma of the Tongue

Squamous cell carcinoma of the tongue is the most common oral carcinoma. Approximately 60% of lesions arise from the anterior two thirds of the tongue, the remainder from the base. Carcinoma of the dorsum of the tongue is now considered to be a rare lesion and usually arises on the basis of a chronic mucosal abnormality such as atrophic glossitis or leukoplakia. Therefore, the majority of the tongue carcinomas occur on the lateral borders of the anterior two thirds of the tongue. Clear separation of this anatomic zone from the floor of the mouth as a site of origin of a particular tumor is not always possible. It is significant that carcinoma of the floor of the mouth is the next most common site for oral carcinoma, indicating that it is the relatively poorly keratinized mucosa of the sides and ventral surface of the tongue that are most susceptible to carcinomatous transformation. The increased susceptibility of this poorly keratinized mucosa emphasizes the role that local physical and chemical agents (tobacco smoke, alcohol, dental trauma, xerostomia) play in the etiology of oral cancer both in humans and in experimental animals, and suggests a reason for the increased prevalence of carcinoma of the dorsum in patients with long-standing atrophic glossitis.

Carcinoma of the tongue is a disease of the middle and later decades of life with the median age at presentation being about 60 years. While the percentage of cases of tongue carcinoma in females has increased twofold in the last 30 years (paralleling similar increases in other tumors, for example, primary lung carcinoma), it is still predominantly a disease of males. Thirty percent of carcinomas of the anterior two thirds and 20% of carcinomas of the posterior third occur in women.

In general, there is an increased prevalence of less well-differentiated tumors toward the more posterior aspects of the tongue, although anaplastic tumors and well-differentiated tumors may be found in both locations. Perhaps because of their location and their tendency to be less well differentiated, carcinomas arising on the posterior third of the tongue as a group, in comparison with carcinomas of the anterior two thirds, are larger on initial diagnosis, are more often found to have invaded neighboring structures, and are more likely to be associated with fixation of the tongue (*i.e.*, evidence of an advanced infiltrating tumor). The incidence of cervical node metastasis is directly proportional to the size and stage of the primary tongue tumor, and as might be expected, more posterior tongue carcinomas (75%) present with regional node involvement at the time of initial diagnosis than do those of the anterior two thirds (30%).

Etiology

The etiology of human lingual carcinoma is not clearly established. Epidermoid carcinomas can be produced in experimental animals, usually rodents, by repeated application of a variety of chemical carcinogens. The effectiveness of these stimuli is increased when they are confined and remain in concentrated form for longer periods of time, as when they are applied to the hamster cheek pouch or to xerostomic oral mucosa. Experimental models for tongue cancer implicate physical trauma, alcohol, tobacco smoke, and candidiasis, at least as co-carcinogens. Additional information relating to the etiology of human tongue carcinoma is derived from epidemiologic associations. Based on this type of evidence, lingual carcinoma is traditionally associated with syphilis, sepsis, alcohol, and tobacco, and there is additional evidence that dietary deficiencies, iron deficiency, local trauma, infection with *Candida albicans*, and food additives play a role.

As far as *syphilis* is concerned, there once existed an increased risk of 3 to 1 for tongue cancer in patients with serologically confirmed syphilis, and there was a greater incidence of syphilis in patients with oral cancer than there was in patients with oral leukoplakia or malignant tumors elsewhere in the body. This increased incidence of tongue carcinoma was related to the occurrence of atrophic glossitis as a late manifestation of syphilis in man, and the tongue carcinomas involved were located on the dorsum. Since this time, tertiary syphilis, luetic atrophic glossitis, and carcinoma of the dorsum have all become rare, and the virtual disappearance of carcinoma of this type may partly account for the observed increase of carcinoma of the anterior two thirds in women.

The association between *chronic dental trauma (and sepsis)* and lingual carcinoma is based largely on the clinical observation that patients presenting with malignancies often have advanced dental disease with stained, fractured teeth, heavy salivary accretions, and periodontal disease and the fact that chronic oral ulcerative lesions and leukoplakia that are noted to be in contact with chronic dental irritants at times undergo malignant transformation.

While *alcohol* alone is not a carcinogen, chronic alcohol intake bears a definite relationship to predisposition to oral carcinoma. The effect may be only partly local and may also involve associated dietary deficiencies and cirrhosis of the liver. Cirrhosis of the liver has been clearly associated with an increased risk of oral cancer and a much poorer survival rate from oral cancer. The effect of alcohol is difficult to separate from the carcinogenic effects of smoking because heavy smoking and heavy use of alcohol are themselves strongly associated.

Tobacco use (cigarette and cigar smoking and betel nut, tobacco, and snuff chewing) is strongly related to the prevalence of both leukoplakia and all oral carcinomas, including carcinoma of the tongue. Leukoplakia is a well-established precancerous lesion with a 5% to 20% chance of malignant transformation over 20 years. In addition, malignant transformation in established leukoplakia is five times as great in those who smoke than in those who do not, justifying the value of stopping tobacco use in patients who already have leukoplakia, but who often argue "why stop now?"

The prevalence of infection with *Candida albicans* is increased in all intraoral epithelial disease, but notably in the case of the "speckled" variety of leukoplakia, which is commonly accepted as a precancerous lesion. *Candida albicans* is also found to be more prevalent in oral malignant disease than in nonmalignant epithelial lesions. While this organism can induce epithelial proliferation on the chorioallantoic egg membrane, its role as an experimental carcinogen has not been clearly established. Chronic *Candida albicans* infection is associated with central papillary atrophy of the tongue and possibly with some cases of atrophic glossitis, but these lesions as currently seen do not appear to undergo malignant transformation with any frequency.

Iron deficiency (sideropenia), as described earlier in relation to the Plummer–Vinson syndrome, predisposes strongly to atrophic glossitis and carcinoma of the dorsum and lateral surfaces of the anterior two thirds of the tongue and also of the posterior surface of the tongue and the pharynx.

The role of *virus infection* in lingual carcinoma is not at all clear. Infection with herpes simplex virus type 1 is not epidemiologically related to oral carcinoma at any site, although patients with malignant oral epithelial tumors demonstrate a decreased lymphocytic stimulation index to herpes simplex virus. Infection with herpes simplex type 2, which has epidemiologic associations with cancer of the uterine cervix, occurs only rarely in the oral cavity and has not been related to oral carcinoma. An anaplastic variant of epidermoid carcinoma referred to as *lymphoepithelioma* (because of the admixture of lymphoid cells and poorly differentiated malignant epithelial cells) occurs on the posterior third of the tongue, although less frequently than it occurs elsewhere (in Waldeyer's ring and in the nasopharynx). In these locations, where it is now usually referred to as nasopharyngeal carcinoma, an epidemiologic association between Epstein–Barr virus (the agent of infectious mononucleosis and non-Hodgkin's lymphoma of the Burkitt type) and this tumor has been established, particularly in Chinese males. Its role in the etiology of lingual lymphoepithelioma has not been established.

Treatment

Early carcinoma of the tongue (T1 and small T2 categories of the TNM staging system; see Chap. 9) responds equally well to treatment by surgical excision or by radiation. Fifty to seventy percent of patients with tumors in this category who are adequately treated are alive and well after 5 years. Advanced T3 stage lingual carcinomas respond poorly to either treatment, unless they are of the relatively uncommon but highly radiosensitive lymphoepithelioma type. Combined surgical and radiation therapy of T3 lingual carcinomas does not provide a greatly increased cure rate, although this form of treatment is currently most commonly used. Five-year survival rates for treated advanced stage lingual carcinoma vary from 10% to 30%.

Where the lesion on biopsy is staged as T1 or T2 and there is no evidence of lymph node metastasis, surgical treatment is usually restricted to partial glossectomy. If it is T2 or T3 without clinical node involvement, prophylactic neck dissection is often advised. Treatment of carcinoma of the anterior two thirds with evidence of node involvement may include radical neck dissection, partial mandibulectomy, and intraoral dissection ("commando operation") in addition to glossectomy. In the case of carcinoma of the base of the tongue, surgery may be more extensive. Where combined surgery and radiation therapy are used, treatments may be separate (with the hope of limiting tumor spread by radiation prior to surgery) or continuous. Complications of these radical procedures are often serious and include secondary infection, poor healing, erosion and "blow out" of the carotid vessels, osteoradionecrosis, salivary fistulae, and medical crises because the patient with oral cancer is usually old, often cirrhotic, and with compromised cardiovascular and pulmonary status.

Efforts to obtain better cure rates with treatment of lingual carcinoma include combined chemotherapy (cis-platinum and bleomycin)–surgery–radiation approaches, use of neutron irradiation, immunotherapy, and transoral laser resection for accessible early-stage carcinomas.

The devastating effects of lingual carcinoma itself (if untreated, the patient will usually die in prolonged misery with a foul and excessively painful oral tumor that prevents swallowing and eventually leads to death from starvation, aspiration pneumonia, invasion of the carotid sheath, or the effects of more distant metastases), the poor survival rate except for early T1 and T2 lesions of the anterior two thirds, and the mutilating nature of both surgical and radiation treatment fully justify every effort to increase the frequency of both self-administered and thorough routine oral examinations in the dental office, with prompt and adequate biopsy of any suspected lesions. A strong case for elimination of smoking, tobacco chewing, and heavy alcohol use can also be made very easily on the same grounds.

Benign Tumors of the Tongue Simulating Epidermoid Carcinoma

The apparent decrease in the frequency of carcinoma of the dorsum of the tongue over the past two decades has stimulated a number of reviews of biopsy specimens obtained before the 1950s. In some instances, benign lesions have been found to be misdiagnosed as carcinoma, a problem that still occurs today when the examining pathologist is not familiar with the full range of lesions that can involve the tongue. Prominent in this regard are those lesions that exhibit extensive pseudoepitheliomatous hyperplasia, cross-sections through the elongated rete pegs in this benign condition often resembling nests of carcinoma cells. Pseudoepitheliomatous hyperplasia is a characteristic component of the

lesion known as the *granular cell myoblastoma* of the tongue (see Chap. 8), and the occurrence in the same section of aggregations of large "myoblast" type granular cells and apparent "epidermoid carcinoma" should alert the pathologist to the need for additional sections to see whether the suspected carcinoma is not simply a florid epithelial hyperplasia. Pseudoepitheliomatous hyperplasia is also an important diagnostic feature of the viral-induced *keratoacanthoma* (see Chap. 8), which can occur as single or multiple lesions on the tongue. Tongue papillomas and irritation "fibromas" may exhibit the same type of epithelial hyperplasia. The presence or absence of cellular atypia is the single most important criterion in the separation of these hyperplasias from carcinoma.

A diagnosis of carcinoma *in situ* of the tongue (*i.e.*, the presence of significant cellular and nuclear atypia distributed vertically throughout the thickness of the epithelium but without any evidence of disruption of the basement membrane and invasion of the submucosa) poses a particular problem. Because the prognosis of invasive carcinoma of the tongue is poor, it is important that lesions are treated adequately and as early as possible. Carcinoma *in situ* is commonly seen on the margins of invasive oral carcinomas, and it is therefore extremely important for the pathologist to be sure that the specimen he has received is representative of the entire clinically apparent lesion. A diagnosis of carcinoma *in situ* of the tongue almost always indicates the need for additional biopsy of adjacent tissue, and in many cases the surgeon will proceed with hemiglossectomy even though repeated biopsy fails to locate invasive carcinoma. Such an approach is certainly justified where there are multiple nodules or an extensively ulcerated area on the tongue. Differentiation between leukoplakia with extensive dyskeratosis and carcinoma *in situ* of the tongue may also be very difficult. For these reasons, the wisdom of using the term *carcinoma in situ* for lesions of the tongue in any situation has been questioned by a number of authors.

The opportunity for incorrect diagnosis of epidermoid carcinoma to be made is always greater where small biopsy specimens are submitted and no guidance is given to the pathologist regarding the orientation of the specimen and its relationship to the clinical lesions. While the presence of some degree of cellular atypia is usually needed for a diagnosis of carcinoma, accurate interpretation of small nests of cells that appear to lie deeply in the submucosal tissues with no connection to overlying mucosa may be impossible. When fragments of a papillated tissue such as the tongue dorsum are sectioned at an angle, these cell nests may represent either cross-sections of elongated rete pegs or invasive carcinoma. Tattooing of the biopsy and adjacent marginal tissue or placement of a suture to mark an important landmark are useful techniques for orienting a specimen.

Conversely, chronic ulcers, particularly on the ventral surface of the tongue, are often underdiagnosed clinically. Their indolent, apparently unchanged clinical appearance over many years, despite antifungal and steroid therapy and removal of obvious dental irritants, may disguise their true nature. In the face of repeated biopsies read as "acute and chronic inflammation," "changes compatible with lichen planus," or "no atypia seen in section," the clinician may well postpone further biopsy and in doing so miss an early carcinoma. To some extent, the poor prognosis of lingual carcinoma does arise from too casual an attitude to chronic lingual ulceration and red lesions of the ventral surface, and the clinician should always be encouraged to biopsy a tongue lesion if there is any question of carcinoma in his mind at all. Overdiagnosis may lead to unnecessary surgical deformity or irradiation, but delayed treatment of lingual carcinoma leads in many cases to far more radical surgery and increased mortality.

MANAGEMENT CONSIDERATIONS FOR TONGUE DISORDERS

The almost constant activity of the tongue that occurs during the day, and for many patients at night as well, means that opportunities for immobilization or rest for this organ are very limited. The constant contact of the surfaces of the tongue with rough teeth, dental restorations, and prostheses also provides a poor environment for re-epithelization and healing of superficial lesions of the tongue. Like the rest of the oral mucosa, the tongue is constantly bathed in a heavily contaminated fluid medium, and when limited in its movements in any way, rapidly develops a heavy coat of indigenous microorganisms on the dorsum. Each of these factors require attention for adequate management of tongue lesions.

Some limitation of muscular activity in the tongue can be achieved by fabricating a plastic "night guard," a thin acrylic or vinyl plate made to fit accurately over either the upper or lower dental arch. With this in place and the jaws slightly opened beyond centric position, the opportunity for thrusting and wedging the tongue against the teeth is reduced, and signs of this such as crenation and ulceration of the tongue margins often rapidly subside. Night guards for this purpose (also referred to as *nonfunctional bite splints*) should cover all the occlusal surfaces of one arch completely and have matching indentations for the cusps of the opposing arch. Attention to this detail and prompt repair of fractured night guards and a general recommendation that they not be worn for more than 12 hours a day will prevent any deformity of the dental arch developing secondary to the night guard and effectively control symptoms of burning and tingling of the anterior third, when they are essentially caused by abrasion of the tongue against the dental arch. Myofunctional therapy administered with or without biofeedback control may also be helpful for some patients for the same reason.

Similar approaches (night guards, control of tongue muscle-tension) will also help reduce abrasion of the tongue by replacing the rough lingual surface of a dental arch with a smooth plastic surface in the case of the night guard and by reducing the number of times the tongue is forced against these rough surfaces in the case of muscle-control techniques. Attention should also be given to eliminating cusps or restorations that feel sharp to the examiner's finger and to polishing rough surfaces on prostheses, teeth, and restorations.

Both antibacterial and antifungal antibiotics also have an important place in the management of tongue lesions, as it is often only by concomitant reduction in the oral flora that healing of ulcers and other superficial lesions can be achieved. Mention has already been made of the role of *Candida* both in glossitis and leukoplakia of the tongue and the rapid change in appearance of a tongue (or other oral mucosal lesion) that often can be observed after 1 week's use of a topical antifungal rinse such as Mycostatin. Topical tetracycline for 4 to 5 days may also be useful in encouraging healing of ulcers of the tongue; longer use, however, usually results in development of a resistant bacterial flora or superinfection with *Candida* that may negate the benefit already achieved.

For control of the severe and destructive grinding jaw movements that occur with severe brain damage, special splints that depress the tongue out of the way of the occlusal table can be constructed and wired in place. Specially designed appliances may also be needed to help minimize the marked abrasion of the tongue that can occur in tardive dyskinesia and other neuromuscular disorders accompanied by rapid, continuous darting and thrusting movements of the tongue. Recommendations for constructing these appliances, many of which have to be customized to a patient's particular problem, are contained in a number of dental publications (some are cited in the bibliography of this chapter).

The resources of dental technology and clinical dentistry play an essential role in the management of tongue disorders, and medications or surgery alone often do not fully answer a patient's needs in this instance. Topically applied analgesics are commonly used to control burning and pain on the anterior two thirds of the tongue. Viscous xylocaine or other types of local analgesics are commonly prescribed. Similar effects can be produced by 0.5% aqueous solutions of a number of antihistamines (*e.g.*, diphenhydramine hydrochloride or dyclonine hydrochloride), which can be mixed with crushed ice and sipped as a cocktail; the antihistamine provides an additional sedative effect if swallowed. Allergic reactions following repeated use of these medications appear to be far less common than they were when novocaine and its derivatives were used for this purpose. Prescription of these medications should carry the warning that excessive use may produce dysfunction of the pharyngeal sphincter with the hazard of choking, particularly in the elderly or in patients with oropharyngeal muscular weakness.

BIBLIOGRAPHY

Anatomy and Functions of the Tongue

Arey LB et al: The numerical and topographical relations of taste buds to human circumvallate papille throughout the life span. Anat Rec 64:9, 1935

Arvidson K: Location and variation in number of taste buds in human fungiform papillae. Scand J Dent Res 87:435, 1979

Arvidson K, Friberg U: Human taste: Response and taste bud number in fungiform papillae. Science 209:807, 1980

Boshell JL et al: A correlative light microscopic, transmission and scanning electron microscopic study of the dorsum of the human tongue. Scan Electron Microsc 3:505, 1980

Gibbons RJ, van Houte J: Bacterial adherence in oral microbial ecology. Ann Rev Microbial 29:19, 1975

Halpern BP: Functional Anatomy of the Tongue and Mouth of Mammals. In Weijnen JAWM and Mendelson J (eds): Drinking Behavior: Oral Stimulation, Reinforcement and Preference, Chap I. New York, Plenum Publishing, 1976

Hamosh M: The role of lingual lipase in neonatal fat digestion. Ciba Found Symp 18:69, 1979

Hellekant G: Circulation of the tongue. In Oral Physiology. Proc. 2nd Wenner–Gren Symposium, Oxford Pergamon Press, 1972

Lowe AA: The neural regulation of tongue movements. Progr Neurobiol 15:295, 1980

Nolte WA (ed): Oral Microbiology with Basic Microbiology and Immunology, 4th ed. St. Louis, CV Mosby, 1982

Weerkamp AH: Adherence of *Streptococcus salivarius* HB and HB-7 to oral surfaces or saliva coated hydroxyapatite. Infect Immunol 30:150, 1980

Examination of the Tongue

Dworkin JP: Tongue strength measurement in patients with amyotrophic lateral sclerosis: Qualitative versus quantitative procedures. Arch Phys Med Rehabil 61:422, 1980

Frantzell A et al: Examination of tongue: clinical and photographic study. Acta Med Scand 122:207, 1945

Ishii T: Capillary microscopic observations of the fungiform papillae in humans. 1. Variations due to age, differences in sex, number, shape and terminal vessel of papillae. 2. The changes in papillae in case with resection of the chorda tympani nerve. J Otol Japan 82:271, 1979

Krudy AG et al: Arteriographic localization of parathyroid adenoma in the presence of lingual thyroid. Am J Radiol 136:1227, 1981

Mettler FA et al: Gray-scale ultrasonography in the evaluation of neoplastic invasion of the tongue. Radiology 133:781, 1979

Myers DE et al: Evaluation of lingual artery hemodynamics in stroke victims using Doppler ultrasound. Oral Surg 51:252, 1981

Naidich TP et al: Case Report: Hypoglossal palsy: Computed tomography demonstration of denervation hemiatrophy of the tongue associated with glomus jugulare tumor. J Comput Assist Tomogr 2:630, 1978

Sauerland EK et al: Non-invasive electromyography of the human genioglossal (tongue) activity. Electromyogr Clin Neurophysiol 21:279, 1981

Inherited, Congenital and Developmental Anomalies

Arneson MA et al: A new form of Ehlers–Danlos syndrome; Fibronectin corrects defective platelet function. JAMA 244:144, 1980

Baughman RA: Median rhomboid glossitis: A developmental anomaly? Oral Surg 31:56, 1971

Corlee R (Chm), Joint Committee on Dentistry and Speech Pathology—Audiology Am Speech and Hearing Assoc: Position statement on tongue thrust and bibliography on tongue thrust. AHSA, J Am Speech and Hearing Assoc. 17:331, 1975

DePorte JV, Parkhurst E: Congenital malformations and birth injuries among the children born in New York City in 1940-1942. NY State J Med 45:1097, 1945

Gellin ME: Digital sucking and tongue thrusting in children. Dent Clin North Am 22:603, 1978

Gorlin RJ, Pindborg JJ: Syndromes of the Head and Neck, 2nd ed. New York, McGraw-Hill, 1979

Gold BM et al: Radiologic manifestations of Cowden disease. Am J Radiol 135:385, 1980

Halperin V et al: The occurrence of Fordyce spots, benign migratory glossitis, median rhomboid glossitis and fissured tongue in 2,478 dental patients. Oral Surg 6:1072, 1953

Leider AS et al: Sebaceous choristoma of the thyroglossal duct. Oral Surg 44:261, 1977

Machida K et al: Aberrant thyroid gland demonstrated by computed tomography. J Comput Assist Tomogr 3:689, 1979

Nevin NC et al: Ankyloglossum superius syndrome. Oral Surg 50:254, 1980

Noyek AM et al: Thyroglossal duct and ectopic thyroid disorders. Otolaryngol Clin North Am 14:187, 1981

Pearson J et al: The tongue and taste in familial dysautonomia. Pediatrics 45:739, 1970

Scully C: Orofacial manifestations in tuberous sclerosis. J Oral Surg 44:706, 1977

Soames JV: A review of the histology of the tongue in the region of the foramen cecum. Oral Surg 36:220, 1973

Tobias N: Scrotal tongue and its inheritance. Arch Dermatol Syph 52:266, 1945

Wright BA: Median rhomboid glossitis: Not a misnomer. Review of the literature and histological study of 28 cases. Oral Surg 46:806, 1978

Young EC, Sacks GK: Examining for tongue tie. Clin Pediatr 18:298, 1979

Disorders of the Lingual Mucosa

Ackerman AB: Differential Diagnosis in Dermatopathology. Philadelphia, Lea & Febiger, 1982

Bakos L et al: Botfly infestation of the tongue. Br J Dermatol 100:223, 1979

Bollet AJ: The conquest of pellagra III. The contribution of Joseph H. Goldberger. Resident Staff Phys pp 25–28, 1982

Dawson TAJ: Tongue lesions in generalized pustular psoriasis. Br J Dermatol 91:419, 1974

Dreizen S: Oral indications of the deficiency states. Postgrad Med 54:97, 1971

Farman AG et al: Central papillary atrophy of the tongue and denture stomatitis. J Prosthet Dent 40:253, 1978

Fredrikzon B et al: Lingual lipase: An important lipase in the digestion of dietary lipids in cystic fibrosis. Pediatr Res 14:1387, 1980

Fujibayashi T et al: Tuberculosis of the tongue. Oral Surg 47:427, 1979

Gandola C et al: Septicemia caused by Capnocytophaga in a granulocytopenic patient with glossitis. Arch Intern Med 140:851, 1980

Halbreich U, Steiner JE: An interaction between hyperbaric pressure and taste in man. Arch Oral Biol 22:287, 1977

Helfman RJ: The treatment of geographic tongue with topical Retin-A solution. Cutis 24:179, 1979

Hoexter DL: Erythema circinata migrans—ectopic geographic tongue. NY State Dent J 46:350, 1980

Krutchik AN et al: Pigmentation of the tongue and mucous membranes associated with cancer chemotherapy. South Med J 72:1615, 1979

Kuepper RC et al: Actinomycosis of the tongue: Report of a case. J Oral Surg 37:123, 1979

Meskin LH et al: Incidence of geographic tongue among 3,668 students at the University of Minnesota. J Dent Res 42:895, 1963

Mukherjle A et al: The histopathology of tongue lesions in leprosy. Leprosy Rev 50:37, 1979

Nicholls MG et al: Ulceration of the tongue: A complication of captopril therapy. Ann Intern Med 94:659, 1981

Peck GL et al: Prolonged remissions of cystic and conglobate acne with 13-cis-retinoic acid. N Engl J Med 300:329, 1979

Plackova A, Skach M: The ultrastructure of geographic tongue. Oral Surg 40:760, 1975

Rahamimoff P, Muhsam HV: Some observations on 1246 cases of geographic tongue. Am J Dis Child 93:519, 1957

San Joaquin VH et al: Acute glossitis and septicemia owing to Hemophilus influenzae Type B. Am J Dis Child 134:91, 1980

Schultz LW, Vazirani SJ: Burns of the oral cavity. Oral Surg 14:143, 1961

Skoda–Türk R: Injured tongue due to bite of fer-de-lance. Laryngol Microbiol Otol 58:470, 1979

Spies TD et al: Recent observations on treatment of six hundred pellagrins with special emphasis on the use of nicotinic acid in prophylaxis. Southern Med J 31:1231, 1938

Stauffer JL et al: Cleft tongue and ulceration of the hard palate: Complications of oral intubation. Chest 74:317, 1978

Svejda J et al: Micromorphology of papillae filiformes of the human tongue in congenital heart disease in the scanning electron microscope. Zahn Mund Kieferheilkd 68:43, 1980

Tang TT et al: Ulcerative eosinophilic granuloma of the tongue, a light and electron microscopic study. Am J Clin Pathol 75:420, 1981

Wright BA et al: Candidiasis and atrophic tongue lesions. Oral Surg 51:55, 1981

Diseases Affecting the Body of the Tongue

Bear SE et al: Sleep apnea syndrome: Correction with surgical advancement of the mandible. Oral Surg 38:543, 1980

Boy-duk N: An anatomic basis for the neck–tongue syndrome. J Neurol Neurosurg Psychiatry 44:202, 1981

Breiser M et al: Amyloidosis of Waldeyer's ring: A clinical and ultrastructural report. Acta Otolaryngol 89:562, 1980

Brouillette RT et al: Control of genioglossus muscle inspiratory activity. J Appl Physiol 49:801, 1980

Brown AM: A comparative study of the elastic membranes of two muscular arteries. IADR 48th Gen Mtg 1970, Preprinted abstract #398

Brunsting LA, MacDonald ID: Primary systema-tized amyloidosis with macroglossia. J Invest Dermatol 8:145, 1947

Dreizen S et al: Human lingual atherosclerosis. Arch Oral Biol 19:813, 1974

Guillerminault C et al: The sleep apnea syndromes. Annu Rev Med 27:465, 1976

Mallory SB et al: Glossoptosis revisited: On the development and resolution of airway obstruction in the Pierre Robin Syndrome. Pediatrics 64:946, 1979

Rapoport DM et al: Reversal of the "Pickwickian Syndrome" by long term use of nocturnal nasal-airway pressure. N Engl J Med 307:931, 1982

Roller NW et al: Amyotrophic lateral sclerosis. Oral Surg 37:46, 1974

Simpson GM, Kline NS: Tardive dyskinesia: Manifestations, incidence, etiology and treatment. In Yahn MD (ed): The Basal Ganglia, Res. Publ Assoc Res Nerv Ment Dis 55:427, 1976

Smith JD: Treatment of airway obstruction in Pierre Robin syndrome. A modified lip-tongue adhesion. Arch Otolaryngol 107:419, 1981

Sofferman RA: Lingual infarction in cranial arteritis. JAMA 243:2422, 1980

Yamaguchi A et al: Amyloid deposits in the aged tongue: A postmortem study of 107 individuals over 60 years of age. J Oral Pathol 11:237, 1982

Malignant Tumors of the Tongue

Ackerman LV, McGavan MH: Proliferating benign and malignant epithelial lesions of the oral cavity. J Oral Surg 16:400, 1958

Batsakis JG: Tumors of the Head and Neck, 2nd ed. Baltimore, Williams & Wilkins, 1979

Cassileth BR, Cassileth P: Clinical Care of the Terminal Cancer Patient. Philadelphia, Lea & Febiger, 1982

Garrett WS et al: Keratoacanthoma. Arch Surg 94:853, 1967

Hatziotis MC et al: Metastatic tumors of the oral soft tissues. Oral Surg 36:544, 1973

Kim RY et al: Metastatic carcinoma to the tongue—a report of two cases and a review of the literature. Cancer 43:386, 1979

Kornblut AD et al: The clinical diagnosis of oral malignant tumors. Otolaryngol Clin North Am 12:57, 1979

Ogus HD, Bennett MH: Carcinoma of the dorsum of the tongue: a rarity or misdiagnosis. Br J Oral Surg 16:115, 1978–79

Sellars SL: Epidemiology of oral cancer. Otolaryngol Clin North Am 12:45, 1979

Strong EW: Carcinoma of the tongue. Otolaryngol Clin North Am 12:107, 1979

Tiger N et al: Cirrhosis and other predisposing factors in carcinoma of the tongue. Cancer 11:357, 1958

Zegarelli DJ et al: Metastatic tumor to the tongue. Report of twelve cases. Oral Surg 35:202, 1973

Management Considerations for Disorders of the Tongue

Barishman H: Controlling pernicious biting of lips, cheeks, and tongue. NY Univ J Dent 15:146, 1957

Hanson GE et al: A tongue stent for prevention of oral trauma in the comatose patient. Crit Care Med 3:200, 1975

Henricsson V et al: Palliative treatment of geographic tongue. Sved Dent J 4:129, 1980

Jackson MJ: The use of tongue-depressing stents for neuropathologic chewing. J Prosthet Dent 40:309, 1978

Jebreil K: Palliative dental treatment in primary amyloidosis. J Prosthet Dent 44:552, 1980

Lanciello FR et al: Prosthodontic and speech rehabilitation after partial and complete glossectomy. J Prosthet Dent 43:204, 1980

Thompson GA, Jr et al: Operant control of pathological tongue thrust in spastic cerebral palsy. J Appl Behav Anal 12:325, 1979

11

Salivary Gland Disease

MARTIN S. GREENBERG

DEVELOPMENTAL ANOMALIES

Aberrant Salivary Glands

An aberrant (or ectopic) salivary gland is salivary gland tissue that develops at a site where it is not normally found. Ectopic salivary gland tissue is sometimes confused with normal minor salivary gland tissue, which is found in the submucosal tissue all over the oral cavity.

True aberrant salivary glands are most frequently reported in the cervical region near the parotid gland or the body of the mandible. The salivary gland tissue in the mandible is found posterior to the first molars and often has a small communication with the major salivary glands. Stene and Pedersen reported a case that appeared as a distinct radiolucency in the bicuspid region. A total of seven cases of salivary gland tissue located in the anterior portion of the mandible have been reported.

Ectopic glands are reported as a single anomaly or in combination with other facial anomalies. Sinha described a patient with multiple anomalies including unilateral tonsillar aplasia, absence of a normal external auditory meatus, and an ectopic salivary gland in the tongue.

Most aberrant salivary glands of the neck occur in the upper portion of the neck in the area of brachial cleft and bronchial cleft cysts. It is rare to find salivary gland tissue in the lower portion of the neck, but several cases have been reported. Adams described a patient with salivary gland tissue in the midline of the lower neck, 2 cm above the suprasternal notch. He theorized that the tissue arose from the ectodermal lining of precervical sinus. Even less frequent is the presence of salivary gland tissue below the neck. Marwah reported a lesion of the vulva, a chorstoma, that contained salivary gland tissue.

Aplasia and Hypoplasia

Total aplasia of the major salivary glands is rare. It may occur alone or in combination with other congenital anomalies such as cleft palate or mandibulofacial dysostosis. The major symptom is severe xerostomia that interferes with eating and leads to severe dental caries if a continuous careful oral hygiene regimen is not followed. These patients require continuous dental supervision and use of fluoride during tooth development as well as topical fluoride indefinitely in an attempt to maintain the dentition.

Hypoplasia of the parotid glands has been reported to be present in patients with Melkersson–Rosenthal syndrome, which chiefly consists of facial paralysis, facial edema, and fissured tongue. It is unclear whether the hypoplasia is caused by a defect in the salivary glands themselves or by atrophy secondary to a neurologic defect.

Accessory Ducts

Accessory parotid ducts are common. Rauch studied 450 salivary glands and found an accessory parotid duct in over one half of the cases. This accessory duct was most frequently found superior and anterior to the normal Stensen's duct orifice.

Diverticuli

Diverticuli are small pouches or outpocketings of the ductal system of one of the major salivary glands and their presence leads to repeated episodes of acute parotitis. Diagnosis is made by sialogram.

SIALOLITHIASIS

Sialoliths are calcified and organic matter that develop in the parenchyma or ducts of the major or minor salivary glands. The composition of the stones has been studied, and they appear laminated with layers of organic material covered with concentric shells of calcified matter. The crystalline structure is chiefly hydroxyapatite and contains octacalcium phosphate. The chemical composition is principally calcium phosphate and carbon with traces of magnesium, potassium chloride, and ammonium.

The etiology of sialolith formation is still debated, but several factors are thought to play a significant role; these include inflammation, local irritants, or drugs that cause stasis leading to build-up of an organic nidus that calcifies. Several workers have theorized that disorders of calcium and phosphorus metabolism lead to sialoliths, but studies of serum calcium and phosphorus levels in patients with sialoliths have demonstrated normal levels of these elements.

Sialoliths occur most frequently in the submandibular duct. Investigators differ on the exact percentages, but approximately 80% to 90% occur in the submandibular gland or duct, 5% to 15% occur in the parotid, and 2% to 5% in the sublingual and minor salivary glands. Multiple calculi occur in close to 20% of cases. Sialoliths are occasionally described in children, but occur most frequently in middle age adults.

Clinical Manifestations

The most common symptom of sialolithiasis is painful intermittent swelling in the area of a major salivary gland, which worsens during eating and resolves after meals. The pain originates from the back-up of saliva behind the stone. This stasis may lead to infection and eventual fibrous and atrophy of glandular parenchyma. Sinus tracts and fistulas may also form in chronic cases, and cases have been described in which the mucosa ulcerates over the stone.

Sialoliths of Stensen's duct or Wharton's duct will be palpable if present in the peripheral portion of the duct. It is believed that more stones form in the submandibular gland duct because Wharton's duct is longer and has more bends and curves than do the ducts of the other salivary glands. Sialoliths of the minor salivary glands appear to occur more frequently than was previously believed. Jensen reported 47 cases of minor salivary gland calculi and the most common site of occurrence was the buccal mucosa. The typical clinical presentation was of an asymptomatic well-circumscribed, freely movable, draining swelling.

Diagnosis is made with the benefit of a properly positioned x-ray film, but the clinician must remember that at least 20% of sialoliths are poorly calcified and will not show up on radiographs. Lateral jaw films are useless in making the diagnosis of parotid stones because of the superimposition of the facial bones. The proper radiographs are an anterior posterior view of the face and a periapical or occlusal x-ray placed inside the mouth in the region of the duct (see Fig. 11-1). Sialography will aid in the diagnosis in cases where the radiographs are negative and will demonstrate a filling defect, narrowing of the duct at the site of the stone, and dilation of the duct proximal to the stone.

Treatment

Management of sialolithiasis includes treatment of acute infections with antibiotics. Stones in the distal portion of the duct may be manually removed; if this is not possible, surgery is performed. In cases of repeated sialoliths, removal of the involved gland may be necessary.

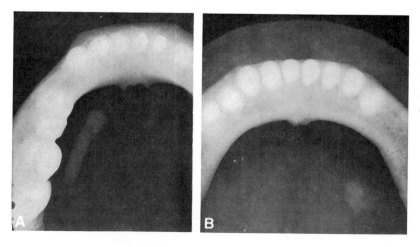

Fig. 11-1 A, Roentgenogram demonstrating a long oval calcareous obstruction in Wharton's duct. B, Roentgenogram demonstrating a nodular calcareous deposit in Wharton's duct.

MUCOCELE

Mucocele is a term used to describe swelling caused by the pooling of saliva at the site of an injured minor salivary gland duct. The majority of these common lesions occur on the lower lip, but they may be present anywhere minor salivary glands are found, including the floor of the mouth and tongue.

Mucoceles may be divided into a mucus-extravasation type and a mucus-retention type. The mucus-extravasation type is the common mucocele and is caused by the laceration of a minor salivary gland duct by trauma. Saliva leaks into the submucosal tissues causing pooling of mucus, resulting in inflammation and formation of granulation tissue. The mucus-retention type is less common and is caused by obstruction of a minor salivary gland duct which causes a back-up of saliva. This continual pressure dilates the duct and forms a cystlike lesion. These lesions have been confused with true cysts of the salivary glands because they are lined with the epithelium of the dilated duct.

Clinical Manifestations

The clinical appearance of the mucocele depends on the location of the pooled saliva. Superficial lesions appear as thin-walled, bluish lesions that rupture easily; they resemble bullae (Fig. 11-2). Lesions may range in size from 3 mm to 4 mm to over 1 centimeter in diameter. Deeper lesions are well-circumscribed swellings covered by normal-appearing mucosa. Unless treated, the deep lesions may last for long periods of time.

A special type of mucocele is the so-called ranula, which occurs on the floor of the mouth from trauma of a sublingual or submandibular gland duct (see Fig. 11-3). These are slowly growing unilateral lesions that were named after their resemblance to the belly of a frog. These lesions may be superficial or deep to the mylohyoid muscle; they are soft and freely movable.

Treatment

The treatment of deep mucoceles or recurring superficial mucoceles is surgical removal of the lesion. A problem in management is that

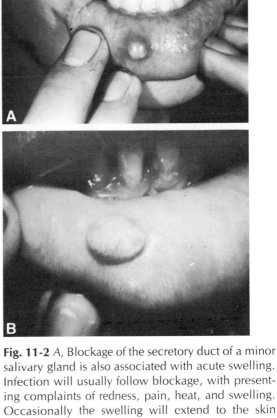

Fig. 11-2 *A*, Blockage of the secretory duct of a minor salivary gland is also associated with acute swelling. Infection will usually follow blockage, with presenting complaints of redness, pain, heat, and swelling. Occasionally the swelling will extend to the skin surface of the lip if the infection and its tissue response are acute. Secretion from the gland duct orifice cannot be observed, but a purulent discharge may be present in the convalescent period. *B*, With time, fibrosis occurs, replacing the acinar functional cells with connective tissues; the inflammatory components disappear, and a sessile, firm mass is observed on the lower lip with normal mucous membrane.

surgery to remove mucoceles may be responsible for the formation of new lesions by causing trauma to other minor salivary gland ducts. Large ranulas are often successfully managed by marsupialization rather than surgical removal. Wilcox and Hickory reported success in treating mucoceles by injecting corticosteroid solution into the lesion; they suggest this should be tried before surgery is attempted.

Fig. 11-3 *A,* Blockage of Wharton's duct at the salivary orifice on the lingual frenum induces acute cystic dilatation of the proximal portion of the duct as the secretory pressure from a functional gland is directed at the point of blockage. The ranula may be caused by blockage of this duct and is manifested by acute swelling in the floor of the mouth. *B,* When blockage is extensive and complete, the swollen mass extends posteriorly throughout the course of the submandibular salivary duct. The tongue may be elevated by this fluctuant mass, with associated pain and discomfort. Note the prominent vasculature, indicating the stretching of the sublingual tissues. *C,* Frequently some form of drainage is spontaneously achieved, but the cystic enlargement of the distal section of duct proximal to the blockage persists, with changes in the tissue architecture of the entire sublingual space.

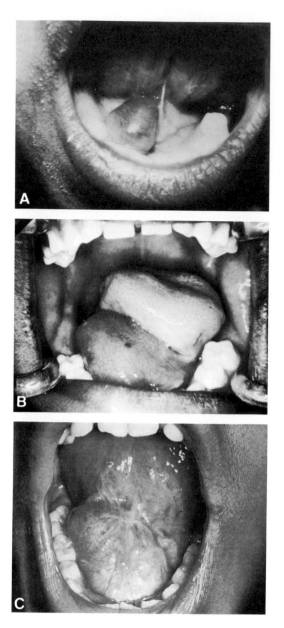

NECROTIZING SIALOMETAPLASIA

Necrotizing sialometaplasia is an inflammatory lesion of unknown etiology that affects the minor salivary glands. Many theorize that trauma causing ischemia of the minor salivary glands leads to the onset of the disease. The disorder occurs most frequently in males, particularly in the fifth and sixth decades of life. This benign, self-healing lesion has been often confused with malignancy causing unnecessary surgery.

Clinical Manifestations

The lesion begins as a large ulcer or ulcerated nodule. The ulcers are well demarcated from surrounding normal tissue and often have an inflammatory reaction around the edge of the lesion (see Fig. 11-4). The disease occurs primarily on the palate, although cases of the lip and retromolar pad have also been reported. A similar type of lesion has been reported in the major salivary glands. If the patient with the lesion is otherwise healthy, routine laboratory tests are within normal limits. The clinical impression is frequently mucoepidermoid carcinoma, adenoid cystic carcinoma, or squamous cell carcinoma. Biopsy of the lesion will show no evidence of malignant cells and is characterized by necrosis of some lobules of the involved gland, squamous metaplasia of the ducts and mucous acini, inflammation, and an overlying pseudoepitheliomatous hyperplasia. An inexperienced pathologist may confuse the histologic picture with mucoepidermoid carcinoma or an invasive squamous cell carcinoma. It is therefore important that when the clinician suspects this disease that a sufficient tissue specimen be taken so that representative tissue might be examined adequately by the pathologist.

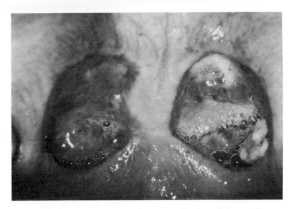

Fig. 11-4 Necrotizing sialometaplasia of the palate. (Courtesy of James Sciubba, D.M.D., Ph.D., New York, NY)

Treatment

Conservative therapy consisting of debridement of the lesion is all that is necessary for management. The lesion will usually heal in 6 to 12 weeks without recurrence.

INFLAMMATORY DISORDERS

Inflammation of the salivary glands (sialadenitis) is characterized by a painful swelling of the affected gland with varying degrees of alteration in function, depending on the nature and severity of the inflammatory reaction.

Inflammation as a result of bacterial or virus infections comprises the most common group of diseases affecting the salivary glands; however, inflammatory reactions secondary to allergic reactions or as a manifestation of systemic disease have also been reported. The flow rate in sialadenitis is usually reduced, and the saliva increases in viscosity and turbidity; with a decrease in flow, the possibility of ascending infections becomes greater. The parotid gland appears to be affected more frequently.

Viral Infections

Mumps

Mumps (epidemic parotitis) is caused by a paramyxovirus. It primarily affects the salivary glands, but also affects the gonads and central nervous system. Fifty percent of the cases of mumps occur between 5 and 9 years of age; 90% occur before 14 years.

In 1967 an attenuated live vaccine was developed and distributed; it was over 95% effective for at least 5 years. Since widespread use of the vaccine, the number of cases of mumps has dropped dramatically. In the United States, the incidence of the disease has been reduced by 90%. Many other countries do not recommend universal vaccination because a relatively benign childhood infection may be replaced by a more severe adult infection. Many patients are still susceptible to mumps, and twenty thousand cases a year still occur in the United States. Therefore, mumps still must be considered as a possible cause of acute nonsuppurative salivary adenitis in noninoculated individuals or patients without a history of the disease.

Clinical Manifestations. The major sign of mumps is sudden onset of salivary gland swelling without purulent discharge from the salivary gland ducts, accompanied by mild generalized signs of fever, malaise, and anorexia (Fig. 11-5). The parotid gland is involved in most cases. Both parotid glands may be involved simultaneously, but more commonly, one parotid swells 24 to 48 hours after the other. The enlarged glands are tender, and pain is experienced when eating sour foods. Submandibular salivary glands may also become enlarged, although they are less noticeable and cause less pain. In approximately 10% of cases, enlargement of the submandibular glands occurs without parotid involvement.

Salivary gland enlargement is accompanied by edema of the skin over the glands and inflammation around Stensen's or Wharton's duct orifice.

Most cases of mumps are self-limiting, with salivary gland enlargement subsiding within a week. The more frequent complications of mumps are meningitis and encephalitis, although most cases are mild. In postpubertal males, orchitis and epididymitis may result. Deafness, myocarditis, thyroiditis, pancreatitis, and oophoritis have also been reported. Diagnosis of the disease is rarely difficult in children. In adults with nonsuppurative parotitis the diagnosis is

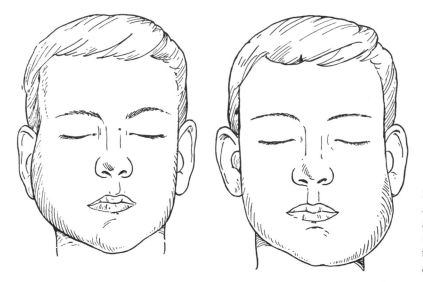

Fig. 11-5 (*Left*) Typical location and configuration of swelling associated with mumps. (*Right*) Usual location and configuration of swelling associated with abscessed mandibular molars.

more complex. The patient should have a negative history of mumps or mumps vaccination and a fourfold rise in antibody titers from acute to convalescent serum. During the acute phase of the disease the serum amylase level may be elevated.

Treatment Treatment of mumps salivary adenitis is supportive. Prevention with live attenuated vaccine is the best method of controlling the disease.

Cytomegalic Inclusion Disease

Cytomegalic inclusion disease (CID) is caused by cytomegalovirus, a herpesvirus similar to herpes simplex virus and varicella zoster virus. Infection with the virus is common, but clinical disease is unusual except in newborns or immunosuppressed adults. Eighty percent of normal adults have been shown to have serum antibody to the virus; 1% of normal infants are born with evidence of virus in the urine. It is believed that many patients acquire the infection transplacentally and the virus remains latent. This is similar to the current theory regarding latent infection with other herpesviruses. Virus has been cultured from saliva, urine, breast milk, blood, and feces. It is believed that in adults the virus may spread by saliva or urine. Cases of infection as a result of blood transfusions have also been reported.

Clinical Manifestations. In newborns and young children the infection is generalized and is usually fatal. Involvement of the liver, lung, and central nervous system is common, although the virus may be isolated from all organ systems. Infants who survive the infection may have permanent central nervous system involvement including mental retardation and seizures. Congenital infection with the virus has been associated with an increased rate of congenital anomalies.

In adults the infection may be caused by a reactivation of latent virus or contact with a carrier. Disseminated infection in adults occurs in immunosuppressed patients, including patients with hematologic malignancies such as leukemia and lymphoma, as well as patients on immunosuppressive drug therapy. Acute pneumonia is the most common manifestation in adults, but involvement of liver, heart, and peripheral nerves has also been reported. An acute febrile illness, cytomegalovirus mononucleosis, has also been described by Klemola and Kääriäimen. This disease clinically resembles infectious mononucleosis, but the heterophil antibody is negative. A rising titer of antibody to cytomegalovirus is detected in the serum.

Infection with cytomegalovirus may cause clinical disease of the salivary glands. Wong and Warner studied 14 adults with CID; most had lung, adrenal, and liver involvement and 2 of the 14 had salivary gland enlargement.

Cunningham suggested that cytomegalovirus may be responsible for salivary gland tumors. He observed salivary gland neoplasms develop in four mice after intraglandular inoculation of cytomegalovirus.

Other Viral Infections

Acute nonsuppurative parotitis has been attributed to viruses other than mumps or cytomegalovirus. Zollar and Mufson observed parotid enlargement associated with parainfluenza type 3 infection in two children. One, a 4-year-old patient, had bilateral parotid involvement; an 8-year-old had unilateral involvement. Both infections subsided in just over a week. Buckley and colleagues isolated parainfluenza type 3 from the parotid fluid of a patient with parotitis. Howlett and co-workers reported four cases of parotitis accompanied by oral ulcers and vesicles in four adults; coxsackie A was isolated from these patients.

Lymphocytic choriomeningitis virus is a common cause of latent infections in mice. Baum and associates reported cases of mumpslike disease in patients infected with the virus. The cases occurred in geographic areas where infected mice were found or in laboratory workers handling the mice. Humans can become infected by inhalation or ingestion of dried mucosa, feces, or urine.

Echoviruses, parainfluenza type 1, and influenza viruses have also been implicated as occasional causes of acute nonsuppurative salivary gland enlargement.

Bacterial Infections

Bacterial infections of the salivary glands may be acute or recurrent. Infection of the parotid is far more frequent than submandibular gland involvement. The infections are potentially lethal, especially in debilitated patients.

Acute Bacterial Sialadenitis

This disorder, also called acute suppurative parotitis and known for centuries, is associated with decreased salivary flow in dehydrated, debilitated patients. Most cases occur in adults, but a neonatal and childhood form of the disease also exists. The infection is most common after surgery or chronic disease. When use of antibiotics was first begun in the 1940s, the incidence of parotitis was lowered considerably, but in 1962 a study of 161 cases by Krippaehne, Hunt, and Dunphy demonstrated that the prevalence of acute parotitis was increasing. It is believed that the increase in cases of acute parotitis primarily resulted from a combination of factors: the development of antibiotic-resistant bacteria and increased use of drugs that decrease salivary flow. Ragheb reported three cases of acute parotitis that developed in patients with xerostomia secondary to the use of tranquilizers. Walker and co-workers reported two patients who developed acute parotitis while taking anti-Parkinson's drugs. These drugs are known to cause decreased salivary flow. Diuretics and antihistamines have also been reported as contributory factors.

Acute bacterial parotitis most frequently occurs in older debilitated patients. Yonkers reported 11 patients with postsurgical parotitis. The mean age of the patients was 70. Penicillin-resistant *Staphylococcus aureus* was the infecting organism in all cases. Dehydration and poor oral hygiene were considered important contributory factors by Yonkers. Speirs and Mason reported 36 cases of acute parotitis; all patients were over 77 years of age, and four of them died. Penicillin-resistant *Staphylococcus aureus* was the most prevalent organism, but *Streptococcus viridans* was also implicated in a few instances. The tubercle bacillus was isolated from a single infected salivary gland. Carlson and Glas reported 28 cases of acute parotitis; 75% of the patients were over 70 years of age, and 26 of the 28 cases were caused by *Staphylococcus aureus*. Five cases of acute parotid actinomycosis have been reported by Sazama. In 1973, Hopkins reported an additional case of parotid actinomycosis.

Clinical Manifestations. Of the reported cases of acute bacterial parotitis, 80% to 90% are unilateral. The patient complains of a sudden onset of pain at the angle of the jaw, which worsens when the mouth is opened for eating or speaking. The pain becomes intense when extensive infection is contained within the confines of the parotid capsule.

Examination reveals a tender, enlarged

gland (Fig. 11-6). The overlying skin is characteristically warm and red. The diagnosis is confirmed when purulent material is milked from Stensen's duct orifice by pressure over the gland (Fig. 11-7). The localized symptoms are accompanied by fever, leukocytosis, and other generalized signs and symptoms of acute bacterial infection. Actinomycosis of the salivary glands is accompanied by sulfur granules in the purulent discharge appearing as gram-positive, granulated branching threads on microscopic examination.

Treatment. Acute suppurative sialadenitis must be treated aggressively because even with antibiotics, death can result in debilitated patients. Specimens of purulent discharge taken directly from the salivary gland duct should be sent immediately to the laboratory for culture and sensitivity, but in severe cases, the clinician should not wait for results before beginning treatment with high doses of parenteral antibiotics active against penicillin-resistant staphylococcus. If necessary, the antibiotic can be changed when the results of the culture and sensitivity are known. The patient must be adequately hydrated and the electrolyte balance properly maintained with intravenous fluids. Salivation should be stimulated to facilitate drainage by the sucking of sour hard candy. Oral hygiene should be maintained by debridement and irrigation. If improvement is not apparent promptly, surgical drainage of the affected gland should be performed by a sur-

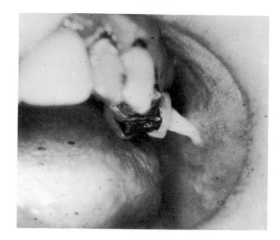

Fig. 11-7 Acute suppurative parotitis caused by a streptococcal organism. Pain, tenderness, inflammation of the duct orifice, and the presence of pus at the orifice of the gland on the buccal mucosa are the key diagnostic features. Culture and sensitivity testing will produce guidance to appropriate antibiotics, but sialography is contraindicated while acute infection is present.

geon who is experienced with surgical techniques now utilized to avoid facial nerve damage.

Chronic Bacterial Sialadenitis

Acute parotitis occurs most frequently in debilitated older adults. Chronic or recurrent forms of parotitis are seen in otherwise normal children, as well as in adults. Virtually all cases of chronic sialadenitis not associated with salivary stones occur in the parotid gland.

The childhood form of the disease commonly begins between the ages of 3 and 5 years. Half the cases affect one gland only, whereas the bilateral cases affect each parotid gland at different times. Some cases can be traced to duct obstruction, congenital stenosis, Sjögren's syndrome, or previous viral infection or allergy, but most cases are idiopathic. Maynard described a theory for the etiology of recurrent parotitis related to metaplasia of ductal epithelium causing formation of mucus-secreting cells in Stensen's duct and resultant blockage.

The bacteria isolated from recurrent childhood parotitis are characteristically *Streptococcus viridans. Escherichia coli, Proteus,* and

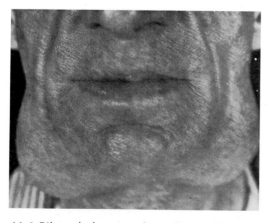

Fig. 11-6 Bilateral chronic submaxillary sialadenitis in a terminal patient. (King HA, Koerner TA: JAMA 167:1813)

pneumococci have been implicated in some cases.

Many cases of chronic childhood parotitis disappear at puberty.

Clinical Manifestations. The major sign of recurrent parotitis is sudden onset of unilateral swelling at the angle of the jaw in a patient with a history of similar occurrences. The symptoms are not as dramatic as those seen in acute bacterial parotitis since the organism is of low virulence, but purulent material may still be expressed from Stensen's duct orifice. This helps to distinguish the disorder from viral or allergic parotitis. Fever, as well as leukocytosis, is absent or mild. Pain is minimal, and antibiotic therapy will resolve the infection within a week. Symptom-free periods last from weeks to months. After several recurrences, decreased salivary flow may result from fibrosis of glandular parenchyma. Sialectasia can be visualized by use of sialography.

Treatment. Many forms of therapy have been suggested for the treatment of recurrent bacterial parotitis. Radiation therapy was formerly utilized extensively to cause fibrosis of the affected gland, but the incidence of head and neck tumors developing in radiated sites reported by Ju and others has placed this form of treatment in disrepute. Surgeons have recommended total removal of the parotid gland in intractable cases, but the risk of facial nerve section causing facial paralysis has resulted in a decrease in enthusiasm for this technique.

Conservative management is in order for childhood cases, since many will disappear at puberty; antibiotic therapy is sufficient in many cases. Use of sialography will help promote drainage in chronic cases. Quinn recommends the use of intraductal erythromycin or tetracycline. He cannulates the duct and anesthetizes the area with an infusion of lidocaine directly into the duct system; this is followed by infusion of the antibiotic into the duct at a concentration of 15 mg/ml. This procedure is repeated for 5 days. Other techniques have been developed to replace radiation or parotidectomy. Ligation of Stensen's duct is a relatively simple procedure and can lead to fibrosis. Drawbacks include severe pain due to backup of saliva and the formation of an extraoral fistula. In order to decrease the incidence of these complications, the technique of tympanic neurectomy has been developed. This technique consists of sectioning the secretomotor nerve supply to the parotid as it passes through the middle ear. Morgan reported good results in six cases using this technique along with ligation. Resouly attempted the technique in three patients and reported poor results in two of the three cases.

Allergic Sialadenitis

Cases of salivary gland enlargement related to allergic reactions to drugs or other allergens have occasionally been reported. Some of the reported cases may not be true hypersensitivity reactions but rather are toxic or idiosyncratic reactions to drugs that cause a decreased salivary flow resulting in secondary infection. Other cases appear to be true allergies, especially when accompanied by angioedema, skin rash, or other signs of allergy.

Nidus and Field reported a case of bilateral parotid gland enlargement when sulfisoxazole was administered for a urinary tract infection. Rothstein reported acute swelling of the parotid glands, conjunctivitis, and a skin rash within hours of instituting phenothiazine therapy. A similar episode occurred on subsequent administration of the same drug. Carter reported angioedema plus painful swelling of all major salivary glands in two cases after treatment with an iodine-containing compound. Koch and associates observed bilateral parotitis within 30 minutes of intravenous injection of a radiopaque dye for urography. A case of enlargement of parotid and submandibular glands associated with hay fever was reported by Banks. The enlargement could be relieved by expressing mucus plugs from the duct orifices.

The diagnosis of allergic sialadenitis should be made cautiously. If there are no associated signs of allergy, such as angioedema or skin rashes, the diagnosis should be accompanied by a healthy dose of skepticism, and the possibility of infection or collagen disease should be ruled out.

Allergic sialadenitis is a self-limiting disease, although secondary bacterial infection has been reported and has developed into chronic salivary gland infection.

Sarcoid Sialadenitis

Sarcoidosis, a systemic, granulomatous disease, affects the parotid gland in approximately 1 out of 20 patients with the disease. The etiology and pathogenesis of sarcoidosis is unknown. *Heerfordt's syndrome,* or uveoparotid fever, is a special form of the disease characterized by inflammation of the uveal tract of the eye, parotid swelling, and facial palsy. Uveoparotid fever may develop in the absence of systemic sarcoidosis.

Clinical Manifestations. The disease usually develops in the third or fourth decade of life. Salivary gland involvement is characterized by bilateral, firm, painless enlargement, but unilateral as well as asymmetric involvement may develop (see Fig. 11-8). Decreased or

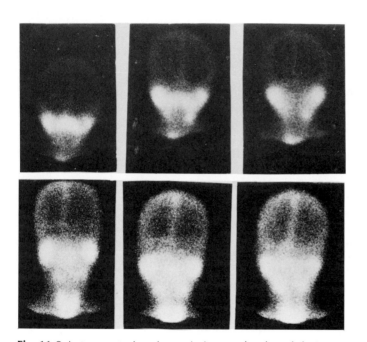

Fig. 11-8 Anteroposterior view scintigrams developed during sequential salivary scintigraphy of the parotid gland for a normal patient (*top row*) and a patient with acute sialadenitis following administration of phenylbutazone (*bottom row*). Both illustrations on the left are at 10 minutes postintravenous injection of ⁹⁹ᵐTc pertechnetate, those in the middle at 30 minutes, and those on the right at 60 minutes. At 10 minutes, the isotope is already concentrated in the parotid and submandibular areas in contrast to that in the bloodstream as reflected in the fainter outline of the cranium and sagittal venous sinuses. The thyroid gland which also concentrates the isotope is also intensely marked at the base of each scintigram. Normal and abnormal scintigrams show little difference at the time. In the normal scintigram at 30 minutes, an additional spot has appeared between the two parotid spots, corresponding to the secretion and accumulation of secreted isotope in the mouth and pharynx. By contrast, in the patient with acute sialadenitis, who had markedly diminished salivary secretion, the parotid spots have intensified without development of a central spot. At 60 minutes, the xerostomia patient still retains a high level of radioactivity in the glands without a central secretory spot, whereas in the normal, the parotid spots are fading in contrast to the central spot. Because of the short half-life of this isotope of 6 hours, all radioactivity will have essentially disappeared from the scintigram by the next day, allowing the technique to be repeated if necessary. (Garfunkel AA et al: Oral Surg 38:223, 1974)

absent salivation is characteristic of the affected gland.

Granulomatous invasion of the salivary gland leads to atrophy and eventual fibrosis of salivary tissues. Sialography of the affected gland will reflect the extent of the atrophy and will vary with the severity of the involvement. Sarcoid involvement of adjacent lymph nodes can also cause pressure on the affected gland, causing further atrophy.

Diagnosis is based on the results of biopsy, preferably of a cervical lymph node. Characteristic are numerous noncaseated, epithelioid granulomas.

Treatment. Treatment of the disease is largely symptomatic, since well over 50% of the patients are either asymptomatic or have undergone spontaneous remission. Corticosteroids are effective during acute exacerbations; the symptomatology is generally proportional to the extent of systemic involvement of the granulomatous process (see also Chap. 18).

Sialadenosis

The sialadenoses (sialoses) are characterized by a nonneoplastic, noninflammatory enlargement of the salivary glands. The enlargement is usually bilateral and may present a course of recurrent, painless enlargement of the glands. The parotid glands are more frequently affected than are the submandibular glands. The condition is more common in women, although some reports do not show this sex distribution. Swelling of the preauricular portion of the parotid gland is the most common symptom, but the retromandibular portion of the gland may also be affected. The histology of sialadenosis is characteristic regardless of the cause of the enlargement and presents as acinar cell hypertrophy, edema of the interstitial supporting tissue, and atrophy of the striated ducts. A characteristic alteration in the chemical constituents of the saliva is a distinguishing feature of the sialadenoses; significant elevations of salivary potassium and concomitant decreases in salivary sodium are observed. Although the magnitude of the alterations varies according to the cause of the enlargement, its presence is a diagnostic fea-ture of the sialadenoses. The cause of sialadenosis is unknown.

Sialadenosis may occur in a variety of conditions. *Hormonal sialadenosis* has been described in association with menarche, menses, pregnancy, menopause, gynecomastia, hypogenitalism, and following ovariectomy. Diabetic sialosis, characterized by retromandibular enlargement of the parotid gland, has also been reported.

Sialadenosis associated with *alcoholic cirrhosis* is a common finding and may in fact precede the development of the systemic symptoms associated with cirrhosis (see Fig. 11-9). Other forms of cirrhosis may also lead to parotid enlargement. Similarly, diseases of the pancreas and kidneys have also been shown to create sialadenosis (see Fig. 11-10).

Symmetrical enlargement of the parotid gland is also associated with *malnutrition,* especially in those states of acute protein deprivation.

Drug administration can also cause glandular enlargement and has been reported with

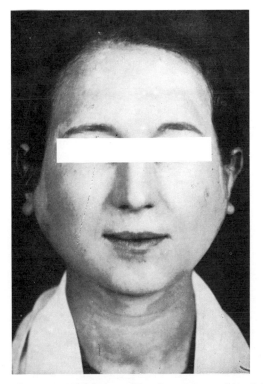

Fig. 11-9 Bilateral swelling in uveoparotitis. (Michelson HE, Becker FT: Arch Dermatol Syph 39:329)

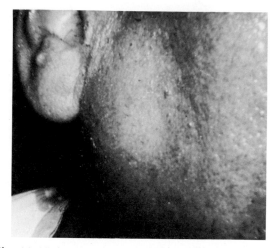

Fig. 11-10 Asymptomatic parotid swelling in an alcoholic. Salivary secretion is abnormal.

iodine-containing drugs, phenylbutazone, and norepinephrine derivatives.

SJÖGREN'S SYNDROME

The first detailed description of this disorder, made in 1933 by Henrik Sjögren, described a series of 19 cases. Sjögren's syndrome is divided into a primary and secondary form, and the localized form of the disease, once called *Mikulicz's disease*, is primary Sjögren's syndrome. This disorder affects the exocrine glands only, primarily the lacrimal and salivary glands. Secondary Sjögren's syndrome consists of lacrimal and salivary involvement with an associated connective tissue disease. Approximately 50% of Sjögren's patients have the primary form, and 50% have the secondary form. The associated connective tissue disease is rheumatoid arthritis in over 50% of patients. Systemic lupus erythematosus, scleroderma, or polymyositis is present less frequently. A study by Alarcon–Segovia suggests that Sjögren's accompanies systemic lupus more frequently than was previously believed. Sjögren's has also been associated with lymphoma, "pseudolymphoma," Waldenstrom's macroglobulinemia, primary biliary cirrhosis, and chronic hepatitis.

The etiology of the disease is unknown, but the large number of abnormal antibodies and the association with collagen disease has led most immunologists to include Sjögren's in the list of "autoimmune" diseases. Cummings studied Sjögren's syndrome with associated rheumatoid arthritis and found serum antibodies directed against salivary duct antigen in 70% of the patients. Feldkamp found similar antisalivary gland antibodies in the Sjögren's patients he studied. Alspaugh demonstrated that a high percentage of Sjögren's patients have precipitating antibody to an extract of human lymphocytes. Talal measured B_2 microglobulin by means of radioimmunoassay in saliva and synovial fluid. He found an increase of this globulin in both fluids of Sjögren's patients and also that the level of B_2 microglobulin reflected the level of disease activity.

General immune abnormalities observed by many workers include hypergammaglobulinemia, rheumatoid factor, antinuclear antibody, anti-DNA antibodies, and an increased erythrocyte sedimentation rate (ESR). These findings are consistent with a disease that should be grouped with the immune disorders.

Talal in 1970 presented a working model for the etiology of Sjögren's syndrome based on his studies with New Zealand mice. He proposed that a genetic predisposition exists among certain individuals causing an abnormal immune reaction to a virus. The theory of genetic predisposition has been strengthened by the association of Sjögren's with certain human leukocytic antigen (HLA) alloantigens.

Clinical Manifestations. Sjögren's syndrome occurs most frequently between 40 and 60 years of age; 80% to 90% of patients are females. A form of the disease that occurs in children closely resembles the adult disorder. Cummings reported in 1971 that in 90% of cases the connective tissue disease appears first with a slow development of dryness of the mouth or eyes. In 10% of cases the eye and oral signs precede the generalized collagen disease.

Lacrimal gland enlargement is an uncommon sign of disease, but complaints of dry eyes may be the first distressing symptoms of disease in a patient with or without collagen disease. Patients complain of a continued feeling of dirt or other foreign body in the eye. Continuous, severe, lacrimal gland involvement may lead to corneal ulceration as well as conjunctivitis.

Dryness of the pharynx, larynx, and nose is noted by some patients. This complaint, caused by a lack of secretions in the upper respiratory tract, may lead to pneumonia. Vaginal dryness is a complaint of 5% of females with the disorder.

Xerostomia is a major complaint in most patients, but a history of salivary gland enlargement varies. The dry mouth may be accompanied by bilateral enlargement of the parotid glands, unilateral enlargement, or no enlargement. Enlargement of the submandibular glands may also occur. Absence of salivary gland enlargement does not exclude Sjögren's syndrome as a possible cause of xerostomia. Intermittent salivary gland enlargement is experienced by some Sjögren's patients; others have continuous slight enlargement with periodic severe enlargement.

Daniels and colleagues studied 100 patients (82 females, 18 males) suspected of having Sjögren's syndrome; 82% had an oral problem as the chief complaint. The oral complaints encountered included inability to chew or swallow or wear dentures owing to a lack of saliva; the necessity of sipping water in order to swallow; dry cracked lips; and dry buccal mucosa and tongue. The lack of oral secretions may lead to secondary oral diseases such as candidiasis or an increase in dental caries.

Other symptoms and signs of Sjögren's syndrome depend chiefly on the associated collagen disease and include the wide variety of joint, muscle, and skin findings seen in rheumatoid arthritis, progressive systemic sclerosis (generalized scleroderma), systemic lupus erythematosus, or polymyositis.

In some patients, Sjögren's may be associated with diffuse enlargement of the lymph nodes, which is especially marked in the cervical region. This develops into lymphoma in some patients. The lymph node involvement is thought to be a reaction to the generalized increase in activity by the reticuloendothelial system. The name *pseudolymphoma* refers to benign cases of lymph node enlargement.

Laboratory Findings. Ophthalmologists use three tests to evaluate lacrimal gland function in suspected Sjögren's patients: the Schirmer test, the break-up time, and the quantitative rose-bengal dye test. The Schirmer test consists of placing a strip of filter paper in the lower conjunctival sac. Normal patients will wet 15 mm of filter paper in 5 minutes. Patients with Sjögren's syndrome will wet less than 5 mm of filter paper. The break-up time (BUT) is performed using a slit lamp and noting the interval between a complete blink and the appearance of a dry spot on the cornea. The rose-bengal dye test is used to detect damaged and denuded areas of the cornea. If two of the three tests are abnormal, the patient is considered to have keratoconjunctivitis sicca.

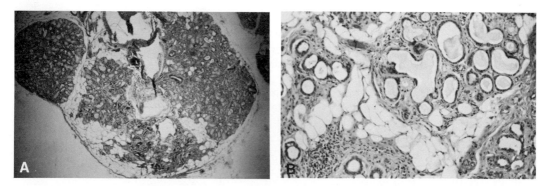

Fig. 11-11 Histologic section of biopsy of minor salivary gland from lip of patient with complaints of dry, sore mouth, persistent salty taste, and evidence of chronic pansialadenitis, diabetes mellitus and Type II hyperlipoproteinemia. H & E stain. *A*, Low-power view showing chronic sialadenitis affecting entire gland with fatty replacement of some area fibrosis and atrophy of the gland parenchyma and cystic dilatation of ducts. *B*, High-power view to illustrate the same features.

Salivary gland function in suspected Sjögren's is now measured chiefly by three tests: parotid flow rate, minor salivary gland biopsy, and salivary scintigraphy.

The measurement of parotid flow rate is accomplished by placing a Lashley, Carlson-Crittenden, or other specially fabricated cup over Stensen's duct orifice. Saliva can be collected stimulated or unstimulated. Daniels and co-workers have reported good results by maximal stimulation of the gland with lemon juice every 30 seconds for 10 minutes. The normal range using this technique is considered to be at least 5 ml of secretion per gland.

Salivary glands affected with Sjögren's syndrome have a chronic inflammatory infiltrate of lymphocytes, plasma cells, and histiocytes (see Fig. 11-11). The major salivary glands are difficult to biopsy and may result, with parotid biopsy, in facial nerve paralysis. Biopsy of the minor salivary glands is considerably less complex and demonstrates histologic evidence of disease. Minor salivary gland tissue may be obtained from the palate or lip. Palatal glands may be biopsied easily with a "punch" biopsy, but labial biopsies can be more easily performed with a scalpel and closed primarily with sutures, causing little patient discomfort. The biopsy specimens are rated 0 to 4+ according to the degree of chronic inflammatory cell infiltrate. Asofsky as well as Greenspan and colleagues have discussed the details of this histologic technique.

Sequential salivary scintigraphy consists of recording the uptake, concentration, and excretion of ^{99m}Tc-pertechnetate by the salivary glands using a gamma scintillation camera (see Fig. 11-12). Ten millicuries of the radioactive isotope is injected intravenously. Photographs are taken every 2 minutes for the first 10 minutes and then every 10 minutes for 1 hour. Sjögren's patients demonstrate a decrease in total uptake of the isotope by the salivary glands, slow uptake, or slow excretion of the isotope into saliva. Abnormal results of two of the three tests described above is considered diagnostic for salivary gland involvement. Recent work has suggested that sialochemistry may be helpful in distinguishing Sjögren's from other causes of xerostomia. Ben-Aryeh and co-workers found significantly higher levels of sodium and

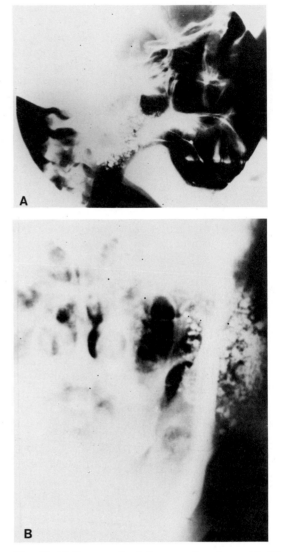

Fig. 11-12 Retrograde sialogram of patient with Sjögren's syndrome. *A,* Lateral view; *B,* Anteroposterior view. Note absence of fine arborization, and the presence of many larger dye-filled spaces (sialectasis). Also note dilatation of major intraglandular duct in lateral view. (Nichols CN, Brightman VJ: J Oral Pathol 6:51, 1977)

potassium in whole unstimulated saliva from Sjögren's patients than from patients with other causes of xerostomia.

Sialography, the injection of a radiopaque dye into the parotid ducts, in advanced cases shows changes consistent with Sjögren's, such as decrease in ductules and punctate or globular sialectasis (see Fig. 11-13). This technique is no longer considered as desirable as

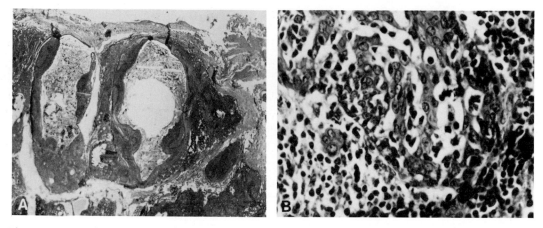

Fig. 11-13 Histologic section of excised parotid gland from patient with Sjögren syndrome; H & E stain. *A,* Low-power view of two cystlike spaces with development of lymphoid follicles in their walls. Elsewhere parotid gland parenchyema is obliterated and replaced by lymphoid tissue. *B,* High-power view of lymphoepithelial proliferation within an area of lymphoid infiltration. (Nichols CN, Brightman VJ: J Oral Pathol 6:51, 1977)

the three techniques described above for diagnosis of Sjögren's, since there is some danger of glandular damage by the injected dye, and in patients with severe Sjögren's the dye will remain in the gland interfering with future tests.

General laboratory changes seen in patients with collagen diseases are seen in patients with Sjögren's syndrome. This includes positive serum rheumatoid factor, positive LE test, and presence of antinuclear antibody. None of these tests is specific for Sjögren's.

Treatment. The goal of treatment for patients with Sjögren's syndrome is to minimize the secondary effects of decreased exocrine secretion. Patients at risk of developing pneumococcal pneumonia due to decreased secretions of the tracheobronchial tree should be vaccinated against common strains of pneumococci. The patient should be examined regularly by an ophthalmologist to decrease the risk of ocular damage and should be encouraged to have routine physical evaluations to detect early signs of lymphoma.

The symptoms of xerostomia can be treated with topical methyl cellulose, glycerin, or a saliva substitute (Oralube). The saliva substitute has certain advantages because it contains sodium fluoride, which minimizes the risk of dental caries.

Bromhexine, which has been used in Europe to increase bronchial secretions in patients with chronic bronchitis, has been recently advocated as a treatment for Sjögren's syndrome. Bromhexine is said to increase lacrimal and perhaps salivary secretions. The use of this drug is controversial, and at least one controlled clinical trial showed no benefit.

Patients with severe Sjögren's syndrome may be treated with systemic corticosteroids or immunosuppressive drugs. In milder cases the risk of these drugs outweigh the benefits.

Dental Considerations. The dentist should emphasize proper care of the teeth, since lack of saliva is often accompanied by an increase in caries. Daily home use of topical fluoride will help control the caries rate. Oral candidiasis, which may develop in Sjögren's patients can be successfully treated by use of topical rinses of nystatin suspension. Be aware that patients with Sjögren's syndrome may be taking systemic corticosteroids or immunosuppressive drugs for treatment of their generalized collagen disease, especially if it is systemic lupus erythematosus. Take precaution against infection preceding oral surgical procedures. Saliva substitutes such as Xerolube or glycerin are helpful in reducing the severity of xerostomia.

BIBLIOGRAPHY

Sialolithiasis

Bahn SL, Tabachnick TT: Sialolithiasis of minor salivary glands. Oral Surg 32:371, 1971

Barnett ML: Sialolithiasis of a labial gland. Oral Surg 32:22, 1971

Blair GS: Hydrostatic sialography—An analysis of a technique. Oral Surg 36:116, 1973

Bruns WT et al: Submandibular sialolithiasis in a cystic fibrosis patient. Am J Dis Child 126:685, 1973

Bullock KN: Salivary duct calculi presenting as trismus in a child. Br J Med 280:1357, 1980

Burstein LS et al: The crystal chemistry of submandibular and parotid salivary gland stones. J Oral Pathol 8:284, 1979

El Deeb M, Holte N, Gorlin RJ: Submandibular salivary gland sialoliths perforated through the oral floor. Oral Surg 51:134, 1981

Hiraide F, Nomura Y: The fine surface structure and composition of salivary calculi. Laryngology 9:152, 1980

Holst E: The clinical entity of sialolithiasis of the minor salivary gland. Acta Odontol Scand 29:75, 1971

Jensen JL et al: Minor salivary gland calculi. A clinicopathologic study of forty-seven new cases. Oral Surg 47:44, 1979

Langlais RP et al: Sialolithiasis: The radiolucent ones. Oral Surg 40:686, 1975

Noehren AH: Multiple calculi in Stensen's duct. JAMA 80:25, 1923

Perrotta RJ, Williams JR, Selfe RW: Simultaneous bilateral parotid and submandibular gland calculi. Arch Otolaryngol 104:469, 1978

Suleiman SI, Hobsley M: Radiological appearances of parotid duct calculi. Br J Surg 67:879, 1980

Yune HY, Klatte EC: Current status of sialography. Am J Roentgenol Radium Ther Nucl Med 115:420, 1972

Mucoceles

Redpath TH: Congenital ranula. Oral Surg 28:542, 1969

Sela J, Ulmansky M: Mucous retention cyst of salivary glands. J Oral Surg 27:15, 1969

Wilcox JW, Hickory R: Nonsurgical resolution of mucoceles. J Oral Surg 36:478, 1978

Sialadenosis

Blomfield J et al: Flow rate and inorganic components of submandibular saliva in cystic fibrosis. Arch Dis Child 48:267, 1973

Gardner AF: Diseases and Neoplasms of the Salivary Glands. Chicago, Year Book Medical Publishers, 1966

Garfunkel AA et al: Phenylbutazone—induced sialadenitis. Oral Surg 38:223, 1974

Hall HD: Diagnosis of diseases of the salivary glands. J Oral Surg 27:15, 1969

Krolls SO et al: Salivary gland lesions in children. Cancer 30:459, 1972

Mandel ID et al: Salivary studies in cystic fibrosis. Am J Dis Child 113:431, 1967

Mandel L, Baurmash H: Parotid enlargement due to alcoholism. J Am Dent Assoc 82:369, 1971

Mason DK, Chisholm D: Salivary Glands in Health and Disease. London, WB Saunders, 1975

Minaire Y et al: Chronic pancreatitis, alcoholic cirrhosis, and salivary secretion. Digestion 12:57, 1975

Rothbell EN, Duggan JJ: Enlargement of the parotid gland in disease of the liver. Am J Med 22:367, 1957

Wintrobe M et al (eds): Harrison's Principles of Internal Medicine, 7th ed. New York, McGraw-Hill, 1974

Wotman S et al: Salivary indicators of systemic disease. Postgrad Med 53:73, 1973

Yoel J: Pathology and Surgery of the Salivary Glands. Springfield, IL, Charles C Thomas, 1975

Developmental Abnormalities

Adams WP, Donahoe PK: Salivary gland heterotopia in the lower part of the neck. Arch Surg 114:79, 1979

Entin MA: Reconstruction in congenital deformity of the temporo-mandibular complex. Plastic Reconstr Surg 21:461, 1958

Hughes RD, Syrop HW: A familial study of the agenesis of the parotid gland duct. In Proceedings of the Tenth International Congress of Genetics, p. 128. Montreal, University of Toronto Press, 1959

Jernstrom P, Prietto C: Accessory parotid gland tissue at the base of the neck. Arch Pathol 73:473, 1962

McKenzie J, Craig J: Mandibulo-facial dysostosis (Treacher-Collins syndrome). Arch Dis Child 30:391, 1955

Marwah S, Berman ML: Ectopic salivary gland in the vulva (chorestoma): Report of a case and review of the literature. Obstet Gynecol 56:389, 1980

Parsons RW: Heterotrophic cervical salivary gland, case report. Plastic Reconstr Surg 49:464, 1972

Rauch S, Gorlin RJ: Diseases of the salivary glands. In Gorlin RJ, Goldman HM (eds): Thoma's Oral Pathology, 2nd ed. St. Louis, CV Mosby, 1944

Sinha SN, Singh AK: Ipsilateral absence of tonsil and microtia with ectopic salivary gland. J Laryngol Otol 92:1147, 1978

Steggerda FR: Observations in the water intake of man with dysfunctioning salivary glands. Am J Physiol 132:517, 1941

Stene T, Pedersen KN: Aberrant salivary gland tissue in the anterior mandible. Oral Surg 44:75, 1977

Salivary Gland Infections

Baum JG: Epidemic non meningitic lymphocytic—Choreomeningitis virus infection. N Engl J Med 274:934, 1966

Brunell PA et al: Parotitis in children who had previously received mumps vaccine. Pediatrics 50:441, 1972

Buckely JM et al: Parotitis and parainfluenza 3 virus. Am J Dis Child 124:789, 1972

Carlson RG, Glas WW: Acute suppurative parotitis. Arch Surg 86:163, 1963

Clizer EE: Cytomegalovirus mononucleosis. JAMA 228:606, 1974

Cunningham BD et al: Murine tumor induction by cytomegalovirus. Oral Surg 40:130, 1975

Duff TB: Parotitis, parotid abscess and facial palsy. J Laryngol Otol 86:161, 1972

Editorial: Br Med J 281:1231, 1980

Garvar LR, Kringstein GJ: Recurrent parotitis in childhood. J Oral Surg 32:373, 1974

Hemenway WG, English GM: Surgical treatment of acute bacterial parotitis. Postgrad Med 50:114, 1971

Hopkins R: Primary actinomycosis of the parotid gland. Br J Oral Surg 11:131, 1973

Howlett JG et al: A new syndrome of parotitis with herpangina caused by the coxsackie virus. Can Med Assoc J 77:5, 1957

Ju DMC: Salivary gland tumors occurring after radiation of the head and neck area. Am J Surg 116:518, 1968

Kaban LB, Donoff RB, Guralnick WC: Acute parotitis; Report of a complex and unusual case. J Oral Surg 31:377, 1973

Keis AFR, Mitchell OG: Cytomegalovirus in the submandibular and sublingual glands of the southern grasshopper mouse. J Dent Res 54:626, 1975

Klemola E, Kääriäinen L: Cytomegalovirus as a possible cause of a disease resembling mononucleosis. Br Med J 2:1099, 1965

Krippaehne WW, Hunt TK, Dunphy JE: Acute suppurative parotitis: A study of 161 cases. Ann Surg 156:251, 1962

Lary BG: Postoperative suppurative parotitis. Arch Surg 89:653, 1964

Leake DL, Krakowiak FJ, Leake RC: Suppurative parotitis in children. Oral Surg 31:174, 1971

Lewis JM, Utz JP: Orchitis, parotitis, and meningoencephalitis due to lymphocytic choriomeningitis virus. N Engl J Med 265:776, 1961

Maynard JD: Recurrent parotid enlargement. Br J Surg 52:784, 1965

Modlin JF, Orenstein WA, Brandling–Bennett AD: Current status of mumps in the U.S. J Infect Dis 132:106, 1975

Morgan WR: Parotid duct ligation and tympanic neurectomy in chronic recurrent parotiditis. Arch Otolaryngol 98:179, 1973

Quinn JH, Graham R: Recurrent suppurative parotitis treated by intraductal antibiotics. J Oral Surg 31:36, 1973

Ragheb M: Parotid infection caused by dryness of mouth—Report of 3 cases after the use of tranquilizers. Geriatics 18:627, 1963

Resouly A: The role of tympanic neurectomy in recurrent parotitis. J Laryngol Otol 87:497, 1973

Saunders HF: Wind parotitis. N Engl J Med 289:698, 1973

Sazama L: Actinomycosis of the parotid gland. Oral Surg 19:197, 1965

Speirs CF, Mason DK: Acute septic parotitis: Incidence, etiology and management. Scott Med J 17:62, 1972

Spratt JS: The etiology and therapy of acute pyogenic parotitis. Surg Gynecol Obstet 112:391, 1961

Walker LG, Hubert T, Smyth NPD: Acute suppurative parotitis associated with certain drugs in the treatment of parkinsonism. Med Ann DC, 31:586, 1962

Weller TH: The cytomegaloviruses: Ubiquitous agents with protean clinical manifestations (Parts I and II). N Engl J Med 285:203; 267, 1971

Wong T, Warner NE: Cytomegalic inclusion disease in adults. Arch Pathol 74:17, 1962

Yonkers AJ, Krous HF, Yarington CT: Surgical parotitis. Laryngoscope 82:1239, 1972

Zollar LM, Mufson MA: Acute parotitis associated with parainfluenza 3 virus infection. Am J Dis Child 119:147, 1970

Allergic Sialadenitis

Banks P: Hypersensitivity and drug reactions involving the parotid gland. Br J Oral Surg 5:60, 1967

Carter JE: Iodide "Mumps." N Engl J Med 264:987, 1961

Gross L: Oxyphenbutazone-induced parotitis. Ann Intern Med 70:1229, 1969

Koch RL, Byl FM, Firpo JJ: Parotid swelling with facial paralysis: A complication of intravenous urography. Radiology 92:1043, 1969

Nidus BD, Field M, Rammelkamp CH: Salivary

gland enlargement caused by sulfisoxazole. Ann Intern Med 63:663, 1965

Pearson RSB: Recurrent swelling of the parotid gland. Gut 2:210, 1961

Rothstein E: Allergic reaction to thioridazine. N Engl J Med 290:521, 1974

Waldbott GL, Shea JJ: Allergic parotitis. J Allergy 18:51, 1947

Sialadenitis

Epker BN: Obstructive and inflammatory diseases of the major salivary glands. Oral Surg 33:2, 1972

Harden RM: Submandibular adenitis due to iodine administration. Br Med J 1:160, 1968

Mardh PA et al: Sialadenitis following treatment with alpha methyldopa. Acta Med Scand 195:333, 1974

Necrotizing Sialometaplasia

Dunley RE, Jacoway JR: Necrotizing sialometaplasia. Oral Surg 47:169, 1979

Fechner RE: Necrotizing sialometaplasia. A source of confusion with carcinoma of the palate. Am J Clin Pathol 67:315, 1977

Forney SK, Foley JM, Sugg WE, Oatis GW: Necrotizing sialometaplasia of the mandible. Oral Surg 43:720, 1977

Lynch DP, Crago CA, Martinez MG: Necrotizing sialometaplasia. Oral Surg 47:63, 1979

Matilla A, Flores T, Nogales F, Galera H: Necrotizing sialometaplasia affecting minor labial glands. Oral Surg 47:161, 1979

Murphy J, Giunta J, Meyer I, Robinson K: Necrotizing sialometaplasia. Oral Surg 44:419, 1977

Sjögren's Syndrome

Akin RK et al: Sjögren's syndrome. J Oral Surg 33:27, 1975

Alarcon-Segovia D: Sjögren's syndrome in prodrome in primary biliary cirrhosis. Ann Intern Med 79:31, 1973

Alarcon–Segovia D: Sjögren's syndrome in progressive systemic sclerosis (scleroderma). Am J Med 57:78, 1974

Alarcon–Segovia D et al: Sjögren's syndrome in systemic lupus erythematosus. Ann Intern Med 81:577, 1974

Alspaugh MA, Tan EM: Antibodies to cellular antigens in Sjögren's syndrome. J Clin Invest 55:1067, 1973

Ben–Aryeh H et al: Sialochemistry for diagnosis of Sjögren's syndrome in xerostomic patients. Oral Surg 52:487, 1981

Chudwin DS et al: Spectrum of Sjögren's syndrome in children. J Pediatr 98:213, 1981

Cipoletti JF et al: Sjögren's syndrome in progressive systemic sclerosis. Ann Intern Med 87:535, 1977

Cummings NA et al: Sjögren's syndrome—newer aspects of research, diagnosis and therapy. Ann Intern Med 75:937, 1971

Daniels TE et al: The oral component of Sjögren's syndrome. Oral Surg 39:875, 1975

Feldkamp TEW, Van Rossum AC: Antibodies to salivary duct cells and other autoantibodies in patients with Sjögren's syndrome and other idiopathic autoimmune diseases. Clin Exp Immunol 3:1, 1968

Frost–Larsen K, Isager H, Manthorpe R: Sjögren's syndrome treated with bromhexine: A randomized clinical study. Br Med J 1:1579, 1978

Golding PL et al: Sicca complex in liver disease. Br Med J 2:340, 1970

Greenspan JS et al: The histopathology of Sjögren's syndrome in labial salivary gland biopsies. Oral Surg 37:217, 1974

Hemenway WG: Chronic punctate parotitis. Boulder, Colorado Associated University Press, 1971

Karsh J, Pavlidis N, Moutsopoulos M: Immunization of patients with Sjögren's syndrome with pneumococcal polysaccharide vaccine. Arthritis Rheum 23:1294, 1980

Katz WA, Ehrlich GE: Acute salivary gland inflammation associated with systemic lupus erythematosus. Ann Intern Med 74:55, 1971

Klestov AC et al: Treatment of xerostomia: A double blind trial in 108 patients with Sjögren's syndrome. Oral Surg 51:594, 1981

Leban SG, Strategos GT: Benign lymphoepithelial sialoadenopathies. Oral Surg 38:735, 1974

Manthorpe R et al: Sjögren's syndrome. A review with emphasis on immunological features. Allergy 36:139, 1981

Sapiro SM, Eisenberg E: Sjögren's syndrome (sicca complex). Oral Surg 45:591, 1978

Talal N: Immunologic and viral factors in the pathogenesis of systemic lupus erythematosus. Arthritis Rheum 13:887, 1970

Talal N et al: Elevated salivary and synovial fluid B_2—Microglobulin in Sjögren's syndrome and rheumatoid arthritis. Science 187:1196, 1975

Tannenbaum H et al: Immunological characterization of the mononuclear cell infiltrates in rheumatoid synovia, in rheumatoid nodules and in lip biopsies from patients with Sjögren's syndrome. Arthritis Rheum 18:305, 1975

Tapper–Jones LM et al: Sjögren's syndrome treated with bromhexine: A reassessment. Br Med J 280:1356, 1980

12
Disorders of the Temporomandibular Joint and Myofascial Pain Dysfunction Syndrome

PHILIP S. SPRINGER

MARTIN S. GREENBERG

A clear understanding of facial pain related to disorders of the temporomandibular joint (TMJ) and the muscles of mastication has unfortunately been hindered by a lack of well-designed objective investigations. Historically, from the time Costen popularized the ill-conceived syndrome bearing his name, diagnosis and treatment of pain of this area have commonly been based on personal observations, uncontrolled studies, and subjective conclusions. Facial pain related to the TMJ is not monolithic; its causes must be considered individually if proper treatment is to be rendered.

An important concept that has classically been emphasized in presenting this topic is the distinction between disorders of the muscles of mastication, primarily myofascial pain dysfunction syndrome, and derangements within the TMJ *per se*. In recent years, the interrelationship of the TMJ and its associated musculature has been highlighted. Skiba and Laskin have noted that ". . .degenerative changes as well as other pathologic processes in the TMJ may precede, accompany or even result from the syndrome." Soft tissue derangement of the TMJ is another aspect that has recently received attention primarily because of the use of arthrography.

ANATOMY

The primary components of the temporomandibular joint are the mandibular condyle, the articular surfaces of the temporal bone, the articular disc, and the joint capsule (see Fig. 12-1). The superior portion of the lateral pterygoid muscle is considered by some to be part of the joint because the disc is a direct extension of it; the inferior portion of the muscle attaches to the condyle. The temporomandibular joint contrasts with other joints of the body in that its articular surfaces are primarily composed of collagen instead of hyaline cartilage.

The disc is a dense fibrous plate that separates the joint into superior and inferior compartments. It is characterized by a thin, avascular central portion and a thicker, vascular posterior region. The elasticity in the posterior attachment of the disc to the tympanic plate is important for translation of the condyle. The disc is normally tightly bound to the medial and lateral poles of the condyle and its main functions are stabilization during condylar movement and shock absorption during mastication. The joint capsule consists of fibrous tissue that attaches to the periphery of the articular eminence of the temporal bone and to the condyle. Synovial membrane lines the capsule and helps lubricate the joint. The capsule is reinforced on the lateral aspect by the temporomandibular ligament, which provides some limitation to mandibular movement. The articular eminence, not the glenoid fossa, is the primary functional area of the temporal bone during mandibular movements. This is indicated by the thin bone and fibrous covering of the fossa area (see Fig. 12-2).

The major sensory innervation of the temporomandibular joint is derived from branches of the auriculotemporal nerve with branches of the masseteric and posterior deep temporal nerves making a smaller contribution. The superficial temporal artery is the primary blood supply to the joint.

The two condylar movements during mandibular function are rotation and translation. The superior joint space is associated with the anterior gliding movements of translation, whereas the inferior joint space is associated with condylar rotation. Because both temporomandibular joints are joined by a single bone, movement in one joint cannot occur without either similar coordinating or dissimilar reactive movements in the other joint. Opening, closing, protrusion, and retraction are bilateral symmetrical movements. Lateral excursions are bilateral asymmetrical movements.

Mandibular opening is produced by contraction of the lateral pterygoid muscles with assistance from the digastric, geniohyoid, and mylohyoid muscles. The masseter, medial pterygoid, and anterior fibers of the temporalis muscles are involved in mandibular closing. Protrusion of the mandible is accomplished by the lateral pterygoid muscles, whereas retruded position is produced by contraction of the posterior fibers of the temporalis muscles. Sideward movement of the mandible occurs when the contralateral lateral pterygoid muscle contracts.

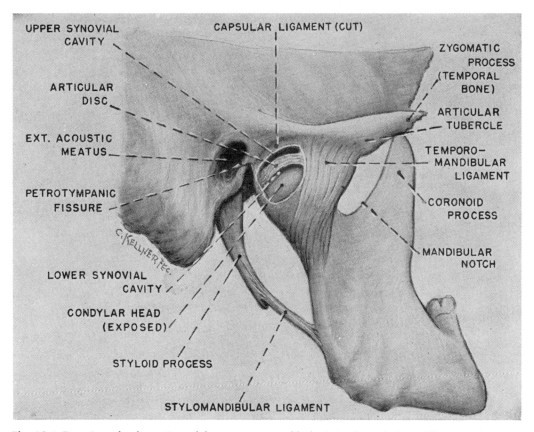

Fig. 12-1 Drawing of a dissection of the temporomandibular joint (lateral view). The capsular ligament has been opened. (Shapiro HH: Applied Anatomy of the Head and Neck, p 109. Philadelphia, JB Lippincott, 1947)

PATIENT HISTORY

The information obtained by carefully listening to the patient with a history of facial pain often is the most significant aspect of the diagnostic process. The patient's description of the location, duration, and characteristics of the pain greatly helps in distinguishing between disorders with similar symptoms and physical findings. It is always an advantage for the practitioner to be a good, empathetic listener when treating patients with facial pain. Allowing patients the time to candidly talk about their problems is often in itself therapeutic. The importance of the doctor–patient relationship in the successful management of myofascial pain dysfunction syndrome (MPDS) has been established by several studies and will be discussed later in the chapter.

In initiating the process of history taking, the chief complaint should succinctly express the problem and its duration in the patient's own terms. This is elaborated upon in the history of the present illness, which provides a chronologic narrative of the disorder from the onset of symptoms until the present. Previous treatments for the disorder and their effect should be recorded.

Information concerning the location of the pain and its characteristics should be elicited from the patient. The location of the pain should be confirmed by asking the patient to indicate where it hurts by pointing to it. This often helps differentiate between a true joint problem, in which the patient usually localizes the discomfort in the pretragus region and a muscular disorder. It is also important to note whether the pain is unilateral or bilateral.

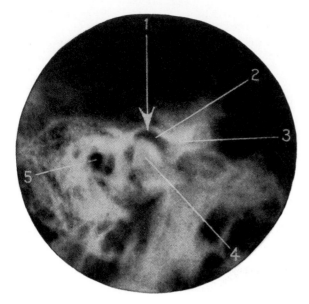

Fig. 12-2 Radiograph of the temporomandibular joint (lateral view). (1) glenoid fossa; (2) space occupied by the articular disc and joint spaces; (3) articular eminence; (4) condylar head; and (5) external auditory meatus. (Shapiro HH: Applied Anatomy of the Head and Neck, p 111. Philadelphia, JB Lippincott, 1947)

The nature of the pain should be described as completely as possible. Questions that should be asked include the following:

1. Is the pain sharp and lancinating or a dull aching and throbbing?
2. Does the pain occur spontaneously or do certain activities cause it?
3. Is the pain constant or periodic?
4. Does the pain gradually build in intensity or is it paroxysmal?
5. Is the pain worse at any time of the day?
6. Is the pain of short duration (seconds; minutes) or long (hours; days)?

The pain associated with myofascial pain dysfunction is most often described as being a dull, unilateral ache that is often worse on awakening. TMJ pain may be dull or sharp, and usually there is increasing discomfort with increasing function.

Jaw and joint symptoms should also be discussed with the patient:

1. Has the patient noted clicking or popping in the TMJ on opening or closing?
2. Has there been any limitation in movement or deviation of the lower jaw on opening?
3. Has the jaw ever locked or dislocated on opening?
4. Has the patient experienced pain and dysfunction in other joints of the body?

Any oral habits that the patient is aware of should be described in this section of the history.

The past medical history should always be reviewed. The patient is questioned about previous illnesses particularly rheumatoid arthritis and degenerative joint disease. It is important to note any trauma to the head and neck, such as an injury from a motor vehicle or bicycle accident. Injuries to the side of the face and chin should be described in detail because they are often responsible for temporomandibular joint problems. Whiplash injuries and the cervical braces used to treat them may contribute to myofascial pain or joint disease. It always is necessary to consider that some patients experiencing accident-related facial pain may actually be suffering from "litigation pain."

Past hospitalizations and surgeries must also be reviewed when taking the history. Allergies to medications and any medications presently being taken and their dosage should be recorded.

Included in the history should be information concerning the patient's dental experience. Recent dental procedures, especially those associated with the onset of symptoms or treatment for the disorder, should be discussed in detail.

The review of systems section of the history involves determining those symptoms the patient has experienced that may or may not be linked to the present illness. For patients with facial pain, an emphasis is placed on the head, ears, eyes, nose, and throat (HEENT) and neurologic and musculoskeletal aspects of the review of systems. Particularly important is recent pain in other joints. Symptoms of stress, anxiety, and depression, which are often associated with psychosomatic disorders, should also be accented.

In the family history, it is essential to specifically ask about rheumatoid arthritis, other connective tissue diseases, and osteoarthritis. The social history is important in determining stress-producing situations at home or work and other occurrences that might contribute to the etiology of MPDS.

CLINICAL EXAMINATION

The clinical examination for a patient with possible temporomandibular joint (TMJ) or myofascial pain should supplement the routine regional head and neck examination. The symmetry of the face is initially assessed. Although mild to moderate asymmetry is common, gross asymmetry may reflect a growth disturbance. This is often seen in patients who during childhood experienced trauma to the chin that resulted in TMJ ankylosis and abnormal facial bone growth. Hypertrophy of the masseter muscles may indicate clenching or other oral habits.

The maximum interincisal opening of the mandible should be determined (see Fig. 12-3). Measurements should also be recorded for the degree of opening when pain or clicking occur. Any deviation and its severity should be noted in examining mandibular opening. It is not uncommon to see an s-shaped opening of the mandible; this can be related to either a muscular or a true joint derangement.

Another significant aspect of the clinical examination is palpation of the pretragus areas. The patient should be requested to slowly open and close the mouth while the practitioner bilaterally palpates the pretragus depression with his index fingers. Similarly, intra-auricular palpation also is performed by inserting the small fingers into the ear canal and pressing anteriorly. It is important to perceive during pretragus and intra-auricular palpation whether the condyles move symmetrically with both the rotation and translation phases being evident. When unilateral problems exist, the mandible will always be seen to deviate to the side with the limited condylar movement. In addition to limitation of joint movement, palpation of these areas is also used to detect clicking and crepitus. Subluxation of the joints should be noted, although it has been demonstrated to be a variation of normal function.

The regional muscles are examined for tenderness and spasm using digital palpation. The temporalis, medial, and lateral pterygoids, masseter, trapezius, and sternocleidomastoid are the primary muscles included in the clinical evaluation. The masseter muscles are most effectively examined by simultaneously pressing from inside and outside the mouth in the process of bimanual palpation. The lateral pterygoids are evaluated by inserting a finger behind the tuberosity region, whereas the medial pterygoids are checked by running a finger in a anteroposterior direction along the medial aspect of the mandible in the floor of the mouth.

The clinical examination must include an evaluation of missing teeth, occlusion classification, occlusal interferences, the periodontal and decay status, and the integrity of fixed and removable prostheses. Because parafunction plays a significant role in the pathogenesis of MPDS and may be involved in certain degenerative changes of the TMJ, any evidence of oral habits, such as wear facets, should be noted.

DIFFERENTIAL DIAGNOSIS

Unfortunately, patients with facial pain are often treated inappropriately for many years before an accurate diagnosis is made. For example, it is not unusual for a patient to have several vital, normal teeth endodontically treated or extracted when the problem is actually myofascial pain dysfunction syndrome. Before treatment of MPDS or TMJ pain begins, it is necessary to exclude other disorders that might present with similar symptoms.

The process of formulating a differential

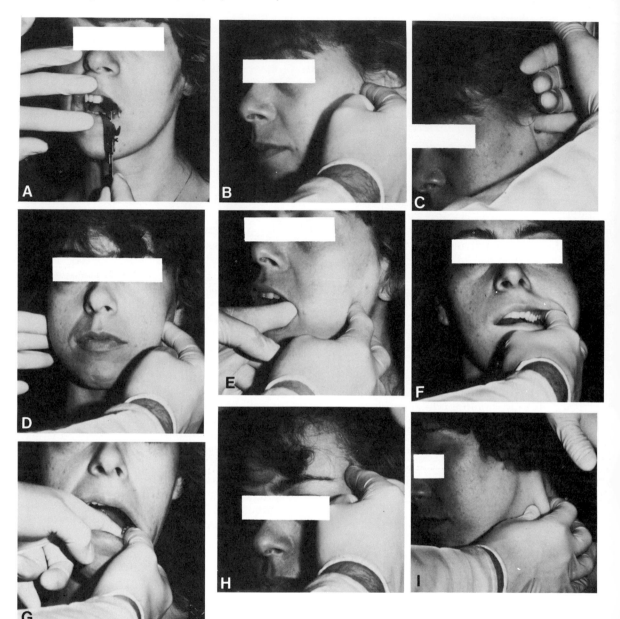

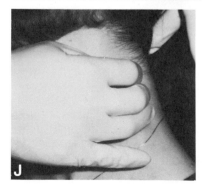

Fig. 12-3 The clinical examination. *A,* Measuring maximum interincisal opening. *B,* Palpation of the pretrogus area. *C,* Intraauricular palpation. *D,* Palpation of the masseter muscles. *E,* Bimanual palpation of the masseter muscle. *F,* Palpation of the lateral pterygoid muscle. *G,* Palpation of the medial pterygoid muscle. *H,* Palpation of the temporalis muscle. *I,* Palpation of the sternocleidomastoid muscle. *J,* Palpation of the trapezius muscle.

diagnosis begins with carefully evaluating the patient's statements and emotional status during the history. In listening, it is important to discern whether the pain is limited to an area innervated by one nerve. Certain disorders are almost always unilateral, and therefore they can be ruled out in making a diagnosis if the patient gives a history of pain crossing the midline. If the pain the patient is experiencing seems anatomically inappropriate it can also help you determine whether the pain is organic or psychogenic in origin (see Table 12-1).

Differentiating between the disorders can usually be facilitated by determining the location, stimulus, and characteristics of the pain. Knowledge of the age and sex predilections of each disorder can also be helpful.

Trigeminal Neuralgia. Also known as *tic douloureux*, trigeminal neuralgia is an extremely debilitating disorder usually involving areas innervated by the second and third division of the trigeminal nerve. Its features include lancinating unilateral pain of short duration (seconds to minutes) provoked by light touch or even a breeze to trigger zones around the

Table 12-1. Major Disorders That May Involve Facial Pain

ORIGIN	DISORDER
Neural	Trigeminal neuralgia (tic douloureux)
	Multiple sclerosis
	Glossopharyngeal neuralgia
Vascular	Temporal arteritis
	Migraine headaches
	Cluster headaches
	Angina pectoris
Musculoskeletal	TMJ disorders
	Myofascial pain dysfunction syndrome (MPDS)
	Elongated styloid process (Eagle's syndrome)
Oral/Salivary	Dental (pulpal, periodontal)
	Salivary gland inflammation or infection, duct blockage, or gland tumors
ENT-related	Otitis
	Sinusitis
Psychogenic	Atypical facial pain

mouth or skin of the face. The pain is of such severity that people unfortunate enough to have this disorder will often be seen protecting these trigger zones by placing their hands just over the area. Trigeminal neuralgia occurs more frequently in women (3:2), and its onset is usually about the fifth decade of life. Although the etiology of trigeminal neuralgia remains unknown, some theories prevail. One theory asserts that pain emanates from compression of the trigeminal root or gasserian ganglion by blood vessels. Proliferative and degenerative changes in the myelin sheaths of the large fibers of the trigeminal ganglion have also been implicated as a possible cause of trigeminal neuralgia.

In 1979, Ratner reported excellent results in the relief of trigeminal pain by curetting bony cavities that were found to remain in the jaws months to years after extractions. This finding promotes the theory that trigeminal pain is a peripheral sensory nerve problem, not a central cranial nerve disorder.

Multiple Sclerosis. Patients having multiple sclerosis, a disease causing demyelination of nerves, often have facial pain similar to trigeminal neuralgia as an early symptom. The average age of these patients is usually between the second and third decades; it is therefore important to consider multiple sclerosis as a possible diagnosis in any young patient with trigeminal neuralgialike symptoms especially if problems in gait and vision are also noticed.

Glossopharyngeal Neuralgia. Glossopharyngeal neuralgia has features similar to trigeminal neuralgia. As its name implies, the areas involved (the throat, tongue, and ears) are innervated by the glossopharyngeal (IX) nerve. The short-duration, unilateral pain of glossopharyngeal neuralgia is most often seen in older males.

Temporal Arteritis. A chronic granulomatous inflammation involving the temporal arteries or any cerebral vessel, temporal arteritis is a rare disorder occurring in older individuals. The pain associated with temporal arteritis has been described as an intense pounding that becomes worse on stooping or lying down. It is localized to the temporal, ear, and facial areas. Elevated and nodular temporal arteries may be noted in these patients. Diagnosis of temporal arteritis is aided by finding an elevated white blood cell count and erythrocyte sedimentation rate. Definitive diagnosis can only be made by arterial biopsy. Visual defects often leading to blindness are a common symptom in temporal arteritis because the ophthalmic branch of the internal carotid artery may be involved.

Migraine Headaches. Migraine headaches are a common disorder involving arterial dilation of the extracranial arteries often at times of anxiety and stress. They are characterized by a unilateral, severe throbbing behind the eye that may last from hours to days. Patients may have prodromal signs of migraine headaches including visual disturbances and numbness followed by tingling of the lips, tongue, and hand.

Cluster headaches may be considered a variation of migraines. They last 1 to 2 hours but recur in rapid succession for days or weeks especially in spring and fall. Flushing and lacrimation are commonly associated with symptoms. The histamine level has been shown to be increased in cluster headaches, and therefore, they are sometimes referred to as histamine headaches.

Angina Pectoris. Angina pectoris often is caused by disease of the coronary arteries. Atherosclerotic plaques deposited in the arteries cause a narrowing of the arterial lumen, which results in a decreased blood flow and oxygenation to the myocardium. This ischemia causes pain sensation or paresthesia in the chest, left arm, neck, or lower jaw. Anginal pain that is referred to the mandible is usually confused with dental pain from teeth in the lower left quadrant. If dental causes of jaw pain are ruled out, the practitioner must consider the heart as a source of referred pain.

Elongated Styloid Process. The pain associated with an elongated styloid process, also known as Eagle's syndrome, has been characterized as severe, unilateral pain radiating from ear to neck. The pain is most commonly brought on by swallowing or by turning the head. The patient may express the feeling that a foreign object is lodged in the throat. A radiograph that shows an elongated styloid process in a symptomatic patient confirms the diagnosis.

Dental Disorders. Facial pain of dental etiology is extremely variable. It may occur as a dull ache or an extreme lancinating pain; the pain may be constant or intermittent, spontaneous, or brought on by mastication, percussion, hot, cold, sweets, or air. To determine whether a dental cause for facial pain exists, x-ray films and a careful examination of the area looking for decay, inflammation, swelling, or exudate are basic. Testing for pain on percussion of a tooth and also sensitivity to cold, heat, or air are standard procedures. The use of an electric pulp tester to determine the neurologic vitality of the pulp can also be extremely valuable in localizing pain and in making a diagnosis.

Salivary Disorders. Pain associated with a disorder of a major salivary gland may be localized to the gland or may radiate from the ear to the neck. Pain related to blockage of a duct, with resulting retention and swelling, is usually greatest during eating. The submandibular gland is most commonly involved with salivary stones. Radiographs and palpation are helpful in making a diagnosis.

Ear, Nose, and Throat-related Disorders. Inflammation and infection of the ear must be considered when pain is localized to that region. If other disorders are ruled out, you are obligated to refer the patient to an otorhinolaryngologist for an evaluation (this is also true for sinusitis). Pain in the region of the maxillary, frontal, ethmoid, or sphenoid sinuses should be followed up by a sinus exam and x-ray films. Sinus headaches are manifested by a deep dull pain that occurs most frequently in the morning.

Psychogenic Disorders. Psychogenic pain is difficult to diagnose because there is a psychological component to all pain perception. Atypical facial pain, a catchall term for pain that commonly does not follow classical nerve distribution, is often bilateral, and cannot be definitely diagnosed. The onset of atypical facial pain is frequently linked with postmenopausal depression. It is sometimes necessary to refer a patient with facial pain for psychiatric evaluation, especially when depression appears to be the cause of the pain. Antidepressant medications and psychological support are often beneficial for these patients.

DIAGNOSTIC STUDIES

Radiography

Radiography is the most important diagnostic aid in distinguishing among the disorders that may affect the temporomandibular joint. Although a routine TMJ series including transorbital and transcranial views probably remains the most requested form of radiographs of the TMJ, its limitations have been emphasized in recent years (see Figs. 12-4 and 12-5). Dunn and associates have stressed that it is necessary to have 30% to 60% addition or subtraction of calcified elements for changes to become apparent on routine x-ray films. Eckerdal and Lundberg also noted that conventional radiographs of the TMJ repro-

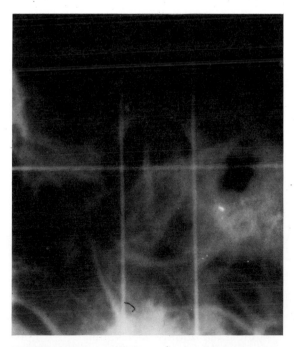

Fig. 12-4 Transcranial view of normal temporomandibular joint in clenched position.

duce a very limited aspect that may not accurately reflect the joint components and their spatial relations. These inherent limitations are thought to lead to an underdiagnosing of joint defects and an increase in the time between the initiation of the disease process and radiographic detection.

Tomography

Most radiologists agree that tomograms are superior to conventional radiographs because of their ability to depict a greater portion of the joint (see Fig. 12-6). By providing a series of sectional radiographs, tomography can reproduce small changes in the central portion of the TMJ and therefore decrease false-negative interpretations. Although tomograms may supply superior diagnostic information, patients undergoing tomography are exposed to substantially more radiation, and the difference in cost is considerable.

Arthrography

Routine radiography and tomography of the TMJ only provide information concerning the osseous components. With increasing interest in soft tissue derangements of the TMJ, arthrography has assumed an important role in the diagnosis of joint disorders. Defects in the position or structure of the joint disc and its attachments can be determined using arthrography. Derangements that are detectable with arthrography include displacement or perforation of the disc, irregularities in the posterior attachment of the disc, adhesions, and possibly synovial proliferations.

Blashke and associates noted that patients who are candidates for arthrography are most commonly individuals who have had progressive TMJ incoordination and locking with normal findings on routine TMJ radiographs and tomograms. Arthrography of the TMJ is performed by injecting a water-soluble, iodine-containing contrast material into the lower joint space (see Fig. 12-7). Lateral or anteroposterior radiographs or tomograms are subsequently taken (see Fig. 12-8). Cinefluoroscopy, essentially a movie produced with relatively low levels of radiation and providing a dynamic depiction of soft tissue

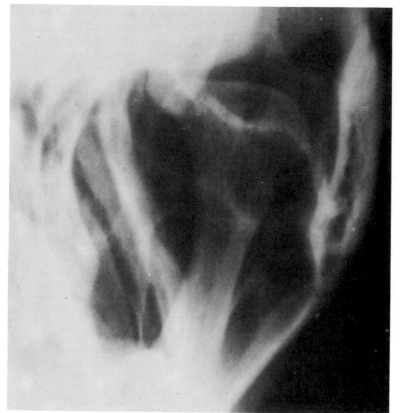

Fig. 12-5 Transorbital view of normal condyle.

components of the joint while in function, has also been used.

Arthrography of the TMJ has been determined to be a safe technique with hypersensitivity to iodine being the only contraindication. Its reliability has also been demonstrated. Bronstein and associates found a 97% correlation between arthrographic diagnosis and subsequent surgical findings in 34 procedures. The most common soft tissue derangement of the TMJ has been shown in several studies using arthrography to be anterior disc displacement.

Electromyography

It is generally accepted that one of the major criteria in diagnosing MPDS is finding tenderness to palpation in one or more of the muscles of mastication related to the increased muscle activity. Electromyography (EMG) provides an objective means of monitoring changes in muscle activity and there-fore can be a valuable aid in diagnosing MPDS and in evaluating the effectiveness of treatment. Although demonstrating increased muscle activity by EMG may help confirm an impression of MPDS in patients with facial pain, it should be remembered that the converse is not necessarily true; not all patients with increased activity in the muscles of mastication have facial pain.

EMG is an important component of biofeedback treatment for MPDS. Auditory or visual electromyographic feedback supplies information to the patient concerning muscle activity. This allows individuals to be aware of muscular changes not normally discernible and helps them control hyperactivity.

It was initially shown by Bessette in 1971 and subsequently confirmed by other investigators that most MPD patients have prolonged masseteric silent periods. The muscles most commonly seen to have prolonged EMG silent periods in MPD patients are the temporalis and the masseter. The silent periods, which are reflexive pauses in muscle activity, were found to become longer with increasing MPD symptom severity and to revert to normal when symptoms were relieved following treatment.

Studies using EMG monitoring have verified the physiological effectiveness of occlusal splints. MPD patients who use occlusal splints usually show a decrease in muscle activity.

Arthroscopy

Although arthroscopy has been a fundamental and routine procedure in diagnosing various orthopedic derangements, it has not historically been used for investigating disorders of the temporomandibular joint; however, recent studies on animals have demonstrated the applicability of arthroscopy in examining the TMJ. Williams and Laskin produced a variety of disorders in the TM joints of rabbits and evaluated their ability to diagnose the induced defects by using arthroscopy. Ste-

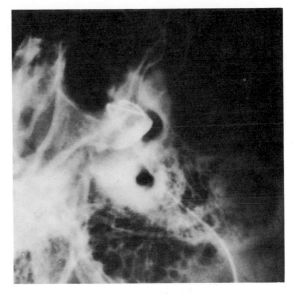

Fig. 12-7 Catheter in place for the injection of contrast media into lower joint space for arthrography.

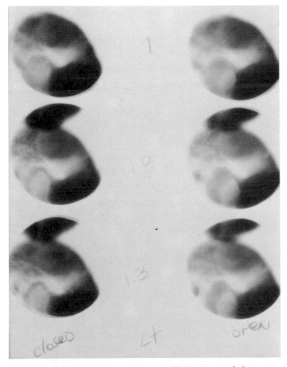

Fig. 12-6 Tomograms showing flattening of the condylar head and increased cortication of the articular eminence indicative of degenerative joint disease.

roid-induced arthropathy, chronic inflammatory changes in the synovium, acute inflammatory disease, and gross damage to the condyle and disc could all be visualized and diagnosed using arthroscopy in their study. They concluded that arthroscopy is a relatively noninvasive diagnostic technique for use in TMJ disorders. Its use in the diagnosis of human TMJ disorders is presently being developed.

MYOFASCIAL PAIN DYSFUNCTION SYNDROME

The theory that skeletal muscles in spasm could be a source of pain was initially published in the medical literature during the 1940s by Travell. Schwartz, noting that only a small percentage of the patients he examined had organic disorders of the TMJ, adapted Travell's work and postulated the TMJ pain dysfunction syndrome. He asserted that the vast majority of patients with pain in the region of the temporomandibular joint were suffering from a functional disorder involving a painful, self-perpetuating spasm of the masticatory muscles. Schwartz was the first to implicate the psychological make-up of the patient as a predisposing factor in the

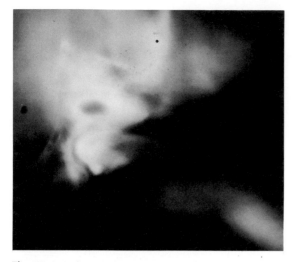

Fig. 12-8 Arthrotomogram.

pain dysfunction syndrome. He hypothesized that stress was a significant cause of the clenching and grinding habits, which resulted in spasm of the muscles of mastication. Schwartz's work was also important because it relegated occlusal abnormalities to a secondary role in the etiology of the pain syndrome.

The next significant advance towards understanding this aspect of facial pain occurred when Laskin presented a more comprehensive explanation of the problem and proposed his psychophysiologic theory in 1969. Stating that *temporomandibular joint pain dysfunction syndrome* was a misnomer because the disorder was primarily related to masticatory muscle spasm and usually not pathologic changes in the joint, he proposed the substitute term *myofascial pain dysfunction syndrome.* The signs and symptoms of MPDS as outlined by Laskin included the following:

1. Unilateral, dull pain in the ear or preauricular region that is commonly worse on awakening
2. Tenderness of one or more muscles of mastication on palpation
3. Clicking or popping noise in the TMJ
4. Limitation or deviation of the mandible on opening

Laskin also emphasized that there should be no evidence of organic changes in the TMJ on radiographic, clinical, or biochemical examination during the initial stages of MPDS. What is commonly overlooked is that Laskin

conjectured that the functional disorder of MPDS could lead to organic changes in the TMJ if the problem became chronic. The interrelationship has since been confirmed by Toller who noted degenerative changes in the joints of patients with long-standing MPDS.

Laskin's psychophysiologic theory, an outgrowth of the work of Schwartz, was based on the premise that MPDS is primarily a result of emotional rather than occlusal and mechanical factors. The main pathway that culminates in the muscle spasm and pain of MPDS, according to the concept, begins with stress. The theory states that stress can cause clenching and grinding, which in turn can lead to muscle fatigue and finally spasm. A self-perpetuating cycle of stress-pain-stress can be created. The muscles most often found to be involved in MPDS are the lateral pterygoid and masseter muscles.

Yemm and Christensen have demonstrated that in chronic cases of MPDS an inflammatory stage may occur in the affected muscles of mastication following the classic spasms. This myositis may perpetuate the symptoms of pain and dysfunction even though the spastic activity and shortening of the muscles have ended.

The emphasis placed on stress and tension as the main antecedents to MPDS has been supported by various studies. Evaskus and Laskin determined that MPD patients have significantly higher levels of steroids and catecholamines than is normal. Several investigations, including some that have used the Minnesota Multiphasic Personality Index (MMPI), have shown that patients with MPDS tend to react to stress by somatization and repression. Treatment of MPDS, therefore, must accent emotional support and stress reduction as well as physically therapeutic techniques.

Irregularities in occlusion appear to be the precipitating factor in the pathogenesis of MPDS in only a minority of cases. Occlusal interferences, posterior bite collapse, and deep overbite–overjet relationships may predispose patients to increase parafunctional activity. Certain types of malocclusion may also tend to restrict freedom of mandibular movement. The overuse of selected muscles of mastication may occur and may result in muscle fatigue and MPDS.

Initial evidence that nocturnal parafunction

may be involved in MPDS stemmed from the observation that jaw pain and limitation of movement were often noted to be worse on awakening. Trenouth performed a computer analysis of nocturnal tooth contacts and found that patients with MPDS kept their teeth in contact for considerably longer periods of time than do normal subjects. He also noted that the control group demonstrated tooth contacts in regular 60- to 90-minute intervals, while the MPDS group of patients exhibited an irregular cycle of tooth contact. General signs of bruxism may include tooth wear, tooth mobility, and thickening of the periodontal ligament noted on radiographs.

Clicking within the TMJ is generally considered to be related to a lack of coordination between the position of the articular disc and the position of the condyle. In acute cases associated with MPDS, the clicking may be attributed to incoordination of upper and lower portions of the lateral pterygoid muscle; the upper portion attaches to the meniscus, whereas the lower portion attaches to the mandibular neck. Other possible causes of clicking are laxity in the posterior attachment fibers of the disc and irregularities of the articular surfaces.

Treatment

To relieve the symptoms of MPDS it is necessary to treat the emotional as well as the physical components of the disorder. Conservative noninvasive treatment is usually successful in alleviating the pain and dysfunction especially in the acute stages.

Treatment of MPDS should begin by showing concern and empathy when reviewing the history of a patient's problem. This will often lead to a strong doctor–patient relationship and an improvement in symptoms. The importance of the doctor–patient relationship in the successful management of MPDS has been demonstrated by a series of studies by Greene, Laskin, and Goodman. They achieved 40% to 64% success in substantially or totally relieving pain and dysfunction by using only practitioner suggestion and placebo drugs, splints, or occlusal equilibration. Part of the initial therapy that also involves the emotional aspect of MPDS is patient reassurance. Patients should be told that they

are not suffering from a more serious, life-threatening disorder such as a malignancy. It is often beneficial in describing the pathogenesis of MPDS to make an analogy between the spasm and pain of the masticatory muscles and common "cramping" of skeletal muscles due to overuse.

Conservative treatment and recommendations at the initial visit should also include the following:

1. The patient should attempt to limit parafunctional habits by becoming more aware of clenching and grinding of the teeth during the day.
2. Warm-to-hot, moist compresses should be applied over the involved muscles about three times a day for 15 to 20 minutes.
3. A relatively soft diet should be advised. The patient should also be told to limit wide opening such as in eating a thick sandwich.
4. Aspirin or nonsteroidal anti-inflammatory drugs should be recommended for the analgesic and anti-inflammatory actions.
5. Injecting the trigger points of muscles that are in spasm with a local anesthetic not containing epinephrine is often beneficial in breaking up the spasm and in disrupting the stress-pain-stress cycle.
6. The skin overlying the affected muscles can be sprayed with ethyl chloride, or ultrasound can be used in an attempt to relieve muscle spasms. The effectiveness of local anesthetic injections, ethyl chloride refrigerant spray, and ultrasound in allowing patients to open wide without pain may be noted immediately following treatment.
7. Jaw exercises, such as placing the tip of the tongue to the back of the palate and then opening and closing, may help in retraining spastic muscles; isometric exercises are often beneficial.
8. The use of diazepam (2 mg three times daily and 5 mg at bedtime) during a 2-week trial period is commonly advocated for its anxiety-reducing and muscle-relaxing properties.

Occlusal Splints

If pain and dysfunction persist without improvement following the treatment and recommendations of the initial visit, an occlusal splint should be fabricated. The splint most often used is a maxillary nightguard made of hard, processed acrylic. A Hawley appliance with an anterior platform has been recommended by some practitioners; however, it can cause extrusion of posterior teeth and result in an anterior open bite if the patient wears the appliance for longer than intended.

The effectiveness of occlusal splints in decreasing the symptoms of MPDS has been demonstrated in many studies. Clark, Solberg, and Kawazoe each noted an objective decrease in masticatory muscle activity as measured by electromyography in most of the MPDS patients they treated following the use of occlusal splints. Clark's findings also indicated that muscle activity reverts to the higher pretreatment levels when splint therapy is discontinued. He therefore has recommended long-term use of the appliances. The benefits derived from occlusal splints have most commonly been attributed to greater freedom in mandibular movement and to an increase in muscle balance. The fact that about 40% of the patients treated with splints may show significant improvement related to a placebo effect must be considered in evaluating the actual effectiveness of the appliances.

Occlusal adjustments for the treatment of MPDS should only be performed when obvious interferences exist and appear to contribute to a specific oral habit or limitation of mandibular movement. Alleviation of symptoms should always be attempted by noninvasive, conservative treatment before doing an occlusal adjustment.

Patients suffering from MPDS from months to years usually do not respond as readily to the conservative treatment that has been outlined. Alternative modes of therapy should be considered when initial attempts to decrease pain and dysfunction have failed. Because degenerative changes within the joint may result from chronic MPDS, it is necessary to consider internal derangements as possibly contributing to the facial pain.

Biofeedback

Biofeedback may be helpful when the primary reason for the failure in initial treatment appears to be the inability to control stress and anxiety. Biofeedback provides patients with information concerning bodily functions that are usually not discernible or controllable. It has been used successfully in treating tension headaches and in controlling blood pressure and heart rate.

Kardachi and Clarke found that when using a biofeedback system they could instruct patients to significantly reduce nocturnal bruxism, with a subsequent decrease in facial pain. Similarly, Dohrman noted a significant reduction in the mean masseteric EMG levels with concurrent reduction in symptoms for patients using biofeedback. He emphasized that biofeedback is a valuable therapeutic aid that permits patients to treat themselves while decreasing their dependence on therapists.

Nerve Stimulation

Transcutaneous electrical nerve stimulation (TENS) has been successfully used in the treatment of phantom limb pain, peripheral nerve injury, lower back pain, cervical pain, joint pain, and a variety of other disorders. The electrical stimulus is typically generated from a portable battery-operated device and transmitted to the patient by electrodes applied to the facial skin. The frequency, intensity, and repetition rate of the stimulus usually varies. TENS treatment appears to be more effective in alleviating chronic pain than acute pain.

The mode of action of TENS in reducing pain is uncertain but has been attributed to neurologic, physiolgic, pharmacologic, and psychologic effects. The neurologic action of TENS is based on Melzack and Wall's gate-control theory of pain. TENS supposedly blocks pain signals being carried over the small, unmyelinated C-fibers by forcing the large, myelinated A-fibers to carry a light touch sensation. TENS may provide pain relief by the physiologic effects of rhythmic muscle movement. The fasciculation of muscles may result in an increase in circulation, a decrease in edema, and a decrease in resting muscle activity. The pharmacologic action of TENS may involve the stimulated release of endorphins, which are endogenous morphinelike substances. The probable placebo effects of TENS in relieving pain must also be considered.

Other Treatments

Acupuncture has also been used in the treatment of chronic MPDS with varying success. In acupuncture, brief intense stimulation is applied to designated points using needles with or without electrical current. The release of endorphins may also be involved in the pain relief associated with acupuncture treatment. Hypnosis may also be used as an adjunct to other treatment in mediating the pain of chronic MPDS. Psychological counseling and antidepressant drugs are indicated in the treatment of MPDS if anxiety or neurotic behavior appears to be a significant component of the facial pain.

INTERNAL DISORDERS OF THE TMJ

Internal derangements of the temporomandibular joint may involve abnormalities of the bony or soft tissue structures. In the past, osseous changes in the articular surfaces of the condyle and temporal bone were emphasized in discussions of intracapsular defects. In recent years, however, the role of soft tissue defects has become more prominent owing to the advances made in TMJ arthrography. Information concerning the position and integrity of the joint disc and its attachments can be provided by arthrography. It was noted earlier that internal derangements may occur separate from, in conjunction with, or secondary to the muscular disorder of MPDS.

The pathogenesis of intracapsular defects may involve degenerative processes, inflammatory disorders, infections, developmental disturbances, trauma, metabolic problems, neoplasia, and drug-induced changes (see Table 12-2).

Degenerative Joint Disease

The most common intracapsular disorder of the temporomandibular joint is degenerative joint disease. Degenerative joint disease, also referred to as osteoarthrosis, osteoarthritis, and degenerative arthritis, is primarily a noninflammatory process involving deterioration of the articular soft tissues and remodeling of the underlying bone. It is essentially a re-

Table 12-2. Internal Derangements of the Temporomandibular Joint

SOURCE	DISORDER
Degenerative	Degenerative joint disease
Inflammatory	Rheumatoid arthritis (and other collagen diseases) Psoriatic arthritis
Infections	Spread from contiguous site Gonorrhea Tuberculosis Syphilis
Developmental	Condylar hyperplasia, hypoplasia, and agenesis
Traumatic	Condylar fracture Ankylosis Dislocation Disc displacement
Metabolic	Gout
Neoplasia	Malignant Benign
Drug-induced	Steroid

sponse of the joint to chronic microtrauma or pressure. The microtrauma may be in the form of continuous abrasion of the articular surfaces as in natural wear associated with age or as increased loading forces possibly related to chronic parafunctional activity.

Degenerative joint disease may be categorized as primary or secondary, although both are similar on histopathologic examination. Primary degenerative joint disease is considered to be a relatively asymptomatic by-product of natural wear and is commonly seen in patients in their 50s and older. Secondary degenerative joint disease usually involves acute pain in younger patients and is associated with some form of stress placed on the joint, such as chronic myofascial pain dysfunction. Toller has confirmed that there is a direct relationship between long-standing MPDS and degenerative changes of the condyle.

Obërg examined temporomandibular joints on autopsy and noted 22% of the joints from subjects older than 20 years of age displayed degenerative changes. The incidence of degenerative changes was observed to increase with age and was rarely seen in subjects less than 40 years old. These findings agreed with the work of Blackwood, who noted degenerative changes in 40% of the temporomandibular joints taken from cadavers over 40 years old. Richards and Brown observed a direct relationship, irrespective of age, between the rate and extent of dental attrition and degenerative disease of the temporomandibular joints in cadavers of aboriginal man. They also noted that the temporal bone exhibited more changes than did the condyle.

An important conclusion that can be made in considering these investigations is that degenerative changes in the temporomandibular joint found on radiographic examination may be incidental and not responsible for facial pain symptoms; however, some degenerative changes may actually be underdiagnosed by conventional radiography because the defects are confined to the articular soft tissue. Perforation and displacement of the articular disc are examples of changes that are detectable with arthrography but not with conventional radiography.

Clinical Manifestations

Major symptoms of degenerative joint disease of the TMJ include unilateral pain directly over the condyle, limitation of mandibular opening, crepitus, and a feeling of stiffness after a period of inactivity. Examination reveals pain and crepitus on intra-auricular and pretragus palpation with deviation of the mandible to the painful side.

Radiographic findings in degenerative joint disease may include narrowing of the joint space, irregular joint space, flattening of the articular surfaces, osteophytic formation, anterior lipping of the condyle, and the presence of Ely's cysts (see Fig. 12-9).

Treatment

Degenerative joint disease of the temporomandibular joint can usually be managed by conservative treatment. Toller noted a significant improvement in many patients after 9 months and observed a burning out of many cases after one year. It seems prudent to manage a patient with conservative treatment for a year before considering surgery; conservative therapy includes nonsteroidal, anti-in-

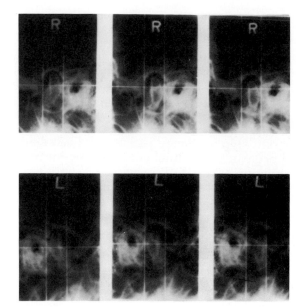

Fig. 12-9 Transcranial temporomandibular joint series showing degenerative remodeling of (*left*) glenoid fossa.

flammatory medications; heat; soft diet; rest; and occlusal splints. It may also be necessary to concomitantly treat myofascial pain. Intraarticular steroids can be used once a year during acute episodes, but repeated injections may cause degenerative bony changes.

When pain is persistent and there is distinct radiographic evidence of degenerative joint changes, surgery is indicated. An arthroplasty, which limits surgery to the removal of osteophytes and erosive areas, is commonly performed. High condylectomies with and without the use of Silastic to restore the vertical dimension are also used to treat more generalized degenerative changes of the temporomandibular joint.

Synovial Chondromatosis of the Temporomandibular Joint (Chondrometaplasia)

Synovial chondromatosis is metaplasia of the synovial membrane resulting in the formation of small foci of hyaline cartilage. In this disorder, cartilage develops from the connective tissue in the synovial membrane. Pieces of the cartilage are pinched off and released into the joint space causing a secondary degenerative joint disease. The joint most commonly involved with synovial chondromatosis is the knee, but there have been several reports of this disorder in the temporomandibular joint. Miller and associates reported a case in a 61-year-old female who had been complaining of swelling and crepitus in the TMJ region. Initially, this swelling was confused with a parotid tumor. Radiographs showed calcified nodules in the joint. Ronald and colleagues reported several cases from the Mayo Clinic. The patients ranged in age from 40 to 60 with an increased incidence in women. Symptoms included pain, limitation of opening, deviation to the affected side, crepitus, and swelling. The presence of swelling helps to distinguish the disorder from degenerative joint disease. Radiographic findings include an irregular joint surface and the presence of loose calcified cartilage in the region of the joint. In addition, Noyek and associates reported sclerosis of the glenoid fossa and mandibular condyle.

Treatment

Proper treatment of this disorder is surgical removal of the metaplastic tissue.

Rheumatoid Arthritis

The systemic inflammatory process of rheumatoid arthritis involves the temporomandibular joints in a majority of cases. The disease process starts as a vasculitis of the synovial membrane. It progresses to chronic inflammation marked by an intense round cell infiltrate and subsequent formation of granulation tissue. The cellular infiltrate spreads from the articular surfaces to eventually cause an erosion of the underlying bone.

Clinical Manifestations

The temporomandibular joints are usually bilaterally involved in rheumatoid arthritis. The most common symptoms mentioned by patients include deep, dull pain in the joints and limitation of mandibular opening. Pain is usually associated with the early, acute phases of the disease but is not a common complaint in later stages. Other symptoms often noted include morning stiffness, joint sounds, and tenderness and swelling over

the joint area. The symptoms are usually transient in nature, and only a small percentage of patients with rheumatoid arthritis of the temporomandibular joints will experience permanent, serious disability.

The most consistent clinical findings include pain on palpation of the joints and limitation of opening. Crepitus may also be evident. Micrognathia and an anterior open bite are commonly seen in patients with juvenile rheumatoid arthritis. Larheim and associates attribute the micrognathia to a combination of direct injury to the condylar head and altered orofacial muscular activity. Ankylosis of the temporomandibular joint related to rheumatoid arthritis is rare. Radiographic changes in the temporomandibular joint associated with rheumatoid arthritis may include a narrow joint space, destructive lesions of the condyle, and limited condylar movement. There is little evidence of marginal proliferation or other reparative activity in rheumatoid arthritis in contrast to the radiographic changes often observed in degenerative joint disease.

Treatment

Involvement of the temporomandibular joint by rheumatoid arthritis is usually treated by anti-inflammatory drugs in conjunction with the therapy for other affected joints. The patient should be placed on a soft diet during acute exacerbation of the disease process, but intermaxillary fixation is to be avoided because of the risk of fibrous ankylosis. An exercise program to increase mandibular movement should be instituted as soon as possible after the acute symptoms subside. When patients have severe symptoms, the use of intra-articular steroids should be considered.

Surgical treatment of the joint is indicated in patients with inactive disease who have severe functional impairment. A high condylectomy, often with the insertion of alloplastic materials such as Silastic, is the technique most often used.

Psoriatic Arthritis

Psoriatic arthritis is a rare cause of temporomandibular joint disease. Diagnosis usually is based on the occurrence of arthritis in a patient who has psoriasis and a negative rheumatoid factor.

Clinical Manifestations

The symptoms of psoriatic arthritis of the temporomandibular joint are similar to those noted in rheumatoid arthritis except that the pain usually is unilateral. Limitation of mandibular movement, deviation to the side of the pain, and tenderness directly over the joint may be observed on examination. Radiographic changes in psoriatic arthritis are not specific and tend to resemble the findings associated with rheumatoid arthritis.

Treatment

The management of psoriatic arthritis is similar to the treatment of rheumatoid arthritis, with an emphasis on physical therapy and salicylates. Antimalarial drugs should not be used because they may cause severe skin reactions in patients with psoriasis. Immunosuppressive drugs, particularly methotrexate, are used for patients with severe disease that does not respond to conservative treatment.

Septic Arthritis

Septic arthritis of the TMJ most commonly results from blood-borne bacterial infection; it may also be caused by trauma directly to the joint or by extension of infection from adjacent sites such as the middle ear, maxillary molars, and parotid gland.

Gonococcus is the primary causative agent of septic arthritis of the TMJ. Streptococcal, staphylococcal, and pneumococcal infections, in addition to viral infections such as measles and influenza, have also been reported to involve the joint.

Clinical Symptoms

Symptoms of septic arthritis of the temporomandibular joint include severe pain on movement and an inability to occlude the teeth owing to the presence of infection in the joint space. Examination reveals redness and swelling in the region of the involved joint. In some cases the swelling may be fluc-

tuant and extend beyond the region of the joint. Large, tender cervical lymph nodes are frequently observed on the side of the infection; this helps to distinguish septic arthritis from more common types of TMJ disorders.

Serious sequelae including ankylosis and facial asymmetry may accompany septic arthritis of the temporomandibular joint, especially when it occurs in children. Of the 44 cases of ankylosis of the temporomandibular joint reviewed by Topazian, 17 resulted from infection. The primary sites of these infections were the middle ear, teeth, and hematologic spread of gonorrhea.

Evaluation of patients with suspected septic arthritis must include a review of signs and symptoms of gonorrhea such as purulent urethral discharge or dysuria. The affected TMJ should be aspirated and the fluid obtained Gram stained and specially cultured for *Neisseria gonorrhoeae*.

Treatment

Treatment of septic arthritis of the TMJ consists of surgical drainage and antibiotics. Prolonged immobilization increases the risk of ankylosis and therefore should be avoided.

Developmental Defects

Developmental disturbances involving the temporomandibular joint may result in anomalies in the size and shape of the condyle. Hyperplasia, hypoplasia, agenesis, and the formation of a bifid condyle may be evident on radiographic examination of the joint. Local factors such as trauma or infection can initiate condylar growth disturbances.

True condylar hyperplasia usually occurs after puberty and is completed by 18 to 25 years of age. Limitation of opening, deviation of the mandible to the side of the enlarged condyle, and facial asymmetry may be observed. Pain is occasionally associated with the hyperplastic condyle on opening.

Facial asymmetry often results from disturbances in condylar growth because the condyle is considered to be a site for compensatory growth and adaptive remodeling. The facial deformities associated with condylar hyperplasia involve the formation of a convex ramus on the affected side and a concave shape on the normal side. If the condylar hyperplasia is detected and surgically corrected at an early stage, the facial deformities may be prevented.

Deviation of the mandible to the affected side and facial deformities are also associated with unilateral agenesis and hypoplasia of the condyle. Rib grafts have been used to replace the missing condyle to minimize the facial asymmetry in agenesis. In hypoplasia, Laskin noted a short wide ramus, shortening of the body of the mandible, and antegonial notching on the affected side with elongation of the mandibular body and flatness of the face on the opposite side. Early surgical intervention is again emphasized to limit facial deformity.

Trauma

Fractures

Fractures of the condylar head and neck often result from a blow to the chin (see Fig. 12-10). The patient with a condylar fracture usually presents with pain and edema over the joint area and limitation and deviation of the mandible to the injured side on opening. Bilateral condylar fractures may result in an anterior open bite. The diagnosis of a condylar fracture is confirmed by radiographic examination. Intracapsular, nondisplaced fractures of the condylar head are usually left untreated. Early mobilization of the mandible is emphasized to prevent bony or fibrous ankylosis.

Dislocation

In dislocation of the mandible, the condyle is positioned anterior to the articular eminence and cannot return to its normal position without assistance. This disorder contrasts with subluxation, in which the condyle moves anterior to the eminence during wide opening but is able to return to the resting position without manipulation. Sheppard has shown that subluxation is a variation of normal function and that the normal range of motion of the condyle is not limited to the fossa.

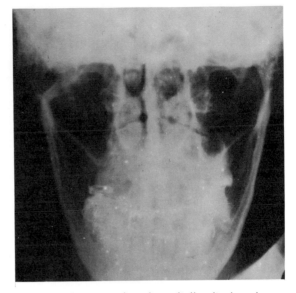

Fig. 12-10 Fractured and medially displaced condyle.

Dislocations of the mandible usually result from muscular incoordination in wide opening during eating or yawning and less commonly, from trauma; they may be unilateral or bilateral. The typical complaints of the patient with dislocation are an inability to close the jaws and pain related to muscle spasm. On clinical examination, a deep depression may be observed in the pretragus region corresponding to the condyle being positioned anterior to the eminence.

The condyle can usually be repositioned without the use of muscle relaxants or general anesthetics. If muscle spasms are severe and reduction is difficult, the use of intravenous diazepam (about 10 mg) can be beneficial. The practitioner who is repositioning the mandible should stand in front of the seated patient and place his thumbs lateral to the mandibular molars on the buccal shelf of bone; the remaining fingers of each hand should be placed under the chin. The condyle is repositioned by a downward and backward movement. This is achieved by simultaneously pressing down on the posterior part of the mandible while raising the chin. As the condyle reaches the height of the eminence, it can usually be guided posterior to its normal position.

Postreduction recommendations consist of

a decrease in mandibular movement and the taking of aspirin or nonsteroidal anti-inflammatory medications to lessen inflammation. The patient should be cautioned not to open wide in eating or yawning because recurrence, especially during the period initially after repositioning, is common. Long periods of immobilization are not advised because of the possible consequences of fibrous ankylosis. .

Chronic, recurring dislocations have been treated with both surgical and nonsurgical approaches. Injections of sclerosing solutions are not used as often now because of difficulty in controlling the extent of fibrosis and condylar limitation. Various surgical procedures have been advocated for treating recurrent dislocations of the mandible; these include bone grafting to the eminence, lateral pterygoid myotomy, eminence reduction, eminence augmentation with implants, shortening the temporalis tendon by intraoral scarification, plication of the joint capsule, and repositioning of the zygomatic arch.

Ankylosis

True bony anklyosis of the temporomandibular joint involves fusion of the head of the condyle to the temporal bone. Trauma to the chin is the most common cause of TMJ ankylosis, although infections may also be involved. Children are more prone to ankylosis because of greater osteogenic potential and less development of the joint disc. Ankylosis frequently results from prolonged immobilization following condylar fracture. Limited mandibular movement, deviation of the mandible to the affected side on opening, and facial asymmetry may be observed in TMJ ankylosis. Osseous deposition may be seen on radiographs.

Laskin has conjectured that traumatic displacement of the articular disc could initiate osseous overgrowth resulting in ankylosis. He advocates the interposition of polymeric silicone (Silastic) to prevent possible fusion in these traumatic cases (see Fig. 12-11). Ankylosis has been treated by several surgical procedures. Gap arthroplasty using interpositional materials between the cut segments is the technique most commonly performed.

Disc Displacement

Trauma to the TMJ, either as acute force or chronic microtrauma, may drive the condyle in a posterosuperior direction resulting in stretching of the posterior attachment of the articular disc and anterior displacement of the disc itself. A lack of coordination of the superior and inferior portions of the lateral pterygoid muscle may also cause anterior disc displacement. Clicking is usually the initial symptom associated with anterior displacement of the disc. As the disc becomes more anteriorly displaced, a closed lock situation may occur where the disc actually blocks translation of the condyle and limitation of mandibular opening is observed. Deviation of the jaw to the affected side will also be noted. Patients with anterior displacement of the disc experience variable pain; muscle spasms secondary to the obstructed condylar path may occur.

Katzberg, Dolwick, and associates found anterior disc displacement to be the most significant finding on arthrography of over 200 patients with unilateral pain and limitation of opening. They emphasized that routine radiographs are ineffective in diagnosing this type of soft tissue derangement. Posterior displacement of the disc is relatively uncommon. Conservative therapy usually is successful in managing the vast majority of patients with mild-to-moderate symptoms associated with disc displacement. A maxillary occlusal splint is often used to aid in repositioning the condyle and the disc. Muscle relaxation therapy, removal of gross occlusal interferences, and treatment of posterior bite collapse by orthodontic or prosthetic therapy is often beneficial.

When symptoms of pain and limitations are severe and not alleviated by conservative therapy, surgery may be indicated. Arthrography is used to corroborate the clinical picture before surgery on the joint is performed.

McCarty and Farrar have advocated the technique of reconstructive arthroplasty and disc repositioning. This involves reduction and smoothing of the condyle and reattachment of the disc to the posterior attachment with the disc placed in its normal position. In 327 surgical procedures over 6 years, they

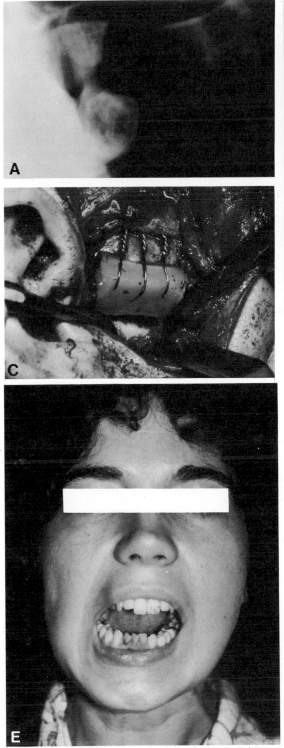

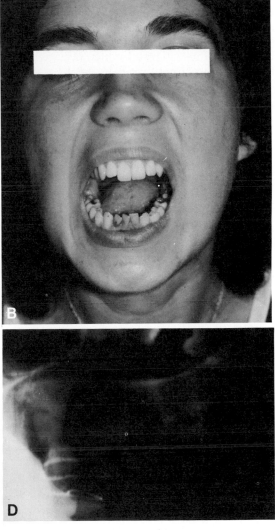

Fig. 12-11 *A,* Condylar hyperplasia and fibrous ankylosis secondary to trauma to chin as a child. *B,* Preoperative clinical appearance showing limited opening and deviation to the affected side. *C,* Gap arthroplasty with insertion of silastic. *D,* Postoperative radiograph. *E,* Postoperative clinical appearance showing increased ability to open and decreased deviation. (Case presentation courtesy of E.S. Moriconi, M.D., Philadelphia, PA)

feel that this surgery for disc displacement has been successful in 94% of the cases. A certain period of pain relief is usually achieved in any surgery involving the TMJ because of the denervation that occurs during the incision of the joint capsule.

Gout

Arthritis related to the metabolic disturbances of gout initially involves the joint capsule and in later stages progresses to degeneration of subchondral bone. Gouty arthritis of the TMJ appears to be very rare in patients having the disease, although crystal deposition may be apparent in tissues adjacent to the joint. In addition to an increase in the serum uric acid, leukocytosis and increase in the erythrocyte sedimentation rate may be associated with acute phases of gout.

BIBLIOGRAPHY

Alderman MM: Disorders of the temporomandibular joint and related structures. Rationale for diagnosis, etiology, management. Alpha Omegan 69:12, 1976

Bell WE: Clinical Management of Temporomandibular Disorders. Springfield, IL, Year Book Medical Publishers, 1982

Bessette R, Bishop B, Mohl N: Duration of masseteric silent period in patients with TMJ syndrome. J Appl Physiol 30:864, 1971

Blackwood IIJJ: Arthritis of the mandibular joint. Br Dent J 115:317, 1963

Blackwood HJJ: Pathology of the temporomandibular joint. J Am Dent Assoc 79:118, 1969

Blaschke DD, Solberg WK, Sanders B: Arthrography of the temporomandibular joint: review of current status. J Am Dent Assoc 100:388, 1980

Bronstein SL, Tomsetti BJ, Ryan DE: Internal derangements of the temporomandibular joint: Correlation of arthrography with surgical findings. J Oral Surg 39:572, 1981

Brooke RI, Stenn PG: Postinjury myofascial pain dysfunction syndrome: Its etiology and prognosis. Oral Surg 45:846, 1978

Burke RH, McNamara JA: Effect of lateral pterygoid myotomy on the structures of the temporomandibular joint: A histological study. J Oral Surg 37:548, 1979

Carlsson GE: Neuromuscular problems in the orofacial region: Aetiology and organic pathology. Int Dent J 31:198, 1981

Choy E, Smith DE: The prevalence of temporomandibular joint disturbances in complete denture patients. J Oral Rehabil 7:331, 1980

Christensen LV: Facial pains and the jaw muscles. A review. J Oral Rehabil 8:193, 1981

Clark GT: Management of muscular hyperactivity. Int Dent J 31:216, 1981

Clark GT, Beemsterboer PL, Solberg WK, Rugh JD: Nocturnal electromyographic evaluation of myofascial pain dysfunction in patients undergoing occlusal splint therapy. J Am Dent Assoc 99:607, 1979

Clarke NG: Occlusion and myofascial pain dysfunction: Is there a relationship? J Am Dent Assoc 104:443, 1982

Clarke NG, Kardachi BJ: The treatment of myofascial pain dysfunction syndrome using the biofeedback principle. J Periodontol 48:643, 1977

Dohrmann RJ, Laskin DM: An evaluation of electromyographic biofeedback in the treatment of myofascial pain dysfunction syndrome. J Am Dent Assoc 96:656, 1978

Dolwick MF, Katzberg RW, Helms CA, Boles DJ: Arthrotomographic evaluation of the temporomandibular joint. J Oral Surg 37:793, 1979

Dunn MJ, Rabinov K, Hayes C, Jennings S: Polycycloidal corrected tomography of the temporomandibular joint. Oral Surg 51:375, 1981

Eckerdal O, Lundberg M: The structural situation in temporomandibular joints. A comparison between conventional oblique transcranial radiographs, tomograms, and histologic sections. Dentomaxillofacial Radiol 8:42, 1979

Edmiston GF, Laskin DM: Changes in consistency of occlusal contact in myofascial pain dysfunction (MPD) syndrome. J Dent Res 57:27, 1978

Evaskus DS, Laskin DM: A biochemical measure of stress in patients with myofascial pain-dysfunction syndrome. IADR Abstracts 46th General Meeting. Abstract #610

Goodman P, Greene CS, Laskin DM: Response of patients with myofascial pain-dysfunction syndrome to mock equilibration. J Am Dent Assoc 92:755, 1976

Gould JF: Shortening of the temporalis tendon for hypermobility of the temporomandibular joint. J Oral Surg 36:781, 1978

Greene CS, Laskin DM: Splint therapy for the myofascial pain-dysfunction (MPD) syndrome: a comparative study. J Am Dent Assoc 84:624, 1972

Guralnick W, Kaban LB, Merrill RG: Temporomandibular joint afflictions. N Engl J Med 299:123, 1978

Heloe B, Heiberg AW, Krogstad BS: A multiprofessional study of patients with myofascial pain dysfunction syndrome. Acta Odontol Scand 38:109, 1980

Henny FA: Surgical treatment of the painful temporomandibular joint. J Am Dent Assoc 79:171, 1969

Howe AG, Kent JN, Farrell CD, Poidmore SJ: Implant of articular eminence for recurrent dislocation of the temporomandibular joint. J Oral Surg 36:523, 1978

Kaban LB, Belfer ML: Temporomandibular joint dysfunction: An occasional manifestation of serious psychopathology. J Oral Surg 39:742, 1981

Katzberg RW, Dolwick MF, Kerth DA et al: New observations with routine and CT-assisted arthrography in suspected internal derangements of the temporomandibular joint. Oral Surg 51:569, 1981

Kawazoe Y, Kotani H, Hamada T, Yamada S: Effect of occlusal splints on the electromyographic activities of masseter muscles during maximum clenching in patients with myofascial pain dysfunction syndrome. J Prosthet Dent 43:578, 1980

Klineberg I, Lillie J: Regional nerve block of the temporomandibular joint capsule: a technique for clinical research and differential diagnosis. J Dent Res 59:1930, 1980

Kreutziger KL, Mahan PL: Temporomandibular degenerative joint disease. Part I Anatomy, physiology and clinical description. Oral Surg 40:165, 1975

Kreutziger KL, Mahan PL: Temporomandibular degenerative joint disease. Part II Diagnostic procedure and comprehensive management. Oral Surg 40:297, 1975

Larheim TA: Comparison between three radiographic techniques for examination of the temporomandibular joints in juvenile rheumatoid arthritis. Acta Radiol (Diagn) (Stockh) 22:195, 1981

Larheim TA, Haamaes HR, Ruud AF: Mandibular growth, temporomandibular joint changes, and dental occlusion in juvenile rheumatoid arthritis. Scand J Rheumatol 10:225, 1981

Laskin DM: Etiology of the pain-dysfunction syndrome. J Am Dent Assoc 79:147, 1969

Laskin DM: Role of the meniscus in the etiology of posttraumatic temporomandibular joint ankylosis. Int J Oral Surg 7:340, 1978

Laskin DM, Greene CS: Influence of the doctor-patient relationship on placebo therapy for patients with myofascial pain-dysfunction (MPD) syndrome. J Am Dent Assoc 85:692, 1972

Lawlor MG: Recurrent dislocation of the mandible: Treatment of ten cases by the Dautrey procedure. Br J Oral Surg 20:14, 1982

Lindvall A, Helkimo E, Hollender L, Carlsson GE: Radiographic examination of the temporomandibular joint. A comparison between radiographic findings and gross and microscopic observations. Dentomaxillofacial Radiol 5:24, 1976

Lowry JC: Psoriatic arthritis involving the temporomandibular joint. J Oral Surg 33:206, 1975

Magnusson T, Carlsson GE: Changes in recurrent headaches and mandibular dysfunction after various types of dental treatment. Acta Odontol Scand 38:311, 1980

Manns A, Miralles R, Adrian H: The application of audiostimulation and electromyographic biofeedback to bruxism and myofascial pain dysfunction syndrome. Oral Surg 52:247, 1981

Marbach JJ: Arthritis of the temporomandibular joints and facial pain. Bull Rheum Dis 27:918, 1976

Markovic MA, Rosenberg HM: Tomographic evaluation of 100 patients with temporomandibular joint symptoms. Oral Surg 42:838, 1976

Mayne JG, Hatch GS: Arthritis of the temporomandibular joint. J Am Dent Assoc 79:125, 1969

McCall WD, Jr, Uthman AA, Mohl ND: TMJ symptom severity and EMG silent periods. J Dent Res 57:709, 1978

McCall WD, Gale EN, Uthman AA: The variability of EMG silent periods in TMJ patients. J Oral Rehabil 8:103, 1981

McCarty WL, Farrar WB: Surgery for internal derangements of the temporomandibular joint. J Prosthet Dent 42:191, 1979

Mercuri LG: The specificity of response to experimental stress in patients with myofascial pain dysfunction syndrome. J Dent Res 58:1866, 1979

Mercuro AR: Nervous control of occlusion. Dent Clin North Am 25:381, 1981

Miller AS, Harwick RD, Daley DJ: Temporomandibular joint synovial chondromatosis: Report of case. J Oral Surg 36:467, 1978

Miller GA, Page HL, Jr, Griffith CR: Temporomandibular joint ankylosis: Review of the literature and report of two cases of bilateral involvement. J Oral Surg 33:292, 1975

Millstein–Prentky S, Olson RE: Predictability of treatment outcome in patients with myofascial pain dysfunction (MPD) syndrome. J Dent Res 58:1341, 1979

Moody PM, Calhoun TC, Okeson JP, Kemper JT: Stress-pain relationship in MPD patients and non-MPD syndrome patients. J Prosthet Dent 45:84, 1981

Nelson CL, Hutton CE: Condylectomy for temporomandibular joint dysfunction. A survey of seventeen postoperative patients. Oral Surg 51:351, 1981

Noyek AM et al: The radiologic findings in synovial chondromatosis of the temporomandibular joint. J Otolaryngol 6:45, 1977

Obërg T, Carlsson GE, Fajers CM: The temporomandibular joint. A morphologic study on a human autopsy material. Acta Ondontol Scand 29:349, 1971

Olson RE, Laskin DM: Relationship between allergy and bruxism in patients with myofascial pain dysfunction syndrome. J Am Dent Assoc 100:209, 1980

Rasmussen OC: Semiopaque arthrography of the temporomandibular joint. Scand J Dent Res 88:521, 1980

Ratner EJ, Person P, Kleinman DJ et al: Jawbone cavities and trigeminal and atypical facial neuralgias. Oral Surg 48:3, 1979

Richards LC, Brown T: Dental attrition and degenerative arthritis of the temporomandibular joint. J Oral Rehabil 8:293, 1981

Ronald JB, Keller EE, Welland LH: Synovial chondromatosis of the temporomandibular joint. J Oral Surg 36:13, 1978

Rowe NL: Surgery of the temporomandibular joint. Proc R Soc Med 65:383, 1972

Sanders B, Brady FA, Adams D: Silastic cap temporomandibular joint prosthesis. J Oral Surg 35:933, 1977

Schwartz LL: Pain associated with the temporomandibular joint. J Am Dent Assoc 51:394, 1955

Schwartz LL, Chayes CM (eds): Facial Pain and Mandibular Dysfunction. Philadelphia, WB Saunders, 1968

Schwartz RA, Greene CS, Laskin DM: Personality characteristics of patients with myofascial pain dysfunction (MPD) syndrome unresponsive to conventional therapy. J Dent Res 58:1435, 1979

Scott DS: Treatment of the myofascial pain dysfunction syndrome: Psychological aspects. J Am Dent Assoc 101:611, 1980

Sheppard IM, Sheppard SM: Subluxation of the temporomandibular joint. Oral Surg 44:821, 1977

Sicher H: Structure and functional basis for disorders of the temporomandibular joint articulation. J Oral Surg 13:275, 1955

Sicher H: Functional anatomy of the temporomandibular joint. In Sarnat BG (ed): The Temporomandibular Joint. St Louis, Charles C Thomas, 1964

Skiba TJ, Laskin DM: Masticatory muscle silent periods in patients with MPD syndrome before and after treatment. J Dent Res 60:699, 1981

Solberg WK: Neuromuscular problems in the orofacial region: Diagnosis, classification, signs and symptoms. Int Dent J 31:206, 1981

Solberg WK, Clark GT (eds): Temporomandibular Joint Problems: Biologic Diagnosis and Treatment. Chicago, Quintessence Publishing, 1980

Speculand B: Unilateral condylar hypoplasia with ankylosis: Radiographic findings. Br J Oral Surg 20:1, 1982

Standlee, JP, Caputo AA, Ralph JP: The condyle as a stress-distributing component of the temporomandibular joint. J Oral Rehabil 8:391, 1981

Toller PA: Osteoarthrosis of the mandibular condyle. Br Dent J 134:223, 1973

Toller PA: Ultrastructure of the condylar articular surface in severe mandibular pain-dysfunction syndrome. Int J Oral Surg 6:297, 1977

Toller PA: Use and misuse of intra-articular corticosteroids in treatment of temporomandibular joint pain. Proc R Soc Med 70:461, 1977

Topazian RG: Etiology of ankylosis of the temporomandibular joint: Analysis of 44 cases. J Oral Surg 22:227, 1964

Travell J: Temporomandibular joint pain referred from muscles of the head and neck. J Prosthet Dent 10:745, 1960

Travell J, Rinzler SH: The myofascial genesis of pain. Postgrad Med 11:425, 1952

Trenouth MJ: Computer analysis of noctural tooth contact patterns in relation to bruxism and mandibular joint dysfunction in man. Arch Oral Biol 23:821, 1978

Trenouth MJ: The relationship between bruxism and temporomandibular joint dysfunction as shown by computer analysis of nocturnal tooth contact patterns. J Oral Rehabil 6:81, 1979

Weissberg GA, Carroll WL, Dinham R, Wolford LM: Transcutaneous electrical stimulation as an adjunct in the management of myofascial pain-dysfunction syndrome. J Prosthet Dent 45:307, 1981

Wenneberg B, Sigvard K: Short term effect of intra-articular injections of a corticosteroid on temporomandibular joint pain and dysfunction. Swed Dent J 2:189, 1978

Williams RA, Laskin DM: Arthroscopic examinations of experimentally induced pathologic conditions of the rabbit temporomandibular joint. J Oral Surg 38:652, 1980

Yemm R: Neurophysiologic studies of TMJ dysfunction. In Zarb GA, Carlsson GE (eds): Temporomandibular Joint—Function and Dysfunction. St. Louis, CV Mosby, 1979

Zarb GL, Carlsson GE (eds): Temporomandibular Joint-Function and Dysfunction. St. Louis, CV Mosby, 1979

13

Ionizing Radiation

ROBERT W. BEIDEMAN

JAMES C. PETTIGREW, JR.

VARIABLES ASSOCIATED WITH RADIATION CHANGES

All ionizing radiations are potentially capable of producing both localized and systemic changes. This chapter focuses on those changes associated with x-ray radiation in the dental diagnostic energy range. An abundance of information is available in the medical literature dealing with much higher x-ray energy ranges, and interested readers are referred to the appropriate sources for in-depth discussions of those subjects.

Radiation-induced changes are directly related to the type of ionizing radiation, the amount and rate of exposure, cell types and ages of exposed cells, and certain individual differences of radiation sensitivity. It must be remembered that radiation-induced changes may or may not be reversible and may or may not produce cell, tissue, or clinically observable changes depending on the above variables. It is well known that the effects of x-ray radiation are cumulative, that is, the subliminal effects of repeated small doses of x-ray radiation may produce clinical changes over time. This concept implies that unobservable changes at the atomic or cellular lev-

els might occur with low-dose exposures, and with repeated exposures these changes may become clinically visible. For example, a cubic centimeter of oral mucosa containing one million cells may be exposed to 200 millirems during a typical intraoral dental radiographic procedure (Fig. 13-1). Of the one million cells, 100 may be altered in some way; of the 100 altered cells, perhaps ten will be permanently altered and 90 will recover. At each subsequent serial exposure this same event may occur, building up a "bank" of permanently altered cells. At some point this bank of cells becomes large enough to clinically alter the function of the host tissue. This scenario is clinically most difficult to prove, but in controlled laboratory studies by Lurie and others such changes can be demonstrated with dental radiation doses repeated at very frequent intervals.

RADIATION ASSOCIATED WITH DIAGNOSTIC DENTAL RADIOLOGIC EXAMINATION

The Biological Effects of Ionizing Radiation III report stated that the dose and effect curves of radiation will be considered at least

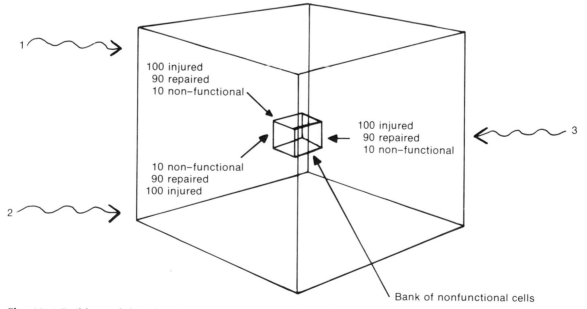

Fig. 13-1 Build-up of the "bank" of nonfunctional cells with serial exposures to a cubic centimeter of tissue.

linear down to zero until proven otherwise (Fig. 13-2). This statement requires dentists to consider the known effects of ionizing radiation when exposing patients so that maximum diagnostic benefits will be obtained from the least amount of exposure. Dental radiographs should be obtained only after a careful history and clinical examination have indicated the need for specific views. X-ray equipment should be in proper working order and used by experienced knowledgeable personnel. Adequate radiologic quality assurance procedures should be followed at all times.

Recently there has been increasing concern expressed by a variety of professional and lay individuals regarding the potential risks associated with diagnostic oral radiology. This has taken the form of newspaper and magazine copy and has resulted in formal discussions by members of the dental profession on the appropriate attitude to be taken toward both the values and risks of dental x-rays. A reasonable consensus has not yet emerged. The public has thus become both aware and concerned about long-range effects of even the small exposures involved in the dental office. Accordingly, the dentist must pay more attention to these values and should be aware of the following methods of reducing radiation exposure:

1. Use of protective neck shields for children to guard against thyroidal absorption and of lead aprons for all patients especially through childbearing age to protect against gonadal and bone marrow absorption.
2. The use of proper collimation of the beam
3. Test of the x-ray unit for scatter radiation
4. Use of adequate filtration of the beam
5. Use of (D- or E-speed) ultrafast films

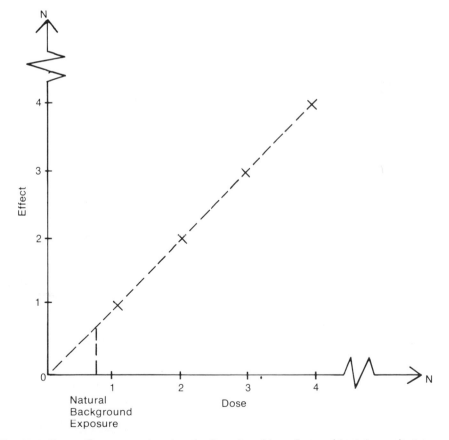

Fig. 13-2 Dose-effect curve showing the linearity of low doses of ionizing radiation.

6. Adequate attention to proper developing procedure

Judgment must be applied in those circumstances in which the patient has previously received therapeutic radiation doses to the face or jaws and now requires dental treatment. Although the principle of minimal radiation exposure may have theoretic validity, it is incumbent upon the dentist, as previously stated, to apply the most valid and effective diagnostic methods to prevent dental disease in these patients. Certainly, routine radiography should be avoided, and each film exposed should be justified in terms of specific diagnostic information. In this manner the incompatibility between minimal exposure and maximal diagnostic validity is somewhat resolved—and in the best long-range interests of the patient.

CHANGES ASSOCIATED WITH RADIATION

Radiation effects are known at the atomic, cellular, and tissue levels. Specific reactions for specific x-ray doses are not known because of the variables already mentioned. At the atomic level, x-ray radiation may react with orbital electrons by either the photoelectric or Compton reaction in diagnostic dental x-ray energy ranges. These reactions may cause several cellular level changes. Formation of hydroperoxides is cytotoxic. The physical changes of heat production may alter enzyme functions or cell permeability. If cellular level changes are great enough, then tissue function may be altered. Somatic tissue effects include reddening, swelling, flaking, alopecia, ulceration, and malignancy, particularly leukemia induction and thyroid cancer. Genetic changes may include several genetic mutations as the result of altered RNA and DNA structures. It is deemed improbable but not impossible that repeated exposure from low-dose x-ray radiation sources can lead to some of these known changes, which are seen at high-dose (therapeutic) ranges of several thousand rem. In 1957, Richards calculated that the radiation dose to the gonads for a full mouth series (20 films) would be

0.0001 of the dose to the head. This would be about 0.0005 rem. The 1964, U.S. Public Health Service x-ray exposure study estimated that the mean dose from all dental films was less than 0.1 mrad. This amount of exposure is extremely small in comparison to the 3 to 5 rem each person receives during a 30-year period from general background radiation; nevertheless, the American Dental Association (ADA) recommends gonadal shielding during dental radiologic procedures.

THERAPEUTIC RADIATION DOSES TO THE HEAD AND NECK

Dentists are at times called upon to treat patients who will have or who have had intraoral therapeutic doses of ionizing radiation to the head or neck (1500 rem to 8000 rem). A major complication of dental treatment for these patients is osteoradionecrosis. Changes in the jaw bones after irradiation result from damage to the bone as well as from impaired vascularity. The ready access of a highly varied microbial flora to heavily irradiated tissue is an important factor in the production of osteoradionecrosis of the jaws. Gowgiel found that in experimental osteoradionecrosis the gross necrotic lesion always began in the interdental papilla of the mandibular molar that was in the center of the field of radiation. The necrosis then extended to the cervical gingiva, the attached gingiva, and the cheek mucosa.

In the early stages of osteoradionecrosis the chief complaint of the patient may be related to the teeth rather than the jaws. The patient may experience a transient proprioceptive or thermal sensitivity of the teeth, or perhaps a continuous dull toothache. Teeth have been observed to spontaneously resorb or apparently become much more brittle following radiation therapy. Spontaneous death of the pulps in erupted teeth has been noted. A peculiar type of dental caries involving primarily the cervical areas of the teeth is explained by a decrease in salivary flow and a lowered salivary pH.

Xerostomia is a frequent complaint of patients who have received radiation. Failure to adequately shield the salivary glands results in rapid atrophy and functional incapacity. Increase in viscosity and marked reduction in stimulated flow result in increased retention of food debris and plaque on the teeth. In some patients, the pattern of circumferential dental caries at the cervical margin require early and aggressive crown application and frequent fluoride treatments to prevent tooth loss with its associated risk of complications.

Pain in the jaws may become continuous and severe. Maintenance of nutrition then becomes a serious problem because of the pain and the patient's inability to open the jaws. Edentulous patients may complain of a constant, gradually increasing pain without any clinical or radiographic explanation for this symptom. After varying periods of time, radiologic changes may be manifested compatible with a diagnosis of osteoradionecrosis, and eventually there may be a breakdown of the soft tissue.

All trauma should be avoided in irradiated areas to minimize the possibility of the development of osteoradionecrosis; this applies not only to procedures performed relatively soon following irradiation but also years later. Severe osteoradionecrosis has followed dental prophylaxis performed many years after the irradiation therapy. Deep gingival curettage is contraindicated, and endodontic therapy is preferable to extraction.

The vitality of the irradiated tissue is permanently altered, although no specific lesions are observed. It is safest never to place dentures over irradiated intraoral tissues; however, carefully fitted dentures may be inserted a minimum of 24 months after radiation therapy if the patient is advised of the possible consequences, of how to maintain good oral hygiene, and of the necessity for frequent dental check-ups. Both the dentist and the radiologist should warn patients of the potential danger of mechanical, thermal, or chemical trauma to the tissues. Patients should be cautioned about gingival and mucosal lacerations caused by food.

Accordingly, even the simple, daily hygienic practices of the patient who has head or neck radiotherapy must be adapted to the tissue deficits, and an individualized therapeutic program should be written out and scrupulously adhered to by the dentist and the patient. This program should include frequent visits for careful prophylaxis and fluoride treatments, avoidance of injury to soft and hard tissues, preventive maintenance of the teeth and periodontal tissues, frequent but modified toothbrushing, and stimulating irrigation procedures. Daily self-administered fluoride rinses have proven effective in reducing or eliminating postradiation caries. Use of electric toothbrushes should be avoided because the irradiated tissues have lost the normal healing responses to even minor traumatic abrasions and contusions; although rubber-tipped interproximal stimulators may be preferable to those made of wood, the patient must be carefully instructed in their proper use.

Water jets and sprays may be helpful hygienic adjuncts but must be used at the lowest force and only where the mouth has been regularly kept free of calculus and where deep periodontal pockets do not exist. Injuries from rotating dental instruments, matrix bands, copper bands, and temporary crowns may initiate tissue necrosis and infection that can take months, if not years, to resolve. More than any other oral circumstance, the patient with radiation changes in the oral tissues must be educated to oral maintenance procedures, and the dental office must be willing to provide the special services required for management. The dangerous triad of irradiated tissue, trauma, and infection must be avoided to prevent osteoradionecrosis.

Because there are so many variable factors involved in the development of osteoradionecrosis, no "safe" roentgen dosage can be established. Radiation doses of 2000 rem or more can be considered as resulting in a potentially hazardous condition.

TREATMENT OF OSTEORADIONECROSIS

Osteoradionecrosis is more easily prevented than treated. Whenever possible, the jaws, teeth, and oral mucosal tissues should be shielded before radiation therapy in the area, or better yet, any unhealthy teeth should be removed before radiation therapy. As a general rule, teeth in the field of primary radiation should be rendered healthy enough to require little or no treatment for 5 years after radiation therapy; however, some therapists espouse the removal of all teeth before therapy. In some instances, the dentist can be of assistance in the fabrication of shields for each patient before therapy to protect the jaw bones.

There is no simple effective treatment for osteoradionecrosis. Surgical intervention is usually contraindicated except for the careful removal of sequestra that may develop. Antibiotic therapy may reduce the secondary infection of the debilitated tissues by the microbial flora of the mouth; however, because in most cases the normal vascularization of the affected area has been greatly diminished, systemic antibiotic treatment may be fruitless. Newer techniques of hyperbaric therapy have been developed whereby a patient is placed in a pressurized chamber to force oxygenation of still vital tissues that are unable to receive oxygen in the normal physiologic manner. Staged sequential hyperbaric treatments along with progressive surgical procedures have been very effective in treating osteoradionecrosis.

While prophylactic antibiotics are indicated to avoid tissue infections, the risk of candidal infections as well as the development of antibiotic-resistant organisms is a constant problem. Irradiated tissues may not demonstrate the typical features of infection (redness, swelling, pain); necrosis, ulceration, and sensitivity may be the only presenting findings. When infection is suspected, cultures and smears should be submitted for microbiologic examination in order to determine the most appropriate antibiotic for specific use in each episode. Slow healing in irradiated tissues may also present complications because the effects of antibiotics on the oral microbial ecology may present opportunities for reinfection by another organism following successful management of the initial infection.

The prognosis of this condition is variable but in general not encouraging. Even though osteoradionecrosis can be difficult to treat, proper considerations by the dental practitioner before and after therapy can reduce the number of demonstrated cases well below the 5% to 10% of those patients receiving therapeutic doses.

EXTRACTION OF TEETH IN IRRADIATED AREAS

As already mentioned, before therapeutic irradiation of the cervicofacial area, all teeth in the field of radiation should be removed or placed in a state of health so that no dental treatment will be required for 5 years after therapy. Unfortunately, the dentist may be called upon to administer to a patient with odontalgia or to remove teeth from an area that has already received therapeutic radiation. The removal of teeth under these circumstances is a hazardous procedure and is likely to be followed by osteoradionecrosis. The radiologist should be informed that the complications that may arise are more likely to be related to the original inadequate treatment planning than to the present surgery.

If routine extraction techniques are to be used, the patient should receive prophylactic antibiotic therapy. The teeth should be removed with the absolute minimum of trauma. Every effort should be made to prevent portals of entry of the oral microbial flora to the tooth sockets. All sharp edges of bone should be rounded or smoothed with a bone file, and the soft tissue should be carefully sutured to cover completely and firmly any exposed bone and the socket areas. Vigorous antibiotic therapy should be continued for 7 to 10 days.

THE DENTAL PRACTITIONER'S ROLE

Dentists should be consulted when radiation therapy is being planned. Following extractions, wounds should be carefully debrided and soft tissues approximated. Niebel and Neenan recommended that an alveolectomy be performed when teeth are removed just prior to radiation to minimize the size of the blood clot. The early blood clot is extremely sensitive to radiation and thus prone to break down. Traditionally, many dentists believe that at least 10 days should elapse between the extraction of the teeth and the start of radiation therapy, and most clinicians advise a delay of 2 weeks if possible; however, the general indications for radiation therapy may not permit this time interval before therapy.

Because radiation reactions do not develop

for approximately 2 weeks after the start of the therapeutic program, all necessary dental and oral procedures except surgery may be performed simultaneously with the initial radiation treatment, and valuable time need not be lost. A comprehensive dental evaluation including radiographs must be performed, and each phase of indicated dental need should be listed in terms of tissue damage and prognosis. Direct communication with the radiation therapist is necessary so that an accurate estimate of the radiation dose to be applied to different parts of the mouth can be determined. Construction of both intraoral and extraoral shielding devices can be done in the dental office so that the healthy tissues will receive minimal exposure. Programming of surgical and other dental procedures must be documented in the context of anticipated irradiation effect.

Never, under any circumstances, should the dentist attempt to give radiation therapy with the regular dental radiologic equipment. This apparatus is not adequately powered, shielded, and controlled for therapeutic purposes, and its use may result in serious harm to both the patient and the operator.

PRESENT AND FUTURE RADIOLOGIC DEVELOPMENTS

As a result of concern over unnecessary use of ionizing radiation, new equipment designed to yield more accurate diagnostic information or to reduce patient exposure is being developed. Most of these systems are presently used in the field of medical radiology but are finding new applications to dental medicine.

One system is xeroradiography, which uses a charged selenium plate instead of x-ray films as the image receptor. This plate is more x-ray sensitive and thus requires less patient exposure to obtain diagnostic images. Special processing equipment is needed to produce images from the selenium plates, however. Computerized tomography (CT) is being adapted for dental medicine. CT allows hard and soft tissue visualization, but expensive and complex computer technology is required for its use. The images formed by relatively low radiation doses are enhanced by computers; these images are detailed then projected onto television screens (or photographed for permanent copy), and thus patient dose is reduced. Body sections are able to be viewed instead of full thicknesses of body parts. Medicine at this time is attempting to define CT usage; outgrowths of CT are emission computed tomography (ECT) and positron emission tomography (PET). Both measure functional variables not possible with CT, but have little dental application at this time.

Even more recently, nuclear magnetic resonance (NMR) has been developed. This is the first imaging system that does not use ionizing radiation. Specific body tissues are placed in high-magnetic fields causing the hydrogen nuclei in those tissues to be polarized. When the magnetic fields are turned off, the nuclei return to specific formations. NMR measures the return times, computes tissue density differences, and generates an image from this data. At this time, research is under way to develop this system in medicine. Dental application is still further away.

These radiologic developments point to the future of examining body structures not clinically visible. In some way, all are designed to obtain more diagnostic information while minimizing potential risks to patients and operating personnel.

BIBLIOGRAPHY

Biological Effects of Ionizing Radiation Advisory Committee: The effects on population of exposure to low levels of ionizing radiation. Washington, DC, National Academy of Science, 1980

Brown JM: Linearity vs. non-linearity of dose response for radiation carcinogenesis. Health Phys 31:231, 1976

Carpenter JS: Dental care for children who have received head and neck therapeutic radiation. J Pedodontics 3:36, 1978

Goaz PW, White SC (eds): Oral Radiology—Principles and Interpretation. St. Louis, CV Mosby, 1982

Gowgiel TM: Experimental radio-osteonecrosis of the jaws. J Dent Res 39:176, 1960

Lurie AG, Cutler LS: Effects of low-level x-radiation on DMBA-induced lingual tumorigenesis in Syrian hamsters. J Natl Cancer Inst 63:147, 1979

Mansfield MJ et al: Hyperbaric oxygen as an adjunct in the treatment of osteoradionecrosis of the mandible. J Oral Surg 39:585, 1981

Marciani RD, Plezia RA: Osteoradionecrosis of the mandible. J Oral Surg 32:435, 1974

Marx RE: A new concept in the treatment of osteoradionecrosis. Maxillofacial Surg 41:355, 1983

Murray CG et al: The relationships between dental disease and radiation necrosis of the mandible. Oral Surg 49:99, 1980

Niebel HH et al: Removal of the teeth from irradiated tissue. J Oral Surg 15:313, 1957

Niebel HH, Neeman EW: Dental aspects of osteonecrosis. Oral Surg 10:1011, 1957

Population dose from x-rays, U.S., 1964. HEW Publication No. 2001, Washington, DC, 1969

Rankow RW, Weisman B: Osteoradionecrosis of the mandible. Ann Otol Rhinol Laryngol 80:603, 1971

Recommendations in radiographic practices, 1981. Council on Dental Materials, Instruments, and Equipment. J Am Dent Assoc 103:103, 1981

Richards AG: Roentgen ray radiation and the dental patient. J Am Dent Assoc 54:476, 1957

Rubin RL, Doku HC: Therapeutic radiology—The modalities and their effects on oral tissues. J Am Dent Assoc 92:731, 1976

Sanders B et al: Advanced osteoradionecrosis of the mandible. J Oral Med 33:73, 1978

Schofield IOF et al: Osteoradionecrosis of the mandible. Oral Surg 45:692, 1978

Valachovic RW, Lurie AG: Risk—Benefit considerations in pedodontic radiology. Pediatr Dent 2:128, 1980

White S, Rose T: Absorbed bone marrow dose from dental radiographic techniques. J Am Dent Assoc 98:553, 1979

Wilson TJ et al: Osteoradionecrosis is a common result of radiation therapy. J Missouri Dent Assoc 61:13, 1981

14

Odontologic Diseases

RONALD JOHNSON

A majority of the bizarre and unusual anomalies of human teeth become evident during the childhood years. In many cases, the family dentist is usually called upon to make a diagnosis and perform whatever immediate treatment may be required. Too often, hereditary conditions are incorrectly diagnosed and dismissed as being the result of "fever" or "faulty nutrition," and parents may thus feel unnecessarily guilty about circumstances over which they have had no control; therefore, it is a source of satisfaction to the practitioner when he is able to pinpoint the nature of a particular anomaly. In circumstances where abnormalities are to be found only in the teeth, it is frequently the dentist who first recognizes their existence. When the dental defects are part of a greater systemic involvement, the dentist may be called upon to act as a member of the medical team investigating the disturbances and developing an overall health care program for the individual. A classification and review of anomalies of the dentition can be of value to the clinician seeking information useful in making a diagnosis.

ANOMALIES OF TOOTH SIZE

Microdontia

Microdontia describes teeth that are smaller than normal (see Fig. 14-1). Three types of microdontia are recognized:

1. True-generalized or generalized proportional microdontia, where all the teeth are normally formed but smaller than normal. This condition occurs in some rare cases of pituitary dwarfism but otherwise is exceedingly rare.
2. Relatively generalized or generalized disproportional microdontia in which normal or slightly smaller than normal teeth are present in jaws that are somewhat larger than normal; there is an illusion of true microdontia. When the parents are evaluated the role of hereditary factors becomes obvious.
3. Localized microdontia involving a single tooth is by far the most frequent variation in the size of teeth. It affects most often

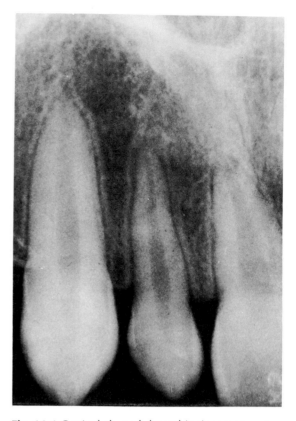

Fig. 14-1 Conical-shaped, lateral incisor represents a form of localized microdontia.

maxillary lateral incisors and third molars. These teeth are often congenitally missing. Supernumerary teeth are frequently of smaller size. Hypoplastic maxillary laterals are a variable expression of the gene for congenitally missing lateral incisors. The condition may involve the presence of a tooth that is a major replica of the normal shape, but more commonly the small tooth is of the rudimentary or conical peg shape variation.

Macrodontia (Megadontia)

Teeth that are larger than normal can be classified as follows. True-generalized or generalized proportional macrodontia is a condition in which the teeth are larger than normal and has been associated with pituitary gigantism and hemihypertrophy. Secretion of an abnormally high level of growth hormone results in increased size of all body tissues including teeth and jaws. Relative-generalized or generalized disproportional macrodontia is the result of the presence of normal or slightly larger than normal teeth in small jaws. This disparity in size gives the illusion of macrodontia and produces crowding and irregular alignment of the dentition. Localized macrodontia is a condition in which one or a few large teeth exist in relation to an otherwise normal dentition and body size. It is relatively rare, of unknown etiology, and usually involves the mandibular third molar. This tooth may appear normal in every aspect except in size. True macrodontia of a single tooth should not be confused with conjoined teeth, in which the union of two or more teeth results in a single large tooth. Localized macrodontia is occasionally seen in cases of hemihypertrophy of the face, in which the teeth of the involved side may be considerably larger than those of the unaffected side.

ANOMALIES OF THE SHAPE OF TEETH

Fusion

Fusion represents the embryonic union of normally separate tooth germs, and reports have been made of two or three teeth fusing. If fusion takes place before calcification, the developing teeth will unite to form a single tooth of almost normal size. If it occurs late in development, the result is a tooth almost twice the normal size or a tooth with a bifid crown. Fusion may occur between the normal complement of teeth or between a normal and a supernumerary tooth. The process is said to be more common in primary than in permanent teeth, is almost always limited to anterior teeth, and may follow a familial tendency. Radiographs of this condition may show that the process is limited to the crowns and roots with separate pulp chambers and pulp canals (see Fig. 14-2). It is thought to form under the pressure of trauma or crowding. Histologically, there is a union of the dentin of one tooth with that of another; they may be joined throughout the entire length or may present as a single wide crown that is supported by two separate roots and two root canals. There may also be a broad root

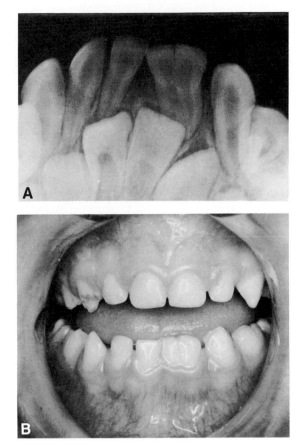

Fig. 14-2 *A,* Fusion is seen in the primary incisor region with a separate pulp chamber and pulp canal. *B,* An abnormally wide tooth is seen in an area where a tooth is missing.

with separate canals. Both gemination and fusion occur most often in the mandibular incisor region of the primary dentition. They are difficult to distinguish; however, when an abnormally wide tooth is seen in an area where a tooth is missing, fusion must be suspected. Racial variations have been noted with a 5% incidence in Japanese and less than 0.5% in Caucasians. The genetic cause is probably autosomal dominant with reduced penetrance.

Gemination

Gemination refers to the process whereby a single tooth germ invaginates, resulting in incomplete formation of two teeth that may appear as a bifid crown on a single root (see

Fig. 14-3). There is a common pulp canal and either a single or partially divided pulp chamber. Gemination does not increase or decrease the number of teeth normally present in the arch. The crown is usually wider than normal, with a shallow groove extending from the incisal edge to the cervical region. The anomaly may follow a hereditary pattern and probably occurs more frequently in primary teeth. Treatment of a permanent anterior geminated tooth may involve reduction of the mesial-distal width of the tooth to allow normal development of the occlusion. Periodic disking and final jacket crown preparation should be considered.

Twinning

Where gemination is a partial attempt of a single tooth germ to divide, twinning indicates that the cleavage of the tooth germ is complete, resulting in the formation of a supernumerary tooth that is the mirror image or a near image of the tooth from which it has developed. Hereditary factors for both gemination and twinning are similar to those for hyperdontia.

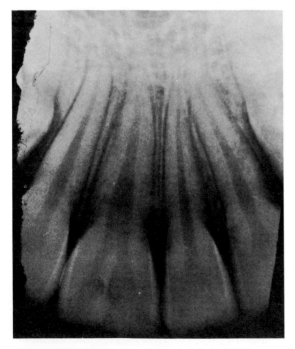

Fig. 14-3 Gemination represented by a bifid crown on a single root.

Concrescence

Concrescence is a form of fusion that occurs after the roots and other major parts of the involved teeth are formed. The roots of two or more teeth must be in close proximity to allow the firm union of one to the other by cementum. The condition is thought to arise from traumatic injury or crowding of teeth with resorption of the interdental bone so that the two roots are approximated and become fused by the deposition of cementum between them. It may occur before or after the teeth have erupted; and although it usually involves only two teeth, there is at least one case on record of three teeth united by cementum. The teeth most frequently involved are the maxillary second and third molars, and the condition appears to be a predisposition of the natural distal inclination of the maxillary molar crowns. If these teeth remain confined within the configuration of the tuberosity, this results in a corresponding crowding and approximation of their roots.

No special treatment is necessary simply because of the concrescence. When extraction is necessary in the maxillary molar region and the condition has not been diagnosed in advance by radiographic examination, an attempted forceps removal of one of the fused teeth can lead inadvertently to the extraction of both teeth. This occurrence may sometimes be further complicated by simultaneous fracture and removal of the bone of the associated maxillary tuberosity. Surgical exposure, separation, and removal of the tooth requiring extraction is the treatment of choice. The possibility of an abnormal union of this type should always be kept in mind when considering the extraction of teeth in the region of the maxillary tuberosity.

Dens in Dente

Dens invaginatus. Originally, *dens invaginatus* was applied to a severe invagination of the enamel organ that gave the appearance of a tooth within a tooth (see Fig. 14-4). In the mildest form of this condition there may simply be a deep pit in the cingulum; in more severe forms, a pocket of enamel is formed within the tooth with dentin at the periphery.

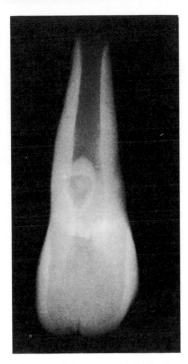

Fig. 14-4 A pocket of enamel is formed within the tooth representing dens in vaginatus.

Dens Evaginatus. In this condition a cone-shaped elevation of enamel is situated in the central groove or the lingual ridge of the buccal cusp of a permanent premolar or molar. It has been referred to as tuberculated teeth or accessory cusps. A tubercle usually consists of all three dental tissues. The incidence among Mongoloid people ranges from 1% to 4.3%. A 15% incidence was observed in an Eskimo population. Autosomal dominance with decreased penetrance is most likely the inheritance.

Paramolar Tubercles or Bolk Cusp

This structure, which appears as a nodular elevation, is seen most frequently on the buccal surface of the mesial buccal cusps in permanent and primary molars. Exaggerated paramolars may result in a supernumerary structure in the interproximal space of the molars, which had been termed a *paramolar tooth*. The structure is almost never seen in white or black peoples, but the trait was found in 2% to 3% of Malaysians and American Indians.

Enamel Pearls, Nodules, or Droplets

Pearl or *droplet* describes a small button or nodule of enamel, usually about 1 mm or 2 mm in diameter, that forms on the root or at the bifurcation of multirooted teeth (see Fig. 14-5). They arise from local activity of remnants of the Hertwig epithelial root sheath before it is reduced to the rests of Malassez. The lesion may occur on the root of any tooth, but most frequently involves the maxillary molars, of which it is estimated that 2% are affected in comparison to only 0.3% of equivalent mandibular teeth. Histologically, the overgrowth may be simply a cap of enamel sitting on the dentin and replacing cementum in the area, or it may consist of a cap of enamel overlying a localized outgrowth of dentin.

Rarely, a small pulpal extension may reach into the center of the nodule and thereby constitutes an additional hazard if any attempt is made to smooth the root by removal of the enamel pearl. Occasionally, the tiny nodule may be sufficiently close to the gingival margin to become involved in periodon-

The opening to the surface is usually constricted or remains open, and food debris may become packed in this area with resultant caries and infection of the pulp, occasionally even before the tooth has completely erupted. The most severe forms may exhibit an invagination extending nearly to the apex of the root. As soon as possible the tooth should be restored and the opening of the defect sealed.

Dens invaginatus has been reported as occurring in 1.8% to 5.1% of white Americans. The condition is rare in the black population; there have been no sex differences noted. The condition can occur in primary and permanent teeth; however, it is most often seen in the permanent maxillary lateral incisors. Anterior teeth with dens are usually of normal size and shape. In other areas of the mouth, however, the tooth can have an anomalous appearance; thus, dens is characterized by an invagination lined with enamel and the presence of a foramen cecum with the probability of a communication between the cavity of the invagination and the pulp chamber.

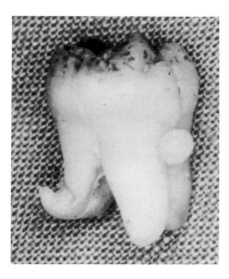

Fig. 14-5 An enamel pearl or nodule of enamel is located near the bifurcation of this multirooted tooth.

tal pocket formation, and its uneven surface may cause additional difficulty in effective cleaning of the area.

Dilaceration

Dilaceration presents as an angulation or sharp bend or curve in the root or crown of a formed tooth. It is thought to result from trauma during the time the tooth is forming. As a result the position of the calcified portion of the tooth is changed, and the remainder of the tooth is formed at an angle. The curve or bend may occur anywhere along the length of the tooth, sometimes at the cervical portion, other times midway along the root or at its apex. Caution should be exercised when extracting these teeth.

Hutchinson's Incisor

Hutchinson's incisor is the term given to anterior teeth characteristically affected by congenital syphilis. The quality of the enamel usually appears to be normal, but the center of the incisal edge shows a typical notching. The most dramatically affected teeth are the permanent incisors and first molars. Affected incisors are characteristically screwdriver-shaped, with tapering marginal ridges converging toward the incisal edge. Although the maxillary central incisors are most dra-

matically affected, all incisors may be similarly involved. Others have indicated that these teeth possess a barrel-shaped outline because of the rounding of the incisal edge.

Moon Molars

Moon molars is the name given to a characteristic syphilitic lesion of the posterior teeth, of which the first molar is the most noticeably affected. The greatest changes affect the quantity of the enamel in the tooth morphology. The cusps of the teeth show exaggerated rounded or nodular shapes. The appearance of the teeth is often grossly distorted, usually narrowed mesiodistally with loss of angulation of the occlusal edge, which may give the cusps a squashed-in appearance.

Mulberry Molars

Mulberry molars is the name given to a characteristic syphilitic lesion of the posterior teeth in which hyperplastic enamel develops with spherical aggregates or globules on the surface of the dentin.

Conical Incisors (Peg-Shaped Laterals)

A rudimentary form of localized microdontia, *conical incisors* most commonly affects the maxillary lateral incisor and to a lesser extent the maxillary third molar. The crown is narrow and tapered to a single cusp or conical, pointed shape.

Globodontia

This globular deformity of the crowns of premolars and molar teeth can be seen in the upper and lower jaws. The teeth have a round globular or clover-leaf appearance. It is characteristic of the otodental syndrome, in which there is a high frequency of deafness from childhood. Other dental anomalies associated with this syndrome are fusion of molar and premolar teeth and double pulp chambers.

Accessory (Supernumerary) Cusps and Ridges

Accessory cusps and ridges are additional tooth structures found on incisors, canines, premolars, and molar teeth (see Fig. 14-6).

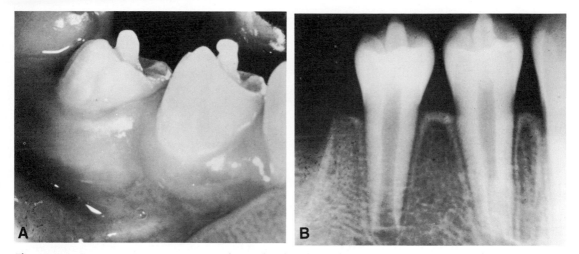

Fig. 14-6 *A,* Accessory cusps are seen on the occlusal surface of the premolars. *B,* Radiography reveals a pulpal extension into the center of the structure.

Accessory or abnormal cusps formed on incisors and canines are recognized as an enlargement of the lingual tubercle, which resembles a fully formed cusp. The marginal ridges may link the accessory cusp with the incisal edge, giving a triangular appearance to the crown; this occurs most frequently in the upper lateral incisors or in the mesiodens.

Carabelli's Cusp or Trait

This accessory lingual cusp is located on the mesiopalatine cusp of the maxillary second primary molar and first, second, or third permanent molars. It was originally considered to be an anomaly; however, this normal trait is seen as a micro form in 90% of Caucasians. The condition is rare in Eskimos of pure ancestry, Chinese, and Japanese. These cusps may be unilateral or bilateral with marked deviations in size.

Accessory Roots

Additional roots occur not infrequently and are often normal in size and shape. They occasionally develop as slender outgrowths at the center of the furcation areas of molar teeth and assume significant clinical importance only during tooth removal or root canal therapy.

Taurodontism

This condition is described as an apical-occlusal extension of the pulp chamber, which appears to have enlarged at the expense of the roots (see Fig. 14-7). The pulp chamber is elongated and extends deeply into the area normally occupied by the roots. A similar condition is seen in the teeth of the cud-chewing animals, such as the ox (Latin: taurus). It is thought to arise when the Hertwig epithelial root sheath fails to invaginate at the proper time. The condition is found rarely in modern Caucasians but occurs among certain modern populations who have lived under relatively primitive conditions in the recent past. There is some evidence the condition is a genetically determined trait offering a selective advantage in populations who use their teeth as tools.

DISTURBANCES IN NUMBER OF TEETH

Anodontia

Anodontia is a rare condition defined as total absence of teeth. It has been reported in most severe forms of ectodermal dysplasia. This absence predisposes to lack of growth of the alveolar process and makes the construction of dentures complicated.

Oligodontia (Hypodontia)

Oligodontia and *hypodontia* refer to a congenital absence of one or a few teeth in the primary or permanent dentition. Specific definitions of these terms are as follows: hypodontia is the absence of one or a few teeth; oligodontia refers to agenesis of numerous teeth.

Congenital absence of primary teeth is relatively rare. Children with a number of missing primary and permanent teeth may have some or all of the signs of ectodermal dysplasia. The size of the primary teeth that are present may be normal or reduced, and anterior teeth often have a conical shape. The primary molars without permanent successors have an unexplained tendency to become ankylosed.

Supernumerary Teeth

Mesiodens. Mesiodens is a special type of supernumerary tooth that is usually conically shaped and located at or near the midline in the incisal region of the maxilla between the central incisors (see Fig. 14-8). The condition may cause retarded eruption, dislocation, or disruption of the root of the existing and regular incisors. When it erupts, it is normally found either palatal to or between the central

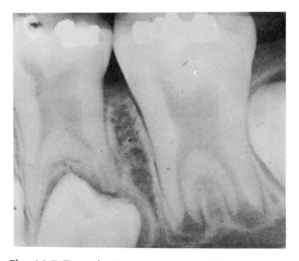

Fig. 14-7 Taurodontism is represented by an elongated pulp chamber that extends deeply into the area normally occupied by the roots.

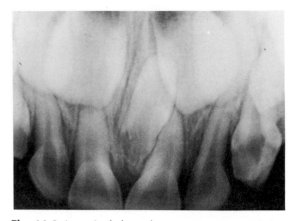

Fig. 14-8 A conical-shaped supernumerary tooth located in the midline of the maxillary incisor region is termed *mesiodens*.

incisors and frequently causes an improper alignment. The sex ratio is 2 to 1, favoring males.

Distomolar. Distomolars are found in the molar region frequently located distal to the third molars. Generally these teeth are smaller in size than are the normal second and third molars, and their general crown morphology is highly abnormal.

Paramolar. Paramolars are usually located in the interproximal space or buccal to the regular molars.

Supplemental Tooth. This type of supernumerary tooth is almost identical in shape to the associated tooth in the arch. Because of its normal shape it is difficult to differentiate from the normal tooth, thus making surgical removal and orthodontic movement somewhat of a problem. The arch in these situations is usually complemented.

Accessory Tooth. This type of supernumerary tooth does not resemble the normal tooth form for the particular location of the dental arch.

Predeciduous Tooth. This is a toothlike structure that develops prematurely and is located in a position resembling natal or neonatal teeth. These rudimentary structures appear to have abnormally formed tooth elements.

Prediduous Dentition

Natal Teeth. Natal teeth are the premature eruption of teeth or toothlike structures that are present at birth (see Fig. 14-9). This rare early eruption seems to be familial. Approximately 90% are primary teeth (85% of which are mandibular incisors), and 10% are supernumerary calcified structures frequently referred to as prediduous teeth. Natal teeth appear more frequently than do neonatal teeth, although they are an expression of the same characteristic. Familial occurrences have been most characteristic of an autosomal dominant trait. One report found 15% of the children with natal or neonatal teeth had parents, siblings, or other near relatives with a similar history. It has been estimated that one in every 2,000 to 3,500 newborn children have erupted teeth already present in the oral cavity.

Most prematurely erupted teeth are hypermobile because of their limited root development. Some teeth may be mobile to the extent that there is danger of displacement and possible aspiration, and in this case removal is indicated. In exceptionally rare cases in which the sharp incisal edge of the tooth may cause laceration of the lingual surface of the tongue or interfere with nursing, the tooth may have to be removed. The more desirable approach is to leave the tooth in place and explain to the parents the desirability of maintaining this tooth in the mouth because of its importance in the growth and uncomplicated eruption of adjacent teeth. Within a relatively short time the prematurely erupted tooth will become stabilized, and the other teeth in the arch will erupt.

Neonatal Teeth. Neonatal teeth are teeth or toothlike structures that erupt prematurely during the neonatal period, from birth to 30 days.

Riga-Fede Disease. This condition is observed in infants who are nursing. It is characterized by ulceration on the ventral surface of the tongue due to irritation by the incisal edges of lower incisors during nursing or sucking. The condition is particularly common in infants with natal or neonatal teeth. Treatment consists of removing the offending

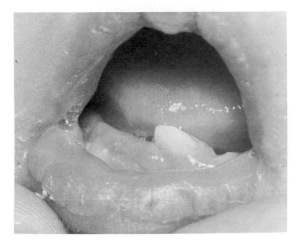

Fig. 14-9 Premature eruption of a tooth in this newborn is referred to as *natal tooth.*

structures, or smoothing or covering the sharp incisal edges to protect the soft tissues during nursing.

DISTURBANCES OF THE STRUCTURE AND TEXTURE OF TEETH

Enamel Disturbances

Enamel Hypoplasia

Localized. *Localized enamel hypoplasia* refers to individual teeth (usually permanent) that have hypoplastic, hypocalcified, or hypomineralized areas on the clinical crown resulting from infection or trauma. Turner first described this localized type of hypoplasia; thus, enamel hypoplasia caused by local infection or trauma is referred to as *Turner's hypoplasia.* The extent and nature of hypoplasia can vary from a mild to a severe form in which pitting and irregularity may be extensive in the crown. The extent of the defect depends on the severity of the periapical infection of the primary predecessor or on the degree of disturbance to the developing tooth bud after trauma to the primary tooth. The amount of hypoplasia also depends on the stage of development of the permanent tooth at the time of trauma or infection.

A traumatic injury to an anterior primary tooth that causes an apical displacement can interfere with matrix formation or calcification of the underlying permanent tooth. The retention of infected primary teeth, even though they are asymptomatic, is unjustifiable. The development of hypoplastic defects on the permanent tooth, its deflection from a normal path of eruption because of the pressure of the inflammatory exudate, or even death of the developing tooth may result.

Prenatal. A marked enamel hypoplasia affects the incisal two thirds of the enamel on maxillary primary incisors, which serves as evidence of a severe metabolic disturbance in fetal life, probably during the second and third trimesters of pregnancy. This condition is also seen in children with cerebral palsy.

Neonatal. A wide band or line of enamel hypoplasia affects the primary teeth of children associated with premature birth or low birth weight. Immature babies suffer considerable metabolic disturbance during the neonatal period that is often reflected in defective amelogenesis. Tetracycline exposure can also be implicated.

Infantile. A wide band of hypoplasia affects the maxillary and mandibular permanent incisors and canines and is felt to be caused by systemic disturbances during infancy.

Hypoplasia Caused by Nutritional Deficiency. Deficiency states, particularly those related to deficiencies in vitamins A, C and D, calcium, and phosphorus, have been related to the occurrence of enamel hypoplasia. Approximately two thirds of the hypoplastic disturbances occur during the infancy period (birth to the end of the first year); approximately another third of these hypoplasias have been found in the portion of teeth formed during the early childhood period (13 to 34 months). Fewer than 2% of enamel defects have been found to originate during the late childhood period (35 to 80 months). Insufficient quantities of vitamin D can cause rickets, a phenomenon resulting from a lack of proper calcification of enamel matrix. Of children suffering from rickets, approxi-

mately 50% will also show signs of enamel hypoplasia. Horizontal pitting occurs in rows on the teeth undergoing matrix formation at the time of a dietary deficiency or during the course of a febrile episode. The extent of the pitting is proportional to the length of time the dietary deficiency persists. The pitting characteristically picks up stains and discolorations.

Enamel hypoplasias have also been demonstrated in the following conditions: brain injury and neurologic defects, nephrotic syndrome, allergies, chronic lead poisoning, excessive x-ray radiation, hypothyroidism, and in a high percentage of children affected *in utero* with rubella.

Hypoplasia Associated with Exanthematous Diseases. Many of the so-called diseases of childhood are accompanied by temporary elevation in body temperature. The temperature may remain elevated for prolonged periods, and under these circumstances the ameloblasts may be adversely affected. The result can be an enamel hypoplasia that is clinically identical to the pitted hypoplasia seen in nutritional deficiencies.

Hypoplasia Caused by Fluoride Ingestion. A disturbance of enamel may be related to excessive ingestion of fluoride during critical stages of dental development (see Fig. 14-10). In its mildest form it affects the ameloblasts during the appositional stage of enamel formation. With extremely high fluoride levels

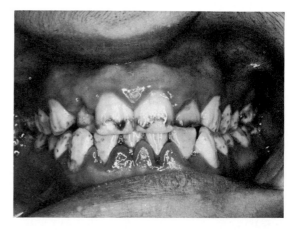

Fig. 14-10 A type of hypoplasia related to the ingestion of high levels of fluoride.

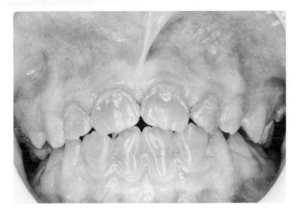

Fig. 14-11 A type of hypoplasia related to the ingestion of tetracycline during the period of tooth formation.

there may also be interference with the calcification process. The fluorosis is characterized by a lusterless opaque appearance to the enamel, which is white in the mild form and yellow to brown in more severe forms. the enamel is mottled and pitted to varying degrees, largely dependent on the amount of fluoride ingested. In its most severe form, fluorosis can grossly alter the morphology of the crown. It occurs symmetrically in dental arches but sometimes with extensive variability in the hypoplasia of individual teeth.

Hypoplasia Associated with Tetracycline Ingestion. Tetracycline may be incorporated in the calcifying enamel matrix by formation of a tetracycline-calcium orthophosphate complex. Upon tooth eruption and exposure to ultraviolet light (sunlight), a discoloration may result, ranging from light yellow to brown. Varying degrees of hypocalcification may also coexist (see Fig. 14-11). Physicians and dentists should avoid prescribing tetracycline (except when no viable alternative exists) during pregnancy and until the child reaches 8 years of age so that incorporation into the developing matrix will be avoided. The dose, time of administration, and type of drug all influence the nature and extent of the discoloration. Permanent teeth are usually less intensely but more diffusely stained than primary teeth. If teeth are stained from tetracycline incorporation, an ultraviolet light applied to the suspected teeth will cause fluorescence.

TYPES OF TETRACYCLINE AND THEIR STAINING

1. Chlortetracycline (Aureomycin)—gray to brown
2. Demeclocycline (Declomycin)—yellow
3. Oxytetracycline (Terramycin)—yellow (least discoloring)
4. Tetracycline (Acromycin)—yellow
5. Doxycycline (Vibramycin)—no change

Preeruptive Caries (Idiopathic Internal Resorption)

Defects seen on the crowns of unerupted and developing permanent teeth may be evident radiographically (appear as carious lesions) (see Fig. 14-12). This condition may occur even though no infection of the associated primary tooth is apparent. The lesion should be carefully checked periodically, and if it increases in size, the associated primary tooth should be removed, the crown of the developing tooth should be exposed, and a temporary restoration placed in the defect on the permanent tooth.

Amelogenesis Imperfecta

Hypoplastic. The hypoplastic forms of amelogenesis imperfecta include disorders in which all or part of the enamel does not reach normal thickness during development. It appears as thin enamel on teeth that do not contact each other mesiodistally, as pits in

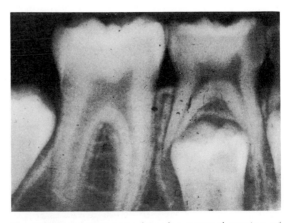

Fig. 14-12 A lesion noted in the coronal portion of an unerupted and developing premolar is diagnosed as *preeruptive caries*.

the enamel, or as vertical or horizontal enamel fissures. The autosomal dominant form appears as a pitted enamel hypoplasia in both the primary and secondary dentition. It usually approaches normal thickness with pinpoint to pinhead pits randomly distributed over the surface. The enamel on newly erupted teeth is hard with a normal yellow-white color. Staining of the pits frequently occurs after exposure to the oral environment, giving the teeth a black, pockmarked appearance. Usually both dentitions are affected; however, in some cases the primary teeth present smooth thin enamel.

Autosomal Dominant, Local. In this type of defect, a horizontal row of depressions or one large hypoplastic area with hypocalcification adjacent to and below the hypoplastic area is found. These defects are most prominent on the buccal surfaces of the teeth, involving the middle third of the enamel. In some cases, the lesion is located closer to the incisal or occlusal, while the lingual aspect may also be involved. The incisal edge or occlusal surface is usually not involved. Primary teeth or teeth in both dentitions may be affected. When all teeth are affected, persons within affected kindreds usually show variation in the number of teeth involved and in the severity of the lesions. The pattern does not present with specific time in the development of teeth as seen in tetracycline or other environmental insults. Changes are usually found on the buccal surfaces of primary molars and premolars. In mildly affected adults the lesion may be represented by only minor defects and hypocalcified areas in the middle third of the buccal surface.

Autosomal Dominant, Smooth. In this condition the enamel is thin, hard, and glossy with a smooth surface. When these teeth are newly erupted they have a yellow color, but may vary from opaque white to translucent brown. The enamel is one fourth to one eighth its normal thickness as if the teeth had been prepared for jacket crowns; the teeth do not meet at the contact points. Some of the enamel may be missing on newly erupted teeth, especially on the incisal or occlusal third, and may be chalky in the interproximal areas. The loss of enamel may be caused by

resorption of the enamel before eruption; thus, delay and failure of eruption occur with resorption of the teeth in the alveolus. Some teeth may be congenitally missing. Radiographically, the enamel may be either missing or represented by a faint, narrow, radiodense outline of the crown. Pulpal calcifications may be present in both erupted and unerupted teeth. Multiple teeth may undergo resorption within the alveolus.

Autosomal Dominant, Rough. In this condition the enamel is hard with a rough granular surface that may chip from the underlying dentin rather than abrade away as seen with the smooth type. The teeth are white to yellow-white when newly erupted and not as subject to attrition as are those with the smooth form. The enamel is one fourth to one eighth its normal thickness, giving the appearance of teeth prepared for jacket crowns, and occasionally a tooth may have thicker enamel at the cervical area. The teeth do not meet at the contact points, but they retain more of the normal tooth outline than do teeth with the smooth form, which have more nearly parallel sides without the normal mesial and distal bulges. Both primary and secondary teeth are affected. Radiographically there is a thin but distinct line of enamel covering the teeth that is easily discerned from the dentin. Impacted or partially resorbed teeth are less frequently seen with this type of defect but do occur.

Autosomal Recessive, Rough. In this condition the teeth when newly erupted have a distinct yellow color like that of normal dentin. The surface is rough and granular resembling ground glass. There is a nearly complete lack of enamel formation detectable clinically or radiographically. The teeth are widely spaced and do not meet at the contact points. All patients with this form of enamel defect have an anterior open bite. Numerous teeth are missing in the erupted dentition and represent radiographically as unerupted teeth undergoing resorption. Both dentitions are usually affected.

Radiographs show no evidence of enamel. Many permanent teeth remain impacted and undergo partial resorption within the alveolus. The teeth have normal-appearing roots and pulp chambers. Areas of impacted teeth are covered by a layer of calcified cuticle with atypical enamel organ remnants arranged in a cystic pattern over the crown and small round calcified bodies in the enamel epithelium.

Hypomaturation Amelogenesis Imperfecta. This form of amelogenesis imperfecta is characterized by enamel that is mottled brown-yellow or white and generally of normal thickness so that the teeth meet at contact points. The enamel is softer than normal and tends to chip from the dentin.

Autosomal Dominant. The most striking feature of this particular condition is found in affected males. The permanent teeth are a mottled yellow-white color but may darken with absorption of stains. The enamel approaches normal thickness but in severely affected males it is occasionally slightly thinner. In most cases the teeth meet at the contact points and have a normal contour. The enamel at the cervical aspect of the tooth crowns tends to be better formed; it is softer than normal, and the point of an explorer can be forced into the tooth structure. Although these teeth chip and abrade more easily than normal, the loss of enamel does not proceed as rapidly as seen with the hypocalcified forms. The primary teeth of affected males have a ground glass, opaque white appearance. A patient occasionally shows a slight yellow cast to the enamel structure.

The color of enamel in primary teeth can best be described as opaque white with translucent white mottling. The surface is moderately smooth, not shiny, as seen with the smooth hypoplastic forms, or rough and granular, as seen with the rough hypoplastic forms, but approaches that of normal teeth. In females, both primary and permanent teeth show alternating vertical bands of white opaque and normal translucent enamel. These vary in width and are randomly distributed over the crown. Radiographs of the teeth of affected females show a uniform radiodensity of enamel and dentin.

Autosomal Recessive, Pigmented. In this condition both the primary and secondary dentitions are affected. The enamel has a milky to shiny agar-brown color on newly erupted teeth but may become more deeply stained on contact with exogenous agents. The teeth are of normal thickness, and the enamel tends to chip away from the dentin, especially around restorations. Resorption of the incisal or occlusal enamel may occur before eruption of teeth. Patients with this condition tend to form large amounts of calculus and may show a type of calculus that contains a pigment-forming organism. On radiographs the enamel is less radiodense than normal and does not contrast well with the dentin. Root and pulp structure appears normal, and the teeth may be seen undergoing resorption within the alveolus.

Snow-Capped Teeth. In this condition varying amounts of enamel on the incisal or occlusal aspects of the crowns have an opaque-white appearance. The opacity may be solid or flecked, and may appear to involve only the surface of the enamel, resembling the appearance seen in white spots. The junction line of opaque-white and translucent enamel is often sharp. The pattern of affected teeth has a distinct anteroposterior relationship and does not correlate with the chronologic order of tooth development. Maxillary teeth tend to be more severely involved than do mandibular. The pattern of the defect on teeth, anterior to posterior, resembles that which would be obtained if a denture were dipped into white paint. In some affected individuals, the incisors through second molars show opaque enamel on the incisal or occlusal third to eighth of the crown. In others only incisors through first molars or incisors through second premolars are affected, so that in mildly affected individuals the defect shows only on central or lateral incisors. The opaque-white enamel does not have the iridescent sheen of the white-frosted ridge enamel seen with mild fluorosis. Both primary and secondary teeth are affected but it is not known whether a person with affected primary teeth will have succedaneous permanent teeth also affected.

Hypocalcified Amelogenesis Imperfecta. In autosomal dominant hypocalcified amelogenesis imperfecta the enamel on newly erupted teeth and unerupted and unresorbed teeth is of normal thickness, although occasional areas of hypoplasia are seen on the middle third of the labial surface. The enamel is so soft that it may be lost soon after eruption leaving a crown composed only of dentin. The enamel has a cheesy consistency and can be scraped from the dentin with an instrument or penetrated easily with a dental explorer. The enamel of the cervical portion of the crown is often better calcified than that on the other portions of the crown. Newly erupted teeth are covered with a dull lusterless, opaque-white, honey-colored, or yellow-orange-brown enamel. The enamel is lost rapidly in the softer supracervical areas, leaving places where dentin is exposed; these areas may be hypersensitive. Numerous teeth may fail to erupt or have marked delay in eruption. Anterior open bite has been recorded in approximately 60% of the cases observed. Patients with this condition are prone to form calculus rapidly, even to a greater extent than are patients with the autosomal recessive hypomaturation type of defect. Radiographically, the enamel fails to contrast with the dentin, and often the dentin is more radiodense than the enamel. The teeth have a moth-eaten appearance on radiograph. Occasionally unerupted teeth can be seen on the radiographs undergoing resorption.

Amelogenesis imperfecta of all types occurs in the general population at a ratio of approximately 1:14,000 to 1:16,000. The most common type is the autosomal-dominant inherited hypocalcification of enamel, which occurs in a ratio of approximately 1:20,000. The modes of inheritance of amelogenesis imperfecta are as follows: hypocalcified has been recorded as autosomal dominant and autosomal recessive; hypomaturation has occurred as sex-linked recessive, autosomal recessive, and autosomal dominant; and hypoplastic has been recorded as autosomal dominant and sex-linked dominant.

Dentin Disturbances

Abnormalities of dentin formation may be classified as follows: dentinogenesis imperfecta (DI) with three variations (Shields type I, Shields type II, and Shields type III) and dentin dysplasia, which occurs as Shields type I and Shields type II.

Other conditions categorized in this area would be odontodysplasia and hereditary dysplasia of enamel and dentin. Three syndromes have been associated with diseases of dentin. They are vitamin-D resistant rickets (hereditary hypophosphatemic rickets), Albright hereditary osteodystrophy, and Ehlers–Danlos syndrome.

Dentinogenesis Imperfecta

Shields Type I. This condition is one of several manifestations of a generalized skeletal disease called *osteogenesis imperfecta.* The features of this condition are multiple bone fractures, hyperextensible joints, blue sclerae, progressive deafness, and dentinogenesis imperfecta. Two types of osteogenesis imperfecta are recognized depending on age of onset and severity: congenita and tarda; in both types the teeth may show a dentin defect. All of the observed abnormalities occur in tissues with major collagen components, and the fundamental defect has been suggested to reside in the collagen matrix. Whether this condition is actually a primary disease of dentin or bone is uncertain.

An amber translucency of both the primary and the permanent dentition is usually seen. There is considerable variation in the expression ranging from all teeth affected to only a few showing mild discoloration. Those that are discolored often have enamel that chips and fractures, which results in rapid attrition of the exposed dentin. Radiographs show that both dentitions may have teeth with accelerated pulp obliteration occurring before eruption or soon after eruption. Short constricted roots are observed in both dentitions.

The dentin enamel junction shows scalloping, but a normal layer of peripheral or mantel dentin may be seen (teeth with no normal dentin have been noted). Dysplastic dentin proliferates to cause obliteration of the pulp chamber and canals. Light microscopic examination of this abnormal dentin shows that it is often atubular or distinctly abnormal with an interglobular type of calcification.

Type I dentinogenesis imperfecta can present as an autosomal dominant trait with variable expressivity in most families with osteogenesis imperfecta. Osteogenesis imperfecta also has been documented to be an autosomal recessive trait with some families showing the most severe and even lethal form of this disorder. The inheritance of the dentin defect follows that of the skeletal defect and may appear as either a dominant or a recessive trait.

Shields Type II (Hereditary Opalescent Dentin). The clinical, radiographic, and histopathologic features are essentially the same as Shields type I. The principle reasons for recognizing this condition as a separate entity are as follows: many families have been reported in which several members exhibited dentinogenesis imperfecta with none of the features of osteogenesis imperfecta; there is a high correlation within families of severity, coloration, and attrition, whereas there is considerable phenotype variation in type I DI; and both dentitions are equally affected. Clinical and radiographic examination never reveal completely normal teeth. By contrast, in type I DI the primary teeth are always more severely affected than are the permanent teeth.

Type II DI represents one of the most common dominantly inherited disorders in humans, affecting approximately 1 in every 8,000 persons. Sporadic cases are virtually unreported, which suggests that the mutation rate is low. Dentin dysplasia and tetracycline-stained teeth may have a clinical appearance similar to hereditary opalescent dentin. These conditions do occur in a sporadic fashion; therefore, any report of a sporadic type II DI or of an affected person with both parents normal who does not have clinical, radiographic, and histopathologic data to confirm the diagnosis is open to serious doubt.

Shields Type III (Brandywine Type). Teeth with Shields type III dentinogenesis imperfecta resemble those with type I and II DI in both coloration and shape; however, considerable phenotypic variability is noted. The most common clinical characteristics are opalescent color, involvement of both dentitions, and bell-shaped crowns.

In primary teeth, there is high variability in radiographic appearance, ranging from normal to that typically observed in type II

DI. The unique feature seems to be the appearance of so-called shell teeth, a term used to describe teeth in which dentin formation did not occur until after the mantel layer of dentin was formed. This unusual situation was observed in 8 of 252 individuals in a Brandywine, Maryland population. This condition seems unusual enough to justify a separate classification of type III DI because there have been no instances of shell teeth observed in all the cases of type II DI.

A third unique radiographic finding of this type of dentinogenesis is occurrence of multiple pulp exposures in the primary dentition. Such a finding is essentially nonexistent in type II DI but perhaps not so remote for type I, in which some teeth can show relatively normal pulp chambers and canals. The pedigree information indicates a possible autosomal dominant trait.

Dentin Dysplasia, Shields Type I

Type I dentin dysplasia appears in the literature under a variety of descriptive terms including *rootless teeth, nonopalescent and opalescent dentin,* and *radicular dentin dysplasia.* Rootless teeth are a significant descriptive feature of the disorder, but over the years *dentin dysplasia* has become the term of choice. The permanent and primary teeth are of normal size, shape, and consistency, although affected teeth are occasionally slightly amber and translucent. The most striking clinical feature is malalignment and malpositioning of teeth due to extreme mobility, which is the result of a failure to form normal root structure. Even minor trauma may result in exfoliation.

Affected teeth have short roots with sharp, conical, apical constrictions. Associated with these short or blunted roots are multiple periapical radiolucencies that when seen in noncarious teeth are of great value in making the diagnosis of dentin dysplasia. Obliteration of the pulp is a significant feature of this disorder, which occurs preeruptively in the permanent dentition and produces a crescent-shaped pulp remnant that is visible radiographically but typically only in permanent teeth. Total pulpal chamber obliteration and absence of root canals is a common feature of the primary dentition. Occasionally calcified masses can be observed in the pulp, but most often these are fused into a single mass continuous with root dentin.

Type I dentin dysplasia is rare, estimated to have a population frequency of about 1 in 100,000. Only some 30 cases have been reported in the literature. Several pedigrees show a dominant mode of inheritance with examples of male-to-male transmission. There appears to be a low mutation rate with lack of sporadic cases.

Dentin Dysplasia, Shields Type II

In type II dentin dysplasia there is a significant color difference in the two dentitions. Primary teeth have an amber translucent appearance, whereas permanent teeth are of normal color. There are no other distinctive clinical features that characterize this disorder, and no unusual attrition rate has been observed in affected primary teeth. Obliteration of the pulp chamber is seen in the primary dentition by 5 to 6 years of age. Some pulp chambers are still evident at 2 years of age, and obliteration never occurs before eruption. The radiographic appearance of the permanent dentition shows evidence of pulp chambers in all teeth, although obliteration has been noted in incisors by 14 years of age. The anterior teeth and premolars typically have a pulp chamber and root canal that are thistle-tube in shape because of the radicular extension of the pulp chamber. Almost all teeth show multiple accumulations of pulp stones in these unusually shaped pulp chambers. By contrast with type I, multiple periapical radiolucencies are not a feature of type II dentin dysplasia.

The primary teeth have a normal appearing layer of coronal dentin with a sudden transition to amorphous and atubular dentin in the radicular portion. Permanent teeth show essentially normal coronal dentin but with interglobular dentin in the pulpal third. Root canals are reduced in dimension. Multiple denticles have been noted in the permanent dentition with some false but most of the true variety. These findings suggest that a more complete and severe dysplasia of dentin is affecting the primary dentition whereas the permanent teeth, although clearly affected, have a more normal and less severe picture.

This rare condition appears to have an autosomal dominant mode of inheritance with a high degree of penetrance, possibly as high as 100%.

Enamel and Dentin Disturbances

Odontodysplasia. Odontodysplasia represents a localized arrest in tooth development. Clinically, a single tooth or even several teeth in the same quadrant may have moderate to severe hypoplasia of the crowns (see Fig. 14-13A, B). One case has been reported in which three of four quadrants of teeth were involved. Affected teeth are often discolored depending on the severity of the enamel defect and are especially susceptible to caries, with local infection a common complication. When primary teeth are affected, the per-

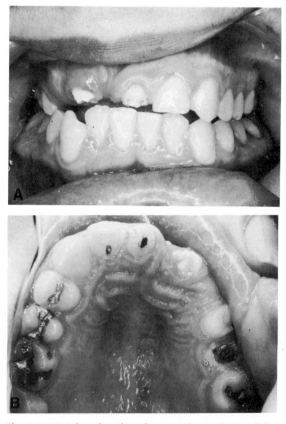

Fig. 14-13 A localized and severe hypoplasia of the crowns of a few teeth in a quadrant can be diagnosed as odontodysplasia.

manent successors are also often involved. Affected permanent teeth may be observed underlying normal primary predecessors. Defective teeth are often unerupted or delayed in their eruption.

Radiographically, these teeth have large pulps, little dentin, and only a thin layer of enamel. A ghostlike appearance is often used to describe the radiographic picture. The roots are poorly outlined and typically shortened. Microscopic examination reveals irregular dentin, false denticles, and normal cementum. The cause of this disorder is unknown, and no familial cases have been reported. This observation, coupled with the localized nature of the defect, makes a hereditary basis unlikely. Evaluations of teeth and tooth development clearly exclude explanations such as nutritional deficiency, trauma, infection, and radiation. One might expect that such a defect in primary dental structures could be transmitted to permanent structures, thereby affecting both dentitions, a situation noted in several cases. At present, it is impossible to say in which structure the primary defect resides. Radiographs confirm a generalized lack of enamel on the primary dentition, some enamel with reduced density, and thickness on the permanent teeth. Multiple periapical radiolucencies have been observed at the apices of some of the teeth with exposed pulps. Pulp chambers and root canals appear to be large. Teeth are usually not missing, and the alveolar bone is normal in appearance. Several teeth show enamel to have an amorphous appearance and to be without enamel structure. There appears to be a relatively thin layer of normal mantle dentin, and the remaining dentin is grossly abnormal. The dentin tubules are reduced in number and irregular.

Case histories suggest an autosomal dominant trait of this rather rare condition with vertical (three generations affected) and male-to-male transmission.

Odontoma. *Odontoma* refers to a benign tumor of tooth structures, composed of a mixture of tissues that form a tooth (see Fig. 14-14). Odontomas may include enamel, dentin, predentin, cementum, pulp, periodontal tissues, and epithelial rests. It may be formed as a result of continued budding of the pri-

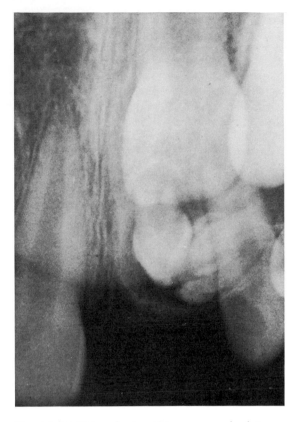

Fig. 14-14 This odontoma is composed of tissues arranged in various combinations that form what appears to be small teeth or toothlike structures.

mary or permanent tooth germ or abnormal proliferation of cells of the tooth germ, in which case an odontoma replaces the normal tooth.

The etiology of the odontoma is unknown. They may occur in any location in the dental arches and are often seen in young children. Odontomas seldom exceed the size of the teeth, but when they do become large, they may expand the jaw. The type that forms many, small, toothlike masses is the most common; it is an asymptomatic condition.

The lesions are principally radiopaque with some areas of radiolucency, and at the periphery there is usually a radiolucent border. Frequently, they are associated with unerupted teeth. The developing lesion may present a diagnostic problem when discovered prior to significant mineralization. In some instances they appear on radiograph as a radiolucent area with some radiopaque foci.

The odontoma may develop a cystic area similar to one developing around the crown of an impacted tooth.

Compound Odontoma (Compound Composite Odontoma). This odontogenic tumor is composed of a multiplicity of tiny teeth or denticles, often many dozen in number. The denticles are usually small replicas, sometimes rudimentary peg-shaped teeth. Within each tiny denticle the arrangement of the individual tissues is comparatively normal with mature enamel capping a tiny tooth-shaped aggregate of dentin, which contains a central pulp and includes a root formation covered by cementum. Each little denticle is enclosed separately in its own individual fibrous tooth sac, and the whole aggregate is separated from the surrounding bone by a fibrous capsule; thus, this calcified mass has some anatomic similarity to normal teeth. This is a more common lesion, occurring twice as frequently as the complex odontoma. There is seldom any difficulty in the radiographic diagnosis of the compound odontoma because of the resemblance of the components to miniature teeth.

Complex Odontoma (Complex Composite Odontoma). This odontogenic tumor contains a mixture of enamel, dentin, cementum, and pulp in which the interrelationship of these tissues is grossly abnormal. The bulk of the tumor may exceed that of a normal tooth. The individual dental tissues are scattered throughout, and the entire overgrowth is surrounded by a fibrous capsule. The compound and complex odontomas are not clear-cut entities. The typical forms of the two lesions constitute the extreme ends of a merging spectrum.

All odontomas should be surgically removed and submitted for microscopic examination in order to be certain of the diagnosis. The lesions tend not to recur.

Vitamin-D-Resistant Rickets (Hereditary Hypophosphatemic Rickets). Vitamin D promotes the absorption of calcium and phosphorus from the intestinal tract; therefore, a diet deficient in vitamin D produces a negative calcium balance that in turn leads to undermineralization of the skeletal system. When such undermineralization is severe enough to produce clinical and radiographic changes, it is identified as rickets. The organic matrix of bone in a person with rickets is essentially normal and eventually may become normally mineralized if calcium and phosphorus are supplied to this tissue in adequate amounts and proper proportions (calcium phosphorus concentrations sufficient for mineralization to occur); thus, rickets is caused by a lack of calcification of cartilage and osteoid tissues.

It has been recognized that certain patients with the classical features of rickets do not respond to ordinary replacement doses of vitamin D therapy, which was typically curative for this disorder. Albright in 1937 demonstrated that these patients would respond to massive doses of vitamin D. The prime features of this disorder are familial recurrence, lowered serum phosphate levels associated with decreased renal resorption of phosphate, and lack of response to physiologic doses of vitamin D. Familial inheritance does not adequately describe this disorder because the hereditary basis is well documented as an X-linked dominant trait. It is characterized by a decreased level of inorganic phosphate in the plasma as a result of failure of reabsorption by defective renal tubules.

Affected children are of short stature and often demonstrate significant bowing of the legs. Bony outgrowths at the site of muscular attachments and around joints may limit motion. Rachitic rosary, seen in classic vitamin-D-dependent rickets, may occur also. The disease is first recognized in young children about the time they begin to walk. At this time the only abnormalities are a shortened stature, an abnormally low serum phosphate, and an elevated serum alkaline phosphatase. Defects in the skeleton vary from mere decrease in height to severe skeletal deformity. Dental lesions have included gross reduction in the amount and quality of dentin. This results in an abnormally wide root canal and large pulp chamber with faulty calcification and marked interglobular spaces in the dentin. Tracts are frequently present leading from the pulp to the dentinoenamel junction or even to the outer enamel surface. These tracts remain patent and may result in early pulpal infection developing in the absence of carious lesions. As a result, apical lesions are sometimes seen in otherwise intact noncarious teeth.

The skeleton shows active rickets with short stature and bowed legs, which persist into adult life. The radiographic picture in adults is of postrachitic deformities and pseudofractures. The serum phosphate levels remain persistently low, and the serum alkaline phosphatase activity ranges from normal to high. This is an X-linked dominant disorder, meaning the affected males (assuming they are married to unaffected females) can have only normal sons and affected daughters.

It behooves the dentist to be especially aware of this disorder because the dental signs and symptoms are largely unknown to the medical profession. Dental changes may produce the first overt symptoms of the disease that cause the patient to seek dental attention leading to a subsequent medical evaluation. Both primary and permanent dentitions are usually involved. The clinical evidence may be draining periapical abscesses and fistulas about the primary teeth, but the permanent teeth are less often affected and present only a nonvital pulp test on routine examination. Radiographic examination of symptomatic teeth often reveals enlarged pulp chambers and extension of the pulp horns into the cusp tips. Periapical pathology is often seen on these affected teeth. Clinical and radiographic signs are seen in teeth that do not demonstrate any causative factors such as dental caries, periodontal disease, or fracture. A routine finding with vitamin-D-resistant rickets is a severe hypoplasia of the incisal or occlusal enamel with radiographs showing dentin changes such as large pulp chambers and delayed closure of root apices. Enamel changes are usually absent in the vitamin-D-resistant form of rickets, and dental changes are confined principally to the dentin. In the region of pulp horns, tubular defects of the dentin extend to the dentinoenamel junction and sometimes into the cusp tips and under the incisal edges; thus, open cracks in the surface enamel may extend into the pulp, offering an avenue for pulpal infection. Prenatal interglobular dentin is another discriminating feature between dependent and resistant vita-

min D disorders because in the dependent form the mother's normal vitamin D metabolism appears to protect the fetus from dental insult.

The primary problem of this condition is a failure of end-organ responsiveness to parathyroid hormone. The condition is characterized by hypocalcemia and hyperphosphatemia as is seen in hypoparathyroidism. The condition is inherited as an X-linked dominant trait. Male-to-male transmission is observed, and females are affected twice as often as males.

Defects of the primary dental structures are as follows: a dull white appearance to the enamel with pitting of its surface, small crowns and short roots with blunt apices, and large pulp chambers and unusual histopathologic changes in the dentin. The dentin shows irregular dentin tubules with sharp bends, while the cementum is thick and of a cellular variety. The pulp chambers are filled with calcified material in a whorl-like pattern.

DISTURBANCES IN COLOR OF TEETH

Black Stain

Stains on teeth sometimes develop as a result of contact with certain metallic elements such as silver, iron, and lead. Black stain may appear as a thin black line running approximately 1 mm or so above the gingival margin; it may occur on both the facial and lingual surfaces of the teeth. The stain is firmly attached to the surface but remains extrinsic; thus, it must be removed by the use of brush and abrasives. It tends to recur quickly, is found more frequently in females than in males, and sometimes in mouths that have excellent oral hygiene. Its cause is unknown, but is thought to form as a result of the activity of chromogenic bacteria.

Green Stain

Green stain is seen frequently and usually occurs as a thick deposit involving the cervical one third of the facial surface of the maxillary incisors of young children. It affects boys 50% more frequently than girls. The condition is associated with poor oral hygiene, and decalcification is sometimes present in enamel underlying the deposit. The nature of the pigment is unknown; however, it may represent the metabolic products of chromogenic bacteria or fungi or it may be caused by bacterial action on blood pigments associated with inflammatory exudate from adjacent gingival inflammation. It may also result from bacterial action on remnants of the enamel cuticle remaining in a region of stagnation. Green stain is extrinsic and may be removed by simple brushing and abrasives.

Orange Stain

Orange stain occurs infrequently and usually involves both facial and lingual surfaces of the incisors. It is more easily removed than green stain and its cause is unknown, but it is believed to result from the action of chromogenic bacteria. It is probably associated with poor oral hygiene. The stain is extrinsic and is easily removed by the use of brushes and abrasives.

Brown Stain

Brown stain is the second most common type of stain and may be seen in nonsmokers. It is usually lighter brown than that of tobacco stain and forms a tenacious but delicate film on the surface of the teeth. It is usually most pronounced on the lingual surfaces of the lower incisors and the buccal surfaces of the maxillary molar teeth. The true nature of brown stain is not certainly known, but it is believed to form as a pellicle-type deposit and to be derived from altered salivary mucins that have undergone change through the action of bacterial enzymes. The stain always remains extrinsic and is easily removed by brush and abrasives.

Erythroblastosis Fetalis

Erythroblastosis fetalis is characterized by an excessive destruction of erythrocytes. The peripheral blood has many nucleated red cells, and anemia develops from excessive hemolysis. The condition develops from immunization of the Rh-negative mother by Rh-positive red cells of the fetus or by previous transfusion of Rh-positive blood cells. The Rh factors are a series of isoantigens that are normally present on the red cell membranes in the blood of the rhesus monkey. They are also found in 85% of humans, leaving 15% of the population Rh-negative and therefore likely to produce antibodies if exposed to Rh-positive blood. Because the Rh antibodies are capable of crossing the placenta, a potentially dangerous situation arises when union of an Rh-negative female and a Rh-positive male produces an Rh-positive fetus. Sensitization of the Rh-negative female may occur through leakage of small amounts of Rh antigen across the placenta into the maternal circulation. This results in production of circulating Rh antibodies that may in turn cross the placenta and produce hemolysis of fetal red cells.

Hemolytic complications found in Rh-factor incompatibilities are estimated to affect approximately 1 in 200 births. In an initial pregnancy, the level of circulating antibodies often is minimal and produces little clinical effect, but subsequent pregnancies tend to reinforce antibody production and to result in increasingly high levels, with correspondingly severe fetal hemolysis. The clinical severity may range from minimal cases in which the child is relatively normal and merely shows a somewhat more severe degree of jaundice (icterus gravis neonatorum) than that which accompanies many normal births. In more severe cases, the child may be born alive but be suffering from a severe hemolytic anemia (erythroblastosis fetalis). In the most severe cases the fetus may have suffered circulatory failure from the hemolytic anemia, become water-logged, and died *in utero* (hydrops fetalis).

Visible lesions of the teeth result from two different causes. First, the severe generalized metabolic upset may produce a systemic pattern of enamel hypocalcification or hypoplasia that becomes progressively more severe as the antibody level builds up during the latter part of the pregnancy; however, if the infant survives, the enamel formation rapidly reverts to normal shortly after birth when hemolysis ceases. This timing sequence means that the upset produces its maximum effect in the primary crowns, with the permanent series being spared. A second cause of abnormality in the forming tooth results through the high level of circulating bilirubin that is an end product of the red cell hemolysis. Pigment is deposited throughout all tissue, producing the severe jaundice that is seen in the skin and frequently results in a greenish yellow discoloration of developing enamel and dentin. The histopathology of the lesion may range through hypocalcification to hypoplasia or even aplasia of enamel, and the underlying dentin may show disturbances.

Both parents and child should be reassured that the malformed and discolored primary teeth are a transient situation that usually will correct itself with eruption of the permanent successors. One can reasonably expect the permanent teeth to be intact.

Porphyria

Porphyria is a group of disorders in which there is a defective metabolism of the pyrrole compounds (Greek: porphyria = purple). This often results in the production of burgundy-colored urine in effected persons because of the excessive production of reduced uroporphyrins.

Classification of the different disease types depends on the particular organ system affected. There is generally a separation into two forms: erythropoietic and hepatic. Most forms of porphyria are genetically determined as autosomal dominant. It commonly appears after adolescence and lasts for the remainder of life. Acquired forms of hepatic porphyria have been reported. Other clinical manifestations include photophobia, hypertrichosis, skin lesions, and intrinsic reddish brown staining of teeth. The skin is photosensitive, and exposure to sunlight triggers vesicles, bullae, and edema. Neuropsychiatric peculiarities may be displayed.

The symptoms of porphyria may be exacerbated by intake of alcohol and barbiturates; thus, these drugs should be avoided by affected persons. The staining of primary and permanent teeth by uroporphyrins can be confirmed by ultraviolet light, which produces red fluorescence. Bullous erosive lesions of the oral mucosa can occur and may be triggered by certain exogenous sources

(*i.e.* phenobarbital) and possibly by sunlight, heat, or trauma.

DISTURBANCES OF ERUPTION AND EXFOLIATION

Ectopic Eruption

Teeth erupt ectopically in the mandibular permanent incisor region about 75% of the time. Removal of primary incisors with no root resorption should be done judiciously. If primary teeth in the lower anterior region are removed prematurely, many will produce an anterior arch perimeter collapse, overeruption of succedaneous incisors, and increased vertical overlap of anterior teeth.

The eruption of the permanent first molar into the roots of the primary second molar (2% to 3% prevalence) usually corrects itself and may result in destruction of the distal root of the primary second molar. Critical examination of periapical and bite-wing radiographs is important before the time of eruption of the first permanent molars in order to detect ectopic eruption. The permanent molar may become hopelessly locked and cause premature exfoliation of the second primary molar or make it necessary to extract the affected tooth. Ectopically erupting first permanent molars may eventually turn upright and erupt into a normal position after causing only minor destruction of the primary molar. Ectopic eruption has been reported to occur in approximately 1 in 50 children. It occasionally occurs in more than one quadrant in the same mouth but has been most often observed in the maxilla. The anomaly has been observed more frequently in boys than in girls. It was reported that 66% of the ectopically erupted molars finally erupted into their essentially normal position without need of corrective treatment.

Pulver describes one or more of the following factors accompanying or related to ectopic eruption: larger than normal mean sizes of all maxillary primary and permanent teeth, larger affected first permanent molars and second primary molars, smaller maxillae, posterior position of the maxillae in relation to the cranial base, abnormal angulation of eruption of the maxillary first permanent molar, delayed calcification of some affected first permanent molars. After the occlusal surface of the first permanent molar becomes exposed in the oral cavity, the eruption path of the impacted tooth can often be favorably influenced by inserting a 0.026-inch brass ligature wire at the site of contact between the molars. The brass ligature is completely looped through the contact area and is tightened with pliers. The primary canine is frequently lost prematurely at the time of eruption of the permanent lateral incisor; this condition is generally referred to as *ectopic eruption*.

Delayed Eruption

Individual permanent teeth are often observed to be delayed in their development and consequently in their eruption. It is not uncommon to observe partially impacted permanent teeth or deviation in the eruption path that results in abnormally delayed eruption, and in cases of this type, it is generally necessary to extract the primary tooth, construct a space maintainer, and allow the permanent tooth to erupt and assume its normal position. Although many theories have been advanced, the factors responsible for the eruption of teeth are not fully understood.

The developmental processes and factors that have been related to the eruption of teeth include elongation of the root, forces exerted by the vascular tissues around and beneath the root, growth of the alveolar bone, growth of dentin, pulpal constriction, growth and pull of the periodontal membrane, pressure from the muscular action, and resorption of the alveolar crest. A radiographic study demonstrated that each tooth starts to move toward occlusion at approximately the time of crown completion. The interval between crown completion and the beginning of eruption until the tooth is in full occlusion is approximately 5 years for permanent teeth.

Gron observed in her study of 874 Boston children that tooth emergence appeared to be more closely associated with the stage of root formation than with the chronologic or skeletal age of the child. By the time of clinical emergence approximately three quarters of root formation had occurred. Teeth reach occlusion before the root development is

complete. Posen reviewed the records of children in the Burlington study who had undergone extraction of primary molars and made the following conclusions. Eruption of the premolar teeth will be delayed in children who lose primary molars at 4 or 5 years of age and before. If extraction of the primary molars occurs between 5 and 8 years there will be a decrease in delay of premolar eruption. Between 8 and 10 years of age, premolar eruption caused by premature loss of primary teeth is greatly accelerated.

Submergence (Ankylosed Teeth)

An ankylosed tooth is one in which the hard tissue of the tooth has fused with at least a portion of the surrounding alveolar bone. It is considered an aberration of eruption in which the continuity of the periodontal ligament has been compromised. There is progressive loss of occlusal direction. The incidence has been reported to be approximately 1.3%. Via concluded that the occurrence of ankylosed primary teeth has a definite familial tendency and is probably an inherited trait. The mandibular second primary molar is the tooth most often observed to be ankylosed. Ankylosis of the anterior primary teeth does not occur unless there has been a traumatic injury. A small number of teeth fail to erupt in the absence of any obvious hindrance or barrier, and these are spoken of as *embedded teeth*.

Transposition

The eruption of a tooth into an abnormal sequence position in the dental arch is called transposition. An example would be the eruption of a lateral incisor into the premolar region (see Fig. 14-15).

Eruption Cyst

An eruption cyst is a form of dentigerous cyst that appears as a swelling of the alveolar mucosa. It is seen in association with erupting primary and permanent teeth (see Fig. 14-16). Treatment is usually unnecessary because the lesion is small and the tooth breaks through causing the swelling to subside. The lesion is more frequently seen in primary sec-

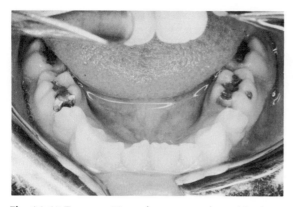

Fig. 14-15 Transposition of permanent lateral incisors into the first premolar position.

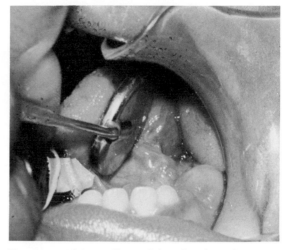

Fig. 14-16 This swelling of the alveolar ridge associated with an erupting primary tooth can be diagnosed as an eruption cyst.

ond molar or first permanent molar regions. This substantiates the conclusion that the condition develops as a result of trauma. When treatment becomes necessary, it consists of excising the overlying soft tissue to expose the crown of the tooth and draining the accumulated fluid.

Eruption Hematoma

The eruption cyst is occasionally filled with blood resulting in a bluish purple elevated mass of tissue; treatment is similar to that used for eruption cyst.

Eruption Sequestra

A tiny spicule of bone overlying the crown of an erupting permanent molar just before or immediately after emergence of the tips of the cusps through the oral mucosa is an eruption sequestra. Generally, the position of the fragment of bone is directly overlying the central occlusal fossa but contoured within the soft tissue. As the tooth continues to erupt and the cusps emerge, the fragment of bone sequestrates through the mucosa.

Premature (Precocious) Exfoliation

Variations in the time of eruption of the primary teeth and in the time of exfoliation are frequently observed in the child patient. A variation of the exfoliation time of primary teeth of as much as 18 months may be considered normal. The widespread loss of sup-

porting alveolar bone with loosening, migration, and spontaneous loss of teeth or the necessity for premature extraction is characteristic of the following conditions:

Papillon–Lefèvre Syndrome. In Papillon–Lefèvre syndrome, affected individuals exhibit the following clinical signs, usually between 2 and 4 years of age: reddened, scaly, and rough palms and soles; inflamed gingivae; and horizontal alveolar bone destruction, usually beginning after eruption of the second primary molars. The first two features are directly related to the hyperkeratosis. Once the primary dentition has been shed owing to the periodontal bone loss, the gingival tissue returns to normal until the permanent dentition makes its appearance; the inflammation and degenerative processes are then repeated. This rare syndrome is inherited as an autosomal recessive trait; the typical affected family consists of normal parents and a negative family history for this condition other than the affected individual himself and possibly some siblings. Treatment is symptomatic and palliative. Full dentures are usually worn by the time the individual reaches puberty.

Familial Juvenile Periodontitis (Familial Juvenile Periodontosis). Familial juvenile periodontitis, formerly known as familial juvenile peridontosis, is a condition in which alveolar bone loss is vertical and more selective than the periodontitis of Papillon–Lefèvre syndrome. It occurs principally around the permanent first molars and the central and lateral incisors. Those affected with this condition lose their teeth early in life but usually not before early adulthood. The disease has been frequently observed as a single, isolated instance in a family. Such observations make genetic hypotheses difficult.

Vitamin D-resistant Rickets (Familial Hypophasphatemic Rickets; *see page 550)*

Reticuloendothelioses (Histiocytosis X). This condition represents a group of metabolic diseases of the reticuloendothelial system for which there is no known etiology. The three diseases included in this group are *Letterer–Siwe disease, Hand–Schüller–Christian disease,* and *eosinophilic granuloma of bone.* Most authorities regard these as a single disease entity with the three forms of the disease representing only a variable clinical expression. Letterer–Siwe disease is an acute fulminating form of the disease that chiefly affects infants and young children; typically these patients develop lesions of the spleen, liver, lymph nodes, skin, and skeleton manifested by hepatosplenomegaly, lymphadenopathy, skin nodules, and destructive lesions of bone, including the jaws. Fever and malaise are commonly present. The lesions themselves consist basically of the accumulation and proliferation of large numbers of histiocytes, often intermingled with focal collections of eosinophils. The intracellular accumulation of the lipid cholesterol within the histiocytes is usually not as prominent as it is in the other two forms of histiocytosis X.

Lesions of the jaws are characterized by a diffuse destruction of bone, usually resulting in loosening and premature exfoliation of teeth. The clinical and roentgenographic appearance of the jaw lesions is not characteristic, however, because many other diseases may produce a similar destruction of bone and loss of teeth. Ulceration of oral tissues and pain are also common findings. Letterer–Siwe disease has a poor prognosis because of its fulminating course. Most individuals with the disease die within a relatively short time. Hand–Schüller–Christian disease is an-

other variation of the same basic disease. It occurs in somewhat older children and young adolescents, has a more subacute course, and presents a more favorable prognosis. Clinically, visceral involvement similar to that in Letterer–Siwe disease occurs but is not usually as diffuse and widespread. A somewhat more common finding is skeletal involvement, although the extent of such involvement varies markedly. Skull involvement is particularly common, often resulting in dyspituitarism and ensuing diabetes insipidus. Retro-orbital involvement producing exophthalmos is also common. The jaws are involved as in Letterer–Siwe disease, with severe destruction of bone and loosening and premature loss of teeth. Extensive oral ulceration with pain, fetid breath, and excessive salivation are also common. The prognosis of Hand–Schüller–Christian disease is somewhat better than for Letterer–Siwe disease, although many individuals with the former die. Prognosis appears to depend chiefly on the extent of the disease with respect to organ and skeletal involvement. X-ray radiation and corticosteroid therapy are both of definite value in treatment.

Eosinophilic granuloma of bone is a third form of histiocytosis X disease. It occurs chiefly in young adults, runs a chronic course, and is limited in extent, often involving only one bone. Because of this limitation, the disease has an excellent prognosis. Any bone in the skeleton may be involved, and lesions of the jaws are common. These lesions are often asymptomatic and are discovered during routine radiographic examination. Some lesions produce mild swelling and occasional pain. Loss of superficial alveolar bone, often mimicking juvenile periodontitis or localized periodontitis, is a common early manifestation of the disease.

Acrodynia. The exposure of young children to minute amounts of mercury may produce a condition referred to as acrodynia or *pink disease.* Ointments, diaper rinses, and medications are the usual sources of the mercury. The clinical features of the disease include fever, anorexia, desquamation of the soles and palms, sweating, tachycardia, gastrointestinal disturbances, and hypotonia. The oral findings include inflammation and ulcerations of the mucous membrane, excessive salivation, loss of alveolar bone, and premature exfoliation of teeth.

Familial Fibrous Dysplasia. Familial fibrous dysplasia (cherubism) is a rare condition of the jaws that may occur in childhood. Although the etiology has not been clearly established, the disease may follow a familial pattern and may present a local disturbance in the embryonic development of tissues. Symmetric or asymmetric enlargement of the jaws may be noted at an early age. Numerous sharp, well-defined multilocular areas of bone destruction and thinning of the cortical plate are evident on the radiograph. Teeth in the involved area are frequently exfoliated prematurely as a result of the loss of support or root resorption (in permanent teeth, as a result of an interference in development of roots). Spontaneous loss of teeth may occur or the child may pick the teeth out of the soft tissue.

Hypophosphatasia. Hypophosphatasia can be characterized by premature exfoliation of the anterior primary teeth. The loss of teeth in a young child may be spontaneous or may result from a slight traumatic injury. There may be absence of gingival inflammation and loss of alveolar bone limited to the anterior region. The disease is believed to be inherited through the action of an autosomal recessive gene, so the diagnostic tests should include determination of serum alkaline phosphatase levels for parents and siblings.

Cyclic Neutropenia. An unusual form of agranulocytosis, cyclic neutropenia is characterized by a periodic or cyclic diminution in polymorphonuclear neutrophilic leukocytes and is accompanied by mild clinical manifestations. This condition spontaneously regresses, only to recur subsequently in a rhythmic pattern. The etiology of the disease is unknown. Although the role of hormonal factors in the etiology of the disease has been suggested, there is no sound evidence to indicate that this is the case. Similarly, a hereditary feature has been suggested but has not been proven.

The condition occurs at any age, and numerous cases have been reported in children. The patients manifest a fever, malaise, sore throat, stomatitis, regional lymphadenopathy, as well as headache, cutaneous infection and conjunctivitis. A bacterial infection is not a serious feature, presumably because the neutrophil count is low for such a short time. Children will exhibit severe gingivitis with ulceration. With the return of the neutrophil count to normal, the gingivae assume a nearly normal clinical appearance. In children with repeated insults of the infection there will be considerable loss of supporting bone around the teeth, and loss of bone around multiple teeth has sometimes been termed *prepuberal periodontitis.* Severe loss of bone may also be seen in the patients with leukemia and diabetes.

Epstein Pearls

This condition is characterized by small white or grayish white lesions formed along the midpalatal raphe of the newborn (see Fig. 14-17). The lesions may be multiple and do not increase in size. They are considered remnants of epithelial tissue trapped along the raphe as the fetus grows. No treatment is indicated because the lesions will be spontaneously shed a few weeks after birth.

Bohn's Nodules

These small white or grayish white lesions form along the buccal and lingual aspects of the dental ridges and on the palate away

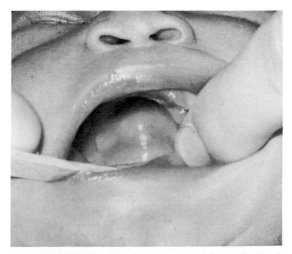

Fig. 14-17 Small white lesions along the midpalatal raphe of the newborn can be diagnosed as Epstein pearls.

from the raphe of the newborn. The nodules are considered to be remnants of mucous gland tissue.

Dental Lamina Cysts

These small white lesions are found on the crest of the maxillary and mandibular dental ridges. The cysts originate from remnants of the dental lamina.

ELECTRIC CORD BURNS

Electric cord burns occur frequently at the commissure region of the lips (see Fig. 14-18). Two main types of electrical burns (contact and arc) have been described. A contact burn occurs when the patient is grounded and the body acts as a conductor, with current passing through it along the path of least resistance; these burns can be fatal. An arc burn is sustained when arcs or sparks appear in the gap between a live wire and tissue. The tissue is burned by thermal changes at the entrance and exit sites of the current. Heat is estimated to be as high as 2,500°C to

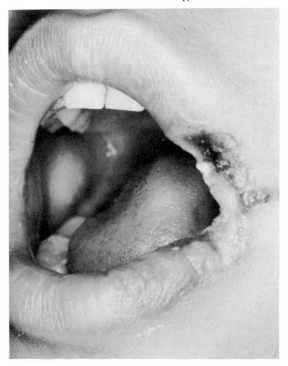

Fig. 14-18 Electric cord burn at the commissure of the lips.

3000°C. The extent of injury with both types of burns is highly variable and largely depends on factors such as the quality, intensity, duration, and location of the stimulus.

Electrical burns in the mouth have commonly been associated with children under 4 years of age. The most commonly reported causes of these burns have been sucking or chewing the live end of an extension cord or chewing through the insulation of a live wire. The child may gnaw at the junction of an extension cord; saliva reaching the metal junction acts as a conductor.

The clinical appearance of an electric burn is a gray-white tissue, surrounded by a narrow rim of erythema. The center of the lesion may be depressed and the margins raised. It has been observed that usually the tissue begins to swell within the first few hours of injury, the margins of the wound become irregular, the lips protrude, and the control of saliva is diminished. Swelling is prominent for 7 to 10 days. It is difficult in the first 2 weeks to differentiate between viable and nonviable tissues. Because there is destruction of neural tissues, the lesions are usually painless, and some sensory and motor loss may result in the surrounding tissues. Necrotic tissues can slough within a few days, but this usually occurs between 2 and 4 weeks following the burn accident. Following sloughing an irregular ulceration may be observed. The chief cause of the tissue necrosis is reported to be ischemia. It is possible for teeth on the direct arc of current to be devitalized. Heat necrosis, the result of electrical trauma, is characterized by coagulation of protein, liquefaction of fat, and vaporization of tissue fluids.

A variety of infrequent complications such as cardiac arrest and secondary shock have been reported. The most common complication is bleeding of the labial artery, which can be controlled with pressure and epinephrine-soaked sponges or in severe cases, by the use of transfusions or vessel ligation. Hospitalization is recommended until the eschar is sloughed.

Recovery from an electrical commissural burn differs from other types of burns: the eschar sloughs later; healing that occurs by secondary intention is slower. One view is that when surgery is not performed, the opposing lips may adhere to each other; when this occurs concomitant with contraction and scarring, asymmetrical facial appearance may result. A conservative attitude is usually adopted in the treatment of superficial electrical burns. When severe tissue damage occurs, surgery has been the recommended treatment. Some surgeons feel the optimal time for surgery is before healing takes place; however, most prefer waiting until the eschar sloughs and the wound heals. With both approaches, the contracture of severe wounds often results in an asymmetrical facial appearance. Scarring may mar the patient's appearance and lead to multiple surgical procedures. In an attempt to reduce the number of surgical approaches and improve oral symmetry, removable and fixed intraoral splinting appliances have been recommended.

The appliances (see Fig. 14-19) have two ovoid acrylic posts that extend from the mouth and flare laterally. The posts are extended to maintain the commissural regions equally distant from the midline. The removable appliance should be worn continuously for 6 months, followed by nocturnal wearing for another year. A fixed maxillary appliance consists of a labial arch wire supporting two acrylic posts. Stainless steel bands are fitted to the primary maxillary second molars and central incisors. The fixed appliance should be worn for 10 months. Subsequently, a removable appliance is constructed for nocturnal wearing.

Critical to the success of the appliance is the establishment of the post position. The vertical position is determined by measuring the location of the unaffected commissure in relation to the incisor teeth. The horizontal dimension is obtained by measuring the distance of the uninjured commissure from the midline. Better results are obtained when healing occurs in an optimal position. Wright feels the commissural distance to the midline must be maintained on both injured and uninjured sides. Because the orbicularis oris is affected, this sphincterlike muscle bundle must be maintained at two points. The splint must be placed before wound healing occurs. The objective is to prevent or minimize contracture during healing. Patients under 3 years of age can be particularly difficult to treat with the removable appliance. If a young patient's second primary molars are unerupted, an extraoral headgear appliance may be an asset for improving retention.

BIBLIOGRAPHY

Bhaskar SN: Synopsis of Oral Pathology, 3rd ed. St. Louis, CV Mosby, 1969

Davis JM et al: An Atlas of Pedodontics, 2nd ed. Philadelphia, WB Saunders, 1981

Fromm A: Epstein's pearls, Bohn's nodules and inclusion cysts of the oral cavity. J Dent Child 34:275–287, 1967

Gron AMP: Prediction of tooth emergence. J Dent Res 41:573–585, 1962

Larson TH: Splinting oral electric burns in children. Report of two cases. J Dent Child 44:30–32, 1977

McDonald RE, Avery DR: Dentistry for the Child and Adolescent. St. Louis, CV Mosby, 1978

Posen AL: The effect of premature loss of deciduous molars on premolar eruption. Angle Orthod 35:249–252, 1965

Pulver F: The etiology and prevalence of ectopic eruption of the maxillary first permanent molar. J Dent Child 35:138–146, 1968

Rapp R, Winter GB: Color Atlas of Clinical Conditions in Pedodontics. Chicago, Year Book Medical Publishers, 1979

Spouge JD: Oral Pathology. St. Louis, CV Mosby, 1973

Stewart RE et al: Pediatric Dentistry Scientific Foundation and Clinical Practice. St. Louis, CV Mosby, 1982

Via WF, Jr: Submerged deciduous molars: Familial tendencies. J Am Dent Assoc 69:128–129, 1964

Wright GZ et al: Electric burns to the commissure of the lips. J Dent Child 44:25–29, 1977

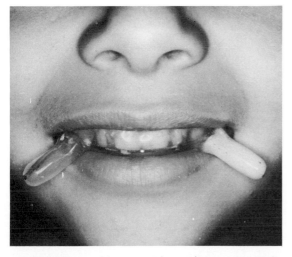

Fig. 14-19 An appliance with acrylic posts to assist healing and limit scar formation.

15

Geriatric Dentistry

SAMUEL J. WYCOFF

SIDNEY EPSTEIN

In the early decades of the twentieth century, public health efforts were mobilized toward combating the diseases of infancy and the communicable diseases of adulthood, such as tuberculosis, typhus, smallpox, and venereal diseases. As urban sanitation has improved and with the development of vaccines and antibiotics to prevent or treat many infectious diseases, public health problems have dramatically changed in character. Today, people live longer than at any other time in history, and the leading causes of death are chronic illness related to stress, the environment, or personal lifestyle—heart disease, cancer, and stroke.

At the turn of the century only 4% of the American population was age 65 years or older. In 1980 approximately 10% of the population was over age 65. By the year 2020, over 50 million Americans will be over age 65. The elderly are the fastest growing age group in the population.

The shift in age demographics is sometimes referred to as "the greying of America." The phenomenal reduction in the incidence of infectious disease in childhood and adulthood bears on the dental health of older Americans because they are living longer and will experience more dental problems because the dentition is longer at risk.

With the introduction of fluorides, improved nutrition, and extensive preventive education, the incidence of dental caries among children has decreased. Although there is no definitive data on the effects of fluorides on the incidence of caries in the elderly, some clinical evidence suggests that elders benefit from topical applications of fluorides. Although the prevalence of dental caries is decreasing, there is no evidence that a decrease in periodontal disease in younger or older people comparable to the preventable infectious diseases noted above has occurred. Oral cancer, too, which constitutes 3% of all cancers, is increasingly observed in older people. Of the more than 24,000 cases found each year, more than 90% occurs in persons over age 45, with a mean age at diagnosis of 60 years.

Older people are dentally underserved. This is the primary reason that it is incumbent to address their oral health needs. Chronic dental disease is more prevalent in older people than among persons in any other age group.

Current statistics show that by almost every measure, older persons are in greater need of dental services than are their younger counterparts in the general population. In one study conducted in 1978, almost two thirds of the subjects between ages 65 and 74 had periodontal disease. The same study found an incidence rate of periodontal disease of 41% in the general population. Older persons have an average of 22.5 decayed, missing, or filled teeth; this is nine more than the average score of younger persons. The presence and severity of periodontal disease and gingivitis also increases steadily with age. Approximately 50% of Americans have lost some of their teeth by age 65, and over two thirds are edentulous by the time they reach age 75. Persons 60 years of age and older are more than four times as likely as younger persons to have lost their natural teeth; 45.5% of elders are edentulous, compared with 10.7% of the general population.

The consequences of poor oral health for physical health in general are quite clear. Older people with chronic dental disease tend to select a diet that is low in protein and high in carbohydrates and fats. Such poor nutrition compounds the risk of cardiovascular disease and other health problems. The problems of poor oral health and insufficient dental care may be particularly acute among restricted elders. For instance, research by Morris and Bhaskar suggests that even though only 5% of the older population is institutionalized, oral pathosis is common in such settings. Indeed, institutionalization in long-term care facilities may significantly contribute to oral disease among elders owing to lack of routine care and preventive education.

ATTITUDES TOWARD ORAL HEALTH

Evidence of elders' lack of knowledge of oral health is found in statistics related to oral health. In 1969 it was estimated that approximately 76% of older people received no dental care. In 1971 45% of persons between the ages of 65 and 74 and 60% of those 75 and older were edentulous. In addition, with increasing age, there is a corresponding increase in periodontal disease, tooth loss, caries, and other oral diseases; yet, many of these problems are avoidable through proper dental care.

It has been noted by many dental researchers that oral disease and tooth loss are not necessarily concomitants of the aging process; instead, they are attributable to inadequate dental hygiene in childhood and adulthood. Fishman suggests that psychosocial care is the most important feature of dentistry for older people. He proposes that if elders' attitudes toward receiving care and their beliefs about disease prevention could be modified, the deterioration of oral health and many subsequent medical problems could be prevented.

The elderly are more likely than younger people to believe that the deterioration of health with age is unavoidable. Most older people agree with the view that one must expect more illness and aches and pains as one gets older. The elderly are generally less interested than are their younger counterparts in preventive care; they report that they take good care of their health and that they are satisfied with the amount of dental care they receive, even when the care is objectively minimal. These findings suggest that older Americans are generally resigned and passive with respect to their oral health needs.

Dental care must be viewed as a continuum in the context of a comprehensive program of general health care services. Elders' health is often characterized by multiple, chronic and progressive disabilities. It is important to emphasize that such disease is not necessarily a function of aging *per se*; instead, it may be an indication of inadequate health services and unmet dental and medical needs. The quality and quantity of health care is markedly influenced by socioeconomic factors that affect the availability of services as well as the individual's willingness to receive treatment.

Like people of all ages, the elderly can be classified according to their physical capacity or level of independence. A model based on four levels of dependence or autonomy is proposed. Each level requires a different kind of care, and services must be coordinated among all four levels. The largest group is composed of vigorous, vital, self-sufficient, and self-caring individuals who are wholly ambulatory; they want and deserve total dental care. The second group consists of individuals who are physically or emotionally debilitated; in great measure, they depend on others to provide for their care and to make all pertinent decisions for them. They may or may not be completely ambulatory. Both groups are readily treatable in private dental offices and clinics. The adequacy of care that is delivered depends on the patient's ability to receive or afford treatment.

The third group consists of individuals confined to nursing homes, acute care hospitals or similar residential institutions. While only about 4% of the general population is confined to extended care facilities at any one time, it is estimated that 20% of those individuals who reach age 65 may spend some time in a nursing home. The fourth group of elders is homebound. They have minimal outside contact and very limited access to treatment. Many homebound people have serious dental problems, and lack of care nearly always has severe human consequences. Unfortunately, homebound elders and nursing home residents frequently must experience intense pain, facial disfigurement, and even systemic spread of oral infection before care is rendered.

Prevention of dental disease and maintenance of existing natural dentition should be the primary focus of comprehensive oral health care. In order for these goals to be achieved, the myth that tooth loss is a necessary consequence of aging must be overcome. In point of fact, edentulousness is not inevitable nor should it be acceptable as part of the emotional and physical deterioration of the individual. To overcome this entrenched attitude toward edentulousness, educators must expose students to the broad base of knowledge about normal and pathologic aging processes. Students also must be made aware of the psychological changes that occur in middle age and old age, especially regarding self-concept and social view. In addition, students, educators, researchers, and practitioners need to understand how agism, social isolation, and poverty affect all aspects of elders' lives, including their relationships with the community, family members, friends, and dental professionals.

In reviewing the literature describing health older persons' oral physiology and the pathologic compromises of normal function imposed by disease, the authors have relied extensively on Baum's careful evaluation of many currently accepted "truths" about the aging oral cavity. He reviewed earlier studies that considered aging-related changes in oral mucosa, the prevalence of dental caries, oral motor function, salivary gland function and saliva production, and sensory–gustatory function. He pointed out that there are many existing information gaps within geriatric dentistry and indicated the directions for further research (see Table 15-1).

THE AGING ORAL CAVITY

Like many other areas of geriatrics, dentistry faces a host of generalizations about the effects of aging on the oral cavity. For instance, while many elders experience good oral health, it is commonly assumed that as part of the normal aging process, elders will experience tooth loss, atrophy of the oral mucosa, high prevalence of cervical caries, atrophy of the orofacial musculature, alterations in the amount and composition of saliva, wear of hard tissues, and decreases in the sensory functions of taste, smell, and touch. Some of these generalizations accurately describe the majority of elders, while others are patent myths or have not been adequately investigated.

Oral Mucosa

Shklar has suggested that significant differences in oral mucosa exist between individuals younger than 16 years and those older than 60 years. In a study conducted during the mid-1960s, he found that the older group had thinner epithelium, more keratinization, and increased levels of epithelial carbohydrate. No gender differences were evident.

Nedelman and Bernick reported histologic changes in the oral mucosa covering edentulous alveolar ridges based on eight necropsy specimens from individuals between ages 72 and 92. The changes reported are similar to Shklar's findings. In addition, these authors noted frequent arteriosclerotic changes in mucosal arteries; however, the biopsies studied were from mucosa overlying edentulous bone, which was probably not normal mucosal tissues.

Baum observes that atrophic changes occur in older persons' oral mucosa. The clinical appearance tends to be pale, and dry tissues

Table 15-1. Prevalent myths about dental health and aging

MYTH	FACT
The deterioration of oral health with old age is inevitable.	Preventive dental care and a sound diet can help elders maintain optimal oral health.
Oral mucosa in older persons is characterized by atrophic changes.	There is insufficient clinical research to document the effect of aging on oral mucosal tissues.
Dental caries are an insignificant problem in older persons.	Elders have a higher prevalence of caries than do most other adult age groups; it is mostly secondary caries.
The orofacial musculature atrophies with increased age.	Although decreased motor function has been observed among elders, it is not known at present whether these changes are the result of disease processes or normal physiology.
There is a significant decrease in stimulated saliva production in the elderly.	There is no empirical documentation of decreased saliva production in older people.
Gustatory function is diminished in older people.	In elders, threshold data changes only moderately for some tastants and not at all for others. There is not adequate data to evaluate changes in suprathreshold taste function in older people.

apparently are more "abradable" by physical stress. Some uncomfortable symptoms that have been associated with these alterations, especially among postmenopausal women, include mouth dryness and sensations of pain or burning on the tongue and buccal mucosa. Among restricted populations, most of whom are female, oral mucosal changes have also been observed. The frequency of these changes is unclear. Whether they are caused by disease or physiological menopause is not known. Baum concludes that there is a paucity of useful or reliable data describing the effects of aging on oral mucosa, in part, because comparisons are often made between different age groups without appropriate controls. Furthermore, there is insufficient reliable baseline data to define the existence of a clinical problem. It is difficult to determine whether aging *per se* has an effect on oral mucosal tissues. The conditions reported in the literature could be caused by disease, inadequate nutrition, or pharmacologic agents.

Dental Caries

Dental caries in older people is often not considered to be a serious oral health concern, even though dental researchers recognize that cervical caries is more prevalent among elders than younger people. Failure to consider dental caries a legitimate oral health problem of elders is misleading and detrimental to oral health-planning efforts. It also affects the quality of care that is delivered.

Available epidemiologic data suggest that older persons have a consequential level of caries per available tooth. Whether coronal or cervical, new or recurrent, caries represents a significant dental treatment effort. Both major dental disease entities, caries and periodontal disease, are usually bacterial in origin; yet, there are few studies that address the oral bacterial ecology of older people.

Available data describe the incidence of cervical caries to the virtual exclusion of coronal caries. Chauncey and others have pointed out that if the prevalence of coronal caries (both new surface and recurrent) is calculated based on the number of teeth present, older individuals actually have a higher prevalence of caries than most other adult age groups. Their data were based on a "healthy" sample of urban males. Unfortunately, the study did not include cervical caries, which probably means that the caries prevalence was underestimated.

Little is known about the etiology of cervical caries; one can hypothesize that differences exist between coronal and cervical carious processes. There has been only limited study of the microbial ecology of elders' oral cavities. Some differences between the bacteria isolated from cervical and coronal lesions have been noted, but apparently, similarities also exist; hence, no definite conclusions can be drawn about the etiology of either disease process.

Oral Motor Function

It is commonly believed that the orofacial musculature atrophies with increased age. Reduced muscle tone and diminished function of the muscles of mastication and deglutition are frequently associated with aging. In fact, there are no reliable data to support these claims.

The orofacial musculature participates in a number of daily functions important to both dentulous and edentulous individuals, including swallowing, chewing, and speech. Subtle impairments in the performance of any of these functions can have marked consequences for an individual's overall health. Feldman and colleagues reported a study on masticatory performance in healthy males of different ages. Among individuals with comparable dentition, masticatory effort was unaffected by age; however, there was a significant change in chewing efficiency as a significant increase in preparative time was observed in the older subjects. Tooth loss correlated with an increase in the food particle size that a subject was willing to swallow. Among edentulous and partially dentate individuals, this could conceivably lead to an increased incidence of choking.

Baum suggests that there is a higher prevalence of altered motor function among older people. For example, lip posture impairment, which is associated with drooling and chronic inflammation of the labial fornices, is found much more frequently in older individuals than among younger people. Impairment of swallowing, however, is found only somewhat more frequently among elders. Whether such changes are caused by disease processes or the normal physiology of aging cannot be ascertained at present.

Salivary Glands and Saliva

The primary function of the salivary glands is the exocrine production of saliva. Saliva is critical to maintaining good oral health. Any qualitative or quantitative impairment in saliva production can result in diminished oral health.

Many studies have reported age-related changes in the morphology of human salivary glands. There is general agreement that the following changes accompany aging: increased infiltration of gland parenchyma by fat and connective tissue, accumulation of autophagic (lipofuscin) granules, and presence of oncocytes and altered, benign cell type. There is relatively little reliable research and even less agreement on the functional correlates of these changes.

An early paper by Meyer and Necheles pointed out the difficulty in considering the many problems in interpreting available data on salivary gland function in elders. The authors examined 29 persons between the ages of 60 and 90. Most of the subjects were residents of a long-term care facility and were described as having "showed one or another of the infirmities of old age." They were compared with a control group of 32 persons between the ages of 12 and 60. The younger controls were characterized as "suitable clinic patients, interns, and graduate students." Whole saliva from both groups was examined following a masticatory stimulus. The older subjects were found to have a significant decrease in stimulated saliva production.

Baum indicates several flaws in the design of this study that make it impossible to interpret the findings accurately. First, the subjects studied were probably not suitable for an investigation of normal salivary gland function. Their health status was not well described, and one can only assume that like most institutionalized elders, they had numerous pathoses. Given such a sample, no description of normal physiology can result. Second, based on the descriptions provided,

subjects in the control group were in all likelihood relatively healthy. This makes data from the control group essentially meaningless. The only kind of control group that would be meaningful is one whose members were in every way similar to the older subjects, except for their chronologic age. Third, the method used for salivary gland stimulation is the muscular coordinating mechanism responsible for mastication and expectoration. Rather than demonstrating salivary function, this method may actually measure oral motor behavior. Because diminution of these oral motor functions may be more frequent among older individuals, this route of stimulation is invalid for making age group comparisons.

A fourth methodologic problem concerns the fact that Meyer and Necheles analyzed expectorated whole saliva. It is particularly difficult to measure this mixed secretion accurately because a centrifugation step is required to remove debris; in addition, sputum can contaminate samples. It is difficult to reach conclusions about individual gland functions from whole saliva.

Several additional concerns, which were unknown to the investigators at the time of the study, are recognized at present (e.g., regulating collection times and postprandial times, consideration of menstrual status, and so forth). For these reasons, the conclusion of this study that there is a significant decrease in stimulated saliva production in older individuals is questionable.

Bertram compared the unstimulated output of whole saliva from three groups of subjects. He found a decrease in average output in the older groups in general, and an even greater decrease in the diseased group than in the healthy group. The range of secretion for the healthy older sample was approximately ten times the range for individuals who had xerostomia. Although unstimulated whole saliva production may be diminished in older persons, the diminution does not ordinarily bring about symptoms. Bertram concluded that xerostomia is most often a symptom of systemic disease, rather than a function of aging per se.

Baum investigated stimulated parotid saliva flow rate in healthy, nonmedicated, community-dwelling subjects. He found that young and old men and women were equally competent at producing stimulated parotid fluid. Postmenopausal women were purportedly most affected by decreased salivary flow and symptoms of dry mouth. Nonmedicated postmenopausal women had levels of stimulated parotid saliva secretion comparable to their premenopausal counterparts. Medicated postmenopausal women, however, showed flow rates that were diminished by approximately 25%; this suggests that earlier observations of diminished salivary flow in elders may actually have resulted from pathoses or pharmacologic agents.

Sensory Functions

Many studies have suggested that gustatory function is diminished in older people. In 1935 Arey and others reported that the number of taste buds on circumvallate papillae decreased with increased age. Although this data has been used to support the thesis that taste acuity decreases with aging, it is unknown how many taste buds or circumvallate papilla actually are required for adequate gustatory function; thus, the clinical and functional significance of this finding is unclear.

In studying possible taste deficiencies in older persons, one should consider whether threshold measures are meaningful estimates of taste perception. Bartoshuk stated that thresholds are inadequate to define real taste function, suggesting instead that evaluation be by "suprathreshold" measures. Taste thresholds measure, in effect, a molecular event—the lowest concentration of a tastant necessary to support taste bud stimulation and allow discrimination of a tastant solution from water alone. This is very different than the level and quality of tastes we perceive in daily life. On the other hand, suprathreshold concentrations estimate tastes that are approximately 100 times greater than threshold concentrations.

Grzegorczyk and others have examined the threshold for tasting sodium chloride in individuals of varying ages. They observed quite modest increases in sodium chloride thresholds with age, much *lower* than previously reported thresholds. This discrepancy reflects methodologic problems in the earlier

studies that have subsequently been resolved.

Studies by Baum and others use methodologies that are similar to Grzegorczyk's. They have also observed a modest increase in sodium chloride taste threshold with age. In addition, they observed a slight increase among elders in quinine sulfate (bitter) taste thresholds, but no differences between younger and older people in sour (citric acid) or sweet (sucrose) taste thresholds. These studies indicate no general diminution in suprathreshold taste function with age; however, among older women, a significant alteration in the perceived intensity of suprathreshold concentrations of sodium chloride and sucrose was found.

Schiffman examined elders' ability to recognize certain foods. In a study comparing 29 older subjects and 27 young college students, she reported a significant decrease in the older subjects' ability to correctly identify a series of blended foods. Although many of the older subjects were residents of a retirement home, they were described as being healthy.

There is inadequate support for the generalization that gustatory function decreases with age. Taste function must be evaluated on at least two levels: threshold and suprathreshold. Current research on older persons suggests that threshold data change only modestly for some tastants and not at all for others.

Review of the literature suggests that, in fact, very little is known about the physiology of the oral tissues across the adult age spectrum. This makes it difficult to appreciate the problems imposed by oral pathoses in elders. Nevertheless, it is important to remember that dental disease is not an inevitable consequence of aging. As pointed out, generalizations and myths about dental health and illness in elders, based on erroneous stereotypes or unreliable research, often have resulted in a confusing picture.

It is easy to criticize studies conducted 20 or 40 years ago because in recent years, methodologic and conceptual advances have rapidly moved the field ahead. Such progress, however, carries the responsibility of learning from and building on earlier research. This responsibility has not been met fully in the field of geriatric dentistry. Rigorous investigation is needed of individuals whose health status is well documented. Research methods must be developed to anticipate new problem areas. Valid and reliable tools for data analysis should be used or if need be, devised. Reliable epidemiologic data are especially needed to describe the status of the oral cavity in older persons and to provide a sound basis for health care planning. Many research problems must be solved.

Even if response differences between groups of adults are identified and elders are found to have certain decreased functions, we cannot reduce such differences to the status of negative changes or pathoses. Physiologic systems are adaptive; what is normal for a 25-year-old is probably not normal for a 75-year-old. Further, when a response difference is defined, one must ask whether it is an actual oral health concern for older persons. If it is, how can it be managed? Can it be prevented?

In the next section of this chapter, preventive oral health care is discussed. The role of dentistry in preventing and screening systemic disease with oral manifestations, dentures, and some dental office hazards to which elders are especially vulnerable will also be reviewed. Epidemiologic and clinical evidence demonstrates conclusively that dental disease varies in type, in onset, and in severity with patient age. Indeed age is the most patent predictor (outweighing even socioeconomic status) of the two major dental diseases—dental caries and periodontal disease.

These major dental diseases and others are to a large extent preventable using present basic techniques—fluoride therapy; mechanical prophylaxis such as brushing, flossing, and professional prophylaxis; dietary modification; pit and fissure sealants; orthodontic adjustment; and patient education and motivation. If these measures are to be effective, they must be directed toward specific populations at specific times. No preventive strategy can succeed if it is directed to the population as a whole without taking into account particular groups' special needs.

The field of preventive dentistry largely reflects the youth orientation of our society. For the most part, efforts are concentrated on preventing caries in children and periodontal disease in adults through the clinical application of research on fluorides and the role of plaque in oral disease. Although children and adolescents can probably benefit most by primary prevention and early detection measures, middle-aged and elderly persons stand to benefit greatly from timely preventive interventions. In a broad sense, preventive dentistry includes any measure to save all or any part of a patient's natural dentition; therefore, elders can benefit greatly by dentists recognizing the needs of people of all ages.

PREVENTIVE DENTISTRY

Caries Prevention

Caries is often characterized as a disease of young people that stabilizes during the mid-20s and remains dormant until gingival recession or periodontal surgery exposes the cemental surfaces. Predictably, root caries then appears. Although there is a paucity of current data on the attack rate of caries in the older population, some recent information suggests that the prevalence of caries *changes* with age; the problem does not disappear.

Axelsson and Lindhe studied the effect of 6 years of controlled oral hygiene on caries and periodontal disease in adults. The control subjects over age 50 in their sample exhibited a substantial level of decay; their mean number of decayed and filled surfaces was 11.9, of which 4.2 were new lesions and 7.7 were recurrent caries. Most of the new lesions were bucco lingual, and most of the recurrent lesions were proximal. Chauncey and associates reported similar findings in their longitudinal study of older patients at the Veterans Administration outpatient clinic in Boston. They found that "contrary to popular belief there is a significant increase in caries incidence associated with aging: mostly secondary caries."

In a review of the literature on root caries, Banting and Ellen described three separate studies in which about 60% of the subjects between 50 and 59 years of age exhibited root surface caries. In the group over age 60, the incidence rate rose to 70%. A similar pattern was reported by Baum for subjects in the Baltimore longitudinal aging study.

Most root caries lesions are found in molars. About 70% of the cavities are proximal, 20% are facial, and 10% are lingual. Restoration is often extremely difficult, and prevention of both root caries and recurrent proximal caries is an important consideration in caring for older persons.

Fluorides

Presently, no definitive clinical data document the effects on caries prevention in elders of routinely applied fluorides; however, it is likely that older persons would profit from using fluoride dentifrices, mouth rinses, and gels. Appropriate fluoride forms should be prescribed according to an individual's anticipated susceptibility to decay and their ability to manage the regimen. For instance, in disabled patients a controlled release device might be considered. Patients with xerostomia caused by irradiation or salivary gland disease, as well as a large number of elders who use medications that cause reduced salivary flow, run a high risk of caries; both groups of individuals would benefit from artificial saliva preparations containing fluoride or fluoride gels.

Stamm and Banting reported that in Canada, the occurrence of root caries in adults who have lived all their lives in areas with fluoridated water was 50% less than in nonfluoridated areas. This is not surprising in view of the high concentrations of fluoride found in gingival crevice fluid and the high uptake of fluoride by cementum and dentin. Experiments *in vitro* show an 80% reduction in acid solubility when acidulated fluorophosphate or stannous fluoride gels are applied to the teeth. The daily use of fluorides can prevent caries even in severely compromised adults who have minimal salivary flow caused by various problems such as irradiation for head and neck cancer.

The latest studies predict that as a result of routine preventive programs, older persons in the next decade are likely to retain more of their natural teeth than the current generation of elders, so the emphasis on dental care for older people will probably change direction. Dentists will need to reassess concepts and attitudes that full dentures are the ultimate resolution of elders' oral health problems and develop and emphasize to a more comprehensive, preventive, therapeutic, and restorative approach.

Abrasion and Erosion

An older population with longer tooth retention and greater cementum and dentin exposure is at increased risk for tooth destruction by abrasion and erosion. In individuals with reduced salivary flow, a diminution in the mucin level in the oral cavity will result in less lubrication and a less protective pellicle. These conditions create an even greater risk of erosion and abrasion.

Abrasion. The most common form of abrasion is caused by overzealous and improper toothbrushing with a hard-bristle brush; therefore, preventing abrasion is largely a matter of instructing the patient in an appropriate method of brushing, selecting a soft-bristle toothbrush, and using a minimally abrasive dentifrice. Toothbrushing habits that produce minimal damage to enamel can be harmful once cementum is exposed. Reviewing toothbrushing and oral hygiene habits should be an ongoing component of dental practice.

Erosion. The most common causes of erosion are overuse of fruit and fruit juices and sucking candies that contain phosphoric or citric acid. Lemons are particularly damaging, although any fruit or juice with a low *p*H can eventually erode tooth enamel if it is consumed excessively or retained in the mouth for prolonged periods. The cause of tooth erosion can usually be identified by taking a careful history. Patients with reduced salivary flow are especially prone to erosion because a common self-treatment for dry mouth is sucking hard candies (*e.g.*, lemon drops), which provides a gustatory stimulus. Substitution of sugar-free candies or sugar-free chewing gum is helpful.

Hypersensitivity

Dentinal hypersensitivity is a common result of abrasion, erosion, or a combination of the two. Dentifrices containing potassium nitrate and strontium chloride may offer relief; however, there is limited definitive clinical data supporting the use of these dentifrice compounds. Fluoride gels and fluoride rinses are probably even more effective. The use of multiple fluorides to prevent root caries should have the additional benefit of reducing dentinal hypersensitivity.

Restorative dental procedures are particularly important for older patients. Secondary caries is a commonplace occurrence. Because of dehydration of teeth and large restorations, there is a high incidence of fractured cusps of posterior teeth. In addition to the concern with recurrent caries and restoring fractured teeth, the dentist must avoid overhanging restorations that accumulate plaque and exacerbate periodontal disease resulting in increased bone loss in the area adjacent to the overhanging restoration.

PERIODONTAL DISEASE

A number of studies have shown that periodontal disease occurs at an accelerated rate in elders. For instance, one study showed that gingivitis developed more rapidly in old than in young individuals during an experimental period of oral hygiene abstinence. Plaque accumulation also was greater for the older subjects than the younger controls during this period. A second study supported the observation of greater plaque accumulation and also suggested that the microbial composition of plaque is qualitatively different in older persons. In addition, a 6-year study in Malmo, Sweden showed that the rate of bone loss for subjects over age 60 was much greater than for younger age groups. In the Axelsson and Lindhe study, the control subjects over age 50 exhibited a greater rate of attachment loss than did the younger subjects. On the basis of these data, plaque control and periodontal health maintenance programs for elders should be even more vigorous than comparable programs targeted toward younger patient populations.

Grön conducted a preventive dental health program for elders that successfully halted this increased tendency toward plaque accumulation. The program, which had 75 subjects, combined frequent plaque removal (every 2 to 4 weeks), scaling as needed, and home-care education. At the end of 1 year he found a significant reduction in gingivitis and only rare bleeding from periodontal pockets on probing. The reduction in gingival index was accompanied by reduced pocket depth. When attached levels were examined at the end of the study, there was no change in buccal or lingual measurements and an actual attachment gain interproximally. This latter finding probably reflects a reduction in inflammation. At the baseline examination, the probe may have passed beyond the epithelial attachment. This is a common occurrence in the presence of inflammation that explains the interproximal gain.

This study provides impressive clinical data about the efficacy of preventive care for older persons. In dental clinics with limited resources, patients at high risk could be screened and targeted for intensive preventive care. A number of indicators of "high risk" are currently being examined in various laboratories and clinical centers; however, there is still no agreement about reliable determinants. This is an active research area that should become part of preventive dentistry in the future.

Techniques for personal plaque control often have to be modified for elders with disabilities because conditions such as stroke, arthritis, and palsies decrease the ability to brush and floss effectively. In selected cases an electric toothbrush and oral irrigator can be useful. For individuals with partial disabilities, the toothbrush often can be modified to facilitate brushing. Nursing staff can modify or enlarge a toothbrush in the following ways:

1. Fitting a large styrofoam ball, bicycle handle grip, or soft rubber ball over the end of the toothbrush handle
2. Gluing a piece of plastic tubing to the handle
3. Wrapping an Ace bandage or aluminum foil around the handle to achieve a suitable thickness
4. Bending the toothbrush handle to achieve a more effective angle
5. Taping an elastic band to the handle or using a "universal cuff" that permits the patient to slip his or her hand under the elastic to hold the brush more securely
6. Extending the length of the handle for individuals with limited arm movements; for flossing, a floss holder often is helpful in using dental floss

Patient education is an important component of plaque control programs in particular and of preventive dentistry in general. This is especially true for the elderly because service utilization studies show that "almost more than half of the older population has not sought dental care in five years or more as opposed to 11% of those under 35 years of age." Dental health education materials should be directed to the specific needs of older people. Wesson has pointed out that in addition to informational content, the print size, color, and paper stock must be carefully selected to ensure visual accessibility. For instance, pamphlets should be printed in large black type on orange, yellow, or gold no-glare paper.

ORAL CANCER

With increased age, there is a gradual reduction in tissue growth and repair processes of the oral epithelium, causing increased susceptibility to irritation that can result in hyperplasias, ulcerations, and keratoses. The most serious problem is the increased risk of oral cancer.

In the United States, oral cancer accounts for 5% of all cancer in males, 2% of all cancer in females, and 2.5% of all cancer deaths. In 1975, more than 23,000 new cases were discovered, and some 8,200 deaths were reported. Nearly 90% of all oral cancers occur in persons over age 45; the mean age at diagnosis is 60. Oral cancer is a more serious threat to the elderly than to any other age group.

The increased incidence of oral cancer with age and the tendency for many elders, especially the edentulous, to visit the dentist at infrequent intervals places an extra responsibility beyond routine examination on the prevention-oriented dentist. Because early detection results in 5-year survival rates well above 50%, a thorough oral examination is essential for all older patients. A preventive program for oral cancer should include patient education and definitive management of suspicious areas. As part of routine practice, the floor of the mouth may be examined by retracting the tongue. Observe for masses,

ulcers, inflammation, lesions, and developmental aberrations.

Oral cancer is increasing in both males and females. The tongue is the most frequent site of oral cancers, of which over 90% are squamous cell carcinomas. Although oral cancer may appear as an ulcer, white or red patch, or exophytic growth, the erythroplastic type is the most invasive. Red or white lesions that change size, bleed, ulcerate, and demonstrate induration on palpation should be biopsied for examination. Most oral cancers are painless until they become large, at which time regional metastases are likely to appear.

Patients with dentures frequently develop denture ulcers that are circumscribed or linear inflammatory lesions of variable size that are contiguous with the border of the denture. These are decubitus ulcers, which result from trauma or pressure atrophy. If they do not disappear within a short time after the denture has been adjusted or modified, biopsy examination is indicated.

Patient education programs should emphasize the following points:

1. The relationship between cancer, cigarette smoking, tobacco chewing, and excessive alcohol consumption. These are well-established, strong risk factors in cancer of the mouth and pharynx. Alcohol and tobacco are estimated to account for approximately three fourths of all cancers of the oral cavity in males in the United States.
2. The importance of a balanced diet and adequate intake of all vitamins and minerals.
3. The need for regular dental care to reduce irritation and mechanical injury and to check oral tissues and alveolar bone for primary and metastatic lesions.
4. The importance of watching for the five warning signs in the mouth that may indicate oral cancer: swelling, lumps, or growths; erythematous or white, scaly patches; a sore that does not heal; persistent numbness or pain; and persistent bleeding.
5. Patients who are exposed to direct sunlight for long periods should use a protective screening or lotion on the face and lips. Excessive exposure to the sun is an established factor in lip cancer. Blacks and other dark-skinned people and Asians are

at less risk than whites of this form of cancer. When suspicious lesions are discovered, visual examination should be followed by a biopsy. If the examining dentist is not comfortable performing the biopsy, the patient should be referred to an oral surgeon, oncologist, or institution that can perform the surgery and the appropriate therapy if a positive diagnosis is made. The examining dentist should maintain contact with the patient after a referral is made.

The dentist should teach patients over age 60 to perform oral self-examination. A simplified technique for self-examination of the oral cavity and head and neck has been developed. Neglect, poor oral hygiene, and lack of dental care increase the risk of oral cancer. Routine dental examinations and a careful home regimen are the most important preventive measures for people of all ages.

ORAL MANIFESTATIONS OF SYSTEMIC DISEASE

It has been said that the mouth is a mirror that reflects the entire body's health. The mouth's unique sensitivity and remarkable vascularity make it a diagnostic touchstone for the body. The World Health Organization's International Classification of Diseases Application to Dentistry and Stomatology lists more than 120 specific systemic diseases, distributed in ten or more classifications, that manifest in the oral cavity. The diagnosis and treatment of stomatologic processes and oral pathology in older persons is discussed elsewhere in this book; therefore, we attempt neither to enumerate nor describe in detail local or systemic oral pathologic entities.

It has become the dentist's moral and legal responsibility to diagnose and treat oral manifestations of systemic disturbances or to refer patients presenting with symptoms for appropriate medical treatment. In order to discuss medical problems that might influence dental treatment, it is essential to take a thorough medical history. Pulse and blood pressure readings, lymph node palpation, and a thorough examination of the soft tissues of the oral cavity have become standard procedures in dental practices. Regular dental visits, therefore, can be viewed as a valuable adjunct to public health screening programs for heart and vascular disease, diabetes, venereal disease, cancer, osteoporosis, arthritis, and nutritional deficiencies.

Generally, except for advice on good nutrition and hygiene, there is little that dentists can do to prevent many of these diseases. Early diagnosis offers the maximum therapeutic benefit; therefore, all dental examinations must include specific attention to the lips, tongue, and all oral mucous membranes, as well as the teeth and gingivae. Attention should be given to all abnormalities, not only to symptoms associated with oral cancer or precancerous lesions.

There are as many medical as dental implications in treating the geriatric patient. It is important to distinguish between disease and changes resulting from the aging process. Many fundamental decrements are not the result of disease. Decrease in functional capacities are related to aging. Many dental problems may be affected by the use of medications. The elderly have many reactions to medications owing to multiple pathologic problems that are made more complex by polypharmacology and increased drug sensitivity.

The dentist must often share knowledge of drugs that the patient may be taking. A careful current drug history is important as well as an awareness of the sources of drugs or medications that are being used, namely, multiple prescriptions, overcounter preparations, and shared drugs of family and friends. Pharmacokinetics in elderly are affected by absorption, disturbances in tissues, metabolism, renal clearance, and environmental factors (e.g., smoking, caffeine, alcohol, altered diet).

About 75% of elderly are receiving some form of medications; about 10% have iatrogenic problems related to drugs. Two principal dental problems that are drug related are xerostomia—dry mouth caused by the suppressive effects on salivary gland secretions by approximately 400 different preparations.

Special attention should be given to diseases of the salivary glands in older people.

Autoimmune diseases, for instance, Sjögren's syndrome, increase in incidence with age. Postmenopausal women are especially vulnerable. Techniques such as sialochemistry, salivary flow rate, sialography, and labial gland biopsy can help to establish the diagnosis of Sjögren's. Patients using medications that cause diminished salivary flow rate are at a higher risk of developing chronic recurrent sialadenitis, especially parotiditis. Here too, sialochemistry is a valuable diagnostic tool and an excellent means of following recovery.

OFFICE HAZARDS

Concerns about dental office hazards usually focus on the vulnerability of the dentist and the dental staff; however, older patients may face special risks. Dentists are particularly vulnerable to exposure to hepatitis and must be checked periodically to determine whether they are carriers (between 1% and 3% of dentists are estimated to be carriers). If a dentist is found to be a carrier, a careful set of precautions must be developed, including gloves, masks, disposable needles, and properly sterilized instruments.

Some older patients may use immunosuppressive drugs, which increase their susceptibility to hepatitis. Patients with heart valve pathoses or cardiovascular prostheses are also at risk of complications caused by transient bacteremias from periodontal, endodontic, or surgical treatments (this is also a risk for patients with an orthopedic replacement); therefore, appropriate prophylactic antibiotics are indicated before and after dental treatment.

Other hazards that should be considered are interference with cardiac pacemakers by electronic equipment. Ultrasonic handpieces that apply an electric current directly to the patient can interfere with a pacemaker. Placing patients in a recumbent position in a contour chair may cause ischemia or restrict the ability to breathe. Using anesthetic and prescribing medications require taking a careful pharmacologic history and extreme caution. Slippery floors, loose rugs, flimsy chairs, and poor lighting may also be office hazards.

DENTURES AND HEALTH

Current statistics indicate that about 85% of all edentulous persons in the United States are 45 years of age and older. Almost a third of all persons over age 45 are without any teeth. The number of edentulous persons increases rapidly with age, which may be a striking predictor of tooth loss. On the other hand, gender and geographic area of residence are relatively insignificant predictors.

There are significant socioeconomics and racial differences between edentulous persons and those retaining their natural teeth. The percentage of edentulous white persons over age 45 is 8.6% greater than the percentage of edentulous colored peoples. Education and income also are accurate predictors of tooth loss. Persons with fewer than 9 years of education and an annual income of $5,000 or less are three times more likely to lose all of their teeth than are persons with 12 or more years of education and an annual family income of $10,000 or more. These findings are not surprising because often, the least expensive and most expedient dental care is extraction of a damaged tooth.

Dentures not only increase local tissue irritation, but they are also associated with a number of oral health and systemic health problems. One common oral problem is denture stomatitis (chronic atrophic candidiasis). This condition manifests when the yeast *Candida albicans* oversteps its normal ecologic bounds and grows out of control. In a survey of patients who visited dental schools for prosthetic treatment, denture stomatitis was found in between 40% and 60% of the patients who wore complete dentures. One British study showed that 50% of denture wearers had some form of denture-induced pathosis that required either conservative or surgical treatment.

Poor nutrition is common among older patients wearing dentures. Research shows that the impaired ability to masticate food leads to nutritional deficiencies. Inadequate protein, or vitamin and mineral intake can accelerate resorption of underlying bone and compromise the ability of oral soft tissue to heal. The result is a vicious cycle of denture irritation, painful mastication, poor nutrition, increased tissue irritation, and sometimes more serious oral and systemic health problems. For the denture patient, regular dental visits, correctly designed and modified prosthodontic appliances, and appropriate dietary counseling are essential for prevention and early detection of oral pathosis.

The potential effectiveness for preventive dentistry is becoming greater than ever before. The technology now exists to virtually eliminate the two major dental diseases in the United States, dental caries and periodontal disease. Yet both problems remain rampant. Dental caries affects more than 95% of the population; roughly 80% of all middle-aged adults have destructive periodontitis; and nearly 50% of all Americans age 65 and over have lost all of their teeth. Indeed, dental disease is the most widespread degenerative disease in the United States. The question is why? If the two major forms of dental disease are preventable, why are they not being prevented? Pain, altered appearance, loss of function, poor dietary habits, and more serious systemic problems caused by dental disease affect both the health and the quality of life of many Americans. The problem is can more effective dental educational and preventive programs be developed?

The solutions to these questions are complex. They are bound in the attitudes and actions of individuals, the dental profession, and the government. Individuals of all ages are often uninformed about dental disease and the need for effective oral hygiene. One study of American adults revealed that only 24% had ever heard of or read about dental plaque, and only 20% had ever been instructed in a dental office to assure that they were cleansing their teeth correctly. Another study showed that only 40% of the respondents had ever attempted flossing. Even so, knowledge of good dental practice, does not always lead to a healthy regimen.

Poor responses to dental health education are generally attributed to beliefs about the likelihood and seriousness of dental disease. Recent surveys show that tooth decay is viewed by the general public as inevitable but not serious. Periodontal disease, on the other hand, is perceived as fairly serious but not very likely. Although most of the survey respondents believed that dental disease could be prevented, there seemed to be little connection in their thinking and attitudes between prevention and regular dental examinations. Only 50% of the total survey sample believed that regular dental visits and early detection were of preventive value.

The responsibility for changing attitudes toward dental hygiene and disease belongs not only to individuals, but to the dental profession because the dental profession is the chief channel of information about state-of-the-art preventive measures. Historically, American dentistry has been instrumental in both developing and promoting preventive technology. Water fluoridation and emphasis on nutritional modifications are examples of strong professional support for preventive measures at the public health level; however, adequate data are lacking about the nature, extent, and effectiveness of preventive practices in private dental offices.

Unfortunately, at the governmental level, dental health is perennially a low-priority issue. Dental health is pushed off center stage by more "serious," more "pressing," and more "emotional" or politically "popular" health issues. It has received only passing attention in several areas, including providing and financing dental services, protecting consumers in areas such as food content and food labeling (particularly with regard to sugar) and allocating resources for dental research. In high-level government discussions about services to be covered under national health insurance, dentistry assumes a low profile in comparison with medical services. Although dental services coverage is included in most current legislative proposals for national health insurance, inadequate description and analysis of the nature and costs of coverage are a stumbling block to informed policy decisions.

There are no simple solutions at the levels of public policy, the profession, or the individual. No single approach by itself can address the complex problems that prevent people of all ages from attaining maximum dental health; however, several programmatic and research directions can be recommended as a point of departure. There is need for comprehensive public dental health outreach programs that are easily accessible to older people at *all* levels of functioning, especially those who are the most underserved. Serious thought should be given to how geriatric treatment centers, senior centers, nutrition projects, and other community programs could incorporate a continuum of dental services including screening and preventive education. There is also need for data about the focus and extent of preventive practices in private dental offices and clinics, as well as the teaching of preventive modalities in dental schools. Multidisciplinary efforts of dental and medical health providers would be useful in reaching the most vulnerable elders to develop comprehensive preventive health services and to press for public policy reform that responds to vital real human needs—particularly the elderly.

BIBLIOGRAPHY

Abelson DC: Denture plaque and denture cleansers. J Prosthet Dent 45:376–379, 1981

Andrew W: Comparison of age changes in salivary glands of man and rat. J Gerontol 7:178–190, 1952

Arey LB, Tremaine MJ, Monzingo FL: The numerical and topographical relations of taste buds to circumvallate papillae throughout the life span. Anat Rec 64:9–25, 1935

Axelsson P, Lindhe J: Effect of controlled oral hygiene procedures on caries and periodontal disease in adults: Results after six years. J Clin Periodontol 8:239–249, 1981

Azen EA: Salivary peroxidase activity and thiocyanate concentration in human subjects with genetic variants of salivary peroxidase. Arch Oral Biol 23:801–805, 1978

Banting DW, Courtright PN: Distribution and natural history of carious lesions on the roots of teeth. J Can Dent Assoc 41:45–49, 1975

Banting DW, Ellen R: Carious lesions on the roots of the teeth: A review. J Can Dent Assoc 42:496–502, 1971

Bartoshuk LM: The psychophysics of taste. Am J Clin Nutr 31:1068–1077, 1978

Baum BJ: In Bryant P, Gale E, Rugh J (eds): Oral Motor Behavior: Impact on Oral Conditions and Dental Treatment, pp 244–252. Bethesda, MD, NIH Publication, No. 79-1845, 1979

Baum BJ: Evaluation of stimulated parotid saliva flow rate in different age groups. J Dent Res 60:1292–1296, 1981

Becks H: Human saliva, XIV. Total calcium content of resting saliva in 650 individuals. J Dent Res 22:397–402, 1943

Berman CL et al: High blood pressure detection: A new public health measure for the profession. J Am Dent Assoc 92:116–119, 1976

Bertram U: Xerostomia. Acta Odontol Scand (Suppl 49) 25:1–126, 1967

Bjorn AL: Dental health in relation to age and dental care. Odontol Rev (Suppl 29) 25, 1974

Chauncey HH et al: The incidence of coronal caries in normal aging male adults. J Dent Res (Special Issue A) 57:148, 1978

Chauncey HS et al: Parotid fluid composition in a study of healthy aging males. J Dent Res (Special Issue) 54:57, 1975

Dreizen S et al: Prevention of xerostomia-related dental caries in irradiated cancer patients. J Dent Res 56:99–104, 1977

Fann WE, Shannon IL: A treatment for dry mouth in psychiatric patients. Am J Psychiatry 135:251–252, 1978

Feldman RS et al: Aging and mastication: Changes in performance and in the swallowing threshold with natural dentition. J Am Geriatr Soc 28:97–103, 1980

Glass RT: Teaching self-examination of the head and neck: Another aspect of preventive dentistry. J Am Dent Assoc 90:1265–1268, 1975

Goldberg J et al: Cross-sectional clinical evaluation of recurrent enamel caries, restoration of marginal integrity and oral hygiene status. J Am Dent Assoc 102:635–641, 1981

Grad B: Diurnal, age, and sex changes in sodium and potassium concentration of human saliva. J Gerontol 9:276–286, 1954

Grön P: Preventive dental health program for the elderly. Spec Care Dent 1:129–132, 1981

Grzegorczyk PB, Jones SW, Mistretta CM: Age-related differences in salt taste activity. J Gerontol 34:834–840, 1979

Hakkarainen K, Ainamo J: Influence of overhanging posterior tooth restorations on alveolar bone adults. J Clin Periodontol 7:114–120, 1980

Hancock EB: Determination of periodontal disease activity. J Periodontol 52:492–499, 1981

Helfman PM, Price PA: Human parotid alpha-amylase—A test of the error theory of aging. Exp Gerontol 9:209–214, 1974

Holm–Pedersen P et al: Experimental gingivitis in young and elderly gingivitis. J Clin Periodontol 2:14–24, 1975

Holm–Pedersen P et al: Composition and metabolic activity of dental plaque from healthy young and elderly individuals. J Dent Res 59:771–776, 1980

Jordan HV, Hammond BF: Filmentous bacteria isolated from human root surface caries. Arch Oral Biol 17:1333–1342, 1972

Kiyak HA, Miller RR: Age differences in oral health attitudes and dental service utilization. J Public Health Dent 42:29–40, 1982

Levin ML et al: Hepatitis B transmission by dentists. JAMA 228:1139–1140, 1974

Mandel ID: What is preventive dentistry? J Prevent Dent 1:25–29, 1974

Mandel ID: Sialochemistry in diseases and clinical situations affecting salivary glands. CRC Crit Rev Clin Lab Sci 12:321–366, 1980

Mandel ID, Wotman S: The salivary secretions in health and disease. Oral Sci Rev 8:25–47, 1976

Meyer J, Necheles H: Studies in old age: Clinical significance of salivary, gastric, and pancreative secretion in old age. JAMA 115:2050–2053, 1940

Meyer J, Spier E, Neuwelt F: Basal secretion of digestive enzymes in old age. Arch Intern Med 65:171–177, 1940

Murphy C: In Han S, Coons D (eds): The effect of age on taste sensitivity. In Special Senses in Aging: A Current Biological Assessment. Ann Arbor, University of Michigan Press, 1980

Nedelman CI, Bernick S: The significance of age changes in human alveolar mucosa and bone. J Prosthet Dent 39:495–501, 1978

Rauald N, Hamp SE: Prediction of root surface caries in patients treated for advanced periodontal disease. J Clin Periodontol 8:400–414, 1981

Rezais FR: Dental treatment of patients with a cardiac pacemaker. Oral Surg 44:662–665, 1977

Rissen L et al: Effect of age and removable partial dentures on gingivitis and periodontal disease. J Prosthet Dent 42:217–223, 1979

Rothstein S et al: Hepatitis B virus: An overview for dentists. J Am Dent Assoc 102:173–176, 1981

Rowe JW et al: The effect of age on creatinine clearance in man: A cross-sectional and longitudinal study. J Gerontol 31:155–163, 1976

Rubin R et al: Infected total hip replacement after dental procedures. Oral Surg 41:18–23, 1976

Schiffman S: Food recognition by the elderly. J Gerontol 32:586–592, 1977

Scott J: Quantitative age changes in the histological structure of human submandibular salivary glands. Arch Oral Biol 22:221–227, 1977

Shannon IL: Fluoride treatment programs for high-caries-risk patients. Clin Prevent Dent 4:11–20, 1982

Shannon IL, Edmonds EJ: Reactions of tooth surfaces to three fluoride gels. NY State Dent J 46:426–429, 1980

Shklar G: The effects of aging upon oral mucosa. J Invest Dermatol 47:115–120, 1966

Socransky SS, Manganiello SE: The oral microbiota of man from birth to senility. J Periodontol 42:485–496, 1971

Special Report on Aging, 1979. NIH Publication No. 80-1907, February, 1980

Stamm JW, Banting DW: The occurrence of root caries in adults with a lifelong history of fluoridated water consumption. J Dent Res (Special Issue A) 57:149, 1978

Sumney DL, Jordan HV, Englander HR: The prevalence of root surface caries in selected populations. J Periodontol 44:500–504, 1973

Syed SA et al: Predominant cultivable flora isolated from human root surface caries plaque. Infect Immunol 11:727–731, 1975

Vratsanos S, Mandel ID: The effect of sucrose and hexitol-containing chewing gum on plaque acidogenesis in vivo. Pharmacol Ther Dent 6:87–92, 1981

Wainwright WW: Human saliva, XIV: Total calcium content of resting saliva in 650 healthy individuals. J Dent Res 22:403–414, 1943

Wesson SS: A preventive dentistry program for the elderly. Spec Care Dent 1:133–135, 1981

Westcott WB et al: Chemical protection against postirradiation caries. Oral Surg 40:709–719, 1975

16

Chronic Oral Sensory Disorders— Pain and Dysgeusia

VERNON J. BRIGHTMAN

CHRONIC ORAL SENSORY DISORDERS

This chapter is mainly concerned with the patient who requests diagnosis and treatment for a complaint of pain, bad taste, diminished ability to taste, dryness of the oral cavity, burning sensation in the tongue, or other oral sensory abnormality that has been present for some time and is now sufficiently intense or of sufficiently long duration to cause the patient to seek medical or dental assistance for the problem. In general, such symptoms (pain in particular) are of lower intensity than those experienced, for example, during dental treatment or as the result of trauma or acute infectious processes involving the pulp and periodontal membrane. Although pain relief for such acute problems is not the concern of this chapter, much of the following discussion on the pathophysiology and psychology of chronic oral sensory disorders is also applicable to the understanding of acute pain.

The majority of oral lesions first attract a patient's attention because of some alteration in stimuli transmitted by the sensory nerves of the orofacial region. Only a small number of lesions develop insidiously and with such negligible symptoms that they first become evident as a visually noticeable change in the appearance of the patient's mouth or face. The high concentration of peripheral nerve endings in the mouth and the long phylogenetic development of this region of the body as an organ of perception ensure that some sensory signals will be received by the individual whenever the mouth is involved by a pathologic process. Indeed we clearly benefit by this "early warning system" in the mouth, but the sensitivity that it confers on the mouth also creates clinical problems, particularly in regard to diagnosis and management of chronic oral sensory disorders.

Individuals appear to differ in what they perceive to be significant variations in oral sensation. Some patients undoubtedly tolerate abnormal oral sensations longer and with greater equanimity than others before they seek medical or dental care for the problem. Dental caries, periodontal disease, and oral carcinoma (several characteristically "insidious" oral diseases) may be well developed before the patient seeks treatment, but such delay is perhaps more often due to the patient's neglecting or denying oral sensory signals, rather than to failure of the pathologic process to induce them. Differences in perception of the intensity and nature of abnormal oral sensations are most easily appreciated when such patients who have delayed seeking treatment for oral disease are compared with those at the other end of the scale, who seek repeated consultations for signs or symptoms that they fear to be cancer but that in reality have already been accurately identified by several dentists as either normal oral structures or minor inflammatory lesions with no neoplastic potential. The capacity for the tongue to magnify the size of an oral lesion, the disproportionate representation of the mouth in the cerebral cortex, and the influence of anxiety and previous sensory experience on pain and other sensory stimuli transmitted to the central nervous system are all factors affecting the patient's perception of abnormality within his oral cavity. Thus, both sensory stimuli caused by a lesion and the patient's perception (or interpretation of the significance) of those stimuli must be considered by the clinician who is called upon to evaluate a patient's sensory complaint.

Oral sensations include the perception of touch, temperature, moisture (and possibly texture) at the surface of the oral mucosa, pressure and kinesthetic sensation in the deeper tissue, pain in both superficial and deep locations, and taste within the oral cavity (and on the extended tongue). These sensations are mediated by the somatic sensory branches of cranial nerves V, VII, IX, and X and of cervical spinal nerves C1 to C3, afferents of the cervical sympathetic nerves associated with cranial blood vessels and special sensory fibers for taste carried in branches of cranial nerves VII, IX, and X. (Pain sensations might conceivably also be carried in cranial parasympathetic fibers in branches of III, V, VII, and IX.)

Despite this variety of sensations that we all recognize in the oral cavity (and which can be separated to some extent by experimental sensory testing techniques), patients usually focus their complaints of abnormal oral sensations on two modalities, pain and taste. On occasion, patients specifically seek assistance for other oral sensory complaints, such as burning or dryness, and even more rarely for what are probably abnormalities of textural sensation (*e.g.,* "the lining of my mouth feels rough"). Also, when tested by questionnaire, many patients with chronic oral pain will admit to a mixture of oral sensory abnormalities, such as burning, dryness, or altered taste, in addition to pain. But *pain* and *disordered taste (dysgeusia)* are the two presenting complaints that constitute the bulk of chronic oral sensory abnormalities for which patients overtly seek medical and dental care. (Patients who complain of a swelling, lump, loose tooth, hemorrhage, or ulcer are excluded from this discussion because such symptoms usually can be readily confirmed objectively, and the diagnostic process then becomes identified with the physical abnormality rather than with the sensory complaint.)

Pain and taste sensations, in general, are caused by different oral stimuli and are transmitted by way of separate peripheral and central nervous system pathways (see Figs. 16-1 and 16-2). It is usual to discuss the diagnosis of pain and the diagnosis of dysgeusia as separate clinical problems, and that approach will also be followed in this chapter; however, there are several considerations regarding the interpretation of a patient's sensory complaints that apply to both pain and dysgeusia, as well as the other less frequent oral sensory disorders. These considerations are appropriately discussed at this point, before the various clinical pain and taste syndromes are described. Interactions between the various oral sensory systems are also included in this discussion because likewise they may influence the way in which oral sensory abnormalities are manifested.

In evaluating a patient for an oral sensory complaint, it is reasonable to start with the assumptions that pain or burning results from noxious stimulation of specific receptors in a particular region of the mouth, that a taste complaint is caused by changes affecting the gustatory branches of cranial nerves VII, IX, and X, and that a dry mouth results from some salivary gland dysfunction. Unfortunately, this simple relationship does not always hold true, and the clinician must be aware of a variety of physiological, psycho-

logical, and even linguistic phenomena that condition oral sensory complaints. The discussion that follows does not imply a lack of concern on the part of the doctor for the discomfort and unhappiness that patients certainly experience with chronic oral sensory disorders. Rather, it is intended to help the diagnostician look beyond the complaint (pain, dryness, bad taste, etc.) that often dominates the clinical situation and to inquire in a variety of ways as to the exact nature of the patient's problem. The capacity for pain to evoke both anxiety and depression, the patient's past experience of pain, and his perception of his current painful problem influence the intensity of his pain and require that the physician and dentist evaluate the patient carefully as to both the likely cause of his pain, its intensity and character, and whether they are reasonably connected. Similar considerations also apply to the evaluation of other oral sensory complaints.

FACTORS CONDITIONING ORAL SENSORY COMPLAINTS

Subjectivity. Although attempts have been made to define what a patient means when he speaks of the sensation of pain (*e.g.,* as Melzack and Torgerson have done by the use of a series of words relating to different qualities and intensities of sensory experience), *pain, like all sensations, remains a subjective experience, and the word "pain" may be used by different individuals to refer to a variety of different noxious or aversive sensations.*

There are no specific, anatomically distinct pain receptors. Pain sensations are carried by a variety of nerve fibers of different dimensions; with increasing intensity, hot and cold touch and pressure stimuli are likely to be reported as pain sensations by most individuals. There is also evidence that efferent neural circuits extend from the higher cerebral centers to inhibit both pain and other somatosensory stimuli reaching the spinomedullary pain center for the orofacial area. If this inhibition does not occur, quite normal somatosensory stimuli from the oral cavity that are otherwise not perceived by the patient or are accepted as normal oral sensations may be identified as pain. The patient's

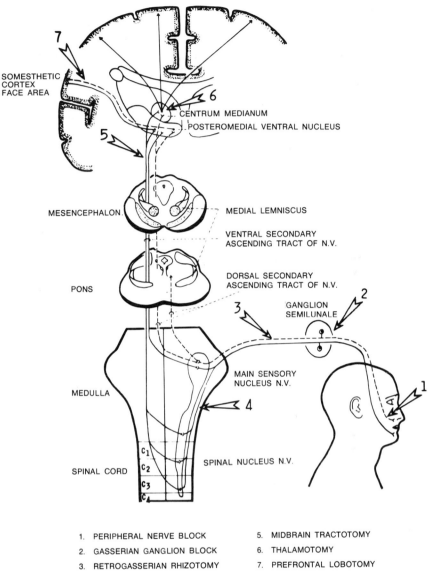

Somesthetic Cortex Face Area

6 Centrum Medianum

Posteromedial Ventral Nucleus

5

Mesencephalon

Medial Lemniscus

Ventral Secondary Ascending Tract of N.V.

Pons

Dorsal Secondary Ascending Tract of N.V.

2 Ganglion Semilunale

3

Main Sensory Nucleus N.V.

4

Medulla

1

Spinal Cord c_1 c_2 c_3 c_4

Spinal Nucleus N.V.

1. PERIPHERAL NERVE BLOCK	5. MIDBRAIN TRACTOTOMY
2. GASSERIAN GANGLION BLOCK	6. THALAMOTOMY
3. RETROGASSERIAN RHIZOTOMY	7. PREFRONTAL LOBOTOMY
4. TRIGEMINAL TRACTOTOMY	

Fig. 16-1 Diagram of facial pain pathways and sites for pain blocking. (Kawamura Y: Fundamental considerations relating to facial pain in pathological conditions. In Alling CC (ed): Facial Pain. Philadelphia, Lea & Febiger, 1968)

past experience, conditioning, and emotional state probably contribute to these inhibitory circuits and determine which sensations are reported as pain and which as touch, pressure, or other experiences.

Other Pain-Associated Sensory Abnormalities. There is also a long-established link between a suffering patient and a doctor, which

results in *communication between doctor and patient usually being in terms of pain* ("Where do you hurt? . . . where is your discomfort?") *rather than in terms of another sensory abnormality.* Complaints of altered taste, dry mouth, and burning are likely to be considered minor disorders and even laughable complaints by both the patient's friends and the physician, dentist, or auxiliary whom he consults. In

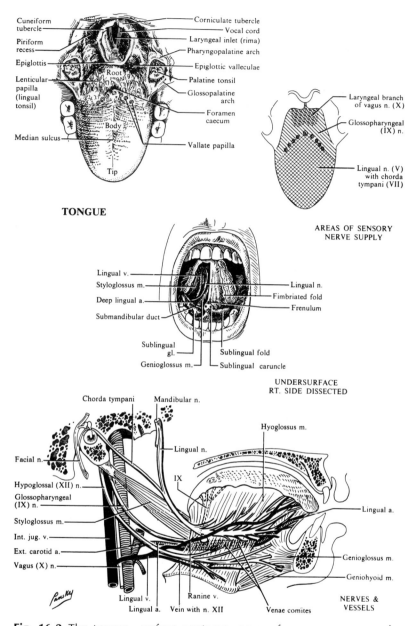

Fig. 16-2 The tongue—surface anatomy, areas of sensory nerve supply, and extracranial relationships of the cranial nerves carrying gustatory (VII and IX) and general sensory (V) stimuli from the surface of the tongue. (Pansky B, House EL: Review of Gross Anatomy. A Dynamic Approach. New York, Macmillan, 1964)

many languages there is also a paucity of words to describe the individual oral sensations, and a patient's attempts at explaining his symptoms may result in bizarre statements that are more likely to be considered signs of a neurosis than of a specific oral lesion (*e.g.*, "My mouth feels sticky"; "I have pieces of saliva in my mouth"; "My mouth feels as though I have just eaten an unripe persimmon"; or "The side of my face feels swollen," or "tight," when there is no objective evidence of such a swelling [a common complaint of patients with temporomandibular joint myofascial dysfunction]). There is thus a good likelihood that a patient will tend to identify his altered oral sensory experience as noxious or painful and not attempt to separate out the individual oral sensory abnormality contributing to his "dis-ease."

General Emotional Discomfort. Very rarely, patients may express their emotional discomfort in terms of specific oral symptoms (see Chap. 18). An emotional problem should certainly be accepted as the cause of a patient's oral symptoms only when there is other evidence of emotional disturbance, but its existence underlies the *interaction between affective state and oral symptoms that occurs in all patients* and can lead to overemphasis of one symptom (*e.g.*, pain, dysgeusia) to the exclusion of others.

All these factors increase the likelihood that a patient's oral complaints will be verbalized in terms of pain rather than in terms of some concomitant symptom or emotion, and they help explain why pain is the most prevalent oral clinical sensory disorder in man. As far as *dysgeusia* (the next most common oral sensory complaint) is concerned, other factors including the following provide additional confusion for the clinician.

Interaction with Other Sensory Pathways. Nerve fibers transmitting somatic sensory information and those transmitting gustatory information, though anatomically distinct, are closely related both in the oral mucosa and in the larger branches of cranial nerves V, VII, and IX. There is also a submucosal plexus on the dorsum of the tongue in which the terminal branches of many nerves anastomose, and interaction between gustatory and somatic sensory nerves at this level may also occur (see Fig. 16-2). *Pathologic lesions affecting these nerves often affect both somatic sensory and special sensory units, and mixed symptomatology (pain, dryness, dysgeusia, and other abnormal oral sensations) results.* Frequently, one of these sensations takes precedence as the patient's chief complaint, although all clearly have diagnostic importance. Stimulation of taste receptors also stimulates reflex secretion of both major and minor salivary glands, and dysgeusia and dryness may

sometimes be linked by a physiological pathway.

Sensation and Perception of Taste. "Taste" like "pain," unfortunately has many meanings, *and a complaint of altered taste sensation does not always signify an abnormality involving a gustatory nerve.* "Taste" may be used in a figurative sense (as, for example, "a man of good taste" and "Taste and see that the Lord is good"), and complaints that "things [?life] no longer taste good," when reported by a depressed patient, must be analyzed as to whether they refer to a psychologic or specific oral sensory discomfort. In addition, usages vary with regard to the use of "taste" for ingested substances: on the one hand, the word may be used with a physiological bias to refer to the pure sensations (usually classified as sweet, sour, bitter, and salty) arising from direct stimulation of taste bud receptors by substances dissolved in saliva. In everyday use, "taste" more often refers to the full range of sensations that accompany the introduction in the mouth, mastication, and swallowing of food or drink. The first of these nonfigurative usages we might call *the sensation of taste;* the second usage, because it includes not only the conscious sensation of taste but also other sensory information occasioned by ingestion of food that the individual may not consciously associate with specific gustatory stimuli, we might call appropriately the *perception of taste* (*e.g.*, information, such as that resulting from olfactory stimulation by volatile components before and during mastication, from tactile and temperature stimulation of oral mucosal receptors, as well as kinesthetic sensations arising from mechanoreceptors in the masticatory muscles, jaw joints, and periodontal membrane).

The complaints that patients bring concerning aberration of taste are often difficult to interpret because some are probably related to the perception of taste and others to the "pure sensations of taste" arising in specific taste receptors. The tongue as an organ of taste is probably more accurately described as an organ of taste perception rather than one of taste sensation. It is not surprising that a wide variety of unusual sensations arising in this organ are apt to be reported clinically as taste aberrations, even when the gustatory nerves are not specifically affected.

Gustatory-Olfactory Confusion. Finally, it must be realized that what is commonly spoken of loosely as the *"taste or flavor of food" includes both gustatory and olfactory sensations.* Loss of olfactory stimulation by way of the first cranial nerve (as often occurs with a cold or other nasal obstruction preventing access of volatile components of food to the olfactory receptors in the upper part of the nasal cavity) alters the "taste of food" greatly because oral chemoreception then becomes the main sensation associated with eating. Damage to the maxillary branch of the trigeminal nerve may also produce diminished taste sensation in the same way, since nonspecific stimulation of receptors of the 5th nerve throughout the nasal mucosa, by heat and pungent volatile components, also contributes to the "taste of food." Evaluation of dysgeusia, therefore, must always include an examination of cranial nerves I and V, as well as VII and IX nerve functions.

EVALUATION OF PAIN AND DYSGEUSIA

History—Presenting Complaint

It is clear from the preceding discussion that the history of a patient's chronic oral sensory complaint is very important and must be recorded in detail and carefully evaluated by the physician or dentist who wishes to make an accurate diagnosis of the problem and expects to provide relief for the patient when others have failed to do so. Many patients with chronic oral sensory complaints consult a variety of medical and dental specialists about their problem, yet review of their available records often reveals only a brief description of the nature of the complaint.

With the development of Pain Control Centers in recent years, many institutions have developed standardized forms and questionnaires designed to collect as much pertinent information as possible about a patient's symptoms. Many of these questionnaires also include numerical or verbal scales that the patient can use to describe the intensity and quality of his symptoms (see Fig. 16-3). Repeated use of such scales, while diagnosis and therapy proceed, can provide a semiquantitative estimate of change in a patient's symptoms that is a useful adjunct to the doctor's own record of the patient's progress.

Items designed to evaluate a patient's psychiatric and general medical status are also sometimes included in these questionnaires, or alternatively, more extensive and time-tested schedules such as the Cornell Medical Index and the Minnesota Multiphasic Personality Inventory are administered together with the pain questionnaire. The details of some of these pain questionnaires have been published; others will often be readily made available to the interested physician or dentist who requests copies from a pain control unit in a regional medical center or teaching hospital. Several centers have also experimented with computerized history and examination data for orofacial pain and have compared the results of diagnoses obtained by computerized analyses with those provided by history and examination carried out by an individual physician or dentist.

Regardless of the manner in which the information is collected, the essential facts that need to be obtained concerning a patient's complaint of chronic orofacial pain can be organized in terms of the four questions that follow.

When Does It Hurt? Details are recorded concerning the onset, temporal features, and periodicity of the symptoms, including information on the time and occasion the symptoms were first noticed; subsequent episodes of pain; trauma, illness, and occupational or other activity associated with onset; frequency of recurrence and events, illness, and so on, associated with recurrence; length of episodes and length of pain-free periods; and if pain is of variable intensity, length of periods of worst pain.

Where Does It Hurt? A detailed description of the location of the pain as it is first experienced is elicited and because it may have changed with time, is elicited as it changes during an episode. The patient should be asked to point to the area affected and outline the way in which pain may spread to affect other areas. He should be asked whether the pain is felt to be superficial or deep. If certain activities consistently produce the pain, the patient can be requested to initiate the pain cautiously and indicate when he feels the symptoms. This is not advisable in cases of suspected trigeminal neuralgia or in other syndromes with trigger zones (see below); in these cases, the painful episodes are so severe that the patient guards intensely against accidental stimuli likely to initiate an episode and often may even deny permission for an oral examination.

How Much Does It Hurt? Pain varies in both quality and intensity, and a record of a patient's past pain, as well as that experienced at each consultation, should include some measure of both of these features. The quality of the pain (throbbing, burning, shooting, aching, pulling, etc) may be recorded in the patient's own words or by having him check appropriate words on a standardized schedule. Intensity may be recorded verbally or by some scaling method (*e.g.*, 0 to 5 on a linear series ranging from none, 0, through worst, 5); checking of a scale marked on a card; or by hand compression of a dynamometer. Calibration of the patient's scale of pain intensity can be carried out by comparison of the pain of the presenting complaint, and the patient's worst experience with other painful disorders (such as toothache, headache, stomachache, bone fracture, childbirth, etc) as appropriate. A comparison of the pain the patient is experiencing at the time of consultation with the same pain at its worst and least is also important information because it provides a measure of the effect of the pain on the patient's behavior. Modification of behavior that the patient attributes to the pain and use of analgesics can also be useful measures of intensity (see below under Associated Phenomena).

If pain is not present at the time of consultation, focusing of the patient's response on his *last* painful episode may provide more accurate information than allowing him to range freely over a history of recurrent or continuous pain of some months' duration. Specific identification of whether the pain is continuous, intermittent and brief, or per-

sisting is important, because these temporal criteria frequently influence the patient's evaluation of the intensity of his symptoms. When multiple oral symptoms, pain of varying character, or pain in two or more locations is described, the temporal character, location, and intensity of each should be recorded separately until a decision has been made as to whether they represent different manifestations of a single problem or independent but temporally related abnormalities.

Are There Associated Phenomena? Details of symptoms or signs that the patient has noted preceding the onset of the orofacial pain (prodromata), as well as those experienced in association with the pain, are frequently useful in defining a particular pain syndrome and should be recorded. These phenomena, as well as various factors that the patient has noted as modifying his symptoms, can also assist in identifying the etiology of a problem; factors that initiate the pain, those that augment the pain and those that diminish it (including treatment and medications) should be evaluated. Pain can also produce objectively evident phenomena such as grimaces and other facial expressions, muscle tensing, grasping and pressing, and other attempts at splinting or immobilizing the affected area. Involuntary activity of this type, as well as hyperkinesia and other evidence of suffering, can often be distinguished from consciously simulated motor activity and may also help identify pain of considerable intensity in an otherwise stoic patient. Vascular flushing, pallor, and an anxious expression may also indicate autonomic phenomena that are often associated with acute pain. A depressed affect or an anxious expression can accompany chronic pain.

Alteration in behavior that is attributable to the pain can also be a useful measure of its intensity. Unwillingness to eat, change to a soft diet, avoidance of social and sexual activity, decreased oral hygiene, and absence from work all evidence the patient's perception that he is ill or suffering. Physical examination often confirms that such behavior is a reasonable physiological response to a diagnosable pain-producing lesion. Patients'

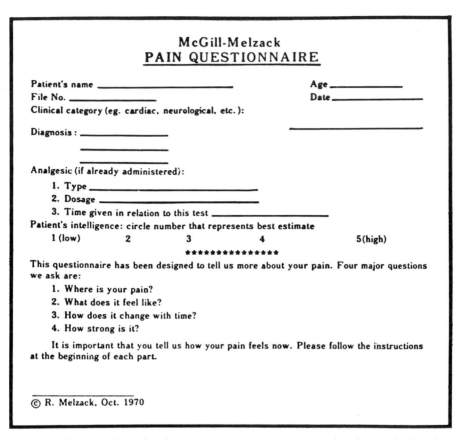

Fig. 16-3 The McGill–Melzack pain questionnaire. An example of a standardized questionnaire for recording qualitative and quantitative features of pain symptoms. (Melzack R: Pain I:227, 1975)

perceptions of the efficacy of local and systemic analgesics and the value of such medications for the relief of various painful states do vary, but a history of a chronic orofacial pain that the patient describes as the worst pain he has ever experienced, yet for which he does not need analgesics, should suggest pain of low intensity or brief duration or some secondary gain to the patient from the painful experience. Conversely, the ease with which patients may become habituated to narcotics and other analgesics prevents the clinician from viewing a patient's recourse to these agents as an accurate measure of pain intensity unless the patient's response to previous painful episodes is known. Behavioral responses to pain are closely related to the patient's family and cultural orientation to pain, as well as to his previous pain experi-

ence; these factors also should be evaluated when the patient is interviewed. Thus, in the evaluation of an orofacial sensory complaint, as in the evaluation of any neurological problem, "No examination can be complete without a history, and no history can be too complete."

Medical and Dental History

In addition to a history of the patient's presenting complaint, it is also essential that *the patient's medical and dental history be reviewed in detail.* Because this is a basic principle of medical history-taking (see Chap. 2), it may seem redundant to stress the need for the taking of another thorough medical and dental history; however, a patient's description of his presenting oral complaint may be quite

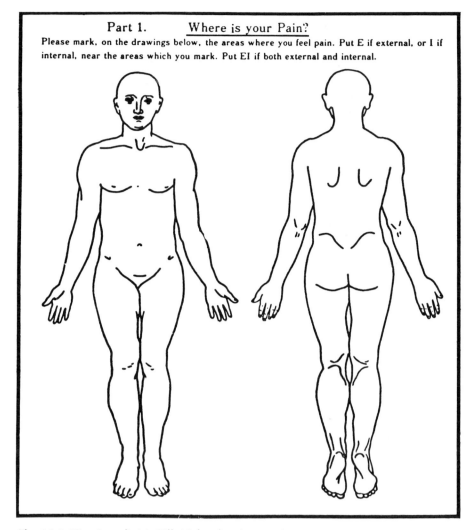

Fig. 16-3 (*Continued*). McGill–Melzack pain questionnaire.

detailed and lengthy, and the accompanying medical and dental history understandably will be brief unless the dentist has been thoroughly trained in the importance of not giving undue emphasis to any one symptom in recording a history. Well-balanced histories from patients with chronic oral sensory problems that give equal emphasis to the presenting complaint and to other systems are not usual outside of neurologic practice, and the use of standardized forms and questionnaires is perhaps to be encouraged in the evaluation of orofacial pain.

Other historical information, not usually included in the medical history, that may be important to record for the patient with chronic orofacial pain includes operative reports where they relate to the affected area, including details of dental anesthetic injections related to onset of the problem; records describing the response to earlier treatment for the problem; records of any psychiatric treatment; and details of treatment provided outside the conventional medical and dental environment (*e.g.*, manipulative, homeopathic, and chiropractic treatment; faith healing; and galvanic and diathermy treatment).

Examination

Although the diagnosis of some neurologic disorders may be made on the basis of char-

---

Part 2.   What Does Your Pain Feel Like?

Some of the words below describe your present pain. Circle ONLY those words that best describe it. Leave out any category that is not suitable. Use only a single word in each appropriate category—the one that applies best.

1	2	3	4
Flickering	Jumping	Pricking	Sharp
Quivering	Flashing	Boring	Cutting
Pulsing	Shooting	Drilling	Lacerating
Throbbing		Stabbing	
Beating		Lancinating	
Pounding			

5	6	7	8
Pinching	Tugging	Hot	Tingling
Pressing	Pulling	Burning	Itchy
Gnawing	Wrenching	Scalding	Smarting
Cramping		Searing	Stinging
Crushing			

9	10	11	12
Dull	Tender	Tiring	Sickening
Sore	Taut	Exhausting	Suffocating
Hurting	Rasping		
Aching	Splitting		
Heavy			

13	14	15	16
Fearful	Punishing	Wretched	Annoying
Frightful	Gruelling	Blinding	Troublesome
Terrifying	Cruel		Miserable
	Vicious		Intense
	Killing		Unbearable

17	18	19	20
Spreading	Tight	Cool	Nagging
Radiating	Numb	Cold	Nauseating
Penetrating	Drawing	Freezing	Agonizing
Piercing	Squeezing		Dreadful
	Tearing		Torturing

Fig. 16-3 (*Continued*). McGill–Melzack pain questionnaire.

acteristic features in the patient's history, *no evaluation for an oral sensory complaint is complete without a thorough physical examination of the head and neck.* The procedure for such an examination (including an examination of cranial nerve function) is outlined in Chapter 2, and it would again be redundant to stress the need for this, except for the number of patients who are referred for evaluation of undiagnosed chronic oral sensory complaints without a thorough dental examination having been recorded. A thorough oral examination (charting of all teeth, restorations, cavities, and periodontal pockets; a full-mouth periapical radiographic series and panoramic dental films; examination of temporomandibular joint (TMJ) function and occlusion; pulp testing; and palpation of intraoral structures,

masticatory muscles, salivary glands, lymph nodes, and perioral soft tissues) may require more than one appointment. A report of "no evidence of an oral cause" for a patient's complaint of orofacial pain should not be made by the dentist until all these procedures have been carried out.

When the dentist finds it necessary to remove artificial crowns and restorations and to observe the response to sedative dental dressings over some weeks before he is sure there is no evidence of dental disease contributing to the patient's pain, he should inform the patient of the reason for the delay and offer appropriate temporary analgesic and sedative medication, rather than refer the patient to another specialist who may assume that the dental examination is com-

Part 3.   How Does Your Pain Change With Time?

1. Which word or words would you use to describe the pattern of your pain?

1	2	3
Continuous	Rhythmic	Brief
Steady	Periodic	Momentary
Constant	Intermittent	Transient

2. What kind of things relieve your pain?

3. What kind of things increase your pain?

Part 4.   How Strong Is Your Pain?

People agree that the following 5 words represent pain of increasing intensity. They are:

1	2	3	4	5
Mild	Discomforting	Distressing	Horrible	Excruciating

To answer each question below, write the number of the most appropriate word in the space beside the question.

1. Which word describes your pain right now?   _____
2. Which word describes it at its worst?   _____
3. Which word describes it when it is least?   _____
4. Which word describes the worst toothache you ever had?   _____
5. Which word describes the worst headache you ever had?   _____
6. Which word describes the worst stomach-ache you ever had?   _____

Fig. 16-3 (Continued). McGill–Melzack pain questionnaire.

plete. If such a referral becomes necessary, such as from pressures generated by an acutely anxious patient with orofacial pain, the referral note should specify that the dental examination is incomplete.

Additional Studies

On the basis of history and physical examination as outlined above, a differential diagnosis of a patient's complaint of chronic orofacial pain can usually be made. Further radiographic examination, laboratory testing, and examination by other medical specialists (internist, neurologist, otorhinolaryngologist, vascular disease specialist, rheumatologist) are sometimes needed and should be sought; the patient should be referred, together with full details of history, examina-tion findings, radiographs, laboratory testing, and the results of treatment.

Evaluation of Dysgeusia

In general, the evaluation of the patient with other chronic oral sensory problems (*e.g.,* dysgeusia, burning, dryness) follows the same pattern as that described for orofacial pain. Additional information that should be collected in the evaluation of patients with dysgeusia is discussed below.

Presenting Complaint. A record of the presenting complaint should include an accurate description of the taste abnormality. Does the patient have complete loss of taste (*ageusia*), diminished perception of taste (*hypogeusia*) for one or more of the four standard taste qualities (sweet, salty, sour, and bitter), or a persistent abnormal taste? Distinction should also be made between an abnormal taste that is present only part of the time and does not always exclude other taste sensation (*parageusia*) and one that is severe enough to prevent normal tasting and is experienced as a continuous, unpleasant sensation (*cacogeusia*). An attempt should be made to have the patient characterize the unpleasant taste, which is often fixed in his mind in terms of some unusual and vividly described experience. Hypogeusia should also be described in terms of the particular quality of taste sensation that is affected. Unfortunately, no clear relationship has been established between particular taste complaints and the various disease states giving rise to them, and much could be gained in our understanding of these problems if they were better described clinically.

Some measure of the intensity of a taste complaint can be gained from inquiring whether the problem persists when the patient eats or whether particular foods mask the problem; some parageusias are reported to occur following ingestion of certain foods. Animal experimentation suggests that loss of taste (and even both taste and olfactory) sensation is unlikely to affect the amount of food a patient consumes, but such loss can be expected to affect the selection of various foods in the diet.

A record of dietary changes that the patient associates with the problem or any other interference with ingestive behavior (*e.g.*, unwillingness to eat out, use of chewing gum, mouthrinses or lozenges to mask unpleasant tastes, and involuntary ingestion of spoiled food) can indicate a problem of some severity. Other modifications of behavior such as absenteeism, diminished social and sexual activity, inability to cope with housework and other responsibilities that are sometimes reported by patients as accompanying their dysgeusia, are also a measure of the severity of the problem, or at least of the depression that often accompanies chronic oral sensory complaints. Some consistent method of scaling the intensity of the problem (as described earlier for chronic orofacial pain) is desirable if improvement or worsening of the dysgeusic symptom is to be distinguished from

changes in general well-being versus illness because dysgeusia, like pain, is usually identified as evidence of "dis-ease" by the patient who seeks help for the problem.

In view of the previously discussed confusion between olfactory and gustatory sensations that combine to give us the familiar tastes we associate with many foods, a history of a dysgeusic patient must include past and present olfactory disorders. Foods such as chocolate are distinguished from other soft, sweet substances largely by their characteristic volatile components, and ability to distinguish a cup of hot chocolate from hot sweetened coffee can be a measure of olfactory (first cranial nerve) function. The response of the patient to strongly irritating volatile compounds such as those contained in onions and smelling salts can be a measure of general sensory function in the nose and conjunctiva, and the absence of sneezing, lacrimation, and nasal irritability with exposure to such compounds suggests diminished trigeminal function, which may cause abnormality of taste perception.

A history of the manner in which the dysgeusia developed is always helpful and may immediately suggest the probable etiology of the dysgeusia. Associated oral sensory abnormalities such as numbness, burning, and pain may be only a minor problem for the patient in comparison with the dysgeusia, but they may indicate the presence of a neuropathy affecting cranial nerves V, VII, or IX. In patients with Bell's palsy, the dysgeusia (which is most often unilateral) is accompanied by paralysis of facial muscles on the same side.

General Medical History. The general medical history for the dysgeusic patient should include a detailed drug history that lists current medications as well as those taken prior to the onset of the problem. Over 250 proprietary preparations listed in the *Physicians' Desk Reference* are described as causing dysgeusia and xerostomia as side-effects, and both transient and persistent taste abnormalities may follow use of these drugs. Radiation to the head and neck likewise may lead to xerostomia complicated by dysgeusia. Some industrial metallic poisonings are associated with dysgeusia, and occupational exposure to unusual compounds including halogens, arsenic, selenium, and chromium should be noted.

Other symptoms suggestive of altered cranial nerve function (*e.g.*, headache, diplopia, dizziness, deafness, muscle weakness, and numbness) should also be covered in taking the history because dysgeusia may occasionally occur as the result of neoplasia of the central nervous system.

Physical Examination. The physical examination should stress careful evaluation of cranial nerve function (as described in Chap. 2) with particular attention to cranial nerves I, V, VII, and IX. Since the evaluation of taste function usually receives only cursory attention even when the cranial nerve examination is carried out by a neurologist, this procedure should be performed with care and the results included in the patient's record as confirmation of a detectable alteration in taste sensation. It is true that taste testing depends as much on the subjective response of the patient as does the history of his dysgeusic complaint, but when carried out in a consistent manner and with adequate controls that minimize the effect of bias by the patient, psychophysiologic taste testing often helps confirm the presence or absence of a sensory deficit for various taste qualities. Parageusic patients may be unaware of such sensory loss; other patients complaining of ageusia or hypogeusia may have no detectable abnormality to taste testing.

Taste Testing. A variety of techniques that differ in their degree of sophistication are available for taste testing.

The midline of the tongue and the V-shaped row of vallate papillae separate the tongue into four quadrants, the anterior two of which bear fungiform papillae with gustatory receptors connected via the right and left lingual branches of the 5th cranial nerve to the chorda tympani and the facial nerve. The posterior two quadrants include the right and left vallates and the pharyngeal surface of the tongue, innervated by gustatory (and general sensory) fibers of the lingual branches of the right and left glossopharyngeal and possibly, the vagus nerves.

Testing of these four quadrants thus allows

separation of abnormalities of the right and left side and 5th versus 9th cranial nerve function. To achieve this, the tongue must be dried or rinsed between each application of tastant, and it must be held in the extruded position from the time of each application until the patient gives his response. Cards on which the four taste qualities and the comments "no taste" and "plain water" are printed allow the patient to respond while keeping his tongue extended. Some techniques make use of crystals of the four tastants and rely on the lingual salivary secretions or a small drop of water applied to the quadrant under test to dissolve the molecules and make them available to the lingual chemoreceptors.

In general, there is less likelihood of bias on the part of the patient, if the identity of each tastant is not revealed until the test on that quadrant is completed. The response of the patient to a drop of water (no added tastant) applied to each quadrant should also be noted. If solutions of the tastants are used, these should be maintained at room or body temperature to minimize the effect of temperature stimuli. The drops of solution are best applied with a pipette rather than with a cotton swab to avoid heavy tactile stimuli. The patient should be allowed to rinse his mouth with tap water from time to time and to retract his tongue and relax between tests.

Such testing using crystals of tastant or a single solution of each tastant at a concentration well above the minimum concentration detectable by the majority of individuals (threshold concentration) is designed to detect gross abnormalities in taste function and may fail to detect minor degrees of diminished taste sensitivity (hypogeusia). When the gross test detects an abnormality or when an abnormality is suspected despite a normal gross test, further testing with graded dilutions of one or more of the four tastant solutions should follow.

Unfortunately, little is known about the psychophysiology of taste in comparison with what is known concerning auditory function, for example, and taste testing at near threshold concentrations lacks the precision of audiologic testing. Moreover, there is still controversy over the theoretical basis of the taste-testing technique to be used, and few attempts have been made to compare the results of different testing techniques or to measure the accuracy and reproducibility of particular techniques. Our own measurements of the success with which our taste-testing procedures can predict individuals who have taste abnormalities in a group of patients with chronic oral sensory problems suggest that the taste system is very complex and not easily adapted to psychophysiologic tests that have a high degree of clinical accuracy. Detailed taste testing of patients with particular taste syndromes or diseases with a high frequency of taste abnormality has often produced contradictory results when the tests are carried out by different investigators using both similar and different techniques.

Techniques that attempt to measure taste sensitivity rather than gross taste abnormality include the three-drop forced-choice method of Henkin, the rinsing technique based on signal-detection theory developed at the Monell Chemical Senses Center by Desor and Maller, and a threshold-detection technique described by Steiner. Each of these techniques may require an hour or longer to perform, and they are really still suitable only for research studies. A simpler technique applicable to the clinical situation of an individual patient with a persistant taste problem is that described by Bornstein. This technique uses "high, medium, and low" concentrations of sodium chloride (salt), sucrose (sweet), acetic or hydrochloric acid (sour), and urea or quinine sulfate (bitter) and may be modified to detect some degree of hypogeusia in all four tongue quadrants. Taste sensation on the palate and in the pharynx, though normally contributing to the taste of ingested food, is not usually tested clinically. Likewise, most taste-testing techniques require the patient to try and identify individual taste sensations and do not concern themselves with taste perception.

Yet another approach to clinical taste testing is the procedure known as electrogustometry by which the gustatory nerves (and to some extent, the general sensory nerves in the area tested) are stimulated with a galvanic current of low intensity. Instruments for this purpose are available commercially (*e.g.,* the Elgustometer) or they can be fabricated from simple components by an electronics techni-

cian. They have been used fairly widely in the evaluation of chorda tympani function in patients with Bell's palsy or other damage to the 7th nerve.

Testing of olfactory and nonspecific trigeminal function as outlined earlier under History—Presenting Complaint should also be confirmed, if possible, by clinical testing. Adequate olfactory testing with scaling of the response requires considerable effort, special equipment, and olfactant solutions, and is usually not attempted outside of research investigations. Testing of trigeminal function should include the use of substances such as smelling salts and careful testing of tactile sensitivity on oral mucosa, skin, and nasal mucosa if second division abnormalities are suspected.

Oral Examination. The oral examination usually includes careful examination for caries and periodontal pockets in which food and plaque may be retained as exogenous sources of malodor and bad taste. This should be accompanied by a search for cryptic tonsils, postnasal discharge, rhinitis, and sinusitis with retention of nasal secretions. The dorsum of the tongue and the seating surfaces of dentures should be inspected for retained food particles and heavy bacterial coatings, and the oral mucosa for evidence of candidiasis (an alleged cause of metallic taste and other taste anomalies). The dorsum of the tongue should also be checked for the presence of a reasonably normal complement of fungiform, vallate, and foliate papillae and the absence of extensive mucosal lesions such as lichen planus, leukoplakia, and glossitis. The side of the tongue, floor of the mouth, and mylohyoid area should be examined for evidence of damage to the lingual branch of nerve V, and the pharyngeal surface of the tongue inspected for masses that may affect the lingual branch of cranial nerve IX.

Techniques for estimating salivary function should be used when the history or the character of the oral mucous membrane and the degree of moisture and amount of saliva seen following palpation of the major glands suggest the presence of xerostomia. Biopsy of a sample of the minor salivary glands from the lip or palate may indicate the presence of a fairly widespread sialadenitis, and sequential salivary scintigraphy may reveal diminished uptake or clearance of technetium by the major salivary glands.

Laboratory Test. Laboratory tests that may indicate the presence of problems sometimes associated with dysgeusia include 2-hour postprandial blood glucose estimations and the glucose tolerance test (also important tests for any patient with chronic oral sensory disability); serum triglycerides and lipoprotein electrophoresis; blood urea nitrogen; thyroid function studies; and possibly, 24-hour urinary excretion of zinc and serum zinc levels.

CLASSIFICATION OF ORAL SENSORY DISORDERS

When possible, it is clearly desirable to identify the cause of a patient's oral sensory abnormalities and to treat the presenting problem (*e.g.,* pain, dysgeusia, or other complaint) by eliminating or controlling the cause. Specific treatment of the symptoms (*e.g.,* with analgesics) may also be needed, especially in the early stages of treatment before the cause is definitely identified and effectively controlled.

If the cause of a patient's oral sensory disorder is identified as a particular problem arising outside of and only secondarily affecting some portion of a peripheral nerve (*e.g.,* pulpitis or acute necrotizing ulcerative gingivitis-causing pain, or an exudate from chronic periodontal pockets causing dysgeusia), it is customary to refer to the patient as having pulpitis, acute necrotizing gingivitis, or chronic periodontitis, as the case may be, rather than pain or dysgeusia of dental or periodontal origin. When similar symptoms are caused by a lesion that primarily involves the terminal receptors or axons of a peripheral nerve, it is more usual to refer to the problem as a sensory disorder (*e.g.,* paresthesia or dysgeusia caused by trauma to a particular nerve), the term here referring to a disorder of a specific sensory nerve.

Abnormal oral sensations can also arise from disease processes located in the central nervous system that affect the perception of oral stimuli reaching the brain in such a way that the patient feels pain, bad taste, or other symptoms in the mouth even though there is no local oral lesion. As mentioned earlier, emotionally disturbed individuals may perceive severe pain in the mouth even though there is no local oral lesion likely to cause such severe pain, and no other abnormality of the central or peripheral nervous system can be identified (psychological pain).

The terminology that different authors use to describe these varied types of oral sensory disorders is confused, and some of the difficulty in understanding and diagnosing oral sensory disorders stems from this confusion and the lack of rigid definitions for the various terms. An attempt was made at the Workshop on Oral Facial Pain, sponsored by the National Institute of Dental Research (NIDR) Pain Control and Behavioral Studies Branch in 1974, to outline a Classification of Oral Facial Pain consistent with current knowledge of the physiopathology and psychology of pain and the procedures available for the diagnosis of pain in the orofacial area. Continued development of this classification has been entrusted to a group on the Taxonomy of Oral Facial Pain of the International Association for the Study of Pain. This classification will be followed in this chapter as far as orofacial pain is concerned; a similar approach to the classification of dysgeusia has also been used in this chapter.

In both of these classifications an attempt has been made to use terms that do not imply a particular pathologic process but simply serve as a label to identify a group of symptoms or signs that currently define a particular clinical syndrome. The classification is thus taxonomic rather than etiologic. This approach is preferred in our current state of ignorance concerning the etiology of many oral sensory disorders, as one that is less likely to give rise to unjustified conclusions regarding etiology and treatment of symptoms, the nature of which can only be speculated on.

It would be desirable if all patients complaining of oral sensory disorders could be contained within one or another of the various categories described in this chapter. Unfortunately, many patients with chronic oral sensory disorders cannot be categorized in this fashion unless certain of their symptoms are neglected and the diagnosis made on the basis of a selected group of signs and symptoms (*e.g.*, those of most concern to the patient at a particular time); clinicians will obviously disagree on the diagnosis to be used for such patients. In the author's opinion, much is to be gained by the use of the nonspecific term *disordered oral sensation* to categorize these patients who usually report rather ill-defined chronic oral sensory problems, usually of mixed symptomatology, and for whom specific anatomic diagnoses are hard to find.

Chronic oral sensory disorders in which pain or dysgeusia are the major presenting complaints and for which a reasonable explanation can usually be found are the concern of the remainder of this chapter. Complaints of dryness (xerostomia) and the diseases of the salivary glands likely to cause this symptom were described in Chapter 11. Complaints of burning and other less frequent but sometimes equally intense and chronic oral sensory complaints are considered in Chapter 17. This organization reflects the fact that such complaints more often than not appear to be without reasonable explanation. This general problem of oral symptoms without apparent physical abnormality being the major topic in Chapter 17, which also considers patients with orofacial pain, dysgeusia, and xerostomia for which there is no clear diagnosis and those in whom the particular oral symptoms appear unreasonable or otherwise atypical (*e.g.*, atypical facial pain).

In the 1974 NIDR Workshop classification, orofacial pain was divided as follows:

1. **Neuropathic pain** (orofacial pain associated with a clinically demonstrable nerve dysfunction, or an observed abnormality in or of a peripheral nerve)
2. **Non-neuropathic pain** (orofacial pain occurring in the absence of disease primarily involving those nerves likely to be associated with the pain and subdivided into that caused by *changes in the central nervous system* and that caused by *extraneural causes*).
3. **Pain of unknown nature**
   Most pain (and dysgeusia) the dentist treats is thus extra-neural, nonneuropathic because it arises outside the peripheral

nerves and only affects the nerves and their receptors secondarily (*e.g.*, pain of dental caries, periodontal disease, and mouth ulcers). Treatment of such pain, as mentioned before, is largely the treatment of the pain-producing disease process itself (even though specific pain-control measures may also be needed). The clinical features and management of some of the diseases causing extraneural nonneuropathic orofacial pain are described elsewhere in this text and are referred to here only to enable a differential diagnosis of orofacial pains to be established (consult Chaps. 5 through 14; see also bibliographies for titles of appropriate texts on operative dentistry, endodontics and periodontics for further details).

Accurate diagnosis of chronic pain, dysgeusia, and other sensory abnormalities is important not only to achieve prompt and permanent relief of the patient's symptoms but also to identify those rarer conditions in which neuropathies (*i.e.*, a disease or dysfunction of a nerve) or lesions of the central nervous system are responsible for oral symptoms. Such lesions, although not always caused by neoplastic processes, because of their deeper locations have the potential for signaling the existence of more widespread and more disabling disorders than those associated with symptoms of extraneural nonneuropathic origin.

CONDITIONS TO CONSIDER IN THE DIFFERENTIAL DIAGNOSIS OF CHRONIC OROFACIAL PAIN

In the following review, it is assumed that a complete history of the patient's problem as well as a thorough oral examination and review of systems (see Chap. 2) have been carried out. The following additional procedures may provide useful information in arriving at a diagnosis:

1. Examination of cranial nerve function (see Chap. 2)
2. Temperature record, palpation of lymph nodes, total and differential white blood cell count, and sedimentation rate to detect evidence of inflammatory processes
3. Recording of pulp responses to hot, cold,

and electric pulp-testing as well as responses of teeth to percussion and cutting of dentin

4. Palpation of masticatory muscles and other investigations of occlusal and TMJ function (see Chap. 12)

5. Diagnostic injections to determine the location of pain-producing stimuli

6. Response to treatment (*e.g.*, to pulp canal therapy or placement of a dental restoration) to corticosteroids or to tranquilizing agents and muscle relaxants versus analgesics

Further details of the conditions that of necessity are described only briefly in this review may be found in several recent excellent texts and articles dealing with orofacial pain. Other useful references on the physiology and psychology of pain are also listed in the bibliography for this chapter.

Non-neuropathic Orofacial Pain of Extraneural Origin

Dental. The large number of causes of pain of dental origin include dental caries; exposed dentin and cementum; pulpal and periapical disease; periodontal disease; pericoronitis; impacted food; ANUG; faulty dental restorations; fractured teeth; traumatic occlusion; tooth eruption and exfoliation; unerupted and impacted teeth; retained roots; dental cysts; postoperative pain following placement of dental restorations and excavation of caries; postsurgical pain; postinjection pain; other direct trauma to teeth; and aerodontalgia.

Alveolar and Adjacent Tissue Origin. Alveolar osteitis (dry socket), sinusitis, miscellaneous neoplastic and non-neoplastic osteolytic lesions, Paget's disease, multiple myeloma, and soft tissue tumors fall under this category.

Musculoskeletal. Deep somatic pain arising from musculoskeletal structures may be caused by TMJ arthralgia, TMJ myofascial dysfunction, myositis, muscle spasm and trismus, cervical muscle spasm, osteoarthritis and arthralgias of the cervical spine, and tension headache.

Pain of TMJ myofascial dysfunction and the less common intracapsular disorders of the TMJ, which form the major topics for Chapter 12, are the musculoskeletal pains most commonly encountered in the orofacial region. Pain of this type frequently exhibits clinical characteristics that identify its deep somatic origin and distinguish it from pain of dental origin, vascular pain, and pain from other extraneural causes. These characteristics include a dull depressing quality to the pain, which is diffusely located and often referred to other head and neck structures (see discussion on referred pain that follows); exacerbations of sharper pain when the affected muscle is stretched and an association between symptoms and muscle activity; localized areas of palpable muscle tenderness and myofascial trigger areas from which pain spreads (or is referred) to relatively constant reference zones (see Fig. 16-4); and a variety of abnormal sensations of "fullness," "tenderness," "numbness," and "swelling" over the affected areas in addition to the diffuse pain, but without objective evidence of sensory loss in the overlying skin.

Vascular. Pain originating in demonstrable structural or functional vascular abnormality may be caused by vascular headache including migraine and cluster headache (*e.g.*, Horton's headache, histamine headache, Sluder's syndrome); toxic and metabolic vascular headache; hypertensive vascular changes; arterial diseases such as aneurysms, emboli, and atheromatous occlusion; cranial arteritis (including giant cell arteritis, polymyalgia rheumatica, and immune arteritis); thrombophlebitis; and carotidynia.

Except in the case of cluster headache, which is identified on the basis of symptoms and the occurrence of various associated autonomic dysfunctions, it is probably undesirable for a diagnosis of vascular pain to be made unless there is objective evidence of structural or functional vascular abnormality, preferably in the area of the pain but at least in a closely related vessel. Such evidence may be the finding of an acutely tender area or nodules along the course of a major vessel, angiographic evidence of occlusion, or biopsy of a lesion affecting the vessel.

The value of this approach is apparent in

HEAD AND NECK

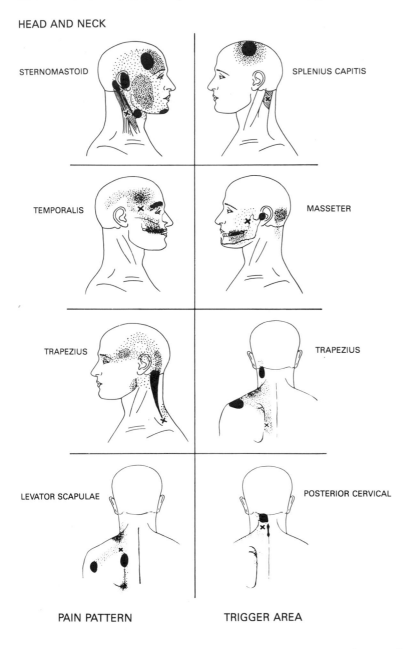

STERNOMASTOID

SPLENIUS CAPITIS

TEMPORALIS

MASSETER

TRAPEZIUS

TRAPEZIUS

LEVATOR SCAPULAE

POSTERIOR CERVICAL

PAIN PATTERN   TRIGGER AREA

Fig. 16-4 Pain reference pattern of myofascial trigger areas in most commonly involved skeletal muscles of head and neck. "Essential" zones (*solid black*) are areas which were involved in 100% of patients. "Spill-over" zones (*stippled*) are those areas which were not involved in all patients. (Travell J, Rinzsler: Postgrad Med 11:425)

the progress that has been made in the understanding of *giant cell arteritis* and the associated disease, *polymyalgia rheumatica*, once the diagnosis of these diseases became based on histologic evidence. Biopsy also serves to separate these diseases from arteritis affecting the temporal and facial arteries as a result of polyarteritis nodosa and other immune phenomena. A raised sedimentation rate is also considered an important diagnostic criteria for polymyalgia rheumatica, which may

not always be associated throughout its course with clinically detectable nodules or pain over the temporal artery.

An exception to this rule is often made in the case of hypertensive vascular disease and vascular changes caused by metabolic diseases such as diabetes mellitus, which may be widespread throughout the body. Where lesions affecting similar-sized vessels elsewhere in the body have been unequivocally demonstrated, it is probably not necessary to repeat the diagnostic procedure (usually angiography) in the orofacial area to explain orofacial pain; however, in the absence of such demonstrations elsewhere in the body, it is unjustified to make the diagnosis of hypertensive or diabetic orofacial pain simply because the patient is hypertensive or known to be diabetic.

The treatment of pain of vascular origin varies, depending on the nature of the vascular lesions involved. The pain associated with inflammatory lesions (arteritis) frequently responds to systemic corticosteroids, but this approach should not be expected to be successful where pain is the result of atheroma or other occlusions associated with hypertension. Vasoconstrictors such as ergotamine tartrate and methysergide are often effective for the treatment of migraine and cluster headache, and various serotonin and histamine antagonists have been used for the treatment of head and facial pain thought to be caused by unusual sensitivity to these intermediates. The literature also contains reports of successful treatment of carotidynia and other facial pain of vascular origin by ligation or resection of a portion of a vessel, or by perivascular stripping of the carotid or its branches, but such procedures are not in common use.

Pain Referred From Outside the Orofacial Area. Otitis media and other inflammatory or neoplastic diseases of the ear; disease of major salivary glands (calculus and other obstructions, cysts, and tumors); lesions of nasal and sinus mucosa; and myocardial ischemia may all cause pain in the orofacial area, often at some distance from the focus of disease. Pain from pulpitis and other local dental disease may also be experienced elsewhere in the head and neck (see Fig. 16-5). In either case, the term *referred pain* is used.

Referred pain describes pain that is felt in a part of the body that is considerably removed from the tissue (or focus) producing the painful stimuli. Although surface pain is sometimes referred in this way, the pain is more often initiated in an organ or other "deep" structure such as a muscle. Such pain is not due to retrograde transmission of stimuli but to synapses in the spinal cord and thalamus between neurons supplying the two areas involved (focus and painful area),

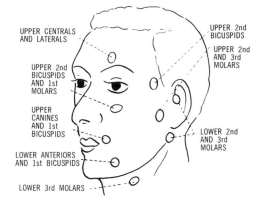

Fig. 16-5 Focal points of referred pain from teeth (after description by Head).
Upper incisors—supraorbital region
Upper second premolar—zygomaticofacial area
Upper first molar or second molar—infraorbital region
Upper second, third molars—anterior to the auricle
Upper canine or first premolar—lateral and inferior to the ala of the nose
Lower incisors, canine or first premolar—lateral and inferior to the corner of the mouth
Lower second or third molar—external auditory meatus parotid region
Lower third molar—submandibular area.
(Shapiro HH: Applied Anatomy of the Head and Neck, 2nd ed. Philadelphia, JB Lippincott, 1947)

such that the person has the *feeling* that the sensations arise in the painful area as well as or instead of in the focus.

In general, referred pain will occur within the same dermatome supplied by the various branches of that nerve, and the focus generating the painful stimuli will occur on the same side of the body as that on which the pain is experienced. Intranasal lesions and lesions of the nasal sinuses are important sources of referred pain to the upper jaw because of the extensive area of nasal and sinus mucosa supplied by branches of the maxillary nerve. Often such pain is referred to the teeth of the upper jaw.

Experimental evidence for the existence of such referred pain has been obtained during otorhinolaryngologic surgery. Pain arising from pulpal, periodontal, and alveolar inflammation in the lower jaw may also be referred to the ear on the same side. It is neurologically possible for any deep pain source in the head and neck (frequently of myofascial origin) to be referred to the teeth and felt as toothache, but it is unusual for toothache to be the only pain complaint in such cases, and local tenderness at least can often be elicited at the focus generating the pain.

Pain referred to the jaw from the lower part of the trigeminal nucleus in the cervical cord by stimuli carried by thoracic spinal nerves from areas of myocardial ischemia is likewise usually accompanied by other pain in more characteristic "cardiac" locations (e.g., left arm, neck, and substernal pain). Such jaw pain may accompany attacks of angina pectoris. It is usually not relieved by local anesthetic infiltration or regional block of the mandibular nerve, but does respond to nitroglycerine and administration of oxygen.

Stimulation of nasopalatine branches of the trigeminal nerve in the roof of the mouth (particularly with cold) may cause severe pain in other segments of the maxillary branch of the trigeminal nerve, frequently in the lower frontal region. The "ice-cream" headache is a common example of this phenomenon that may be mistaken by a patient for a chronic pain syndrome—a mouthful of warm water relieves the symptoms.

Referral of patients with pain thought to be caused by sinusitis does not always provide an explanation for the pain, despite thorough otorhinolaryngologic and radiographic examination. Most sinus pain, however, does diminish or resolve with application of hot moist towels to the face, and it is possible that vascular changes in the sinus mucosa as the result of inhaled irritants may cause this type of pain (particularly in patients otherwise subject to episodes of allergic rhinitis), even in the absence of evidence of chronic sinusitis.

Non-neuropathic Orofacial Pain of Central Origin

In separating pain into neuropathic (i.e., pain associated with a clinically demonstrable dysfunction of a peripheral nerve) and nonneuropathic categories, the entrance point of the dorsal roots of the cranial nerves into the brain is chosen as the dividing line between peripheral and central nervous systems. Pains caused by lesions affecting the intracranial but extrapontine or extramedullary portions of cranial nerves V, VII, IX, and X are classified as of neuropathic origin; those caused by pathologic processes in the brain and cord (i.e., the central nervous system) are referred to as nonneuropathic pains of central origin. Thus, if the lesion in trigeminal neuralgia is accepted as being in the gasserian ganglion or dorsal root of the 5th nerve, trigeminal neuralgia is classified as a neuropathic pain.

Much of the orofacial pain that results from intracranial tumors is also classified as neuropathic because it is usually only when tumors affect the cranial nerves and meninges that pain syndromes arise from this cause. As will be discussed below, space-occupying and vascular lesions within the brain do not usually produce classical orofacial syndromes even though they often cause other motor and sensory neurologic abnormalities in the orofacial area.

Neuronal Damage. Pain of central origin includes orofacial pain that is thought to result from neuronal damage in the central nervous system secondary to traumatic injury (and possibly other types of injury) to peripheral nerves. Evidence to support this etiology for chronic orofacial pain apparently not associated with a current extraneural painful focus comes from experiments in which section of sensory branches of the trigeminal nerve both distally and proximally to the gasserian ganglion was shown to lead to degenerative changes in neurons in the gasserian ganglion and in the sensory nucleus of the 5th nerve in the brain stem.

Although severed peripheral nerves usually regenerate grossly, selective loss of larger ganglion cells and their centrally projected fibers may still occur and cause loss of afferent inhibition of pain impulses carried by the intact smaller fiber components. Central pain of this type thus owes its origin to an original neuropathic process, but the pathologic state that results in the chronic pain experienced long after damage to the peripheral nerve has resolved resides at least partially in the brain stem.

Phantom Limb Pain. Phantom limb pain and causalgia (a persistent, burning sensation resulting from peripheral nerve trauma; associated with various phenomena and curable by stellate ganglion block) are thought to be examples of this type of nonneuropathic pain of central origin. Causalgia affecting the mouth and face is also referred to as minor reflex sympathetic dystrophy; it may follow quite minor oral surgery. Posttraumatic trigeminal neuralgias and some cases of atypical facial pain (see Chap. 17) have been postulated as having a similar pathogenesis.

Brain Tumor and Central Lesions. The possibility of a brain tumor or other central lesion should always be considered in the diagnosis of chronic orofacial pain, particularly if it is associated with other focal neurologic symptoms that gradually increase in severity and appear to involve multiple cranial nerves. However, orofacial pain is a quite infrequent presenting complaint for a central lesion, and it is only when a tumor spreads to involve the cranial nerves or actually arises in one of the cranial nerves that orofacial pain is likely to be experienced.

The classical triad of symptoms for a brain tumor are headache, vomiting, and choked disc, also referred to as *papilledema* (*i.e.,* swelling of the head of the optic nerve with engorgement of vessels and hemorrhage in the surrounding portion of the retina). These symptoms usually occur in association with other evidence of increased intracranial pressure, often with convulsive seizures, abnormal states of consciousness, mental symptoms, visual changes, and vasomotor phenomena as associated findings. The headache that affects 90% of patients with brain tumors is not specific for that diagnosis either by nature or location, but it rarely affects the lower half of the face. Such headache is also thought not to be caused by destruction of nerve pathways within the brain but by pressure and traction on intracranial blood vessels and the roots of the cranial nerves.

Tumors, vascular lesions, and other destructive lesions of the brain stem, pons, thalamus, and cerebrum, however, may cause other focal neurologic abnormalities in the orofacial area, and the physician or dentist called on to evaluate oral sensory and motor abnormalities of the orofacial region should be well aware of the possibility of central lesions when the patient presents with oral or facial hypesthesia, paresthesia or anesthesia, dysgeusia (see below), or paralysis of facial, masticatory and oropharyngeal muscles, whether these symptoms occur alone or in association with orofacial pain.

Other Causes of Pain of Central Origin. The lesions of the central nervous system that are associated with pain in the distribution of the trigeminal nerve include the *thalamic syndrome of Dejerine and Roussy,* which results from small tumors of the thalamus or vascular occlusion of the posterior inferior cerebral artery and is characterized by widely distributed sensory and motor abnormalities on the opposite side of the body to the lesion, as well as episodes of spontaneous and severe pain that can affect the orofacial area and are often accompanied by dysgeusia. *Wallenberg's syndrome,* caused by vascular occlusion of the posterior cerebellar artery, usually involves cranial nerves V, IX, and X; *syringobulbia,* tubelike cavitation affecting the medulla and cord, may interfere with pain fiber tracts; *tertiary neurosyphilis* or *tabes dorsalis,* is often associated with destruction of neurons and fiber tracts over wide areas of the brain and cord. *Multiple sclerosis* and the *Guillain–Barré syndrome,* if it affects the upper spinal cord are also associated with pain in the distribution of the trigeminal nerve.

These lesions constitute the rare exceptions to the general rule that lesions confined to the brain stem, pons, and various fiber tracts through to the cortex are only rarely associated with painful symptoms. Pain from these different lesions has no constant quality and often is described as "severe discomfort from mild stimuli," or an alteration of pain perception, rather than in terms of specific qualities. Specific orofacial pain syndromes are characteristically associated with these central lesions *only* when the pathologic process involves the centrally directed fibers arising in the gasserian ganglion, as they pass by way of the dorsal trigeminal root into the pons.

Orofacial Pain of Neuropathic Origin

A review of the literature on trigeminal sensory neuropathies reveals a long list of infectious, metabolic, immunologic (connective tissue diseases), traumatic, neoplastic, and toxic disease states that have been associated with chronic neuralgias of the orofacial area (see Table 16-1). Although less well studied and certainly rarer, neuralgias of cranial nerves VII, IX, and X probably have an equally extensive set of etiologies. The term *neuralgia* is used here to refer to any form of painful neuropathy (*i.e.*, chronic pain associated with a clinically demonstrable dysfunction of a sensory nerve supplying the affected area) and not to pain with any specific quality or temporal character. Some neuralgias are paroxysmal (*i.e.*, pain occurring in clearly defined episodes of sudden onset that are separated by pain-free periods), such as classical tic douloureux, also commonly referred to as *trigeminal neuralgia* (a practice that has led to the term *neuralgia* sometimes being restricted to the type of severe pain associated with that condition—a usage that is avoided here and in Chap. 17); others are nonparoxysmal. In general, there is no clear etiologic differentiation of a trigeminal neuralgia in terms of whether it is paroxysmal, classical tic douloureux, for example, being seen as either an essential or primary condition (*i.e.*, one that is not secondary to another lesion) or as secondary to an identifiable lesion or etiology. (The word *neuritis*, and the associated adjective, *neuritic*, both of which are also commonly used in describing pain of this type, should preferably be restricted to conditions in which inflammation of the nerve is clearly demonstrated.) *Tic*, as used in this context, refers to the dramatic onset and spasmodic quality of the pain in paroxysmal trigeminal neuralgias and to the reflex tensing of the facial musculature of the patient as he experiences the paroxysm. It does not imply an affection of motor nerves in addition to the primary sensory (pain fiber) abnormality.

Paroxysmal Pain of Neuropathic Origin

This type of pain may affect cranial nerves V, VII, IX, and X. There is much in common among these conditions (which are therefore sometimes grouped as the "major neuralgias") irrespective of the nerve involved. Since these pains usually affect the trigeminal nerve, the following discussion is focused on

Table 16-1. Disease States Associated with Orofacial Pain of Neuropathic Origin Affecting the Trigeminal Nerve

	DISEASE STATE
Connective Tissue Disease	Rheumatoid arthritis
	Sjögren's syndrome
	Polyarteritis nodosa
	Disseminated lupus erythematosus
	Scleroderma
	Progressive hemifacial atrophy
	Amyloidosis
Infectious Disease	Neurosyphilis
	Leprosy
	Herpes zoster
	Fungus infections
	Sarcoidosis
Metabolic Disease	Diabetes mellitus
	Hypovitaminosis B
	Chronic alcoholism
	Pernicious anemia
Intoxications	Heavy metal poisoning (As, Pb, Hg, Cd)
	Drug intoxications (digitalis, penicillin, steroids, stilbamadine)
	Acute alcoholic intoxication
	Organic chemical intoxications (acrylamide, aminopyrine, phenylbutazone)
Tumors	Trigeminal neurinoma
	Meningioma
	Metastatic neoplasia
	Neurofibromatosis
	Neurilemmoma including acoustic neurinoma
	Tuberculoma
Trauma	Anesthesia dolorosa
	Traumatic neuroma
	Extracranial nerve trauma

(Modified from Gregg JM: Post-traumatic pain: Experimental trigeminal neuropathy. J Oral Surg 29:260, 1971. This paper includes an extensive bibliography on trigeminal sensory neuropathy.)

paroxysmal trigeminal neuralgia or tic douloureux, with brief comments following on paroxysmal neuralgias of cranial nerves VII, IX, and X.

Tic Douloureux. Tic douloureux is a particularly well-defined pain syndrome, the severe and dramatic nature of which usually results in its rapid diagnosis and treatment by a neurologist, neurosurgeon, or general medical practitioner. In fact, the availability of medications for the control of this condition appears to have reduced the number of patients who are referred to specialty clinics because of this condition; and those that are referred often have an atypical form of the syndrome, have not responded well to medication, or require additional psychiatric or medical management. In its classical form, tic douloureux has the following features:

1. It is a pain with a characteristic quality. It is a recurrent pain of great severity and intensity that causes the patient extreme agony and obliterates all other concerns while it is present; but it is also a pain of short duration. It is described as like an electric shock and as one of the worst pains that can be experienced. It may be preceded on occasions by brief, minor electric shocklike intimations, but the intense paroxysm of pain itself is abrupt in onset. Some residual mild aching or burning may follow the paroxysm, and the patient is usually exhausted and in a shocklike state for some time after the episode. The characteristic feature is that between the brief episodes the patient is completely free of pain, often for days or months at a time.

2. The pain is limited to the anatomic distribution of the affected nerve (although more than one division of the trigeminal nerve may be affected simultaneously), and between episodes no motor or sensory deficit should be demonstrable in the affected nerve, provided the condition has not previously been treated by nerve section or injection of anesthetic or sclerosing agents.

3. The pain episodes are often initiated by minor sensory stimuli to the skin or mucous membrane supplied by the affected nerve. Small areas that consistently give rise to paroxysms of pain when stimulated in this fashion are referred to as *trigger zones,* and although not always present in tic douloureux, they are almost diagnostic when they are present. Trigger zones should, however, be clearly distinguished from areas of point tenderness over unabsorbed, postsurgical bony spicules of the alveolus and from tender nodules along the superficial course of a nerve,

palpation of which often produces a sharp, shooting pain along the nerve. Such pain, although abrupt in onset and often severe enough to cause the patient to jerk away or to bring tears to his eyes, lacks the severity of the paroxysm experienced in tic douloureux.

4. Many cases of tic douloureux respond quite well to treatment with carbamazepine (Tegretol), but the course of the disease is unpredictable and pain of increasing frequency and longer duration may develop over the years in some patients. Current practice is to attempt treatment with carbamazepine, phenytoin (Dilantin), and various psychotropic drugs (see Chap. 17) and to resort to anesthetic injections about the gasserian ganglion or to surgical section of the nerve, only when nonsurgical measures fail.

Paroxysmal trigeminal neuralgia of this type may be either idiopathic or symptomatic (*i.e.,* the result of a tumor, vascular abnormality, or other process affecting the root of the 5th nerve). Such tumors may arise intracranially or they may be the result of metastasis or direct spread of a nasopharyngeal carcinoma, for example.

Pain that is indistinguishable from that of tic douloureux is reported in multiple sclerosis and is believed to be caused by sclerotic changes about the centrally directed fibers of the 5th nerve as they enter the pons. It follows, therefore, that the differential diagnosis of tic douloureux should include the long list of conditions that can damage the root of the 5th nerve, and alcohol injections or surgery should not be carried out until a full investigation to rule out these possibilities has been completed.

Unfortunately, as emphasized in Chapter 17, small carcinomas may be virtually undetectable in the nasal sinuses and may invade the cranial cavity and produce trigeminal neuralgia before being detected. As often as not, however, intracranial neoplasms will cause other cranial nerve abnormalities in addition to the symptoms of tic douloureux. Lesions confined to the brain stem and pons do not cause tic douloureux.

Considerable controversy still exists concerning the pathogenesis of "idiopathic" tic douloureux (*i.e.,* tic douloureux with no obvious cause) and whether the focus causing the characteristic paroxysms of severe pain is located in the gasserian ganglion, in the dorsal root of the 5th nerve, or in the thalamus or brain stem. There is, however, a strong body of evidence to support a peripheral (*i.e.,* intracranial, but not within the central nervous system) location for the focus. Some neurosurgeons who use an approach that allows them to visualize the dorsal root of the trigeminal nerve in the posterior cranial fossa, rather than the more conventional approach through the middle cranial fossa, report that all patients with this problem have been found to have a vascular abnormality, neoplasm, or sclerotic lesion compressing or distorting the dorsal root at its entry into the pons. Others have noted a demyelinating lesion within the ganglion and dorsal root that possibly allows short-circuiting of impulses that may cause the characteristic episodes of acute flashing pain.

Treatment. Carbamazepine (Tegretol) anticonvulsant appears to have a specific effect on the pain of tic douloureux, which because of its severity, abrupt onset, and brief duration is not amenable to treatment with analgesics or psychotropic medications. The success rate of treatment with carbamazepine is quoted as 65% to 100%, depending on whether the series of patients were those referred to a neurologist or those treated by general practitioners, the latter generally reporting better success rates. This drug does not cure the disease; it only prevents the episodes of severe convulsive pain, so as a rule, administration must be continued throughout the patient's life.

Opinions seem to vary as to the relapse rate under treatment, although it is often stated that carbamazepine appears to be less successful for this condition than it was first thought to be when introduced in the early 1960s. Dizziness, nausea, somnolence, skin rashes, and especially leukopenia may complicate and even prevent its use for some patients. In young patients who may need to use the drug for 20 years or more, surgical treatment is often considered more desirable.

Surgical treatment includes injection of hot water and alcohol into the region of the gasserian ganglion, as well as percutaneous radiofrequency treatment of the ganglion. Recurrences of the problem after an initial period of freedom from pain are common with these forms of treatment, and recourse is often made to section of the affected branch of the trigeminal nerve as it leaves the cranium or to rhizotomy or retrogasserian section of the dorsal root. In either case, anesthesia of a considerable part of the face and oral cavity develops, a problem that some patients tolerate very poorly. Factitial, destructive lesions often result from this approach because of the inability of the patient to avoid picking or chewing the permanently numb area. The consistent finding of a lesion compressing the dorsal root as a result of the posterior fossa approach has reawakened interest in the effectiveness of decompression techniques that leave the dorsal root and trigeminal sensation more or less intact.

Geniculate Neuralgia. Geniculate neuralgia (*i.e.,* paroxysmal neuralgia affecting the nervus intermedius, the sensory root of cranial nerve VII) is said to be characterized by pain with the quality of tic douloureux that is localized deep in the ear. It is an exceptionally rare condition according to most authors.

Glossopharyngeal Neuralgia. Glossopharyngeal neuralgia (9th nerve tic), by contrast, has a definite literature describing it, although it is a much less frequent problem than is paroxysmal trigeminal neuralgia. The paroxysmal pain in this case is felt in the ear, tonsil, side of the tongue, and lateral wall of larynx and pharynx and is usually triggered by swallowing or yawning. Palpation of the oropharynx may initiate an episode. Pain of similar character is also described in *styloid process syndrome,* thought to be caused by pressure on the glossopharyngeal nerve by an elongated or a fractured styloid process. Surgical reduction of the styloid process via the lateral wall of the pharynx is sometimes undertaken in this condition. It should be pointed out, however, that inequalities in the length of the right and left styloid processes are common, and the finding of an elongated styloid process does not necessarily mean it is the cause of pain of this type.

Similar pain may be associated with tumors

and stones in the submandibular gland, tumors in the wall of the pharynx, and with temporomandibular myofascial dysfunction. The possibility of these conditions must be eliminated before a diagnosis of glossopharyngeal neuralgia is accepted. Local application of strong topical anesthetic agents to the trigger zone may aid these patients. Section of the 9th nerve produces ageusia and anesthesia to the posterior third of the tongue on the affected side and may cause difficulty in deglutition. Glossopharyngeal neuralgia may be accompanied by symptoms related to the vagus (cranial nerve X), and syncope and even cardiac arrest may accompany the episodes of pain.

Superior laryngeal neuralgia is another rare form of paroxysmal neuralgia affecting a branch of the 10th cranial nerve, with symptoms localized in the upper part of the larynx, as well as the zygoma, ear, and upper thorax.

Nonparoxysmal Pain of Neuropathic Origin

Pain that lacks the temporal and electric shocklike qualities of tic douloureux is referred to as nonparoxysmal pain. Such pains, when of neuropathic origin, are usually well localized, and the patient can identify the affected area consistently and accurately. Infiltrations and regional blocking with local anesthetic solutions usually allow the site of the painful focus to be identified; however, trigger zones are not a feature of these pains. Such pains are to be distinguished from the poorly localized, deep dull aching sensations commonly associated with many atypical facial pains (see Chap. 17), the throbbing pain of vascular origin, and the pain of myofascial origin, many of which are referred away from the primary painful focus. In the tongue, they must be distinguished from the continuous burning sensation of glossodynia (also described in Chap. 17).

Nonparoxysmal pain of neuropathic origin may develop over a long period of time in patients with tic douloureux as episodes get longer and more frequent and gradually merge, but such a history is unusual. Nonparoxysmal neuropathic pain usually develops following clearly defined episodes such as surgical or other trauma involving branches of the trigeminal nerves, viral infections, use of particular drugs, or heavy metal intoxication. Other cases bear a clear relationship to the development of tumors, granulomatous lesions, or other infiltrations that can be shown to involve branches of the trigeminal nerve. Others occur in patients with evidences of neuropathy elsewhere in the body, as a result of diabetes mellitus, chronic alcoholism, or other intoxications.

Depending on the particular etiology involved, nonparoxysmal neuropathic pain may be continuous or subject to periods of more severe exacerbation. Such periods of increased severity may relate to the particular lesion involved (*e.g.,* the wearing of a denture in a patient with a superficial neuroma or easily traumatized branch of the mental nerve on the crest of a heavily resorbed mandibular alveolus) or to psychological factors affecting tolerance for such pain when it is of long standing. However, even when the clinical situation is complicated by either anxiety or depression, the remarkable nature of nonparoxysmal neuropathic pain is its reasonableness, the clear association of stimulus, region of nerve damage, and anatomical distribution of symptoms.

Diagnosis of pain of this category requires clinical demonstration of a dysfunction involving the affected nerve. Such evidence may be a clinical history of decreased sensation, numbness, or pricking sensation in an anatomically related area; a complaint of taste aberration related to the anterior half of the tongue on the same side when the lingual nerve is involved; or a similar evidence of altered nerve function obtained by sensory nerve testing or taste testing (see Chap. 2). Palpation of the superficial course of the nerve may detect a nodule that can represent scar formation, a neuroma, or other lesion involving the nerve.

Radiographic examination of the jaws may demonstrate the presence of a lesion involving the mandibular nerve or its branches, or the history may include convincing evidence of trauma to the nerve, such as surgical exploration of the retromolar triangle, jaw fracture, removal of a deeply impacted tooth, curettage of a periapical lesion, or injury to the lingual nerve during dental treatment. Diagnostic nerve blocking usually also produces clear-cut evidence for the location of the painful focus (compare with atypical facial pain, see Chap. 17).

Posttraumatic Pain. Posttraumatic pain frequently exhibits the characteristic features just outlined for nonparoxysmal pain of neuropathic origin and represents the largest subcategory (over 30% of one series) within this grouping. The majority of patients give a history of a prior dental surgical procedure that is described as difficult or with subsequent complication. Usually the pain involves only one division of the trigeminal nerve, unless the trauma was such that the likelihood of involvement of both maxillary and mandibular branches is great.

Posttraumatic pain follows removal of impacted teeth with such frequency that patients should be warned of the close anatomic relationship of the mandibular nerve and the roots of the mandibular teeth and the risk of this complication. The damage to the nerve may result in little more than prolonged paresthesia and a pins-and-needles sensation, although alteration in taste sensation and sensation of temperature changes or dryness in the lip and cheek may be experienced. Even when unaccompanied by pain, such symptoms, if chronic, can be sufficiently distressing to cause the patient to seek repeated consultation.

Not all complaints of this type are caused by detectable neuroma formation (*i.e.* proliferative changes involving nerve elements and sheath cells at the site of nerve damage), and radiographic examination of the mandible will only occasionally reveal a bony lesion that can account for the neuropathy. In the absence of clear evidence for the presence of a lesion impinging on the nerve, exploratory surgery, such as examination of the retromolar fossa or repeated curettage of an apparently well-healed tooth socket, is rarely justified and frequently further complicates both diagnosis and treatment.

Many sensory abnormalities of this type gradually improve, with slow disappearance of the pain and increased paresthesia and tingling often signaling return to normal sensation. Small areas of numbness may be the sole abnormality after several months have passed. Loss of sensation in the lower lip produces a functional abnormality similar to that seen following the usual mandibular block regional anesthetic injection. Loss of proprioceptive sensation prevents the lip being closely adapted to the teeth, and apparent drooping or laxness of the lip may be mistakenly interpreted as a facial paralysis. Areas of diminished sensation to pinprick or graded von Frey hairs may be detected by comparing skin and mucous membrane on the affected and unaffected sides.

The terms *causalgia* and *posttraumatic pain* are often used interchangeably; however, causalgia usually implies the presence of some associated autonomic phenomena that are not usually a feature of posttraumatic pain (*i.e.*, all pain that follows trauma is not necessarily accurately classified as posttraumatic pain). Anesthetic blocking of the superior cervical ganglion (stellate ganglion block) is described as specific treatment for causalgia. Posttraumatic pain, if mild, is treated with local electric or mechanical stimulation to the affected area, with systemically administered analgesics, hypnosis, acupuncture, and even a course with carbamazepine, phenytoin, or tricyclic antidepressants if the pain is prolonged and accompanied by a noticeable depressive reaction.

In rare cases, section of the affected nerve proximal to the suspected painful focus may be attempted. As discussed earlier (see Nonneuropathic Pain of Central Origin), some posttraumatic pain may include abnormal sensation arising from a lesion affecting neurons in the central nervous system that resulted from an original traumatic episode to a peripheral nerve. In such cases, section of the nerve may not be successful in completely removing the pain.

Postviral Orofacial Pain. A variety of oral sensory abnormalities including quite severe pain, usually of a nonparoxysmal type, can occur during or following viral infections and are thought to be caused by direct neuronal damage by the virus. Viruses such as herpes zoster and herpes simplex produce these and other neurologic problems (*e.g.*, encephalitis) so frequently, that they are sometimes classified as *neurotrophic viruses.*

The term *postherpetic pain* refers to the occurrence of pain over the distribution of a branch of a related sensory nerve (usually the 5th nerve in the orofacial area, but occasionally the 7th nerve also, producing a geniculate neuralgia) that commences during an episode of herpes zoster or a short time thereafter. Classically, the skin and mucous membrane vesicles that identify herpes zoster are arranged along the superficial distribution of the sensory branch of a nerve, and this picture may be seen in trigeminal zoster (see Fig. 16-6). The focus of viral reproduction for this infection is the associated trigeminal sensory ganglion.

Postherpetic pain of this type, whether experienced (more commonly) in association with zoster of a spinal nerve or as trigeminal zoster, is frequently a very severe and continuously aching pain that may continue in this fashion for several weeks or months. Narcotic analgesics are often required to control pain of this type, particularly in adults. Postherpetic pain is surprisingly rare in children with zoster or the related infection, chickenpox. Herpes zoster is usually a nonrecurrent infection except in immunologically compromised patients; however, episodes of postherpetic pain do recur in immunologically competent individuals, and persistent infection or damage to the ganglion cells is accepted as the explanation for repeated and more or less identical episodes of pain even if only the first episode was associated with skin lesions of herpes zoster.

Pain of very similar character can also complicate oral infections with herpes simplex virus (primary herpetic gingivostomatitis, recurrent herpes labialis, and recurrent intraoral herpes). Recent studies of excised sensory ganglia (including the trigeminal ganglion) maintained in organ culture have confirmed that ganglion cells are a likely source of herpes simplex virus for recurrent herpetic infections. At the time of such recurrences, the virus rapidly travels along perineuronal lymphatics to the oral mucosa and skin and becomes manifest as skin vesicles or tiny clustered mouth ulcers or is simply excreted in the oral cavity. It is therefore not difficult to understand why patients occasionally complain of pain along the distribution of one of the branches of the trigeminal nerve with an episode of oral herpes, viral infection of the trigeminal ganglion presumably causing the pain. However, recurrent oral herpes is a very prevalent infection, and it is risky to identify a neuralgia as postherpetic simply because the patient gets recurrent herpes from time to time. Additional evidence, such as the occurrence of vesicles or characteristic mouth ulcers along with the episodes of pain or demonstration of herpes simplex virus in oral secretions at this time is needed to make a definite diagnosis.

Nonparoxysmal Pain of Neuropathic Origin Due to a Neoplasm. Facial neuralgia should always be thought of as possibly the result of a hidden neoplasm, until some other convincing explanation is found and a thorough search has been made to rule out the existence of such a lesion. Pain as a result of pressure on or invasion of a branch of the trigeminal nerve has no characteristic quality except that it is unlikely to be paroxysmal unless the sensory root of the trigeminal nerve is involved. More often than not, once the lesion is identified and the extent of involvement of the nerve clearly defined, the distribution of the pain will be found to be logical. However, small tumors of unknown location, especially those involving the intracranial and immediate extracranial course of

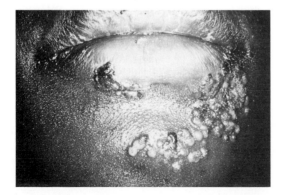

Fig. 16-6 Herpes zoster affecting the mandibular branch of the 5th cranial nerve. The crop of vesicles is often associated with severe neuralgic pain originating in sensory neurons of the 5th nerve in the gasserian ganglion that are infected with the neurotropic varicella virus. Episodes of neuralgic pain may continue for many months after healing of the skin lesion.

the 5th nerve, may produce quite inexplicable symptoms. Lesions in the following locations, in particular, are commonly associated with trigeminal pain of neuropathic origin.

Tumors of the Parotid Gland. Tumors in the deeper portion of the parotid gland may extend medially and upward to involve branches of the trigeminal nerve, often with no damage to the facial nerve, which runs a superficial course over the lateral surface of the gland. Usually, retrograde sialography or sometimes sequential salivary scintigraphy will reveal such a lesion.

Tumors of the Nasopharynx. These small tumors of the upper nasopharynx may be quite difficult to detect, and only when they lead to bony destruction will they become apparent in tomographic radiographs. By this time, damage to the trigeminal nerve as it leaves the cranium, or even intracranial spread of the tumor, may have occurred. It is not unusual for repeated otorhinologic consultations to be normal and for the trigeminal neuralgia or associated chronic sensory abnormality to be the only evidence of such tumors until they reach considerable size with local invasion and even metastasis. Similar symptoms may arise from nonneoplastic granulomatous masses and infiltrations such as amyloidosis, sarcoidosis and tuberculosis if they develop in association with the trigeminal nerve.

Cerebellopontine Angle Tumors. These tumors (acoustic neurinomas) are usually neurofibromas or neurilemmomas of the 8th (auditory) nerve, the various terms often being used interchangeably. The majority of these tumors develop within the temporal bone along the course of the vestibular division of the auditory nerve, from where they spread intracranially to occupy the space between the brain and cranium. Because of the close anatomic relationship of the roots of the cranial nerves (Cr) 5, 6, 7, 8, and 9 (see Fig. 16-7), several nerves are usually affected by the tumor, which will also compress the brain stem and cerebellum as it enlarges. Cerebellopontine angle tumors are usually histologically benign and slow growing, and symptoms are often present for many months or years before the diagnosis is made.

Acoustic neurinomas can occur as solitary lesions (usually with onset of symptoms in the third to sixth decades and with a tendency to female predominance) or as part of a generalized neurofibromatosis (see Chap. 8). The most common symptoms reported by patients with this tumor are deafness, headache, tinnitus, and loss of balance (nerve involvement of Cr 8), but hypesthesias and paresthesias of the face (Cr 5) and blurred or double vision (Cr 6) are also experienced. The 5th cranial nerve is affected in about 50% of cases, and careful neurologic testing will often show evidence of hypesthesia of the trigeminal sensory areas or weakness of the masticatory muscles. Severe neuralgia or tic douloureux are not common symptoms, and only rarely is pain in the trigeminal area a presenting symptom. Involvement of cranial nerve IX produces gustatory abnormality as well as sensory loss in the oropharynx and posterior two-thirds of the tongue.

Similar symptoms (cerebellopontine angle syndrome) may be produced by other tumors in this location (*e.g.*, meningiomas, gliomas) as well as cysts and aneurysms. Acoustic neurinomas, like nerve sheath cell tumors elsewhere, are not radiosensitive, and the only successful treatment is surgical excision of the lesion either in part or in toto, with surgical anastomosis of cranial nerves VII and XII to correct deformity caused by facial paralysis (as is sometimes done in the treatment of facial paralysis from other causes, such as Bell's palsy).

CONDITIONS TO CONSIDER IN THE DIFFERENTIAL DIAGNOSIS OF DYSGEUSIA

Dysgeusic syndromes (*i.e.*, conditions causing complaints such as complete loss of taste, diminished taste sensitivity, altered taste, and persistent bad tastes) will be discussed here.

Dysgeusia of Non-neuropathic Origin

Non-neuropathic Dysgeusia of Extraneural Origin

This type of dysgeusia is caused by abnormal compounds in mixed saliva in the oral cavity. Since the sensation of taste in humans is

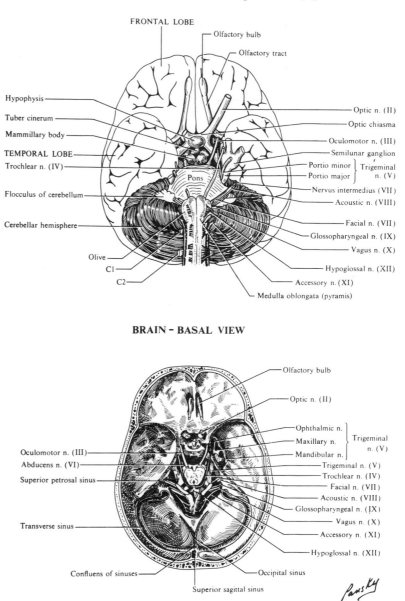

FRONTAL LOBE

Olfactory bulb

Olfactory tract

Hypophysis

Tuber cinerum

Mammillary body

TEMPORAL LOBE

Trochlear n. (IV)

Flocculus of cerebellum

Cerebellar hemisphere

Olive

C1

C2

Pons

Optic n. (II)

Optic chiasma

Oculomotor n. (III)

Semilunar ganglion

Portio minor

Portio major

Trigeminal n. (V)

Nervus intermedius (VII)

Acoustic n. (VIII)

Facial n. (VII)

Glossopharyngeal n. (IX)

Vagus n. (X)

Hypoglossal n. (XII)

Accessory n. (XI)

Medulla oblongata (pyramis)

BRAIN – BASAL VIEW

Olfactory bulb

Optic n. (II)

Ophthalmic n.

Maxillary n.

Mandibular n.

Trigeminal n. (V)

Oculomotor n. (III)

Abducens n. (VI)

Superior petrosal sinus

Transverse sinus

Confluens of sinuses

Superior sagittal sinus

Trigeminal n. (V)

Trochlear n. (IV)

Facial n. (VII)

Acoustic n. (VIII)

Glossopharyngeal n. (IX)

Vagus n. (X)

Accessory n. (XI)

Hypoglossal n. (XII)

Occipital sinus

Fig. 16-7 Basal view of the brain showing the origins of the cranial nerves and the close relationship of the roots of cranial nerves V, VII, X, and XII. (Pansky B, House EL: Review of Gross Anatomy, A Dynamic Approach. New York, Macmillan, 1964)

BRAIN STEM AND CRANIAL NERVES
IN RELATION TO SKULL

largely concerned with substances introduced into the mouth (rather than with those contacted by the extruded tongue), the unexpected development of an unusual or unpleasant taste that is not directly associated with ingestion or introduction of some object into the mouth will usually be perceived as an abnormality, and if it persists, as evidence of a disease state. Such dysgeusic symptoms may, of course, develop as a result of damage to those parts of the peripheral and central nervous systems concerned with taste sensation, but they are equally likely to result from the appearance of abnormal compounds in the saliva. It is the belief that their dysgeusia arises from some such compound and the expectation that dental treatment will remove it, that seems to motivate many dysgeusic patients to consult a dentist for their problem. Substances with unpleasant or unusual tastes are produced in the mouth as the result of bacterial fermentations in dental plaque and the gingival crevice, but they are certainly not restricted to this source. A more complete list of potential sources includes the following:

1. Abnormal oral secretions (crevicular fluid and exudates from periodontal pockets; fluids discharged from cysts and abscesses; exudates from extraction sockets and surgical wounds; nasal, tonsillar, and other respiratory secretions that enter the oral cavity)
2. Alterations in the oral microbial flora associated with specific endogenous infections such as candidiasis and acute necrotizing gingivostomatitis and nonspecific bacterial proliferations such as coated tongue
3. Abnormal secretions from major or minor salivary glands as the result of xerostomia; sialadenitis; and drugs, metabolic intermediates and other compounds excreted in saliva or rapidly transferred across the oral mucosa from the local vasculature (e.g., iodides, certain industrial metallic poisons, glucose, urea, saccharin, and calcium gluconate)
4. Metallic dental restorations or prostheses that contribute silver and mercuric salts to saliva or create a sensation of a metallic taste by galvanic stimulation of taste receptors from contact between dissimilar metals
5. Blocking of palatal taste receptors by full dentures (diminished taste sensitivity often reported by full denture wearers may be due more to the decreased oral handling time for food that is characteristic of denture wearers than to blocking of taste receptors, however)

The literature contains case reports attesting to this wide range of oral abnormalities that may be associated with dysgeusic symptoms. The complaints of patients with these problems do not always specify the presence of a persistent bad taste, and equally frequently the complaint may be one of diminished taste sensitivity for familiar foods. The majority of these conditions have received only scanty investigation, however, and it is not known in what way the presence of unusual substances interferes with the physiology of taste sensation.

If removal of the suspected offending substance is followed by disappearance of the symptom, it is generally assumed that it has been acting only through an extraneural mechanism. Such arguments, however, do not eliminate the possibility that many such substances, especially when they circulate in the bloodstream, may have a transient effect on the neurologic components of the taste system as well. The sensitivity of the taste system is also probably under involuntary control, so that maximal attention can be given to the perception of familiar substances in foods and little attention paid to the taste of saliva in the oral cavity.

No doubt this system may also allow minor persistent unusual tastes to be tolerated and not even perceived by some patients. The existence of such a tuning mechanism in the taste system seems necessary to explain the ability of many to tolerate a dentition that is thickly covered with plaque and calculus and surrounded by draining periodontal pockets.

The symptoms reported by patients whose dysgeusia appears to arise through this extraneural mechanism are variable. Complete loss of taste (ageusia) does not usually appear to be due to this cause, but loss of taste for particular qualities (e.g., sweet, salt) is sometimes reported. Here again, clinical testing data are rarely available to confirm whether such complaints are associated with specific diminished taste sensitivity under controlled taste-testing conditions.

Patients may complain that the unusual taste is foreign and not usually one associated with food, but a persistent sweet, salty, sour, or bitter taste that is experienced irrespective of the presence or absence of food may also be perceived as dysgeusia by the patient. In a few cases, specific association of a characteristic taste and a particular source seems to exist (e.g., the metallic taste caused by iodides), but there are inadequate data to allow a diagnosis of the cause of the dysgeusia to be made from its reported quality. The complaint may also be that a particular food or drink has acquired a specific unpleasant taste. This phenomena may be noted with extraneural, nonneuropathic dysgeusia associated with use of some drugs, but for the majority of the 250 or more proprietary medications reported to cause dysgeusia or xerostomia, data to suggest a consistent association between a specific dysgeusic symptom and one of a family of drugs do not appear to exist.

A dental consultation concerning a complaint of dysgeusia should include a review of each of these possible causes of an extraneural problem, and where plaque, dental caries, gingivitis, periodontal disease, candidiasis, or other potential oral source for the complaint is present, it should be eliminated and the effect on the symptom noted. Oral examination should include the salivary glands and oropharynx, and where a nasal or bronchial source is suspected, appropriate medical consultation should be made.

Nonneuropathic Dysgeusia of Central Origin

The central pathways of the gustatory branches of cranial nerves VII, IX, and X involve synapses at three levels within the brain: the medulla, the thalamus, and the cerebral cortex. At the level of the medulla and the thalamus in man (see Fig. 16-8), there is little interaction between the afferent fibers and second-order neurons on one side of the brain and those on the other; however, in passing to the cortex (where two principal taste areas have been identified), the third-order neurons pass to both the ipsilateral and contralateral sides of the cortex. Small lesions of the thalamus and medulla that affect the gustatory fiber tracts may be associated with taste loss affecting a single quadrant of the tongue; cortical lesions affecting taste are more likely to result in a more uniform defect of all taste areas. The cortical taste area is closely associated with the cortical olfactory area, and lesions of the cortex (usually temporal lobe lesions that result from trauma) may lead to loss of both olfactory and gustatory acuity or to unusual sensations of both taste and odor.

Hypogeusia and parageusia are rarely presenting complaints that lead to the recognition of brain damage, although the literature does contain occasional references to cases in which some dysgeusic symptom was the clue that led to a confirmed diagnosis of brain damage (e.g., the case of Cohen, in whom dysgeusia led to a diagnosis of multiple scle-

rosis). More frequently, dysgeusia is one of several symptoms that appear together or in sequence as the central nervous system (CNS) disease progresses. The onset of the dysgeusic symptoms may be quite dramatic, as following head trauma, brain surgery, a seizure or cerebrovascular accident, or they may develop gradually with the patient unaware for some time of decreased taste acuity. The importance of taste sensation to many people is underlined by the fact that patients with chronic neurologic problems will sometimes seek specific treatment for their dysgeusia or ageusia even though it is only one of several sensory or motor deficits they have.

Certainly the diagnostician must always consider the possibility that a patient's dysgeusic symptoms may arise from some CNS disease; and his index of suspicion will always be higher if the patient has other evidence of CNS disease or has evidence in his history of events (e.g., head trauma) or other diseases (e.g., syphilis, tuberculosis, vasculitis) that may be complicated by lesions of the CNS. On occasion, it may be difficult to confirm the existence of a lesion in a specific part of the CNS that would justify the patient's symptoms, even though all evidence points to the existence of such a lesion.

Among the diseases of the central nervous system that are often associated with dysgeusia, mention should be made of head trauma, particularly when it leads to damage to the temporal lobes of the cortex; vascular diseases such as strokes, cerebral arteriosclerosis and occlusions and infarcts of the thalamus (see discussion of thalamic syndrome earlier in this chapter); brain tumors; tertiary syphilis; multiple sclerosis; and a particular form of epilepsy referred to as uncinate seizures.

Both gustatory and olfactory abnormalities can follow severe head trauma, and it is difficult to explain the simultaneous appearance of these two sensory anomalies on the basis of intracranial damage to specific cranial nerves because of the anatomic separation of the peripheral nerves concerned with taste and smell. (We are not concerned here with the apparent loss of taste that many complain of as a result of olfactory damage, but with patients in whom detailed olfactory and gus-

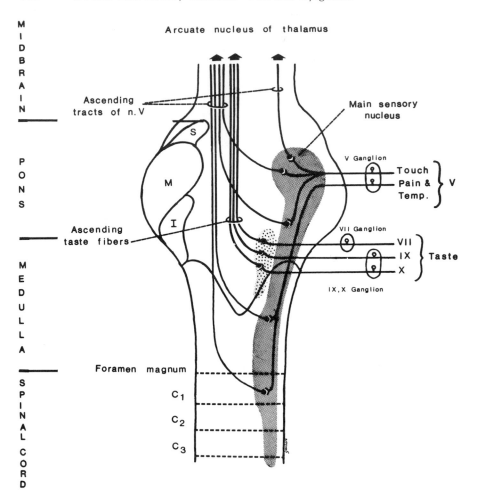

Fig. 16-8 Diagrammatic representation of afferent nerves (for taste, touch, pain, and temperature sensations) from oral mucosa to their first synapse in the brain stem and spinal cord. The spinal nucleus of the trigeminal nerve is darkly shaded and extends from the main sensory nucleus in the pons caudally to approximately the level of C3 or C4. The nucleus Solitarius, shaded lightly, contains the first synapse for afferent taste fibers. S,M,I-superior, middle, and inferior cerebellar peduncles. (Farbman AI, Allgood JP: Innervation, sensory receptors and sensitivity of the oral mucosa. In Squier CA, Meyer J [eds]: Current Concepts of the Histology of the Oral Mucosa. Springfield, Ill., Charles C Thomas, 1971)

tatory testing reveals diminished sensitivity in both systems.) Lesions that lead to combined loss of olfactory and gustatory sensitivity are usually located in the temporal lobe, which may be damaged during head injury by pressure against the greater wing of the sphenoid bone or directly as the result of penetrating wounds in the side of the head.

Trauma, vascular lesions, and small tumors that affect this part of the temporal lobe of the cerebral cortex (which is referred to as the *uncinate gyrus*) may result in an unusual form of epilepsy characterized by the sensation of peculiar odors and tastes. Known as uncinate epilepsy, the problem is usually of petit mal type, and the patient may not lose consciousness with the seizure. Sometimes involuntary movements of the tongue and lips are described, as though the patient were savoring the taste of something in the mouth.

Alternatively, the peculiar odor and taste sensation may come as an aura or prelude to the seizure. The peculiar odor and taste may have a familiar association for the patient (*e.g.*, the odor of burning food; taste of spoiled milk) but is usually not described in terms of a single taste quality. Treatment of the patient with phenytoin or other anticonvulsant medications usually decreases the frequency of seizures and may eliminate the problem. Symptoms of this type justify a thorough search for small tumors or vascular lesions in the temporal lobe.

The treatment of dysgeusic symptoms that result from brain lesions is essentially the treatment of the lesion itself. In many cases, such symptoms are not curable, even when the lesion is discrete and amenable to surgical removal.

Dysgeusia of Neuropathic Origin

Specific gustatory sensations are transmitted by well-defined branches of only three cranial nerves (VII, IX, and X) or four, if the trigeminal nerve is included. (The lingual branch of nerve V carries within its sheath but does not anastomose with the gustatory fibers from the anterior third of the tongue that pass into the chorda tympani.) Lesions affecting these nerves usually produce fairly well-localized taste abnormalities. There is little anastomosis between the nerves supplying the right and left sides of the anterior third of the tongue, but some communication in the midline area of the vallate papillae is described in humans. Anteroposterior anastomoses across the row of vallate papillae are unusual.

Dysgeusia of neuropathic origin therefore includes lesions of the taste receptors on the dorsum of the tongue and to a lesser extent on the soft palate and oropharynx; lesions of the lingual nerve; lesions of the chorda tympani and facial nerve, and lesions of the glossopharyngeal and vagus nerves. (The clinician also must always be aware of the possibility that a complaint of altered taste sensation is in reality due to an olfactory problem, to loss of general trigeminal sensation, or to nongustatory stimulation of lingual sensory receptors, as was discussed earlier in this chapter. Neuropathy affecting the olfactory and trigeminal nerves, other than

the lingual branch of the trigeminal is not considered here.)

As a result of the well-localized nature of many dysgeusias of neuropathic origin, the patient may be only faintly aware of or completely unaware of altered taste sensitivity. In general, the perception of taste is concerned with a complex of sensations from various parts of the mouth, which combine to provide an appreciation of taste for the portions of food taken into the mouth, as well as for the bolus of food and saliva. During eating, food is moved about in the mouth, and the entire oral cavity is quickly coated with tastant molecules dissolved in saliva, so that decreased sensitivity in one area may not be appreciated by the patient when taste sensations elsewhere in the mouth continue to be strong. Likewise, clinical taste testing in such patients may fail to reveal an abnormality if a rinsing technique is used or if the patient is allowed to mix the drops of tastant with saliva before reporting the taste sensation experienced. Some patients seem able to analyze their oral sensations with more accuracy, and they may notice and seek diagnosis and treatment for quite localized hypogeusia.

Anomalies of Taste Receptors

Anomalies of taste receptors can be either congenital or acquired. The best known example of congenital ageusia is that associated with *familial dysautonomia*, a relatively rare disorder, more common in Jews, in which the inability to taste is only one of a series of abnormalities related to defective metabolism of acetylcholine. Affected children are usually hypotonic, easily disturbed, and exhibit excessive sweat and mucus production. The tongues of these children show a characteristic anomaly of absent vallate and fungiform papillae, the tongue being devoid of taste receptors.

Congenital abnormality of the taste buds is also postulated in the rare syndrome known as *aglycogeusia* (in which the affected individual is unable to distinguish sugar solutions from water), which has also been linked by some authors with the defective taste sensitivity sometimes reported by patients with *pseudohypoparathyroidism*. Patients with gonadal dysgenesis and various other congenitally acquired syndromes involving facial hypoplasia and palatal clefts are also reported to experience hypogeusia, but the taste bud has not been confirmed as the site of the lesion underlying these problems.

Taste bud cells are continually being replaced in the lingual epithelium as the result of a trophic influence from the gustatory nerve, and section of the gustatory nerve (the various causes of which are discussed in the following paragraphs) leads to atrophy and disappearance of taste buds.

A variety of lesions affecting the tongue may also result in destruction of taste buds. Glossitis, as a result of vitamin B deficiency, iron deficiency, and extensive white lesions of the oral mucosa (such as lichen planus and leukoplakia) may produce such changes. Xerostomia, whether drug-induced or the result of salivary gland disease, is commonly associated with a complaint of dysgeusia, partly as a result of destruction of taste buds in the dry atrophic mucosa and partly as a result of nonneuropathic causes, such as the absence of saliva to dissolve tastant molecules and development of thrush.

The stomatitis that follows irradiation treatment of the head and neck for cancer is almost always complicated by hypogeusia (sometimes referred to as "taste blindness" in this context) and various parageusic symptoms, which arise partly on the basis of xerostomia but also as the result of direct damage to taste buds by the radiation. Some improvement in these symptoms may occur as the stomatitis subsides, provided the relatively radiation-resistant peripheral taste nerves have not been injured. No adequate trials have been carried out to determine whether the use of frequent mouthwashes, salivary stimulants, or artificial saliva provides relief for these patients, and the relative contribution of dryness, taste-bud cell destruction, and candidiasis to these symptoms is unknown. Dysgeusia following the use of chemotherapeutic agents also probably results from interference in the replacement of taste bud cells, and a variety of other drugs producing dysgeusia (*e.g.,* penicillamine) may also operate at this level.

The number of taste buds (particularly those in the vallate and foliate papillae) decreases with age, and a rapid decrease often occurs after 70 years of age. This rather well-documented change possibly accounts for the decreased taste sensitivity that has been demonstrated as a normal age change, but the possibility that it results from arteriosclerotic or other specific changes that only secondarily affect the taste bud has not been carefully explored. Examination of vallate papillae at autopsy reveals many morbid changes in their structure and that of the surrounding tongue dorsum, the etiology o which is largely unknown, and further study of this area is needed before the full range of lesions contributing to taste bud loss is known.

The taste bud has also been postulated as the site of the lesion causing dysgeusia in a variety of systemic metabolic abnormalities. The evidence for this is largely hypothetical, however, and we really have no clear idea of the cause of the dysgeusia that often complicates long-term corticosteroid therapy, adrenal dysfunction, hypothyroidism, cancer, and diabetes mellitus. A syndrome referred to as *idiopathic dysgeusia,* which has been postulated as a zinc-deficiency syndrome, is also described as resulting from defective taste bud function secondary to zinc deficiency.

Provided that the gustatory nerve supplying an area of taste buds is intact or regenerates after injury, regeneration of damaged taste buds can be expected along with gradual reduction of the dysgeusia. Where extensive damage of the lingual mucosa leads to scarring (*e.g.,* in erosive lichen planus) or where permanent section of the gustatory nerve prevents taste bud regeneration, symptoms can be expected to be permanent. Currently, there are no medications available that will influence the rate of taste bud regeneration or correct dysgeusic symptoms caused by taste bud abnormalities.

Systemically administered zinc sulphate is widely used for the treatment of patients with idiopathic dysgeusia (as well as dysgeusia due to other causes), but there are no double-blind trials confirming the efficacy of this form of treatment. Although some benefit was apparent when this compound was tested in dysgeusic patients, the opportunities for bias in the evaluation of dysgeusia and in the selection of patients for treatment in the open trials that have been reported raise some doubt as to its therapeutic effectiveness. The absence of proven therapies for dysgeusia and the lack of any known metabolic intermediates in the process of reception and transduction of the taste stimulus that might be tested in controlled trials make the management of dysgeusia very difficult.

Lesions of the Lingual Nerve

Lesions of the lingual nerve usually result from surgical trauma to the nerve as it passes from the retromolar space along the lingual aspect of the mandible below the mylohyoid ridge and across to the ventral aspect of the tongue. Such trauma may be a complication of regional blocking of the nerve, extraction of mandibular molar teeth, jaw fracture, probing or removal of a stone in the submaxillary gland duct, or accidental laceration of the ventral surface of the tongue during dental restorative treatment. As this nerve carries both general sensory and gustatory fibers to the anterior third of the tongue, various sensations of pain, burning, and numbness in that area caused by damage to the general sensory fibers usually accompany the dysgeusic symptoms.

Lesions of the Chorda Tympani

Lesions of the chorda tympani often follow middle ear surgery because the nerve passes immediately behind the eardrum in the middle ear and must be disturbed to gain access to the ear ossicles. Chronic inflammation and tumors of the middle ear (carcinoma, meningioma, cholesteatoma), temporal bone, and parotid gland may also impinge on the chorda tympani and produce unilateral anterior third dysgeusia. In patients with Bell's palsy and other diseases affecting the 7th nerve, the lesion may be sufficiently proximal to affect the chorda tympani. Dysfunction of salivation (and lacrimation) on the affected side may also accompany damage to the 7th nerve. Lesions of the nerve near its point of origin in the facial canal or in the region of the geniculate ganglion are accompanied by a paralysis of motor, gustatory, and autonomic functions of the nerve; lesions between the geniculate ganglion and the point

of separation of the chorda tympani produce the same dysfunction as that of injury in the region of the geniculate ganglion, except that the lacrimal secretion is not affected; and involvement of the nerve at the level of the stylomastoid foramen results only in paralysis of the facial muscles without dysgeusia. Thus, in uveoparotid fever (sarcoidosis of the parotid) and the Melkersson–Rosenthal syndrome, facial palsy but not dysgeusia is the rule.

The dysgeusia associated with damage to the chorda tympani disappears with repair of the damage to the nerve, and changes in the threshold for tongue stimulation with the electrogustometer are sometimes used as an index of recovery. Decompression of the facial nerve in the facial canal in the temporal bone is claimed to speed recovery of both motor and gustatory defects associated with Bell's palsy. Anastomosis of the damaged portions of the facial nerve may be performed when spontaneous recovery of an extracranial neuropathy of the 7th nerve does not occur. Such operations are frequently successful in reestablishing gustatory as well as motor and autonomic function in the nerve.

When the lesion occurs intracranially or within the temporal bone and end-to-end anastomosis is impossible, some improvement can still be obtained by anastomosing the 7th nerve with either cranial nerve XI or XII. This procedure effectively corrects the facial paralysis (and painful muscle spasm that sometimes complicates the palsy) but not the dysgeusia. Atrophy and paralysis of the sternomastoid and upper trapezius or one half of the lingual musculature will result from the operation, but this apparently poses less of a problem for most patients than the considerable cosmetic deformity of permanent unilateral facial muscle paralysis.

Lesions of the Glossopharyngeal Nerve

Lesions of the extracranial portion of the glossopharyngeal nerve are unusual, but damage to this nerve may result from removal of pharyngeal tumors and repeated tonsillectomy or cauterization of the tonsillar bed. Transient dysgeusia, in fact, often follows tonsillectomy. Dysgeusia restricted to one side of the posterior two thirds of the tongue is an unusual but not impossible presenting complaint for a neoplasm arising in or invading the lateral pharyngeal wall. Loss of gag reflex on the same side will usually accompany these symptoms. As mentioned earlier in the chapter, section of the 9th nerve for intractable glossopharyngeal neuralgia abolishes taste sensation on the posterior lingual surface, palate, and pharynx on the affected side.

Extracranial lesions of the vagus nerve do not cause dysgeusia, although motor abnormality (paralysis of the soft palate with deviation of the uvula to the opposite side on speaking) may be detected on oral examination, and dysphagia may be present. Intracranial lesions affecting the roots of the vagus nerve may cause some dysgeusia because it is likely that some of the special sensory fibers of the 9th nerve enter the medulla by means of anastomosis with the roots of the 10th nerve. In practice, however, such lesions will also affect the adjacent roots of cranial nerve IX, and the intracranial connections of the roots of the cranial nerves IX and X are largely a question of anatomic rather than clinical interest.

Cranial nerves VII and IX may also be affected by diphtheritic neuritis caused by spread of toxin from the pharyngeal infection in nonimmunized individuals.

Intracranial Lesions of Nerves VII, IX, and X

Within the skull, cranial nerves VII, IX, and X may be affected by neoplasms (metastatic carcinoma, meningioma, glioma, neurofibroma), aneurysms, granulomas, and infectious processes, with symptoms of dysgeusia appearing together with various motor and sensory abnormalities characteristic of the nerve affected. Because of the close anatomic association of these three nerves and the roots of cranial nerves V, VI, and VIII, multiple cranial neuropathy is the usual feature of many of the syndromes that result from intracranial lesions in the region of the pons and brainstem.

The facial nerve in its intracranial course is most commonly affected by metastatic carcinoma, meningitis, Paget's disease of the temporal bone, or aneurysms. Cranial nerve IX may be involved by a cerebellopontine angle

tumor, and dysgeusia of the posterior two thirds of the tongue may accompany but is rarely the presenting complaint for a tumor in this location. The roots of these nerves may also be damaged during surgical treatment of other intracranial lesions.

BIBLIOGRAPHY

Alling CC III (ed): Facial Pain. Philadelphia, Lea & Febiger, 1968

Bell WE: Orofacial Pains, Differential Diagnosis. Dallas, Denedco, 1973

Bond M: Pain: Its Nature, Analysis and Treatment. Edinburgh, Churchill–Livingstone, 1979

Brain WJ, Walton JN: Brain's Diseases of the Nervous System, 7th ed. Fair Lawn, NJ, Oxford University Press, 1969

Browning E: Toxicity of Industrial Metals. London, Butterworths, 1961

Curro FA (ed): Symposium on pain. Dent Clin North Am 22, January 1978

Dallesio DJ: Wolff's Headache and Other Head Pain, 3rd ed. Fair Lawn, NJ, Oxford University Press, 1972

Farbman AI, Allgood JP: Innervation, sensory receptors and sensitivity of the oral mucosa. In Squier CA, Meyer J (eds): Current Concepts of the Histology of the Oral Mucosa. Springfield, IL, Charles C Thomas, 1971

Freese AS: Pain. New York, Penguin Books, 1975

Grossman RC, Hattis BF: Oral mucosa sensory innervation and sensory experience—A review. In Bosma JF (ed): Symposium on Oral Sensation and Perception. Springfield, IL, Charles C Thomas, 1967

Henkin RI: The role of taste in disease and nutrition. Bordens Rev Nutr Res 28:71, 1967

Knighton RS, Dumke PR (eds): Pain. Boston, Little, Brown, 1966

Melzack R, Casey M: Model of Pain. In Kenshalo DR (ed): First International Symposium on the Skin Senses. Springfield, IL, Charles C Thomas, 1968

Merritt HH: Textbook of Neurology, 5th ed. Philadelphia, Lea & Febiger, 1975

Proceedings First World Congress of the International Association for the Study of Pain. Florence, Italy, September 1975

Sillito AM: Taste and olfaction. In Lavelle CLB (ed): Applied Physiology of the Mouth. Bristol, J. Wright & Sons Ltd, 1975

Sternbach RA: Pain Patients: Traits and Treatments. New York, Academic Press, 1974

Warfield CA, Stein JM: Chronic pain: Contributory factors. Hosp Pract 17:49, 1982

Youmans JR (ed): Neurological Surgery: A Comprehensive Reference Guide to the Diagnosis and Management of Neurosurgical Problems. Philadelphia, WB Saunders, 1973

Evaluation of Pain and Dysgeusia

Alpers BJ, Mancall EL: Essentials of the Neurological Examination. Philadelphia, FA Davis, 1971

Bornstein WJ: Cortical representation of taste in man and monkey II: Localization of the cortical taste area in man and a method for measuring impairment of taste in man. Yale J Biol Med 13:133, 1940-41

Brightman VJ: Disordered oral sensation and appetite. In Proceedings Second International Conference on Chemical Senses and Nutrition. Chap. 15. Philadelphia, Monell Chemical Senses Center, June 1976. New York, Academic Press, 1977

Desor JA, Maller O: Taste correlates of disease states: Cystic fibrosis. J Pediatr 87:93, 1975

Dixon AD: Nerve plexuses in the oral mucosa. Arch Oral Biol 8:435, 1963

Henkin RI, Christiansen RL: Taste localization on the tongue, palate, and pharynx of normal man. J Appl Physiol 22:316, 1967

Henkin RI, Graziadei PPG, Bradley DF: NIH clinical staff conference. The molecular basis of taste and its disorders. Ann Intern Med 71:791, 1969

Huff BB (ed): Physicians' Desk Reference, 31st ed. Oradell, NJ, Medical Economics, 1977

Leonard MS et al: Automated diagnosis of craniofacial pain. J Dent Res 52:1297, 1973

Melzack R: The perception of pain. Psychobiology, The Biological Bases of Behavior. IX. Determinants of Perception, Readings from the Scientific American. San Francisco, WH Freeman, 1967

Melzack R: The McGill pain questionnaire: Major properties and scoring methods. Pain 1:277, 1975

Melzack R, Perry C: Self-regulation of pain: The use of alpha-feedback and hypnotic training for the control of chronic pain. Exp Neurol 46:452, 1975

Peiris OA, Miles DW: Galvanic stimulation of the tongue as a prognostic index in Bell's Palsy. Br Med J 71:1162, 1965

Pilling LF: Psychosomatic aspects of facial pain. In Alling CC (ed): Facial Pain. Philadelphia, Lea & Febiger, 1968

Steiner JE et al: Taste perception in depressive illness. Isr Ann Psychiatry 7:223, 1969

Nonneuropathic Orofacial Pain of Extraneural Origin

Anderson LG, Bayles TB: Polymyalgia rheumatica and giant cell arteritis. DM January, 1974

Carlsson SG, Gale EN, Öhman A: Treatment of temporomandibular joint syndrome with biofeedback. J Am Dent Assoc 91:602, 1975

Das AK, Laskin DM: Temporal arteritis of the facial artery. J Oral Surg 24:226, 1966

Dickey DM: Evaluation of pain of dentoalveolar origin. In Symposium on Dental Emergencies. Dent Clin North Am 17:391, 1973

Duquette P, Goebel WM: Pulpitis simulating the myofascial pain dysfunction syndrome: Report of three cases. J Am Dent Assoc 87:1237, 1973

Freese AS: Temporomandibular joint and myofascial trigger areas in the dental diagnosis of pain. J Am Dent Assoc 59:448, 1959

Glick DH: The interpretation of pain of dental origin. In Symposium on Endodontics. Dent Clin North Am p. 535, November 1967

Greene CS, Laskin DM: Splint therapy for the myofascial pain-dysfunction (MPD) syndrome: A comparative study. J Am Dent Assoc 84:624, 1972

Greene CS et al: The TMJ pain-dysfunction syndrome: heterogeneity of the patient population. J Am Dent Assoc 79:1168, 1969

Hamilton CR, Jr, Shelley WM, Tumulty PA: Giant cell arteritis: Including temporal arteritis and polymyalgia rheumatica. Medicine 50:1, 1971

Harris WE: Endodontic pain referred across the midline: Report of a case. J Am Dent Assoc 87:1240, 1973

Horton BT: Use of histamine in the treatment of specific types of headache. JAMA 116:377, 1941

Jackson R: The Cervical Syndrome, 3rd ed. Springfield, IL, Charles C Thomas, 1976

Kern WA: Painful carotid artery. Ann Intern Med 80:417, 1974

Laskin DM (ed): Derangements of the temporomandibular joint. Conf. Am. Soc. Oral Surgeons. Chicago, July, 1968. J Am Dent Assoc 79:92, 1969

Paine R: Vascular facial pain. In Alling CC (ed): Facial Pain. Philadelphia, Lea & Febiger, 1968

Rood JP: Chest pain of dental origin. A case report. Br Dent J 133:110, 1972

Travell J: Temporomandibular joint pain referred from muscles of the head and neck. J Prosthet Dent 10:745, 1960

Travell J, Rinzler SH: Scientific exhibit: Myofascial genesis of pain. Postgrad Med 11:425, 1952

Nonneuropathic Pain of Central Origin

Albert ML: Carbamazepine for painful posttraumatic paresthesia. N Engl J Med 290:693, 1974

Fisher CM, Mohr JP, Adams RD: Cerebrovascular diseases. In Wintrobe MM et al (eds): Harrison's Textbook of Internal Medicine, 7th ed. New York, McGraw–Hill, 1974

Gregg JM: Posttraumatic pain: Experimental trigeminal neuropathy. J Oral Surg 29:260, 1971

Lapresle J, Haguenau M: Anatomicoclinical correlation in focal thalamic lesions. Z Neurol 205:29, 1973

Melzack R, Wall PD: Pain mechanisms: A new theory. Science 150:971, 1965

Editorial: Brain tumor: Current status of treatment and its complications. Arch Neurol 32:781, 1975

Potts DG: Brain tumors: Radiographic localization and diagnosis. Radiol Clin North Am 3:511, 1965

Orofacial Pain of Neuropathic Origin

Alderman MM: Management of oral and facial pain in the hospital environment. In Symposium on Hospital Dental Practice. Dent Clin North Am 19:657, 1975

Aring CD: Pain in multiple sclerosis. JAMA 223:547, 1973

Baddour HM et al: Eagle's syndrome. Oral Surg 46:486, 1978

Baringer JR, Swoveland P: Recovery of herpes-simplex virus from human trigeminal ganglions. N Engl J Med 288:648, 1973

Bohm E, Höjeberg S: Follow-up investigation of one hundred and eleven cases of trigeminal neuralgia treated by the decompression operation between 1952-1954. Acta Neurochir 6:1, 1958

Bohm E, Strang RR: Glossopharyngeal neuralgia. Brain 85:371, 1962

Burgoon CF, Jr, Burgoon JS, Baldridge GD: The natural history of herpes zoster. JAMA 164:265, 1957

DeJong RH: Defining pain terms. JAMA 244:143, 1980

Devine KD et al: Diagnostic problems in surgery of the head and neck. Surg Clin North Am 41:1049, 1961

Douglas BL, Huebsch RF: Atypical facial neuralgia resulting from fractured styloid process of the temporal bone. Oral Surg 6:1199, 1953

Eagle WW: Symptomatic elongated styloid process; report of 2 cases of styloid process carotid artery syndrome with operation. Arch Otolaryngol 49:490, 1949

Ecker A, Perl T: Precise alcoholic Gaserian injection for tic douloureux. J Neurol Neurosurg Psychiatr 28:65, 1965

Gardner WJ: Trigeminal neuralgia. In Hassler R, Walker AE (eds): Trigeminal Neuralgia, Pathogenesis and Pathophysiology. Philadelphia, WB Saunders, 1970

Gold E: Serologic and virus-isolation studies of patients with varicella or herpes-zoster infection. N Engl J Med 274:181, 1966

Hassler R, Walker AE (eds): Trigeminal Neuralgia, Pathogenesis and Pathophysiology. Philadelphia, WB Saunders, 1970

Jaeger R: The results of injecting hot water into the gasserian ganglion for the relief of tic douloureux. J Neurosurg 16:656, 1959

Jannetta PJ et al: The Neurosurgical Approach to the Relief from Pain. Curr Prob Surg February 1973

Janetta PJ: Microsurgical approach to the trigeminal nerve for tic douloureux. Progr Neurol Surg 7:180, 1976

Kerr FWL: Peripheral versus central factors in trigeminal neuralgia. In Hassler R, Walker AE (eds): Trigeminal Neuralgia, Pathogenesis and Pathophysiology. Philadelphia, WB Saunders, 1970

Kerr FWL, Miller RH: The pathology of trigeminal neuralgia: Electron microscopic studies. Arch Neurol 15:308, 1966

Lazar ML: Current treatment of tic douloureux. Oral Surg 50:504, 1980

Lundborg T: Diagnostic problems concerning acoustic tumors: Study of 300 verified cases and Békésy audiogram in differential diagnosis. Acta Otolaryngol (Suppl) 99:1, 1952

Mruthyunjaya B et al: Trigeminal neuralgia: A comparative evaluation of four treatment procedures. Oral Surg 52:126, 1981

Nichol CS: Four-year double blind study of Tegretol in facial pain. Headache 9:54, 1969

Rand RW, Poulos DA, Sweet WH: Surgical treatment of trigeminal neuralgia. In Morley TP (ed): Current Controversies in Neurosurgery. Philadelphia, WB Saunders, 1976

Ratner EJ et al: Jaw bone cavities and trigeminal and atypical facial neuralgia. Oral Surg 48:3, 1979

Robinson M, Slavkin HC: Dental amputation neuromas. J Am Dent Assoc 70:662, 1965

Sanger RG et al: Referred oral facial pain from brain abscess. Oral Surg 53:131, 1982

Shaber EP, Krol AJ: Trigeminal neuralgia—A new treatment concept. Oral Surg 49:286, 1980

Stalker WH: Facial neuralgia associated with recurrent herpes simplex. Oral Surg 49:502, 1980

Sugar O, Bucy PC: Postherpetic trigeminal neuralgia. Arch Neurol Psychiatry 65:131, 1951

Svien HJ et al: Partial glossopharyngeal neuralgia associated with syncope. J Neurosrug 14:452, 1957

Swanson HH: Traumatic neuromas: A review of the literature. Oral Surg 14:317, 1961

Theobald W, Krupp P, Levin P: Neuropharmacologic aspects of the therapeutic action of carbamazepine. In Hassler R, Walker AE (eds): Trigeminal Neuralgia, Pathogenesis and Pathophysiology. Philadelphia, WB Saunders, 1970

Thomas JE, Waltz AS: Neurological manifestations of nasopharyngeal malignant tumors. JAMA 192:95, 1965

Trodahl JN, Carroll GW: Traumatic neuroma of

the mandibular ridge: Report of a case. Oral Surg 24:563, 1967

Voorhies R, Patterson RH: Management of trigeminal neuralgia (tic douloureux). JAMA 245:2521, 1981

Wilson AA: Geniculate neuralgia: Report of a case relieved by intracranial section of the nerve of Wrisberg. J Neurosurg 7:473, 1950

Dysgeusia of Nonneuropathic Origin

Box HK: Necrotic Gingivitis. Toronto, University of Toronto Press, 1930

Cohen L: Disturbance of taste as a symptom of multiple sclerosis. Br J Oral Surg 2:184, 1965

Dale JW, Wing S: Clinical and technical examination of a tonsillolith: A case report. Aust. Dent J 19:84, 1974

Giddon DB et al: Relative abilities of natural and artificial denture patients for judging the sweetness of solid foods. J Prosthet Dent 4:263, 1954

Guggenheimer J, Brightman VJ, Ship II: Effect of chlortetracycline mouth rinses on the healing of recurrent aphthous ulcers: A double-blind controlled trial. J Oral Ther Pharmacol 4:406, 1968

Henkin RI, Christiansen RL: Taste thresholds in patients with dentures J Am Dent Assoc 75:118, 1967

Maw RB, McKean TW: Hand–Schüller–Christian disease: Report of a case. J Am Dent Assoc 85:1353, 1972

Moncrieff RW: The Chemical Senses, p 150. London, Leonard Hill, 1951

Shenkin HA, Lewey FH: Taste aura preceding convulsions in a lesion of the parietal operculum. J Nerv Ment Dis 100:352, 1944

Sumner D: Posttraumatic ageusia. Brain J Neurol 90:187, 1967

Dysgeusia of Neuropathic Origin

Axelrod FB, Nachtigal R, Dancis J: Familial dysautonomia: Diagnosis, pathogenesis and management. Adv Pediatr 21:75, 1974

Brody HA, Prendergast JJ, Silverman S, Jr: The relationship between oral symptoms, insulin release and glucose intolerance. Oral Surg 31:777, 1971

Cohen T, Gitman L: Oral complaints and taste perception in the aged. J Gerontol 12:294, 1959

Conger AD: Loss and recovery of taste acuity in patients irradiated to the oral cavity. Radiat Res 53:338, 1973

DeWys WD: A spectrum of organ systems that respond to the presence of cancer. Abnormalities of taste as a remote effect of a neoplasm. Ann NY Acad Sci 230:427, 1974

Henkin RI: Abnormalities of taste and olfaction in patients with chromatin negative gonadal dysgenesis. J Clin Endocrinol Metab 27:1436, 1967

Henkin RI: Impairment of olfaction and of the tastes of sour and bitter in pseudohypoparathyroidism. J Clin Endocrinol Metab 28:624, 1968

Henkin RI: A double-blind study of the effects of zinc sulphate on taste and smell dysfunction. Am J Med Sci 272:285, 1976

Henkin RI et al: Idiopathic hypogeusia with dysgeusia, hyposmia and dysosmia: A new syndrome. JAMA 217:434, 1971

Henkin RI, Shallenberger RS: Aglycogeusia: The inability to recognize sweetness and its possible molecular basis. Nature 227:965, 1970

Henkin RI et al: Abnormalities of taste and smell in Sjögrens Syndrome. Ann Intern Med 76:375, 1972

MacCarthy–Leventhal EM: Post-radiation mouth blindness. Lancet 2:1138, 1959

Pearson J, Finegold MJ, Budzilovich G: The tongue and taste in familial dysautonomia. Pediatrics 45:739, 1970

Revilla AG: Neurinomas of the cerebellopontile recess: A clinical study of 610 cases including operative mortality and end results. Johns Hopkins Hosp Bull 80:254, 1947

Schelling JL et al: Abnormal taste threshold in diabetes. Lancet 1:508, 1965

Scott PJ: Glossitis with complete loss of taste sensation during dindevan treatment. Report of a case. NZ Med J 59:296, 1960

Tarab S: Troubles de la gustation après tonsillectomie. Pract Otorhinolaryngol 17:260, 1955

17

Oral Symptoms Without Apparent Physical Abnormality

VERNON J. BRIGHTMAN

One of the most difficult problems in oral medicine is the patient who consistently complains of a symptom or a sign that he interprets as abnormal, but for which the dentist or physician can find no convincing physical explanation. Many problems of this type center about complaints of chronic sensory abnormality, such as pain, burning sensations, dysgeusia, and sensations of dryness or swelling (*i.e.*, complaints regarding a subjectively experienced sensation); others concern patients' anxieties regarding anatomic structures they can see or feel in their mouths and that they identify as abnormal and possibly evidence of disease. Such "lesions" may or may not be associated with symptoms. Despite the failure of quite competent diagnosticians to identify the cause of these symptoms and despite repeated assurance that the "lesion" the patient associates with these symptoms is a "harmless," normal, anatomic structure, patients with chronic complaints of this type frequently continue their search for a diagnosis and specific treatment through a long series of consultations, which involves many dental and medical specialists whom they hope will solve their problems and provide relief from their symptoms and attendant anxieties.

These problems are not restricted to the oral cavity or to the speciality or oral medicine, and all who practice medicine or dentistry usually become aware of them early in their careers. Such problem patients are seen with greater frequency in specialists practices, simply because unsolved problems commonly lead to referral for further diagnostic testing. In fact, for the young resident in speciality training one of the most sobering discoveries is that his chosen career will involve a considerable number of patients with such problems and that his practice will not always be concerned with patients with clearly defined pathologic states that are amenable to treatment. Unexplained oral sensory abnormality, in particular, is a reality in both dental and medical practice, and even when a reasonable diagnostic search fails to find an explanation for such symptoms, the patient still requires management and some form of treatment. Adequate training in oral medicine and the various surgical specialities

concerned with the mouth (oral surgery, endodontics, periodontics and otorhinolaryngology) should include a consideration of these problem patients and appropriate procedures for their management.

This chapter does not contain any new solution to these problem patients; however, it does attempt to set out the pitfalls involved, and it may reduce some of the frustration that is commonly experienced by both patient and doctor who are involved with unsolved oral symptoms.

The assumption underlying all diagnostic investigations is that an explanation will be found for the patient's complaint of pain, swelling, dryness, or other abnormal sensation in the discovery of an extraneural or neuropathic, inflammatory, degenerative, or neoplastic process that provides a focus for these symptoms. When extensive and reasonably adequate diagnostic investigations fail to find such an explanation, the initial response by both patient and doctor is that further testing that may probe for more unusual conditions is needed. When this approach also fails, the doctor may reasonably begin to assume that the patient's symptoms are not real and that they represent malingering (*i.e.*, overemphasis or exaggeration of a symptom for the purpose of some secondary gain) or a psychiatric abnormality. Alternatively, the doctor, again not unreasonably, may begin to doubt his own judgment. He may wonder whether the borderline abnormality he noted in sensory evaluation, by palpation, or radiographic study might not be more serious than he had at first considered and possibly evidence of a lesion to explain the patient's symptoms.

Both of these responses on the doctor's part, although perfectly reasonable considerations under the circumstances, can also be exaggerated and become unreasonable responses. As such, they represent two of the major pitfalls that can complicate the management of these problem patients. On the one hand, to accept that the symptoms are simply evidence of psychiatric abnormality and deny the patient the opportunity for further diagnostic testing that in months ahead may provide the solution to the unusual symptoms; on the other hand, to proceed with surgical treatment even when there are only minimal physical findings to justify risks complicating the diagnostic situation with the side-effects of the surgical procedure. All clinicians, no doubt, will at sometime make one or the other of these errors in treating a particular patient. Awareness of these pitfalls at all times, however, does help prevent such extremes of response on the doctor's part.

The patient will respond to the failure of his doctor to provide explanation and relief for his symptoms. This may be in the form of his request for further tests or for further consultation to be initiated by his doctor or by his privately seeking consultations from other dental or medical practitioners. Considering the wide variety of training and traditions that the health professions encompass, it is relatively easy for the patient to find a practitioner who will provide some treatment that he believes may relieve his symptoms. If his own doctor will not carry out the surgical procedure he feels may help him the patient can usually, by further consultation, find someone who will. Multiple consultation and heavy use of surgical services are characteristic features of patients with chronic disorders, and these features are even more marked among those with unexplained symptoms.

Among one series of 19 patients referred to the Oral Medicine Research Clinic at The Philadelphia General Hospital* for diagnosis and treatment of recurrent mouth ulcers with an average duration of 10 years, the average number of prior consultations per patient was 3.8 (with some patients having seen over a dozen doctors about their problem); among 22 patients with unexplained oral sensory abnormalities with an average duration of only 3 years, the number of prior consultations was already 4.2. The honest statement, "I don't know what is the cause of your symptoms" when made by a patient's doctor logically leads to the patient's seeking further consultation. Diagnosed and clearly evident disease (*e.g.,* mouth ulcers), even if inadequately treated, less frequently causes the pa-

tient to seek a new doctor. Management of the patient with unexplained oral symptoms, therefore, must involve a clear understanding between patient and doctor concerning the difficult nature of the symptoms, the need for carefully selected diagnostic studies and surgical intervention at the appropriate time as well as frequent communication between the various health professionals the patient has consulted for treatment of his problem.

Chronic symptoms for which a doctor cannot provide relief certainly justify the patient's seeking help elsewhere but no consultant can provide assistance for the patient until a measure of trust is established between the consultants and the patient that will allow for diagnostic studies and treatment that all will feel to be in the patient's best interest. The extent of surgical procedures, dental restorations, and diagnostic testing to which many of these problem patients submit justifies the consultant's requesting that the patient place himself in one doctor's care at least for a given period of time to see what can be accomplished.

IMPORTANCE OF FOLLOW-UP AND REPEATED EXAMINATION AND TESTING

Of prime importance in the management of patients with unexplained oral symptoms is the recognition that identification of the cause of these symptoms may only come with time. Several studies of chronic oral sensory complaints (*e.g.,* those of Rushton and Gibilisco concerning atypical facial pain, as well as our own at The Philadelphia General Hospital) have shown that with time, approximately one half of those patients with unexplained orofacial pain will be found to have specific pathologic diagnoses that reasonably explain their symptoms, *provided repeated examination and diagnostic testing are continued beyond the initial period of consultation.*

The success of the referral clinic in managing problems of this type possibly stems more from a program of continued surveillance of the patient with a coordinated group of consultants than it does from the availability of sophisticated diagnostic equipment.

* Studies of patients with oral sensory abnormalities at The Philadelphia General Hospital that are described in this chapter were carried out with support from USPHS DE03764 and RR-107.

With time, small lesions such as tumors in the nasopharynx, parotid gland, and infratemporal fossa that can impinge on oral sensory and motor nerves will increase in size and become apparent through the development of other abnormalities, and systemic neurologic disease such as diabetes mellitus and multiple sclerosis will develop from a prodromal stage where only unusual oral symptoms are present, to one where a variety of tests will reveal the presence of the disease and explain the patient's oral symptoms.

The literature contains numerous references to patients whose oral symptoms remained unexplained for long periods of time until further growth of a tumor revealed the focus for the patient's symptoms. Alderman recently described a case that was diagnosed as temporomandibular joint (TMJ) dysfunction and atypical facial pain for some 5 years before repeated biopsy of the nasopharynx led to discovery of a cylindroma of the parotid, which had already spread to the base of the skull. Thomas and Waltz have reviewed a large series of cases with cranial neurologic involvement secondary to nasopharyngeal tumors.

ORAL SYMPTOMS AS A PRODROME OF SYSTEMIC DISEASE

Many systemic diseases may also manifest through oral symptoms. *Pernicious anemia* and *chronic iron-deficiency anemia* are said to cause painful burning sensations frequently in the tongue, and deficiency of nicotinic acid is also associated with these symptoms. *Multiple myeloma* is recognized as a strong suspect for unexplained chronic bone pain in all parts of the skeleton. In the jaws, such pain is usually associated with the presence of osteolytic defects, which are easily detected by radiologic examination, but the case of Arm and Brightman underscores the fact that atypical facial pains can result from this cause even when radiologic examination fails to reveal these bony defects. *Paget's disease*, in its osteoblastic phase, by producing occlusion of bony foramina may also cause neuralgic symptoms that seem to have no explanation until other evidences of bone deformity begin

to appear. Likewise, other diseases that affect the jaw bone and eventually produce destructive lesions (*e.g.*, cysts, metastatic carcinoma, lymphosarcoma, hyperparathyroidism, histiocytosis) may in their early stages be associated with jaw pain, numbness, and other sensory abnormalities well before there is convincing radiologic evidence of their presence in the jaws.

Degenerative changes of the peripheral nerves and nerve receptors (*diabetic neuropathy*) are recognized as complications of diabetes mellitus that may lead to permanent sensory deficits. This association of diabetes and neuropathy is well known, and the dental literature makes frequent reference to the need for a search for diabetes mellitus in patients with a variety of sensory disorders, notably, unexplained symptoms of pain, burning, dryness, and altered taste perception. Despite this frequently stated relationship between diabetes mellitus and various oral sensory disorders, however, it should be noted that there are few published experimental data to explain the role of diabetes in these problems.

Brody, Prendergast, and Silverman noted a high incidence of diabetes (1 in 3) among patients attending an oral medicine clinic, evidence of the disease being found with about the same frequency among those with chronic unexplained oral sensory complaints as among those with visible oral mucosal lesions or periodontal disease. In a group of patients referred to The Philadelphia General Hospital, blood glucose abnormalities were detected in 42% of those with oral sensory abnormalities that could be explained on the basis of traumatic neuropathy, vascular disease, or TMJ myofascial dysfunction and at the same high level among an age-matched group with unexplained oral sensory complaints. Additional abnormalities of blood lipids among these patients raised the total incidence of blood glucose and blood lipid abnormalities to over 50% in both groups. Diabetes mellitus, therefore, does not have any specific relationship with *unexplained* oral symptoms, but it is found very frequently among patients with chronic oral disease, particularly those with chronic oral sensory complaints.

Other investigators of serum lipid abnormalities have also noted the high incidence of these abnormalities among patients attending a variety of referral clinics for chronic complaints elsewhere in the body. One explanation for this association of blood glucose and lipid abnormalities and chronic oral sensory disease is that in its early stages, the peripheral vascular damage that occurs in diabetes mellitus predisposes the patient to chronic peripheral neurologic problems from a variety of sources well before other evidence of advanced peripheral vascular disease occurs. In such patients, nerve damage from obvious and identifiable causes such as trauma and virus infection, as well as other minor or unrecognized causes, produces permanent rather than transient neurologic symptoms. Patients with chronic oral sensory complaints developing without obvious cause and those with complaints persisting long after the normal processes of healing should have eradicated the problem, should be thoroughly investigated for evidence of blood glucose or blood lipid abnormalities.

Opinions differ as to the desirability of treating patients in whom no additional physical evidence of diabetes or other lipid abnormality can be detected, but early treatment of their metabolic problem revealed in abnormal blood glucose or lipid values should be recommended both as a means of controlling oral complaints and as a hope of preventing further permanent neurologic damage. Careful testing of oral sensory function as described in Chapters 2 and 16 may provide additional evidence of abnormality of the trigeminal nerve in these patients and encourage early treatment.

For most of those systemic diseases that manifest in the oral cavity, there is little information on the frequency with which signs and symptoms identified in the oral cavity lead to the recognition of the presence of the systemic disease. The dentist who recognizes an oral lesion that leads to the diagnosis of a systemic process probably feels a sense of accomplishment and may publish a case report. The literature, therefore, becomes a poor guide to the likelihood of finding evidence implicating a previously undiagnosed systemic disease process as the cause of the patient's unexplained oral symptoms. Diseases such as diabetes mellitus, hyperuri-

cemia, and Paget's disease (which occur with some frequency in the older general population) will often be found.

Evidence associating the systemic disease and the oral symptoms, however, may be harder to find. In our experience, clinical investigation of the majority of patients referred following initial evaluation by the dentists and physicians in their community for an unsolved oral complaint only rarely detects previously undiagnosed systemic disease. More often, abnormal blood lipid and glucose levels have been noted at earlier examinations, and a decision has been made not to treat the abnormality, so its possible association with the oral symptom has gone unrecognized. Alternatively, both patient and physician are aware of the presence of the systemic disease, but the methods used to control it have been inadequate. Referral consultations for unexplained oral complaints may thus result in recommendations for additional treatment of systemic disease noted at the time of consultation, but in many cases these recommendations are not specifically related to the oral complaint.

Despite the time and money invested in extensive searches for systemic disease that only rarely find a possible cause of a patient's unexplained oral symptoms, such searches are probably justified. Unexplained chronic oral symptoms generate considerable anxiety in addition to the discomfort experienced by the patient, and a "leave no stone unturned" approach often seems necessary to allay these anxieties. For the indigent patient, unfortunately, the cost of these investigations often prohibits them because even those patients with third party insurance find it difficult to obtain reimbursement for the continued evaluation of symptoms that have no specific disease as their basis. When the cost of repeated testing is not a consideration, patients with these problems accept and sometimes even demand a continued battery of more and more sophisticated studies. In these circumstances, the clinician's judgment is needed to control the laboratory and physical examinations to be carried out in order to prevent unnecessary repetition of tests and to advise the patient on the likelihood of a particular procedure providing additional useful diagnostic information. The clinician has the responsibility to help the patient avoid unnecessary diagnostic procedures, just as he does to guide him in submitting only to those surgical or dental rehabilitative procedures that are likely to benefit his oral problem.

ORAL SYMPTOMS OUT OF PROPORTION TO RECOGNIZED ORAL LESIONS

It is unrealistic to assume that all patients with unexplained oral symptoms present to the clinician with an oral cavity that is completely free of dental, periodontal, and mucosal lesions that must be considered as possible causes for the unusual symptoms. On the contrary, evaluation of these patients commonly involves decisions as to whether a degenerating pulp, a coarsely fissured tongue, or muscle tension as a result of a malocclusion, for example, may explain complaints of chronic pain or burning and painful tongue. Where possible, treatment of the abnormality by root canal therapy, increased oral and tongue hygiene, correction of the malocclusion, or administration of muscle relaxants in the situations just described may answer the question. However, when symptoms persist in the face of apparently adequate treatment, the clinician must attempt to determine whether the patient's symptoms arise from another cause or whether they simply represent an exaggerated response to the particular oral abnormality that has been found and presumably adequately treated.

Among the patients with unexplained oral symptoms who have been referred to us, there is undoubtedly a group whose symptoms are explained as far as the painful focus is concerned. The unusual feature of their problem is their atypical or exaggerated response to the pain focus and perhaps also the length of time their symptoms have persisted. In defining patients with atypical facial pain, therefore, we must include not only those whose symptoms are unusual and unexplained by the usual anatomic pain pathways (see following section) but also those whose response to an identifiable and often minor chronic pain focus is atypical.

It is helpful to identify the patient whose problem appears to be his inability to handle minor oral sensory abnormality and who reacts to chronic low-grade pain in the same manner as to pain of greater intensity. Although this decision must be made very cautiously and reviewed from time to time as treatment progresses, it does help focus treatment on the emotional component of the patient's pain problem and helps reduce continued and unnecessary diagnostic search for another obscure physical cause of the symptoms.

Psychological and Emotional Factors

Because pain is a subjective sensory experience, psychological factors enter into all painful and abnormal sensory states. The relative proportions of psychological factors and physical factors (i.e., pathologic tissue changes) involved varies considerably from patient to patient. It is common experience that similar traumatic episodes will evoke varied emotional responses in different individuals even under the same conditions; and pathologic states in and about the mouth likewise trigger a wide range of emotional responses. In fact, considering the importance of the oral cavity in the emotional development and maintenance of the individual organism (see discussion to follow), it should be expected that psychological factors will complicate orofacial pain. No painful experience is without its psychological correlates, and both anxiety and depression to some extent always accompany pain.

Figure 17-1 is a graphic representation of this phenomenon. The bulk of the population falls within the elliptical curve that is itself determined by two curves—one for those who hyperreact to pain and one for those who are defined as hyporeactors in comparison with assumed population norms. Patients who exhibit high psychological factors in response to low levels of physical factors are termed type I or hyperreactors; type II patients are those with mild problems in which neither psychological nor physical factors feature strongly and who may not even seek help for their problem; type III patients are hyporeactors; type IV patients are those with evidence of severe physical abnormality

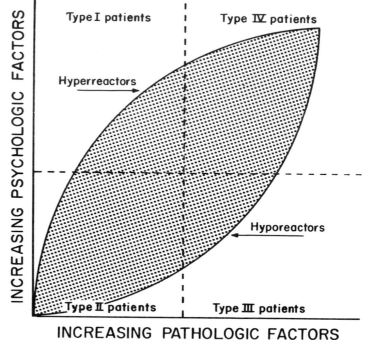

Fig. 17-1 Diagram of the distribution of patients in a given population to illustrate the interaction of psychologic and pathologic factors in the production of pain. Further details are given in the text.

with maximal psychological involvement to complicate the pathologic process.

Identification of a given patient as type I through IV is the result of the process of history-taking together with the findings of physical and laboratory studies (including radiographic and biopsy information where applicable). The assessment process may include the evaluation of the effect of the pain on work and social activity, help-seeking behavior in various forms (consultation, use of analgesics and other modes of therapy), and the use of psychological inventories and pain-rating scales as described in Chapter 16. Although much of this information can be obtained by the dentist who is interested in and committed to the treatment of patients with chronic pain problems, on occasion the service of a psychiatrist or other individual skilled in psychological interviewing (e.g., clinical psychologist or psychiatric social worker) may be advantageous in obtaining information that can define the extent to which psychological factors are involved in the patient's complaint of pain.

Clues that a patient may be reacting in an unusual fashion to abnormal sensory stimuli of low intensity can come from a variety of inquiries developed during the dentist's own diagnostic interview. For instance, at one extreme the dentist will recognize those patients who reveal evidence of thought disorder during the interview: inability to provide clear and consistent statements about symptoms or events that the dentist can check with reasonable certainty; persistent and obvious verbal confusion between symptoms and an emotionally charged event or personal relationship; use of bizarre, mechanical, or animalistic explanations for oral symptoms, revealing the patient's inability to separate himself from either real or imaginary objects or persons. The dentist will also recognize those who express marked paranoia (e.g., that the pain is due to an object purposely left behind by the surgeon, who is acting as the agent of a god or an enemy of the patient) or severe depression about symptoms (see section that follows).

Although none of these phenomena alone substantiates a diagnosis of mental disease (and specific diagnoses such as schizophrenia and paranoia and depression made by the dentist on this basis are completely unjustified), a dentist who becomes aware of any type of compromised mental ability in his patient should consider the likelihood that abnormal psychological factors may be complicating the diagnostic situation. Whether such mental confusions involve organic or functional mental disease of a particular type may be more difficult to determine; however, in these extreme cases the ability of the dentist to help the patient at all depends on a better understanding of the patient's mental and psychiatric states; consultation with the family physician or psychiatrist about the patient will be necessary. At times, review of records of prior hospital admissions and detailed enquiry into medications the patient has used may provide evidence of earlier mental problems or treatment for mental disease. Occasionally, the family history will reveal an inheritable mental problem, and the social and occupational history can identify the extreme social misfit.

Mental disease, mental retardation, and inability to conform to society do not produce oral symptoms, but they may affect the individual's ability to handle sensory abnormality. Conversely, pain and other abnormal oral sensations are also experienced by the mentally ill in response to physical causes, and the clinician must always be on guard not to discount oral symptoms in the mentally ill in favor of a psychological explanation without thorough examination of the patient.

Emotional Factors

The majority of patients in whom emotional factors obviously complicate their oral symptoms do not have diagnosable mental disease, although they are often erroneously branded as "crazy." Periods of increased emotional stress, whether brought about by interpersonal conflicts, external pressure of work or family, or an individual's own physical and personal drives, are normal for everyone, but such episodes also frequently reduce pain tolerance and the patient's ability to handle chronic low-grade sensory abnormality. To the observer, the influence of the patient's emotions on his oral symptoms may at times be quite evident; for the patient, clear separation of the psychological and physical factors in his problem may be impossible, and he may not be able to control either factor

without assistance from the clinician. Patients frequently provide the clue to this relationship by the setting of their story, by clearly describing the time of onset or aggravation of the problem in a period of increased personal, family, or work stress. At other times, the patient will volunteer this information when the clinician makes specific enquiry. Occasionally, the patient will deny such an association in the face of clear evidence of a situation in which any normal person might be expected to be extremely uncomfortable. (In referral clinics, as compared to community practice, the percentage of patients with diagnosable psychiatric abnormality may be higher; psychiatric interviews carried out on a series of patients attending the Oral Medicine Clinic at The Philadelphia General Hospital revealed that over a third were abnormal, the most common diagnoses being depression [20%], anxiety, character defect, schizophrenia, and stress reaction.)

By means of the medical history, the dentist may identify the patient whose medical and dental treatments over the years have been unusually extensive and perhaps characterized by multiple surgical procedures and the use of many medications (often despite minimal evidence of organic disease). Although often able to tolerate considerable pain from surgical procedures, individuals who customarily rely heavily on physicians, dentists, and other health professionals may also report a level of symptoms as "dis-ease" that other more robust individuals tolerate as part of life. The person who shows this pattern (sometimes referred to as *increased help-seeking behavior*) presumably senses that he is ill more often than others and will tend to identify a particular unusual oral sensation as evidence of disease more readily than others. Further enquiry into the daily life of such a patient often suggests ways in which the patient may gain psychologically from being "ill" and from the "help-seeking behavior" of which the oral problem appears to be a part. Because a patient's report of his personal involvements always contains some degree of bias, temptations to inquire further and to point out such suspicions might prudently be avoided by the clinician who does not have special psychiatric training. Once again, the clinician needs to be especially careful with these patients not to accept a symptom as imaginary, simply because in the past, investigations of the patient's complaints have revealed little physical abnormality.

Pain tolerance may also be markedly affected by medications. Certain patients show unusual and almost idiosyncratic reaction, particularly to narcotic analgesics and to barbiturates. These patients appear to tolerate pain and other abnormal oral sensations less well when they are using these medications. The narcotic addict also may describe both acute and chronic pain symptoms far in excess of what might be expected from the extent of any detectable oral lesion. Presumably his distorted belief is that such symptoms will cause the dentist or physician to prescribe narcotics, barbiturates, or other addicting medication, or even hospitalization and surgery with further justification for heavy drug treatment. However, addicts also may have physical explanations for their oral symptoms, which unfortunately may be missed if the oral examination is not complete.

Patients who have been free of oral disease until adulthood and who then need restorative or other dental procedures often respond with more anxiety and emotional reaction than those who have learned to tolerate such procedures earlier in life. Young adults suddenly becoming aware of the effects of either heavy emotional or physical tension on the musculoskeletal system may also report considerable discomfort despite evidence of only mild myofascial inflammation. The need to recognize such responses is emphasized in Chapter 12, which deals with disease of the temporomandibular joint. Paradoxically, those who have suffered painful traumatic and surgical episodes in childhood may also become intolerant of the discomfort associated with dental procedures or minor dental pain.

At the other end of the spectrum of emotional states contributing to the overemphasis of oral symptoms is the normal individual who under the stress of the death of a close relative or discovery of a serious disease in a friend, acquaintance, or relative becomes anxious that he too may be experiencing an "early warning sign" of a similar disease. Under such circumstances, the patient may become convinced that a mild symptom or a small nodule, ulcer, or mucosal lesion is not a transient inconsequential event but is evidence of serious disease. Normal anatomic structures may be thought of as potential signs of disease, and by introspection about his oral sensations, the patient may bring to conscious level sensations associated with normal oral function of which he was not previously aware. Sensations of roughness, dryness, altered taste, burning, and even pain may be brought to the dentist's attention under these conditions. Such functional symptoms need to be distinguished from similar sensations arising from physical changes affecting the oral cavity. Alternatively, there may be no increase in the sensation of which the patient may have been consciously aware for some time; it may be simply the patient's awareness of how long a chronic symptom or other abnormality should be tolerated before seeking dental or medical assistance that has changed in the light of the anxiety generated by a friend's death. A catalogue of recent deaths among family and acquaintances is a common feature of both medical and dental histories.

Normal oral structures often mistakenly identified as physical abnormalities by the patient under these conditions and consequently often identified as the cause of unexplained oral symptoms include tongue papillae, fissures, and median rhomboid glossitis; pharyngeal and palatal mucosal lymphoid nodules; benign migratory glossitis; Fordyce spots; minor salivary glands and the orifices of parotid and submandibular glands; sublingual varicosities; and palatal and mandibular tori. These structures are described elsewhere in this text. There is no evidence that any of these are associated with symptoms in a cause-and-effect relationship, although symptomatic lesions may arise from other causes in mouths that feature these structures prominently. Their presence should not blind the examiner to the need for a thorough oral examination. In general, patients should be informed of their presence and reassured of their asymptomatic and harmless nature.

All patients with apparently unexplained oral symptoms, irrespective of the dentist's perception of a multitude of psychological factors influencing the symptoms, deserve a thorough oral examination (see Chaps. 2 and 16) to determine the extent of physical abnormality which may be contributing to the symptoms. It is only through such an examination, repeated in detail each time the patient is evaluated, that a convincing diagnosis of psychological pain or "oral symptoms aggravated by psychologic (or emotional) factors" can be established. Such a diagnosis cannot be accepted simply because the patient is mentally ill or shows other evidence of irrational behavior; oral examination findings, which include all approaches appropriate to the particular oral complaint, must be shown to be minimal or nonexistent and to remain so on repeated evaluation.

The oral examination also allows the clinician an opportunity to observe the patient's response to manipulation of oral and facial tissues. The nature of the patient's response to palpation or percussion of the painful area, when he is aware it is being explored and at other times when he does not know exactly what the dentist is examining in his mouth, may indicate a high level of psychological involvement. Repeated use of scaling techniques (see Chap. 16) helps characterize the intensity of the pain and to some extent allows separation of the painful sensation from the patient's emotional response to the pain. Patients with psychiatric problems may be unable to comply with this requirement in any consistent fashion and may also be unable to complete the standard psychiatric questionnaires (*e.g.*, Cornell Medical Index; MMPI).

In the absence of recognizable physical abnormalities to explain the patient's symptoms, a diagnosis of psychological pain should not be made without clear evidence of psychiatric abnormality. Except where there is a preexisting diagnosis of mental disease, the diagnosis of psychological pain can only be confirmed by psychiatric evaluation of the patient. In our experience, the assistance of a psychiatrist who works closely with the oral medicine diagnostic unit and who is familiar with oral disease and psychological problems associated with the oral cavity is invaluable in the evaluation of suspected psychologic oral problems as well as in the identification and management of den-

tal patients in whom emotional factors complicate their physical oral problems.

Even when no physical abnormality can be found to explain a patient's oral pain and when there is evidence of psychiatric abnormality and the diagnosis of psychological pain seems justified, it should not be thought that the pain the patient experiences is any less real than that felt, for instance, by a patient with an acute alveolar abscess. Pain is undoubtedly felt by both these patients; the difference is that in our present state of knowledge, the pain in the first case is better understood in terms of psychological rather than pathophysiologic mechanisms. The term *psychological pain* rather than *psychogenic pain* is preferred because the latter implies that the pain arises from psychological causes; there is no evidence to support such an origin for pain.

ORAL FUNCTION AND SYMBOLISM

In considering the role that psychological factors can play in oral disease, it is useful to review the various important functions served by the oral cavity. Many of these functions are concerned with preservation of the organism and are linked to intense natural desires that the majority of humans seem obliged to fulfill. From most of these functions, we derive considerable pleasure (hedonic stimulation) in addition to the physiological needs they satisfy. It is not surprising that limitations of oral function or a threat of limitation of oral function by a chronic oral sensory abnormality can lead to strong emotional reaction, anxiety, and depression. A brief review of oral physiological and psychological functions follows; concern about the loss of some of these functions presumably occurs whenever there is chronic oral pain or other sensory abnormality.

In all species having an oral cavity, the mouth is the means by which the organism obtains food. In man, the oral functions of grasping and prehension may be dispensed with, but masticatory function, salivation, and oral somatic sensory and chemoreception are needed to prepare a bolus for swallowing, which lingual and pharyngeal neuromuscular mechanisms in turn control. Oral sensation provides the individual with some perception of what he is eating, as well as with many pleasurable sensations. When the oral ingestive route is severely compromised, life can be maintained artificially in man by liquid foods obtained by mouth or introduced by an intragastric or intravenous route, but both common experience and psychiatric studies tell us that life under such conditions is unpleasant and emotionally unsatisfying.

Because the mouth serves mostly as a resonating chamber and a device for modulating rather than producing speech, oral disorders have less effect on the communicatory function of the mouth than do, for example, laryngeal lesions; however, chronic oral pain, facial paralysis, loss of teeth, and a variety of other oral problems can significantly affect speech, particularly in persons who rely heavily on their voices in their daily lives. Facial expressions also play a large part in nonverbal communication, and the tendency to avoid social occasions, which is often reported by patients with chronic orofacial sensory and motor abnormalities, may be the result of their inability to communicate effectively in this way. Appearance can likewise be affected by oral disease, and anxiety about facial disfigurement is an important emotional response of patients threatened by real or imagined surgical procedures on the mouth and face.

In humans, the mouth features prominently in a variety of sexual encounters in infants, children, and adults alike. Inability to fulfill these desires and to satisfy the needs for oral psychosexual stimulation undoubtedly produces emotional stresses.

In addition to these real physiological functions that the oral cavity performs and that satisfy essential hedonic as well as physiological demands, a number of imagined or symbolic functions are traditionally assigned tc the mouth. Although largely unsupported by the facts of physiology and anatomy, these "functions" feature prominently in our language and thoughts, and they are sometimes as strongly associated in a patient's mind with threats to oral function as are those functions having their bases in anatomic reality. The following examples of these images are suggested:

1. The oral cavity as the "mouthpiece of the mind." The mouth is the source of pleasant, complimentary, encouraging, and virtuous statements as well as smiles, laughs, and blessings; such are the product of the healthy, wholesome mouth. By contrast, invective, imprecations, critical tight-lipped comments, scowls, and curses arise from a dirty, unwholesome, and diseased mouth.

2. The oral cavity as "an organ of perception." The mouth allows us to distinguish pleasurable from aversive foods and by extension it allows us to taste the pleasurable and unhappy aspects of life. Loss of taste sensation implies not only loss of specific chemoreception but also of the ability to experience and critically evaluate the joys and sorrows of life.

3. The oral cavity as "a source of pleasure" and as the "gate of hell." The mouth can provide kisses and caresses or it can be the mark of an aggressive, devouring personality. In the one case it is pictured as clean, soft, moist and warm, in the other as filthy, like that of a ravaging beast, scarred, broken, and with steaming, noisome breath.

The extent to which these traditional images exist in the thoughts of patients with oral disease is largely undocumented and probably could be revealed only by psychoanalysis; however, comments patients make in regard to their oral symptoms during regular diagnostic interviews suggest that such symbolism is a very common accompaniment to oral disease. It is important that the clinician recognize these psychological interactions because it allows him to distinguish between complaints that are essentially psychological in nature and those which more directly concern altered physiological states. The treatment for one is quite different from treatment for the other. Simultaneous treatment for both problems may be needed. It is also an error to consider that the patient who uses symbolic images in relating his oral problems is necessarily psychologically abnormal, even when the images appear to be somewhat bizarre and overly graphic. It is likely that oral symbolism is normally quite well developed in most minds, and concern about oral pain and discomfort simply allows patients to be somewhat less reserved about expressing their thoughts than they might usually be.

ATYPICAL OROFACIAL PAIN

Atypical orofacial pain refers to pain that does not conform to recognized anatomic pathways in its distribution. The following are therefore included within this definition:

1. Orofacial pain that cannot be relieved by interruption of trigeminal or glossopharyngeal pathways
2. Orofacial pain that has no identifiable neuropathic or nonneuropathic (extraneural or central) focus
3. Orofacial pain that is associated with a potential pain-producing focus but that is out of proportion to the focus or not strictly related to it in terms of recognized anatomic pathways and physiological mechanisms

Because all of these features are negative, it follows that the diagnosis of atypical facial pain is often made by exclusion. Furthermore, as pointed out earlier, with time and repeated clinical investigation, a pathophysiologic explanation is found for many pains that have been placed in the category of atypical facial pain. For this reason, many authors refer to atypical orofacial pain as a grab-bag category or a syndrome with multiple etiologies. Two features (the steady, diffuse, aching and poorly localized quality of the pain and the commonly associated depression) occur with such frequency in many patients with this "diagnosis" that there is some practicality in discussing them as a group, particularly from the standpoint of current management. Psychological factors are also prominent in this group of patients, and it is difficult to distinguish the category of atypical facial pain clearly from what other authors may refer to as psychogenic or psychological pain. TMJ myofascial dysfunction, orofacial pain of vascular origin, and referred pains in the head and neck all show some resemblance to atypical facial pain, and this term has been used on occasion to include these conditions. Whenever these conditions are

diagnosed there should be specific information available to justify such a diagnosis that will exclude that patient from the atypical facial pain category (see Chap. 16).

Attempts have also been made to distinguish between atypical facial pain and atypical facial neuralgia (*i.e.*, pain of atypical quality but of neuropathic origin) on the basis of the ability to temporarily relieve the symptoms of steady aching pain in the latter by peripheral nerve block. As has been pointed out in Chapter 16, orofacial pain of neuropathic origin possesses no one quality and may be either episodic as in tic douloureux or of a steady, aching quality; therefore, any pain that is interrupted by nerve block presumably arises from a pathologic focus in or about the segment of the nerve that is distal to the block and should be labeled either extraneural nonneuropathic or neuropathic and should not be included in the category of atypical facial pain. In this regard, it must also be realized that the opportunity for symptoms to be altered by suggestibility is quite high in patients with atypical facial pain, and the results of diagnostic nerve blocking may be open to question unless it is carried out in a blind-controlled fashion. Moreover, where pain is diffuse and crosses anatomic boundaries and the patient's account of its location and intensity is vague and inconsistent, it may be impossible to design a useful trial of nerve blocking.

The feature that most commonly suggests to the clinician that he may be dealing with a patient with atypical facial pain is the inability of the patient to be precise in defining the location and quality of the pain. Descriptions such as "deep, dull ache" are frequently used by the patient, and requests to point out the location of the pain rarely narrow the area affected to the extent that a patient with pulpitis or pain caused by a traumatic nerve injury can achieve. A tendency to discursive, wandering replies is often also noted in these patients, adding significantly to the frustration of the clinician trying to document a clear history of the patient's pain problem. These two features are noteworthy, first because they can be clues to the dentist that he may be dealing with atypical facial pain and because they should alert the dentist to the likelihood that he will be less attentive to this patient and even somewhat cursory in his oral examination unless he makes a conscious effort to complete his interview and examination in a systematic fashion. This patient should be examined on more than one occasion and should be recalled for further evaluation at regular intervals if a diagnosis of atypical facial pain is made.

Not uncommonly, patients with these problems describe other oral sensory problems such as burning, dryness, and taste aberrations. Questionnaires that ask about these various oral sensory abnormalities frequently elicit evidence of mixed symptomatology in these patients; the patient may or may not include them in his chief complaint and may mention them only if specifically asked. When these patients are followed for many years, it is often noticed that one chronic oral symptom replaces another, with diagnosis and treatment at one time focussed on pain and at another on suspected salivary gland disease or glossodynia.

Although the patient with atypical facial pain may be imprecise about his symptoms, there is usually no doubt that he is suffering. The pain may be described as dull and not particularly intense, but it will often be categorized as the worst pain the patient has ever had, and emotional breakdowns, tears, and hysteria are not uncommon features of the diagnostic interview for these patients. Relatives are also impressed with this aspect of the patient's problem and will often seek aid for the patient for this cause. When asked why he cries with the pain, the patient will often be able to distinguish the fact that he is upset by the chronicity of the pain and his frustration over it and that he has had more severe (i.e., intense) pains at other times. Objective evidence of intense pain is rarely present, and episodes during which the patient grimaces, clutches the affected area, and becomes pale or sweaty, for example, are noticeably absent.

It may therefore seem surprising when the patient relates that this long-standing pain interferes seriously with his work and home-life and that he has discontinued particular activities (e.g., a hobby, social outings, even work) on account of the pain. These patients also have usually consulted a series of health services and specialists about their problem

and may have subjected themselves to extensive and even potentially dangerous diagnostic and therapeutic procedures in the hope of gaining relief.

Many of these features will be recognized as those sometimes seen in depressed patients, and further questioning often reveals other evidence suggestive of such a diagnosis (e.g., disturbance of sleep pattern, loss of appetite, loss of weight, loss of interest in a variety of activities, fatigue, irritability, and agitation). The patient's appearance may also suggest such a diagnosis; a sad, unhappy face, inability to respond in a positive, happy way to any question, often with the explanation that all would be all right if only the pain would go away.

Depression of some degree has been shown to accompany all chronic pain. (Anxiety is a normal response to acute pain and will recur from time to time whenever pain persists; in time depression usually becomes the major psychological change irrespective of the etiology of the pain.) However, depression occurs with such consistency in patients with atypical facial pain and treatment of the depression is so frequently followed by alleviation of the complaint of pain that now a large body of literature identifies atypical facial pain as a manifestation of depression and specifies its treatment as that for depression, namely by means of tricyclic antidepressants or monoamine oxidase inhibitors, by electroshock, or by psychotherapy.

Most authors who have dealt with this subject in the last 10 years have supported the above approach, although others have noted that similar orofacial pain complaints may occur in association with other psychiatric diagnoses, namely, anxiety, obsessional neurosis, and hysteria. To some extent these disagreements can be attributed to changing patterns of diagnostic categories in psychiatry, but they also emphasize the fact that treatment of atypical facial pain with antidepressant medications without skilled psychiatric assistance may produce undesirable effects and severe emotional disturbance of the patient.

Consideration is also given in the literature to the possibility of atypical facial pain occurring as a depressive equivalent (i.e., to its being the only manifestation of the depression, the other symptoms of which are masked or otherwise atypical). In view of the risk that patients with atypical facial pain may be inadequately examined or may be dropped from follow-up schedules if they are treated solely for depression on the basis of orofacial pain being the only manifestation of that psychiatric problem, it is essential that a search for other confirmatory evidence for depression be made by a psychiatrist before that diagnosis is accepted. Even then, a diagnosis of atypical facial pain as a depressive equivalent is a dangerous diagnosis and should be re-evaluated at least every 6 to 12 months with appropriate reexamination clinically, radiographically, and with laboratory aids to ensure that a previously unrecognized lesion or underlying systemic problem is not the cause of the patient's chronic orofacial pain. In similar fashion, patients with atypical facial pain and a clear diagnosis of depression should be re-evaluated at regular intervals to ensure that they do not also have a physical lesion to explain their pain.

Differential Diagnosis

The differential diagnosis for atypical facial pain should include temporomandibular myofascial dysfunction syndrome and TMJ disease because pain in these conditions may also be deep and diffuse and occasionally not readily controlled by diagnostic block unless the localized focus of muscle tenderness is carefully infiltrated with local anesthetic. Referred pain may also be poorly localized, and pain of vascular origin in the head may be hard to separate from atypical facial pain unless an area of tenderness or a nodule can be detected along the course of a vessel or the pain exacerbated by palpation of a vessel. By definition, atypical facial pain is not associated with trigger zones and is also relatively easily separated from tic douloureux because of its continuous, nonparoxysmal quality. There is some suggestion in the literature, however, that tic douloureux of many years' standing, or following treatment with carbamazepine (Tegretol), may gradually convert to a chronic, more nearly continuous and less intense pain that may be hard to distinguish from atypical facial pain. As stressed in the preceding text, all patients with atypical facial

pain should be thought of as potentially having pain with a recognizable focus that may be too small and well hidden to be detected at the time or that may have been missed during the various examination procedures.

As a minimum requirement, patients with atypical facial pain should receive a thorough examination of nose and pharynx from an otorhinolaryngologist; a radiographic examination of the jaws, accessory nasal sinuses, and base of the skull (with additional tomographic studies of poorly defined areas); and a thorough oral examination as described in Chapter 16. Consideration should be given at this time to the large number of extraneural nonneuropathic causes of orofacial pain listed in Chapter 16, to rule out the possibility that one of them is the cause of the patient's chronic pain. In addition to a complete blood count and SMA-12 laboratory studies, a protein electrophoresis to eliminate the possibility of multiple myeloma and a glucose tolerance test to detect early diabetes should be carried out. Some of these procedures, at least, should be repeated each year if the pain persists. A thorough neurologic evaluation including careful examination of cranial nerve function should also be repeated. Careful palpation of the parotid gland may reveal a nodule, discovery of which should be followed by sialographic examination. Cranial arteriography, brain scans, and computerized axial tomography may offer additional help in selected cases.

Treatment of atypical facial pain, as defined in this section, is by treatment of the associated depression. Treatment of depression should be carried out with the assistance of the patient's general physician or internist. In many cases, the service of a psychiatrist is also desirable. Tranquilizers and muscle relaxants such as diazepam (Valium) and thioridazine (Mellaril) usually have no effect on atypical facial pain and may also induce further psychological disturbance.

GLOSSODYNIA (GLOSSALGIA, GLOSSOPYROSIS)

Painful, burning sensations localized in the tongue or affecting other areas of the oral mucosa (stomatopyrosis) are relatively common complaints of dental patients. Although the general dental and medical literature contains multiple references to this problem and to the difficulties of treating it, the neurologic literature gives it minimal consideration. The description of the symptom varies from patient to patient, some referring to "pain," others to "burning," "tingling," or "numbness" in the organ. Melzack (see Fig. 16-3) includes a burning sensation as one descriptor of pain, placing it as greater than "hot" and less than "scalding and searing," in ascending order of intensity. Patients with glossodynia are often surprisingly precise in their selection of words from among the 20 categories of pain qualities on the Melzack questionnaire and may circle only one word in the "sensory-thermal" category out of the 97 words available. Glossodynia may occur in this fashion as an isolated symptom; in other patients it may be one of a group of oral symptoms that often include dull, deep, continous pain of the atypical facial pain variety.

Patients with glossodynia are classically divided into those who have symptoms associated with clinically observable changes in the tongue and those without observable clinical change. That the anatomic association of lesion and symptoms in the tongue is not necessarily an etiologic one, however, has been well established in studies of the development of symptomatology in geographic tongue. Where an abnormality of the surface mucosa is present in as obvious a region as the tongue, there is a strong possibility that any symptoms experienced in that organ will be attributed to the mucosal abnormality, irrespective of the cause of the symptoms. The constant mobility of the tongue and its importance in speech, eating, and sexual encounters also ensure that even minor affections of this organ, whether or not they are associated with lesions, will be experienced as a significant and continuous disability. Etiologic studies of glossodynia are therefore difficult to evaluate, and the validity of some classical associations of systemic disease and glossodynia may be questioned.

Dental evaluation of the patient with a complaint of glossodynia usually begins with examination for and elimination of any obvious local irritants (rough teeth, restorations, appliances, dentures, or calculus, as well as irritating foods, oral muscular habits,

and heavy smoking). Where the shape of a lesion on the tongue closely matches the suspected irritant, its etiologic role seems more certain. The lack of close assocation between lesions, symptoms, and the presence of irritants, however, suggests that muscular tension in the tongue may be important as well.

The role of muscular tension is also frequently invoked where glossodynia is considered to be associated with decreased (and increased) vertical dimension or a component of the myofascial pain dysfunction syndrome and where individuals with glossodynia exhibit obviously exaggerated or aberrant oral muscle habits. That symptoms of glossodynia may on occasion respond to myofunctional therapy also suggests an important role for muscular tension.

Allergies to denture base materials, metallic restorations, and particular foods, medications, mouthwashes, and dentifrices are often blamed, but symptoms do not always resolve when these agents, as well as local dental irritants, are eliminated. Burning may be an early symptom of oral candidiasis (see Chap. 6).

Observable changes in the lingual mucosa are described as components of several systemic diseases as well as a variety of deficiency states. Untreated pernicious anemia, and the Plummer–Vinson syndrome are associated with atrophy of the lingual epithelium and obvious changes in color and appearance of the dorsum, as is deficiency of nicotinic acid (pellagra). Symptoms of soreness, tenderness, and burning frequently accompany these findings, but such symptoms are not specific for these conditions, and it must be quite rare for glossodynia to be the presenting complaint and the only clinical evidence for the deficiency state.

The lack of specificity of these symptoms is indicated, for example, by the fact that one author recorded oral complaints such as soreness, burning, irritation, and low tolerance to dentures as well as mucosal atrophy in 30% of patients with achlorhydria confirmed by gastric analysis, but similar signs and symptoms were also recorded in 20% of patients with normal gastric analyses. The development of lingual filiform papillary atrophy has also been observed in cancer patients, normal volunteers, and prisoners of war maintained on protein- and vitamin-deficient diets. Objective changes in the tongue occurred after about 1 month on these grossly deficient diets, with subjective complaints of discomfort in swallowing, burning of the tongue and lips, and sensations of dryness and taste disturbance occurring after 2 to 3 months of continuous deficiency. With return to normal diet, both objective and subjective changes disappeared.

Glossodynia may occur with diabetes mellitus, either as a result of oral candidiasis or perhaps from peripheral neuropathy. That such symptoms may be a prodrome of diabetes remains controversial, however (see description earlier in this chapter). Other systemic problems that should be considered as an explanation for glossodynia include amyloidosis, multiple myeloma, and malignant lesions metastatic to the tongue.

Burning sensations in the tongue secondary to neuropathy of the lingual nerve should also be distinguished from the orolingual pain that arises from the various causes just described. The quality of pain described by these patients may be no different, but there is usually a history of an episode that could have damaged the lingual nerve (e.g., removal of submaxillary gland calculus, a difficult third molar extraction, jaw fracture, or laceration of the side of the tongue during a dental procedure) with almost immediate onset of the abnormal sensation. Diagnostic nerve blocking proximal to the suspected site of nerve damage will also usually allow the focus of the symptoms to be identified and their neuropathic nature to be confirmed. Such symptoms sometimes resolve with time, but some residual numbness and sensitivity often remain on an isolated area of the anterior third of the tongue. Episodic pain in the posterior part of the tongue may also be reported by patients with glossopharyngeal neuralgia (see Chap. 16), but the paroxysmal nature of that pain, its location, and its association with other symptoms of nerve dysfunction separate it from glossodynia.

Finally, there is a group of patients in whom no cause can be found for the glossodynia. Many of these resemble patients with atypical facial pain in many respects (namely, the diffuse, poorly localized quality of their tongue symptoms, their discursiveness and depressed affect), and there is some indication in the literature to support the idea

that glossodynia of this idiopathic variety is simply a variant of atypical orofacial pain.

Despite the prevalence of patients with glossodynia, the literature is composed largely of case reports, and very few critical studies have been carried out on the etiology or treatment of this condition. When the cause of the glossodynia is recognized as one of the mechanisms described above, treatment follows logically and includes removal of local oral irritants; construction of plastic retainers to cover irregularities of the occlusion that magnify the side-effects of tongue habits; treatment of the muscular tension by correction of the malocclusion or by muscle-relaxants such as diazepam; or treatment of the systemic disease such as diabetes mellitus. Surgical exploration of glossodynia of neuropathic origin may relieve some of the more distressing symptoms, especially if there is a nodule of scar tissue or neuroma formation at the site of damage to the lingual nerve, but some numbness and even burning will usually persist.

Some relief from symptoms is also usually obtained from the use of topical analgesics such as 0.5% aqueous diphenhydramine (Benadryl) alone or mixed with 0.5% dyclonine (Dyclone), or lidocaine or other analgesic ointments applied to the affected area. Concern has recently been expressed that excessive use of such medications that are swallowed may cause some inhibition of the gag reflex and may contribute to food aspiration ("café coronaries"). Patients should be cautioned in this regard, particularly if they use alcoholic beverages.

Where local irritants such as an irregular dental arch (which could not be corrected without major orthodontic rehabilitation) and muscular tension are prominent factors, small doses of muscle relaxants are often very effective in controlling these symptoms. For the idiopathic problem associated with depression, treatment of the depression frequently also controls the lingual symptoms as it does the symptoms of atypical facial pain. With the exception of patients in whom there is other evidence of a nutritional deficiency, vitamin and protein supplements are unlikely to have anything other than a placebo effect on the tongue symptoms (and also do not usually correct areas of papillary atrophy).

Cancerphobia (an excessive fear of cancer) may be a prominent feature of patients with idiopathic glossodynia and is also considered a depressive equivalent. (See following discussion on depression.)

SUBJECTIVE XEROSTOMIA

Unlike pain, dryness might be expected to be a sensation that is detected equally well by the patient and a trained observer examining his mouth. For severely affected patients, this assumption is true: individuals with marked degrees of xerostomia not only feel dry and require quantities of fluid to ingest a meal, their oral mucosae are also red and dry on inspection, and objects such as a dental mirror or a tongue blade adhere tightly to the poorly lubricated surface. With minor degrees of xerostomia, however, this association of subjective and objective findings is not always evident. Slowly developing xerostomia may progress insidiously in a patient to the extent that his mouth appears dry to the observer, even though the patient may be unaware of any subjective sensations of dryness.

More often, the dentist is confronted with the patient who complains of severe dryness and inability to swallow, yet inspection of the mouth and salivary ducts reveals no apparent diminution of salivary flow. A situation such as this is sometimes encountered in patients with atypical facial pain, but unexplained sensations of dryness may also occur without other oral symptoms. Where the patient's complaint does not appear to be confirmed by inspection of the oral cavity and the finding of a dry mucosa and reduced salivary flow, the term *subjective xerostomia* is appropriate.

In some cases, measurement of salivary flow rates (total mixed salivary flow and right and left parotid flow or mixed sublingual, submandibular salivary flow under "resting" and lemon-stimulated conditions) provides evidence of diminished salivary function, and the qualifying adjective "subjective" can be removed from the diagnosis. Under these circumstances, the differential diagnosis should include the long list of local and systemic problems and medications that can af-

fect the salivary glands (see Chap. 11). When these fairly standardized tests and additional investigations (such as minor salivary gland biopsy, sequential salivary scintigraphy, and even retrograde sialography) fail to reveal any abnormality of the salivary glands, it is usually concluded that the patient has a problem analogous to atypical facial pain. This impression is also generally supported by the finding of depressive symptoms in these patients.

In the same category we place those patients who complain of any of an array of oral sensory abnormalities that are difficult to explain in terms of recognized oral sensory modalities and that have no objective findings to confirm them (*e.g.,* complaints of lumpy, gritty, or particulate saliva; roughness of the lining of the mouth; *idiopathic dysgeusia*; areas of numbness or swelling that cannot be identified by changes in pinprick or tactile sensitivity or by inspection of the oral cavity). Depressive symptoms frequently can be noted during interview of these patients, and treatment of the depression not uncommonly reduces the severity or eliminates these complaints. Like patients with atypical facial pain, these patients also must receive adequate follow-up examinations to detect changes in symptoms and any signs of a physical lesion that may explain the apparently bizarre symptoms. These symptoms have also been noted to appear as depressive equivalents in some patients described in the literature.

DEPRESSION

The term *depression* is used in everyday language to refer to a passing mood of unhappiness, sadness, or the blues that all of us experience from time to time as part of the normal pattern of life. The same word is used also to describe a clinical state that may be similar to such mood changes but also encompasses a broader range of symptoms and signs that on occasion severely limit an individual's ability to function. In this text and in the clinical literature in general, depression has this latter meaning and defines one of the major categories of mental illness. No clear line of separation can be drawn between clinical depression and transient mood swings, and some authors still debate whether depression is a disease; however, severely depressed patients often become increasingly unable to carry out their customary daily tasks and work and maintain satisfactory relationships with their friends and relatives. They certainly experience suffering as part of their problem, and in some cases they also appear to develop secondary physical changes such as loss of weight, increased susceptibility to disease, and altered function of a variety of bodily systems. In many, specific treatment for the depression alleviates many of these symptoms. From a functional point of view, therefore, there is considerable practical value in considering clinical depression as a disease and providing treatment for patients with this problem.

Depression of various degrees frequently accompanies chronic illness, and as discussed earlier in this chapter, it is very common in patients with chronic oral pain and other oral sensory disorders, irrespective of the cause of the sensory abnormality. The dentist or physician who treats patients with chronic oral disease is therefore often involved with a depressed patient. Depressed patients show excessive concern about various bodily functions (including oral function and appearance), and a dentist should expect to find depressed patients among those who repeatedly seek the most extensive forms of dental treatment. In general, the treatment of oral disease in a depressed patient will have an unsatisfactory outcome regardless of whether the patient's oral problem is dental caries, periodontal disease, TMJ myofascial dysfunction, recurrent mouth ulcers, chronic orofacial pain, or unsatisfactory dentures. It is very important that the dentist be able to recognize the depressed patient and obtain appropriate treatment for him, if he is to succeed in managing the patient's oral problem.

Depression is one of the more prevalent forms of mental illness which the dentist is likely to encounter in his patients (one estimate suggests that 5% of the population will experience significant depression at some age), and it is also a problem that is less likely to result in hospitalization or admission to an institution than are problems such as schizophrenia. It may therefore be less prominent in the patient's medical history than are other forms of mental illness. The depressed patient may make a strong effort to deny or cover up his depression, and hidden depressive symptoms must also be watched for carefully. It is unfortunate, because of the continuing philosophical debate about the nature of depression, that there is often a tendency on the part of both clinicians and families to avoid the problem of a patient's depression, even when the symptoms and the patient's inability to function are quite obvious. Failure to recognize and treat the patient's depression not infrequently causes considerable frustration and suffering as well as wasted time and effort for both doctor and patient.

Ability to recognize the presence of depressive symptoms should not be confused with the making of a psychiatric diagnosis of depression. Depressive symptoms may accompany many types of mental illness such as schizophrenia and also may result from brain damage and the use of drugs such as reserpine, phenothiazides, and other tranquilizing agents. Depression may be a reasonable response to death of a loved one or to chronic illness and disability.

To the psychiatrist, depression is not a single disease but one which is recognized in a variety of forms, the categorization of which has led to one of the most prolonged debates in psychiatry. One category of depression consists of cases that are described as endogenous (i.e., caused primarily by some biological derangement; for example, those diagnosed as biphasic or manic-depressive psychoses or involutional melancholia); the other major category is reactive depression, thought to be caused primarily by some external stress such as bereavement, financial loss, or unemployment (e.g., those diagnosed as psychogenic or neurotic depression).

Continued biochemical studies of the role of catecholamines and other intermediates in central nervous system function suggest that some biochemical abnormality may be present in all types of depression, but no unifying hypothesis to explain all depressive illness has appeared. Consequently, the diagnosis of the nature of the patient's psychiatric problem and whether he indeed has a mental illness remains in the hands of the psychiatrist, who should be consulted, if at all possible, when the dentist recognizes significant depression in his patient.

Symptomatology

The major changes occurring in depression are characterized in terms of alteration in mood (*e.g.*, sadness, loneliness, apathy), a negative self-image (*e.g.*, feeling guilty and taking blame), regressive activity (*e.g.*, desires to escape, hide, or die), vegetative changes (*e.g.*, anorexia, insomnia, and loss of libido), and change in activity level (*e.g.*, tiredness or agitation). Symptoms of depression, in general, follow this pattern as summarized below.

SIGNS AND SYMPTOMS OF DEPRESSION*

- **Mood**
    Sad, unhappy, blue
    Crying

- **Thought**
    Pessimism
    Ideas of guilt
    Self-denigration
    Loss of interest and motivation
    Decrease in efficiency and concentration

- **Behavior and Appearance**
    Neglect of personal appearance
    Psychomotor retardation
    Agitation

- **Somatic**
    Loss of appetite
    Loss of weight
    Constipation
    Poor sleep
    Aches and pains
    Menstrual changes
    Loss of libido

- **Anxiety Features**
- **Suicidal Behavior**
    Thoughts
    Threats
    Attempts

* Mendels, J: Concepts of Depression. New York, John Wiley & Sons, 1970)

Emotional manifestations such as a mood of dejection, misery, or unhappiness may be prominent symptoms of the depressed patient, particularly when they seem inappropriate to the somatic symptoms or situations to which the patient attributes them. Emotional response must be evaluated carefully in terms of what the dentist might consider the normal range of patient behavior and if possible in terms also of the behavior the patient has previously shown under similar circumstances. At times, the depressed patient may be unable to give a reason for his unhappiness; often, though, in the context of the consulting room, he will attribute it to his chronic oral problem. The patient's mood may be obvious to the examiner; alternatively, it may be expressed by the patient affectively ("I feel depressed") or in somatic terms ("I have a lump in my throat," "Things no longer have any taste"; see discussion on dysgeusia in Chap. 16). Crying spells may punctuate the process of obtaining the history; alternatively, with the added attention and concern expressed by the clinician, the patient's mood may improve, a phenomenon often occurring when a depressed patient is demonstrated to a class of students.

Although perfectly rational to himself, the depressed patient's thought processes may seem quite abnormal to the clinician. Such cognitive manifestations of depression in general reflect abnormality in the patient's thoughts about himself, his achievements, his abilities and his relationship to his family and work associates, and his customary responsibilities at home and at work. Not uncommonly, a depressed patient will associate difficulties in any of these spheres with chronic oral symptoms and will express the feeling that all of his problems would be solved if only the oral symptoms would be cured. Oral symptoms do cause considerable difficulty with a variety of oral functions as described earlier, but the depressed patient's reponse to his oral symptoms can often be quite extreme (*e.g.*, loss of employment blamed on ill-fitting dentures or halitosis; decreased social visiting blamed on loss of taste; inactivity and lack of interest in family, friends, work, or hobbies blamed on chronic low-grade oral pain). Loss of gratification from work, family, and home may be expressed in a variety of ways by the depressed patient (even when it appears to bear no obvious relationship to oral symptoms) as well as feelings of guilt, loss of affection, pessimism, and hopelessness. In extreme cases, patients will relate their thoughts contemplating suicide that have stemmed from chronic oral symptoms.

Other cognitive problems in depression include lack of motivation and indecisiveness (difficulties that often become apparent when a dentist embarks on a complicated plan of dental treatment requiring decisions by the patient on the design, expense, and appearance of a prosthetic restoration) and increased dependence on others that may be directed to medical personnel as well as to family and friends. Such dependence in depressed patients can often be recognized as a *desire* by the patient for help rather than a clear *need* for help, and the plea for help is often patently misdirected. In such situations, a dentist must be able to recognize his limitations and attempt to provide only the assistance that is appropriate to the patient's demonstrated oral problems. The terms *help-seeking behavior* and *orality* refer to related aspects of dependence that are often discussed in regard to depression. Both terms reflect the role of the mouth as a means of expression of a patient's thoughts and emotions and emphasize the important relationship between depression and oral symptomatology.

The vegetative or physical manifestations of depression have been stressed by some authors because their existence suggests that depression (and other mental disorders in which they occur) may be a basic autonomic or hypothalamic disturbance with widespread biochemical effects. Such manifestations include symptoms of easy or excessive fatigability, disturbances of sleep pattern, loss of appetite and loss of interest in sexual activities, as well as constipation, aches and pains, and menstrual changes. Such symptoms, however, have been shown to correlate poorly with the severity of depression and may also reflect other organic abnormality accompanying the depression. Diminished salivary flow and hypogeusia are two oral symptoms that are often described as vegetative manifestations of depression, but careful studies of the former, at least, have so far failed to confirm this association. Accurate testing of such hypotheses is compromised by the difficulty of finding a large series of patients with untreated depression and by the fact that the drugs commonly used to treat depression cause xerostomia.

Patients with severe depression may experience delusions and even psychotic hallucinations. Although not restricted to somatic content, such delusions may focus on oral function (taste in particular) and may feature overemphasis of the symbolic oral functions described earlier as part of normal psychological experience. These somatic delusions may be brought to the dentist's attention while he is taking a history; otherwise, the characteristic delusions of depression regarding worthlessness, crime and punishment, poverty, and death are unlikely to be related to him other than by a fairly disturbed patient.

None of the foregoing symptoms either alone or in twos or threes can be considered diagnostic of depression. Each to some degree is part of normal experience for both normal individuals and for those who have at some time been depressed but who have recovered from the episode. It is only when many of these symptoms represent persistent behavior for a given patient that there is a strong chance that they are evidence of clinical depression rather than of a transient mood or personality change. Alternatively, fewer symptoms, with each present to a severe degree, may be indicative of depression. Under either circumstance, a dentist would be justified in considering the possibility of depression in his patient and in seeking appropriate assistance before embarking on a plan of dental treatment. Experience in a given field of dentistry, plus some social and emotional maturity and an awareness of the wide range of normal behavior will aid the clinician in evaluating a patient's symptoms in this regard. The MMPI and Cornell Medical Index as well as questionnaires designed specifically for the detection of depression (such as those of Beck and Zung) are also useful in the identification of the depressed patient. Routine use of these questionnaires is common in pain-control clinics and clinics concerned with chronic illness.

Management of the Depressed Patient

Three treatment modalities are currently available for use in depression: electroconvulsive shock therapy, psychotherapy, and antidepressant medication. With the exception of antidepressant medication, treatment for depression is usually provided by a psychiatrist. Antidepressant medications, however, are probably used equally frequently by general medical practitioners and internists. The selection of the appropriate method of treatment depends very much on the diagnosis of the particular form of depression involved as well as on the psychiatrist's preference. Because of the untoward effects of antidepressant medications on patients with psychotic, paranoid, and manic tendencies, they should not be prescribed by anyone who is ill-equipped to recognize such potential problems or unable to handle them when they develop. Tricyclic antidepressants have strong anticholinergic effects and should not be prescribed for patients with anterior angle glaucoma; they also strongly inhibit salivary secretion, the onset of a dry mouth usually being used as an index of the maximum therapeutic dose allowable. The use of monoamine oxidase (MAO) inhibitors for treatment of depression is further complicated by the possibility of severe hypertensive episodes developing when the medication is taken in conjunction with certain cheeses and other foods with a high tyramine content, other MAO inhibitors, and sympathomimetics such as amphetamines and various dopamines.

For the dentist, the main problem is usually the referral of a patient whom he suspects may be depressed and whom he wishes to get to a physician who will be able to confirm his suspicions and organize appropriate treatment. In general, little is gained by the dentist's telling a patient that his problem does not seem to be a physical one and that he should perhaps consult a psychiatrist. Unless he has been severely frightened by thoughts of suicide, a depressed patient will often deny his emotional problems in favor of a physical diagnosis and will simply take himself to another doctor. The patient who believes he needs a psychiatrist will usually consult one directly rather than wait for the dentist's referral. Two exceptions to this that are sometimes seen and should be looked for are the patient who has had previous treatment for depression and is aware of the help this treatment gave him on an earlier occasion and the patient who realizes that he has emotional problems beyond his own control, but who just needs the added stimulus of the dentist's recommendation to actually seek out a psychiatrist.

In our own experience, many depressed patients will accept referral to a psychiatrist and willingly undertake whatever treatment he prescribes, provided there is no overt acknowledgement of this in the dentist's or his own family's discussions of it. Where a psychiatrist is part of the oral medicine team, such referrals can be made quite comfortably with the euphemism that "I wish to refer you to a physician who works with us and who is specially trained in the management of chronic oral problems." The patient who wishes to know whether this doctor is a psychiatrist will then ask the psychiatrist at the time of consultation. Many patients never ask, yet readily accept psychiatric care. The availability of medication for the treatment of depression in appropriate cases also has eased some of the problems of these referrals because electroshock therapy and psychoanlysis provide a far greater threat to patients.

On occasion, a patient will thank the dentist for making a forthright statement that he felt the patient needed psychiatric help and will admit that he had realized for some time that he needed such help. The dentist had simply been consulted at the end of a series of other doctors in the faint hope that an oral symptom might have had a somatic dental explanation.

Referral of the patient to a trusted family medical practitioner or internist can sometimes also be a useful route. The physician may be willing to investigate the problem and undertake the necessary treatment or provide additional guidance in the selection of an internist or psychiatrist who will. Where good rapport exists between the dentist and the patient's physician or the psychiatrist, continued management of the problem and adjustment of the dose of antidepressant medication can sometimes be handled by the dentist under the guidance of the psychiatrist. Such an arrangement allows treatment to be focused on the oral symptoms, which is often the primary concern for the patient.

Discussion of the patient's oral problem as a manifestation of stress or muscle tension where such factors have a logical part in the complex etiology of a complaint of burning tongue or atypical orofacial pain may also be tolerated more comfortably by the patient in speaking with his dentist than would the use of terms such as "depression," or "anxiety," which have a stronger psychiatric association. In fact, at the time the dentist sees the patient, he is usually without evidence to confirm his suspicion of depression, and it is quite inappropriate for him to use diagnostic terms that imply a mental illness. Muscle relaxation techniques (which are now more commonly administered with the aid of electromyographic biofeedback equipment) are also a familiar method of treatment used by some psychiatrists. Referral for this specific form of treatment can serve as the patient's introduction to the psychiatrist, if the patient's problem has already been discussed by the dentist in terms of "stress-reactions."

For the most part, depression is a passing episode. About 70% to 95% of cases recover completely (although there are recurrences), with the chance of recovery improving, the younger the patient; however, there seems to be no information to indicate whether this recovery rate is specifically reflected in the patients who present with oral symptoms associated with their depression that the dentist is likely to see. After an initial attack of depression, one half to three fourths of the patients will have a recurrence sometime in their lives, hence the importance of a detailed medical history that covers significant past psychiatric problems. Endogenous depression with manic phases is more likely to be recurrent.

Approximately 5% of patients who have been hospitalized with manic-depression subsequently commit suicide. This outcome should always be considered with any de-pressed patient, despite the relative rarity with which it occurs. It is difficult to separate myth from reality in regard to suicidal threats, but those who have attempted to manage patients with chronic orofacial pain can usually document cases where such threats have been related to them by depressed patients. Because the communication of suicidal intent is the best single predictor of a successful suicidal attempt, it is imperative that the dentist make every effort to obtain psychiatric care for such patients as soon as possible.

Depressive Equivalents and Cancerphobia

The term *depressive equivalent* (also referred to as masked, latent, or incomplete depression) was introduced about 20 years ago to describe patients who had various somatic complaints but who showed no apparent mood depression. Various vegetative symptoms of depression may be present, such as disturbance of sleep cycle or loss of appetite and energy; these symptoms together with the response of the previously intractable somatic symptoms to electroconvulsive therapy or antidepressant medications constitute the basis for diagnosis of a depressive equivalent. Atypical facial pain, glossodynia, subjective xerostomia, and idiopathic dysgeusia when unaccompanied by evidence of a depressed mood have been considered in some cases as depressive equivalents. If such somatic symptoms do disappear with appropriate antidepressant therapy, the critical test for the diagnosis of a depressive equivalent would seem to have been achieved.

As pointed out earlier, however, the very vagueness of the evidence on which a diagnosis of depressive equivalent is made can allow it to be stretched to cover practically any somatic syndrome that has no apparent physical abnormality to explain it. Great care, therefore, must be used in managing patients with this tentative diagnosis (and I believe it must always be a tentative diagnosis, even when the symptoms appear to respond to antidepressant therapy), so that an apparently minor physical abnormality is not overlooked. *Thorough re-examination of these patients at least every 6 months is essential.*

An excessive and unreasonable fear of cancer (*cancerphobia*) when unaccompanied by other symptoms of depression has been referred to by some authors as a depressive equivalent. Such anxieties are quite real for many patients, particularly if a relative or friend has developed oral cancer or if they themselves have a chronic oral lesion such as an ulcer, white patch, or growth that defies diagnosis or surgical treatment. In such cases, the term *cancerphobia* should perhaps not be used; it is applicable, however, where there are no chronic lesions to alarm the patient and where repeated oral examination and reassuring the patient that no lesion is present fail to satisfy his anxiety. Management of such patients as recommended for other depressed patients with unexplained oral symptoms can provide some relief from these persistent anxieties. It is important to remember, however, that cancerphobia is no prevention for cancer and that thorough and repeated oral examinations constitute a necessary part of the dental management of these patients. The depressed patient with unexplained oral symptoms should not be lost to dental follow-up simply because he has accepted referral to the psychiatrist.

Dental Disease Secondary to Depression and Antidepressant Therapy

Most antidepressant medications as well as certain other drugs used to alter mood (*e.g.*, tranquilizing drugs such as thioridazine, chlorpromazine [Thorazine], prochlorperazine [Compazine], and perphenazine [Trilafon]) and possibly depression itself lead to significant reduction in salivary flow. Because the disease and its therapy in particular may last from months to years, this diminished salivary flow can have disastrous effects on the dentition. Depression is also likely to be compounded by poor oral hygiene in times of emotional stress, and these patients often use candy to control xerostomic and dysgeusic symptoms. Rampant dental caries analogous to that seen after therapeutic radiation

to the oral cavity thus often results from an episode of depression.

Unfortunately, if the depression continues or as often happens, if the patient suffers a serious financial setback as the result of this severe illness, he will be poorly situated to have the necessary dental restorative treatment he needs. Depressed patients are usually unable to tolerate lengthy dental appointments or an extended treatment plan, and considerable dissatisfaction on both sides and even malpractice suits result when complex treatment is begun for the depressed patient. Where such treatment is needed, the dentist should be in consultation with the patient's psychiatrist, and a clear statement of the time, effort, money, and oral discomfort likely to be involved in each component of the dental treatment should be discussed with both patient and psychiatrist before the work is begun. A similar caveat applies to prosthetic or surgical treatment planned for the depressed patient.

BIBLIOGRAPHY*

Atypical Orofacial Pain

Alderman MM: Disorders of the temporomandibular joint & related structures. Rationale for diagnosis, etiology, management. Alpha Omegan (Scientific Issue) December pp. 12–17, 1976

Braun C: Diagnostic procedures and tests for neurologic diseases and evaluation of specific neurologic complaints. In Halstead JA (ed): The Laboratory in Clinical Medicine, Chaps. 31 and 32. Philadelphia, WB Saunders, 1976

Brightman V, Arm RA: Multiple myeloma presenting as atypical facial pain. Oral Surg [In press.]

Brody HA, Prendergast JJ, Silverman S, JR: The relationship between oral symptoms, insulin release and glucose intolerance. Oral Surg 37:777, 1971

Engel GL: Primary atypical facial neuralgia: Hysterical conversion syndrome. Psychosomat Med 13:375, 1951

Frazier H: Atypical neuralgia: Unsuccessful attempts to relieve patients by operations on the

* See also Chapter 16 for references dealing with many of the conditions to be considered in the differential diagnosis of atypical facial pain, glossodynia, subjective xerostomia and idiopathic dysgeusia and hypogeusia.

cervical sympathetic system. Arch Neurol 19:650, 1928

Glaser MA: Atypical neuralgia, so-called; critical analysis of 143 cases. Arch Neurol Psychiatry 20:537, 1928

Laband P: Use of "time" as a tool to diagnose facial pain. Dent Survey 50:29, 1974

Ledley RS et al: Computerized transaxial x-ray tomography of the human body. Science 186:207, 1974

Rushton JS, Gibilisco JA: Atypical facial pain. JAMA 171:545, 1959

Thomas JE, Waltz AG: Neurological manifestations of nasopharyngeal malignant tumors. JAMA 192:95, 1965

Glossodynia (Glossalgia, Glossopyrosis)

Barry RE: Coeliac disease. The clinical presentation. Clin Gastroenterol 3:55, 1974

Brody HA, Nesbitt WR: Psychosomatic oral problems. J Oral Med 22:43, 1967

Drum W: Burning sensation under new dentures. Quintessence Int 1:38, 1970

Engman MF: Burning tongue. Arch Dermatol Syph 1:137, 1920

Garliner D: Myofunctional Therapy in Dental Practice. Brooklyn, Bartel Dental Book Co, 1971

Harris M: Psychogenic aspects of facial pain. Br Dent J 136:199, 1974

Hjørting–Hansen E, Bertram U: Oral aspects of pernicious anemia. Br Dent J 125:266, 1968

Kutscher AH, Chilton NW: Dolorimetric evaluation of idiopathic glossodynia. NY Dent J 18:31, 1952

McLeod RDM: Abnormal tongue appearances and vitamin status of the elderly—A double-blind trial. Age Ageing 1:99, 1972

Redman RS, Meslin L, Gorlin RJ: Psychological component in the etiology of geographic tongue. J Dent Res 45:1403, 1966

Redman RS, Shapiro BL, Gorlin RJ: Hereditary component in the etiology of benign migratory glossitis. Am J Human Genet 24:124, 1972

Schetman D: The Plummer–Vinson syndrome. A cutaneous manifestation of internal disease. Arch Dermatol 105:720, 1972

Schoenberg B et al: Chronic idiopathic orolingual pain. NY State J Med 71:1832, 1971

Sharp GS: The hot tongue syndrome. Arch Otolaryngol 5:90, 1967

Sharp GS, Helsper JT: Oral manifestations of systemic disease. Regimen of treatment. Oral Surg 23:737, 1967

Ziskin DE, Moulton R: Glossodynia: A study of idiopathic orolingual pain. J Am Dent Assoc 33:1432, 1946

Zucker AH: A psychiatric appraisal of tongue symptoms. J Am Dent Assoc 85:649, 1972

Xerostomia

Bates JF, Adams D: The influence of mental stress on the flow of saliva in man. Arch Oral Biol 13:593, 1968

Bertram U: Xerostomia. Clinical aspects, pathology and pathogenesis. Acta Odontol Scand 25 (Suppl. 49): 1, 1967

Busfield BL, Wechsler H: Salivation rate; a physiologic correlate of improvement in hospitalized depressed patients treated with three antidepressant medications. Psychosomat Med 24:337, 1962

Busfield BL, Wechsler H, Barnum WJ: Studies of salivation in depression. II. Physiological differentiation of reactive and endogenous depression. Arch Gen Psychiatry 5:472, 1961

Cheraskin E, Ringsdorf WM: The edentulous patient. I. Xerostomia and the serum cholesterol level; II Xerostomia and the blood sugar level. J Am Geriatr Soc 17:962, 962, 1969

Conner S, Iranpour B, Mills J: Alteration in parotid salivary flow in diabetes mellitus. Oral Surg 30:55, 1970

Elfenbaum A: The dry mouth. NY J Dentistry 38:400, 1968

Gottlieb G, Paulsen G: Salivation in depressed patients. Arch Gen Psychiatry 5:468, 1961

Lantz HJ: Xerostomia and the edentulous geriatric patient. Bull Phila County Dent Soc 36:10, 1961

Palmai G et al: Patterns of salivary flow in depressive illness and during treatment. Br J Psychiatry 113:1297, 1967

Peck RE: The SHP Test—Aid in the detection and measurement of depression. Arch Gen Psychiatry 1:35, 1939

Uthman AA: Plummer–Vinson syndrome. Report of a case. Oral Surg 20:449, 1965

Idiopathic Dysgeusia

Cooper RM, Bilash I, Zubek JP: The effect of age on taste sensitivity. J Gerontol 14:56, 1959

Hart HH: Bad taste (cacogeusia). Arch Neurol Psychiatry 39:771, 1938

Henkin RI et al: Idiopathic hypogeusia with dysgeusia, hyposmia and dysosmia: A new syndrome. JAMA 217:434, 1971

Linker E, Moore ME, Galanter E: Taste thresholds, detection models and disparate results. J Exp Psychol 67:59, 1964

Schelling J et al: Abnormal taste thresholds in diabetes. Lancet 1:508, 1965

Simon N: The Last of the Red Hot Lovers—Act III. The Comedy of Neil Simon, pp 585–657. New York, Random House, 1971

Steiner JE, Rosenthal–Zifroni A, Edelstein EL: Taste perception in depressive illness. Israel Ann Psychiatry 7:223, 1969

Depression, Psychological Pain, and Other Unexplained Oral Symptoms

Bahn SC: Drug-related dental destruction. Oral Surg 33:49, 1972

Beck AT: Depression, Causes and Treatment. Philadelphia, University of Pennsylvania Press, 1967

Brand D: Beyond the blues. Mental depression afflicts more in the U.S. No one is sure why. New York, The Wall Streeet Journal CLXXIX #69 Apr. 7, 1972

Cowen J, Friedman WW: Psychological considerations in long-term dental care. Dent Survey 47:34, 1971

Dalessio DJ: Chronic pain syndromes and disordered cortical inhibition: Effect of tricyclic compounds. Dis Nerv Syst 28:325, 1967

Dalessio DJ: Some reflections on the etiologic role of depression in head pain. Headache 8:28, 1968

Gayford JJ: The aetiology of atypical facial pain and its relation to prognosis and treatment. Br J Oral Surg 7:202, 1970

Gessel AH, Alderman MM: Management of myofascial pain dysfunction syndrome of the temporomandibular joint by tension control training. Psychosomatics 12:302, 1971

Hollister LE: Mental disorders—antipsychotic and antimanic drugs, and —antianxiety and antidepressant drugs. N Engl J Med 286:984, 1195, 1971

Lascelles RG: Atypical facial pain and depression. Br J Psychiatry 112:651, 1966

Lefer L: Psychic stress and the oral cavity. Postgrad Med 49:171, 1971

Lesse S: Atypical facial pain syndromes of psychogenic origin, complications of their misdiagnosis. J Nerv Ment Dis 124:346, 1956

Mendels J: Concepts of Depression. New York, John Wiley & Sons, 1970

Moulton RE: Psychiatric considerations in maxillofacial pain. J Am Dent Assoc 51:408, 1955

Pilling LF: Psychosomatic aspects of facial pain. In Alling CC (ed): Facial Pain, pp 107–119. Philadelphia, Lea & Febiger, 1968

Rabkin JG, Struening EL: Life events, stress and illness. Science 194:1013, 1976

Russell–Taylor AH: A comparative determination of side effects associated with oral use of three anticholinergic-psychotropic drugs. Int Z Klin Pharmakol Ther Toxikol 3:1, 1970

Sandler S: Depression masking organic diseases and organic diseases masking depression. J Med Soc NJ 45:108, 1948

Scopp IW, Heyman, RA: Significance of dryness of the mouth caused by chlorpromazine J Oral Therap 2:399, 1966

Tully TA: Drug induced xerostomia and severe dental pathology: The role of psychotropic drugs. J Hosp Dent Pract 5:122, 1971

Webb HE, Lascelles RG: Treatment of facial and head pain associated with depression. Lancet 1:355, 1962

Winer JA, Bahn S: Loss of teeth with antidepressant drug therapy. Arch Gen Psychiatry 16:239, 1967

Part III

SYSTEMIC DISEASE

18

Diseases of the Respiratory System

MALCOLM A. LYNCH

UPPER RESPIRATORY INFECTIONS

The Common Cold

The common cold (acute rhinitis-coryza) is an acute infection of the upper respiratory tract caused by one or more of several hundred viruses known to attack these passages. It is estimated that up to 10% of upper respiratory infections are caused by more than one virus, and the symptoms are not uniquely related to the particular virus or viruses causing the disease. The nose and pharynx are the anatomic sites most commonly involved, with laryngeal involvement sometimes occurring. Most commonly implicated is a group of viruses known as the rhinovirus of which there are more than 90 antigenic subtypes. Other viruses implicated include coxsackievirus A21, respiratory syncytial virus, and the parainfluenza viruses.

Respiratory illnesses occur more commonly in the winter, and it has been estimated that half of the population will develop a cold sometime during the winter season. In contrast, only about one fifth of the population will develop a summer cold. Children younger than 6 years of age and their parents seem to be more susceptible to colds and have on the average about six colds a year. The average adult has only two to three colds a year. Studies by Aronson and associates demonstrated a highly significant correlation between cigarette smoking and the occurrence and severity of acute respiratory tract illnesses. Smokers had more respiratory tract infections of longer duration and had a greater likelihood of an upper respiratory infection developing into a lower respiratory tract infection than did nonsmokers.

The average cold lasts from 5 to 7 days. The method of spread is person to person by means of aerosol droplets and hand-to-hand and body-to-body contact. When aerosol droplets are involved, it is thought that viruses in droplets 5 microns or larger lodge in the upper respiratory tract while smaller droplets go further down into the respiratory tract and cause lower respiratory infection (pneumonitis, bronchiolitis, and bronchitis). The incubation period is short varying from 2 to 4 days.

Symptoms

Symptoms vary depending on the part of the respiratory tract involved, but almost all patients have nasal discharge (rhinorrhea), nasal obstruction (congestion), and a sore throat. The sore throat may precede the nasal symptoms and subside as the nasal symptoms worsen. Three-fourths of patients complain of headache and cough. Other less common symptoms are feverishness, myalgia and headache.

Diagnosis

The common cold is diagnosed on the basis of symptoms and the absence of signs of involvement of the lower respiratory tract.

Treatment

Treatment is symptomatic. Antibiotics have no known or proven value in viral upper respiratory infections, and the efficacy of vitamin C both in prevention and cure is highly questionable. Antihistamines are effective in decreasing nasal secretions, and sympathomimetic amines (such as phenylpropanolamine) given topically or systemically may provide temporary relief of nasal congestion. Sympathomimetic amines are also sometimes beneficial in reducing lymphoid swelling around the nasopharyngeal opening of the eustachian tube, thereby decreasing the chance of a bacterial middle ear infection developing secondary to eustachian tube obstruction. *Topical* use of the sympathomimetic amines, as in nose drops or nasal sprays, for periods exceeding 2 or 3 days is not recommended because of the rebound that is seen on discontinuing their use and the tendency for patients to become habituated to them. Aspirin and acetaminophen are useful for the antipyritic and analgesic effects. Adequate fluid intake is necessary to prevent dehydration with subsequent drying and bacterial infection of the respiratory passages.

Oral Manifestations

Recurrent herpes labialis is sometimes seen in association with upper respiratory infections.

Dental Considerations

An upper respiratory tract infection interferes seriously with a dentist's professional duties. He should not operate on patients during the early stage of infection unless a surgical mask is worn and even then some patients think they are being exposed unnecessarily. Although a dentist can hardly refuse a patient who has a cold, he can tactfully suggest that dental treatment be postponed until a later date. A considerate dentist or patient will not run the risk of giving the other a cold.

Sinusitis

Sinusitis is an acute inflammation caused by viral or bacterial infections of the mucosa of the paranasal sinuses. It is sometimes a complication of the common cold initiated by a virus. Bacterial infection then supervenes. The organisms most frequently involved are *Streptococcus pneumoniae*, *Streptococcus pyogenes*, *Staphylococcus aureus*, and, particularly in children, *Hemophilus influenzae*. The maxillary sinus is most frequently involved.

Symptoms

Symptoms of acute sinusitis are headache, severe pain localized in the region of the involved sinus, an elevation of temperature, and malaise. Edema and redness of the malar eminence and beneath the eyes are common symptoms of maxillary sinusitis. The location of the swelling and the referred pain in the maxillary teeth may cause the patient to seek dental treatment. A common symptom of chronic sinusitis is a morning headache that disappears gradually during the day because of better drainage of the sinuses in the upright position. A postnasal discharge is an annoying symptom.

Diagnosis

The diagnosis of maxillary sinusitis is made on the basis of the history, the physical and radiologic findings, and transillumination. Firm pressure over the sinus may give rise to increased pain. The percussion note of an infected maxillary sinus is dull as compared with the resonant note of an aerated sinus. Although a suggestion of maxillary sinus involvement can be obtained from the regular intraoral dental films, occlusal films or preferably a series of radiologic films (commonly called *paranasal sinus films*) is required to make the diagnosis.

Treatment

Because it is not usually possible to differentiate viral sinusitis from bacterial sinusitis on clinical grounds without surgical intervention, antibiotics are the first choice in the treatment of maxillary sinusitis. Penicillin or if the patient is allergic, erythromycin, is the drug of first choice in adults. In young children, more likely to be infected with *H. influenzae*, ampicillin is a preferable first choice antibiotic. Antibiotics should be used in conjunction with the sympathomimetic drugs to help provide drainage from the maxillary sinuses. If the patient does not respond promptly he should be referred to an otolaryngologist, who may elect to establish drainage of the sinus through surgical means. If the patient does not respond to antibiotic therapy and drainage is not established, necrosis of the bony walls of the sinus may occur with resulting septicemia, meningitis, and sometimes death. Approved methods of sinus treatment do *not* require or sanction the removal of a tooth to establish drainage.

Dental Considerations

The roots of the maxillary premolars and molars and the nerves supplying these structures are in close proximity to the maxillary sinus, often being separated only by the sinus mucosa. This relationship explains why dental symptoms are associated frequently with maxillary sinus disease. Alveolar dental abscesses of the maxillary premolar and molar teeth open occasionally into the maxillary sinus and may give rise to sinusitis.

Maxillary sinusitis is more frequently the cause of dental symptoms. The maxillary teeth in close anatomic relation to the infected sinus often ache, feel elongated, and are sensitive to percussion. These symptoms may precede the typical symptoms of sinusitis. Pain in the maxillary premolars and molars that is unaccounted for by local lesions may be caused by maxillary sinusitis.

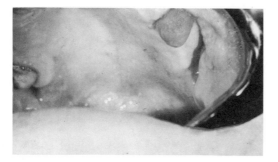

Fig. 18-1 Polyps from maxillary sinus appearing in oral cavity following extraction of maxillary molar.

Occasionally during extraction a root fragment is forced into the maxillary sinus. When this occurs, the patient should be informed of the complication. If the operator has not had experience with similar accidents, the patient should be referred to an oral surgeon for removal of the root fragment.

Following the removal of a tooth near the maxillary sinus, normal healing of the socket occasionally fails to take place. A polypoid mass of friable, often bleeding tissue fills the alveolus and extends into the mouth (Fig. 18-1). If the extraction has been complete, the dentist should suspect the existence of a polyp or more rarely, a neoplastic growth in the sinus.

Dental root cysts of the maxillary premolars and molars may encroach on the sinus and almost obliterate this structure. When infected, these cysts are at times diagnosed incorrectly and treated unsuccessfully as acute sinus infections. Special radiologic studies will permit a correct diagnosis and successful treatment.

Pharyngitis and Tonsillitis

Infection of the mucosa and lymphoid tissue in the pharynx and tonsils is a common complaint and may occur as an isolated incident or coincident with nasal involvement in an upper respiratory infection (see above). The most common etiologic agent in pharyngitis is a virus including those named under the section on upper respiratory infection, herpes simplex virus, and the virus associated with infectious mononucleosis. Bacteria, usually group A beta-hemolytic streptococcus (*S. pyogenes*) and very rarely diphtheria, may sometimes be the etiologic agent. Diag-

nosis is important in bacterial disease because of the possibility of rheumatic fever as a sequela to streptococcus pharyngitis or the high fatality rate associated with diphtheria. The distinction between pharyngitis and tonsillitis is a rather arbitrary one inasmuch as most patients with pharyngeal infections who have tonsils will also have tonsillitis. Likewise, if the tonsils have been removed there will be no tonsillitis.

Symptoms

The patient will complain of a sore throat with dysphagia. There may be associated symptoms of a common cold if the etiologic agent is a virus.

Peritonsillar abscess occurs rarely as a complication of acute tonsillitis and is characterized by a noticeable systemic reaction with extreme pain, marked tonsillar swelling, dysphagia, and a high leukocytosis. This condition is serious because of the possibility of extension of the infection to the deeper structures of the neck, erosion of a large artery, or the spontaneous rupture of the abscess during sleep with aspiration of the infected material. Recurrences are common.

Diagnosis

A differential diagnosis of the etiology includes pharyngitis caused by viruses, bacteria, and that secondary to infectious mononucleosis. A culture of the throat will usually serve to differentiate viral and bacterial disease. In cases suspected to be mononucleosis, because of the additional symptoms of undue fatigue and signs of posterior cervical and anterior cervical lymphadenopathy, diagnostic procedures useful in infectious mononucleosis such as the differential white cell count and one of the several mononucleosis antibody tests (see Chap. 3) should be used.

Treatment

Treatment of pharyngitis and tonsillitis depends on the etiology. When it is viral, treatment is symptomatic and confined to analgesics and when appropriate, decongestants and antihistamines if there are upper respiratory symptoms. Bacterial disease (the most common is group A beta-hemolytic strepto-coccus, *S. pyogenes*) is treated with penicillin or erythromycin in penicillin-allergic patients. For children, in whom the etiologic agent is more likely to be *H. influenzae*, ampicillin is preferable to penicillin V.

Laryngitis

Acute

Acute laryngitis usually results from abnormal use of the vocal cords (as from cheering, or public speaking), irritation due to excessive smoking, or the extension of a viral inflammatory process in the nose and throat. The condition is far less serious than the dramatic symptoms would indicate. With resting of the voice, the symptoms gradually clear up in a few days. Failure to rest the voice will not only prolong convalescence but also cause polyps to form on the vocal cords in some patients, necessitating surgery to remove the polyps.

Chronic

A slowly developing hoarseness may precede by many months the more typical symptoms of carcinoma or more rarely, syphilis or tuberculosis. In tuberculous laryngitis the patient usually experiences acute pain and dysphagia. Carcinoma of the larynx should always be considered in cases of persistent hoarseness in adults. The dentist should refer these patients to an otolaryngologist for examination.

LOWER RESPIRATORY DISEASES

Asthma

Asthma (bronchial asthma) is a spontaneous, reversible spasmodic contraction of the smooth muscle of the bronchioles resulting in bronchiolar narrowing. Such spasm is caused by bronchiolar hyperactivity and is most often due to allergens. Most commonly these allergens are inhaled, such as dusts, pollens, and industrial contaminants in the air, but may on occasion be ingested. One of the most common and potentially serious in-gested allergens is found in patients developing acute asthmatic attacks after taking aspirin. Patients whose asthma results from an allergic cause often have a positive family history of the disease as well as a positive atopic history including hay fever, rose fever, and eczema. The serum levels of IgE are usually elevated, and the patient will have positive skin tests for specific allergens.

Respiratory infections, usually viral, are well-known inciting factors in the asthma patient. Some patients have acute asthma attacks after prolonged exercise, and acute asthma has also been known to occur during emotional states such as nervousness and anxiety. Patients whose asthma does not appear to have an allergic cause often do not have the family history of asthma or an atopic history and have negative skin tests and normal serum IgE levels. It is estimated that 1% to 2% of the population has asthma at one time. It is much more common in children, especially boys, but 50% of children with asthma become symptom-free in adulthood. Death occurs occasionally during an acute asthmatic attack. Secondary cardiac changes may follow asthma of long duration.

Symptoms

Predominating symptoms in an acute asthmatic attack are wheezing, coughing, and labored breathing. With a severe attack, the patient is extremely anxious and agitated.

Diagnosis

Diagnosis of bronchial asthma is based on the symptoms, pulmonary function tests (including a reduced vital capacity and elevated residual volume, arterial blood gas changes of hypoxemia, hypocarbia, and respiratory alkalemia), and the physical findings of expiratory wheezes during the acute attack. Emphysematous changes in the chest film are common with chronic asthma.

Treatment

Treatment of chronic asthma by the physician utilizes drugs such as the beta-adrenergic receptor stimulators ephedrine, isoproterenol, and terbutaline. Other drugs include amino-phylline, tranquilizers, corticosteroids, and cromolyn sodium. Antihistamines are usually not useful because they produce drying and further obstruction of the airway.

Emergency treatment of asthma includes inhalation of a solution containing 0.1 mg isoproterenol or injection of 0.1 ml of 1:1000 epinephrine subcutaneously or inhalation of 1:1000 epinephrine by nebulizer. Terbutaline, a specific beta$_2$ agonist (bronchodilator) does not have the cardiac side-effects of epinephrine or isoproterenol but has a longer onset of action time (30 to 60 minutes) than does epinephrine. Consequently, there is controversy about its usefulness in an acute attack. Continuous oxygen by nasal catheter at 2 to 3 liters per minute is helpful to relieve the hypoxia. Hydration is necessary to mobilize the viscous respiratory secretions and usually must be given intravenously in the form of 5% glucose in water because the patient is unable because of dyspnea to maintain adequate oral fluid intake.

Dental Considerations

Emergency drugs such as those detailed in the preceding paragraph should be available in the dental office for treatment of an acute asthmatic attack. The dentist should avoid inhalation anesthetics or analgesics in asthmatic patients because of the possibility of stimulating an acute asthmatic attack.

Chronic Obstructive Pulmonary Disease (Chronic Bronchitis; Emphysema)

Chronic obstructive pulmonary disease may be defined as a condition in which there is chronic obstruction to air flow secondary to chronic bronchitis or emphysema. The patient may be defined as having chronic bronchitis when there is a mucus-producing cough present for at least 3 months of the year for more than 2 consecutive years. Airway symptoms other than cough may vary in severity from virtually no symptoms to a disabling condition in which the slightest exertion of the patient can cause severe dyspnea. The most common cause of chronic bronchitis is smoking, although other factors such as chronic recurrent infection, air pollution and occupational inhalants may play a part. Emphysema is a distension of the alveolar spaces and rupture of the alveolar septae with resultant loss of pulmonary gaseous diffusion surfaces. Emphysema is usually the result of chronic bronchitis, although some patients may have chronic bronchitis for years with minimal resulting emphysema; conversely, some may exhibit emphysema with minimal chronic bronchitis. This is especially true in the genetic variety of emphysema, in which there is an inherited deficiency of the enzyme alpha$_1$-antitrypsin. The exact mechanism wherein this enzyme deficiency produces emphysema is not known.

Symptoms

The symptoms of chronic obstructive pulmonary disease are wheezing, dyspnea, and cough. Patients with primarily emphysematous changes will have dyspnea without appreciable wheezing or cough.

Diagnosis

A patient is deemed to have chronic bronchitis if symptoms fit those described in the definition given above. Physical examination of the patient with emphysema reveals flat diaphragms and an enlarged chest wall, especially in the anteroposterior diameter. On chest film the chest x-ray confirms the physical findings with an additional finding of increased radiolucency of the lung fields owing to *hyperinflation* (Figs. 18-2 and 18-3). Pulmonary blood gas studies show hypoxemia and hypercarbia.

Treatment

When possible, etiologic factors should be removed; unfortunately this is not often possible especially with heavy cigarette smokers, who despite severe pulmonary dysfunction often persist in their habit. Bronchodilators are particularly effective in relieving the bronchospasm so common in chronic obstructive pulmonary disease. Antibiotic therapy should be initiated at the earliest sign of chest infection because this inordinately exacerbates the dyspneic symptoms in most patients. Oxygen therapy is useful both intermittently on a chronic basis and continuously with an acute exacerbation of the disease.

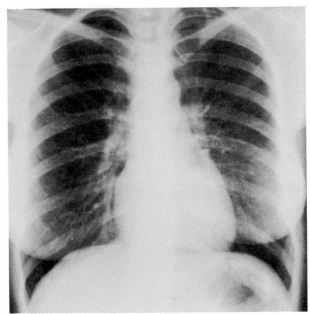

Fig. 18-2 Normal chest x-ray. (Juhl JH (ed): Paul and Juhl's Essentials of Roentgen Interpretation, 4th ed, p 801. Philadelphia, Harper & Row, 1981)

Dental Considerations

Considering the alterations in blood gases in the patient with chronic obstructive pulmonary disease, it should be realized that their tolerance to long treatment sessions is low; this should be taken into consideration when planning dental therapy. The patient's tolerance to partial airway obstructing devices such as a rubber dam should be evaluated carefully, and before obstructing the oral airway the dentist should ascertain that the nasal passages are capable of supplying the patient's respiratory needs. Inhalation analgesics or anesthetics should be given only when absolutely necessary and in conjunction with an anesthesiologist.

Lung Abscess

A lung abscess is a localized area of suppuration and necrosis of the parenchymal tissue. It may be the sequela of acute bronchitis, bronchiectasis, the aspiration of infected material during anesthesia, or secondary pyogenic infections of tubercular cavities. Pulmonary abscesses caused by fusospirochetal organisms produce a particularly foul-smelling lesion. Foreign bodies in the lung, such as buttons, a peanut, dental instruments, or

tooth fragments, also give rise to lung abscesses. The aspiration of infected material from calculus-encrusted teeth and purulent gums during sleep may explain the lung abscesses of "unknown etiology."

The symptoms of lung abscess include an irregular fever, expectoration of large quantities of putrid sputum, and progressive weight loss. Rarely, amyloidosis may develop. The diagnosis is based on the past history, the physical findings, and the radiologic studies (Fig. 18-4).

Dental Considerations

Good oral hygiene is an important prophylactic against lung abscesses. It is also of definite value in preventing recurrent attacks of bronchiectasis. The dentist should be extremely careful that particulate matter is not inadvertently allowed to go from the oral cavity into the respiratory tract.

Pulmonary Foreign Bodies

Foreign bodies occluding or obstructing a main respiratory passage will produce cyanosis and asphyxia. Sudden and violent attacks of coughing accompanied by shortness of breath and chest pain are classic symptoms

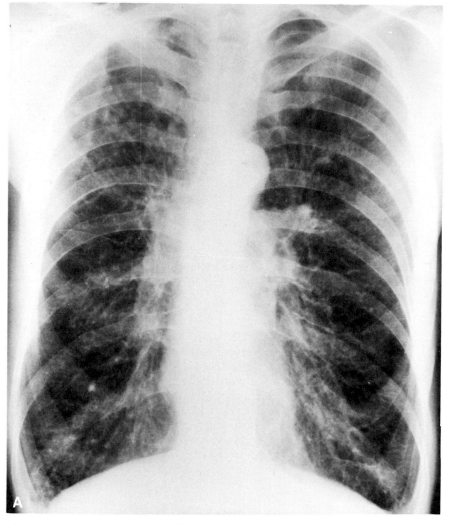

Fig. 18-3 Posteroanterior (*A*) and lateral (*B*) chest x-rays of a 58-year-old man with emphysema. Note flattened diaphragm and increased anteroposterior chest diameter. (Fishman MC, Hoffman AR, Klausner RD et al: Medicine, pp 98, 99. Philadelphia, JB Lippincott, 1981) (continued)

of a pulmonary foreign body. These symptoms are particularly significant if they follow dental extractions or operations. Small foreign bodies at times produce few if any symptoms, and they may be discovered accidentally during chest radiography or after the development of a lung abscess.

Dental Considerations

Dental procedures are directly or indirectly involved in a high percentage of foreign body problems; hence, the cooperation of the dentist is essential for the prevention of these accidents. It is not understood that artificial dentures are an important indirect cause of foreign body accidents. The tactile sense of the denture patient is severely impaired by the dentures, and the foreign body (usually bones) may pass the point of recovery by reflex action before the patient is aware of it. Consequently, maxillary full-denture patients should be warned of this possibility and should be instructed to chew their food twice

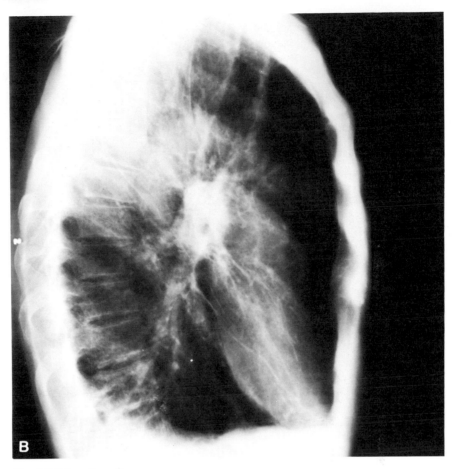

Fig. 18-3 (continued)

as long as when they had their natural teeth, with the objective of detecting unknown hard foreign bodies. Bunker stated that 30% of all foreign bodies in the air and the food passages of persons of all ages are bones; however, in the patient with complete dentures this rises to 85%.

Sherman and associates called attention to the hazard of radiolucent dentures as foreign bodies associated with high-velocity automobile crashes. A real danger exists that the denture base or a portion of it may become embedded in the soft tissues or block the respiratory or alimentary tracts without being detected by x-rays. The materials scientists should devote some of their attention and research efforts to the development of a radiopaque material that is both physically and esthetically acceptable for routine use.

Dental foreign bodies can be placed into the following three main groups: a portion of a tooth, a restoration or an operating instrument that is "lost" during dental treatment; teeth, tooth fragments, or portions of restorations dislodged as a result of manipulation of mouth gags and instruments during surgery; and prostheses "lost" by the patient. Fortunately for both the patient and the dentist, the normal pharyngeal reflexes assist in preventing many accidents.

Anesthesia, either local or general, adds to the risk of aspiration because the cough reflex is either diminished or abolished. Endodontic therapy without the rubber dam is to be condemned both with respect to the technique and to the risk of aspirating or swallowing small instruments. Inlays, crowns, pieces of amalgam, and inlay wax are all potential foreign bodies. When one considers the great number and variety of dental operations per-

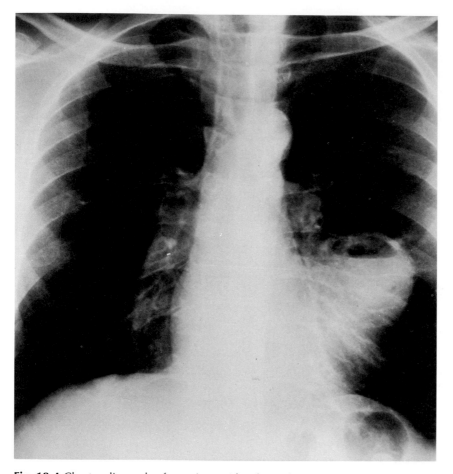

Fig. 18-4 Chest radiograph of a patient with a lung abscess. Note fluid in abscess in left lung field. (Fishman MC, Hoffman AR, Klausner RD et al: Medicine, p 136. Philadelphia, JB Lippincott, 1981)

formed without the rubber dam, it is to the credit of the dentist's technique and the patient's quick pharyngeal reflexes that more accidents of this nature do not occur. The risk of respiratory tract foreign bodies can be eliminated almost entirely by the use of the rubber dam or throat packs.

Partial and complete dentures may of themselves be foreign bodies. Complete and partial dentures should be removed during sleep, unconsciousness from any cause (coma, shock, intoxication), and before surgery. Loose or cracked dentures are also potential foreign bodies.

The clasps on partial dentures make removal difficult should they become lodged in the air passages. Construction of small partial dentures such as those replacing one tooth ("spider" partials) are to be particularly condemned because of the particular ease with which they may become dislodged and inhaled.

Foreign body accidents related to dental treatment or dental objects can be prevented to a large extent by proper preventive procedures and by adequate patient education by the dentist.

Pneumonitis

Pneumonitis or pneumonia is inflammation of the lung tissue usually caused by an infectious agent. The majority of cases of pneumonitis are caused by a virus, although bacterial and rarely, fungal pneumonias do occur. Mycoplasmal pneumonia is probably the most common nonbacterial pneumonia, although viruses such as the respiratory syncytial virus, the parainfluenza viruses, influenza virus, and others are sometimes implicated. Bacterial pneumonias are most commonly caused by *Streptococcus pneumoniae, Klebsiella pneumoniae,* and *Hemophilus influenza.* Less common but prognostically more severe, staphylococcal pneumonia sometimes occurs. Pneumonia caused by *Legionella pneumophilia,* Legionairres' disease, is a recent discovery. In immunosuppressed patients, pneumonia caused by *Pneumocystis carinii* can occur in and is associated with a very poor prognosis.

Lung infection with *Histoplasma* and *Mycobacterium tuberculosis* will be discussed in separate sections in this chapter because these two types of pulmonary infection are chronic and can be associated with oral lesions.

Symptoms

Symptoms of viral and mycoplasmal pneumonia are generally mild and consist of a cough often productive of sputum, mild fever, and on occasion, dyspnea.

The symptoms of bacterial pneumonia are more marked and usually have a sudden onset. The patient appears ill, has a cough productive of purulent sputum, and has a fever and often, pleuritic chest pain.

Diagnosis

The diagnosis is made on the basis of history, physical findings of rales in the chest, and chest x-ray evidence of pulmonary infiltrate or lobar consolidation (Figs. 18-5 and 18-6). In bacterial pneumonias the etiology can often be ascertained from an examination of a Gram-stained sputum specimen.

Treatment

Treatment of viral pneumonias is supportive. Mycoplasmal pneumonia responds readily to tetracycline or erythromycin therapy. Bacterial pneumonias respond to an antibiotic appropriate for the particular organism causing the infection. For this reason it is quite important that the specific etiologic agent be identified in a bacterial pneumonia, both because of the potential seriousness of the disease and the nonresponse to ineffective antibiotic therapy.

Tuberculosis

Although tuberculosis may involve almost any organ in the body, it is discussed in this chapter because it most commonly presents

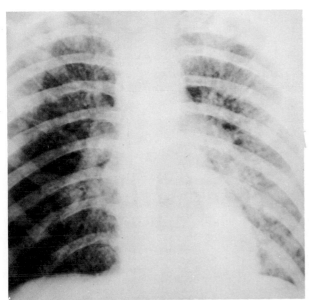

Fig. 18-5 Chest radiograph of a patient with extensive widespread bronchopneumonia. Note the mottled density is more severe on the left side. (Juhl JH [ed]: Paul and Juhl's Essentials of Roentgen Interpretation, 4th ed, p. 844. Philadelphia, Harper & Row, 1981)

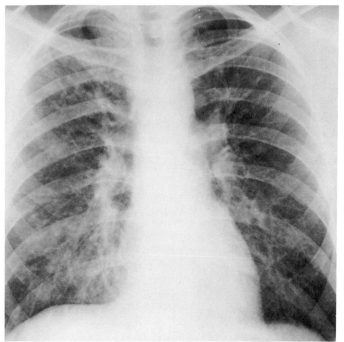

Fig. 18-6 Chest radiograph of a patient with viral pneumonia, more severe on the right side. (Juhl, JH [ed]: Paul and Juhl's Essentials of Roentgen Interpretation, 4th ed, p 852. Philadelphia, Harper & Row, 1981)

in the United States as a pulmonary infection. Tuberculosis is a widespread infectious disease caused by *Mycobacterium tuberculosis* that affects man, animals, and birds. A tuberculous infection is frequently referred to as an *acid-fast infection* because of the staining properties of the tubercle bacillus. The term *acid-fast infection* may be useful when discussing this disease in the presence of the patient.

Human or bovine strains of *M. tuberculosis* can be responsible for the disease in man, but infection with the bovine strain is uncommon in the United States. The American Indian, blacks, and Eskimos are particularly susceptible. When tuberculosis is introduced to primitive peoples, it runs an acute course.

Poor nutrition, general debilitating diseases, overcrowded living conditions, and certain respiratory diseases such as silicosis are important predisposing factors.

While the incidence of tuberculosis in the United States has been declining for the past several decades, this decline has slowed during the past 5 years and in many areas of the country is actually showing a slight increase. This increase is thought to be caused by the presence of immigrants from underdevel-

oped countries where tuberculosis is much more prevalent than it is in the United States.

The disease is transmitted almost exclusively by air droplets less than 8 μ in diameter. In the United States, bovine tuberculosis is usually transmitted by milk. It was formerly thought that fomites were important in transmission of the disease, but this has been shown not to be the case. Dental instruments or objects in the dental office are not implicated in transmission of tuberculosis unless aerosol particles 8 μ or less are produced. It is therefore unlikely that the dentist would play a role in transmission of the disease unless he himself or one of his office personnel has the disease.

Symptoms

The initial symptoms of this disease are subtle and may include loss of weight, mild cough, anorexia, and marked fatigability. A clue to the diagnosis is often found in a pneumonitis that fails to clear on conventional antibiotic therapy. Less commonly seen today is a patient with classic symptoms of a persistent cough accompanied by bloody sputum, an afternoon rise in temperature of 0.5° to 2°F, nightsweats, and a cavitary pneumonia on chest radiographs.

Less frequently, tuberculosis may develop as an acute pulmonary infection or as a generalized infection known as *miliary tuberculosis*. The organs most commonly involved after the lungs are the kidneys, but involvement of the liver, the adrenals, uterus, skin, bone marrow, and lymph nodes may also occur.

The chronicity of these lesions and the lack of marked pain or acute inflammatory symptoms have resulted in the term *cold abscess*. A large cerebral abscess, a tuberculoma, may simulate a brain tumor. Tuberculosis of the adrenal cortex may result in Addison's disease.

A glandular form of the disease, characterized by marked enlargement of the cervical lymph nodes with caseation and frequent breakdown of the glands was formerly fairly common. This form of the disease was usually related to the consumption of raw milk from tuberculous cows. Such tuberculous involvement of the cervical lymph nodes is called *scrofula*. Tuberculous involvement of the spine, usually in childhood, is known as *Pott's disease*. The major salivary glands may be the site of primary or secondary tubercular involvement, with the parotid being affected most frequently. Clinical diagnosis of the true nature of the disease process in the salivary glands is exceedingly difficult and differential diagnosis from benign mixed tumor, syphilis, actinomycosis, and even malignancy is almost impossible on clinical grounds alone.

Diagnosis

Asymptomatic patients are usually detected on the basis of their tuberculin tests (PPD) becoming positive and in the case of pulmonary tuberculosis, x-ray findings suggestive of tuberculosis. The diagnosis in symptomatic patients may be suspected on the basis of the systemic symptoms. In either case, follow-up studies with demonstration of the presence of *M. tuberculosis* are necessary to confirm the diagnosis. In pulmonary tuberculosis, the radiologic findings (Fig. 18-7), the presence of acid-fast bacteria in the sputum smear, and the growth of *M. tuberculosis* on sputum culture serve to prove the diagnosis. In extrapulmonary tuberculosis, biopsy of the organ involved with demonstration of acid-fast organisms on an acid-fast histologic stain and growth of the organism from the macerated tissue is necessary to establish a diagnosis.

Routine chest films are no longer recommended for case finding in tuberculosis inasmuch as the incidence of the disease has decreased markedly, and the harm from radiation probably exceeds the good done by filming the populace. Periodic skin testing in patients who are tuberculin-negative is recommended, especially for health personnel or those exposed to the disease. Skin testing should be done using an intermediate strength (5 tuberculin units) of purified protein derivative (PPD). The multiple puncture tests should not be used because they have both a high rate of negative and positive results. It is thought that these erroneous results are caused by the variation in the

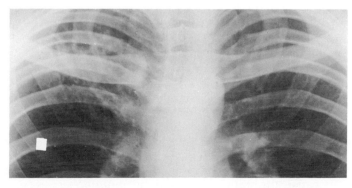

Fig. 18.7 Upper portion of a chest radiograph showing the lung apices. Note the mottled density in the right apical area, which represents apical tuberculosis. (Juhl JH [ed]: Paul and Juhl's Essentials of Roentgen Interpretation, 4th ed, p 878. Philadelphia, Harper & Row, 1981)

amount of antigen that is introduced subcutaneously with the multiple puncture tests. Conversion of the PPD skin test from negative to positive is considered to be evidence of infection with *M. tuberculosis.* Such infection may be symptomatic or asymptomatic.

Treatment

The use of antituberculosis drugs has completely changed the prognosis for tuberculosis. Chemotherapy and antimicrobial therapy with isoniazid, rifampin, ethambutol, streptomycin, and para-aminosalicylic acid (PAS) supplemented by the proved regimens of rest and good nutrition will arrest most cases. Treatment of the patient with active tuberculosis consists of use of at least two of the above drugs. Isoniazid is almost always one of the two drugs and it is combined most commonly with rifampin, although ethambutol is sometimes used. It has been found that in order to complete therapy in less than 18 months both isoniazid and rifampin must be used. When the organism is resistant to rifampin, ethambutol is added to the regimen, but therapy generally takes 18 to 24 months in this case.

For far-advanced disease or disease resistant to the above antimicrobials, streptomycin (which must be given by injection) is usually combined with either isoniazid and ethambutol or with isoniazid and rifampin. Patients who have *no* clinical evidence of the disease, whose only manifestation is a recent (within 2 years) conversion of the tuberculin skin tests are usually treated with isoniazid alone for a year, as are asymptomatic patients who are household or close contacts of active cases.

Surgery is rarely done nowadays because most patients respond to medication. When indicated, surgery is usually for a persisting pulmonary cavity with acid-fast-positive sputum despite 6 months of chemotherapy. The usual type of surgery done is segmental resection of a lung or a complete lobectomy. Extrapulmonary tuberculosis responds more readily to drugs than does advanced pulmonary tuberculosis because with the exception of cavitary renal tuberculosis, the bacterial populations are smaller.

Because the patient is rendered noninfec-

tious shortly after initiation of antituberculosis therapy, long-term hospitalization is no longer required. This has resulted in the closing of numerous state hospitals that existed solely for the treatment of the patient with tuberculosis. Inasmuch as tuberculosis may be considered to be inactivated but not cured, the patient is subject to reactivation of disease when poor health supervenes or resistance is lowered. Steroid therapy is known to be instrumental in reactivating the disease. It has been shown that more cases of symptomatic tuberculosis result from reactivation of previous disease (patients with positive tuberculin tests) than from patients who have never had tuberculosis.

Oral Manifestations

Oral lesions (Figs. 18-8, 18-9, and 18-10) are an infrequent occurrence in tuberculosis and are observed more often in patients having advanced disease. They may on occasion develop in patients without other demonstrable symptoms of this disease. Although lesions may develop as the result of hematogenous seeding or lymphatic spread, they are most often associated with pulmonary tuberculosis and result from contact of the oral tissues with infected sputum.

The infrequent occurrence of oral tuberculosis lesions, considering the number of patients with positive sputum, has been explained in part by the mechanical cleansing action of the saliva and the food. The thickened oral epithelium, when intact, may also minimize the frequency with which lesions

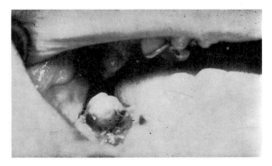

Fig. 18-8. Tuberculous lesion mesial to the lower right second molar. Smears were negative for tubercle bacilli. Repeated biopsy studies and animal inoculations were positive for tuberculosis.

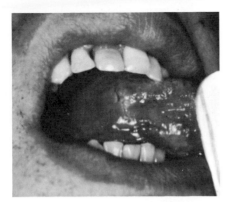

Fig. 18-9. Tuberculous ulcer of the lateral margin of the tongue. The lesion developed where the tongue margin was irritated by a broken-down tooth. (Courtesy Dr. Irving Gruber, New York City)

develop in these tissues. Piasecke–Zeyland and Zeyland have also reported an inhibitory affect of saliva on the tubercle bacillus.

The tongue is the most frequent site of oral lesions, but the cheeks, the lips, and the palate also are involved. Tuberculous involvement of periapical dental granulomata, the salivary glands, and tuberculous periostitis also have been reported; a tuberculous periostitis may pose a difficult diagnostic problem.

The method of inoculation is undetermined in most oral lesions; however, patients with oral tuberculous lesions often give a history of pre-existing trauma. Any area of chronic irritation or inflammatory response may furnish a favorable site for localization of organisms. Darlington and Salman reported 12 instances of tuberculous apical dental granulomata; looseness of the teeth was the outstanding clinical symptom. Cohen described a tuberculous lesion in the buccal sulcus associated with irritation from the flange of a mandibular denture. Tuberculous ulcers at the site of recent tooth extraction have been reported.

Tubercular oral lesions, particularly those of the lips, frequently begin as small tubercles or "pimples" that break down to form a painful ulcer. Additional small tubercles characteristically develop about the periphery of the ulcer, and the process is repeated. The corners of the mouth are common sites of involvement. Characteristically, tuberculous ul-

cers of the cheeks have an irregular, undermined border. Tongue lesions develop commonly where the lateral margin of the tongue rests against rough, sharp, or broken-down teeth, or at the site of other irritants. Deep central ulcers of the tongue are usually typical in appearance with a thick mucous material in the base of the ulcer.

Oral tuberculous lesions are characterized by severe, unremitting and progressive pain that interferes seriously with proper nutrition and rest.

Diagnosis of Oral Lesions. Diagnosis of oral mucosal lesions may be difficult if tuberculosis is not suspected. Oral tuberculosis always should be suspected in the differential diagnosis of oral ulcerations or granulomas. Tuberculous lesions are usually extremely painful. Chancre, gumma, carcinoma, and traumatic and other infectious ulcers must be considered. Staining of biopsy material from suspected lesions for acid-fast organisms is a useful diagnostic procedure. Diagnosis cannot be made on histopathologic findings alone unless acid-fast staining organisms can be demonstrated. Minerals such as silica and beryllium may give rise to a granulomatous reaction simulating tuberculosis, although pain is not so marked in these conditions. Culturing of the tuberculosis organism from an oral lesion in the patient with pulmonary tuberculosis cannot be considered diagnostic of the lesion's tuberculous character, inas-

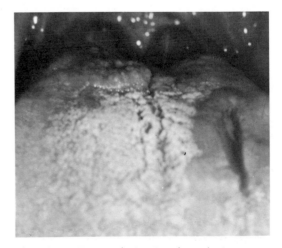

Fig. 18-10. Tongue lesion in tuberculosis.

much as the sputum and saliva may harbor these organisms even if the oral lesion is not tuberculous in origin.

Patients with suspicious oral lesions thought to be tuberculosis should be referred to a physician for evaluation.

Treatment of Oral Lesions. Local palliative treatment of oral lesions is supplemental to the systemic treatment outlined previously. The establishment of good oral hygiene and the elimination of all sources of irritation should be the first phase of treatment. The elimination of traumatic irritation of the mucosa and the tongue minimizes the possibility of the development of oral mucosal lesions.

Dental Considerations. In patients who are not known to have tuberculosis but who may be suspected to harbor the infection because of clinical symptoms, physical appearance or close household contacts, it is prudent for the dentist to wear a face mask during dental treatment. The patient should be persuaded to seek medical attention, and if the symptoms are striking enough (*e.g.*, hacking cough with hemoptysis and fever) the dentist is justified in withholding all but emergency treatment until the patient has been evaluated by his physician. Sterilization procedures adequate to kill the tubercle bacillus should be observed, even though fomites are not an important method of patient-to-dentist or patient-to-patient transmission.

In a patient known to have tuberculosis and to be under treatment, it should be ascertained by consultation with the patient's physician that the patient is responding to treatment and the organism is sensitive to the drugs used. Continuing patient compliance with the medication regimen should be carefully explored because as with any chronic medication, patient compliance with drug therapy has been shown to be relatively poor.

Histoplasmosis

Histoplasmosis is a fungal disease caused by *Histoplasma capsulatum.* It occurs endemically in the United States in the Ohio and Mississippi River valleys. Most cases are mild and

are detected years after the fact by the incidental findings of fibrous hilar node calcification on chest radiographs. Occasionally the disease may become progressive and disseminated resulting in destruction of the lung with cavitation and spreading of the organisms to the adrenals, liver, spleen, and meninges. Oral involvement is usually secondary to pulmonary involvement in patients with the disseminated form of the disease. Histoplasmosis is discussed in more detail, including diagnosis, treatment, and oral manifestations in Chapter 5 under the category, Chronic Ulcerative Lesions of the Oral Cavity.

Wegener's Granulomatosis

Wegener's granulomatosis is a granulomatous involvement of blood vessels resulting in necrosis of tissue. It is of unknown cause and initially involves the nose and the paranasal sinuses with later extension to the lower respiratory tract and eventually to the gut, joints, nervous system, and kidneys. It is considered in this chapter because of the primary involvement of the upper respiratory tract and eventual extension into the lower respiratory tract. Involvement of the kidney is the most common cause of death. Any age or sex may be involved, but persons 45 to 60 years of age are more commonly involved, and males are involved twice as often as females.

Symptoms

The most chronic symptoms of Wegener's granulomatosis are nasal stuffiness with chronic discharge, sometimes bloody. With involvement of other organs, symptoms peculiar to these organs become prominent.

Oral Manifestations

It is not uncommon to see involvement of the oral tissues in Wegener's granulomatosis. Walton reviewed 56 cases of which 21 had oropharyngeal lesions. Of these, seven had tongue involvement and seven had gingival involvement. Initial symptoms of the disease were present in the oral cavity in five of the cases. Involvement of the oral tissues usually consists of swelling, inflammation, and ulceration, but a hemorrhagic gingival enlargement has also been reported to be a presenting feature of Wegener's granulomatosis. Scott and Finch reviewed seven such cases and reported another. They pointed out that the inflammatory process starts in the interdental papillae, spreading rapidly to the remainder of the gingivae and into the periodontium. There are often signs of alveolar bone loss with teeth mobility. The gingivae are enlarged with petechiae and a granular appearance. They emphasized that prompt recognition by the dentist will facilitate an early start to treatment and may thus improve the prognosis. Scott and Finch also pointed out that destruction of the hard palate and alveolar bone by spread of lesions from the nose or sinuses, which is commonly described in midline granulomata (see next section), is quite uncommon in Wegener's granulomatosis. In Wegener's granulomatosis the oral and palatal ulcerations usually arise independently of the nasal lesions.

Diagnosis

Diagnosis should be suspected on the basis of clinical symptoms and findings. Definitive diagnosis is made by histologic examination of a biopsy specimen of infected tissue, which must show the characteristic granulomata involving the arteries and the necrotizing vasculitis. While not diagnostic, it is characteristic of the disease that the Westergren sedimentation rate is always extremely elevated, usually over 100 mm/hr.

Treatment

Treatment is by use of cytotoxic agents such as cyclophosphamide or azathioprine. Remissions of up to 15 years have been reported in over 95% of the patients so treated. Harrison and colleagues reported dramatic improvement in patients within 72 hours following intravenous corticosteroid–cyclophosphamide therapy. This remarkably favorable response to cyclophosphamide therapy represents a true advance in treatment of a disease that was heretofore thought to be uniformly fatal and untreatable.

Midline Granuloma

Midline granuloma affects the midline structures of the face and is characterized by a chronic progressive destructive process. The cause is unknown. In the past it has been classified as a variant of Wegener's granulomatosis, but the consensus today is that it is a different disease entity. Unlike Wegener's granulomatosis, it does *not* affect the lungs or kidneys, and the death that may result is caused by localized destruction of tissue in the midline of the face. Males 20 to 50 years of age are more commonly involved.

Symptoms

Nasal obstruction and discharge are early symptoms, but with involvement of the skin of the nose and maxillary area there is a concurrent progressive loss of facial tissue.

Diagnosis

Diagnosis is made by the presence of characteristic clinical symptoms and by biopsy. Midline granuloma is differentiated from Wegener's granulomatosis in biopsy in that there is no vasculitis in the tissue specimen.

Oral Manifestations

Progressive involvement leads to destruction and perforation of the hard and soft palate as well as other structures contiguous to the midline of the nose. A small percentage of patients will have gingival, oral mucosal, or palatal ulcerations as the primary symptom.

Treatment

Antibiotic therapy is useful only in controlling secondary infection. Radiation therapy, 5000 rad, appears to be the treatment of choice at the present time with some remissions of over 15 years reported. Some benefit has been reported from the use of cytotoxic agents. Surgical intervention does not help and in some cases appears to exacerbate the disease.

Dental Considerations

Midline granuloma should be suspected as a possible diagnosis in any chronic ulceration in the oral cavity or with any perforation of the hard or soft palate of unknown cause. Because of the massive destruction of the tissues of the face, nose, and mouth, the maxillofacial prosthodontist will be of inestimable value to patients in whom radiation therapy is successful.

Sarcoidosis

Sarcoidosis is a disease of unproved etiology involving multiple systems including but not limited to the lungs, skin, eyes, nerves, muscles, liver, spleen, gastrointestinal tract, heart, joints, and kidneys. It is included in this chapter because it presents most frequently with bilateral pulmonary hilar adenopathy and pulmonary infiltration. It is seen twice as often in women as in men and occurs most often in patients 25 to 50 years of age. Blacks in the United States are affected ten times as often as are whites.

Symptoms

Symptoms of sarcoidosis are widespread and depend on the organ system involved. Fever, weight loss, and fatigue are the predominating nonspecific symptoms. Sarcoidosis should be considered in the differential diagnosis of all patients presenting with multiple systems involvement. It is often asymptomatic and detected on routine chest film by the presence of hilar adenopathy.

Oral Manifestations

Sarcoidosis must be considered in the differential diagnosis of cervical lymphadenopathy, parotid enlargement, and Sjögren's syndrome. The latter may result in increased dental caries and ulcerations of the buccal mucosa due to salivary insufficiency. Oral cavity involvement, while quite rare in sarcoidosis, may consist of a painless submucosal nodule with a normal overlying mucosa

as reported by Orlian and Birnbaum or an intraosseous lesion in the maxilla or the mandible as reported by Betten and colleagues.

Diagnosis

Diagnosis is strongly suggested by the multiple system involvement and exclusion of other diseases. Hypercalciuria occurs in about half of the patients. There is no definitive diagnostic procedure, but the one most commonly used is the Kveim–Sitzbach test, which is the intradermal injection of a saline suspension of known human sarcoid tissue used as an antigen into a patient suspected to have sarcoidosis. One month after injection any palpable nodule is excised and examined histologically for evidence of a sarcoid reaction, epitheloid tubercles. These epitheloid tubercles are also diagnostic when found in a lesion biopsy if the patient has other clinical features characteristic of the disease. Diseases with which sarcoid may be confused are Crohn's regional enteritis, primary biliary cirrhosis, tuberculosis, and Hodgkin's disease.

Treatment

Asymptomatic patients require no treatment. In a patient with symptomatic or active inflammatory disease, corticosteroids are the drugs of choice. Oral therapy is begun with high doses of corticosteroids given several times a day slowly tapering over a period of weeks to a maintenance dose of once-a-day therapy. Patients often improve symptomatically in 2 weeks, but therapy should be continued for a minimum of 6 to 8 months. Lifelong therapy may be necessary if the patient's signs and symptoms return subsequent to attempts to discontinue therapy.

Dental Considerations

The patients with sarcoid may require agents to moisten the mouth in the presence of Sjögren's syndrome. There may be osteoporosis, lessened resistance to infection, impaired healing, lowered glucose tolerance, and mental changes in the patient on long-term high-dose steroid therapy.

Cystic Fibrosis

Cystic fibrosis (mucoviscidosis) is an autosomal recessive inherited disease that affects all exocrine glands, its effect being most apparent in the mucus-producing glands. The pancreas and lungs are most prominently involved. Involvement of the pancreas results in a deficiency of pancreatic enzymes and digestive disturbances with malabsorption. Pulmonary involvement is much more serious and is usually the cause of death. The pulmonary involvement consists of generalized bronchiolar obstruction secondary to mucous plugs. This obstruction results in chronic bronchitis, bronchiectasis, and increased susceptibility to respiratory infections. Prognosis, while improving with improved treatment methods, is still poor. Only 5% of patients live to be 20 years of age.

Symptoms

The symptoms of this disease relate primarily to the pancreatic and the pulmonary involvement. The newborn fails to gain weight despite a large appetite and passes large frequent stools. Early pulmonary involvement is evident by tachypnea and a cough.

Diagnosis

Diagnosis is made by use of the sweat test, which is predicated on the patient's having a three- to fivefold increase in the concentration of sodium and chloride in the sweat. In this test, sweat is stimulated by the use of pilocarpine and collected and analyzed for sodium and chloride. A positive sweat test in conjunction with the clinical symptoms suffices to make the diagnosis of the disease.

Treatment

Pancreatic deficiency can be corrected by adding pancreatic extract to the diet. Pulmonary function is aided by having the patient perform postural drainage three to four times daily. There is some evidence that nebulization with agents to decrease the viscosity of pulmonary secretions may be of value. The mainstay of therapy of chronic lung disease involves antibiotic prophylactic therapy; tetracyclines are the drugs most commonly used.

Oral Manifestations

Tetracycline staining of the teeth is commonly seen in cystic fibrosis patients but is a relatively small price to pay for increased longevity. Enamel defects consisting of hypoplasia or hypomineralization are also seen. Paradoxically, these are accompanied by a lower than normal incidence of dental caries. In a study by Primosch of 86 patients with cystic fibrosis, tetracycline discoloration and enamel defects were found in about 25% of the patients. Submandibular gland enlargement has been noted to occur in some patients.

BIBLIOGRAPHY

Abbott JN et al: Recovery of tubercle bacilli from mouth washings of tuberculous dental patients. J Am Dent Assoc 50:49, 1955

Aronson MD et al: Association between cigarette smoking and acute respiratory tract illness in young adults. JAMA 248:181, 1982

Betten D et al: Sarcoidosis with mandibular involvement. Oral Surg 42:731, 1976

Brooke RI: Wegener's granulomatosis involving the gingivae. Br Dent J 127:34, 1969

Brooks BJ et al: Ulcer of the hard palate. JAMA 247:819, 1982

Bunker PG: Foreign body complications. Laryngoscope 71:903, 1961

Cawson RA: Gingival changes in Wegener's granulomatosis. Br Dent J 118:30, 1965

Cohen L: Oral tuberculosis. Oral Surg 12:265, 1959

Cohen PS, Meltzer JA: Strawberry gums, a sign of Wegener's granulomatosis. JAMA 246:2610, 1981

Darlington CG, Salman I: Oral tuberculous lesions. Am Rev Tuberc 35:147, 1937

Donohue WB, Bolden TE: Tuberculosis of the salivary glands. Oral Surg 14:576, 1961

Editorial: Tuberculosis of the mouth. Br Med J 1:333, 1969

Harrison HL et al: Bolus corticosteroids and cyclophosphamide for initial treatment of Wegener's granulomatosis. JAMA 244:1599, 1980

Lagerlof B et al: Tuberculous lesions of the oral mucosa. Oral Surg 17:735, 1964

Meyer G et al: Hodgkin's disease of the oral cavity. Am J Roentgenol 81:430, 1959

Orlian AI, Birnbaum M: Intraoral localized sarcoid lesion. Oral Surg 49:341, 1980

Piaseska–Zeyland E, Zeyland J: On inhibitory effect of human saliva on growth of tubercle bacilli. Tubercle 19:24, 1937

Scott J, Finch LD: Wegener's granulomatosis presenting as gingivitis. Oral Surg 34:920, 1972

Sherman BM et al: Fatal traumatic ingestion of radiolucent dental prosthesis. N Engl J Med 279:1275, 1968

Walton EW: Giant cell granuloma of the respiratory tract (Wegener's granulomatosis). Br Med J 2:265, 1958

19

Diseases of the Cardiovascular System

MALCOLM A. LYNCH

Fatal cardiac emergencies are uncommon in the dental office, but this does not lessen the need for a thorough understanding of the potential problems with which cardiac patients confront the practicing dentist. The wide range of potent drugs now being prescribed for patients with diseases of the cardiovascular system may pose serious problems for the dentist in furnishing dental care for these patients; infections of dental and oral origin may cause or aggravate endocardial heart disease; and in certain cases of heart disease, any operation or anesthesia is a major risk. The dentist also may play a major role in early detection of remedial cardiovascular disease such as hypertension.

CORONARY HEART DISEASE

In diseases of the myocardium secondary to a decreased or inadequate blood supply (coronary heart disease), this impairment of the blood supply may lead to pain (*angina pectoris*) or to death of myocardial tissue (*myocardial infarction*). At the onset it is useful to clarify terminology that is sometimes used incorrectly or interchangeably:

- *Coronary insufficiency*—Inability of the coronary circulation to supply metabolic demands of the heart
- *Myocardial insufficiency*—Inability of the cardiac muscle to pump enough blood to meet the demands of the body
- *Angina pectoris*—Temporary constant short-acting chest pain caused by coronary insufficiency, usually brought on by exertion but sometimes occurring at rest and not lasting longer than 20 minutes.
- *Myocardial infarction*—Death of cardiac muscle tissue caused by coronary insufficiency, usually manifested by angina-like pain lasting longer than 20 minutes and not necessarily brought on by exertion

Coronary heart disease (CHD) may be caused by any one or a combination of the following factors causing coronary insufficiency: coronary atherosclerosis, coronary arterial spasms, aortic valvular disease (with aortic stenosis being more common than aortic insufficiency), dissecting aneurysm, and usually in combination with the above, acute anemia, carbon monoxide poisoning, or tachycardia. CHD is usually seen after 40 years of age, and when it occurs at an earlier age it is usually accompanied by some other predisposing disease such as diabetes or hypertension. It is more common in males than females up to middle age. After menopause, CHD occurs equally in both sexes.

Certain factors are known as the Coronary Risk Profile, which describes an increased susceptibility to coronary heart disease in a particular patient. These are hypertension, diabetes (high-plasma insulinlevels have the greatest predictive value of any risk factor for coronary heart disease), a family history of coronary disease, cigarette smoking, left ventricular hypertrophy on the electrocardiogram, increased serum triglyceride levels, and sex. Clearly some of these factors are alterable by the individual patient; others are not.

Angina Pectoris

Hypoxemia of the cardiac muscle, resulting from an imbalance between the oxygen consumption and oxygen supply of the cardiac muscles is the basic pathophysiologic alteration in angina pectoris. Angina pectoris may be manifested as almost any kind of pain that results from this disproportion between the oxygen requirement and the oxygen supply to the heart muscle. It is commonly associated with coronary artery disease and has been shown to be sometimes caused by coronary artery spasm. Stress, physical or emotional, or use of tobacco may predispose to an attack.

The most common type of angina is classic or Heberden's angina. This is characterized by chest pain provoked by increase in cardiac work and electrocardiographic changes of ST segment *depression* during the painful episodes. The less common type of angina, variant or Prinzmetal's angina, is characterized by pain occurring at rest often nocturnally or during ordinary activity (not exertion) and associated with transient ST segment *elevation.*

Angina pectoris comprises about 25% of all forms of heart disease. It is most common in the age range from 45 to 65 years. The average age of 6,882 patients in one study was 58.8 years; the ratio of males to females was roughly 4:1. Individuals whose occupation is associated with mental stress—the so-called high-pressure business and professional persons—are frequently affected. Death may occur during the initial attack or during a subsequent attack as a result of myocardial infarction or an acute arrhythmia.

Angina may precede a frank myocardial infarction, and in fact when angina lasts longer than 20 minutes, infarction may be considered to have occurred.

The Framingham, Massachusetts study of angina pectoris showed that mortality among angina victims who never develop any other manifestations of CHD is about the same as among patients in the posthospital phase of myocardial infarction. Furthermore, survival in patients with uncomplicated angina is no better than survival after the acute phase of a myocardial infarction in patients whose angina was complicated or concurrent with a myocardial infarction. These data indicate that angina should be considered a more ominous disease than it has been.

A study by Midwall and associates found that angina either before or after myocardial infarction is significantly correlated with the extent of coronary artery disease. Absence of angina both before and after a myocardial infarction correlated strongly with *single* vessel disease while the presence of angina before or after a myocardial infarction correlated with *two* or *three* vessel disease.

Symptoms

The typical attack of classic angina usually follows physical exertion or emotional stress. The patient is seized with a viselike crushing pain in the substernal region. The pain radiates characteristically to the left shoulder and down this arm to the fourth and fifth fingertips, but it may radiate to other areas, including the neck region and even the jaws. Jaw pain has been reported to occur in the absence of precordial or substernal pain. The dentist should be aware of this in patients with no oral or dental lesions who present with jaw pain brought on by exertion and relieved by rest. This crushing pain lasts a few seconds or a few minutes, seldom longer.

There is fear of impending death. In most instances the pain is relieved almost immediately by the cessation of exertion. For this reason, and because of the intense pain, the person commonly maintains a fixed position during an attack.

Severe pain following the ingestion of a hearty meal may represent anginal attacks rather than acute indigestion. During digestion the metabolic rate is increased, and more work is demanded of the heart. Anginal pain bears no constant relation to blood pressure, although hypertensive patients with angina may have amelioration of their symptoms when the blood pressure is brought under control. During the anginal attack there is little variation in the pulse rate.

The typical attack of variant angina occurs during rest, often at night, or during ordinary exercise. The character and distribution of the pain is otherwise similar to that of classic angina.

If anginal pain persists for more than half an hour, myocardial infarction or some acute abdominal condition should be considered.

Diagnosis

The diagnosis of angina pectoris or anginal pain rests on the patient's history, the opportunity of the physician to take an electrocardiogram coincident with the patient's having an anginal attack, or on coronary angiographic studies. In patients having normal electrocardiograms at rest, changes consistent with myocardial hypoxia and angina can sometimes be induced by having the patient take a stress or exercise electrocardiogram. In this procedure, the patient exercises while the electrocardiogram is being taken, and it is sometimes possible to elicit hypoxic changes on the electrocardiogram. Coronary angiographic studies will demonstrate narrowing of the coronary arteries, usually caused by atherosclerosis, in all patients with classic angina and in some patients with variant angina. In patients having the symptoms of variant angina and normal coronary angiographic studies, coronary spasm may be induced for diagnostic purposes by administration of agents such as ergonovine maleate, methacholine, or a combination of propranolol and epinephrine.

Relief of the anginal pain within 3 minutes by treatment with nitroglycerin sublingually or amyl nitrite is considered virtually diagnostic of angina pectoris if the placebo effect is discounted.

Treatment

Treatment of angina pectoris consists of administering short-acting drugs used for an acute attack such as nitroglycerin tablets (sublingually) or amyl nitrite (inhaled). For long-term prevention, prophylactic, long-acting or sustained-action drugs are administered. These include the nitrates such as pentaerythritol tetranitrate and isosorbide dinitrate tablets or capsules to be chewed or swallowed (not sublingual). Long-acting nitrates in the form of nitroglycerin ointment may also be applied to the skin in increments of one half inch; they appear to have a duration of action up to 4 to 6 hours. Adhesive nitroglycerin tablets may be placed under the lip or in the buccal pouch and begin activity in minutes, providing up to 5 hours of effectiveness. Nitroglycerin is also now available in a gel-like matrix attached to an adhesive bandage, which is applied to the skin and used as a transdermal infusion system. The bandage is effective for 24 hours. The nitrate drugs may act by improving the distribution of coronary blood supply to the subendocardium and are effective in reducing ventricular volume by peripheral pooling and reducing cardiac work load by reducing peripheral pressure by arterial dilatation.

A beta-adrenergic blocking drug such as propranolol is another of the group of long-acting drugs effective in angina pectoris. Propranolol prevents the effects of cardiac sympathetic stimulation and reduces myocardial oxygen demand by decreasing heart rate, ventricular systolic pressure, and peripheral arterial pressure. Combined use of a beta-adrenergic blocking drug and a nitrate is frequently effective when one preparation alone is ineffective in the prophylactic treatment of angina pectoris. It should be noted that the use of a beta-adrenergic agent is generally not recommended for variant angina because it has been shown on some occasions to exacerbate rather than ameliorate the symptoms.

The most recent group of drugs to be approved for long-term therapy of angina pectoris are the calcium antagonists (e.g., verapamil, nifedipine), which act as blocking agents to prevent calcium from entering muscle cells such as cardiac or arterial muscle. Calcium entry into these cells is an essential step for activating their contraction. Because the calcium antagonists appear to block entry at a specific location, they are called calcium-slow-channel blockers. They are particularly effective in preventing variant angina (angina at rest), but they have also been shown to be useful in improving exercise tolerance in patients with classic (exercise-induced) angina.

Further treatment of angina consists of limiting the demands of the heart to a degree commensurate with its blood supply by carefully devised work and exercise patterns. Patients with angina pectoris should be managed in this regard in the same way as are post-myocardial infarction patients.

Dental Considerations

Acute anginal attacks may occur as a result of the stress associated with dental services, particularly extractions. They have been experienced when the patient was in the waiting room or sitting in the dental chair before treatment has begun. The pain of angina pectoris is occasionally referred to the jaws and the teeth, causing the patient to seek dental attention. Such a case was recently reported by Graham and Schinbeckler in which a patient presented with acute jaw pain initially thought to be caused by a toothache but subsequently found to be caused by a myocardial infarction. It is speculated that because of the overlapping of the 5th cranial nerve, 3rd cervical nerve, and 1st thoracic nerve, cardiac pain may be transmitted to the jaw and interpreted as dental pain. Anginal jaw pain is characterized by its extreme severity, its onset associated with exertion, and its disappearance with rest. These characteristics serve to differentiate it from the usual pain of dental origin.

If the patient experiences an anginal attack while in the dental chair, a nitroglycerin tablet should be placed immediately under the tongue or the patient should inhale amyl nitrite. These medications are not useful in patients known to be having a myocardial infarction. In a patient with known angina pectoris, either classic or variant, relatively short-acting antianginal drugs such as sublingual isosorbide nitrate tablets are recommended prophylactically (in addition to any long-acting nitrate drugs the patient may be taking) before initiating dental therapy or a particularly stressful phase of dental therapy.

Myocardial Infarction

Symptoms

The pathogenesis and etiology of myocardial infarction is the same as that discussed earlier under Angina Pectoris; however, there may be additional symptoms that will indicate that the patient is having a myocardial infarction rather than an anginal attack. As mentioned earlier, an anginal attack lasting longer than 30 minutes is considered by definition to be a myocardial infarction. An attack of anginalike chest pain accompanied by any of the following symptoms should be considered a myocardial infarction until proven otherwise: nausea and vomiting, tachycardia and grossly irregular pulse, symptoms of shock with pallor and diaphoresis, and pulmonary edema with difficulty in breathing.

In a 20-year study of 5,127 men and women initially free of coronary heart disease, symptomatic myocardial infarctions occurred in 193 men and 53 women. Asymptomatic and unrecognized myocardial infarction occurred in an additional 45 men and 28 women. In this study, it was shown that 30% of patients who had heart attacks had "silent" myocardial infarction. That is, the infarctions were asymptomatic and detected only by biennial electrocardiograms. There was no difference in survival rates for patients with recognized and unrecognized myocardial infarction after the first 3 years.

Diagnosis

The characteristic history of the chest pain and pain radiating to other areas as described for angina may be the only guide. Patients who present with this history must be carefully evaluated because early on in the disease the history may be the only positive finding. The electrocardiogram shows changes characteristic of or compatible with acute myocardial infarction in 80% of the cases; however, it does not show such changes in 20% of early myocardial infarction cases and therefore cannot be relied on to exclude the presence of a myocardial infarction.

Changes in various serum enzymes are particularly helpful in the diagnosis of the myocardial infarction; the creatine phosphokinase (CPK), serum glutamic oxalacetic transaminase (SGOT), aspartate transaminase (AST), and lactic dehydrogenase (LDH). Certain of these enzymes rise earlier than do others in an acute infarction, and the pattern of enzymatic changes can help differentiate myocardial infarction from other clinically similar diseases. (See the chapter on Laboratory Diagnosis for a comprehensive discussion of these enzymatic changes and their usefulness in the diagnosis of myocardial infarction.)

There is often a mild leukocytosis and slight temperature elevation the first several days after a myocardial infarction. The physical examination is sometimes useful later in the acute phase. Some patients develop a physiological aneurysm of the ventricular wall that can be palpated on physical examination. An atrial as well as a ventricular gallop may develop and on occasion heart murmurs may develop consistent with mitral regurgitation secondary to papillary muscle dysfunction or rupture or very rarely, to a ruptured interventricular septum. A pericardial friction rub develops in 20% to 30% of the patients.

Radionuclide techniques have in recent years been able to provide more accurate information about the character and extent of coronary heart disease than was previously possible. In these techniques gamma-emitting radionuclides (usually potassium, thallous chloride, TL-201; or technetium, Tc-99m) are used in making cardiac scintigrams. Normally perfused myocardium is labeled by these radionuclides, and abnormally perfused myocardium is not labeled, producing a "cold" spot on the scintigram. These techniques are generally useful quantitatively in actually measuring myocardial blood flow and qualitatively in providing static images that demonstrate areas of decreased myocardial perfusion and the extent of myocardial infarction. Myocardial scintigrams tend to become abnormal within 10 to 12 hours after infarction, become most abnormal for 24 to 48 hours, and then return to normal after 6 or 7 days.

Positron-emission tomography appears to offer an even more promising technique in the diagnosis of myocardial infarction. The advantage of this technique lies in its ability to show areas of reduced or absent cellular metabolism as opposed to reductions in blood flow or anatomic defects as in radionuclide scintigraphy. In the positron-emission tomographic technique, positron-emitting isotopes such as nitrogen-13, oxygen-15, or carbon-11 are used synthesized with water or sugars, such that when given to human subjects they accurately reflect metabolic activity within the body. Thallium scans show only dead scar tissue, while positron-emission scanning demarcates tissue that is still alive but has reduced metabolism.

Treatment

Newer treatment methods have resulted in an increasing number of survivals in patients treated for cardiac arrest before arriving at the hospital. In a cardiopulmonary arrest, cardiopulmonary resuscitation should be immediately begun. In patients with life-threatening acute arrhythmias, usually premature ventricular contractions or ventricular tachycardia, occurring in the dental office before transportation of the patient to an acute care medical facility, prophylactic 10% lidocaine can be injected intramuscularly in the deltoid muscle at a dose of 4 to 6 mg/kg body weight. Note that this is *not* 2% lidocaine with epinephrine as is found in the usual dental office.

Treatment of myocardial infarction consists of the relief of pain in the early stages of the disease (with morphine sulfate) and absolute mental and physical rest during the prolonged convalescence. Oxygen and the controlled administration of anticoagulants are established therapeutic agents. Nitrous oxide in a concentration of 35% mixed with oxygen has been shown to be quite effective in decreasing the pain of acute myocardial infarction, and no adverse hemodynamic or other adverse effects have been noted. It is most effective in those patients with less severe pain, whereas patients with the most severe pain usually require the addition of more potent analgesics.

The use of anticoagulants is decreasing. Some physicians believe that patients with CHD should be kept on this therapy permanently; others use anticoagulants only for the first 2 weeks while the patient is hospitalized after an acute infarction. The evidence is more convincing that anticoagulation is of greater use in preventing complications of thromboembolism than it is in preventing recurrence or extension of the infarction.

Studies continue to appear in the literature reporting conflicting results on the efficacy of anticoagulation in acute myocardial infarctions. Mutual problems with all these studies include sample size and randomized selection of control and placebo groups.

It has been suggested that aspirin because of its interference with platelet adhesiveness might be effective in reducing mortality in post-myocardial infarction patients. For this reason, a study was conducted over a 3-year period to test whether the regular administration of aspirin in the dose of 1 g per day to post-myocardial infarction men and women would be of any value. Results of this study indicated that there is no significant difference in mortality in the two groups, and aspirin is not recommended for routine use in patients who have survived a myocardial infarction.

The use of beta blocking agents both during the acute and follow-up phases of myocardial infarction has been shown to be promising. One study using propranolol hydrochloride showed a 26% decrease in mortality over 27 months. The use of propranolol in patients with no contraindications to beta-blocking agents who have had a recent myocardial infarction is recommended for at least 3 years.

Prognosis

Between 1968 and 1976, mortality from coronary heart disease declined in the United States by more than 20%. The average annual decline was 3% per year in the 1970s, and about 42% of the cardiovascular mortality decline since 1950 was achieved in the 5-year period from 1972 to 1977. These declines in cardiovascular mortality have been accompanied by favorable changes in dietary habits, smoking, treatment of hypertension, and increased physical activity in the population.

In addition to the general downward trend in cardiovascular mortality over the last decade, there has also been a decrease in mortality in patients after the first myocardial infarction. This improved survival does not occur after discharge from the hospital but rather appears to be almost exclusively related to acute in-hospital care such as that received in coronary care units. Survivals in one study were as follows: 20% of the men who had a first myocardial infarction died within 1 year, and the acute mortality rates for hospitalized infarction patients were appreciably greater in those whose myocardial infarctions were complicated by ventricular fibrillation or cardiac arrest. For patients discharged from the hospital, however, there was no significant difference in long-term survival in those who suffered these complications and those who did not. Men surviving the first year had a 23% increased risk of death over normal during the next 5 years and a 25% cardiovascular mortality for the subsequent 5 years.

In more recent years it appears that improved emergency medical services, coronary bypass surgery, and use of beta blocker drugs may have significantly improved post-hospital survival rates in myocardial infarction patients. A recently reported, well-controlled randomized double-blind study of the use of beta blocking agents as post-myocardial infarction therapy demonstrated a 26% reduction in 24-month mortality in the treated patients.

Dental Management of the Patient with CHD

The dentist is in a unique position to render his patient an important health service by taking a careful history to elicit present symptoms or past history of cardiac disease and by taking the patient's pulse and measuring his blood pressure. The average patient rarely seeks medical care unless he is ill but probably has formed the habit of visiting his dentist twice a year. Thus the dentist has an unusual opportunity of detecting the early signs of cardiovascular disease and referring these individuals for medical supervision at a time when the results of conservative methods of therapy will be most effective.

The management of the patient with cardiovascular disease in the dental office is becoming an increasingly important phase of dental practice. For example, a large segment of our population is at an age when chronic diseases have a greater tendency to develop; of these chronic diseases, those of the cardiovascular system form an important segment. Cardiovascular disease is the number one cause of death in the United States. It is estimated that currently well over 10 million persons in the United States have some form of cardiovascular disease, and this number will probably increase rather than decrease in future decades.

A second reason that patients with cardiovascular disease require special management in the dental office is that they may have decreased ability to withstand stressful situations, and in many cases dental treatment may aggravate already existing cardiovascular disease. In addition, the extensive use of potent therapeutic agents to treat various forms of cardiovascular diseases poses problems in dental patient management. All of these considerations might cause the dentist to hesitate to treat these patients; however, dental treatment should not be denied the patient with cardiovascular disease. It is particularly important for these patients that the oral health be maintained in the best possible condition. Nowhere is this more important than in the increasing number of patients with intracardiac prostheses who are highly susceptible to infection following dental procedures unless the most stringent precautions are taken. The American Dental Association and the American Heart Association have summarized the dental care of cardiovascular patients clearly and concisely in a joint report, *Management of Dental Problems in Patients with Cardiovascular Diseases*, approved by the appropriate group of these two national organizations in 1965. This report has provided the physician and the dentist with an authoritative series of guidelines:

> Generally speaking, a fully ambulatory patient without cardiac symptoms, who can come to the dental office, is suitable for outpatient care. Management of dental problems in patients with cardiovascular disease requires close co-operation between the physician and dentist. The physician must be aware of the dentist's problem, and, in turn, the dentist should know the medical problem and the limitations it imposes. There is need for mutual understanding, respect and cooperation between the physician and the dentist if the best interest of the patient is to be served.

When dealing with patients suspected of having cardiovascular disease, it is imperative that a comprehensive medical history be taken. Periodic re-evaluation of the medical history is especially important in discovering developing cardiovascular disease.

Premedication

It is important to premedicate the patient with CHD with a short-acting barbiturate or other sedative such as diazepam before administering a local anesthetic or performing dental operative procedures. The medication should be given in the waiting room 45 minutes before the dental procedures are contemplated to minimize the stress reactions occurring in the waiting room as well as in the dental chair. Pentobarbital in a dosage of 30 to 60 mg, or seccobarbital in a dosage of 50 to 100 mg, or 5 mg diazepam is satisfactory for most adults. The exact dosage should be determined on an individual basis and with full consideration of other medication the patient is receiving. All patients to whom barbiturates are administered should be accompanied to the dentist's office and should not drive an automobile immediately following the appointment. In patients susceptible to attacks of angina pectoris, especially when stress induced, administration of isosorbide dinitrate sublingual tablets is advised. Onset of action is within 2 to 5 minutes, and duration of action is 1 to 2 hours. This may be used in addition to any other long-acting nitrate preparation the patient may be taking to prevent angina.

The dentist should consult with the patient's physician before administering anti-sialagogues such as atropine or methantheline. The dosage of these drugs as used in dentistry may be associated with tachycardia, which would be undesirable in certain forms of heart disease.

The Patient on Anticoagulant Therapy

Patients on long-term anticoagulant therapy should be given specific instructions, particularly with regard to bleeding, if surgical procedures such as dental extractions become necessary. Frequent periodic prothrombin time determinations should be made by the physician, especially during intercurrent illnesses, and the patient should be cautioned concerning the possible risk of taking drugs such as aspirin and broad-spectrum antibiotics such as tetracycline or ampicillin. Ensor and Peters reported on the complications occurring in 268 patients on active long-term anticoagulant therapy. There were 58 hemorrhagic episodes of which seven consisted of bleeding from the gums. The dentist should specifically ask whether patients requiring surgery are on anticoagulant therapy.

Dental extractions have reportedly been performed successfully with the patient on the usual maintenance dosage of anticoagulant agents. On the other hand, some oral surgeons believe that the anticoagulant dosage should be decreased by the cardiologist or the internist before the surgical procedure. The sudden withdrawal of anticoagulant drugs, especially if any vitamin K preparations are administered, may result in thrombosis or embolism, but the continuance of full dosage of the anticoagulant may cause profound bleeding in some patients.

Much of the confusion in this area has been cleared up by the work of Greenberg and associates, who demonstrated that such confusion in the literature usually resulted from the use of a single test—the prothrombin time—to measure therapeutic anticoagulation. The coumarin drugs exhibit some variation in their depression of clotting Factors VII, IX, II, and X, and one of these, Factor IX, is not measured by the prothrombin time. It is possible for a patient on a coumarin drug to have a prothrombin time within therapeutic limits but with a severely depressed Factor IX level, which could cause bleeding after an oral surgical procedure. Factor IX is measured by the partial thromboplastin time, however, and if both the patient's prothrombin time *and* partial thromboplastin time are within the therapeutic range, it should be possible to carry out all but the most extensive oral surgical and periodontal procedures without altering the patient's usual dose of anticoagulant drug.

Use of Local Anesthesia

Local anesthetic agents properly administered are generally preferred to general anesthetics for patients with cardiovascular disease. There has been much controversy about the maximum of local anesthetic that can be used with relative safety in patients with cardiovascular disease and whether the anesthetic should contain a vasoconstrictor agent. Complete and total anesthesia is essential in these patients to minimize apprehension and the discharge of endogenous epinephrine. The commonly accepted procedures for the administration of local anesthetic agents, particularly aspiration before injection, should be followed carefully.

Sedative premedication is a "must" for the patient with severe cardiovascular disease. The minimum of anesthetic, containing the lowest concentration of vasoconstrictor agent compatible with complete anesthesia, should be used, and the patient should be kept under close observation following the injection. Intravascular injections of anesthetic agent and the commonly used vasoconstrictor agents may be especially dangerous in the patient with cardiovascular disease. For this reason only aspirating-type syringes and needles should be employed. A needle smaller than a 25-gauge should not be used because this often prevents aspiration. If the position of the needle is changed during injection, the operator must reaspirate before continuing the injection. If blood is aspirated, the cartridge should be discarded.

A vasoconstrictor is generally indicated because it aids in more profound anesthesia and limits the rate of absorption of the anesthetic agent. The pain that might result from inadequate anesthesia in a cardiovascular patient might cause release of endogenous epinephrine in excess of the amount that would be given with the local anesthetic. Concentrations of vasoconstrictors normally used in dental local anesthetic solutions are therefore not contraindicated in patients with cardiovascular disease when administered carefully. The following concentrations can be used:

- Epinephrine   1:50,000 to 1:250,000
- Levarterenol   1:30,000
- Levonordefrin   1:20,000
- Phenylephrine   1:2,500

Cheraskin and Prasertsuntarasai found that the systolic, the diastolic, and the mean pulse pressures, as well as the pulse rate, varied little between the preinjection period and 10 minutes after the injection of 2 to 8 ml of a 2% lidocaine hydrochloride solution with or without 1:100,000 epinephrine in normotensive or hypertensive patients who had or had not been sedated with 1.5 grains secobarbital administered orally. The sedated hypertensive patient given epinephrine fared better than did the one who received neither sedation nor a vasoconstrictor. A study by Tolas, however, indicated that after 3 and 5 minutes, arterial plasma epinephrine concentrations in patients given an injection with a standard carpule of 2% lidocaine with 1:100,000 epinephrine increased to more than two times the baseline level.

At times vasoconstrictor agents are used in greater concentrations than the above for gingival retraction or hemostasis. The use of vasoconstrictors for gingival retraction or hemostasis is potentially dangerous and should be avoided in patients with a history of hypertension or in cardiovascular disease predisposing to the development of arrhythmias. If their use cannot be avoided, it is wise to follow the recommendations of Buchannan, who on review of the literature recommended that the retraction system of choice in the hypertensive patient is 8% racemic epinephrine-impregnated retraction cord. Because absorption of this solution could easily lead to significant blood pressure elevation, it should be used sparingly and the patient carefully monitored.

Extent of Dental Procedures to Be Accomplished at One Time

There is no set rule governing the extent of procedures to be undertaken at one time. It requires judgment based on experience. The important consideration is the amount of trauma that may be associated with the intended procedure and the patient's ability to withstand the trauma. This requires consultation with the patient's physician. It is a good general working guide that in patients who develop chest pain, shortness of breath, diaphoresis, pallor, or a rapid or irregular pulse during the dental procedure, the procedure should be terminated. Later, shorter appointments with less extensive traumatic procedures should be scheduled. Medical consultation is indicated, because these patients probably have serious underlying heart disease and need careful monitoring.

Other Considerations

When surgical procedures are necessary for patients with a history of coronary artery disease, the general precautions and procedures summarized earlier in this section should be followed. If general anesthesia is necessary the patient's physician and an anesthesiologist should be consulted about the choice of a general anesthetic.

RHEUMATIC HEART DISEASE AND RHEUMATIC FEVER

Rheumatic fever is believed to be a disease of altered immunologic reaction to group A beta-hemolytic streptococcal infection, usually a pharyngitis. This abnormal reaction to the streptococcal infection causes lesions in the nervous system, the subcutaneous tissues, joints, and most frequently, the heart. The only lesions capable of causing permanent clinical sequelae are those in the heart. Rheumatic fever usually comes on 1 to 3 weeks after the streptococcal infection, but it is not possible to predict which patients with a streptococcal infection will develop rheu-

matic fever. In group A beta-streptococcal epidemics there is a 3% occurrence of rheumatic fever. If a patient has had previous rheumatic fever, the chance of recurrence with a group A beta-streptococcal infection is up to 50% and is more likely to occur with a severe, recurrent streptococcal infection or in a patient who has had previous cardiac damage from an earlier streptococcal infection.

Acute rheumatic fever is mainly a disease of childhood occurring most often between the ages of 6 and 16 years with a peak at 8 years (the "growing pains" of childhood may be symptoms of rheumatic fever). It is particularly common in New England and the Middle Atlantic States. Cold damp weather, rapid changes in temperature, and attacks of tonsillitis predispose to the disease. There appears to be a family predisposition. Its incidence is presently on the decline, although this is difficult to measure because rheumatic fever is not always a reportable nor a reported disease. In any case, in 1950 the crude death rates from acute rheumatic fever and rheumatic heart disease were 14.5/100,000; in 1972 this rate had declined to 6.8/100,000. Considering that deaths from rheumatic heart disease often occur in the older population who have had rheumatic fever as children, one might expect the death rate declines from rheumatic heart disease to be most evident in younger age groups. This appears to be the case. In the age group 25 to 44 years the mortality per 100,000 declined 76% from 1950 to 1972, while in the age group younger than 24 years, the mortality declined 91%.

All of the factors contributing to this decline are not known. Certainly the use of penicillin to control recurrent rheumatic fever plays a big part. Less well understood is the decline in the severity of the cardiac involvement. Other factors such as better treatment and prevention of bacterial endocarditis, cardiac surgery, and improved methods of treating congestive heart failure have also contributed to the decline in mortality.

Symptoms and Signs

Chorea (involuntary movements), the symptoms of acute carditis, rheumatic arthritis, or the typical subcutaneous nodules may be the initial symptoms of rheumatic fever. The child often complains of a sore throat, is listless, and has a temperature of 100°F to 102°F (38°C to 39°C). At times an erythematous skin eruption, erythema marginatum, is present during the acute attack. Rheumatic arthritis is characterized by involvement of successive joints, which are red, tender, and painful. The wrists, ankles, elbows, and knees are most commonly involved. Even the weight of the bedclothes causes severe pain. The rheumatic nodules, small oval fibrous subcutaneous masses, are common on the extensor surfaces of the wrists and on the ankles and are usually painless.

Varying degrees of acute carditis occur in most cases of rheumatic fever, with permanent cardiac lesions resulting in 25% to 50% of the patients, but in recent years, cardiac involvement has been on the decline. Cardiac valvular lesions affect the mitral valve in 97% of the cases, with the aortic valve being the second most commonly involved, resulting in varying degrees of insufficiency and stenosis usually with accompanying murmurs on physical examination. These valves are frequently the site of subsequent subacute bacterial endocarditis. The myocardial lesions produce fibrosis of the myocardium and lessened cardiac reserve.

Diagnosis

In patients with a history typical of a preceding streptococcal infection and predominant manifestations of arthritis and carditis, the diagnosis of rheumatic fever is made relatively easily. In the majority of patients, however, the diagnosis is not nearly so clear-cut. For example, only 50% of patients with acute rheumatic fever have a history of a preceding streptococcal infection. More often than not the symptoms are mild or similar to symptoms of other diseases, and any one symptom is insufficient to make the diagnosis of rheumatic fever. For this reason, in 1944 Jones developed a set of criteria, which were modified in 1955, for the diagnosis of rheumatic fever. He established five major and five minor criteria with the provision that two major or one major and two minor criteria were sufficient evidence for making the diagnosis of rheumatic fever. These criteria are

listed in Table 19-1, and in addition to these criteria, there should be supporting evidence of a preceding streptococcal infection such as a positive throat culture for group A streptococcus or increased antistreptolysin O (ASO) titer or other streptococcal antibodies or a history of recent scarlet fever.

Treatment and Prevention of Recurrence

The treatment of rheumatic fever consists of bedrest and sedation during the acute episode. Salicylates are almost specific for the pain of rheumatic arthritis. Corticosteroid therapy has resulted in remissions of symptoms of this disase, but it is unlikely that it alters the ultimate course of the disease by preventing rheumatic heart disease. Symptoms of the acute attack subside within 6 weeks in about 75% of patients, and within 12 weeks, symptoms will have subsided in 90% of patients. Patients who have had rheumatic fever have a 50% chance of its recurring (with further heart damage) with another group A beta-hemolytic streptococcal infection. For this reason, continued prophylaxis against a beta-streptococcal infection is indicated, to be given in the form of a monthly injection of 1.2 million units of benzathine penicillin G or in 200,000 units of oral penicillin given twice daily, or 1 g of sulfadiazine given orally once a day. Such prophylactic therapy is often discontinued when the patient is 20 or 30 years old, although the American Heart Association recommends that patients with rheumatic heart disease be

Table 19-1. Jones criteria (modified) for diagnosis of rheumatic fever

MAJOR CRITERIA	MINOR CRITERIA
Carditis	Fever
Polyarthritis	Arthralgia
Chorea	Previous rheumatic fever or rheumatic heart disease
Subcutaneous nodules	
Erythema marginatum	Elevated Erthrocyte sedimentation rate or positive C-reactive protein
	Prolonged PR interval

continued on prophylactic therapy for their lifetimes.

The general regimen of the individual with rheumatic heart disease often requires a restriction of normal physical activity. Those who develop cardiac arrhythmias or congestive heart failure must be treated accordingly. Cardiac surgery with prosthetic valve replacement may ultimately be necessary in some patients.

Dental Considerations

Dental management of the patient with rheumatic heart disease is the same as management of the dental patient to prevent endocarditis. It is discussed in the next section under Dental Considerations.

INFECTIVE ENDOCARDITIS AND SUBACUTE BACTERIAL ENDOCARDITIS

Infective endocarditis is a serious disease that is most commonly bacterial in origin but on occasion may be mycotic. It is sometimes acute, especially when the organisms are particularly virulent. In such acute cases, an intact endocardium not damaged by previous disease may be involved. Cases of endocarditis of dental origin are almost always caused by bacteria of low virulence that slowly (subacutely) attack a previously damaged endocardium, causing a subacute bacterial endocarditis.

Subacute bacterial endocarditis may occur at any age but is most common in midlife. It has a marked predisposition for persons with rheumatic or congenital cardiac or vascular defects, and at present 40% to 60% of the patients with infective endocarditis have these underlying cardiac defects that predispose them to the disease. Other cardiac lesions predisposing to endocarditis include a bicuspid aortic valve, luetic aortic valvular disease, idiopathic hypertrophic subaortic stenosis, and mitral valve prolapse (click-murmur syndrome). With increasing use of cardiac surgery and implantation of valvular prostheses, endocarditis superimposed on the valvular transplant site is frequently difficult to determine the immediate causative factors, but surgical trauma and dental ex-

tractions are commonly related chronologically to the onset of the clinical symptoms.

Symptoms

Endocarditis is so insidious that the symptoms may not be recognized for several months. The patient experiences progressive weakness, loss of weight, dyspnea, anorexia, and muscular and joint aches and pains. A low-grade fever is usually present.

Once the microbially involved fibrinous vegetative lesions (thrombi) have developed on the cardiac valves, they serve as foci for the intermittent dissemination of microorganisms throughout the body. These vegetative lesions are extremely friable, and small pieces may break off and form septic emboli. The petechial hemorrhages in the conjunctivae and the oral mucosae, which occur in 20% to 40% of the patients represent phenomena associated with minute septic emboli. Larger emboli lodge occasionally in the spleen, the kidneys, the lungs, and the brain, where they produce symptoms referable to the structures and the organs involved. Some manifestations of the disease are thought to be immunologically mediated. These include musculoskeletal manifestations, some skin manifestations, and most certainly glomerulonephritis, in which immune complexes have been shown to be deposited in the glomeruli and which is associated with a depressed level of serum complement.

Diagnosis

The clinical diagnosis of subacute bacterial endocarditis is frequently made by the elimination of other conditions that may produce mild febrile symptoms, weakness, and loss of weight. This disease should be suspected in any patient with valvular heart disease who has unexplained fever for a week or more or exhibits embolic phenomena or an unexplained anemia. The final diagnosis is made on the physical findings and the demonstration of a positive blood culture.

Treatment

Many patients with streptococcal endocarditis can now be cured with hospitalization for intensive antibiotic therapy, usually up to

20,000,000 units of penicillin a day, intravenously, for 6 weeks. Formerly this disease was almost uniformly fatal.

Dental Considerations

Considerable laboratory and clinical evidence points to the importance of an oral focus for the microorganisms. Twenty papers were published between 1935 and 1975 on the frequency of bacteremia in postextraction blood cultures, and positive cultures were reported in anywhere from 15% to 100% of patients studied. These discrepancies can be accounted for by the numbers of patients in the studies and differences in collecting, handling, and culturing the specimens.

In their study of the etiology of subacute bacterial endocarditis, Okell and Elliot made blood cultures before and following the extraction of teeth under nitrous oxide anesthesia. They demonstrated a transient bacteremia, usually *Streptococcus viridans*, in 76% of the cases. The percentage of positive cultures was related to the state of the oral hygiene. These investigators demonstrated that the organisms responsible for subacute bacterial endocarditis were disseminated commonly through the bloodstream following dental extractions.

Burket and Burn made similar studies, except that the teeth were removed under local anesthesia. The percentage of positive cultures (17%) was lower than that reported by Okell and Elliot (76%), which may be accounted for in part by the local vasoconstrictor in the local anesthetic. By the use of a nonpathogen, *Serratia marcescens*, it was demonstrated later that the gingival sulcus was an important site from which the bacteria gained entrance into the bloodstream. Topical antimicrobial agents were found to be ineffective in rendering this field sterile. Actual cauterization of the gingival crevice before extraction markedly reduced the percentage of transient bacteremias.

Review of the literature by Cawson (1981) estimated that only about 6% to 10% of the cases of infective endocarditis occurred subsequent to dental treatment. It is not possible to know the likelihood of developing endocarditis subsequent to dental therapy in a susceptible patient who has *not* received prophylaxis. Hilson in 1970 estimated that the risk might be as low as 1 in 3,000, and Pogral and Welsby in 1975 indicated that the risk might be as low as 1 in 115,500 dental treatments. Nonetheless, for medicolegal reasons if no other, prophylaxis is currently thought to be both effective and necessary. There is conflicting evidence in the literature as to the influence of the degree and duration of trauma and the amount of oral infection present on the production, frequency, and magnitude of bacteremia. Some studies have suggested a strong positive correlation between these factors, whereas other studies have suggested that these factors play a minimal role. Even in the absence of direct dental manipulation, a bacteremia can be produced secondary to foci in the oral cavity. This has been demonstrated to occur with chewing and in oral irrigating devices using water under pressure. Cases of bacterial endocarditis have been reported in edentulous patients in whom the portal of entry was postulated to be secondary to denture sores. Almost any kind of dental manipulation has been associated with the production of bacteremia, including root canal filling, occlusal cavity preparations in stable teeth, and even placing amalgam restorations in previously prepared teeth. Any dental procedure that results in gingival bleeding, however small, will result in a bacteremia.

Streptococcus viridans was the organism most commonly recovered in bacteremias prior to 1960. Because of the large number of anaerobes in the oral cavity, it was felt that more effort should be made to detect the presence of anaerobes in dental bacteremias. Culture methods for anaerobes were developed and improved, and as a result our knowledge of the spectrum of bacteria isolated from bacteremias originating from the oral cavity has changed considerably. Several investigators have estimated that about 10% of endocarditis cases seen in the general hospitals are caused by anaerobes, and the mouth is an important source of these organisms.

When one considers the extremely serious nature of this disease, it is apparent that every known prophylactic measure should be taken to preclude the possibility of transient bacteremias occurring in patients with known valvular lesions.

Prevention

The following suggestions for prophylactic procedures for the reduction of postextraction bacteremias and the possible development of subacute bacterial endocarditis are simple, and if subacute bacterial endocarditis should develop, one has the satisfaction that prophylactic procedures were taken:

1. Question the patient about a history of rheumatic fever, a known history of "heart disease" with valvular involvement, or a heart murmur.
2. If heart disease predisposing to endocarditis is known to be present (Table 19-2), administer prophylactic antibiotic therapy before dental treatment (see below). If a questionable positive history of heart disease is obtained, consult the patient's physician. Antibiotic prophylaxis should be given to all patients in whom gingival bleeding is likely to result from dental treatment. Ordinarily, simple adjustment of orthodontic appliances does not necessitate premedication as does not the shedding of deciduous teeth. Table 19-2 lists examples of heart disease in which patients need to be premedicated; note that this does *not* include uncomplicated cases of secundum atrial septal defect.
3. Have the patient rinse with an antibacterial mouthwash immediately before dental treatment to help reduce the number of oral microorganisms.
4. Keep dental procedures as atraumatic as possible.
5. All patients who are at risk of developing endocarditis subsequent to dental treatment should be instructed to consult a physician if a febrile illness develops within 3 months of a dental treatment.

Penicillin is the drug of choice for administration to patients with rheumatic or congenital heart disease undergoing dental manipulations or surgical procedures in the oral cavity. Although the exact dosage and duration of therapy are empirical, there is some evidence that for effective prophylaxis, reasonably high concentrations of penicillin must be present at the time of dental procedures and over a period of several days thereafter to prevent organisms from lodging in

Table 19-2. Heart disease necessitating antibiotic prophylaxis before dental treatment

REQUIRE REGIMEN A	REQUIRE REGIMEN B
Congenital heart disease	Prosthetic heart valve
Rheumatic heart disease	
Acquired valvular heart disease	
Idiopathic hypertrophic subaortic stenosis (IHSS)	
Mitral valve prolapse syndrome	

the heart valves or to eradicate them promptly before the formation of a vegetation.

See Table 19-2 for indications for regimens of antibiotic prophylaxis.

Specific antibiotic regimens for prevention of bacterial endocarditis are as follows:

REGIMEN A

For Patients Who Can Take Penicillin
  Parenteral and Oral
    Adults—Aqueous crystalline penicillin G (1,000,000 units) mixed with procaine penicillin G (600,000 units). Give intramuscularly 30 minutes to 1 hour before procedure and then give penicillin V (formerly called phenoxymethyl penicillin) 500 mg orally every 6 hours for 8 dosages.
    Children—Aqueous crystalline penicillin G (30,000 units/kg) mixed with procaine penicillin G (600,000 units) intramuscularly. Timing of doses for children is the same as for adults. For children less than 60 lbs, the dosage of penicillin V is 250 mg orally every 6 hours for 8 dosages.
  Oral only
    Adults—Penicillin V, 2.0 g orally 30 minutes to 1 hour before the procedure and then 500 mg orally every 6 hours for 8 dosages.
    Children—Penicillin V, 2.0 g orally 30 minutes to 1 hour before the procedure

and then 500 mg orally every 6 hours for 8 dosages. For children less than 60 lbs, use 1.0 g orally 30 minutes to 1 hour before the procedure and then 250 mg orally every 6 hours for 8 dosages.

For Patients Allergic to Penicillin

Adults—Erythromycin, 1.0 g orally 1½ to 2 hours before the procedure and then 500 mg orally every 6 hours for 8 dosages.

Children—Erythromycin, 20 mg/kg orally 1½ to 2 hours before the procedure and then 10 mg/kg every 6 hours for 8 dosages.

REGIMEN B

For Patients Who Can Take Penicillin and Streptomycin

Adults—Aqueous crystalline penicillin G (1,000,000 units intramuscularly) mixed with procaine penicillin G (600,000 units intramuscularly) plus streptomycin (1 g intramuscularly) given 30 minutes to 1 hour before the procedure; then penicillin V 500 mg orally every 6 hours for 8 dosages.

Children—Aqueous crystalline penicillin G (30,000 units/kg intramuscularly) plus streptomycin (20 mg/kg intramuscularly). Timing of doses for children is the same as for adults. For children less than 60 lbs, the recommended oral dose of penicillin V is 250 mg every 6 hours for 8 dosages.

For Patients Allergic to Penicillin or Streptomycin

Adults—Vancomycin (1 g intravenously over 30 minutes to 1 hour). Start initial vancomycin infusion ½ to 1 hour before procedure; then erythromycin 500 mg orally every 6 hours for 8 dosages.

Children—Vancomycin (20 mg/kg intravenously over 30 minutes to 1 hour). Timing of doses for children is the same as for adults. Erythromycin dose is 10 mg/kg every 6 hours for 8 dosages.

In instances of delayed healing and subsequent possible prolonged bacteremia, antibiotic prophylaxis should be continued longer than the 2 days indicated. The dosage regimen employed for long-term prophylaxis against group A streptococci to prevent recurrent rheumatic fever is inadequate for preventing bacterial endocarditis. Spencer and co-workers demonstrated that penicillin-resistant gingival organisms occur in patients who are on oral penicillin rheumatic fever chemoprophylaxis. For patients in this group, it is suggested that erythromycin be employed instead of penicillin.

Some workers have been concerned that antibiotic prophylaxis does not achieve the result of sterilizing root abscesses or periodontal lesions and might lead to the emergence of antibiotic-resistant microorganisms, constituting a very difficult therapeutic problem if they became implanted in the valves. Others have speculated that antibiotic prophylaxis too long before dental treatment might also lead to overgrowth of resistant organisms. It has therefore been argued that prophylaxis should not be instituted until shortly before the dental procedure. For this reason the prophylactic regimen as described earlier is considerably shorter than that used before the latest revision of antibiotic prophylaxis was published in 1977.

Patients who have cardiac prostheses or renal transplants have been shown to be unusually susceptible to endocarditis by oral microorganisms as a result of dental manipulation. These patients should be premedicated with larger doses (regimen B) of intramuscular or intravenous antibiotic to prevent infection.

HYPERTENSION

General Considerations

The term *hypertension* (high blood pressure) indicates a disease entity in which the systolic or diastolic pressure, or both, is elevated. Systolic hypertension alone may be seen in elderly patients and is probably the result of decreased distensibility of the arteries. It may also be seen in hyperthyroidism and in congestive failure. In systolic elevation (alone) of the pressure, it is the underlying disease that is treated; when it is the result of decreased distensibility of the arteries in elderly patients, treatment must be monitored carefully in order that cerebral blood flow not be reduced. It was once thought that systolic elevation of the pressure alone should not be treated inasmuch as it was the elevation of the diastolic component that produced the ravages of the disease. In recent years this opinion has been challenged, and more physicians are recognizing that it is probably elevation of the mean blood pressure that has serious systemic consequences. There is no question however, that diastolic elevation of the blood pressure, usually accompanied by systolic elevation, has serious prognostic consequences and must be treated. The definition of the level of pressure considered to be abnormal is rather arbitrary, but a persisting systolic pressure of over 140 mm Hg or 90 mm Hg diastolic is considered to be borderline hypertension. Elevated blood pressure begins at 160/95, but severe cases of systolic pressures of over 250 mm Hg are not unusual.

An estimated 10% of adults in the United States have undetected or untreated hypertension. A survey of the blood pressures of 856 dentists taken in the health screening program at the 1973 American Dental Association (ADA) annual session showed that 16.66% of the group in the third decade of life had diastolic pressures above 90 mm Hg, and 27% of the entire group of dentists (all ages) showed similar diastolic hypertension. Repeated epidemiologic surveys show that 50% to 60% of people with hypertension are unaware of their condition; 25% do not seek care when told of the hypertension, and of those who do seek therapy, 15% to 20% receive inadequate long-term therapy.

Two hallmark reports by the Veterans Administration Cooperative Study Group on antihypertensive agents in 1967 and 1970 definitively demonstrated the absolute necessity for treatment in hypertension. The report in 1970 studied a group of 73 patients whose diastolic blood pressures averaged between 115 and 129 mm Hg and who were treated with antihypertensive drugs. This group was compared to a matched group of equally hypertensive patients treated with placebos. During the period of the study, 27 severe complications and 4 deaths occurred in the placebo group in contrast to 2 complicating

events and no deaths in the actively treated group. The 1967 study disclosed similar differences between treated and placebo groups in patients with mild to moderate hypertension. In one study, 380 men with diastolic blood pressures averaging 90 to 114 mm Hg were randomly assigned to either antihypertensive drugs or placebos. Over an average 3.3-year period, cardiovascular complications occurred in 22 treated patients in contrast to 56 in the control group, and there were only 8 deaths in the treated series compared to 19 in the untreated series.

In view of the above, the National Heart and Lung Institute launched a nationwide program to inform the public about hypertension and to engage health professions in rigorous efforts to screen all patients with the disease. The American Medical Association (AMA) independently established a special committee to review the problem and to outline a series of proposals for effective action. This AMA committee suggested that all patients must have their blood pressures taken routinely by all physicians, dentists and other health personnel. The National Task Force on Hypertension has cosponsored with the ADA two national conferences on the role of dentists in detection of hypertension. Recent dental literature is replete with articles exhorting the dentist to measure blood pressure in his patients. A survey of 800 dentists conducted by *Dental Survey* showed that 80.9% of the respondents felt that dentists *should* measure a patient's blood pressure, but only 30.8% indicated that they actually *did* measure the blood pressure of their patients; 86.3% indicated that they were familiar with the technique of measuring blood pressure; 89.4% indicated that they ask their patients if they are being treated for hypertension, whereas 10.6% did not. There is no reason in modern dentistry why the dentist should not be thoroughly familiar with his patient's blood pressure, and in most instances, the most accurate way to be familiar is to take the pressure in the dental office. Patients with undetected hypertension may account for an occasional sudden death in the dental office.

Most cases (two thirds) of elevated systolic or diastolic pressures are of unknown cause; these are termed *primary* (idiopathic, essential) *hypertension.* The other third are termed *secondary hypertension* and may be caused by factors such as renal parenchymal disease, renal artery disease, adrenal cortical hyperfunction, pheochromocytoma, or a central nervous system lesion.

Essential hypertension is found commonly in those whose occupations are associated with considerable nervous tension and worry. There also appears to be a familial predisposition. The exact mechanism of the increased blood pressure is not entirely known. The harmful influence of obesity is well established, the mortality rate in obese patients being much higher than that in those of average weight or below. Abnormal stimulation of the sympathetic nervous system, either emotionally or by fear or by repression of anger or rage, may be an important predisposing cause.

Hypertension may be present for months or years before symptoms referable to this condition are manifested or recognized. The patient is frequently asymptomatic or at most has the symptoms of congestive heart failure secondary to the hypertension. Frequently recurring and persisting headaches, shortness of breath, general malaise, nosebleeds, and dizziness are not uncommon symptoms. There are no oral symptoms, although odontalgia has occasionally been reported in patients with hypertension for which no local cause could be discovered. Hyperemia of the dental pulp or congestion of this tissue resulting from the increased blood pressure could account for this symptom.

Hypertensive patients may succumb to cerebral hemorrhage, myocardial infarction, cardiac decompensation, or renal failure.

Treatment

The treatment of essential hypertension is temporizing and symptomatic rather than curative. There is no question, however, as reported in the Veterans Administration Study, that treatment significantly lowers morbidity and mortality. Treatment is directed toward lowering the blood pressure to a degree that will minimize the symptoms and the complications. Patients are generally advised to avoid salty foods (*e.g.,* potato chips, pretzels) and to add no salt to food either during cook-

ing or at the table. A wide variety of antihypertensive agents have been developed in recent years. These are listed in Table 19-3. The most commonly used drugs are those in the thiazide group, which are also used as diuretics in patients with congestive heart failure and which have the effect of lowering both body sodium and potassium, the latter being an undesirable side-effect. Other side-effects of the thiazides include hyperuricemia and hyperglycemia.

Beta-adrenergic blocking agents are also sometimes used as the drug of first choice particularly in young people or in those in whom it is thought that excessive adrenergic activity might account for their elevated blood pressure (*e.g.,* highly anxious patients).

In those patients who cannot be controlled by thiazides or with beta-adrenergic blocking agents, other more potent drugs are used. With the exception of the thiazides, which are often used in conjunction with another drug, it is generally desirable to use only a

Table 19-3. Antihypertensives

CATEGORY	NAME
Thiazide diuretics	Chlorothiazide
	Chlorthalidone
	Hydrochlorothiazide
	Metozalone
Loop diuretics	Ethacrynic acid
	Furosemide
Potassium-sparing diuretics	Amiloride
	Spironolactone
	Triameterene
Beta-adrenergic blockers	Atenolol
	Metoprolol
	Nadolol
	Propranolol
	Timolol
Alpha-adrenergic blockers	Phenoxybenzamine
	Prazosin
Ganglionic blocking agents	Guanethidine
	Reserpine
	Trimethaphan
Vasodilators	Hydralazine
	Minoxidil
CNS agents	Clonidine
	Methyldopa
Angiotensin-converting enzyme inhibitors	Captopril

single antihypertensive drug. If a drug is found to be ineffective, the physician discontinues it when substituting another. Many of these potent therapeutic agents are effective in reducing blood pressure; however, they are associated with annoying and at times potentially serious side-reactions. Surgical procedures occasionally may be employed but more often in the treatment of secondary hypertension.

Dental Considerations

The dentist should have equipment (stethoscope and sphygmomanometer) in his office to measure blood pressure. The automatic devices while being easier to use have not yet been well validated for accuracy. Many patients visit a dentist much more frequently than a physician, and the dentist will do his patient an invaluable service if he detects hypertension in the early stages so that it may be treated before a stroke, heart attack, or irreversible renal damage has occurred. All adult patients should have their blood pressure taken on the first visit to the dental office and at least once yearly afterward. Patients with known hypertension should have the pressure taken at each dental visit to assure that there is no risk of harm from the stress of the dental procedure.

All patients on antihypertensive medication should be carefully questioned to ascertain that they have not self-discontinued it. If the blood pressure in a resting patient is persistently 160/95 or greater after being taken two or three times during the same or on closely spaced dental visits, the patient should be referred to his physician for further observation and decision regarding antihypertensive medication.

An elevated blood pressure in a dental patient requires careful consideration in treatment planning, premedication, selection of an anesthetic, and determining the duration and the extent of operative procedures. Anything that results in an elevation of blood pressure, causes nervousness, or creates a stressful situation should be minimized in hypertensive patients. Adequate premedication will materially allay nervousness. Local anesthetics containing 1:50,000 epinephrine may be employed, but patients at high risk

such as those with underlying cardiac disease should be carefully monitored. A study by Tolas and colleagues indicated that after 3 and 5 minutes, arterial plasma epinephrine concentrations increased to more than two times the baseline in patients who were given an injection with a standard carpule of 2% lidocaine with 1:100,000 epinephrine. Patients who received an injection of lidocaine without epinephrine had no significant change of plasma epinephrine. With adequate precautions the extraction of teeth in *well-controlled* hypertensive patients is a fairly safe procedure, and, if cerebral vascular accidents should follow dental extractions, they may as easily be attributed to the natural course of events. Such is not the case if the patient is not well controlled.

Buchanan reviewed the literature on the systemic effects of epinephrine-impregnated retraction cord in fixed partial denture prosthodontics and concluded that all factors considered, in the hypertensive patient the retraction system of choice is the 8% racemic epinephrine-impregnated retraction cord.

Based on experience and observation, there has been an opinion among many clinicans for some time that tooth extraction on an emergency basis in a hypertensive patient who is not well-controlled is often attended by excess postoperative bleeding. Although this has not been documented with an extensive series of cases in the literature, it is the opinion of the author that such excess hemorrhage can and does occur, and when extractions are necessary on an emergency basis, a patient with poorly controlled hypertension should be hospitalized and local hemostatic measures carefully taken to avoid undue hemorrhage. The patient should not be permitted to struggle when using inhalation analgesia or general anesthesia, and adequate oral or parenteral presedation should be used.

Many of the antihypertensive drugs in current use are associated with side-effects of interest to the dentist. The central nervous system agents often cause a dry mouth. Many of the diuretic and antihypertensive drugs such as the alpha-adrenergic and ganglionic blocking agents predispose to orthostatic hypotension, and patients may faint when changed from a relatively supine position in the dental chair to an upright, sitting, or standing position. Methyldopa, the most frequently prescribed nondiuretic antihypertensive in the United States at the present time, has been reported to cause oral mucous membrane lesions in up to 0.8% of patients. These are described as painful persistent oral ulcerations that fail to respond to conventional treatment but resolve slowly over a period of several months after medication is changed. Hay and Reede reviewed and reported 17 such cases in 1978.

CONGENITAL HEART DISEASE

Congenital heart diseases occur in about 0.5% of all live births. The most common congenital cardiac anomalies include atrial and ventricular septal defects; the syndrome of ventricular septal defect, pulmonary stenosis, overriding aorta, and right ventricular hypertrophy known as the tetralogy of Fallot; and a persistent ductus arteriosus.

The clinical manifestations of those anomalies with an appreciable left-to-right shunt in infancy and childhood are those associated with insufficient oxygenation of the blood. In later life they may serve as sites for subacute bacterial endocarditis. In the patients with tetralogy of Fallot studied by Kaner and associates, there was a general bluish red discoloration of the oral mucosa with severe marginal gingivitis and bleeding. The tongue was deeply fissured and edematous. The teeth were structurally normal, but both the deciduous and the permanent teeth were delayed in their eruption.

ARTERIOVENOUS ANASTOMOSES

Arteriovenous anastomoses are abnormal communications between an artery and a vein through which the blood bypasses the capillary network. This malformation results in diminution of blood flow through the capillaries distal to the anastomoses. Because of easier flow into the veins and increased pressure on the veins impeding the return of blood from the capillaries, blood supply is diminished in the affected area. Davies re-

ported a case in which a patient presented with a telangiectatic area on the skin of the face and extensive loss of alveolar bone around the maxillary and mandibular teeth on the same side secondary to an arteriovenous anastomoses.

COARCTATION OF THE AORTA

Coarctation of the aorta is a developmental anomaly characterized by a marked diminution in the caliber of the aortic arch just distal to where the left subclavian artery arises. Because of the altered vascular hemodynamics, the blood pressure in the upper extremities and the head is much higher than that in the lower extremities. The main collateral circulation around this defect in the aorta is through the posterior intercoastal arteries, resulting in marked enlargement of these vessels and the production of defects in the lower borders of the ribs, which can be demonstrated radiographically. There is no cyanosis.

Oral Aspects

The abnormal vascular pressure in the head and the neck during early development of coarctation of the aorta results in a marked enlargement of the mandibular arteries and the branches leading to the individual teeth. The radiolucencies resulting from these enlarged vascular channels are unusually conspicuous in jaw radiograms.

Healy and Daley discovered four cases of coarctation of the aorta on the basis of the dental radiologic changes, which were verified by chest radiographs and other clinical findings. All these patients presented two consistent dental findings: prominence of the circulatory canals in the dental radiographs and prognathism. The chief complaint in one case was arterial hemorrhage following tooth extraction. Pressure over the bleeding socket was ineffective. Kaner and colleagues found that the pulps of the four maxillary incisors were markedly enlarged and funnel-shaped, occupying a great portion of the crowns and roots in patients with coarctation of the aorta. The dental pulps also revealed marked dilation of capillaries.

CRANIAL ARTERITIS

A granulomatous disease of unknown etiology, cranial arteritis might well have been discussed elsewhere in the text, but because of its involving the blood vessels in the head and neck, it is put in this chapter on cardiovascular disease. Cranial arteritis is a better name for the disease than temporal arteritis, which is sometimes used, because other vessels in the head and neck are involved in addition to the temporal artery. There is a distinctive granulomatous histologic lesion in the large and medium-sized arteries of the upper part of the body, especially the temporal vessels. The chief and striking complaint is a severe throbbing headache that often has an abrupt onset, with the pain usually being in one temple but occasionally involving the whole side of the face. The headache may be associated with exquisite hyperesthesia. The most serious complication of cranial arteritis is visual impairment, which may lead to the sudden onset of unilateral or bilateral blindness. Urgent therapy is imperative to prevent such a serious complication, and the practitioner should be aware that the transient episodes of blindness *without pain* may be the first symptom of temporal arteritis.

Oral symptoms were found frequently by Kilbourne and Wolff in patients with cranial arteritis. Of these patients, 50% complained of pain on mastication, and in some cases this was the initial symptom. Redness of the skin and swelling of the tissues overlying the temporal arteries were also present. There is often pain in the teeth, the jaw, and the zygoma region. In a study by Sofferman, 25% of patients admitted with cranial arteritis complained of masticatory or lingual discomfort well in advance of actual recognition of the underlying cranial arteritis. These painful symptoms result from involvement of the internal and the external maxillary arteries. Pain in the tongue associated with blanching and even gangrene has been described in this disorder, probably because of the involvement of the lingual arteries. Sofferman reported three cases of lingual infarction secondary to cranial arteritis. An exacerbation of pain and arterial inflammation have followed the extraction of infected teeth.

Diagnosis

Diagnosis is usually made on the basis of clinical symptoms and a markedly elevated erythrocyte sedimentation rate. Biopsy of the temporal artery is rarely necessary but should be performed without hesitation if it is necessary to make the diagnosis.

Treatment

Cranial arteritis is usually treated by a medical specialist using corticosteroid therapy, which is begun with a high dose and is gradually reduced over a period of weeks to a maintenance dose. In most cases, marked reduction or disappearance of symptoms is noted, but temporal arteritis is a chronic disease and the practitioner should be aware that spontaneous recurrences may appear long after the initial illness.

Dental Considerations

Because of the necessity of prompt steroid therapy for the disease, the dentist who has a patient with symptoms consistent with cranial arteritis should be particularly alert to refer the patient for medical diagnosis and therapy.

SYNCOPE

Syncope (fainting) is a sudden, transient, benign circulatory insufficiency. Fear, profound emotional disturbances, and pain are important predisposing factors. Fatigue, hunger, prolonged standing among crowds, and convalescence from an illness are other causes. More unusual causes of "fainting" include hyperventilation, certain types of heart disease and carotid sinus sensitivity.

Syncope may be precipitated when there is inadequate venous return, insufficient cardiac output, inadequate oxygenation of the blood, or local disorders of the central nervous system. Usually multiple mechanisms are operative in a syncopal attack. Psychological factors also play an important role in fainting in otherwise healthy patients as exemplified by the athlete who faints at the sight of a hypodermic needle. If the patient is carefully observed before the faint, he may be noted to become pale and to sweat profusely. There is a tendency to nausea and profound salivation. A feeling of uneasiness, giddiness, or light-headedness may precede the actual faint. There may be intermittent respirations with frequent sighing. Vision may become blurred. Occasionally the individual will have a few convulsive movements. There may be only a clouding of consciousness. At other times the clinical picture in syncope is startling: deathly pale skin, usually dilated pupils, and no pupillary reflex. Respirations are slow, and the pulse is feeble, usually from 30 to 60 beats per minute.

Dental Considerations

Syncope is common in dental practice. It may be associated with extractions or other painful procedures or merely the stressful situation associated with dental treatment. Hypoglycemia may also contribute. Adequate sedative premedication will allay or minimize the emotional factors that may predispose to syncope. Such premedication is especially recommended for individuals who are susceptible to fainting. Unless the patient is to be given general anesthesia, he should not be treated in the fasting state.

When a patient experiences the first signs of syncope, the dental chair should be placed immediately in a horizontal position with the head slightly lower than the body. This will usually result in increased cerebral circulation and a corresponding improvement in the general condition of the patient. This position is more comfortable for the semiconscious patient than is the head-between-the-knees position. Peripheral stimulation in the form of cold applications to the face and the forehead or inhalation of aromatic spirits of ammonia vapors is also useful. Oxygen may be administered if the patient does not respond within 2 or 3 minutes. The patient should remain in a supine position until fully recovered. When consciousness is regained, the patient can be given from eight to ten drops of aromatic spirits of ammonia in half a glass of water. After the patient revives, he may continue to feel unwell and shaky for a time.

If a satisfactory response to an attempt to bring the patient back to consciousness is not obtained within 2 to 3 minutes, a cardiopulmonary arrest may have occurred. If the patient is not breathing and if there is no palpable pulse, artificial mouth-to-mouth respiration and closed chest cardiac massage should be instituted immediately and a physician summoned. Stimulants injected subcutaneously are of little value because of their poor absorption during the circulatory inefficiency.

CARDIAC ARRHYTHMIAS

Cardiac arrhythmias are manifested by abnormal pulse rates or rhythms and may vary in severity from innocuous to life-threatening. Those associated with ventricular rates over 180 beats per minute are likely to cause vascular collapse or pulmonary edema and are life-threatening emergencies. Because of the diverse etiologic factors, proper diagnosis is essential before definitive treatment, and the electrocardiogram is essential for diagnosis. Specific cardiac arrhythmias include sinus bradycardia, sinus tachycardia, ectopic beats of atrial or ventricular origin, paroxysmal supraventricular tachycardia, paroxysmal ventricular tachycardia, and paroxysmal atrial tachycardia. Some arrhythmias require no treatment, others require mild sedative treatment, and still others require the use of digitalis or antiarrhythmic drugs such as procainamide, quinidine, propranolol, or lidocaine. Implantation of a cardiac pacemaker is necessary for some patients to live functionally.

Dental Considerations

The patient who is noted in the dental office to have an abnormal pulse rate or rhythm should be referred to his physician for appropriate diagnosis and treatment. Patients who lose consciousness because of decreased cardiac output associated with a decreased heart rate may often be helped by direct vigorous thumping on the precordium. Similar symptoms associated with rapid heartbeats may sometimes respond to vagal stimulation such as carotid sinus massage. This is done by first massaging the right carotid sinus for 10 to 20 seconds. If this is ineffective, the left carotid sinus is massaged. Both carotid sinuses should *not* be massaged simultaneously. Having the patient execute a Valsalva maneuver further increases vagal tone. Eyeball pressure should *not* be used because of the possibility of causing retinal detachment. Induction of vomiting is unpleasant and usually not indicated. Emergency measures other than the above rely on the administration of drugs or cardioversion (electrical shock), both of which must be carefully monitored with an electrocardiogram.

Electromagnetic radiation in the dental office interfering with cardiac pacemakers has been the subject of some concern. Simon and others studied this problem and concluded that there is only a small risk that the operation of pacemakers may be affected but any dental equipment that applies an electrical current directly to a patient may interfere with a pacemaker. The pacemakers currently in use operate either at a fixed rate (asynchronous type) or are programmed to stimulate the heart only when the intrinsic heart rate or rhythm is abnormal (synchronous or demand type). Most of the implanted pacemakers fall in the latter category, and it is this category that is more subject to disturbance from an electromagnetic field. Electrocautery in particular has been shown to have a disturbing effect on cardiac pacemakers; however, it is possible that any dental equipment used may have an electrical leakage unsuspected by the dentist that could interfere with the pacemaker. Inasmuch as design of the cardiac pacemakers is constantly changing and there is a wide range of equipment capable of producing electromagnetic radiation in the dental office, it is suggested that the dentist who has a patient with a cardiac pacemaker consult the patient's cardiologist for guidance when treating these patients.

Rezai has suggested certain precautions to lessen the danger of dental treatment in patients with pacemakers. These include asking about a pacemaker on the health questionnaire, checking all line-power devices that can contact the patient for leakage, being sure that electrical connections in appliances are properly grounded, and in consultation with the patient's physician, using beta blocking agents prophylactically to inhibit the effects of epinephrine and norepinephrine in local anesthetic solutions. Should the pacemaker accidentally shut off, all possible electrical sources of interference should be switched off and cardiopulmonary resuscitation should be begun if indicated. Artificial respiration should cause the heart to resume its normal rhythm and the pacemaker to resume its normal function.

CONGESTIVE HEART FAILURE

General Considerations

Congestive heart failure (cardiac decompensation, myocardial insufficiency) is a symptom rather than a disease. It is an indication that the cardiac reserve of the person has been exceeded and that cardiac decompensation has occurred. Under usual circumstances the functional potential of the heart far exceeds the work it is called upon to perform, there being a considerable cardiac reserve. This cardiac reserve may be diminished by degenerative changes in the cardiac musculature resulting from presbycardia or coronary artery disease or by increased work demanded of the heart as a result of cardiac valvular lesions (stenosis or regurgitation), hypertension, or increased metabolic demand, as in hyperthyroidism. The cardiac reserve diminishes gradually until it is no longer sufficient to fulfill the demands made on the heart.

Failure may involve either or both ventricles. Left ventricular failure causes pulmonary venous and pulmonary capillary pressures to rise resulting in pulmonary edema, leaking of a transudate from the pulmonary vasculature into the alveoli. In right ventricular failure the pressure in the veins of the systemic circulation becomes elevated resulting in peripheral edema such as ankle swelling, accumulation of fluid in the peritoneal cavity (ascites), and an enlarged liver.

Increasing breathlessness following moderate exertion is an early symptom of heart failure. Mild pulmonary edema is associated with a chronic productive cough, which is accompanied occasionally by blood-tinged sputum. At times the bluish skin pigmentation associated with argyria may be confused with the cyanosis found in congestive heart failure. Pitting edema of the lower extremities, hepatic enlargement, generalized edema, and congestion of the large veins of the neck are symptoms of more advanced cardiac decompensation. In severe cases the patient is short of breath and wheezes unless he is in a sitting position (cardiac asthma), and such patients may sleep with two, three, or more pillows in order to obtain rest (orthopnea). Anorexia, vomiting, and functional disturbances of the gastrointestinal tract are other common symptoms.

Treatment

The treatment of congestive heart failure consists of rest, limitation of salt and fluid intake, and the administration by the physician of digitalis and diuretics. The diuretics include agents such as the thiazides, furosemide, spironolactone, and triamterene. Other drugs may also be administered depending on the underlying cause of the congestive heart failure. After cardiac compensation has been established, attempts should be made to alter the living regimen of the patient so that the work demanded of the heart will fall within the work potentiality of this organ.

Dental Considerations

The dentist should watch for early signs of congestive heart failure in his patients. Cyanosis of the lips, the tongue, and the oral mucosa is readily detected in mild states of cardiac decompensation, and ankle edema is readily detected as the patient sits in the dental chair.

The dentist should be familiar with the classification of cardiac patients used by the American Heart Association that is based on the overall assessment of various factors in diagnosis and the effect of available therapies on prognosis. Cardiac status is classified as follows:

1. Uncompromised
2. Slightly compromised
3. Moderately compromised
4. Severely compromised

Because serious anatomic and physiological abnormalities caused by congenital or acquired heart disease may exist without compromising cardiac status at the time the patient is classified, but with the ability to do so in the future unless proper therapy is undertaken, there is also a prognosis classification which is as follows:

1. Good
2. Good with therapy
3. Fair with therapy
4. Guarded despite therapy

For example, a patient with minimal valvular disease and no cardiac decompensation who needs antibiotic prophylaxis to prevent endocarditis might be cardiac status 1, prognosis 2.

Cardiac status 1 and 2 patients present no unusual risk of developing cardiac decompensation during any dental procedure. Cardiac status 3 patients may require modification of the usual treatment planning and consultation between the dentist and the physician to prevent further cardiac decompensation. If dental treatment is required in patients with cardiac status 4, it should be of a palliative nature. Necessary extractions can be performed later if the patient is compensated with less risk. Local anesthetics are preferred. Any patient with prognosis other than 1 should have his physician consulted before dental treatment.

VENOUS THROMBOSIS, THROMBOPHLEBITIS, AND PULMONARY EMBOLISM

Thrombosis of the veins is uncommon unless there has been injury to the intimal lining, infection, or abnormal venous stasis. The relative venous stasis of the lower extremities favors thrombosis and thrombophlebitis of the femoral and the iliac vessels. It is generally agreed that the oral contraceptive agents are associated with an increased incidence of thrombophlebitis.

Thrombosis may be a serious and even fatal sequela of abdominal operations. Progressive thrombophlebitis may develop until a crucial vessel is involved, or small portions of the thrombus may break off and circulate as emboli to produce a variety of symptoms, depending on size, number, and location of their lodgment. Pulmonary embolism is the most serious complication and may, if the embolus is large enough, lead to sudden death. It has been speculated to be the most common cause of death in the hospital and reasonable estimates are that fatal pulmonary embolism occurs in 5 of every 1,000 hospitalized patients and nonfatal embolism in 20 of every 1,000 hospitalized patients. Strict adherence to asepsis, good surgical technique, and good postoperative care with early ambulation will minimize the possibility of postoperative thrombophlebitis and embolism. Treatment consists of hospitalization, anticoagulation, usually with heparin, and sometimes surgical intervention in the form of venous ligation or in severe, intractable and life-threatening cases, placing a partially occluding clamp or a filter in the inferior vena cava.

Dental Considerations

The dentist should insist on as early ambulation as possible with his hospitalized patients. Recognition of the patient prone to thrombophlebitis and daily observation of the bedfast patient for early signs or symptoms such as increased heat or tenderness in the calf or thigh is essential. Medical consultation must be obtained promptly with the slightest suspicion that thrombophlebitis may be occurring in order that treatment may be initiated as soon as possible.

CAVERNOUS SINUS THROMBOSIS

Cavernous sinus thrombosis (thrombophlebitis) is a serious condition that results from septic thrombus formation in the cavernous sinus and its numerous communicating branches. Because of the anastomotic drainage of the veins in the maxillary region of the face into the cavernous sinus, infections of the face and mouth may give rise to cavernous sinus thrombosis. The direct extension of antral infections may also give rise to this disease.

Infections of the upper lip, the face, and the nares can reach the cavernous sinus through the communicating angular veins. Cavernous sinus thrombosis is at times a sequela of pimples of the upper lip, especially if these are squeezed or manipulated. Hot moist applications and massive antibiotic therapy are far safer methods of treatment. The common habit of pulling out hairs in the nostrils is also dangerous.

The symptoms of cavernous sinus thrombosis include exophthalmos, edema, and ecchymosis of the eyelids and the sclerae, a septic type of temperature reaction, papilledema, and edema of the conjunctivae. Headache and vomiting may be prominent symptoms. Paralysis of the external ocular muscles is commonly present. Death is caused by pyemia, sepsis, brain abscess, or meningitis. Although the prognosis is better since the advent of antibiotics, a well-established infection in the cavernous sinus still has a high mortality. A few cases are amenable to surgery.

Dental Considerations

Cavernous sinus thrombosis is of interest to the dentist because infectious processes of the face, the jaws, and associated parts may give rise to this serious condition.

Infection from the teeth or the surrounding tissues may reach the cavernous sinus by way of the pterygoid plexus and the emissary veins from the pterygomaxillary space. Infections of the parotid gland are also known to give rise to cavernous sinus thrombosis. The majority of the reported cases of cavernous sinus thrombosis of proved or suspected dental origin arise from infections in the maxillary and the mandibular third molar regions. This results possibly from the intimate relationship of the pterygoid plexus to these areas, which favors the direct extension of infection. Many of these have followed surgical procedures performed during the acute stage of infection or have resulted from infection carried into the deeper tissues during the injection of the local anesthetic. Instances have been recorded, however, in which cavernous sinus thrombosis developed following an abscessed deciduous tooth that was removed without anesthesia.

Although cavernous thrombosis is a rare complication in connection with dental procedures, its seriousness justifies consideration whenever acute infections, particularly in the molar regions, are encountered. It can be prevented in most instances by good surgical judgment in the treatment of dental infections. Prophylactic antibiotic therapy may aid in the prevention of this complication in infections occurring in high-risk locations (*i.e.*, in areas of the face draining into veins that can communicate with the cavernous sinus).

BIBLIOGRAPHY

American Heart Association: Coronary Risk Handbook, New York, American Heart Association, 1973

Anticoagulants in acute myocardial infarction. Results of a cooperative clinical trial. JAMA 225:724, 1973

Aspirin Myocardial Infarction Research Group: A randomized controlled trial of aspirin in persons recovered from myocardial infarction. JAMA 243:661, 1980

Barot AJ: Temporal arteritis without pain. JAMA 243:61, 1980

Behrman SJ, Wright IS: Dental surgery during continuous anticoagulant therapy. JAMA 175:483, 1961

Behrman SJ, Wright IS: Dental surgery during continuous anticoagulant therapy. J Am Dent Assoc 62:171, 1961

Benchimol A et al: Resting electrocardiogram in major coronary artery disease. JAMA 224:1489, 1973

Benter, IB et al: Comparative effects of local and systemic antibiotic therapy in the prevention of post-extraction bacteremia. J Am Dent Assoc 57:54, 1958

Benter IB, Pressman RS: Antibiotic treatment of the gingival sulcus in prevention of postextraction bacteremia. J Oral Surg 14:20, 1956

Berman CL: Screening dental patients for hypertension. Dent Survey 50:46, 1974

Berman CL. Guarino MA, Giovannoli SM: High blood pressure detection by dentists. J Am Dent Assoc 87:359, 1973

Beta Blocker Heart Attack Study Group: The beta blocker heart attack trial. JAMA 246:2073, 1981

Blumberg S: Recurrence of temporal arteritis. JAMA 244:1713, 1980

Buchanan WT: Systemic effects of epinephrine-impregnated retraction cord in fixed partial denture prosthodontics. J Am Dent Assoc 104:482, 1982

Burket LW, Burn CG: Bacteremia following dental extraction. Demonstration of source of bacteria

by means of a nonpathogen. J Dent Res 10:521, 1937

Burnstein V et al: Lidocaine intramuscularly in acute myocardioinfarction. JAMA 219:1027, 1972

Cawson RA: Infective endocarditis as a complication of dental treatment. B Dent J 151:409, 1981

Cheraskin E, Prasertsuntarasai T: Use of epinephrine with local anesthesia in hypertensive patients. J Am Dent Assoc 58:61, 1959

Cutright DE: Survey of blood pressures of 856 dentists. J Am Dent Assoc 94:918, 1977

Davies RM et al: Oral manifestations of an arteriovenous anastomosis. Oral Surg 44:2, 1977

Doyle JT et al: Cigarette smoking and coronary heart disease. N Engl J Med 266:796, 1962

Ebert EV et al: Long-term anticoagulant therapy after myocardial infarction. JAMA 207:2263, 1969

Editorial: JAMA 224:390; 226:561, 1973

Effects of treatment on morbidity in hypertension: Results in patients with diastolic blood pressures averaging 115 through 129 mm. Hg. Veterans Administration Cooperative Study Group on Antihypertensive Agents. JAMA 202:1028, 1967

Effects of treatment on morbidity in hypertension: II. Results in patients with diastolic blood pressure averaging 90 through 114 mm. Hg., Veterans Administration Cooperative Group Study on Antihypertensive Agents. JAMA 213:1143, 1970

Eisenbud L: Subacute bacterial endocarditis precipitated by non-surgical dental procedures. Oral Surg 15:624, 1962

Galen RS, Reiffel JA, Gambino SR: Diagnosis of acute myocardial infarction. Relative efficiency of serum enzyme and isoenzyme measurements. JAMA 232:145, 1975

Goldberg R et al: Acute myocardial infarction prognosis complicated by ventricular fibrillation or cardiac arrest. JAMA 241:2024, 1979

Gordon P, Kannel WB: Premature mortality from coronary heart disease: The Framingham study. JAMA 215:1617, 1971

Gottsegen R, Gorlin RJ: Periarteritis nodosa with involvement of the tongue. Oral Surg 2:1250, 1949

Graham LL, Schinbeckler GA: Oral-facial pain of cardiac origin. J Am Dent Assoc 104:47, 1982

Greenberg MS, Miller MF, Lynch MA: Partial thromboplastin time as a predictor of blood loss in oral surgery patients receiving coumarin anticoagulants. J Am Dent Assoc 84:583, 1972

Harrison DC: Practical guidelines for the use of lidocaine—Prevention and treatment of cardiac arrhythmias. JAMA 233:1202, 1975

Hay KD, Reade PC: Methyldopa as a cause of oral

mucous membrane reactions. B Dent J 145:195, 1978

Healy JC et al: Intraoral diagnostic sign of aortic coarctation. Appollonian 11:167, 1936

Hilson GRF: Is chemoprophylaxis necessary? Proc R Soc Med 63:267, 1970

Hobson FG, Juel–Jensen BE: Teeth, Streptococcus viridans, and subacute bacterial endocarditis. Br Med J 2:1510, 1956

Hutter AM, Moellering RC: Assessment of the patient with suspected endocarditis. JAMA 235, 1603, 1976

Kaner A et al: Oral manifestations of congenital heart disease. J Pediatr 29:269, 1946

Kannel WB: Meaning of the downward trend in cardiovascular mortality. JAMA 247:877, 1982

Kannel, WB et al: Prognosis after initial myocardial infarction. Am J Cardiol 44:63, 1979

Kannel WB, Feinleib M: Natural history of angina pectoris: the Framingham study. Am J Cardiol 154:2929. 1972

Kilbourne ED, Wolff HG: Cranial arteritis: a critical evaluation of the syndrome of "temporal arteritis" with report of a case. Ann Intern Med 24:1, 1946

Kirshenbaum HB et al: The spectrum of coronary artery spasm. JAMA 246:354, 1981

Lopes MG et al: Prognosis in coronary care unit—noninfarction cases. JAMA 228:1558, 1974

Matson MS: Pain in orofacial region associated with coronary insufficiency. Oral Surg 16:284, 1963

Midwall J et al: Angina pectoris before and after myocardial infarction: Angiographic correlations. Chest 81:681, 1982

Myerburg RJ et al: Survivors of pre-hospital cardiac arrest. JAMA 247:1485, 1982

Oglesby P: The medical management of angina pectoris. JAMA 238:1847, 1977

Okell CC, Elliott SD: Bacteremia and oral sepsis with special reference to the etiology of subacute endocarditis. Lancet 2:869, 1935

Pogral MA, Welsby PD: The dentist and prevention of infective endocarditis. Br Dent J 139:12, 1975

Rezai FR: Dental treatment of patient with a cardiac pacemaker. Oral Surg 44:662, 1977

Ritland S, Lygrene T: Comparison of efficacy of three and 12 months' anticoagulant therapy after myocardial infarction. Lancet 1:122, 1969

Simon AB et al: The individual with a pacemaker in the dental environment. J Am Dent Assoc 91:1224, 1975

Sofferman RA: Lingual infarction in cranial arteritis. JAMA 243:2422, 1980

Spencer WH et al: Rheumatic fever, chemoprophylaxis and penicillin-resistant gingival organisms. Ann Intern Med 73:683, 1970

Thompson PL, Lown B: Nitrous oxide as an analgesic in acute myocardial infarction. JAMA 235:924, 1976

Tolas AG et al: Arterial plasma epinephrine concentrations and hemodynamic responses after dental injection of local anesthetic with epinephrine. J Am Dent Assoc 104:41, 1982

Valentine PA et al: Lidocaine in the prevention of sudden death in the prehospital phase of acute infarction. N Engl J Med 291:1327, 1974

Vernale CA: Cardiovascular response to local dental anesthesia with epinephrine in normotensive and hypertensive subjects. Oral Surg 13:942, 1960

Wallace DA: Systemic effects of dental local anesthesia solutions. Oral Surg 9:1297, 1956

Weinblatt E et al: Mortality after first myocardial infarction. JAMA 247:1576, 1982

Ziffer AM et al: Profound bleeding after dental extractions during Dicumarol therapy. N Engl J Med 256:331, 1957

20

Diseases of the Gastrointestinal Tract

MALCOLM A. LYNCH

Diseases of the gastrointestinal tract primarily affecting areas other than the oral cavity will be discussed in this chapter; this is not intended to be a comprehensive discussion of all diseases affecting the gastrointestinal tract. Rather it is limited to those diseases of particular interest to the dentist because of their frequency in the dental patient population, alterations in dental treatment necessitated by the presence of the disease, oral involvement, or finally the infectious nature of the disease, which could be of danger to the dentist or his patients.

DISEASES OF THE ESOPHAGUS

Dysphagia

Dysphagia or difficulty in swallowing is the most likely complaint of esophageal disease to be encountered by the dentist. Dysphagia may result from a mechanical obstruction in the esophagus or from a disorder of the nervous system that prevents the coordinated reflex contraction of the appropriate musculature necessary for normal swallowing. Cranial nerves V, VII, IX, X, and XI are all involved in the neurologic reflexes associated with swallowing, and both smooth and skeletal muscles are utilized. The skeletal muscles include the tongue, larynx, and upper one third of the esophagus, whereas smooth muscle is seen in the lower two thirds of the esophagus. Dysphagia associated with neurologic dysfunction is characterized by inability to swallow both liquids and solids; mechanical obstruction, at least early in the disease, is more often associated with inability to swallow liquids developing later in the disease. Diseases associated with neurologic dysfunction include poliomyelitis, myasthenia gravis (see Chap. 27), myotonic dystrophy, sarcoidosis, scleroderma, systemic lupus erythematosus, and multiple sclerosis. Diseases causing mechanical lesions include those such as obstructing carcinoma paraesophageal lymph node enlargement, or obstruction by a foreign body.

Plummer–Vinson Syndrome

The Plummer–Vinson syndrome is characterized by an esophageal web with resulting dysphagia particularly in the upper segment of the esophagus as well as by atrophic changes in the mucous membranes of the mouth and by a hypochromic microcytic anemia. Esophageal changes may be diagnosed radiographically (see Fig. 20-1, 20-2, and 20-3) as well as by direct endoscopic observation. (See Chap. 22 for a more complete description of this syndrome.)

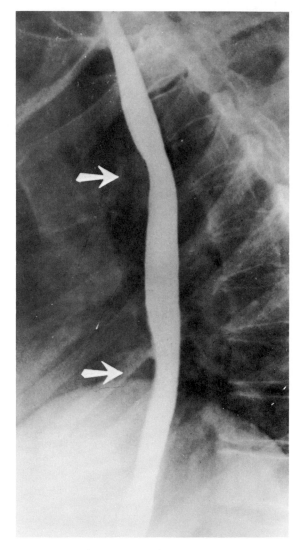

Fig. 20-1 Right posterior oblique view of a barium swallow of a normal esophagus. The upper arrow indicates the indentation produced by the transverse aortic arch, and the lower arrow indicates the slight impression at the level of the left atrium. (Juhl JH [ed]: Paul and Juhl's Essentials of Roentgen Interpretation, 4th ed, p 526. Philadelphia, Harper & Row, 1981)

Esophageal Ulcers

There have been a few case reports of esophageal ulcers associated with tetracycline therapy. These appear to occur more often after dry swallows of the tablets or capsules, especially at bedtime. The patients have usually presented with severe retrosternal burning pain. Patients respond well to symptomatic therapy.

Dental Considerations

The esophageal diseases discussed above will be seen by the dentist primarily on a symptomatic basis referable to the dysphagia. Exceptions are scleroderma and the Plummer–Vinson syndrome, which may produce oral lesions that are described elsewhere in the text. Because of his unique position in treating the oral cavity, the dentist may be the first to detect these conditions and should promptly refer them to the appropriate physician in order that early diagnosis and possible treatment may be undertaken. Treatment of dysphagia depends on the etiology. When treating a patient who is known to have one of the above diseases, proper precautions should be taken to prevent the patient's aspirating material secondary to the dental procedure. In patients complaining of severe retrosternal burning pain who are on tetracycline therapy, the possibility of tetra-

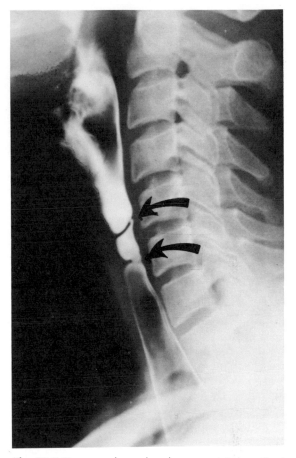

Fig. 20-3 Two esophageal webs present in a patient with Plummer–Vinson syndrome (*arrow*). (Juhl JH [ed]: Paul and Juhl's Essentials of Roentgen Interpretation, 4th ed, p 549. Philadelphia, Harper & Row, 1981)

cycline-induced esophageal ulceration must be considered. Patients who are prescribed tetracycline should be warned to swallow the tablets or capsules with adequate amounts of liquid.

PEPTIC ULCERATION

Ulceration of the mucosa of the gastrointestinal tract caused by the action of protein-digesting pepsin on the mucosa is one of the most common diseases in the gastrointestinal tract and one of the most common diseases to afflict man. The presence of hydrochloric acid in the stomach is necessary for the conversion of the precursor pepsinogen to pep-

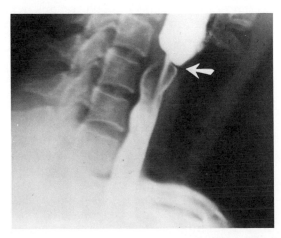

Fig. 20-2 Plummer–Vinson web in the upper end of the esophagus (*arrow*). (Juhl JH [ed]: Paul and Juhl's Essentials of Roentgen Interpretation, 4th ed, p 549. Philadelphia, Harper & Row, 1981)

sin. Because of the necessity for acid, peptic ulcerations ordinarily include the lower one third of the esophagus, the stomach, and the duodenum in increasing frequency. The precise cause of ulceration in a particular patient is not known, although factors contributing to increased stomach acid production are known to be associated with an increased incidence of peptic ulceration.

The normal stimuli for acid secretion include the thought, sight, smell, or taste of food, which mediated by the anterior hypothalamus, acts either by vagal stimulation directly on the mucosa of the stomach to cause acid production or intermediately by the pituitary to produce adrenocorticotropin (ACTH), which stimulates the adrenal cortex to produce corticosteroids, which in turn stimulate the acid-producing cells of the stomach. Hypoglycemia and mental stress also act by means of the same mechanism (anterior hypothalamus) to increase stomach acid production. In addition, the presence of food in the antrum of the stomach will, by the mechanism of distention, cause increased production of the hormone gastrin, which acts directly on the acid-producing cells of the stomach. Therefore, factors such as hypoglycemia, stress, and food, especially coffee and alcohol which have no acid-neutralizing effect, are exacerbating factors in peptic ulceration. Tobacco has also been known to be involved.

Duodenal Ulcer

Eighty to eighty-five percent of peptic ulcers are duodenal, and duodenal ulcers occur 6:1 in males. The precise etiology is not known, but factors such as stress, exogenous steroids, parathyroid disease, malignant carcinoid, cirrhosis, gastrinoma of the pancreas (Zollinger-Ellison disease), polycythemia vera, and chronic lung disease have been associated with a duodenal ulcer. The ulceration is usually located in the first part of the duodenum (see Fig. 20-4), inasmuch as the acid chyme ordinarily becomes alkaline after pancreatic secretions enter the intestine in the second part of the duodenum. The most common symptom is epigastric pain usually occurring either just before eating or 1 to 3 hours after eating. The pain is described as

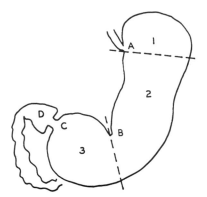

Fig. 20-4 Diagram of the normal stomach to show the major anatomic divisions (1) fundus, (2) body, (3) antrum, (A) anatomic cardia, (B) incisura angularis, (C) pyloric canal, and (D) first portion of the duodenum or duodenal bulb. (Juhl JH [ed]: Paul and Juhl's Essentials of Roentgen Interpretation, 4th ed, p 557. Philadelphia, Harper & Row, 1981)

burning in nature and is sometimes associated with nausea and vomiting. It is characteristically relieved by food. If the ulceration is large enough to erode an artery, bleeding may be the primary symptom. Gastrointestinal bleeding is manifested most commonly by black tarry stools or more rarely, by vomiting of blood. The vomitus appears like "coffee grounds" because of the blood's reaction with acid.

Oral Manifestations. There has been no clear evidence to associate oral ulcerations with peptic ulceration. Gius and associates have described certain vascular formations of the lip found more frequently in patients with peptic ulcer or a history of peptic ulcer than in those without ulcers. These vascular abnormalities occurred in approximately 25% of the patients, increased with age, and were more common in males than in females. The vascular formations were of three types: a small, sharply circumscribed, red dot-type of lesion known as a *microcherry*; a conglomeration of tortuous, thin-walled vessels 1 to 2 mm or more in size (called *glomeruli*, because they resemble the kidney glomerulus); and a dilated submucosal vein resembling a miniature varix, known as *venous lakes*. These lesions are usually seen at the inner surface of the labial commissures.

Diagnosis. Physical examination is usually of little use in the diagnosis of duodenal ulcer unless the ulcer has penetrated the entire intestinal wall causing the contents of the intestine to spill out into the peritoneal cavity. In this rare instance, the abdomen will be exquisitely tender, and the peritonitis if untreated will cause the patient to die of septic complications. The mainstay of diagnosis of a duodenal ulcer is an upper GI radiologic examination, which will demonstrate the presence of an ulcer in up to 90% of patients (see Figs. 20-5 and 20-6). In this procedure, the patient swallows a barium salt (usually barium sulfate) that outlines the lumen and mucosal surface of the gastrointestinal tract. It thereby demonstrates any disruption of the mucosal surface as is found in a duodenal ulcer. In some instances an ulcer crater will not be visible, but there will be a deformed duodenal bulb indicative of ulcer disease with scarring. The procedure is usually performed using fluoroscopic examination and selected films are made of areas which demonstrate the ulcer particularly well. In young patients with characteristic symptoms in whom cancer is not a consideration, it is often advisable to use a therapeutic trial of antiulcer medication (see below) rather than subject the patient to the radiation required in the GI series. If the patient does not promptly respond to therapy, then one can always proceed with the radiologic examination.

In the Zollinger–Ellison syndrome caused by a gastrinoma of the pancreas, specific diagnosis of the etiology is necessary because this disease is treatable and is particularly severe, causing multiple ulcers and debilitating diarrhea. The tumor in the Zollinger–Ellison syndrome secretes gastrin, a potent acid producer, and the diagnosis is made on the basis of extremely high levels of gastric acid and elevated levels of serum gastrin as determined by radioimmunoassay.

Complications. Possible complications of duodenal ulcers include massive bleeding (which if not checked can lead to exsanguination), obstruction (which may have to be surgically corrected), perforation (which *must* be surgically corrected), and intractability to medical treatment (which also requires surgical correction).

Treatment. In the absence of the possible complications listed above, treatment is usually of a medical rather than surgical nature and involves both dietary alterations and drugs. At the present time, there is no good evidence that proscription of coarse or highly seasoned foods is of any value in the treatment of peptic ulceration, although foods which cause obvious discomfort to the patient should be avoided. Food or drugs that have potent acidogenic properties with little ability to neutralize acid should be avoided; among these are alcohol, tobacco, and aspirin. Medical treatment involves four classes

Fig. 20-5 Radiograph of a normal stomach and duodenal bulb; compare with the diagram in Figure 20-4. (Juhl JH [ed]: Paul and Juhl's Essentials of Roentgen Interpretation, 4th ed, p 557. Philadelphia, Harper & Row, 1981)

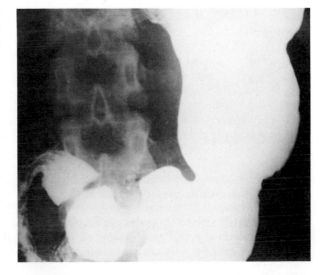

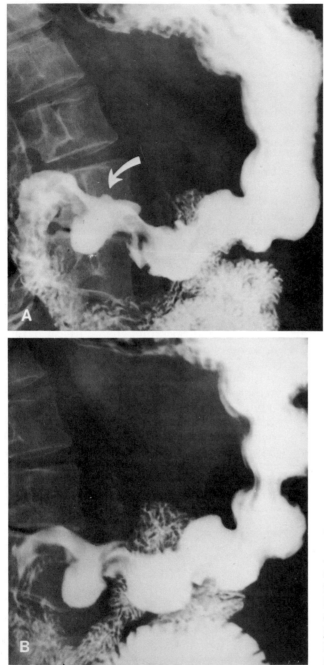

Fig. 20-6 Upper gastrointestinal radiographs using barium in a patient with a duodenal ulcer. *A,* The duodenal bulb is deformed, and there is a small crater projecting as an ulcer niche on the lesser curvature side (*arrow*). *B,* Six weeks later the crater has disappeared, but the contour of the duodenal bulb remains abnormal. (Juhl JH [ed]: Paul and Juhl's Essentials of Roentgen Interpretation, 4th ed, p 602. Philadelphia, Harper & Row, 1981)

of drugs: sedatives to reduce mental stress when this is felt to play an etiologic part in the ulcer, antacids to neutralize the excess acid present in the stomach, anticholinergic drugs to decrease the production of acid by the gastric mucosa, and an H_2 histamine-receptor blocker such as cimetidine or ranitidine. Cimetidine or ranitidine blocks the action of histamine on the gastric parietal cells, thus reducing food-stimulated acid secretion by up to 75%. When antacids are given they usually are prescribed 1 and 3 hours after meals and at bedtime. The liquid form, though less convenient, is more effective than is the tablet form. Most antacids are combinations of calcium carbonate, magnesium hydroxide, and aluminum hydroxide, which are present in a balanced amount to prevent either constipation or diarrhea. In some patients an undesirable side-effect of constipation or diarrhea may still result. In this event, another antacid can be substituted that has less of the undesirable side-effects.

Dental Considerations. The dentist should avoid administering drugs that exacerbate ulceration, the most common of which is aspirin or one of its related compounds. Phenylbutazone is also implicated in gastric irritation but is less commonly used in dental practice. A patient who reacts in a particularly stressful way to dental procedures should be sedated before dental treatment. Dentists should be aware that patients taking anticholinergic drugs often present with dry mouth; this may present some problems because of an increase in the viscosity of the mucus or discomfort in wearing full dentures. The xerostomia has also been shown to lead to an increased incidence of cervical caries. Because many of the antacids contain calcium, magnesium, and aluminum salts that bind both erythromycin and particularly tetracycline, the dentist should be aware that administration of one of these drugs within an hour of such antacid therapy may decrease the absorption of the antibiotic by as much as 75% to 85%. Exogenous steroid administration is likely to exacerbate the ulcer because of the increased production of acid caused by the steroid. Patients who are given oral penicillin should be given penicillin V instead of penicillin G because of the resistance of the former to gastric acid. This is generally a good dictum to follow with all patients but is essential in patients with peptic ulceration.

The dentist should be aware that a patient with a peptic ulcer may have occult bleeding from the ulcer and thereby may have a chronic anemia of which he is unaware. Before extensive oral surgical or periodontal procedures that might entail appreciable blood loss are undertaken, the patient's hemoglobin or hematocrit (packed cell volume) should be determined.

Gastric Ulcer

Gastric ulceration is about one tenth as common as duodenal ulcer in the United States. It is of more concern to the physician because the ulcer may be a malignant ulceration of the gastric mucosa rather than a peptic ulceration; malignant ulceration of the duodenum is virtually unknown. Gastric ulcers occur more often after 50 years of age, and are seen 3:1 in males. The same factors associated with exacerbation of peptic gastric ulcers are present in duodenal ulcers, and the diagnostic procedures are the same as with duodenal ulcers except that urgency is of more importance in diagnosis of a gastric ulcer because of the possibility that one might be dealing with a malignancy. In addition to the radiographic diagnostic studies (see Fig. 20-7) described for duodenal ulcers, gastroscopy (direct visualization of the stomach mucosa with the gastroscope) and cytologic examination of cells obtained from the gastric mucosa are employed. It is essential to obtain gastric acidity levels with ulcers of the stomach inasmuch as a stomach ulcer in the presence of histamine-fast achlorhydria has a very high chance of being a malignant ulcer rather than a peptic one. Treatment for peptic ulcerations of the stomach is the same as for a duodenal ulcer except that surgical treatment is used more often if there is no satisfactory response to medical therapy.

Dental considerations for patients with gastric ulcers are the same as those for patients with duodenal ulcers.

DISEASES OF THE LIVER

The dentist may suspect liver dysfunction or disease by the presence of jaundice of the oral mucosa or the sclerae. Patients with certain forms of liver disease, especially those associated with severe jaundice and hepatic dysfunction, may present with spontaneous bleeding in the oral cavity or severe bleeding following oral surgical or periodontal operations. These patients will require a modification of the usual treatment in the dental

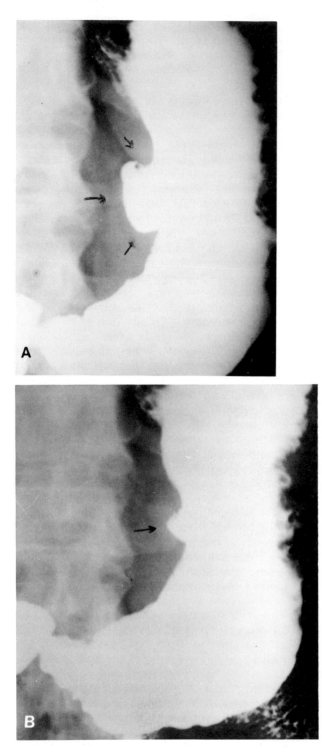

Fig. 20-7 Barium contrast upper gastrointestinal radiograph of a benign gastric ulcer. *A,* Large crater observed on the initial study. *B,* Three weeks later a distinct decrease in the crater's size is evident. The patient had been on medical therapy in the interval. (Juhl JH [ed]: Paul and Juhl's Essentials of Roentgen Interpretation, 4th ed, p 564. Philadelphia, Harper & Row, 1981)

office. In addition, patients with incubating or active hepatitis A, B, or non-A, non-B, or carriers of hepatitis B or non-A, non-B represent a distinct hazard both to the dentist and to other patients. The virus may be transmitted by as little as 0.0004 ml of blood on a dental instrument that has not been properly sterilized. Cold or boiling water sterilization will not kill the virus. Although proper attention to sterilization of instruments may prevent transmission of hepatitis to the dentist's patients, only a careful history for symptoms of incubating, or active hepatitis, examination of a patient for jaundice, or a history of hepatitis B or non-A, non-B will prevent the dentist's becoming infected. There is suggestive evidence that cancer of the mouth occurs more frequently in patients having liver disease, particularly alcoholic cirrhosis.

Jaundice

Jaundice or icterus, which is a symptom rather than a disease, results from an excess of bilirubin in the circulation. This excess bile pigment may be caused by the production of excess bilirubin by hemolysis of red blood cells (hemolytic jaundice), obstruction in the biliary tree preventing excretion of bilirubin (obstructive jaundice), or liver parenchymal disease (hepatocellular jaundice). Very often, obstruction and parenchymal disease are seen concurrently.

Hemolytic Jaundice

Hemolytic jaundice is not a gastrointestinal disease but is discussed here for the sake of completeness in the discussion of jaundice. Hemolytic jaundice results from an excessive hemolysis or destruction of the erythrocytes produced by an inherent abnormality in the cells (*e.g.,* sickle-cell disease, hereditary spherocytosis, thalassemia, glucose-6-phosphate dehydrogenase deficiency), some acute diseases, certain drugs or poisonous agents (*e.g.,* nitrobenzene, toluene, phenacetin), or acquired immune disease (*e.g.,* systemic lupus erythematosus).

Diagnosis of jaundice caused by a hemolytic process is based on the presence of an anemia with a high reticulocyte count, a decreased level of serum haptoglobins, and an elevated serum bilirubin (seldom greater than 8 mg/dl) primarily caused by an increase in the indirect fraction. The specific cause of the increased hemolysis of the red cell is determined by studies such as hemoglobin electrophoresis, erythrocyte fragility studies, and the Coombs' test for antibodies to red cells.

Obstructive Jaundice

Obstructive jaundice is caused by stoppage within the biliary duct system resulting from stones, inspissated bile, or external pressure on the biliary passages associated with infectious or neoplastic lesions. Common bile duct blockage caused by gallstones and pressure from neoplasia, particularly carcinoma of the head of the pancreas, is a common cause of obstructive jaundice.

Hepatocellular Jaundice

Hepatocellular jaundice can be caused by diseases such as hepatitis and alcoholic and postnecrotic cirrhosis.

Hepatitis

Hepatitis may be induced by chemical agents such as phosphorus or carbon tetrachloride, drugs such as alcohol or isoniazid hydrochloride, associated with collagen diseases such as lupus erythematosus, or with bacterial infection such as leptospirosis or syphilis, or it may be viral in origin. Among viral hepatic diseases are those caused by infectious mononucleosis and cytomegalic inclusion virus. Of most interest to the dentist is viral hepatitis caused by the hepatitis A, B, or non-A, non-B virus. Discussion of hepatitis will be limited to hepatitis A, B, and non-A, non-B because these are the most common types and certainly the types of most importance to the dentist.

Symptoms. The symptoms of hepatitis A, B, and non-A, non-B are essentially the same, and the diseases cannot be differentiated on the basis of symptomatology. Generally speaking, hepatitis A has milder symptoms than those of the other types. Antibody studies to detect infections have indicated that more than half of the cases of all the types of hepatitis are either subclinical or mild enough to escape diagnosis.

Prodromal symptoms of general malaise, arthralgia, myalgia, and an upper respiratory infection are common, and the patient develops a striking distaste for cigarettes. There is often a morbilliform skin rash. Acutely, the patient usually experiences anorexia, nausea, and a high fever with tenderness and enlargement of the liver. The urine turns dark and the stools light in color. Jaundice develops in about 5 days after which the fever gradually subsides. Lymphadenopathy and splenomegaly are common.

Oral Manifestations. The only oral manifestation of hepatitis is icterus of the oral mucosa, which is most readily seen on the palate and in the sublingual area.

Hepatitis A

Hepatitis A was formerly known as infectious hepatitis, but this is a misnomer inasmuch as hepatitis A, B, and non-A, non-B are all infectious. The incubation period varies from 15 to 50 days. It has an acute onset with high fever, occurring most frequently before age 35. The virus is virtually always transmitted by means of fecally contaminated food or water but rarely can be transmitted by injection of blood or blood products from an acutely ill patient, as in a dentist's or physician's office. Only 25% of patients with hepatitis A have had known contact with symptomatic persons. Food known to transmit hepatitis A is either uncooked or touched by contaminated human hands after cooking (*e.g.*, potato salad). The period of infectiousness is highest during the week before the onset of clinical symptoms. Little if any virus is present in the stool at the time of the onset of jaundice. The human reservoir of infectious hepatitis has been estimated to be between 0.5% and 6.0% of the population.

Treatment. Treatment is symptomatic. Bedrest during the early weeks of the disease is recommended, activity being resumed gradually. Isolation of stool, urine, and blood-contaminated objects is practiced to prevent spread of the disease to other patients. A high-protein and high-carbohydrate diet is also recommended. Complete recovery is gradual, taking place within 6 to 8 weeks. The mortality rate is very low and chronic hepatitis does not develop.

Prevention. Persons who have had contact with a patient such that they may have ingested minute amounts of fecal material or have been injected with as little as 0.0004 ml of infected blood should be given prophylactic gamma globulin injections. These will often prevent hepatitis A entirely if given early enough or may at the least ameliorate the symptoms and cause anicteric hepatitis. Persons traveling to areas of the world where hepatitis A is endemic should be given gamma globulin (immune serum globulin) prophylactically. Protective effect lasts for about 6 weeks.

Hepatitis B

Hepatitis B virus (HBV) was formerly known as serum hepatitis and was thought to be transmitted only by the parenteral route. HBV is now known to be present in blood, saliva, and semen, although the transmissibility of the disease by the latter two vehicles without blood contamination is not known. It is certainly transmissible by oral means as well as parenterally, but it does not survive transit through the GI tract, and oral transmission appears to occur by absorption of the virus in areas of the gastrointestinal tract proximal to the stomach.

Studies have shown evidence of percutaneous spread of the hepatitis B virus, presumably by small amounts of blood, through skin with minor abrasions or a skin disease. Guadagnino and associates demonstrated that there was a higher risk of infection with hepatitis B in patients with chronic skin diseases. The patients studied had either eczema or psoriasis. They indicated that patients with chronic lesions of the hand should be considered to be at high risk for hepatitis B virus infection. Kashiwagi and others reported an outbreak of hepatitis B in members of a sumo wrestling club, also presumably spread by percutaneous means.

While HBV does not overall appear to be a highly transmissible disease, the rate of infectivity in sexual contacts and to a lesser degree, household contacts does appear to be high. Evidence of the virus (HB_sAg; see section below) is detectable in the serum before the onset of clinical symptoms and remains detectable during the first several weeks after clinical illness. In approximately 10% of the cases it persists in the serum for 1 to 2 years. In 4% to 5% of the cases the chronic carrier state develops and has been shown to last up to 25 years. If the carrier state lasts for more than 12 months, there is a high probability that it might well become persistent. The overall carrier rate in the United States is estimated to be three tenths of a percent.

The following factors appear to be associated with an increased risk of a patient's developing persistent asymptomatic antigenemia: depressed immunologic status, occupation, sexual promiscuity, sharing a household with other chronic carriers, and male sex. At present, it is not clear whether the asymptomatic carrier is capable of transmitting the infectious agent by means other than infected blood. Although the hepatitis B surface antigen has been demonstrated in saliva, feces, semen, urine, and other body secretions, the preponderance of evidence seems to indicate that the contagiousness of carriers by means of these routes is relatively low. The chronic carrier may develop either chronic persistent hepatitis, a benign self-limiting disease, or chronic active hepatitis, a potentially fatal disease.

Treatment. The treatment for hepatitis B is the same as that for hepatitis A.

Prevention. Immune serum globulin prepared in the last decade appears to have higher titers of antihepatitis B antibodies than that prepared earlier. There is also available now, a hyperimmune antihepatitis B gamma globulin. While there is some question about the superiority of this hyperimmune gamma globulin to immune serum globulin, it is recommended that the former be given to all *blood* contacts (*e.g.,* needle or dental instrument) of known patients or carriers with hepatitis B. In other contacts such as sexual contacts, many feel that immune serum globulin prophylaxis is sufficient. The cost of a dose

of hyperimmune gamma globulin is about 50 times that of immune serum globulin.

A vaccine prepared from the plasma of asymptomatic carriers of hepatitis B is now available. The vaccine is composed of noninfectious hepatitis B surface antigen particles. It is recommended for all high-risk groups, including dentists and physicians. Three doses are required over a period of 6 months; the third dose is important in that 75% to 90% immunity is acquired after the two doses, while over 95% immunity is acquired after the third dose.

Hepatitis non-A, non-B

Non-A, non-B hepatitis (NANB) is probably more than one disease, and the term non-A, non-B is one of exclusion in that the usual antigen and antibody tests for hepatitis A and B in a patient with hepatitis NANB are negative. The disease appears to be in most respects more similar to hepatitis B than to hepatitis A. About 90% of post-transfusion hepatitis today is NANB, and this probably the most common mode of transmission of the disease. The reason for transmission by transfusion is that as yet there are no reliable immunologic markers available for use in blood banks to exclude the blood from use. Alter and others have suggested that the incidence of post-transfusion hepatitis could be decreased by 29% by using elevated serum levels of alanine aminotransferase (ALT, formerly SGPT) in donors for exclusion.

Treatment. Treatment is supportive as with hepatitis A and B.

Prevention. There are no known preventive measures, although immune serum globulin might be expected to be useful in the exposed patient.

Diagnosis. On the basis of clinical symptoms and elevated bilirubin and alanine aminotransferase (ALT) levels in the acutely ill patient, the diagnosis of hepatitis can generally be made. Differentiation as to whether the hepatitis is A, B, or non-A, non-B depends on further antigen and antibody studies. The following serologic markers are useful in this regard:

- HB$_s$Ag— This is hepatitis B surface antigen denotes either acute infection or the chronic carrier state; it becomes positive about 6 weeks after exposure.
- Anti-HB$_s$Ag— This antibody to HB$_s$Ag indicates past infection with hepatitis B; it may take up to 3 to 4 months to appear after infection but generally remains positive for life; it denotes immunity of the patient to further hepatitis B infection.
- HB$_e$Ag— The presence of the e antigen denotes carriers who are much more likely to transmit the disease than are HB$_e$Ag-negative carriers.
- Anti-HB$_c$— This antibody to the core antigen of the hepatitis B virus (HB$_c$) appears early in the disease and may last from months to a lifetime; it neither denotes immunity nor excludes it.
- Anti-HAV— These antibodies to hepatitis A indicate present or previous infection with the disease. These antibodies may be fractionated into IgG, which indicates infection with hepatitis A sometime in the past, and IgM, which indicates the infection any time in the period of 1 week to 3 to 4 months. The IgM fraction is used to diagnose acute infection with hepatitis A.

In routine screening of patients to determine whether they are carriers of hepatitis B, the HB$_s$Ag is determined. In the diagnosis of acute hepatitis, laboratory tests can be ordered sequentially depending on the age of the patient. Because a child is more likely to have hepatitis A than are adults, the laboratory test of first choice should be anti-HAV. If positive, anti-HAV should then be fractionated into anti-HAV IgM to determine whether the infection is acute. If the anti-HAV is negative *or* if the IgM fraction is negative, the patient does not have *acute* hepatitis A and should be tested for HB$_s$Ag and anti-HB$_c$. The latter is sometimes positive early in the disease before the HB$_s$ is positive. In an adult, who is more likely to have hepatitis B, it is suggested that the initial tests be HB$_s$Ag and anti-HB$_c$. If these are negative, the tests for hepatitis A are performed. If tests for both hepatitis A and B are negative and other factors point to viral hepatitis as the diagnosis, then the diagnosis of non-A, non-B hepatitis is made.

Dental Considerations

Dental Personnel as a Source of Infection to Patients. Because hepatitis A is transmitted primarily by the oral–fecal route and is not associated with a chronic carrier state, transmission by dental personnel is extremely unlikely; neither have dental personnel been significantly implicated in the spread of non-A, non-B hepatitis. Surveillance data of hepatitis B transmission indicates that transmission of HBV by infected dentists is minimal and is not, in general, a major mode of transmission of the disease; however, dentists who are carriers of HBV can transmit the infection to their patients. Ahtone and Goodman reviewed five such cases of transmission to patients by carrier dentists reported since 1975. They also reviewed three cases of HB$_s$ Ag-positive dentists who were not implicated in spread of the disease to their patients.

Infection of Dental Personnel by Patients. Hepatitis A, not being associated with the chronic carrier state, is unlikely to be spread to dental personnel from an infected patient except in that rare instance where inadvertent inoculation occurs by blood (*e.g.*, finger stick) from an acutely ill patient or a patient late in the incubation period.

Hepatitis B and non-A, non-B can be transmitted to a dentist or his patients from an infected patient during the prodromal or acute phase of the disease, and the hepatitis B surface antigen has been shown to be present in serum up to 2 months *before* the onset of clinical signs and symptoms. The hepatitis B surface antigen was detected by Villarejos and others in saliva in 76% of 41 patients with acute type-B hepatitis. The antigen was also found, although not constantly, in the saliva of carriers. In another study, Ward and coauthors indicated that 51% of patients with antigenemia had the antigen in their saliva. Hepatitis B and non-A, non-B are of particular interest to the dentist because they are the only forms of hepatitis known to be associated with a chronic carrier state. Both oral surgeons and periodontists have been shown to be at a higher risk to develop hepatitis B than the average practitioner because of their increased exposure to blood. At the 1972 annual session of the American Dental Association (ADA) in San Francisco where 1,200 general dentists voluntarily participated in a screening program for serologic evidence of prior infection by the HBV, there was a 13.6% frequency of evidence of prior infection with HBV in these dentists as manifested by the presence of antibodies to HBV. A similar study among 1,192 physicians at two American Medical Association (AMA) conventions showed a rate of prior infection of 18.5%. A study at one dental school by Hollinger and others showed antibody to hepatitis B present in 23% of fourth-year dental students, while a study by Bass and others at another dental school found antibody present in 13% of faculty members but only 8.4% of students.

Preventive Measures. Protection for the dentist should lie in identifying those people most likely to transmit the disease. Several groups are known to have a much higher carrier state than the general population; these include hemodialysis patients, institutionalized mentally retarded patients, immunosuppressed patients, multiple blood transfusion recipients, percutaneous drug abusers, male homosexuals, and recently, Indochinese refugees. A study of 3,626 patients by Tullman at the Louisiana State University School of Dentistry indicated a prevalence rate of 0.61% (22) positive patients for HB$_s$Ag. Eighteen of these 22 positive patients (carriers) had no past history of hepatitis. A study of the reliability of the medical history in identifying patients with hepatitis B conducted by Goebel indicated that 58% of the patients who gave a history of hepatitis A had actually had hepatitis B and 31% of the

patients with possible histories of hepatitis had hepatitis B; 50% of the HB$_s$Ag-positive carriers gave no history of having had hepatitis. All of these factors considered, other than routine testing of all dentist patients for HB$_s$Ag, which is difficult and expensive to accomplish, the dentist has only the history and the knowledge of the high-risk groups to guide in protecting himself and patients from hepatitis. For this reason, routine aseptic techniques and proper sterilization are paramount.

Considering the minute amount of blood needed to transmit hepatitis B, it is significant that Allen and Organ found occult blood under the fingernails of 81% of senior dental students who were treating patients compared with only 20% of second year dental students who were *not* treating patients (who served as controls). They recommended that rubber gloves be worn routinely by the dentist to protect both himself and his patients from hepatitis B. Dentists and dental personnel who treat patients in a high-risk group for transmitting hepatitis are advised to wear gloves while treating these patients, and gloves should be worn while treating all patients when bleeding occurs.

The usefulness of wearing masks is debatable. In a study by Peterson and others in which air samples were collected from the dental operatory during treatment of patients whose blood was positive for HB$_s$Ag, no samples contained HB$_s$Ag-positive blood. They suggested that environmentally mediated transmission of hepatitis B is more likely to occur through contact with contaminated surfaces than through the airborne route.

Dentists who are known carriers should, as recommended by Ahtone and Goodman, do the following: determine whether any factors such as a chronic dermatitis are present that would favor transmission of the disease; obtain informed consent in writing from their patients that they are aware that although full precautions are being taken, the dentist is an HBV carrier; and use barrier techniques involving the use of mask and gloves when performing any dental treatment. If despite these measures there is evidence of transmission of the disease by the dentist, the dentist should discontinue his practice. It is not recommended that practice be discontinued solely on the basis of a dentist's being HB_s Ag-positive if there is no evidence of transmission of disease to patients.

Tests of sterilization shown to be efficacious by epidemiologic data include immersion in 100°C (boiling) water for 30 minutes, exposure to saturated steam at 121°C, and 15 psi pressure for 30 minutes, dry heat at 106°C for 1 hour, or ethylene oxide gas at 10% concentration and carbon dioxide at 55 to 69°C for 8 to 10 hours. The U.S. government Centers for Disease Control has developed an *in vitro* measure for the effectiveness of a disinfectant agent on the HBV. The following additional methods or agents have been shown by this *in vitro* technique to be effective and significant in inactivating HB_s Ag: immersion in 100° C boiling water for 10 minutes or immersion in a 1% solution of sodium hypochlorite for 10 minutes. Solutions of ethyl or isopropyl alcohol and quaternary ammonium compounds are *not* considered to be effective in inactivating the HBV.

One major problem of sterilization in the dental office is that of the dental handpiece. Sanger and others (1978) reviewed the manufacturer's suggestions for sterilization-inactivation of dental handpieces. It was apparent from their study that some models could not be boiled, autoclaved, or sterilized by dry heat or use of ethylene oxide. It was suggested that the practitioner contact the manufacturer regarding sterilization methods for handpieces used and further that this be a consideration before the purchase of a handpiece.

DISEASES OF THE SMALL INTESTINE

Polyps of the small intestine and less commonly of the stomach and colon occur sporadically or as a familial trait associated with pigmentation of the perioral region and of the oral mucosa. This comprises the syndrome known as the Peutz–Jeghers syndrome, which is discussed in Chapter 7, on pigmentation of the oral mucosa. The polyps have been reported to undergo malignant change in about 3% of cases.

INFLAMMATORY BOWEL DISEASE

Chronic inflammatory diseases of the small intestine and large bowel are of interest to the dentist because oral manifestations have been reported in some of these diseases and may be the initial finding. In addition, medications that the patient may be taking for the disease might alter the course of dental therapy. Classification of chronic inflammatory disease of the bowel is at best confusing. Among these diseases are ulcerative colitis, an inflammatory disease that is confined to the mucosa and submucosa of the colon, and regional enteritis (regional ileitis) also known as Crohn's disease of the small bowel, which is an inflammatory disease involving the entire wall of a portion of the small gut. The term *regional enteritis* is preferable to regional ileitis, inasmuch as the disease may involve more of the small intestine than of the ileum.

Other chronic inflammatory diseases of the bowel resemble ulcerative colitis in some respects and regional enteritis in others. It is at this point that classification and differentiation of the diseases becomes confusing. There is a granulomatous colitis of the colon different from ulcerative colitis, which is known as Crohn's disease of the colon. In the latter disease the small bowel is also involved in up to 80% of the cases, whereas in ulcerative colitis the lesions are confined to the colon. Symptoms of the various chronic inflammatory diseases of the intestine are variable, but all include upper or lower abdominal pain, usually cramping in nature, along with fever and episodes of bloody diarrhea. Interenteric and anorectal fistulae develop as do segmental narrowing of the intestinal lumen, toxic megacolon, and rectal bleeding.

Diagnosis. Diagnosis is made on the basis of gastrointestinal radiographs, upper and lower GI series, and sigmoidoscopy, which involves a direct visualization of the colonic mucosa. On occasion rectal biopsy may be necessary to confirm the diagnosis.

Treatment. Medical therapy for chronic inflammatory granulomatous disease of the bowel may include any or all of the following:

salicylazosulfapyridine (Azulfidine), a sulfonamide the metabolites of which are concentrated in the intestinal tissues; corticosteroid therapy (both corticosteroids and ACTH are used); and immunosuppressive therapy. The latter, which includes compounds such as azothioprine and mercaptopurine, are being used with increasing frequency in inflammatory bowel disease. Approximately 15% to 20% of patients with ulcerative colitis require surgery, and approximately 40% to 50% of patients with Crohn's disease require surgery. The high rate of surgery in the latter is because of complications such as abscess or fistula formation, hemorrhage, or obstruction. Surgery is generally more successful in ulcerative colitis because colectomy fully removes the target organ. Other inflammatory bowel diseases tend to recur in the small intestine after a surgical resection of either portions of the small bowel or after resection of the colon.

Oral Manifestations. Crohn's disease either of the colon or the small bowel can affect all regions of the bowel and has been reported to produce oral lesions. Bishop and others reported a patient with Crohn's disease who exhibited an oral granulomatous lesion as the initial manifestation of the disease 1 year before radiologic changes in the terminal ileum. The lesion was described as a nodular mass in the mucobuccal fold that upon biopsy showed chronic inflammatory response with granulation tissue extending to the depths of the biopsy specimen. The numerous large, well-formed, noncaseating granulomata contained epithelial cells, giant cells, and lymphocytes. These histologic findings are compatible with the appearance of lesions of Crohn's disease elsewhere in the gastrointestinal tract.

Other authors have reported lesions resembling aphthous ulcers in Crohn's disease. Whether these represent a manifestation of Crohn's disease or are coincidental is not known, but such aphthouslike ulcerations have been reported to occur in up to 20% of patients with Crohn's disease. Bernstein and McDonald reviewed 22 cases and reported two new cases of oral manifestations of Crohn's disease. They found that there was a predilection for occurrence in certain anatomic areas, and lesion appearance depended on location. The most frequently affected areas were the buccal mucosa, showing a cobblestone pattern; the vestibule, which had linear hyperplastic folds with ulcers; and the lips, which appeared swollen and indurated. Less frequently, granular erythematous lesions appeared on the gingiva and alveolar mucosa and palatal ulcers. Cataldo and others reported on a case of pustular lesions on the oral mucous membrane in a patient with Crohn's disease. They also reviewed 7 other cases with similar lesions who had either colitis or a gastrointestinal disturbance in addition to the oral pustular lesions. In regional enteritis a history of exacerbation of episodes of aphthous ulcers of the mouth may be a prologue to an acute exacerbation of the enteritis.

Dental Considerations. Medical treatment for chronic inflammatory bowel disease may necessitate alterations of dental therapy or special precautions on the part of the dentist. Patients on immunosuppressive therapy might be expected to have changes in the white and red blood cell counts, and patients on Azulfidine therapy may also occasionally have such changes. The enteritis itself may cause an anemia secondary to the effects of chronic illness on the bowel or gastrointestinal bleeding. For these reasons, both the total and differential white blood cell counts and hemoglobin concentration should be ascertained before embarking on surgical procedures on patients with such bowel diseases. Patients on corticosteroid therapy may develop both hyperglycemia and osteoporosis, both of which have adverse effects on contemplated dental therapy.

BIBLIOGRAPHY

Ahtone J, Goodman RA: Hepatitis B and dental personnel: Transmission to patients and prevention issues. J Am Dent Assoc 106:219, 1983

Ahtone J, Maynard JE: Laboratory diagnosis of hepatitis B. JAMA 249:2067, 1983

Allen AL, Organ RJ: Occult blood accumulation under the fingernails: A mechanism for the spread of blood-borne infection. J Am Dent Assoc 105:455, 1982

Alter HJ: Donor transaminase and recipient hepatitis. JAMA 246:630, 1981

Bass BD et al: Quantitation of hepatitis B viral markers in a dental school population. J Am Dent Assoc 104:629, 1982

Bernstein ML, McDonald JS: Oral lesions in Crohn's disease: Report of two cases and update. Oral Surg 46:234, 1978

Bishop RP, Brewster AC, Antonioloi DA: Crohn's disease of the mouth. J Gastroenterol 62:302, 1972

Cataldo E et al: Pyostomatitis vegetans. Oral Surg 52:172, 1981

Cooley RL, Lubow RM: Hepatitis B vaccine: Implications for dental personnel. J Am Dent Assoc 105:47, 1982

Council on Dental Materials, Instruments and Equipment, Current Status of Sterilization Instruments, Devices, and Methods for the Dental Office. J Am Dent Assoc 102:683, 1981

Crowson TD, Head LH, Ferrante WA: Esophageal ulcers associated with tetracycline therapy. JAMA 235:2747, 1976

Denes AE et al: Hepatitis B infection in physicians. JAMA 239:210, 1978

Donaldson RM: The muddle of diets for gastrointestinal disorders. JAMA 225:1243, 1973

Francis DP, Maynard JE: The transmission and outcome of hepatitis A, B and non-A, non-B: A Review. Epidemiol Rev 1:17, 1979

Giger M et al: Tetracycline ulcer of the esophagus. Dtsch Med Wochenschr 103:1038, 1978

Gius JA et al: Vascular formations of the lip and peptic ulcer. JAMA 183:725, 1963

Goebel WM: Reliability of the medical history in identifying patients likely to place dentists at an increased hepatitis risk. J Am Dent Assoc 98:907, 1979

Griffin FM: Hepatitis B antigenemia in apparently healthy blood donors. JAMA 226:753, 1973

Guadagnino V et al: Risk of hepatitis B virus infection in patients with eczema or psoriasis of the hand. Br Med J 284:83, 1982

Heathcote J et al: Hepatitis B antigen in saliva and semen. Lancet 1:71, 1974

Hollinger FD et al: Hepatitis B prevalence within a dental student population. J Am Dent Assoc 94:521, 1977

Kashiwaqi S et al; An outbreak of hepatitis B in members of a high-school sumo wrestling club. JAMA 248:213, 1982.

Kirsner JB: Observations on the medical treatment of inflammatory bowel disease. JAMA 243:557, 1980

Krugman S: The newly licensed hepatitis B vaccine. JAMA 247:2012, 1982

Krugman S et al: Infectious hepatitis. Evidence for two distinctive clinical epidemiological and immunological types of infection. JAMA 200:365, 1967

Krugman S, Giles J: Viral hepatitis. JAMA 212:1019, 1970

Levin ML et al: Hepatitis B transmission by dentists. JAMA 228:1139, 1974

Mosley JW, White E: Viral hepatitis as an occupational hazard of dentists. J Am Dent Assoc 90:992, 1975

Peppercorn MA et al: Esophageal motor dysfunction and systemic lupus erythematosus. JAMA 242:1895, 1979

Petersen NJ et al: Air sampling for hepatitis B surface antigen in a dental operatory. J Am Dent Assoc 99:465, 1979

Rosenberg JL et al: Viral hepatitis: An occupational hazard to surgeons. JAMA 223:395, 1973

Rothstein SS et al: Hepatitis B virus: An overview for dentists. J Am Dent Assoc 102:173, 1981

Sanger RG: An inquiry into the sterilization of dental hand pieces relative to transmission of hepatitis B virus. J Am Dent Assoc 96:621, 1978

Szmuness W: Recent advances in the study of epidemiology of hepatitis B. Am J Pathol 81:629, 1975

Szmuness W et al: Hepatitis B vaccine, demonstration of efficacy in a controlled clinical trial in a high risk population in the United States. N Engl J Med 303:833, 1980

Tullman MJ et al: The threat of hepatitis B from dental school patients. Oral Surg 49:214, 1980

Villarejos VM et al: Role of saliva, urine and feces in the transmission of type B hepatitis. N Engl J Med 291:1375, 1974

Ward R et al: Hepatitis B antigen in saliva and mouthwashing. Lancet 2:726, 1972

21

Renal Disease

S. GARY COHEN

ETIOLOGY

Kidney disease is reportedly the fourth leading health problem in the United States, with a new incidence of end-stage renal disease occurring at a rate of between 60 and 100 new patients per million population or between 10,000 and 18,000 new patients each year. Approximately 8 million Americans are afflicted.

Renal failure can be caused by many diseases. The United States Transplant Registry and the European Dialysis and Transplant Association have generated statistics showing that glomerulonephritis accounts for 55% of all the patients receiving dialysis and transplants. Pyelonephritis is the second most common cause of renal failure with 15%; polycystic renal disease, nephrosclerosis, diabetes, collagen vascular diseases, and other less common disorders make up the remainder (see Table 21-1). Renal failure produces a standard symptom complex, regardless of the underlying cause.

The prognosis of the patient with renal disease has improved significantly during the last decade. The development of dialysis and transplantation techniques has provided patients with the opportunity for survival in the face of complete loss of renal function. The

dental profession has the responsibility of providing oral health care for these patients, who sometimes have complicated management problems. This section reviews the dental management and treatment implications of patients with chronic renal failure and focuses on those patients with end-stage renal disease receiving hemodialysis and kidney transplantation.

Glomerulonephritis

Glomerulonephritis represents a heterogeneous group of diseases of varying etiologies and pathogenesis that produce irreversible impairment of function. Some begin with an attack of acute glomerulonephritis subdivided into either streptococcal or nonstreptococcal. Others may enter the chronic stage from a nephrotic syndrome; the most typical examples of this are idiopathic membranous glomeruleonephritis and membranoproliferative glomerulonephritis. In the largest group, the patients merely present with the featues of chronic renal failure and hypertension or with a chance proteinuria that over the years has progressed to chronic nephritis.

Chronic glomerulonephritis is usually insidious in onset. The course is very slowly but steadily progressive, leading to renal failure and uremia in a period from a few years to as many as 30 years. It is thought to be a disorder of immunologic origin. The continuous nature of the immunologic injury is demonstrated by the recurrence of disease in kidneys transplanted to patients with some type of glomerulonephritis, even after their own kidneys have been removed.

Pyelonephritis

Pyelonephritis refers to the effects of bacterial infection in the kidney. It may present as an acute form with active pyogenic infection or a chronic form where the principal manifestations are caused by an injury sustained during a preceding active infection. Chronic bacterial pyelonephritis can be further subdivided into reactive and inactive forms; one or both kidneys may be affected.

Any lesion that produces obstruction of the urinary tract can predispose to active pyelo-

Table 21-1. Etiology of End-Stage Renal Disease

ETIOLOGY	PERCENTAGE OF ALL DIALYSIS AND KIDNEY TRANSPLANT PATIENTS
Glomerulonephritis	55%
Pyelonephritis	15
Polycystic renal disease	7
Nephrosclerosis	7
Diabetic nephropathy	5
Collagen vascular disease	6

Other diseases
  hereditary neuropathy
  analgesic abuse nephropathy
  obstructive nephropathy
  gouty nephropathy
  neoplastic nephropathy
  unknown nephropathy
	6

nephritis. Pyelonephritis may also occur as part of a generalized sepsis as in patients with bacterial endocarditis or with staphylococcal septicemia.

The clinical picture of acute pyelonephritis may be characteristic; sudden rise of body temperature to 38.9°C to 40.6°C, shaking chills, aching pain in one or both costovertebral areas or flanks, and symptoms of bladder inflammation. Laboratory tests reveal large numbers of pus cells as well as bacteria in the urine and a polymorphonuclear leukocytosis. There are no signs of impaired renal function or acute hypertension as is sometimes seen in acute glomerulonephritis. Patients with chronic active pyelonephritis often suffer from recurrent episodes of acute pyelonephritis or may have persistent smoldering infections that gradually result in end-stage renal failure secondary to destruction from scarring of renal parenchyma. This process may continue for many years. An inability to conserve sodium, a feature in any patient with impaired renal function, is more pronounced in pyelonephritis than in glomerulonephritis. This "salt-losing" defect may be pronounced and may dominate the clinical picture.

Uremic Syndrome

The kidney is responsible for excretory functions and maintaining body homeostasis by its significant role in sodium excretion, acid-base electrolyte, and water balance, along with blood pressure regulation. When renal function is impaired or lost, a wide variety of signs and symptoms may appear that reflect dysfunction or failure of virtually every organ system (see Table 21-2).

Early renal failure simply reflects decreased renal reserve. There may be no symptoms or prominent biochemical disturbances; a decreased creatinine clearance may be the only observable change. As the kidney fails, the nephron population falls. If this progresses, the glomerular filtration rate (GFR) falls, and the blood urea nitrogen (BUN) rises. Among the consequences are mild azotemia (abnormal retention of nitrogen products in the blood), impaired ability to concentrate urine, nocturia, and mild anemia. If this continues, frank renal disease follows with its associated

Table 21-2. Systemic Disturbances in Renal Disease

BODY SYSTEM	MANIFESTATION
Gastrointestinal	Nausea, vomiting, anorexia, ammoniacal taste and smell, stomatitis, parotitis, esophagitis, gastritis, GI bleeding
Neuromuscular	Headaches, peripheral neuropathy, paralysis, myoclonic jerks, seizures, asterixis
Hematologic-immunologic	Normocytic and normochromic anemia, coagulation defect, increased susceptibility to infection, decreased erythropoietin production, lymphocytopenia
Endocrine-metabolic	Renal osteodystrophy (osteomalacia, osteoporosis, osteosclerosis), secondary hyperparathyroidism, impaired growth and development, loss of libido and sexual function, amenorrhea
Cardiovascular	Arterial hypertension, congestive heart failure, cardiomyopathy, pericarditis, arrhythmias
Dermatologic	Pallor, hyperpigmentation, ecchymosis, uremic frost, pruritus, reddish brown distal nail beds

polyuria. The anemia may become severe, and hypocalcemia and hyperphosphatemia may occur along with a metabolic acidosis. This may then progress to uremia. Uremia is a clinical condition that resembles systemic poisoning caused by ingested toxin. Advanced uremia is associated with derangement of function in many major organ systems (*e.g.*, pericarditis and pericardial effusions, neuropathies, metabolic encephalopathy, pronounced azotemia, life-threatening hyperkalemia, bone disease, and bleeding disturbances). Other uremic symptoms include anorexia, nausea, vomiting, weakness, fatigue, irritability, itching, and muscle cramps. The prominence of specific symptoms may vary from patient to patient.

MANIFESTATIONS OF RENAL DISEASE

Gastrointestinal

The gastrointestinal system shows a myriad of symptoms in the uremic syndrome. The more common symptoms include nausea, vomiting, and anorexia. Gastrointestinal inflammations such as gastritis, duodenitis, and esophagitis are common in late renal failure.

Neurologic

Some of the early signs and symptoms of chronic renal failure are related to the neurologic system. The electroencephalogram becomes abnormal with changes commensurate with metabolic encephalopathy. As the disease progresses, asterixis and myoclonic jerks may become evident; central nervous system irritability and eventually, seizures occur. Seizures can also occur secondary to hypertensive encephalopathy, electrolyte disturbances such as hyponatremia, and alkalosis, which induces hypocalcemia.

Along with neurologic hyperirritability, peripheral neuropathy can occur as a result of a disturbance of the conduction mechanism rather than a loss of nerve fiber. The clinical picture is dominated by sensory symptoms and signs. Impairment of vibratory sense and loss of deep tendon reflexes are the earliest, most frequent, and most constant findings. The predominant patient complaint is paresthesia or "burning feet" that may progress to eventual muscle weakness, atrophy, and finally, paralysis; there is a tendency toward increasing incidence with decreasing renal function. This predominantly affects the lower extremities but can affect the upper ones as well; rarely, facial, oral, and paraoral regions can also be affected.

Hematologic

Patients with chronic renal dysfunction will often have hematologic problems, most commonly anemia and bleeding. The anemia associated with renal disease is a function of decreased erythropoiesis in the bone marrow and is usually normocytic-normochromic. It is not uncommon for these patients to have hematocrit levels in the 20% to 35% range. The pathogenesis of the anemia is multifactorial with nutritional deficiencies, iron metabolism abnormalities, and circulating uremic toxins that inhibit erythropoiesis all playing a role. The major factor, however, is the inability of the diseased kidney to produce erythropoietin, which stimulates, through a feedback mechanism, the bone marrow to produce red blood cells. Hypertension, retention of waste products, and altered body fluid pH and electrolyte compositions create a suboptimal environment for living cells; therefore, there may be accelerated destruction of red blood cells contributing to the anemia. Another cause of anemia in many dialyzed patients is the frequent blood sampling and loss of blood in hemodialysis tubing and coils.

Interestingly, these patients tolerate their anemia quite well. Whole blood transfusions are usually unnecessary, with the exception of general anesthesia, expected significant blood loss, or moderate to severe symptoms of anemia. These symptoms of anemia may include pallor, tachycardia, systolic ejection murmur, a widened pulse pressure, and angina pectoris in patients with underlying coronary artery disease. Transfusions may further suppress the production of red blood cells. The risk of hepatitis is increased with the number of transfusions.

It had previously been policy to withhold blood from dialysis patients to prevent sensitizing them to tissue antigens that would make future kidney transplantation more difficult but Opelz and Terasaki provide impressive evidence that the larger the number of pretransplant transfusions the better the chance of graft survival.

Bleeding may be a significant problem, and it has been attributed to an intrinsic coagulation defect, a deficiency in platelet factor 3 (PF3), or the anticoagulants used in conjunction with anticoagulants used in conjunction with dialysis (heparin) and access-site maintenance (coumarin derivatives). The coagulation defect, one of altered platelet adhesiveness, is related to an altered pathway of urea metabolism. This condition is improved by dialysis and may be eliminated after transplantation. Platelets numbers affect bleeding, and it has been shown that mechanical trauma to the platelets during dialysis can cause a decrease of up to 17% in the platelet count. In addition to lowered platelet counts, which is usually not clinically significant, and qualitative platelet defects, the effects of medications on platelets contribute to bleeding episodes. Patients on dialysis will be given heparin to prevent clotting in the dialyzer and tubing. Some patients have a tendency to be hypercoagulable; for these patients a regimen of sodium warfarin (Coumadin) therapy is instituted to maintain a continous anticoagulated state to ensure shunt patency.

Metabolic Renal Osteodystrophy

Renal osteodystrophy refers to the skeletal changes resulting from chronic renal disease and is caused by the disorders in calcium and phosphorus metabolism, abnormal vitamin D metabolism, and increased parathyroid activity. In early renal failure, intestinal absorption of calcium is reduced because the kidneys are unable to convert vitamin D into its active form. The mechanism behind this conversion is as follows: a compound called 7-dehydroxycholesterol is located in the skin; exposure to sunlight converts this compound to cholecalciferol (vitamin D_3); this substance is then metabolized in the liver to a more biologically active form called 25-hydroxycholecalciferol (25-HCC); further conversion to either 1,25-dihydroxycholecalciferol (1-25-DHCC) or 21,25-dihydroxycholecalciferol (21,25-DHCC) then occurs in the kidney parenchyma.

When the serum calcium is high, 25-HCC is metabolized to 21, 25-DHCC; a hypocalcemic state initiates the conversion of 25-HCC to 1,25-DHCC. It is this form which is the most biologically active for absorbing calcium from the digestive tract (see Fig. 21-1). Impaired absorption of calcium because of defective kidney function and the corresponding retention of phosphate cause a decrease in the serum calcium. This is associated with a compensatory hyperactivity of the parathyroid glands (parathyroid hormone production), which increases the urinary excretion of phosphates, decreases

urine calcium excretion, and release augments of calcium from bone.

The most frequently observed changes associated with compensatory hyperparathyroidism are those involving the skeletal system, and these changes can appear before as well as during treatment with hemodialysis. It some cases the renal osteodystrophy becomes worse during hemodialysis. Some of the changes that are accelerated are bone remodeling, osteomalacia, osteitis fibrosa cystica (a rarefying osteitis with fibrous degeneration and cystic spaces that result from hyperfunction of the parathyroid glands), and osteosclerosis.

The bone lesions are usually of the digits, the clavicle, and the acromioclavicular joint. Other lesions that can be seen are mottling of the skull, erosion of the distal clavicle and margins of the symphysis pubis, rib fractures, and necrosis of the femoral head. In children, the predominant lesion is osteomalacia—a deficiency or absence of osteoid mineralization—that is associated with bone softening that leads to deformities of the ribs, pelvis, and femoral neck—*renal rickets*. It should be emphasized that early stages of renal osteodystrophy may be detected histologically or biochemically without the presence of definitive radiographic changes because dependable radiographic evidence of bone disease appears only after 30% of bone mineral contents have been lost.

Osteodystrophy patients are placed on protein restricted diets and phosphate binders (aluminum hydroxide or aluminum carbonate) to keep the serum phosphorus within the normal range (between 3.5 mg/dl and 5.0 mg/dl). They are also given vitamin D supplements (such as 1-25 DHCC). If these measures fail, a parathyroidectomy may be performed, wherein 3.5 of 4 glands are removed leaving residual parathormone-secreting tissue.

Immune Status

Other complications experienced by patients with renal failure can be attributed to their altered host defenses. Uremic patients appear to be in a state of reduced immunocapacity, the cause of which is thought to be a combination of uremic intoxication and en-

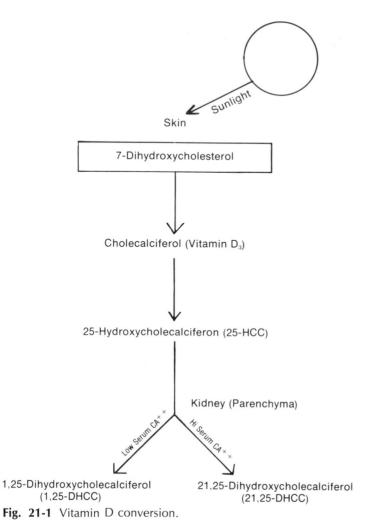

Fig. 21-1 Vitamin D conversion.

suing protein and caloric malnutrition. Uremic plasma contains nondialyzable factors that suppress lymphocyte responses manifested at both the cellular and humoral levels such as granulocyte dysfunction and suppressed cell-mediated immunity; impaired or disrupted mucocutaneous barriers decrease the protection from environmental pathogens. Together, these impairments place uremic patients at a high risk of infection, which is the most common cause of their death and disability.

Oral Manifestations

With impaired renal function, decreased glomerular filtration rate, and the accumulation and retention of various products of renal failure, the oral cavity may show a variety of changes as the body progresses from an azotemic to a uremic state. The dentist must recognize these oral symptoms as part of the patient's systemic disease and not as an isolated occurrence. In studies of renal patients, up to 90% were found to have oral symptoms of uremia. Some of the presenting signs were ammoniacal taste and smell, stomatitis, gingivitis, decreased salivary flow, xerostomia, and parotitis.

As renal failure develops, one of the early symptoms may be patient complaints of bad taste and odor, particularly in the morning. This uremic fetor, an ammoniacal odor, is typical of any uremic patient and is caused by the high concentration of urea in the saliva and its breakdown to ammonia. Salivary urea levels correlate well with the BUN levels, but no fixed, constant relationship exists. An acute rise in the BUN may result in uremic stomatitis, which may appear as an erythemopultaceous form, characterized by red mucosa covered with a thick exudate and a pseudomembrane, or an ulcerative form, characterized by frank ulcerations with redness and a pultaceous coat. In all reported cases, intraoral changes have been related to BUN levels greater than 150 and disappear spontaneously when medical treatment results in a lowered BUN level. Although its exact cause is uncertain, uremic stomatitis can be regarded as a chemical burn or a general loss of tissue resistance and the tissue's inability to withstand normal and traumatic influences.

White plaques called *uremic frost* commonly found on the skin can rarely be found intraorally. This uremic frost results from residual urea crystals left on the epithelial surfaces after perspiration evaporates. A more common oral finding is xerostomia probably caused by a combination of direct involvement of the salivary glands, chemical inflammation, dehydration, and mouth breathing. Salivary adenitis can occasionally be seen.

Other oral manifestations of renal disease are related to the renal osteodystrophy. These manifestations usually become evident late in the course of the disease. The classic signs of hyperparathyroidism (HPTH) of the mandible and maxilla are bone demineralization, loss of trabeculation, ground-glass appearance, total or partial loss of lamina dura, giant cell lesions or brown tumors, and metastatic calcifications (Fig. 21-2). The rarefaction in the mandible and maxilla is secondary to the generalized osteoporosis. The finer trabeculae disappear later leaving a coarser pattern. Small lytic lesions may occur that histologically prove to be giant cell tumors. The compact bone of the jaws may become thinned and eventually disappear. This may be evident as loss of the lower border of the mandible, the cortical margins of the inferior dental canal and floor of the antrum, and lamina dura. Spontaneous fractures may occur with the thinning of these areas of compact bone.

While the skeleton may undergo decalcification, fully developed teeth are not directly affected; however, in the presence of significant skeletal decalcification the teeth will appear more radiopaque. The loss of lamina dura is neither pathognomonic for nor a consistent sign of HPTH. A similar loss of lamina dura may also be seen in Paget's disease, osteomalacia, fibrous dysplasia, sprue, and Cushing's and Addison's diseases. Various studies indicate lamina dura changes in only 40% to 50% of known HPTH patients.

The lesions of HPTH are called *brown tumors* because they contain areas of old hemorrhage and clinically appear brown. As the tumor increases in size, the resultant expansion may involve the cortex, which is eventually destroyed. Although the tumor rarely breaks through the periosteum, gingival swelling may result. The brown tumor lesion contains an abundance of multinucleated giant cells, fibroblasts, and hemosiderin. This histologic appearance is also consistent with central giant cell tumor and giant cell reparative granuloma. Associated bone changes consist of a generalized osteitis fibrosa with patches of osteoclastic resorption on all bone surfaces. This is replaced by a vascular connective tissue that represents an abortive formation of coarse-fibered woven bone. This histologic picture may also be seen in fibrous dysplasia, giant cell reparative granuloma, osteomalacia, and Paget's disease.

Other clinical manifestations of hyperparathyroidism include tooth mobility, malocclusion, and metastatic soft tissue calcifications. Increasing mobility and drifting of teeth with no apparent pathologic periodontal pocket formation may be seen. Periapical radiolucencies and root resorption may also be associated with this gradual loosening of the dentition. The teeth may be painful to percussion and mastication. A positive thermal and electric pulp test response will be elicited. Splinting is a useful adjunct to prevent pain and further drifting and the splint should be maintained until adequate treatment of the hyperparathyroidism results in bone remineralization. Malocclusion may result from the increased mobility and drifting of the dentition. Extreme demineralization and collapse of the temporomandibular and paratemporomandibular bones may also produce a malocclusion.

Metastatic calcification can also occur, particularly when the calcium–phosphate solu-

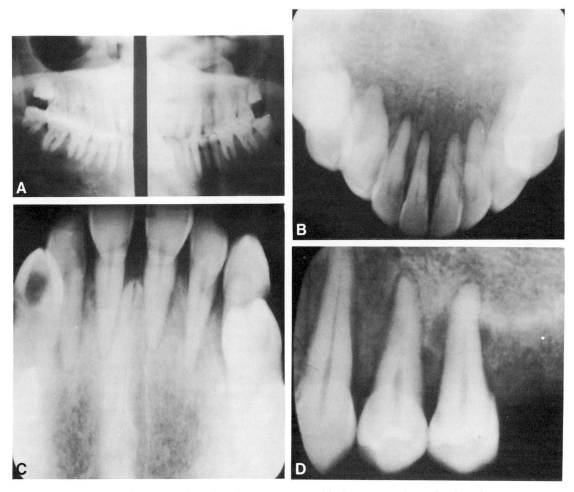

Fig. 21-2 *A,* Panorex showing trabecular changes. *B,* Mandibular anterior loss of trabeculation. *C,* Maxillary anterior loss of trabeculation. *D,* Loss of lamina dura.

bility product (Ca × P) is greater than 70. In normal subjects, a relation exists between plasma calcium and inorganic phosphate. When expressed in terms of total calcium (mg/dl) and inorganic phosphate (mg/dl), the ion product or Ca × P solubility product normally average 35. A rise in the Ca × P ion product in the extracellular fluid may cause metastatic calcifications because of precipitation of calcium phosphate crystals into the soft tissues such as the sclera, corner of the eye, subcutaneous tissue, skeletal and cardiac muscle, and blood vessels. This may also occur in the oral and associated paraoral soft tissues. These calcifications are visible radiographically.

Abnormal bone repair after extraction, ra-diographically characterized by lack of lamina dura resorption and deposition of sclerotic bone in the confines of the lamina dura, has been reported in patients with renal disease, although it is not unique to them. This finding is termed *socket sclerosis* (Fig. 21-3).

Enamel hypoplasia is frequently seen in patients whose renal disease started at a young age. Prolonged corticosteroid administration may also contribute to this deficit (Fig. 21-4). Studies have shown a high correlation between the time of onset of severe renal disease and the time at which the hypoplastic enamel was formed. A 1977 study by Kanekeo and associates showed eruption patterns of permanent teeth to be uneffected by renal disease.

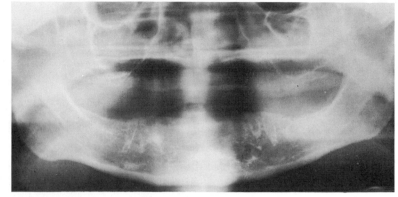

Fig. 21-3 Panoramic radiograph of extraction sites representative of socket sclerosis. Teeth were extracted 6 years before x-ray and 2 years before diagnosis of end-stage renal disease.

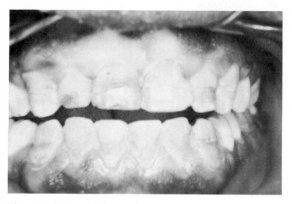

Fig. 21-4 Enamel hypoplasia and tetracycline stains in young patient with end-stage renal disease.

DIALYSIS

Hemodialysis

For patients with irreversible kidney disease, hemodialysis has significantly decreased the mortality of this once invariably fatal disease. Long-term maintenance dialysis therapy has been a reality since 1961. In 1964 there were fewer than 300 patients in the United States receiving hemodialysis. Because of amendments to the Social Security Act in 1972, dialysis therapy was made possible to virtually everybody who developed end-stage renal disease. Today, approximately 55,000 are given treatments with artificial kidneys. It is estimated that 100,000 patients will be suitable candidates for hemodialysis by the late 1980s.

Hemodialysis refers to the removal of nitrogenous and toxic products of metabolism from the blood by means of a dialysis system. Exchange occurs between the patient's plasma and dialysate (the electrolyte composition of which mimics that of extracellular fluid) across a semipermeable membrane that allows uremic toxins to diffuse out of the plasma while retaining the formed elements and protein composition of blood (Fig. 21-5A through D). Dialysis does not provide the same degree of health as does normal renal function because there is no resorptive capability in the dialysis membrane; therefore, valuable nutrients are lost and potential toxic molecules are retained. The usual dialysis system consists of a dialyzer, dialysate production unit, roller blood pump, heparin infusion pump, and various devices to monitor conductivity, temperature, flow rate, and pressure of dialysate and to detect blood leaks and arterial and venous pressures.

Dialysis therapy can be delivered to the patient either in outpatient dialysis centers, where trained personnel administer therapy on a regular basis, or in the home environment, where family members trained in dialysis techniques assist the patient in dialysis therapy. It has been shown that patients performing dialysis at home fare better psychologically, have a better quality of life, and have lower morbidity and mortality than do hospital dialysis patients; it is also less expensive. This home care may not be applicable for all patients because it is more difficult and requires a high degree of motivation not always found in this population.

The frequency and duration of dialysis is related to body size, residual renal function, protein intake, and tolerance to fluid removal. The typical patient undergoes hemodialysis three times per week with each treatment lasting 4 to 6 hours. During treatments

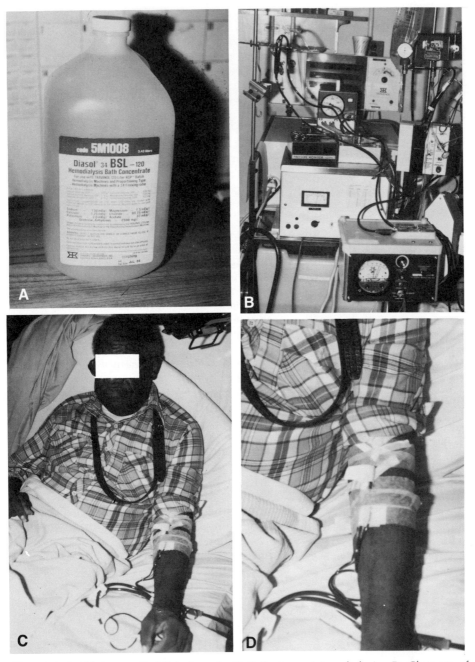

Fig. 21-5 *A*, Dialysate. *B*, Dialysis unit. *C*, Patient receiving dialysis. *D*, Close-up of access.

and for varying amounts of time afterward, anticoagulants are administered by regional or systemic methods.

Vascular access for hemodialysis can be created by a shunt, an external cannula, or by an arteriovenous fistula (an internalized access). The fistula is preferred for long-term treatment. The classic construction is a side-to-side anastomosis between the radial artery and the cephalic vein at the wrist. In patients with very thin veins, it can be technically impossible to create a direct arteriovenous fistula, and in some patients fistulae have clotted in both arms resulting in a demand for other forms of vascular access (sometimes the thigh is used as a site). A great advance with expansion of the access capability was the introduction of subcutaneous artificial arteriovenous grafts beginning with Gore-Tex (W. L. Gore & Assoc. Inc., Flagstaff, AZ) heterografts. Fistulae are now being constructed between arteries and veins by means of saphenous vein autografts, polytetrafluoroethylene grafts, Dacron, and other prosthetic conduits. Hemodialysis is performed by direct cannulation of the graft (Fig. 21-6).

Despite optimal dialysis, these patients remain chronically ill with hematologic, metabolic, neurologic, and cardiovascular problems that are more or less permanent. Growth alterations especially in the very young with renal disease may be seen particularly if they are maintained on hemodialysis. This growth deficiency has been attributed to the poor caloric intake of these patients and the uremic state. Dietary supplements have produced accelerated growth spurts and successful kidney transplantation may also restore a normal growth rate with the major determining factor being the bone age. For patients older than 12 years it is doubtful that significant growth would be attained.

Peritoneal Dialysis

During peritoneal dialysis, 1 to 2 liters of dialysate are placed in the peritoneal cavity and allowed to remain for varying intervals of time. Substances diffuse across the semipermeable peritoneal membrane into the dialysate. Compared to the membranes used for hemodialysis, the peritoneal membrane has greater permeability for high molecular weight species. The Tenckhoff Silastic catheter has made peritoneal puncture for each dialysis unnecessary. The Tenckhoff is a permanent intraperitoneal catheter that has two polyester felt cuffs into which tissue growth occurs. If used with sterile technique, it permits virtually infection-free, long-term access to the peritoneum (Fig. 21-7A through D).

Several regimens can be used with peritoneal dialysis. In one, 2 liters of dialysis fluid are instilled into the peritoneal cavity, allowed to remain for 30 minutes, and then drained out. This is repeated for 8 to 12 hours three to five times per week. Recently, a variation of this has become popular: chronic ambulatory peritoneal dialysis (CAPD), in which 2 liters of dialysate are exchanged every 6 to 8 hours around the clock for 6 to 7 days per week.

Some of the benefits of peritoneal dialysis are that systemic heparinization is unnecessary, and there is no risk of air embolism and blood leaks. These features along with the simplicity, make peritoneal dialysis safe for patients at risk when hemodialysis is used (*e.g.*, the young, the elderly, those with high-risk coronary and cerebral vascular disease, and those with vascular access problems). Some of the problems encountered with peritoneal dialysis are pain, intra-abdominal hemorrhage, inadequate drainage, leakage, and peritonitis.

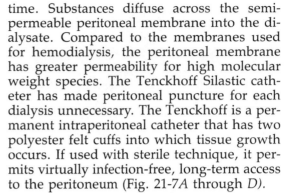

Dental Considerations

Many patients receiving dialysis have conditions of oral neglect. The results of a survey of dental needs of a random sample of 100 renal dialysis patients showed that over 60% needed dental treatment and that the majority of these patients were not aware of the possible complications of dental neglect while on hemodialysis. In addition to the usual excuses for neglecting routine dental treatment, these patients experience nonavailability of dental care because many dentists are reluctant to treat patients with severe systemic diseases. Because most dialysis cen-

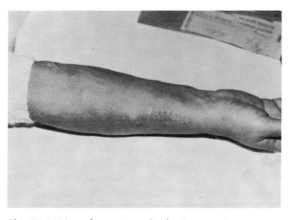

Fig. 21-6 Vascular access site in arm.

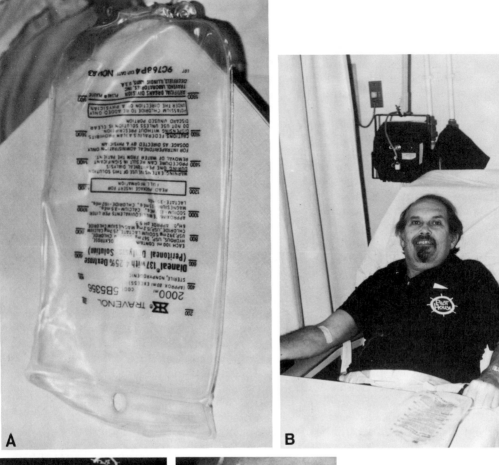

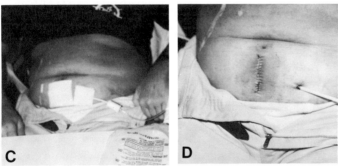

Fig. 21-7 *A*, Dialysate for chronic ambulatory peritoneal dialysis. *B*, Patient receiving peritoneal dialysis. *C*, Close-up of dialysis. *D*, Close-up of peritoneal access.

ters refer their patients to general practitioners for most forms of treatment, it is important that more generalists be familiar with the management problems associated with the dialysis patient.

The following are some of the preoperative considerations in the dental management of the dialysis patient. If time and patient condition permit, dialysis should be part of the preoperative preparation. Dialysis will return the state of hydration, serum electrolytes, urea nitrogen, and creatinine toward normal and will reduce the need for dialysis in the immediate postoperative period. Extractions and other surgery should be done early in the dialysis cycle, when the patient's blood is free from heparin, and there is sufficient time after surgery for clotting to occur before the next dialysis session and reheparinization.

The arteriovenous site should never be jeopardized. That arm should never be used for injection of medication, either intramuscularly or intravenously, nor should the access site itself be used as an injection site. The blood flow through the arm should not be impeded by requiring the patient to assume a cramped position or using that arm to measure blood pressure. When the access site is located in a leg, the patient should avoid sitting for long periods with the leg dependent. Obstructing venous drainage by compression at the groin or behind the knee must be avoided, especially because it tends to occur normally when the patient is in the sitting position. Such patients should be permitted to walk about for a few minutes every hour if a lengthy dental prodedure is required.

The presence of an a access site necessitates consideration of increased susceptibility to infective endocarditis and endarteritis. Sepsis and bacterial endoarteritis occur from infections at the access site by organisms seeded through punctures. More important, there have been three reported cases of infective endocarditis in patients with access-site grafts on hemodialysis after receiving dental treatment. The presence of an arteriovenous shunt or synthetic graft (fistula) sutured in place increases the risk for infective colonization from infection at the suture lines or at the surface discrepancies between normal arterial intima and the so-called prosthetic pseudointima. These sites provide a nidus for intravascular lodgment of bacteria, leading to persistence of an otherwise transient bacteremia (such as one resulting from dental manipulation) with subsequent endarteritis and possible endocardial infection.

A period of high susceptibility to infection is usually seen within the first 3 months after implantation, after which there is a gradual decline possibly caused by an "insulating effect" of the developing pseudointima. Because there is no way to know whether there is a well-developed pseudointima without removal and inspection, antibiotic prophylaxis is important.

The preferred antibiotic depends on many variables, but is primarily based on the type of microorganisms that have been cultured at the site of manipulation. It is noteworthy that in patients reported to have acquired infective endocarditis after dental treatment, either viridans or enterococcus groups of streptococci were the causative agents, therefore indicating the use of a prophylactic regimen of penicillin and streptomycin or a broad spectrum antibiotic such as amoxicillin (for quick blood levels) or vancomycin in patients with hypersensitivity to penicillin or streptomycin. All dosages should be adjusted with regard to the patient's decreased ability to clear the drugs owing to impaired renal function (see Table 21-3).

Infection is a major consideration in the dialysis patient. A majority of septicemic infections have been attributed to the vascular access site, but oral diseases such as periodontal disease, pulpal infection, and oral ulcerations, along with dental treatment may also provide a convenient portal of entry for microorganisms into the circulatory system.

Viral hepatitis B is another dental consideration when treating dialysis patients. Hepatitis B is a complication associated with the large numbers of transfusions and increased exposure of dialysis patients. Many of the patients with renal disease may have viral hepatitis without clinical manifestations; in these patients, the disease tends to run a chronic, persistently active though subclinical course. With the advent of the use of prophylactic immunoglobulin and the hepatitis B vaccine, the number of dialysis unit outbreaks of hepatitis has decreased; however, the dialysis patient should still be considered to be in a high-risk group. Until more sensitive tests with greater reliability are developed, all available precautions should be implemented to avoid the possible transmission of hepatitis B during dental treatment.

Bleeding may also be a problem for dentists treating dialysis patients. The dentist is presented with a patient with a reduced platelet count, increased capillary fragility, decreased platelet adhesiveness, and prolonged bleeding and clotting times, all of which may cause increased loss of blood. Hemorrhagic episodes from the gingiva are not uncommon. Ulcerations and purpural or petechial lesions may be noted on the oral mucosa. Bruising after trauma is common, and hematoma for-

Table 21-3. Drug Therapy in Renal Disease

| DRUG | Normal | ADJUSTMENTS FOR RENAL FAILURE | |
		Moderate Glomerular Filtration Rate 10–50	*Severe* Glomerular Filtration Rate < 10
Antifungal Agents			
Amphotericin	q 24 h	Unchanged	Unchanged
Miconazole	q 8 h	Unchanged	Unchanged
Aminoglycosides			
Gentamicin	q 8 h	q 12–24 h	Avoid if possible
Tobramycin	q 8 h	q 8–24 h	Avoid if possible
Streptomycin	q 12 h	Avoid if possible	Avoid if possible
Other Antimicrobials			
Penicillin G	q 6–8 h	q 8–12 h	q 12–18 h
Erythromycin	q 6 h	Unchanged	Unchanged
Ampicillin	q 6 h	q 6–12 h	q 12–16 h
Amoxicillin	q 8 h	q 8–12 h	q 12–16 h
Cephalothin	q 6 h	Unchanged	q 8–12 h
Carbenicillin	q 4 h	q 8–12 h	Avoid if possible
Analgesics			
Acetaminophen	q 4 h	q 6 h	q 8 h
Acetylsalicylic acid	q 4 h	q 4–6 h	Avoid
Phenacetin (APC)		Avoid	Avoid
Nonsteroidal anti-inflammatories		Avoid	Avoid
Narcotics			
Codeine	q 4 h	Unchanged	Unchanged
Meperidine (Demerol)	q 4 h	Unchanged	Unchanged
Morphine	q 4 h	Unchanged	Unchanged
Pentazocine (Talwin)	q 4–6 h	Unchanged	Unchanged
Propoxyphene (Darvon)	q 4 h	Unchanged	Unchanged
Naloxone (Narcan)	Bolus	Unchanged	Unchanged
Sedatives, Hypnotics, and Tranquilizers			
Chlordiazepoxide (Librium)	q 6–8 h	Unchanged	Unchanged
Diazepam (Valium)	q 8 h	Unchanged	Unchanged
Flurazepam (Dalmane)	q 24 h	Unchanged	Unchanged
Meprobamate (Miltown)	q 6 h	q 9–12 h	q 12–18 h
Methaqualone (Quaalude)	q 8 h	Unchanged	Unchanged
Amitriptyline (Elavil)	q 8 h	Unchanged	Unchanged
Antihistamines			
Chlorpheniramine (Chlortrimeton)	q 4–6 h	Unchanged	Unchanged
Diphenhydramine (Benadryl)	q 6 h	q 6–9 h	q 9–12 h
Corticosteroids			
Cortisone	q 8 h	Unchanged	Unchanged
Hydrocortisone	q 8 h	Unchanged	Unchanged
Prednisone	q 8 h	Unchanged	Unchanged
Neurologic			
Phenytoin (formerly diphenylhydantoin) (Dilantin)	q 8 h	Unchanged	Unchanged
Lidocaine		Unchanged	Unchanged

(Modified from Bennett WM et al: Guidelines for drug therapy in renal failure. Ann Intern Med 86:754, 1977)

mation is to be expected after alveolectomy or periodontal surgery. Though rare, hemorrhagic effusions into the temporomandibular joint space presenting as pain and swelling have been reported in a patient on dialysis and sodium warfarin therapy.

Medication in the dialysis patient is another major consideration. Most drugs are excreted at least partially by the kidney, and renal function affects drug bioavailability, volume of drug distribution, drug metabolism, and rate of drug elimination. The dentist can obviate problems of drug reactions and further renal damage by following simple principles related to drug administration and by altering dosage schedules according to the amount of residual renal function. Many ordinarily safe drugs must not be administered to the uremic patient, and many others must be prescribed in smaller doses or over longer intervals (see Table 21-3). The hydrogen ion, nitrogen, or electrolyte content of medications may be significant in renally diseases patients. Certain drugs may be metabolized to acid and nitrogenous waste or may stimulate tissue catabolism. Nonsteroidal anti-inflammatory drugs may induce sodium retention, impair the action of diuretics, prevent aldosterone production, and cause acidosis. Tetracyclines and steroids are antianabolic, increasing urea nitrogen to about twice the baseline levels. Other drugs such as phenacetin are nephrotoxic and put added strain on an already damaged kidney (see Table 21-4).

For most drugs, it is proper to give a loading dose similar to that given in patients without renal disease. This provides a clinically desirable blood concentration that can be sustained by the necessary dosage adjustments. Whenever reliable blood drug level measurements are available, they can be used to monitor therapy. In the absence of precise blood levels, the best guide to therapy is carefully obtained data on biological half-lives in humans with varying degrees of renal failure.

Fluorides and water fluoridation are another consideration in the dialysis patient. The safety of the fluoridated community water supply for patients in hemodialysis has been questioned as being a contributing factor to the incidence of renal osteodystrophy, fluoride toxicity, and fluorosis; however, there has been only one reported instance

Table 21-4. Drugs to Limit or Avoid When Treating Dialysis Patients

REASON FOR AVOIDANCE/LIMITATION	DRUG
Magnesium content	Antacids (Maalox, Riopan) Laxatives
Potassium content	IV fluids Salt substitutes Massive penicillin therapy (1.7 mEq/million units)
Sodium content	Carbenicillin (4.7 mEq/g) Alka Seltzer (23 mEq/tablet) IV fluid
Acidifying effects	Ascorbic acid Ammonium chloride (in cough syrup) Nonsteroidal anti-inflammatory agents
Catabolic effects	Tetracyclines Steroids
Nephrotoxicity	Phenacetin (APC) Cephalosporins, long term, especially when combined with gentamicin
Alkalosis effect	Absorbed antacids Carbenicillin (large doses) Penicillin (large doses)

(involving eight dialysis patients) of fluoride intoxication since fluoridation of community water supplies began. That instance was related to a spill of hydrofluosilicic acid into the water supply that was then used to mix the dialysates that were not deionized. There is no satisfactory evidence that the fluoride content of fluoridated drinking water is harmful to patients with severe renal disease. Dialysis patients, however, should receive dialysates that are water-purified and deionized. No studies have reported on the dental use of topical fluoride or any related problems in patient with renal disease. If a patient with renal disease needs fluoride supplements for caries control, the preferred delivery route should be fluoride rinses until more definitive studies are carried out. (Many of the precautions necessary with hemodialysis are not necessary with peritoneal dialysis because vascular access is not obtained. This includes antibiotic prophylaxis and anticoagulant problems.)

KIDNEY TRANSPLANTATION

Another method for prolonging life in patients with end-stage renal failure is renal transplantation. Although any improvement in the 5-year prognosis of patients undergoing renal transplantation compared with age and diseased matched patients undergoing maintenance dialysis may be controversial, there is no argument that the quality of life is far better following successful transplantation. Kidney transplants are being performed with increasing success, and mortality appears to be improving as physicians and surgeons become more willing to remove poorly functioning grafts. About 25,000 transplant patients are alive today with 5-year survivals approaching 60%.

Transplantation involves the surgical removal of a kidney from a donor and implantation of the kidney into a recipient. The donor may be from a living first-degree relative such as a sibling, parent, or child or a recently expired source (cadaver donor). Recipients of transplants from nonrelatives have less chance for graft survival. In all cases of transplantation except between monozygotic twins, transplantation rejection will occur, and the rejection reaction is mediated through the lymphocytic system. The antigens that precipitate the rejection reaction are called *histocompatibility antigens* and are located on the surfaces of all nucleated cells. The two major groupings of histocompatibility antigens are the human lymphocyte antigens (HLA) and the mixed lymphocyte culture (MLC) reaction. The immune reaction basically consists of a cell-mediated reaction in which the foreign antigens of a graft are recognized by immunocompetent cells of the recipient, which produce cytotoxic cells capable of destroying the stimulating antigen. A humoral response follows in which specific circulating antibodies are created against the graft, causing it to be rejected.

A definite correlation exists between histocompatibility matching and both graft survival and patient survival in renal transplants. All recipients and donors (including cadaver grafts) are tested for HLA similarity, index of stimulation on the MLC test, and compatibility in ABO blood type. Transplantation cannot successfully be performed when an ABO incompatibility is present.

Kidney transplant patients usually receive a continuous regimen of immunosuppressive medication to ensure graft survival. The usual drug regimen consists of a combination of an immunosuppressive agent and an anti-inflammatory glucocorticoid to prevent transplant rejection. Azathioprine (Imuran), the 5-imidazolyl derivative of 6-mercaptopurine, is the cornerstone of the immunosuppressive regimen, with doses ranging from 50 mg to 200 g per day. This drug produces an increased susceptibility to infection by impairing both humoral and cellular immunity. Clinical experience has shown that most infections are produced by endogenous organisms that cause disease during states of depressed immunologic capability. Patients who receive immunosuppressive drugs are more susceptible to gram-negative fungal and viral infections caused by a reduction in T-lymphocyte competence.

Along with immunosuppressive agents, corticosteroids are used in antirejection therapy. Prednisone is the preferred drug, in doses from 10 mg to 40 mg per day. Steroids may be given on an alterate day regimen that is as effective in graft survival and produces fewer adverse cushingoid effects than with daily use. Other medications and techniques used in order to retain the kidney include alkylating agents (cyclophosphamide), anti-lymphocyte globulin (a horse antihuman lymphocyte serum derivative), and local graft irradiation. The recipient may undergo splenectomy before transplantation to remove a bulk of immunologic tissue; these patients tolerate immunosuppressive therapy with less neutropenia and thrombocytopenia. Recently, deliberate donor-specific blood transfusions, before renal transplantation from a living relative have been used in cases where there is a one-haplotype matched donor with a high lymphocyte culture index to achieve better graft survival.

Clinical Manifestations

The majority of clinical manifestations in transplant patients occur secondary to the immunosuppresive drugs. The steroids are responsible for the cushingoid effects, characterized by a rapidly acquired adiposity about the upper portion of the body, mooning of the face, and a tendency to become round shouldered and develop a "buffalo hump" at the base of the neck. Hypogammaglobulinemia has developed in patients on high-dose steroids while taking immunosuppressive medication. The gamma globulin levels return to normal when dosages are decreased or temporarily discontinued.

Corticosteroids can cause increased susceptibility to fungal infections owing to decreased migration and impaired phagocytic function of leukocytes and macrophages. The diabetogenic effect of steroids may also predispose patients to infection, but steroids mask the normal warning signs of inflammation, such as redness, swelling, and pain. This alteration of normal signs and symptoms may make accurate diagnosis extremely difficult; further diagnostic confusion can arise from the suppressed febrile response, absolute and relative granulocytosis, and lymphopenia. Corticosteroids affect the healing potential. An excessive amount of cortisone inhibits fibroblast proliferation, reticulin deposition, new capillary formation, and synthesis of mucopolysaccharides. Bone matrix formation may be impaired with an interference in mineralization.

Azathioprine therapy may cause the following complications: bone marrow hypoplasia with decreased leukocyte and platelet counts, hepatic toxicity, pancreatitis, skin ulceration, and interference with the body's tumor surveillance mechanism, thereby promoting oncogenesis.

Oral Manifestations

The following are orofacial manifestations of renal transplantation:

- Pale mucosa with diminished color demarcation between attached gingiva and alveolar mucosa
- Enlarged (asymptomatic) salivary glands
- Odor of urea on breath
- Metallic taste
- Decreased salivary flow
- Dry mouth
- Enamel hypoplasia
- Dark brown stains on crowns
    Extrinsic—secondary degrees to liquid ferrous sulfate therapy
    Intrinsic—secondary to tetracycline staining

- Dental malocclusions
- Low caries rate
- Increased calculus formation
- Low-grade gingival inflammation
- Bleeding from gingiva and mouth
- Petechiae and ecchymosis
- Erosive glossitis
- Burning and tenderness with dryness of mucosa
- Candidal infections
- Dehiscence of wounds
- Demineralization of bone
- Loss of bony trabeculation
- Ground glass appearance
- Loss of lamina dura
- Gaint cell lesions—brown tumors
- Socket sclerosis

Azathioprine can produce stomatitis and drug-induced xerostomia. Another oral manifestation is candidal infections of the oral mucosa, which has been attributed to depression of cell-mediated immunity. Treatment consists of nystatin oral rinses or vaginal suppositories dissolved in the mouth four to five times a day. If compliance is a problem, ketoconizole 200 mg to 400 mg once daily can be substituted. More uncommon fungal infections such as mucormycosis and aspergillus have been reported numerous times in transplant patients. Treatment may consist of reduction in immunosuppressive drugs, debridement of infected areas, and judicious use of amphotericin B.

White plaquelike lesions of the oral mucosa have been reported in immunosuppressed renal transplant patients. These lesions resemble acute pseudomembranous candidiasis and can be scraped off, leaving a bleeding surface that fails to respond completely to antifungal therapy. The lesions represent a bacterial overgrowth of nonpathogens and not fungi, and the incidence follows periods of heavy-dosage steroid therapy. Perioral dermatitis, an entity characterized by red papules, small pustules, and some scaling on the chin, upper lip, and nasolabial fold, is also seen in transplant patients. The rapid response to doxycycline indicates an infective etiology in which normal skin flora become pathogenic in an immunologically compromised patient.

A recently attributed oral manifestation of immunosuppressive drug therapy is its rela-

Table 21-5. Review of Preoperative Dental Considerations and Clinical Management of the Patient with Renal Disease

PREOPERATIVE STATUS	MANAGEMENT
Dialysis	Dental treatment should be performed within 24 hours of dialysis to ensure optimal correction of hydration, serum electrolytes, urea nitrogen, creatinine, and coagulation defects.
Shunt	Consider the presence of heparin (which has a half-life of 4 to 6 hours) and its anticoagulation effect.
	Be aware of patient positioning; do not compromise the extremity that has the access site; avoid using the arm with the shunt for blood pressure readings or infusion of medications.
	The possibility of bacterial endocarditis exists.
	Discuss prophylactic antibiotics with patient's physician.
Hepatitis	Regard patient as being at high risk until proven otherwise; wear protective clothing (face mask, double gloves, protective glasses, disposable cap, gown).
	All instruments should be disposable or sterilizable by autoclaving, ethylene oxide, or dry heat.
	Sinks used to clean instruments should be thoroughly disinfected with hypochlorite preparation (at least 10,000 ppm of free chloride) once per day.
	During use, instruments should be placed on a disposable or sterilizable tray.
	Use of rubber dam is encouraged to minimize spread of handpiece aerosol spray.
	Operatory equipment and area should be wiped down with an approved operating room disinfectant after patient treatment.
Hypertension and impaired response	Monitor blood pressure, pre-, intra-, and postoperatively.
	Consider premedication with antianxiety agents.
Anemia and hemorrhage	Severity of anemia is important if general anesthesia is necessary.
	Obtain coagulation profile, including platelet count, prothrombin time, partial thromboplastin time, and bleeding time, because of the possibility of coagulopathy or effect from heparin-warfarin management.
	Anticipate hematoma formation after traumatic procedures (*e.g.*, periodontal surgery or alveolectomy).
	If multiple extractions will be done, consider treating a single or limited area on first visit to determine patient response.
	Anticipate delayed healing and consider keeping sutures in place for longer than usual.
	Dehiscence of wounds is a frequent complication.
Renal osteodystrophy	Recognize that many oral manifestations are associated with renal disease.
	Be aware of possible pathologic or iatrogenic fractures during oral surgery.
Medications	Consult with primary physician for discussion of any drugs to be used in dental treatment.
	Be aware of adverse or synergistic effects with any of the patient's other medications.
Infections	Consider premedication with antimicrobials (there are no established guidelines).

Table 21-5. Review of Preoperative Dental Considerations and Clinical Management of the Patient with Renal Disease

Preoperative Status	Management
	Suggestions
	Nystatin mouthwashes 500,000 units/ml four times per day, the day before dental treatment, the day of, and 2 days after.
	Obtain culture and sensitivity of area to be treated to assure proper antibiotic therapy.
	Start on broad-spectrum antibiotic (*e.g.,* ampicillin 1 g 1 hour before treatment, then 500 mg every 6 hours for eight dosages).
Immunosuppressive drug therapy (for transplant patients)	These patients are prone to infections; therefore, consider premedication with an antimicrobial agent.
	Obtain CBC and differential count to evaluate number of lymphocytes and neutrophils.
	Immunosuppressive therapy decreases granulocytes, T cells, IgG, IgA.
	There is a decreased periodontal response to local etiology and treatment.
Steroid therapy	Anticipate possible hypoadrenal crisis (monitor blood pressure throughout treatment).
	Consider supplemental steroids according to anticipated stress load.
	Observe patient for signs of the diabetogenic aspects of steroid therapy.
	Remember that steroids inhibit the inflammatory response.

tionship to periodontal disease. Studies have shown that persons on immunosuppressive therapy show no correlation between periodontal disease and age, plaque, or calculus and have less gingivitis than do normal patients with similar amounts of dental plaque. This may imply that a low-grade immune response is involved in the perpetuation of periodontal disease.

Dental Considerations

The successful management of the transplant patient begins before transplantation with the preoperative elimination of potential sources of infection. This includes any present or potential inflammatory pathosis of the dental, oral, and maxillofacial region. After transplantation, routine dental treatment should be postponed until maintenance doses of prednisone and azathioprine are reached.

Most transplant patients are ambulatory, and their dental needs can be serviced on an outpatient basis. Close dental supervision is essential in renal transplant patients because the consequences of previous renal disease as well as current medical regimens will affect their dental management (Table 21-5). Many dental problems seen in transplant patients are associated with immune-response alterations and the loss of host resistance secondary to their posttransplant medications.

Kidney transplant patients are placed on continuous regimens of immunosuppressive medication to reduce new organ rejection. These regimens can increase the risk of infection a majority of which are caused by microorganisms that normally are of little or no pathologic significance but that often cause serious or fatal infections in the patient with an impaired immunologic response.

Microorganisms found in the oral flora can cause many of these infections. These microorganisms include gram-negative bacteria such as *Klebsiella, Pseudomonas,* and *Proteus;* fungi such as *Candida, Aspergillus,* and *Mucor;* and viruses such as herpes simplex and herpes zoster. Periodontal disease, pulpal infection, and oral ulcers may cause the spread of these oral microorganisms into the bloodstream, or aspiration may cause them to spread to the respiratory tract. Oral infection in transplant patients has been reported as frequently as pneumonia or urinary tract infection, the most frequently reported infection in these patients. The systemic factors related to the development of oral infection are low lymphocyte count and an extended course of immunosuppressive drug therapy. Other studies have shown correlations between the development of infection and transplant patients with juvenile-onset diabetes. Hyperglycemia from steroid-induced diabetes has also been identified as an important risk factor in the development of infection after transplantation.

Prompt diagnosis of the site and cause of infection in immunosuppressed patients should be an extremely high priority. Identification of the pathogen should be performed with a culture, sensitivity, aspiration technique, or biopsy. This helps ensure proper antibiotic management because a wide variety of organisms may be found in these patients. Surgical drainage should be considered in infections not showing early and rapid improvement, and differential diagnosis must always include unusual or resistant organisms.

The difficult question of whether or not to discontinue immunosuppressive therapy during infection often arises. If a specific, highly effective antimicrobial agent is available to treat the infection in question, perhaps immunosuppression need not be discontinued; however, if such therapy is not available, restoration of the immune system would probably be necessary before control of infection could be acheived.

When kidney transplant patients present for dental treatment the amount of steroid medication they are taking must be considered in their management. Corticosteroid therapy at adrenal suppressive levels increases susceptibility to shock because the body may be unable to cope with the added stress of a dental procedure or the emotional stress associated with it. Dental treatment carries no more risk for the patient with adrenal insufficiency taking steroids than for a normal patient if certain precautions are followed. The amount of stress (physical and/or psychologic) that the patient is going to be subjected to should be considered. For procedures involving minimal stress, no change in steroid dosage need be considered; for short procedures involving mild to moderate stress, the dosage of oral steroids should be doubled the day before, the day of, and 2 days after treatment, or a single 100-mg dose of hydrocortisone hemisuccinate (Solu-Cortef) should be given intramuscularly just before treatment, and an extra 20-mg dose should be given early that evening, with resumption of prior therapy dosage the next day. For major stress (e.g., removal of impacted teeth), 100 mg hydrocortisone hemisuccinate IM is given every 6 hours, with the first dosage being given before the procedure. Adequate fluid, glucose, and electrolyte intakes must be provided. If recovery is satisfactory, the dosage of hydrocortisone should be reduced 50% each day for 3 days until the patient is taking 20 mg orally, twice daily. Hydrocortisone dosage at 20 mg twice daily is continued until the seventh day, and then prior therapy is resumed.

The following steps should be considered to ensure proper management of the renal transplant patient. The patient's physician should be consulted to coordinate treatment. A broad-spectrum antibiotic should be used in the prophylactic medication of the patient before dental treatment because of decreased immune response and the presence (usually) of an access site from previous dialysis. Because prednisone and azathioprine can cause myelosuppression, a complete blood count with differential and platelets should be obtained before any surgical procedure. If surgery is needed, culture and sensitivity testing of the area to be treated should be obtained. Simple operative dentistry can be accomplished in a routine manner, but impaired wound healing and hematoma formation should be expected in transplant patients. An increase in the steroid dose should be considered, and a supplemental dose of steroids should be available for administration, intramuscularly or intravenously, in the event of a hypoadrenal crisis. Vital signs must be monitored during the procedure. Antianxiety agents should be considered. With these precautions, the renal transplant patient can be treated as an outpatient in any dental setting, and reasonable reparative processes can be expected to take place.

BIBLIOGRAPHY

Adams SJ, Davison AM, Cunliffe WJ, Giles GR: Perioral dermatitis in renal transplant recipients maintained on corticosteroids and immunosuppressive therapy. Br J Dermatol 106:589, 1982

Adkins KF, Moule AJ: Drug-induced xerostomia: Cellular changes produced in parotid acinar cells by azathioprine. NZ Dent J 69:112, 1973

Anderson R et al: Fluoride intoxication in a dialysis unit. Maryland MMWR 29:134, 1980

Beaney GPE: Otolaryngeal problems arising during the management of severe renal failure. J Laryngol Otol 78:507, 1964

Bennett WM et al: Guidelines for drug therapy in renal failure. Ann Intern Med 86:754, 1977

Birkeland SA: Uremia as a state of immune deficiency. Scand J Immunol 5:107, 1976

Bookatz BN, Parker TF, Hunt WC: Oral problems related to kidney disease and management and care of patients after establishment of dialysis treatment. Arch Found Thantol 5:221, 1975

Bottomley WK, Cioffi RF, Martin AJ: Dental management of the patient treated by renal transplantation: Preoperative and postoperative considerations. J Am Dent Assoc 85:1330, 1972

Bryny RL: Preventing adrenal insufficiency during surgery. Grad Med 67:219, 1980

Burrell KH, Groepp RA: Abnormal bone repair in jaws, socket sclerosis: A sign of systemic disease. J Am Dent Assoc 87:1206, 1973

Carlin RJ, Seldin R: Oral ulcerations asociated with uremia. NY State Dent J 35:211, 1969

Chow MH, Peterson DS: Dental management for children with chronic renal failure undergoing hemodialysis therapy. Oral Surg 48:34, 1979

Cohen SG, Greenberg MS: Rhinomaxillary mucormycosis in a kidney transplant patient. Oral Surg 50:33, 1980

Cross AS, Steigbigel RT: Infective endocarditis and access site infections in patient on hemodialysis. Medicine 55:453, 1979

Dahlberg W, Sreebny L, King B: Studies of parotid saliva and blood in hemodialysis patients. Soc Appl Physiol 23:100, 1967

Epstein SR, Mandel I, Scopp IW: Salivary composition and calculus formation in patients undergoing hemodialysis. J Periodontol 51:336, 1980

Fletcher PD et al: Oral manifestations of secondary hyperparathyroidism related to long-term hemodialysis therapy. Oral Surg 43:218, 1977

Fluoridated water, hemodialysis, and renal disease. Med Let August 8, p. 67, 1969

Goodman JS et al: Bacterial endocarditis as a possible complication of chronic hemodialysis. N Engl J Med 280:876, 1969

Greenberg MS, Cohen SG: Oral infection in immunosuppressed transplant patients. Oral Surg 43:879, 1977

Gruskin SE, Tolman DE, Wagoner RD: Oral manifestations of uremia. Minn Med 53:495, 1970

Gutman RA, Amara AH: Outcome of therapy to end-stage uremia. Postgrad Med 64:183-184, 1978

Halazonetis J, Harley A: Uremic stomatitis. Oral Surg 23:573, 1967

Heard E, Staples AF, Czerwinski AW: The dental patient with renal disease, precautions and guidelines. J Am Dent Assoc 96:793, 1978

Herman LT, Friedman JM: Management of orofacial infection in patients with chronic renal disease. J Oral Surg 33:942–945, 1975

Holmes JH et al: The relation of salivary flow to the state of hydration in patients with uremia and renal failure. Trans Am Soc Artif Intern Organs 6:152, 1960

Hooley JR, Petersen WM: Dental management of patients with renal failure being treated by hemodialysis. Oral Surg 28:660, 1969

Houston JB et al: Radiography of secondary hyperparathyroidism. Oral Surg 26:746, 1964

Hovinga J, Roodvoets AP, Gaillard J: Some findings in patients with uremic stomatitis. J Maxillofac Surg 3:125–127, 1975

Jaspens MT: Unusual oral lesions in a uremic patient. Oral Surg 39:934, 1975

Kaneko Y et al: Eruption of permanent teeth of handicapped children. Bull Tokyo Dent Coll 18:99, 1977

Kardachi BJR, Newcomb GM: A clinical study of gingival inflammation in renal transplant recipients taking immunosuppressive drugs. J Periodontol 49:307. 1974

Kelly WH, Mirahmadi MK, Simon JH, Gorman JT: Radiographic changes of the jawbones in end-stage renal disease. Oral Surg 50:372, 1980

Krekeler G, Wilms H, Akuamua–Boateng E: Inflammatory pathology in the dental system in renal transplantation. Int J Oral Surg 9:383–386, 1980

Larato DC: Uremic stomatitis: Report of a case. J Periodontol 46:731–733, 1975

Lauttamus A et al: Oral manifestations in uremia. Proc Finn Dent Soc 70:50, 1974

Lieberman JA, Cohen SG: Management and treatment of the immunosuppressed renal transplant patient. J Endodont 6:881–884, 1980

Lindemann RA, Henson JL: The dental management of patients with vascular grafts placed in the treatment of arterial occlusive disease. J Am Dent Assoc 104:625–628, 1982

Merril A, Peterson LJ: Gingival hemorrhage secondary to uremia. Oral Surg 29:530, 1970

Oliver WJ et al: Hypoplastic enamel associated with the nephrotic syndrome. Pediatrics 32:399, 1963

Opelz G, Terasaki PI: International histocompatibility work-shop study on renal transplant. In

Terasaki PI (ed): Histocompatibility Testing 1980, pp 592–624. Los Angeles, CA, University of California Press.

Opelz G, Graver B, Terasaki PI: Induction of kidney graft survival rate for multiple transfusion. Lancet 1:1223, 1981

Oshrain HI, Mender S, Mandel ID: Periodontal status of patients with reduced immunocapacity. J Periodontol 50:185, 1979

Potter JL, Wilson HF: A dental survey of renal dialysis patients. Public Health, London 93:153, 1979

Rehorst ED, DeGroot GW: Preoperative management of glucocorticoid-dependent pedodontic patients. J Am Dent Assoc 93:809, 1976

Reyna J et al: Head and neck infections after renal transplantations. JAMA 247:3337, 1982

Rothstein D et al: Massive neck swelling secondary to uremic submaxillary gland involvement. Oral Surg 27:333, 1969

Salvatierra O et al: Deliberate donor-specific blood transfusions prior to living related renal transplantation. Ann Surg 192:543, 1980

Schuller PD, Freedman HL, Lewis DW: Periodontal status of renal transplant patients receiving immunosuppressive therapy. J Periodontol 44:167, 1973

Schweizer RT, Kountz SL, Belzer FO: Wound complications in recipients of renal transplants. Ann Surg 177:58, 1973

Shinaberger JH, Blumenkranz MJ: Dialysis therapy and transplantation in uremia. Postgrad Med 64:169, 1978

Shustorman S, Fallens FX: The prevalence of enamel defects in childhood nephrotic syndrome. J Dent Child 82:435, 1969

Soderholm G, Lysell L, Svensson A: Changes in the jaws in chronic renal insufficiency and hemodialysis. J Clin Periodontol 1:36, 1974

Sowell SB: Dental care for patients with renal failure and renal transplants. J Am Dent Assoc 104:171, 1982

Stuart FP, Simonian SJ, Hill JL: Special considerations in surgical management of patients on hemodialysis and after successful kidney transplantation. Surg Clin North Am 56:15, 1976

Tollefsen T, Saltvedt E, Koppang HS: The effect of immunosuppressive agents on periodontal disease in man. J Periodont Res 13:240, 1978

Tyldesley WR, Rother E, Sells RA: Oral lesions in renal transplant patients. J Oral Pathol 8:53, 1979

Westbrook SD: Dental management of patients receiving hemodialysis and kidney transplants. J Am Dent Assoc 96:464, 1978

Wyler DJ, Golde DW, Grausz H: Bacterial endocarditis in a patient with a saphenous vein graft A-V fistula receiving dental work. Calif Med 117:75, 1972

22

Hematologic Disease

MARTIN S. GREENBERG

MALCOLM A. LYNCH

LEUKOCYTE DISORDERS

General Considerations

To understand leukocyte disease, several aspects of normal function must be appreciated. Leukocytes originate from either the bone marrow or lymphoid tissue: granulocytes and monocytes are derived from the same stem-cell precursors in the bone marrow, while lymphocytes originate in the lymph nodes. The three types of granulocytes are neutrophils, eosinophils, and basophils. Neutrophils provide the first line of defense against bacterial invasion of the mucous membranes and skin, and three cellular functions must be intact for neutrophils to provide this protection against infection. They must respond to chemotactic stimuli and migrate to the site of tissue damage; they must be capable of phagocytosis; they must destroy bacteria through enzymatic activity. The risk of infection is increased if insufficient numbers of neutrophils are present or if one of the three actions of neutrophils is not intact. Neutrophil function is aided by the presence of immunoglobulins and complement, which help the neutrophils attach to the surface of microorganisms. If these proteins are not present, neutrophil function will decrease. The ability of neutrophils to destroy microorganisms with intracellular enzymes can be evaluated by the nitroblue tetrazolium reduction test (NBT). Normal neutrophils contain enzymes that convert colorless NBT to dark blue granules within the cell. When dark blue granules are not seen, neutrophils will not destroy bacteria.

The function of the other granulocytes, esoinophils and basophils, is not as well understood. Eosinophils may phagocytize foreign substances but cannot kill bacteria. Basophils migrate to tissues and act as mast cells in allergic reactions. Monocytes are immature cells when in the bloodstream and use the bloodstream briefly as a transportation system. Once in the tissues they mature to macrophages and are phagocytes active in the immunologic system. Lymphocytes are the primary cells involved in immunity. Both B and T lymphocytes are seen in the peripheral blood. A description of lymphocyte function is contained in the chapter on immunologic disease.

Peripheral blood contains approximately 4,000 to 11,000 white blood cells per cubic millimeter. The hematology laboratory also reports the differential white blood cell count, which reports the proportion of cell types by percentages. When interpreting the differential white blood cell count the clinician should not rely on the percentage to decide whether a cell type is increased or deficient because this number may be misleading. The clinician should determine the absolute number of each cell type by multiplying the total white count by the percentage. The absolute number is a more accurate reflection of disease because it maintains the relationship of the total to the differential count.

The normal range of the absolute number of white blood cells is as follows:

- Bands 0/mm^3 to 2,000/mm^3)
- Segmented neutrophils (3,000/mm^3 to 6,000/mm^3)
- Lymphocytes (1,500/mm^3 to 4,000/mm^3)
- Monocytes (200/mm^3 to 900/mm^3)
- Eosinophils (100/mm^3 to 700/mm^3)
- Basophils (20/mm^3 to 150/mm^3)

In this chapter, diseases of granulocytes will be described. (Lymphocyte disorders are described in the chapter on immunologic disease.) Diseases of granulocytes are divided into three major types: quantitative, qualitative, and myeloproliferative. Quantitative disorders result from an abnormal number of white cells, qualitative disorders result from poorly functioning cells, and myeloproliferative disease results from abnormal bone marrow cells present in the peripheral blood and includes myelofibrosis, myeloid metaplasia, and leukemia. Leukemia is the myeloproliferative disease described in this chapter.

Quantitative Disorders

Granulocytosis

Increases in the number of white blood cells may result from infection, tissue necrosis, allergic reactions, neoplastic diseases, inflammatory diseases, or any activity that increases epinephrine release such as stress or exercise. A persistent elevation of the white blood cell count with the absolute neutrophil count remaining above 30,000/mm³ is called a *leukemoid reaction*. This reaction, secondary to infection (often a severe viral infection), is distinguished from leukemia because in leukemoid reaction the cells are mature with only an occasional cell less mature than a band. A bone marrow examination is sometimes required to distinguish a leukemoid reaction from leukemia.

Granulocytopenia and Agranulocytosis

Granulocytopenia may occur alone or as part of a generalized suppression of the bone marrow also affecting the erythrocytes and platelets (aplastic anemia). A decrease in granulocytes chiefly results from a decrease in neutrophils, and most cases of granulocytopenia are known as neutropenia. The obvious problem for neutropenic patients is increased susceptibility to infection.

The normal absolute number of neutrophils in the peripheral blood is 3,000/mm³ to 6,000/mm³. Mild neutropenia is present when 1,000/mm³ to 2,000/mm³ neutrophils are present, moderate neutropenia when 500/mm³ to 1,000/mm³ neutrophils are present, and severe neutropenia when fewer than 500/mm³ neutrophils are present in the peripheral blood. The term *agranulocytosis* is used when no neutrophils are seen on a peripheral blood smear.

Neutropenia like anemia is not a disease itself but a sign of underlying disorder; it has a wide range of underlying causes. Certain infections decrease the number of neutrophils in the circulating blood because of increased migration of neutrophils into the tissues, sequestration of neutrophils, or direct toxic effect of the microorganism and its toxins on the blood marrow. Infections with hepatitis A or varicella zoster virus are commonly associated with neutropenia, and overwhelming bacterial infection, particularly septicemia, can be accompanied by neutropenia because the cells are used at rapid rate to overcome the infection. Diseases causing sequestration of neutrophils include systemic lupus erythematosus and Felty's syndrome. Hemodialysis patients experience a decrease in neutrophils owing to destruction by complement activated by the dialysis membrane.

The most common cause of neutropenia is drug reaction. The earliest cases of drug-related neutropenia were reported as reactions to coal tar derivatives and aminopyrine. It is now known that a large number of drugs can cause neutropenia or aplastic anemia. Neutropenia secondary to a drug reaction results from one of two phenomena, toxic or idiosyncratic. Toxic neutropenia occurs predictably in all persons who take the offending drugs at sufficient doses for long enough periods of time. These drugs interfere with DNA synthesis, protein synthesis, or mitosis. Drugs that act to cause toxic neutropenia include drugs used in cancer chemotherapy, benzene, and alcohol. Neutropenia secondary to ionizing radiation also results from a direct toxic effect on the division of bone marrow cells.

Idiosyncratic reactions are not dose related and occur only in a small percentage of individuals taking the drug. Idiosyncratic drug reactions causing neutropenia are thought to be either an immunologic reaction affecting the bone marrow or an inherited inability to properly metabolize the drug. Drugs that have an increased risk of causing idiosyncratic neutropenia include phenothiazides, phenylbutazone, sulfonamides, and chloramphenicol. Cimetidine, a drug that is now widely prescribed for peptic ulcer and other gastrointestinal disorders, has been recently described by several authors as a cause of severe neutropenia.

Clinical Manifestations. The most common complication of neutropenia is infection. The clinician must be aware that the localizing clinical signs of infection may be few or absent owing to a decreased inflammatory reaction. Swelling and pus will be minimal. The most common sign of infection in neutropenic patients is fever. Other common manifestations include mucosal ulcers, acute pharyngitis, and lymphadenopathy. Common sites of infection include the lungs, urinary tract, skin, rectum, and mouth. Acute bacterial infections are the most common and usually are caused by *Staphylococcus aureus* or gram-negative bacilli such as *Klebsiella, Pseudomonas,* and *Proteus.*

Treatment. First, the cause of the neutropenia must be determined. All drugs should be discontinued and the patient carefully observed for signs of infection. At the first sign of infection, cultures must be taken and the patient started on a regimen of combined antibiotics. A combination of carbenicillin, methicillin, and gentamicin is commonly used because of the broad coverage against most organisms known to cause infection in neutropenic patients, such as *Staphylococcus* species and gram-negative bacilli. Some medical centers use reverse isolation or sterile environments such as life islands or laminar flow beds to reduce the risk of infection. Other centers find that the psychological stress engendered by isolation is not worth the slight decrease in the incidence of infection.

Some hematologists treat neutropenia with white blood cell transfusions, but their routine use in neutropenic patients has been questioned by studies that show them to be of marginal value. Other treatment modalities depend on the cause of the neutropenia. Patients with antibodies to neutrophils benefit from corticosteroids; neutropenia associated with Felty's syndrome, a disease where neutrophils sequester in the spleen, benefit from splenectomy; allogeneic bone marrow transplantation has been used to treat patients with severe aplastic anemia when a suitable donor is available.

Oral and Dental Considerations. The most common oral sign of neutropenia is ulceration of the oral mucosa (see Fig. 22-1). Neu-tropenic ulcers differ from other oral ulcers in that they lack surrounding inflammation and are characterized by necrosis. Because the bacteria are poorly opposed by neutrophils the ulcers become large irregular, deep lesions that are extremely painful. The necrotic tissue is often foul smelling, a characteristic of fusospirochetal organisms, although invasion by species of *Staphylococcus*, or gram-negative bacilli is common.

Oral ulcers, advanced periodontal disease, pericoronitis, and pulpal infections in patients with severe neutropenia should be considered potentially life threatening because they may lead to bacteremia and septicemia. The infection must be cultured to determine the predominant organism, and the patient should be placed on the appropriate combination of parenteral antibiotics. Topical application of antibacterial mouth rinses may also be helpful for ulcers. Garfunkel and co-workers recommend the use of an individualized Omnivac splint made from a maxillary study cast. This splint covers the palatal lesions and carries medication in a well that continually bathes the oral ulcers. Combination of topical neomycin, bacitracin, and nystatin have been used to reduce the risk of severe infection. Chlorhexidine oral rinses are recommended by many dentists experienced in the management of neutropenic patients, but it is not approved by the Food and Drug Administration (FDA) for use as an oral rinse in the United States. The pain of the

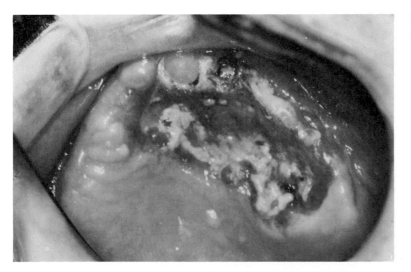

Fig. 22-1 Large palatal ulcer in neutropenic patient.

ulcers is reduced by the use of topical anesthetic mouth rinses. A solution containing 5% dyclonine and 5% diphenhydramine hydrochloride (Benadryl) mixed with magnesium hydroxide (Milk of Magnesia) or kaolin with pectin (Kaopectate) is useful for this purpose. Dental treatment for neutropenic patients is discussed in detail in the section on leukemia.

Cyclic Neutropenia

Cyclic neutropenia is a rare disorder secondary to a periodic failure of the stem cells in the bone marrow. Much of the current understanding of this disease has been deduced from observation of a similar periodic bone marrow failure in gray collie dogs that has served as a model for the human disease. The disease is frequently present during infancy or childhood and both sexes appear to be equally affected. The patient is healthy between neutropenic episodes, but at regular intervals the absolute neutrophil count falls quickly below 500/mm^3; in some patients the neutrophil count falls to 0. The frequency of the neutropenic episodes varies from 2 to 4 weeks with 21 days being the most common. The neutropenic period lasts from 3 to 5 days, after which the peripheral blood is rapidly replenished with mature neutrophils. Normal hematopoiesis is not constant in the bone marrow of patients with cyclic neutropenia, causing fluctuations in marrow platelet and erythrocyte precursors as well as granulocytes.

Clinical Manifestations. The major signs and symptoms of cyclic neutropenia are related to infection occurring during neutropenic episodes. The most common signs are fever, stomatitis, pharyngitis, and skin abscesses. The severity of the infections is related to the severity of the neutropenia. Some patients with severe periodic neutropenia experience few infections owing to a compensatory increase in monocytes, which act as phagocytes to prevent the spread of bacterial infection; less frequently, patients experience lung and urinary tract infections as well as rectal and vaginal ulcers. Cases of amyloidosis occurring in patients with cyclic neutropenia have been described and are thought

to be caused by the repeated increased antigenic stimulation during neutropenic episodes. One patient reportedly died of perforation of the intestine caused by massive amyloid deposition.

Treatment. The universally accepted treatment for most cases of cyclic neutropenia is careful monitoring of the patient for infection during neutropenic periods and vigorous early management of each infection. In some patients, use of corticosteroids, adrenocorticotropin (ACTH) or testosterone modulates the sharp reduction in marrow function. Unfortunately, use of these drugs is not successful for all patients.

Oral and Dental Considerations. Oral lesions are common in cyclic neutropenia and may be the major clinical manifestation of the disease. The two most common oral manifestations are oral mucosal ulcers and periodontal disease. The oral ulcers recur with each new bout of neutropenia and resemble the large, deep scarring ulcers seen in major aphthous stomatitis. The periodontal manifestations range from marginal gingivitis to rapidly advancing periodontal bone loss caused by bacterial infection of the dental supporting structures (see Figs. 22-2, 22-3, and 22-4). It is recommended that patients with major aphthous ulcers or generalized rapidly advancing periodontal disease that cannot be explained by local factors alone should have cyclic neutropenia ruled out as a possible cause. Suspicion of cyclic neutro-

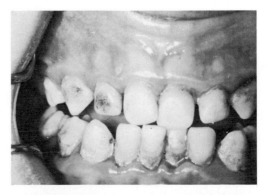

Fig. 22-2 Gingival changes in cyclic neutropenia. (Cohen DW, Morris AL: J Periodont 32:159)

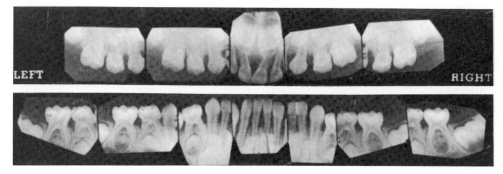

Fig. 22-3 Full-mouth radiographs of a 4-year-old boy with cyclic neutropenia showing resorption of the alveolar and supporting bone. (Cohen DW, Morris AL: J Periodont 32:159)

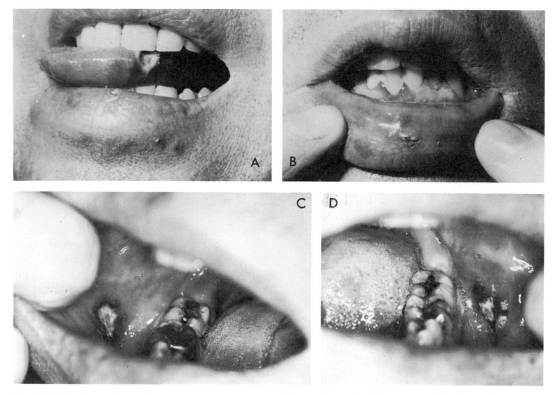

Fig. 22-4 Lesions of cyclic neutropenia on second day of attack: (*A*) tongue, (*B*) lip and gingival margins, (*C, D*) cheek lesions. (Levy EJ, Schetman D: Arch Dermatol 84:432)

penia should be particularly high when either of these oral diseases is seen in children.

The clinician must remember that a single white blood cell count is not sufficient to rule out the diagnosis of cyclic neutropenia because the examination may be performed as the peripheral neutrophils are being replenished. A series of three total and differential white blood cell counts per week for 4 to 6 weeks is necessary to rule out this disease. Patients with known cyclic neutropenia require dental treatment to minimize periodontal disease. Routine treatment should be confined to the periods when the absolute neutrophil count is above 2,000/mm³. A white count taken the day of a dental procedure is a wise precaution because the neutrophil count can rapidly change. Oral hygiene must be carefully maintained, and patients should be recalled for oral hygiene every 2 to 3 months.

Qualitative Leukocyte Disorders

Lazy Leukocyte Syndrome

First described by Miller, Oski, and Harris in 1971, lazy leukocyte syndrome is caused by loss of the chemotactic function of neutrophils. The bone marrow contains normal numbers of mature neutrophils, but the patients have severe neutropenia because the cells are unable to migrate from the marrow to the peripheral blood. The infections observed in these patients result from the neutropenia and the fact that the neutrophils present in the peripheral blood cannot migrate to the site of tissue injury although phagocytic and bactericidal functions remain intact. Pinkerton and co-workers studied the granulocytes from a patient with lazy leukocyte syndrome using scanning electron microscopy and demonstrated alterations on the surface of the cell membrane that were manifest as abnormal knoblike projections. The true incidence of the disease is unknown, because tests of neutrophil chemotaxis are not performed on all children with neutropenia. Yoda and associates described a case of transient lazy leukocyte syndrome that had spontaneous remission at 16 months of age.

Clinical Manifestations. The clinical manifestations of lazy leukocyte syndrome become apparent at age 1 to 2 years when infectious complications begin. The most common infections noted are gingivitis, stomatitis, otitis media, and bronchitis. The total white blood cell count is in the low normal range, but the absolute neutrophil count is as low as $100/mm^3$ to $200/mm^3$. Erythrocytes and platelets are normal. The diagnosis is based on neutrophil mobilization tests showing lack of normal response to epinephrine and piromen (a *Pseudomonas* polysaccharide). Inflammatory stimulation using skin windows will show little neutrophil migration, while tests for phagocytosis and bactericidal activity (nitro-blue tetrazolium dye reduction) will be normal.

Oral and Dental Considerations. Gingivitis and stomatitis are early and common signs described in patients with lazy leukocyte syndrome. The inability of neutrophils to function normally is frequently associated with periodontal disease. Cianciola and co-workers studied patients with idiopathic juvenile periodontitis (periodontosis); the neutrophils from these patients were defective in chemotaxis and phagocytosis.

Chédiak-Higashi Syndrome

First described just over 30 years ago, Chédiak-Higashi syndrome is a congenital, autosomal recessive defect of granule-containing cells such as granulocytes and melanocytes. Abnormal granules have also been observed in renal tubular cells, nerve cells, and fibroblasts. Mice, cats, mink, and cattle as well as man are susceptible to this hereditary defect. The giant melanosomes in skin and hair result in pigment dilution. The abnormal granules seen in all blood granulocytes result in neutrophils with decreased chemotactic and bactericidal ability, although phagocytosis remains intact. The abnormality in bactericidal activity is thought to be caused by an inefficient utilization of lysosomal enzymes.

Clinical Manifestations. Hypopigmentation resulting from the pigment dilution will be noted in skin and hair during infancy. The hair will have gray streaks. The defects of the neutrophils cause recurrent bacterial infections of the skin and respiratory tract, caused chiefly by gram-positive organisms such as *Staphylococcus aureus* and beta-hemolytic *Streptococcus*. This differs from the infections seen in patients neutropenic from leukemia or cancer chemotherapy, in whom gram-negative bacilli cause the majority of infections. Patients usually die of recurrent infections before the age of 10. Patients who survive the recurrent infections experience an accelerated phase of the disease that resembles lymphoma. The lymph nodes, spleen, liver, and bone marrow become infiltrated with lymphohistiocytic cells. This accelerated phase of the disease is generally fatal. Diagnosis of Chédiak-Higashi syndrome is based on the pathognomonic giant blue-gray granules seen in the cytoplasm of granulocytes when examining a peripheral blood smear.

Treatment. Medical management of Chédiak-Higashi syndrome in infants centers on rigorous treatment of infections as soon as they occur. Because gram-positive organisms cause a majority of infections, the infections respond well to antibiotics. An interesting case was reported by Boxer and co-workers, who treated an 11-month-old Chédiak-Higashi patient with 200 mg ascorbic acid daily. The treatment increased the chemotactic and bactericidal capacities of the neutrophils. Vincristine and prednisone therapy has been used to treat the accelerated phase of the disease.

Oral and Dental Considerations. Gingival and periodontal disease are common findings in patients with Chédiak-Higashi syndrome, and early loss of teeth owing to periodontal disease and caries is frequently mentioned. Blum and Wolff described four cases of which three had gingival and periodontal disease; two of the four had all of their teeth extracted in childhood. Temple and colleagues studied the periodontal health of four patients with Chédiak-Higashi syndrome. The two younger patients, ages 10 and 13, exhibited severe gingivitis, periodontal pockets, and mobility of teeth, the older patients, ages 19 and 20, already had all of their teeth removed because of advanced periodontal disease.

Chronic Idiopathic Neutropenia

Reports of long-standing, severe neutropenia with few associated abnormalities have appeared in the literature under a variety of names including familial neutropenia, chronic benign neutropenia, chronic neutropenia, and hypoplastic neutropenia. These cases resemble each other and are described as a group in this section—chronic idiopathic neutropenia (CIN). The etiology of this group of disorders is unknown, but they are characterized by a decreased production of neutrophils in the bone marrow. Some patients have antineutrophil antibodies detectable in

the serum and comprise a subset of patients with so-called chronic immunoneutropenia.

Because the disorder is uncommon, most reports have described only a few cases. One paper by Dale and associates summarized the findings of 29 patients examined at the National Institutes of Health. The cases were predominantly in females; some cases were familial, but they did not differ clinically from cases with no evidence of an inherited disorder. Only one of the patients tested had antibody to neutrophils. The bone marrow of patients with chronic idiopathic neutropenia shows a normal number of immature cells but a decrease in the number of mature neutrophils. This phenomenon has been called *maturation arrest*, but the reason for this problem is unclear. Increased margination of neutrophils has been noted in some cases.

Clinical Manifestations. Many patients with CIN are asymptomatic and free from infections even though the absolute neutrophil count may be below 500/mm^3. This is caused by a compensatory monocytosis, which accounts for a normal number of phagocytes present at the site of a tissue injury. Kyle described 15 CIN patients with absolute neutrophil counts ranging from 0/mm^3 to 696/mm^3; none of the patients experienced any serious sequelae.

A minority of patients do experience recurrent bacterial infections, although these are rarely of a life-threatening nature. The most common infections are recurring upper respiratory tract infections, otitis media, bronchitis, and furunculosis. Oral ulcers, periodontal disease, sinusitis, and perirectal infections also occur.

Treatment. Management of CIN often involves refraining from overtreating patients who are asymptomatic. Patients who develop severe recurrent infections benefit from alternate-day corticosteroid therapy. The bacterial infections that develop are usually gram-positive and respond well to antibiotic therapy. The risk of serious infection remains low in a significant majority of these patients.

Oral and Dental Considerations. There have been many isolated case reports of patients with CIN with oral signs and symptoms.

These patients also had a history of other recurring infections especially of the skin and upper respiratory tract. Deasy and colleagues reported two siblings with CIN: the brother had a history of recurring skin and respiratory infections and also had severe oral signs; the sister had neutropenia but no problem with infections and no increased oral disease.

The most distressing oral problem repeatedly reported in CIN patients is severe, rapidly advancing periodontal disease. The gingivae appear intensely red with granulomatous margins. Severe gingival recession is common, and early severe periodontal disease with advanced bone loss, mobility, denuded roots, and loss of teeth has been described by several authors. These changes occur early in life. One may question the finding of intense red gingiva in patients with few neutrophils. This consistent clinical finding coincides with the observations of Allstrom, who studied the gingiva of neutropenic dogs. The gingiva of the dogs was intensely red owing to an exaggerated vascular response. A second common oral finding in CIN patients is recurring oral ulcers (see Fig. 22-5). In Dale's study, 13 of the 29 patients experienced oral ulcers, and the ulcers did *not* correlate with the severity of the neutropenia. Gates described a case of a 24-year-old CIN patient who developed a severe infection secondary to an oral ulcer.

The dental management of CIN patients

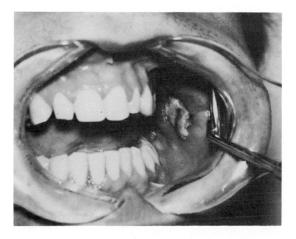

Fig. 22-5 Ulcer of the buccal mucosa in a patient with chronic idiopathic neutropenia. The ulcer was infected with gram-negative enteric bacilli.

should depend on their past history of infections. The dentist should remember that even a CIN patient with severe neutropenia may not be highly susceptible to infection owing to a compensatory monocytosis. If a CIN patient has never experienced an infection, it would not be reasonable to take extraordinary precautions for routine dental procedures.

Leukemia

Leukemia is a malignancy affecting the white blood cells of the bone marrow. The malignant cells replace and turn off the normal marrow elements causing anemia, thrombocytopenia, and a deficiency of normally functioning leukocytes. In time, the leukemic cells infiltrate other body organs destroying normal tissue. Leukemia is classified as either acute or chronic as well as by cell type. The etiology of leukemia is unknown, but several factors that increase the risk of the disease are well established. Radiation in doses over 100 rad is known to significantly increase the risk of leukemia. A high incidence of leukemia was observed in survivors of atomic blasts and in early radiologists. It is controversial whether lower doses of radiation also increase the risk of the disease, but until conclusive evidence is found, it is prudent to minimize radiation exposure to both clinicians and patients.

Exposure to certain chemicals and drugs has been related to an increased risk of leukemia. Benzene has been related to leukemia, and acute leukemia has been reported after the use of the arthritis drug phenylbutazone and the antibiotic chloramphenicol. Patients treated with certain anticancer drugs have an increased risk of developing leukemia; particularly susceptible are patients treated for lymphoma with chemotherapy and radiation.

Viruses are major suspects as etiologic factors because they have been shown to cause cancers in lower animals. No conclusive evidence yet exists for a leukemia virus in man, but genetic diseases have been related to an increased leukemia incidence, particularly Down's syndrome and sex-linked agammaglobulinemia.

Acute Leukemia

The acute leukemias are divided into two major clinical types: acute lymphocytic (ALL) and acute nonlymphocytic (ANLL). The majority of cases of ANLL are acute myelocytic leukemia; other cell types of ANLL include promyelocytic monocytic, myelomonocytic, and rarely erythroleukemia, a malignancy involving the stem cell precursor of both red and white blood cells. The various forms of ANLL are grouped together by clinicians because the treatments are similar.

Clinical Manifestations. Acute leukemia can occur at any age, but ALL is the leukemia commonly found in children while ANLL occurs more frequently in adults. The symptoms and signs of acute leukemia result from either bone marrow suppression or infiltration of leukemic cells into other organs and tissues. The bone marrow changes cause anemia, thrombocytopenia, and a decrease in normally functioning neutrophils. The anemia results in pallor, shortness of breath, and fatigue, which is the most common presenting symptom.

Thrombocytopenia will cause spontaneous bleeding such as petechiae, ecchymoses, epistaxis, melena, increased menstrual bleeding, and gingival bleeding when the platelet count falls below 25,000/mm^3. Approximately 50% of patients have some complaint of purpura or bleeding at the time of diagnosis. Although most bleeding results from decreased numbers of platelets, disseminated intravascular coagulation (DIC) can result from substances released from leukemic cells, which activate coagulation. These patients, who usually have promyelocytic leukemia, have the ironic combination of thrombosis as well as hemorrhage owing to depletion of coagulation factors.

Although leukemic patients often present with a greatly increased number of leukocytes, these leukemic cells do not function normally in migration, phagocytosis, or bactericidal action. Infection is therefore a frequent complication of the disease and is the most common cause of morbidity and mortality. Fever is an early sign of disease owing to recurrent infections of the lungs, urinary tract, skin, mouth, rectum, and upper respiratory tract. Infiltration of organs and tissues by leukemic cells causes lymphadenopathy, hepatomegaly, and splenomegaly. Cells may infiltrate the central nervous system or peripheral nerves leading to cranial nerve palsy, paresthesia, anesthesia, and paralysis. Localized tumors consisting of leukemic cells are called chloromas. The surface of these tumors turns green when exposed to light because of the presence of myeloperoxidase.

The diagnosis of acute leukemia is made with laboratory examination of the peripheral blood and bone marrow. The peripheral white blood cell count is usually elevated, but some cases present with normal or decreased white cell counts; these cases are called *subleukemic* or *aleukemic* leukemia. In most cases significant numbers of immature granulocytic or lymphocytic precursors or even stem cells are present in the peripheral blood accompanied by a significant anemia and thrombocytopenia. Microscopic examination of a bone marrow aspirate finalizes the diagnosis.

Treatment. Use of antileukemic chemotherapeutic drugs is the treatment of choice for patients with acute leukemia. The cytotoxic drugs are used in doses that kill 99% to 99.9% of leukemic cells. When the natural defenses of the body eliminate the remainder of the malignant cells the patient achieves a remission of the disease. Therapy is divided into stages: induction therapy attempts to achieve a remission of disease, while consolidation therapy attempts to maintain the remission.

The chemotherapy used depends on the type of leukemia. The treatment of ALL in children is one of the dramatic success stories of the use of cancer chemotherapy. Previously, ALL patients died in months, but now over 90% of children achieve complete remissions, and 50% of these remissions are prolonged enough to be considered cures. The term *complete remission* is used when the patient is asymptomatic and laboratory tests return to normal. A combination of drugs has been found to be more effective than a single agent. The combination of vincristine and prednisone has been widely used in the treatment of ALL.

The treatment of ANLL has not been as successful, and most patients die within 2 years of diagnosis. A major reason for the high mortality is the toxicity of the combination of drugs used to treat ANLL. A common drug combination used to treat ANLL is daunorubicin, arabinosyl cytosine, and 6-thioguanine (DAT). This highly toxic combination essentially depletes the marrow of normal elements during the induction phase.

In addition to chemotherapy, treatment of acute leukemia includes supportive care during the severe bone marrow aplasia. The use of platelet transfusions has significantly reduced the mortality from hemorrhage; packed red blood cells are widely used to decrease the signs and symptoms of anemia; and heparin is administered to patients with DIC to prevent thrombosis.

Infection, especially with bacteria and fungi, is the major cause of death in leukemic patients because of their increased susceptibility to infection from the disease process itself as well as from the bone marrow aplasia caused by toxic chemotherapy. Infections with gram-negative bacilli, such as *Pseudomonas, Klebsiella,* and *Proteus* are common as are fungal infections with *Candida, Aspergillus,* and *Phycomycetes.* Early diagnosis and prompt treatment of infections of the urinary tract, respiratory tract, rectum, skin, and mouth are necessary. Generalized viral infections, especially with herpes simplex, varicella zoster, and cytomegalovirus are also common complications (see Fig. 22-6).

Chronic Leukemia

Chronic leukemias are characterized by the presence of large numbers of well-differentiated cells in the bone marrow, peripheral blood, and tissues and a prolonged clinical course even without therapy. This distinguishes chronic leukemia from acute leukemia, in which immature cells predominate and the untreated clinical course leads to death in months. The two major types of chronic leukemia are chronic granulocytic and chronic lymphocytic leukemias, which differ in natural history, clinical presentation, prognosis, and treatment.

Chronic Granulocytic Leukemia

Chronic granulocytic leukemia (CGL) was the first type of leukemia identified by physicians in the 1840s, when macroscopic changes in the blood were noted in patients with spenomegaly. CGL is the form of leukemia most closely related to exposure to ionizing radiation and toxic chemicals. The disease is identified by genetic changes seen in the patient's chromosomes: 90% of CGL patients have the Philadelphia chromosome, an acquired genetic defect resulting from translocation of genetic material from chromosome 22 to a

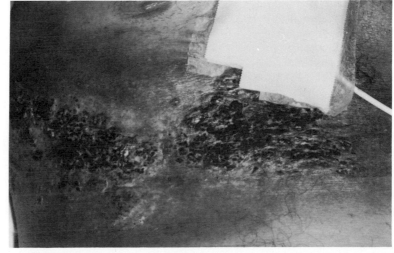

Fig. 22-6 Herpes zoster that developed during chemotherapy of acute leukemia.

second chromosome; another change is the depletion of leukocyte alkaline phosphatase. These two biochemical abnormalities are not present in the other forms of leukemia.

CGL has two phases: chronic and blastic. During the chronic phase, large numbers of granulocytes are present in the bone marrow and peripheral blood, but the cells retain normal functions. It takes between 5 and 8 years after the formation of the first CGL cell for clinical signs and symptoms to develop. The blastic phase, which takes place 2 to 4 years after diagnosis, is characterized by further malignant transformation to immature cells, which act similar to cells in acute leukemia.

Clinical Manifestations. CGL occurs most frequently in patients between the ages of 30 and 50. No symptoms are noted by the patient during the first few years, and the disease may be discovered during a routine examination when splenomegaly or an elevated white blood cell count will be noted. Early signs and symptoms are usually secondary to anemia or the packing of leukocytes into the spleen and bone marrow. The anemia causes weakness, fatigue, and dyspnea on exertion, while bone pain or abdominal pain in the upper left quadrant results from the spleen and bone marrow changes. As the disease progresses, thrombocytopenia can cause petechiae and ecchymosis as well as hemorrhage.

Laboratory tests taken during this stage show a markedly elevated white blood cell count that may reach several hundred thousand leukocytes per cubic millimeter. The bone marrow will be hypercellular. Diagnosis is confirmed by presence of the Philadelphia chromosome in 90% of cases and the absence of leukocyte alkaline phosphatase. The patient often survives for years before the disease enters the blastic phase. Transformation of the blastic phase may occur suddenly or slowly develop over a course of months. The symptoms caused by splenomegaly worsen, and other organs, particularly the liver, lymph nodes, and skin, become involved. Death occurs within months after the blastic phase begins.

Treatment. Control of the chronic phase of CGL is often successful. If the disease is dis-

covered while the patient is asymptomatic, only careful monitoring is necessary. When symptoms begin, the most common treatment is use of busulfan or other alkylating agents; radiation is used to shrink the size of a massively enlarged spleen. The disease is controlled during the chronic phase with chemotherapy and radiation, but true remissions are rare. The blastic phase of the disease is refractory to treatment. Life may be occasionally prolonged by use of chemotherapy protocols used in the treatment of acute leukemia.

Chronic Lymphocytic Leukemia

Chronic lymphocytic leukemia (CLL) results from a slowly progressing malignancy involving the lymphocytes. Most cases involve the B lymphocytes, which are responsible for immunoglobulin synthesis. The CLL B lymphocytes do not carry out their normal immunologic function and do not differentiate into normal immunoglobulin producing plasma cells when exposed to antigen. One reason the disease progresses slowly is that unlike the cells in other forms of leukemia, the CLL cells do not turn off normal marrow cells until late in the course of the disease. Occasional cases of T lymphocytic CLL have been reported.

Clinical Manifestations. CLL occurs most frequently in males over 40, with 60 being the most common age of onset. As a result of the slow natural history, it is not uncommon for the disease to be detected by a routine hemogram before any signs or symptoms are apparent. The peripheral blood will show many small well-differentiated lymphocytes: hundreds of thousands, even millions of cells/mm^3 may be present in the peripheral blood. The asymptomatic phase of the disease may last for years, but eventually signs and symptoms of infiltration of leukemic cells in the bone marrow, lymph nodes, or other tissues will appear. Bone marrow infiltration causes anemia, and thrombocytopenia and results in pallor, weakness, dyspnea, and purpura. Infiltration of other tissues causes lymphadenopathy, splenomegaly, hepatomegaly, and leukemic infiltrates of skin or mucosa. Cervical lymphadenopathy and tonsillar enlargement are frequent head and neck signs of CLL.

CLL patients exhibit some degree of hypogammaglobulinemia with an increased susceptibility to bacterial infection. Infection with varicella zoster virus is also common. Late in the disease, massive lymphadenopathy may cause intestinal or urethral obstruction and obstructive jaundice. Leukemic infiltrates result in skin masses, liver dysfunction, intestinal malabsorption, pulmonary obstruction, or compression of the central or peripheral nervous system. Abnormal immunoglobulins may cause hemolytic anemia or thrombocytopenia.

Treatment. Most oncologists will not treat asymptomatic all CLL patients with chemotherapy because there is presently no convincing evidence that early treatment enhances survival. When signs and symptoms of disease appear, alkylating agents such as chlorambucil or cyclophosphamide are administered. The chemotherapeutic drug may be given in conjunction with corticosteroids, which help to destroy lymphocytes as well as to control the hyperimmune effects on the erythrocytes and platelets. Radiation may also be used in some cases.

Oral and Dental Considerations in Leukemia

The oral manifestations of leukemia depend on the general status of the patient. Bone marrow suppression, effects of chemotherapy, and leukemic infiltrates cause a wide range of oral disease that have been reported by many clinicians. The most common sign of leukemia observed in a region routinely examined by a dentist is cervical lymphadenopathy owing to infiltration of leukemic cells into the lymph nodes. Lynch and Ship reported cervical adenopathy in 44% of patients with acute leukemia and 29% of patients with chronic leukemia. Michaud and associates found cervical lymphadenopathy in 40% of children with ALL.

Thrombocytopenia and anemia caused by marrow suppression from disease and chemotherapy result in pallor of the mucosa, petechiae, and ecchymoses as well as gingival bleeding (see Fig. 22-7). Michaud and co-

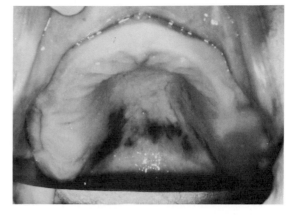

Fig. 22-7 Ecchymosis of the palate in a patient with thrombocytopenia secondary to acute leukemia.

workers detected purpura in 60% and spontaneous gingival bleeding in 20% of ALL patients while Lynch and Ship found purpura reported in 36% of acute leukemic patients (see Fig. 22-8). The extent of gingival bleeding depends on the severity of the thrombocytopenia as well as local irritants. Spontaneous gingival bleeding is common when the platelet count falls below 10,000/mm^3; severe gingival bleeding may frequently be managed successfully with localized treatment, reducing the need for platelet transfusions. The dentist should always weigh the risk of platelet transfusions against their benefit before recommending their use for treatment of oral bleeding. The risks of platelet transfusion include hepatitis, transfusion reactions, and the formation of antiplatelet antibodies, which reduces the usefulness of platelet transfusions during future hemorrhagic episodes.

Topical treatment to stop gingival bleeding should always include removing obvious local irritants and direct pressure. Splints and periodontal packs do not replace finger pressure for controlling acute bleeding. The use of absorbable gelatin sponges with topical thrombin or the placement of microfibrillar collagen held in place by packing, or splints are helpful. Some workers have reported successful management of gingival bleeding with oral rinses of antifibrinolytic agents. If these local measures are not successful in stopping significant gingival hemorrhage, platelet transfusions are necessary. The den-

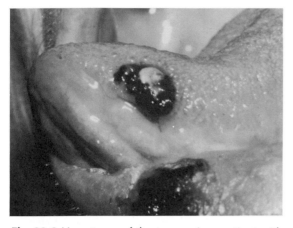

Fig. 22-8 Hematoma of the tongue in a patient with thrombocytopenia secondary to acute leukemia.

tist should remember that a few cases of bleeding will be caused by disseminated intravascular coagulation rather than by thrombocytopenia.

Oral Ulcers. Oral mucosal ulcers are common findings in leukemic patients taking chemotherapy and are frequently caused by the direct effect of chemotherapeutic drugs on the oral mucosal cells. Lockhart and Sonis reported that ulcers secondary to chemotherapy begin approximately 7 days following the start of treatment. Bacterial invasion secondary to severe neutropenia also plays a role in the formation of oral ulcers, and these lesions may be seen as an early sign of disease (see Fig. 22-9). The ulcers are characteristically large, irregular, foul smelling, and surrounded by pale mucosa caused by anemia and a lack of normal inflammatory response. Oral ulcers may also result from viral infection with herpes simplex or herpes zoster, and these lesions tend to be larger and last longer than herpetic lesions seen in normal patients. Some patients develop larg, chronic peretic ulcers (see section on chronic herpes in Chap. 5); use of antiviral agents such as acyclovir should be considered in these cases.

The management of oral ulcers in leukemic patients should prevent the spread of localized infection, minimize bacteremia, promote healing, and reduce pain. The ulcers in hospitalized leukemic patients taking chemotherpy may be infected with organisms not commonly associated with oral infection, particularly gram-negative enteric bacilli. (Dreizen and co-workers have described oral ulcers infected with these organisms). Ulcers infected with *Pseudomonas* were described as raised, dry, nonpurulent lesions, sharply demarcated from the surrounding tissue. Cultures should be obtained of oral ulcers seen in neutropenic leukemic patients so that the appropriate antibiotic treatment can be instituted. Topical antibacterial treatment can be attempted with povidone-iodine solutions, bacitracin-neomycin creams, or tetracycline rinses. The clinician should remember that tetracycline rinses increase the risk of candidiasis and must be accompanied by nystatin rinses. Chlorhexadine has been used extensively, but is not FDA approved for this purpose in the United States. Dyclonine (Dyclone) and diphenhydramine (Benadryl) oral rinses can be used effectively to reduce pain.

Oral Infections. Oral infection is a serious, potentially fatal complication in neutropenic leukemic patients. Candidiasis is a common oral fungal infection, but infections with other fungi such as *Histoplasma*, *Aspergillus*, or Phycomycetes may also begin on the oral tissues. When these lesions are suspected, a biopsy must be taken because a culture is not a reliable test for these organisms.

Diagnosis of dental infection particularly periodontal and pericoronal infections is difficult in neutropenic leukemic patients because normal inflammation is absent. The

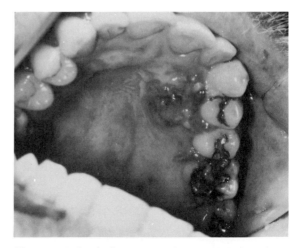

Fig. 22-9 Palatal ulcer as initial presentation of acute nonlymphocytic leukemia.

early diagnosis of oral infection is imperative because it has been demonstrated that oral disease is a significant source of potentially life-threatening infections with gram-positive as well as gram-negative bacilli. Peterson and Overholser carried out a retrospective analysis of 38 charts of ANLL patients showing that 12 of 22 infections were oral; periodontal disease was the most common source of infection. Greenberg, Cohen, and co-workers carried out a prospective study of the oral flora in 33 ANLL patients. The oral flora and oral disease was the most likely source of septicemia in 7 of 12 cases. Dental treatment to eliminate potential sources of oral infection such as pericoronal flaps or teeth with moderate to severe periodontal disease was accompanied by a significant reduction in the rate of septicemia. It is the obligation of dentists to carry out screening examinations and eliminate sources of infection before instituting chemotherapy, although platelet transfusions, intravenous combinations of antibiotics, and in some cases, white blood cell transfusions may be required before dental treatment.

Oral signs may also result from the presence of leukemic infiltrates. These are most frequently reported as gingival infiltrates in patients with myelomonoblastic leukemia or acute promyelocytic leukemia (Figs. 22-10, 22-11, and 22-12). Reports of leukemic infiltrates involving the palate, aleolvar bone, and dental pulp have also been reported. Segelman reported gingival infiltrates in 5 of 25 leukemic patients. These lesions were not proven by biopsy but did regress after chemotherapy. Leukemic infiltrates may cause oral signs and symptoms because of involvement of the 5th and 7th cranial nerves. Disorders of the 5th and 7th cranial nerves have also been reported in leukemic patients as a result of the use of vincristine, a drug commonly used to treat ALL.

Lymphoma

The lymphomas are a group of malignant solid tumors involving cells of the lymphoreticular or immune system, for example, B lymphocytes, T lymphocytes, and monocytes. Lymphomas are divided into two major categories: Hodgkin's disease and non-

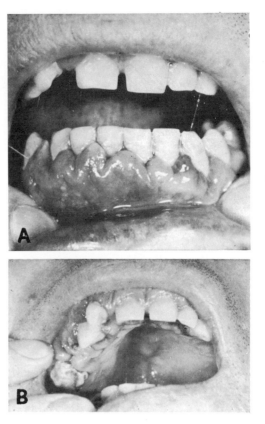

Fig. 22-10 *A,* Gingival hypertrophy associated with myelogenous leukemia. Patient sought dental treatment for hypertrophied gums. WBC 180,000/mm³ with 92% polymorphonuclear leukocytes. *B,* Gingival hypertrophy and necrosis around retained molar roots in the same patient.

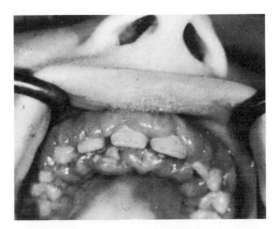

Fig. 22-11 Marked gingival enlargement in monocytic leukemia in 12-year-old patient.

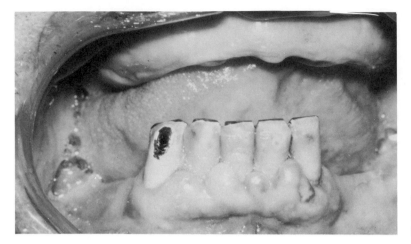

Fig. 22-12 Leukemic gingival infiltrate in a patient with acute myelogenous leukemia.

Hodgkin's lymphomas. These diseases usually begin in the lymph nodes, but may be first diagnosed in extranodal lymphoid tissue.

Hodgkin's Disease

Hodgkin's disease (HD), a malignant lymphatic disease, was first described by the British pathologist Thomas Hodgkin in 1832. The etiology remains unknown, but many infectious agents have been proposed as the likely cause because of the histologic resemblance of the disease to an inflammatory response. The infectious agent theory has been encouraged by several reports of clusters of HD among high school classmates, friends, and relatives. Currently, viruses (particularly herpes and oncorna virus) are being extensively investigated as possible etiologic agents. Evidence for a viral etiology includes viruslike particles seen in electron microscopic studies of tissue cultures of HD tumor cells and elevated antibody titers to Epstein–Barr virus in some HD patients.

HD was a uniformly fatal disease, but modern modes of diagnosis and treatment have given a newly diagnosed patient over 70% chance of cure. One reason for this advance is improved methods of classifying and staging the disease, which improves the opportunity for the patient to be managed properly.

HD is classified histologically according to the Rye system, which lists four major subgroups: lymphocyte predominant, nodular sclerosis, mixed cellularity, and lymphocyte depleted. The lymphocyte predominant type has the best prognosis and lymphocyte depleted the worst. The disease is also staged clinically according to the criteria established in the Ann Arbor conference of 1971 (see Table 22-1). Stage I has the best prognosis and stage IV the worst.

Males have an increased incidence of HD, and the disease has two peaks of highest incidence. The first peak occurs during the second and third decades of life and the second after the fourth decade. Differences in clinical presentation in the two age groups has lead some to speculate that each of these peaks may represent a distinct disease entity.

Clinical Manifestations. The most common presentation of HD is a painless enlargement of the lymph nodes in a patient without other symptoms of disease. The cervical lymph nodes are the initial sites of involvement in two thirds to three quarters of the cases. Early involvement of the axillary and inguinal nodes is also common. On examination the involved nodes are nontender and feel rubbery. The presentation of asymptomatic, enlarged peripheral lymph nodes is most common in younger patients with HD and is consistent with a histologic classification of lymphocyte predominant or nodular sclerosis. In older patients with increased risk of developing the lymphocyte depleted or mixed cellularity histologic pattern, systemic symptoms such as malaise, fever, and night-

Table 22-1. Staging of Hodgkin's Disease: Ann Arbor Staging Classification

CLASSIFICATION	EXTENT OF DISEASE
Stage I	Involvement of one lymph node region or single extranodal site
Stage II	Involvement of multiple lymph node regions on the same side of the diaphragm
Stage III	Involvement of lymph nodes on both sides of the diaphragm
Stage IV	Generalized involvement

sweats may precede noticeable lymphadenopathy.

As the disease progresses, signs and symptoms arise from pressure and obstruction caused by enlarging nodes. Enlarged mediastinal nodes cause dysphagia, while retroperitoneal nodes can cause ureteral obstruction. Further progression of the disease leads to invasion of the bone marrow, lungs, liver, bones, and spinal cord.

Characteristic clinical features of HD include the Pel–Ebstein fever, a cyclic spiking of high fever, and generalized severe pruritus of unknown etiology. Pruritus is a symptom seen most frequently in young women with HD. Many investigators of HD have demonstrated a defective functioning of T lymphocytes that results in a faulty, delayed-type hypersensitivity reaction. Early in the course of HD, this immune deficiency can be demonstrated by a decreased reaction to skin tests and prolonged survival of grafts from noncompatible donors. When the disease is generalized, the immune deficiency leads to increased susceptibility to viral and fungal infections. Diagnosis of HD is always finalized by biopsy of enlarged lymphoid tissue. Demonstration of the characteristic Reed–Sternberg cells is diagnostic, but the nature of this cell is still controversial.

Treatment. The management of HD consists of radiotherapy, chemotherapy, or a combination of both, depending on the stage of the disease at time of diagnosis. Five-year sur-vival of patients with stage I disease exceeds 75%, and the mean 5-year survival exceeds 50% for all stages of the disease. All patients with HD should be referred to medical centers experienced in treating large numbers of lymphoma patients where the disease can be skillfully staged and appropriate treatment carefully planned.

Radiation commonly consists of 3500 rad to 4500 rad delivered to the involved lymph node chain and contiguous areas. Chemotherapy consists of a combination of drugs, the most common combination being nitrogen mustard, vincristine, procarbazine, and prednisone (MOPP). The combination of radiotherapy and chemotherapy is used for advanced disease, but it increases the chance of complications such as bone marrow aplasia and acute leukemia.

Non-Hodgkin's Lymphoma (NHL)

This group of malignant disorders arises from lymphocytes. The classification of these diseases is in a state of evolution owing to the recent use of immunologic techniques to identify receptors on the surface of the cell, but the Rappaport classification is still in common clinical use to predict prognosis. The Rappaport system divides NHL into a nodular and diffuse form based on the general histologic configuration. It also classifies NHL by the presence of lymphocytes and the degree of cellular differentiation. Nodular, lymphocytic, well-differentiated lesions have the best prognosis.

Clinical Manifestations. The most common presentation of NHL is painless enlargement of the lymph nodes, but extranodal lesions occur more commonly than in HD especially in the diffuse form of the disease. NHL lesions may be detected in Waldeyer's ring, the gastrointestinal tract, the spleen, skin, and bone marrow. NHL is more common in patients over age 40, but can occur at any age. In children, NHL may enter a leukemic phase with malignant lymphocytes pouring into the peripheral blood. Signs and symptoms depend on the site of involvement and result from the pressure of enlarged lymph nodes or infiltration. Renal obstruction, neurologic impairment, liver or skin infiltration, as well as bone marrow involvement commonly occur during the course of the disease.

Treatment. Radiation and chemotherapy are the most successful modes of treatment. Localized NHL is highly radiosensitive so will frequently be treated with 3,000 rad to 4,000 rad to the involved area. More disseminated forms of the disease are treated with either chemotherapy or total body radiation, which uses multiple small doses of radiation over the entire body. Combinations of chemotherapeutic drugs have achieved higher rates of remissions and cures than have single agents. Many combinations have been tested and compared. Cyclophosphamide, adriamycin, vincristine, and prednisone are included in many of the commonly used drug protocols.

Burkitt's Lymphoma

During the 1950s, Dennis Burkitt described rapidly growing jaw and abdominal lymphoid tumors in East African children. This neoplasm had a strict geographic distribution and occurred in zones where malaria was endemic. The tumor, named Burkitt's lymphoma (BL), is the human cancer most closely linked with a virus. Epstein–Barr virus is associated with 90% of African patients with BL, but this percentage is considerably lower for BL seen in other parts of the world, and the reason for the association between BL and Epstein–Barr virus remains unknown. The virus may be a prime etiologic agent, a cocarcinogen, or just an innocent passenger. Since the original description by Burkitt, BL has been found in many countries outside Africa including the United States. The primary tumor cell has been shown to be a poorly differentiated B lymphocyte.

Clinical Manifestations. The African form of BL most frequently manifests itself as rapidly growing, extranodal jaw tumors in young children, but it may also be first detected as an abdominal mass involving the kidneys or ovaries. Cases reported in the United States appear to follow a pattern that differs from the African disease. A majority of United States cases are abdominal lesions arising from Peyer's patches or mesenteric lymph nodes. The tumor expands rapidly and may double in size in 1 day, making it the fastest growing human cancer. This rapid growth nullifies the usefulness of the Ann Arbor classification used for other non-Hodgkin's lymphomas, and BL patients are divided into two categories: small tumor burden and large tumor burden.

Treatment. BL lesions have a dramatic response to chemotherapy, particularly cyclophosphamide. The tumor has also been shown to be sensitive to methotrexate, vincristine, and cytarabine. Combinations of drugs have achieved remissions and cures in over 50% of patients.

Oral and Dental Considerations of Lymphoma

Asymptomatic enlargement of the cervical lymph node chains is a common early sign of lymphoma, and the dentist should play a significant role in early detection by routine examination of the neck. It is uncommon for primary lesions of Hodgkin's disease to begin in an extranodal site, so primary jaw lesions are uncommon. Extranodal primary non-Hodgkin's lymphoma is reported more frequently. One common site for extranodal NHL is the lymphoid tissue of Waldeyer's ring; therefore, nontender enlargements of tonsillar tissue in adults should be referred for evaluation by an otolaryngologist.

NHL of the jaws and mouth, particularly the palate, has been reported by several authors. These palatal lesions have been described as slow-growing, painless, bluish, soft masses, and they have been confused with minor salivary gland tumors. Oral NHL also mimics other more common disorders and may present as a gingival mass, tongue mass, or intraosseous lesion. Lesions of the gingiva are frequently treated for months as a pulpal or periodontal problem before the correct diagnosis is finally made by biopsy.

The dentist must remember that tissue from the sockets of isolated mobile teeth should be submitted for histopathologic evaluation to rule out neoplastic disease. When lymphoma is included in the differential diagnosis of an oral disease, the biopsy specimen should be taken from the center of the lesion and sent to a pathologist experienced in evaluating lymphoma. Lymphomas may be confused with benign lymphoepithelial lesions or other benign lymphoproliferative disorders by inexperienced histopathologists.

Multiple Myeloma

Multiple myeloma a malignant neoplasm of the plasma cells of the bone marrow, is of dental interest because of the widespread involvement of the skeletal system, including the jaws and the skull. An excellent review of multiple myeloma has been made by Bayrd and Heck and by Bruce and Royer. It occurs approximately equally in males and females and most often in the age group over 50 years. Skeletal pain, which is associated with motion or pressure over the bony nodules or tumor masses, is an early symptom, and spontaneous pathologic fractures may occur. Many times the disease is detected during radiologic examination for other purposes. The most common radiographic abnormality is the presence of "punched-out," radiolucent lesions (plasmacytomas), but generalized osteoporosis may occur in the absence of these discrete punched-out lesions (see Fig. 22-13).

Proliferation of abnormal plasma cells causes most of the manifestations of the disease. These plasma cells produce abnormal monoclonal immunoglobulins that are very useful in the diagnosis of the disease by their

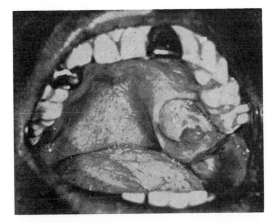

Fig. 22-13 Palatal view of multiple myeloma lesion showing formation of red cap on inferior surface. (Calman HI: Oral Surg 5:1303)

electrophoretic pattern. Bone marrow examination shows the presence of increased numbers of abnormal plasma cells. Bence Jones protein can be demonstrated in the urine of patients who have multiple myeloma and is an excretory product of the abnormal serum globulins. The abnormal globulins may bind with coagulation factors causing a bleeding disorder and also increase blood viscosity. The myeloma patient has a decrease in normal immunoglobulins making him more susceptible to bacterial infection. Hypercalcemia is often present and there is usually an associated anemia. The white cell and platelet counts are usually normal prior to therapy.

Treatment. Treatment of multiple myeloma consists in the use of one of the chemotherapeutic agents such as melphalan or cyclophosphamide (Cytoxan). Local symptomatic lesions are treated with radiotherapy. Average survival with treatment is 2 to 3 years, but with the introduction of newer chemotherapeutic agents this is increasing, some patients having remissions of 6 years or more. A common cause of death is the *myeloma kidney*, in which renal failure is caused by the accumulation of abnormal proteins in the renal tissue.

Oral Manifestations. Approximately 30% of myeloma patients have jaw lesions, and accidental discovery of lesions in the jaws may be the first evidence of this disease. The patient may experience pain, swelling, numbness of the jaws, epulis formation, or unexplained mobility of the teeth. Skull lesions are usually more common than are jaw lesions. Multiple radiolucent lesions of varying size, with ill-defined margins and a lack of circumferential osteosclerotic activity, should suggest this diagnosis (Fig. 22-14).

The mandible is more frequently involved because of its greater content of marrow. Lesions are most common in the region of the angle of the jaw, where red marrow generally is present. In most instances the lesions appear unassociated with the apices of the teeth. Extraosseous lesions also occur in a significant number of patients (Fig. 22-15). A large elevation of the palate with sloughing of the tissues and a clinical picture resem-

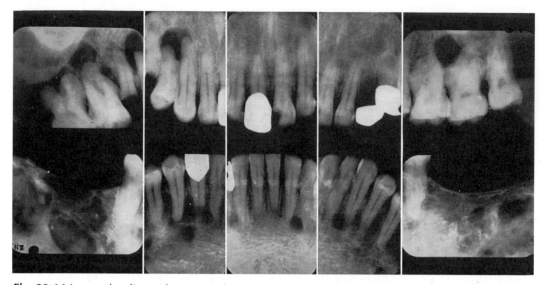

Fig. 22-14 Intraoral radiographic series showing multiple involvement of the maxilla and the mandible in multiple myeloma. (Calman HI: Oral Surg 5:1304)

bling carcinoma were present in one of the cases reported by Thoma.

Cahn has called attention to the development of oral amyloidosis as a complication of this disease. The tongue may be enlarged and studded with small garnet-colored enlargements, including nodes on the cheeks and lips. Amyloidosis occurs in about 7% of patients with multiple myeloma according to Tillman and may be detected in tissue specimens with a Congo red stain. When a dentist is requested to take a gingival biopsy to detect amyloidosis, the biopsy must include muscle tissue from the mucobuccal fold (see Fig. 22-16). Delay in correct diagnosis may ensue when the patient receives treatment for a long period of time for loose teeth, or gingivitis, or a draining sinus before the diagnosis of multiple myeloma is established.

Excessive hemorrhage (oral and elsewhere) may be encountered, caused by a thrombocytopenia secondary to increased proliferation of the plasma cells in the marrow or secondary to uremia—myeloma kidney (see Fig. 22-17). The hemorrhage may also be caused by the abnormal serum protein tying up clotting factors in an inactive complex.

Dental Considerations. For emergency dental care, the patient should be hospitalized in order to control undue hemorrhage should it occur. For routine dental care, the patient's hematologic status should be stable, and there should be consultation with the patient's physician in planning dental procedures, inasmuch as there are transitory periods of leukopenia and thrombocytopenia secondary to the chemotherapeutic agents being used. Dental procedures that involve prolonged periods of time, such as extensive periodontal therapy, are best avoided.

Infectious Mononucleosis

Infectious mononucleosis or glandular fever is a relatively benign disease that occurs predominantly in the 15-year-old to 30-year-old age group. Recent studies have shown Epstein–Barr virus (EB virus: EBV) to be the etiologic agent in the disease. All patients studied who had documented infectious mononucleosis had antibodies to EBV; further, those patients who initially had no EBV antibodies and who became ill with mononucleosis during the course of the study, developed antibodies to EBV.

The disease probably is more common than is generally believed, occurring chiefly between 15 and 30 years of age. It is quite commonly seen on college campuses, and nurses and physicians are said to have the disease

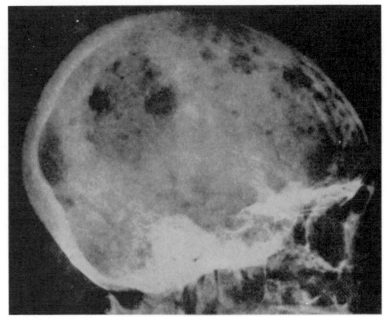

Fig. 22-15 Radiograph of the skull discloses widely distributed lesions in multiple myeloma. (Calman HI: Oral Surg 5:1308)

more commonly than does the population at large. Because of occurrence in the younger adult age group and because of the probability of spread by means of saliva, it has been known as the "kissing" disease.

Infectious mononucleosis is a self-limiting, mild to severely debilitating condition. Symptoms usually last 2 to 6 weeks, with the acute symptoms subsiding in about 2 weeks and the lassitude slowly tapering off within 6 weeks. Because of the abnormal blood smear and lymphadenopathy, the disease may sometimes resemble the leukemias although it is much more common. Complications of infectious mononucleosis are uncommon and may include neurologic manifestations (transitory paralysis), ruptured spleen, mononuclear hepatitis, hemolytic anemia, and thrombocytopenia. Fatalities are extremely rare—fewer than 0.01%—and usually result from respiratory paralysis due to involvement of the respiratory center by lymphocytic infiltration.

Infectious mononucleosis is usually characterized by the acute onset of a sore throat accompanied by a fever—usually 100°F to 103°F—and extreme fatiguability. Physical examination usually shows the palatine tonsils to be enlarged, with a copious amount of cheesy yellow exudate filling the tonsillar crypts. In most patients some or all of the anterior and posterior cervical nodes are enlarged and only slightly tender on palpation. Enlargement of the posterior cervical nodes as well as the anterior nodes in a patient with a pharyngotonsillitis should be a clue that one is dealing with a systemic disease involving the entire lymphopoietic system. There is also splenomegaly in over half of the patients, and lymphadenopathy may occur in any of the groups of nodes in the body; however, cervical lymph node involvement is the most common presenting sign of the disease. Some patients may present with only cervical node enlargement and fatigue without any pharyngotonsillitis. Other uncommon forms of presentation of infectious mononucleosis are a morbilliform skin rash or gastrointestinal symptoms such as nausea, vomiting, or diarrhea.

Diagnosis. The leukocyte count is usually between 4,000/mm³ and 15,000/mm³. Large atypical lymphocytes comprise from 20% to 80% of the differential count and have pseudopodia that project from the cell outline in three or four directions. There is a normal hemoglobin. The abnormal lymphocytes may persist for weeks or even months following the disappearance of clinical symptoms.

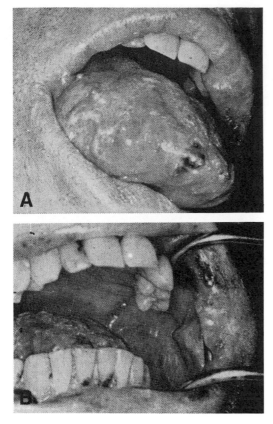

Fig. 22-16 *A,* An enlarged amyloid tongue. Note its grossness and irregular lumping. *B,* Amyloid deposits in the buccal mucosa. There are also some ulcerations of the lips. (Cahn L: Oral Surg 10:740)

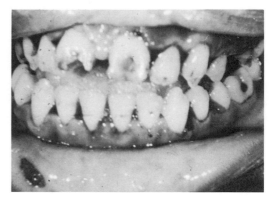

Fig. 22-17 Gingival and mucosal bleeding in thrombocytopenic purpura.

Although the disease is caused by EBV, the nonspecific heterophil antibody test or variation of this test, the Mono-Test (mono-spot test), is still the most common *serologic* basis of diagnosis of the disease. (See Chap. 3.) Specific antibody tests to the EB virus have been developed and are being used with increased frequency as they become available on the clinical level. By the use of these tests, some patients who have the clinical signs and symptoms of infectious mononucleosis but who are negative on heterophil tests are able to be diagnosed. The tests also indicate whether a patient has ever had mononucleosis in the past by the presence of specific IgG antibodies that last for years to a lifetime.

The heterophil antibody test is positive in most patients and along with the atypical lymphocytes and clinical signs and symptoms, makes a diagnostic triad for the dis-

ease. Patients with heterophil-negative results throughout the course of the disease are rare, and heterophil antibodies may persist in the patient's blood long after the disappearance of clinical signs and symptoms. It was believed at one time that a high incidence of biological false-positive reagin tests for syphilis (BFP) occurred in infectious mononucleosis, but there is no sound basis for this belief. The BFP in infectious mononucleosis is about 0.66%.

Other conditions that may be associated with cervical adenopathy, with or without oral or pharyngeal lesions, must be considered in the differential diagnosis. The most common cause of a clinical syndrome identical to infectious mononucleosis but with negative heterophils and EB virus studies is the cytomegalic inclusion virus.

Manifestations. Oral lesions (as distinguished from pharyngeal or tonsillar lesions) are uncommon in infectious mononucleosis and take the form of an aphthouslike stomatitis or a fusospirochetal gingivitis. It is not clear whether these oral lesions are an integral part of the disease or occur as incidental findings in patients debilitated with infectious mononucleosis, although the latter is more probable. Many clinicians consider the presence of petechiae, especially on the palate, to be a significant finding; however, such lesions have been shown to occur in other viral pharyngitides and in streptococcal pharyngitis. In one study, petechiae were observed in all of 28 patients with infectious mononucleosis and were considered to be an important diagnostic sign even when fewer than five petechiae were present. In another study this sign was present in 75% of the patients; the petechiae were roughly related to the duration of the fever.

Treatment. The oral lesions of infectious mononucleosis are treated symptomatically. A topical anesthetic may be used for the painful ulcers, and hydrogen peroxide rinses aid in ameliorating the fusospirochetal gingivitis. With severe pain, oral analgesics may be administered. There is no specific general treatment other than rest. The pharyngitis and fever do not usually persist longer than 10 days to 2 weeks, although the fatigue may last from 6 weeks to 2 months.

Convalescence is gradual, and the patient is often unable to state exactly when the fatigue is no longer present. The course of the disease is determined clinically by how the patient feels. Follow-up blood studies for atypical lymphocytes and heterophil antibodies are of little prognostic value. In patients with a pharyngitis so severe that food intake is difficult, hospitalization for the purpose of enforced rest and intravenous fluid feeding may be necessary. Only about 2% to 5% of patients will need hospitalization. The severe pharyngitides usually respond dramatically to corticosteroid therapy, although the ultimate course of the convalescence (*i.e.*, period of fatigue) does not seem to be affected by the corticosteroid therapy.

RED BLOOD CELL DISORDERS

Increase in Red Blood Cells

Polycythemia

Polycythemia may be defined as an abnormal increase in the concentration of hemoglobin. It is always accompanied by an increase in the erythrocyte count, but the converse is not always true (*e.g.*, there may be a slightly increased number of red cells in early microcytic hypochromic anemia, but because the cells are small, the hemoglobin concentration will be normal to slightly decreased). The polycythemia may be a relative rather than an actual increase in the hemoglobin concentration. This relative polycythemia is caused by the loss of body and intravascular fluid, which may be the result of such diverse conditions as diabetic ketoacidosis, postsurgical dehydration, prolonged vomiting or diarrhea, or rapid diuresis secondary to treatment for congestive heart failure. In relative polycythemia the hemoglobin rarely rises more than 25%, and there are no appreciable oral changes.

When a real polycythemia exists, it may be primary (polycythemia vera, erythremia) resulting from actual neoplastic proliferation of the erythropoietic tissues, or it may be secondary to some other disease.

Secondary Polycythemia

Secondary polycythemia (erythrocytosis) is observed commonly in people living at high altitudes and in patients with congenital heart disease, congestive heart failure, and pulmonary diseases such as emphysema, silicosis, and lung alveolar membrane thickening (*e.g.*, due to mitral stenosis). All these conditions are associated with a lowered blood oxygen concentration, usually less than 90%.

Secondary polycythemia also occurs with some brain tumors (usually vascular), Cushing's syndrome, and renal and lung carcinomas. It is postulated that an erythropoietin-like substance may be elaborated by these tissues and cause the secondary polycythemia.

Treatment of secondary polycythemia is the treatment of the causative disease whenever possible.

Polycythemia Vera

Primary polycythemia is uncommon. It is a condition characterized by a neoplastic erythropoietin-independent increase in the circulating red blood cell mass, the hemoglobin, the leukocyte count, the platelets, and the viscosity of the blood. All these factors favor the thrombotic phenomena that are a prominent feature of this disease. The cause is unknown.

This disease is relatively uncommon in blacks, and Jews seem to have a slight predilection for it. The clinical findings include marked purplish red coloration, especially of the head, neck, feet, and hands, which gives the afflicted individual an extremely angry appearance. The superficial veins are dark and distended, and patients complain of nervousness, headache, tinnitus, and neuralgias. The tips of the fingers usually have a cyanotic appearance. Paresthesias are common, particularly those involving the cranial nerves. They result from localized areas of cerebral anemia caused by the increased viscosity of the blood, hemorrhage, or thrombosis. Hemorrhage commonly occurs most often in the form of bleeding peptic ulcer or epistaxis. There is splenomegaly in over 75% of the patients, often accompanied by a feeling of fullness in the left upper quadrant of the abdomen. Systolic hypertension is a common finding but is not universal.

Surgical procedures in patients with polycythemia vera for coincidental disease appear to be complicated by excessively high morbidity and mortality. Complications are less in controlled patients whose hemoglobin and hematocrit are within the normal range of values, but even when effectively controlled, polycythemia vera predisposes to postoperative hemorrhage and thrombosis, often severe and at times fatal.

Oral Manifestations. The purplish red discoloration of the ears, the oral mucosa, the gingivae, and the tongue is one of the outstanding findings. The tongue may appear as if it had been painted with crystal violet. The gingivae are markedly swollen and frequently bleed spontaneously, but they exhibit no tendency to ulcerate. Petechiae of the oral mucosa are common. Severe hemorrhage may follow dental extractions or periodontal surgery in individuals with polycythemia vera.

Diagnosis. Diagnosis of polycythemia vera is made on the characteristic clinical findings, the history of the disease, and the hematologic findings. Blood oxygen saturation and pulmonary function studies are usually normal. It may also be differentiated from secondary polycythemia and argyrosis on clinical grounds. There are usually 7 million red blood cells/mm^3 or higher; counts of 16 million erythrocytes/mm^3 have been reported. The hemoglobin is elevated, having levels of 18 g/dl to 24 g/dl of blood. The leukocyte and

the platelet counts are also elevated and there is a characteristic basophilia. Nucleated red blood cells and variations in the size and the shape of the cells are noted on the blood smears. The leukocyte alkaline phosphatase is elevated, and there is a hyperuricemia.

Treatment. Venesection (phlebotomy) is indicated when the hematocrit is over 60%. Radiation therapy is of little value because it also tends to depress white blood cell production. Radiophosphorus (^{32}P) therapy may produce a remission of 1 year or more in 75% of the patients and is used to suppress bone marrow function when the hematocrit is above 60% or the platelet count rises appreciably. There is a tendency for leukemia to develop in about 15% of the patients so treated, which has caused this treatment to be used less frequently in recent years. A satisfactory symptomatic and hematologic response has also been achieved following oral administration of an average course of 30 mg triethylenemelamine (TEM), with remissions of 8 to 9 months, but most hematologists feel that ^{32}P is the chemotherapeutic treatment of choice. Considering the oncologic potential of chemotherapy, many prefer to treat the disease with phlebotomy alone.

Oral and Dental Considerations. Each patient should have a hemogram (hemoglobin, total and differential white blood cell counts) and a platelet count before dental procedures involving significant surgery. This is especially true if there has been recent ^{32}P therapy. Oral treatment consists of maintaining good oral hygiene during the acute stage of the disease. Severe hemorrhages have been experienced following extraction during periods when the red cell count was high. A moderate hemorrhage in these patients is not serious.

Decrease in Red Blood Cells (Anemia)

Anemia is present whenever there is a decrease in the normal amount of circulating hemoglobin. This reduction in hemoglobin may result from blood loss, as in common iron-deficiency anemia; from decreased production of red cells, as in pernicious and folic-acid deficiency anemias; from increased destruction of the red blood cells, as in the hemolytic anemias; or from combinations of the first three. When there is a combination of causes, one mechanism usually predominates.

The above is an etiologic classification of anemia. Anemias may also be classified on the basis of the size (microcytic, normocytic, macrocytic) of the red cells or their hemoglobin concentration (hypochromic, normochromic). The term *hyperchromic* is seldom used but refers to a macrocytic cell with normal hemoglobin concentration that because of its large size has an increased hemoglobin content. For further understanding, see the red cell indices: mean corpuscular volume (MCV), mean corpuscular hemoglobin (MCH), and mean corpuscular hemoglobin concentration (MCHC) determinations in the chapter on Laboratory Diagnosis. General symptoms of all anemias include pallor of the skin, palpebral conjunctiva and the nail beds, with dyspnea and easy fatigability. The more common anemias or those with common oral manifestations will be discussed in this chapter.

Blood Loss Anemias

Iron-Deficiency Anemia. Iron-deficiency anemia (blood loss anemia, microcytic hypochromic anemia) is probably the most common of all anemias and may result from chronic blood loss, such as in menstrual or menopausal bleeding, parturition, bleeding hemorrhoids, or a bleeding malignant lesion or ulcer in the gastrointestinal tract. It may also develop in patients from a variety of causes that may decrease the rate of absorption of iron, such as after subtotal or complete gastrectomy, in clay eating, or in the malabsorption syndrome.

An inadequate dietary intake of iron may also be responsible, but the diagnosis of iron deficiency caused by dietary insufficiency must be made with extreme caution. The body zealously guards its iron stores and it has been estimated that the adult male can go 10 years without iron intake before an iron-deficiency anemia develops. Women normally lose about 50 ml of blood with each menstrual period and are thereby more likely to become anemic with an iron-deficient diet. Chronic iron-deficiency anemia is one of the typical findings in gastrointestinal malignancy and in certain forms of parasitic infections. According to the studies of Moore, a positive iron balance is maintained in health by a narrower margin than is generally believed. This margin of iron balance is much less in growing children and menstruating women.

In addition to the symptoms common to all anemias, patients with iron-deficiency anemia also note a tendency of the nails to crack and split. Weakness and dyspnea on exertion and a painful tongue may be present for some time before the development of other clinical signs or symptoms of anemia. Recent clinical investigation has shown lingual signs and symptoms to be much less common than was previously believed.

Oral Manifestations. In addition to the lingual symptoms noted above, angular cheilitis may be present (see Fig. 22-18). Patients may manifest slow healing after oral surgical or periodontal procedures. It is difficult for even the experienced clinician to evaluate the degree of anemia from physical examination alone. The soft palate and the tongue are the oral tissues most likely to show definite pallor.

Diagnosis. Diagnosis is based on finding a lowered hemoglobin in routine blood counts; on a peripheral smear, the cells are microcytic and hypochromic. When the anemia is well-developed there is a decrease in the mean corpuscular hemoglobin, the mean corpuscular hemoglobin concentration, and the mean corpuscular volume. Whenever the hemoglobin value is less than 11g/dl, it is of definite clinical significance. The iron-deficiency anemia patient will have low serum iron concentrations and a high serum iron-binding capacity; serum ferritin levels are markedly reduced. There is a characteristic absence of stainable iron in the bone marrow, which is an early finding in the disease. It is most important that the physician search thoroughly for the source of bleeding, including using radiologic surveys of the gastrointestinal tract, sigmoidoscopy, a gynecologic examination, and a complete menstrual and dietary history.

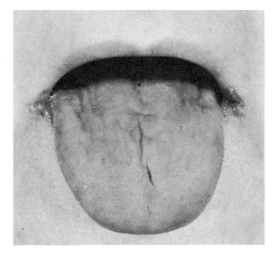

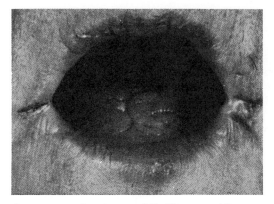

Fig. 22-19 "Carp's mouth"; Plummer–Vinson syndrome. (Hertz J: Oral Surg 9:695)

Fig. 22-18 The painful and atrophic tongue of a patient with severe iron-deficiency anemia. Note the associated cheilitis. These changes are quickly corrected by the oral administration of iron salts. (Monto RW: J Dent Med 12:47)

Oral and Dental Considerations. Dental patients presenting symptoms of anemia or oral signs suggestive of this condition should have routine blood studies. If significantly lowered hemoglobin values are obtained, refer the patient to his physician for more thorough medical history, laboratory diagnosis, and treatment. Do not perform elective oral surgical or periodontal procedures on patients with marked anemia because abnormal bleeding and faulty wound healing may occur. Never treat the patient with iron until the cause of the microcytic hypochromic anemia is found and corrected or until a thorough search for the cause has proved fruitless.

Plummer–Vinson Syndrome. First described by Plummer and Vinson, this syndrome is characterized by dysphagia and a microcytic hypochromic anemia. A smooth and often sore tongue, a dry mouth, spoon-shaped nails, and angular stomatitis are common findings (see Fig. 22-19). There is atrophy of the tongue papillae but less severe than in pernicious anemia. There are atrophic changes in the mucosa of the mouth, the pharynx, the upper esophagus, and the vulva. These tissues are dry, inelastic, and glazed in appearance. In addition, general symptoms include listlessness, pallor, ankle edema, and dyspnea—all related to the anemia.

Many patients with this syndrome are edentulous, having lost their teeth early in life. Complaints of sore mouth and inability to wear dentures are frequent. In addition, patients with Plummer–Vinson syndrome often complain of a "spasm in the throat" or of "food sticking in the throat." The dysphagia, which represents an important feature of this disease, appears to be the result of muscular degeneration in the esophagus and stenoses. or webs of the esophageal mucosa.

The diagnosis of this syndrome can be made on the basis of the history and the hematologic findings. The esophageal lesions are demonstrable radiologically (barium swallow) or by esophagoscopy (see Figs. 20-2 and 20-3). Relative degrees of achlorhydria are usually present. Because many of the symptoms in this syndrome are similar to those observed in vitamin B-complex deficiency and simple hypochromic anemias, treatment of these conditions should be tried. Variable and apparently unpredictable response to therapy can be expected. At times the dysphagia improves following iron therapy.

Plummer–Vinson syndrome is potentially serious because pharyngeal and intraoral carcinoma are more common in these patients. Of 250 patients with carcinoma of the mouth and the upper respiratory tract studied, 70% had Plummer–Vinson syndrome. Follow patients with symptoms of this syndrome at short intervals and be alert for the development of malignant lesions.

Hemolytic Anemias

The hemolytic anemias result from excessive destruction of erythrocytes that may be caused by intracorpuscular defects in the erythrocytes (often hereditary) or by extracorpuscular factors.

Some of the more common causes are as follows:

EXTRACORPUSCULAR FACTORS

1. Overwhelming infections and toxins
2. Cardiac valvular prostheses
3. Hypersplenism
4. Rh factor incompatibility (hemolytic disease of newborn, erythroblastosis fetalis)
5. Chronic liver disease
6. Autoimmune hemolytic disease (*e.g.*, as in systemic lupus erythematosus)
7. Transfusion reactions

INTRACORPUSCULAR DEFECTS

1. Abnormal shape of the erythrocytes
   Hereditary spherocytosis
   Hereditary elliptocytosis
2. Abnormal hemoglobins (hemoglobinopathies)
   Sickle-cell anemia and sickle-cell trait
   Thalassemia
   Other hemoglobinopathies—Hgb C, Hgb F, and so on
3. Erythrocyte enzyme deficiencies
   Glucose-6-phosphate deficiency
   Pyruvate kinase deficiency
4. Erythrocyte defects associated with other diseases
   Chronic granulocytic leukemia
   Folic-acid and B_{12}-deficiency anemias

The bone marrow has a capacity to increase production of erythrocytes by six to seven times, and considerable hemolysis can take place before producing an anemia. Similarly, a small amount of hemolysis can take place without producing jaundice because of the normal liver's ability to excrete increased amounts of bilirubin.

The hemoglobinopathies, exemplified by sickle cell disease and thalassemia, are caused by defects in the globin portion of the hemoglobin molecule. These defects render the erythrocyte containing the abnormal hemoglobin more susceptible to hemolysis. A normal hemoglobin molecule consists of two pairs of amino acid chains, the alpha and beta chains. This normal hemoglobin, hemoglobin A, may be represented by the formula $\alpha_2\beta_2$, indicating that there are two alpha and two beta chains. In the hemoglobinopathies, abnormal hemoglobins are produced either in the form of abnormal chains (*e.g.*, gamma, delta) or of small alterations in the alpha or beta chain. Fetal hemoglobin, normal in the fetus but abnormal if persisting into adult life, is designated hemoglobin F and is represented by the formula $\alpha_2\gamma_2$, indicating that it differs from HgbA in that the beta chains are replaced by two different chains, the gamma chains. Sickle cell disease involves a single amino acid abnormality: the glutamic acid normally found in position 6 of the beta chain is replaced by valine. Thus, the formula for hemoglobin S is $\alpha_2\beta_2 6$ valine.

Over 30 different hemoglobins have at present been identified. Identification is made possible by the use of electrophoresis. Many of the abnormal hemoglobins will show slower or faster electrophoretic mobility than hemoglobin A. Specific identification of the exact biochemical abnormality depends on more sophisticated analysis of the molecule. At present, the specific molecular abnormality in many of the hemoglobinopathies has not been identified.

Diagnosis. Laboratory findings common to all hemolytic anemias are a decreased hemoglobin, increased reticulocytes (young red cells released into the circulation as a result of the marrow's producing more red cells to compensate for the excessive destruction), and an increase in the serum bilirubin, mostly in the indirect (unconjugated, prehepatic) fraction.

Other diagnostic tests that may be useful in certain of the hemolytic anemias include the following:

1. To measure red cell survival time, a small amount of the patient's red cells may be

tagged with radioactive chromium (^{51}Cr) and reinjected. If the hemolysis is caused by an extracorpuscular factor, a compatible donor's red cells, similarly tagged and injected into the patient, should disappear as quickly as do the patient's own red cells; if the hemolysis is caused by intracorpuscular defects, the compatible donor's red cells should survive longer than the patient's red cells when injected into the veins of the patient.

2. Most hemolytic anemias are accompanied by a decrease in the serum haptoglobins, which are globulins with a marked affinity to bind hemoglobin. When hemoglobin is released into the blood by hemolysis, it is quickly bound by haptoglobins, and the haptoglobin-hemoglobin complex is rapidly removed from the circulation by the reticuloendothelial system, thus resulting in a lowered serum haptoglobin level.

3. Although the hemolytic anemias are usually characterized by normocytic, normochromic morphology on a blood smear with normal red cell indices, the cells in hereditary spherocytosis and hereditary elliptocytosis may exhibit an abnormal spherical or elliptical shape. This may be more apparent in wet preparations than in dried smears.

4. The cells in hereditary spherocytosis show increased hemolysis (osmotic fragility) in hypotonic saline solutions, which do not affect normal red cells.

5. The Coombs' test is useful in demonstrating antibodies to the erythrocytes. The direct Coombs' test demonstrates incomplete antibodies attached to the erythrocytes, which require a substance such as antihuman globulin to produce hemolysis. The indirect Coombs' test detects antibodies to the red cells, which are present in the patient's serum.

6. Hemoglobin electrophoresis identifies the abnormal hemoglobins.

Oral and Dental Considerations. Certain oral and physical findings are common to all hemolytic anemias. When sufficient hemolysis has taken place to produce anemia, pallor will result, which is most easily observed in the nail beds and palpebral conjunctiva. Pallor of the oral mucosa—especially evident in the soft palate, tongue, and sublingual tissues—is also observable as the anemia progresses. In contrast to the anemias produced by bleeding or by factor deficiencies, the hemolytic anemias produce jaundice caused by the hyperbilirubinemia secondary to erythrocyte destruction. This is best seen in the sclera, but the skin, soft palate, and tissues of the floor of the mouth also become icteric as the serum bilirubin increases. There is hyperplasia of the erythroid elements of the bone marrow in an attempt to compensate for the anemia. This hyperplasia produces a characteristic appearance on the dental radiograph. Because of the enlargement of the medullary spaces, the trabeculae become more prominent, creating increased bone radiolucency with prominent lamellar striations. Splenomegaly may be seen with some of the hemolytic anemias but is an inconstant finding.

Sickle Cell Disease. In this hemoglobinopathy found almost exclusively in blacks, an abnormality in the beta chain of hemoglobin is present in which valine is substituted for the normal glutamic acid residue on position 6. This relatively minor biochemical change results in profound undesirable physical characteristics in the hemoglobin. In the presence of either a lowered blood oxygen tension or an increased blood pH, the hemoglobin will form a sickle-shaped crystal (a tactoid) within the erythrocyte. This sickling of the erythrocyte leads to stasis and hemolysis of the red cells, especially in end-capillary circulation. The stasis then results in an even lower oxygen tension, increased pH, and further sickling. The disease is hereditary (non-sex-linked) and may manifest itself as either the sickle cell trait or as sickle cell anemia.

In sickle cell anemia, 75% to 100% of the hemoglobin is S hemoglobin, the remainder being F hemoglobin; in sickle cell trait, only 20% to 45% of the hemoglobin is S hemoglobin, whereas the rest is normal hemoglobin A. In sickle cell trait (heterozygous), only one of the beta chains is thought to be abnormal, whereas in sickle cell anemia (homozygous) both beta chains are abnormal.

Patients with sickle cell trait—estimated at 9% of blacks in the United States—are not anemic and have no symptoms of their disease unless they are placed in situations where there is abnormally low oxygen, such as in an unpressurized airplane or with injudicious administration of general anesthesia. On the other hand, patients with sickle cell anemia—about 0.15% of the black population of the United States—usually exhibit marked clinical manifestations.

Clinical Manifestations. Patients with sickle cell anemia show marked underdevelopment and often die before 40 years of age. The clinical manifestations are the results of the basic anemia and hemolytic process (jaundice, pallor and cardiac failure) or result from necrosis following stasis of blood and vaso-occlusion. This latter phenomenon is manifested by splenic infarction, chronic leg ulcers, priapism, cerebral vascular thromboses ("strokes"), and painful attacks of abdominal and bone pain (pain crises). The long bones may present radiodense, sclerotic areas as a residual of small infarcts.

Aplastic crises sometimes develop from infection, hypersensitivity reactions, or unknown causes. In these aplastic crises, the patient becomes acutely ill, red cell production virtually stops, and the hemoglobin drops precipitously. It has been suggested that folic-acid deficiency may develop in these patients because of the increased demand for folic acid as a result of increased erythropoiesis. The folic-acid deficiency may play a part in the genesis of the aplastic crisis.

Oral Manifestations. Other than the jaundice and pallor of the oral mucosa, patients often show delayed eruption and hypoplasia of the dentition secondary to their general underdevelopment. Because of the chronic increased erythropoietic activity and marrow hyperplasia (an attempt to compensate for the hemolysis), increased radiolucency resulting from the decreased number of trabeculae is seen on dental radiographs. This change is noted especially in the alveolar bone between the roots of the teeth where the trabeculae may appear as horizontal rows, creating a ladderlike effect. By contrast, the lamina dura appears dense and distinct. In skull films, the diploë is thickened, and the trabeculae are coarse and tend to run perpendicular to the inner and outer tables, giving a radiographic appearance of "hair on end." The teeth do not present undue mobility. Areas of sclerosis or increased radiopacity represent areas of past thromboses with subsequent bony infarction.

Sickle cell anemia patients, probably because of hypovascularity of the bone marrow secondary to thromboses, are particulary prone to develop osteomyelitis. Inasmuch as the initial radiographic changes in vascular thrombosis and osteomyelitis are quite similar, confusion will likely result in the differential diagnosis of these two conditions, and other supporting data must be used to differentiate the two.

Hays' study of the nuclear characteristics of the buccal mucosa cells in sickle cell anemia showed that in those who were folate deficient there was an increased number of cells with enlarged nuclei. This is not a surprising finding because it is also found in patients who have generalized megaloblastic changes as in pernicious anemia or folic-acid deficiency anemia.

Patients presenting with temporary anesthesia of the mental nerve thought to be secondary to vascular occlusion involving the nerve blood supply have been reported by both Kirson and Friedlander.

Diagnosis. A smear of peripheral blood usually shows normochromic, normocytic cells. Sickling will not often occur until the oxygen tension is lowered. To this end, a sickle-cell preparation was formerly used for diagnosis: fresh blood was sealed in a small chamber of a microscopic slide with sodium metabisulfite (reducing agent) for an hour and then observed for sickling. Hemoglobin electrophoresis is now available and is less expensive, more accurate, and more definitive in the diagnosis of sickle cell disease.

Treatment. There is no treatment for sickle cell disease other than symptomatic treatment. Antibiotics should be used early in the treatment of infection, and analgesic drugs should be used if necessary but with caution to prevent iatrogenic addiction. Neither splenectomy nor antianemic drugs (except possibly, folic acid) are of any value. Transfusions are avoided unless the patient has an aplastic crisis with a resulting extremely low hemoglobin level, because the transfusion effects are transitory and the patients tend to develop antibodies, making it difficult to find suitable donors for future transfusions. There is the ever-present risk of hepatitis with transfusions; and because the patients do not lose the iron portion of the hemoglobin molecule, transfusions can result in iron overload and eventual hemosiderosis.

Many physicians routinely use folic acid dietary supplements for sickle cell anemia patients with increase to therapeutic doses in treating an aplastic crisis. There is no good evidence that folic acid treatment increases the blood hemoglobin level.

Dental Considerations. Do not start prolonged or extensive dental procedures involving the soft tissues unless absolutely necessary because of the chronic anemia and slow healing. Keep the dentition as healthy as possible because there is always the chance that any infection might precipitate an aplastic crisis and kill the patient. Avoid using general anesthesia both in patients with sickle cell trait and those with sickle cell anemia; when used, it is imperative to avoid episodes of hypoxia because of the cerebral or myocardial thrombosis which might result.

Thalassemia. Thalassemia refers to a group of hemolytic anemias involving defects in synthesis of either the *alpha* or the *beta* polypeptide chains of hemoglobin (alpha thalassemia, beta thalassemia). Thalassemia *minor* is the clinical manifestation of patients heterozygous for the disease, while thalassemia *major* is the clinical manifestation of homozygous patients. The homozygous form of beta thalassemia (thalassemia major or Cooley's anemia) exhibits the most severe clinical symptoms and is discussed here because of the marked orofacial defects that patients with this disease manifest. Heterozygous beta thalassemia (beta thalassemia minor) is the most common form of the disease but rarely presents any clinical symptoms other than chronic mild anemia, which may be confused with iron-deficiency anemia. Alexander reported a case of alpha thalassemia minor in which the patient demonstrated anterior maxillary protrusion, splaying of the anterior teeth, and severe generalized alveolar bone loss. It was speculated that these changes, which are often seen in thalassemia major, could have been caused by alpha thalassemia minor.

Thalassemia Major (Cooley's anemia). Beta thalassemia major is seen chiefly in beta people of Mediterranean extraction. The onset of symptoms occurs early in infancy. The patients are severely anemic and have a short life expectancy. Patients with the most severe form of the disease rarely survive into adulthood.

Clinical Manifestations. The dentist will note that the patient is quite small for the chronologic age and has a mongoloid facies. Further clinical examination reveals that the spleen and usually the liver are markedly enlarged, and there are often cardiomegaly and manifestations of congestive heart failure due to the chronic anemia and hypoxia. Radiographs of the long bones reveal osteoporosis resulting from the erythroid hyperplasia. Also evident are increased trabeculation and cortical thinning.

Oral Manifestations. By the second year of life the child with Cooley's anemia begins to develop a mongoloid appearance with prominent frontal and parietal bosses and a marked overdevelopment of the maxilla and the malar bones, which is associated with a short nose having a depressed bridge (see Fig. 22-20). The overdevelopment of the maxilla frequently results in malocclusion, an open bite, and spacing of the teeth of the maxillary arch (Fig. 22-21).

The oral mucosa is pale and has a lemon-yellow tint because of the chronic jaundice. The color is best seen slightly posterior to the termination of the hard palate and in the floor of the mouth.

The radiologic changes in the skull represent one of the most striking and consistent findings in this disease (Fig. 22-22). There is marked thickening and rarefaction of the cranium. The trabeculae joining the inner and the outer tables of the skull are observed on the radiogram as radially arranged calcified spicules, which appear as calcified hairs extending between the inner and outer tables. These are not unlike the changes seen

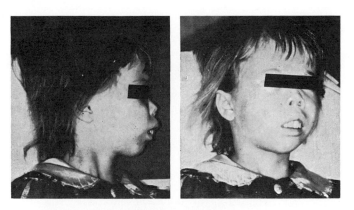

Fig. 22-20 Profile and front views of a 9-year-old girl with Cooley's anemia. (Novak AJ: Am J Orthod 30:542)

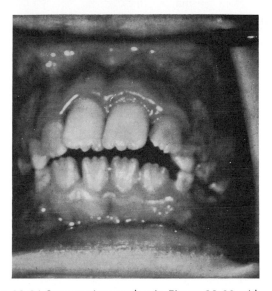

Fig. 22-21 Same patient as that in Figure 22-20 with Cooley's anemia. Open bite and prominent enamel tubercles on the incisal edges of the teeth. (Novak AJ: Am J Orthod 30:542)

in sickle cell anemia. Radiograms of the maxillae reveal a marked increase in the size of these bones with a decreased density and loss of trabecular detail.

Diagnosis. Diagnosis is based on the family history, clinical signs, appearance of the blood smear, and on hemoglobin electrophoresis. Hemoglobin F is present up to a level of 90%. The remaining hemoglobin A is electrophoretically normal, but there may be some defect in its biochemical makeup not affecting electrophoretic mobility, which has not yet been clarified. The red cell morphol-

ogy is microcytic and hypochromic, but the serum iron is high, and many targets cells may be present.

General Treatment. There is no specific drug therapy for thalassemia. Transfusions are often used to keep the patient's hemoglobin as nearly normal as possible in order to abate the symptoms of hypoxia. As with most hemolytic anemias, however, transfusion therapy must be used judiciously and cautiously because it often eventually leads to iron overload and hemosiderosis. This may be ameliorated somewhat by the intravenous administration of desferrioxamine, an iron-chelating agent. The patient may need supplementary folic acid because of the increased requirement for this vitamin owing to the increased erythropoiesis. Because of the hereditary nature of this disease, patients with both thalassemia major and minor should be given genetic counseling.

Dental Considerations. It should be recognized that, as in any patient with a chronic anemia, poor healing may ensue after dental procedures. There is also always the possibility of exacerbating the symptoms of cerebral or cardiac hypoxia if there is substantial bleeding in a patient who is already anemic; however, these patients do not exhibit a bleeding diathesis.

Glucose-6-Phosphate-Dehydrogenase Deficiency. This type of intracorpuscular defect is the most common red blood cell enzyme defect, is found most commonly in American blacks, about 15% of whom are said to be affected, but is known to have a worldwide

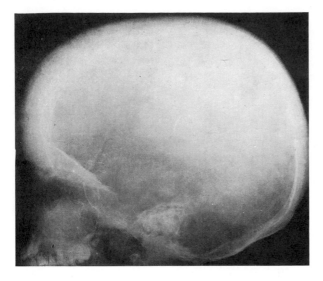

Fig. 22-22 Skull changes in Cooley's anemia. Note the marked thickness of the cortex and a radial arrangement of the bone trabeculae. Same patient as shown in Figure 22-21. (Novak AJ: Am J Orthod 30:542)

distribution. Carried on the X chromosome, it occurs in both males and females. In affected individuals the red blood cell life span is reduced to about two thirds of normal. Ordinarily the bone marrow and liver can compensate for this decreased life span, and the patient exhibits no anemia and no clinical symptoms of pallor or jaundice. There may be acute exacerbation of the hemolysis, however, which may be brought on by infection, diabetic ketoacidosis, or administration of potentially oxidant drugs. The mechanism of the hemolysis is that the G6PD deficiency makes the erythrocyte less able to manufacture glutathione, a reducing agent; lack of glutathione in turn makes the red cell less able to withstand such factors as oxidant compounds, which then denature the hemoglobin and alter the cell membrane, causing hemolysis.

Dental Considerations. This disease is of interest to the dentist because of its relative frequency in the population and because an acute attack of hemolysis may be brought on by dental infection or by the administration of drugs containing phenacetin, which is converted to an oxidant compound in the body.

Anemias of Decreased Red Cell Production

Pernicious Anemia. Pernicious anemia (addisonian anemia) is a chronic disease that results from a deficiency of intrinsic factor, a substance secreted by the parietal cells of the fundus of the stomach. Intrinsic factor is necessary for the absorption of vitamin B_{12} (extrinsic factor), which takes place in the ileum. About 20% of patients with pernicious anemia have a family history of the disease. Pernicious anemia is a disease of late adult life and almost never occurs before 35 years of age. It has an equal incidence in both sexes and is much less common than iron-deficiency anemia. Histologically, there is atrophy of the gastric mucosa. Recent evidence suggests that immunologic mechanisms are responsible for the disease: most patients have been found to have antibodies to their own gastric parietal cells. About half of the patients with pernicious anemia also have antibodies to intrinsic factor. A few cases of pernicious anemia arise secondary to gastric surgery in which the fundus of the stomach is removed.

The clinical manifestations of pernicious anemia are those of any vitamin B_{12} deficiency, but the term *pernicious anemia* should be reserved for patients who have B_{12} deficiency secondary to intrinsic factor deficiency. Other causes of B_{12} deficiency are extremely rare and may be caused by inadequate dietary intake (a diet low in animal or bacterial products), overgrowth of intestinal bacteria that utilize the vitamin, as in the "blind loop syndrome," intestinal disease involving the ileum and interfering with absorption, or intestinal infestation with the fish tapeworm.

Symptoms. Onset of the disease is insidious, and the initial symptoms may be referable to many organ systems, including the oral cavity. The blood is eventually involved in almost 100% of the cases, and neurologic and gastrointestinal involvement are also commonly seen. Gastrointestinal signs and symptoms other than those in the oral cavity are not usually severe and consist of vague epigastric discomfort, constipation, or diarrhea. Oral manifestations will be discussed below. Neurologic changes *precede* those of the anemia in about 10% of patients and usually begin as a tingling sensation in the fingers and toes that eventually progresses to numbness. incoordination, and muscular weakness. The loss of vibration sense is one of the first abnormalities noted on physical examination. Because neurologic involvement can be present without changes in hemoglobin, patients with signs and symptoms suggestive of pernicious anemia should be conclusively evaluated for the disease even if their hemoglobin is normal. Other symptoms of pernicious anemia are the same as for any anemia and include fatigue, pallor, and shortness of breath.

Oral Manifestations. In 1877 Moeller described certain atrophic lingual changes that were believed to be a clincial entity. In 1909 Hunter called attention to the relationship between oral infection and pernicious anemia. In all probability the atrophic lesions described by Moeller and Hunter are a single clinical entity. J. Waldenstrom's hypothesis of the mechanism of the atrophic lingual changes explains the similarity of the clinical lesions that may result from a variety of causes.

The tongue symptoms and changes are prominent and common in pernicious anemia (Fig. 22-23). A painful glossitis and glossopyrosis may be early symptoms of this disease, symptoms that cause the patient to seek dental advice. According to one study, 50% of the patients complained of a sore tongue and difficulty in swallowing. The glossitis associated with pernicious anemia is characterized by its fiery red color and its usual distribution to the tip and the margins of the tongue, with papillary atrophy of the affected areas.

In advanced disease there is diminution of the papillary anatomy of the entire tongue,

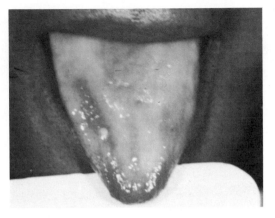

Fig. 22-23 Fiery red glossitis involving the lateral margins and the tip of the tongue in a patient with pernicious anemia. The initial symptom in this patient was the inability to wear full dentures because of the painful tongue and denture-supporting areas.

with a loss of the normal muscle tone. Some patients also complain of a loss of taste sensation. Greenberg reported a case in which the major oral lesions were erythematous macules involving the buccal and labial mucosa (Fig. 22-24). Although the lingual papillae were mildly atrophic and there was localized erythema occasionally present on the tongue, this was a minor feature, and the patient did not have the classic atrophic glossitis commonly associated with pernicious anemia. For this reason the diagnosis in the case was delayed for a year while the patient was treated for a variety of traumatic and allergic disorders.

Patients with pernicious anemia commonly complain of difficulty in wearing dentures, a difficulty that cannot be that explained on the basis of technical factors. These patients, like those with nutritional deficiency, do not have mucosal tissues that can tolerate the additional irritation induced by the dentures.

The oral mucosa also presents the greenish yellow color frequently observed on the skin. This is best seen at the junction of the hard and the soft palates when daylight is used for illumination.

The dental practitioner must differentiate between the glossitis associated with pernicious anemia and simple mechanical irritative lesions; the atrophic glossitis of syphilis; glossopyrosis; glossodynia; psychogenic pain; and possibly allergy. Important points in the

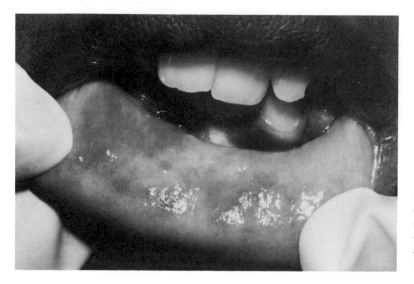

Fig. 22-24 The case of pernicious anemia described by Greenberg in which erythematous macules of the oral mucosa were the predominant oral manifestation.

diagnosis of pernicious anemia include the fiery red appearance of the tongue, the areas involved, and the spontaneous remissions and exacerbations that are usually associated with systemic symptoms. A hemoglobin determination will usually establish the diagnosis of an anemia and should be requested in all cases in which local causes cannot be found for persisting tongue lesions. If an anemia is present, refer the patient to his physician for further evaluation.

Local treatment, other than the removal of all causes of irritation, will give the tongue or the denture-contacting area little relief. Topical application of medicaments does little to relieve the painful symptoms.

Diagnosis. Pernicious anemia should be suspected in any anemic (low hemoglobin) patient with neurologic symptoms such as described above. The first definitive clue that one is dealing with pernicious anemia, however, is the finding of macrocytic, normochromic red cells on the blood smear. The mean corpuscular volume (MCV) will be increased, the mean corpuscular hemoglobin (MCH) will be increased, and the mean corpuscular hemoglobin concentration (MCHC), normal. In addition, there will be considerable variation in the shape of the red cells, abnormally large platelets, and the neutrophils will often be hypersegmented, having as many as six lobes to their nuclei instead

of the usual three. A bone marrow examination will bear out these morphologic changes by the presence of megaloblastic marrow changes. Because folic-acid deficiency may also produce these hematologic changes, further studies are necessary to pinpoint vitamin B_{12} deficency as the cause. This may be done by serum assay for vitamin B_{12} and folate using a microbiologic or radioisotope technique. Once it has been established that a vitamin B_{12} deficiency exists, the mechanism, the deficiency must be determined. To diagnose pernicious anemia, the Schilling test is used. A recently developed test for blocking antibodies to intrinsic factor is positive in up to 75% of patients with pernicious anemia. When positive, it is highly specific for diagnosis of the disease.

In the Schilling test the patient is given a measured, small amount of radioactive vitamin by mouth followed shortly after by a large flushing dose of parenteral, nonradioactive vitamin B_{12}. Because the total dose of vitamin B_{12} far exceeds the renal threshold for this vitamin, the excess will appear in the urine within the next 24 hours. The amount of radioactivity in the urine will be proportional to the amount of the orally administerd vitamin B_{12} that has been absorbed. The normal patient will excrete 7% to 30% of the radioactive B_{12} in 24 hours, whereas the patient with pernicious anemia will excrete no more than 3%. Further studies may be necessary to determine that intestinal disease is not responsible for the malabsorption, and these are carried out by giving the patient suspected of having pernicious anemia a complex of radioactive B_{12} and intrinsic factor. The pernicious anemia patient should then exhibit normal absorption and urine excretion of vitamin B_{12}.

Gastric achlorhydria, even after histamine stimulation, is found in almost all if not all patients with pernicious anemia; however, because it may be found in other diseases, the failure to find achlorhydria is more useful in excluding pernicious anemia than is the presence of achlorhydria in making the diagnosis of pernicious anemia.

Treatment. Although a few patients have been treated with massive oral doses of vitamin B_{12} most patients have to be given vitamin B_{12} parenterally, usually one injection a month. This treatment corrects the hematologic changes but will only arrest, not correct, the neurologic changes. It should be given by the patient's physician and *must be continued for the rest of the patient's life.* Patient who give a history of being treated for anemia for "a while" with B_{12} shots, who no longer take the injections, and who are not anemic, almost certainly do not have pernicious anemia. Almost 100% of pernicious anemia patients will have a relapse within 6 months after discontinuing B_{12} therapy.

Because the hematologic changes of pernicious anemia may be reversed by oral folic acid therapy *without* arresting the neurologic changes, patients who are anemic should never be given folic acid therapy without first ascertaining that they do not have pernicious anemia. To give the patient folic acid removes a valuable diagnostic sign (low hemoglobin) and allows the neurologic changes, which are mostly irreversible even with B_{12} therapy, to progress even further. It is best when prescribing therapeutic vitamins to choose one without folic acid or alternatively, to be sure the hemoglobin is normal before instituting vitamin therapy.

Folic-Acid Deficiency Anemia. One of the two most common causes of a macrocytic anemia with megaloblastic marrow changes is folic-acid deficiency (the other is pernicious anemia). Folic-acid deficiency is found almost exclusively in patients who have an inadequate diet, especially a diet devoid of leafy vegetables, and who have an increased folic-acid requirement. For this reason, it is found in pregnant women in the lower socioeconomic groups and has been called the anemia of pregnancy. It may also be seen in patients with intestinal malabsorption syndromes. The hematologic changes are the same as those of pernicious anemia, but folic-acid deficiency does not cause any specific neurologic symptoms. The gastrointestinal tract may be involved; the symptoms are those of any anemia and include diarrhea. Oral manifestations include angular cheilitis and with severe cases, ulcerative stomatitis and pharyngitis. (Similar oral findings are observed in the oral cavity from cancer chemotherapeutic agents that act as folic-acid antagonists.)

Diagnosis is made by a dietary history, intestinal biopsy, and observation of the hematologic changes (the same as those in pernicious anemia) with a normal Schilling test and serum vitamin B_{12} assays but with low serum assays of folic acid. Treatment of folic-acid deficiency consists of oral folic acid tablets. Oral doses of 1 mg a day are adequate for most patients, and a 5-mg tablet suffices to treat even a patient with intestinal malabsorption.

Aplastic Anemia. Aplastic anemia is a normochromic, normocytic anemia caused by bone marrow failure. Although the cause is frequently unknown, about half of the cases are suspected to be caused by chemical substances (*e.g.,* paint solvents, benzol, chloramphenicol) or exposure to large amounts of x-ray radiation. The term *anemia* is in a sense a misnomer in that all three cellular elements of the marrow are often involved (a pancytopenia), or at least one other cellular element (platelets or white cells) is sometimes involved in addition to the erythrocytes.

Oral Manifestations. As might be expected with a pancytopenia, the oral manifestations include those of a deficiency of all cellular elements in the blood. As with any other anemia, pallor is visible on the oral mucous membranes, and petechiae and purpura of the oral and pharyngeal tissues are also common. The most common oral manifestation is gingival bleeding with no apparent cause (see Fig. 22-25). While not a common initial oral manifestation, ulcers may be present and are characterized, like those of neutropenia, by having little surrounding erythema. In 22 cases observed by Lasser and his colleagues, oral manifestations were the initial chief complaint in 18%. On initial physical examination, 95% of the patients had oral signs secondary to aplastic anemia.

Dental Considerations. The primary problem in management of patients with aplastic anemia is an infection with bleeding being a less common but still significant potential problem. Because bacteremia from oral sources can be a fatal source of infection in these patients, they should at the time of initial diagnosis be examined thoroughly and treatment undertaken to remove sites of current infection and to eliminate potential sites of future infection. As pointed out by Lasser and colleagues, the treatment regimen should meet the following requirements: keep the number of dental procedures to a minimum and make each procedure as definitive as possible; completely eliminate infection; beware of the potentiality of any procedure to cause hemorrhage; and treatment personnel should wear masks to preclude further contamination of the environment by airborne organisms.

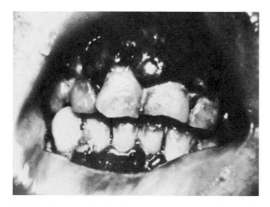

Fig. 22-25 A case of aplastic anemia (pancytopenia) in a 35-year-old woman, in whom the major clinical manifestation was bleeding into the gingival tissues causing gingival hematomas. The direct cause of the bleeding was the thrombocytopenia associated with the aplastic anemia.

Treatment. Bone marrow transplantation is now considered to be the treatment of choice by many hematologic oncologists with success rates of over 70% reported. High doses of corticosteroids and splenectomy are sometimes effective in attenuating the disease temporarily.

Prognosis. The prognosis has improved markedly since the use of marrow transplantation therapy. When it occurs, death is usually due to hemorrhage or overwhelming infection.

BIBLIOGRAPHY

Neutropenia and Neutrophil Dysfunction

Andrews RG et al; Chronic benign neutropenia of childhood with associated oral manifestations. Oral Surg 20:719,1965

Attstrom R, Schroeder HE: Effect of experimental neutropenia on initial gingivitis in dogs. Scand J Dent Res 87:7, 1979

Awbrey JJ, Hibbard ED: Abbreviated case report: Congenital agranulocytosis. Oral Surg 35:526, 1973

Becker FT, Coventry WD, Tivera JL: Recurrent oral and cutaneous infections associated with cyclic neutropenia. Arch Dermatol 80:731, 1959

Blume RS, Wolff SM: The Chediak-Higashi syndrome: Studies in four patients and a review of the literature. Medicine 51:247, 1972

Boxer LA et al: Correction of leukocyte function in Chediak-Higashi syndrome by Ascorbate. N Engl J Med 295:1041, 1976

Carloss HW et al: Cimetidine induced granulocytopenia. Ann Intern Med 93:57, 1980

Cohen DW, Morris AL: Periodontal manifectations of cyclic neutropenia. J Periodontol 32:159, 1961

Dale DC, Guerry D et al: Chronic neutropenia. Medicine 58:128, 1979

Deasy MJ et al: Familial benign chronic neutropenia associated with periodontal disease: A case report. J Periodontol 51:206, 1980

Garfunkel AA, Kaufman E, Galili D, Eldor A: Local therapeutic approach to agranulocytic oral ulcers. Pharmacol Ther Dent 4:21, 1979

Gates GF: Chronic neutropenia presenting with oral lesions. Oral Surg 27:563,1969

Gorlin RJ, Chaudry AP: The oral manifestation of cyclic (periodic) neutropenia. Arch Dermatol 82:344, 1960

Kalkwarf KL, Gutz DP: Periodontal changes associated with chronic idiopathic neutropenia. Pediatr Dent 3:189,1981

Kyle RA: Natural history of chronic idiopathic neutropenia. N Engl J Med 32:908,1980

Lampert F, Fesseler A: Periodontal changes during chronic benign granulocytopenia in childhood: A case report. J Clin Periodontol 2:105, 1975

Levine S: Chronic familial neutropenia with marked periodontal lesions. Oral Surg 12:310, 1959

Miller ME, Oski FA, Harris MB: Lazy-leukocyte syndrome: A new disorder of neutrophil function. Lancet 1:665,1971

Mishkin DJ, Akers JO, Darby CP: Congenital neutropenia: Report of a case and a biorationale for dental management. Oral Surg 42:738, 1976.

Pincus SH, Boxer LA, Stossel TP: Chronic neutropenia in childhood: Analysis of sixteen cases and a review of the literature. Am J Med 61:849, 1976

Pinkerton PH, Robinson JB, Senn JS: Lazy-leukocyte syndrome—disorder of the granulocyte membrane? J Clin Pathol 31:300, 1978

Price TH, Dale DC: The selective neutropenias. Clin Haematol 7:501, 1978

Reichart PA, Dornow H: Gingivo-periodontal manifestations in chronic benign neutropenia. J Clin Periodontol 5:74, 1978

Shiomara T et al: A case of generalized amyloidosis associated with cyclic neutropenia. Blood 54:628, 1979

Tempel TR, Kimball S, Kakehashi S, Amen CR: Host factors in periodontal disease: Periodontal manifestations of Chediak-Higashi syndrome. J Periodont Res 10:26, 1972

Yoda S et al: Transient "lazy leukocyte" syndrome during infancy. Am J Dis Child 134:467, 1980

Leukemia

Carey JA, Checote RR: Dental treatment for the child with acute lymphocytic leukemia. J Dent Child 42:191, 1975

Dreizen S, Bodey GP, Brown LR: Opportunistic gram-negative bacillary infections in leukemia: Oral manifestations during myelosuppression. Postgrad Med 55:133, 1974

Dreizen S, Bodey GP, Rodriguez V: Oral complications of cancer chemotherapy. Postgrad Med 58:75, 1975

Ferguson MM, Stephen KW, Dagg JH, Hunter IP: The presentation and management of oral lesions in leukemia. J Dent 6:201, 1974

Goepferd JJ: Leukemia and its dental implications. J Dent Handicap 4:44, 1979

Goodstein DB, Himmelfarb R: Allopurinol-induced mandibular neuropathy. Oral Surg 39:51, 1975

Greenberg MS, Cohen SG, McKitrick JC, Casseleth PA: The oral flora as a source of septicemia in patients with acute leukemia. Oral Surg 53:32, 1982

Guggenheimer J et al: Clinicopathologic effects of cancer chemotherapeutic agents on human buccal mucsa. Oral Surg 44:58, 1977

Limogelli WA, Clark MS, Williams AC: Noma like lesion in a patient with chronic lymphocytic leukemia. Oral Surg 41:40, 1976

Lockhart PB, Sonis ST: Relationship of oral complication to peripheral blood leukocyte and platelet counts in patients receiving cancer chemotherapy. Oral Surg 48:21, 1979

Lynch MA, Ship II: Initial oral manifestations of leukemia. J Am Dent Assoc 75:932, 1967

McGoroan DA, Gorman JM, Otridge BW: Intensive dental care in adult leukemia. Dent Practit 20:239, 1970

Michaud M, Baehner RL, Bixler D, Kafrawey AH: Oral manifestations of acute leukemia in children. J Am Dent Assoc 95:1145, 1977

Peterson DE, Overholser CD: Increased morbidity associated with oral infection in patients with acute nonlymphocytic leukemia. Oral Surg 51:390, 1981

Segelman AE, Doku HC: Treatment of the oral complications of leukemia. Oral Surg 35:469, 1977

Sinrod HS: Leukemia as a dental problem. J Am Dent Assoc 55:809, 1957

Smillie AC, Cowman SC: Pulp and periapical involvement in leukemia. NZ Dent J 65:32, 1969

Weistein RA, Choukas NC, Wood WS: Cancrum oris-like lesion associated with acute myelogenous leukemia. Oral Surg 38:10, 1974

Worth HM: Some significant abnormal radiologic appearances in young jaws. Oral Surg 21:609, 1966

Lymphoma

Abaza NA, Iczkovitz ML, Henefer EP: American Burkitt's lymphoma manifested in a solitary submandibular lymph node. Oral Surg 51:121, 1981

Bathard–Smith PJ, Coonar HS, Markus AF: Hodgkin's disease presenting intraorally. Br J Oral Surg 16:64, 1978

Blok P, van Delden L, van der Waal I: Non-Hodgkin's lymphoma of the hard palate. Oral Surg 47:445, 1979

Cline RE, Stenger TG: Histiocyte lymphoma (reticulum-cell sarcoma). Oral Surg 43:422, 1977

Lehrer S, Roswit B, Federman Q: The presentation of malignant lymphoma in the oral cavity and pharynx. Oral Surg 41:441, 1976

Long JC: The immunopathology of Hodgkin's disease. Clin Haematol 8:531, 1979

Mittelman D, Kaban LB: Recurrent "non-Hodgkin's lymphoma" presenting with gingival enlargement. Oral Surg 42:792, 1976

Smith DB et al: Soft swelling of the hard palate. J Am Dent Assoc 102:199, 1981

Steg RF et al: Malignant lymphoma of the mandible and maxillary region. Oral Surg 12:128, 1959

Symposium: Staging in Hodgkin's disease. Ann Arbor, Michigan. Cancer Res 31:1707, 1971

Tomich CE, Shafer WG: Lymphoproliferative disease of the hard palate: A clinicopathologic entity. A study of twenty-one cases. Oral Surg 39:754, 1975

Vickery IM, Midda M: Dental complications of cytotoxic therapy in Hodgkin's disease: A case report. Br J Oral Surg 13:282, 1976

Ziegler JL: Burkitt's lymphoma. N Engl J Med 305:735, 1981

Multiple Myeloma

Akin RK, Barton K, Walter PJ: Amyloidosis, macroglossia and carpal tunnel syndrome associated with myeloma. J Oral Surg 33:690, 1975

Bayrd ED, Heck FJ: Multiple myeloma: A review of 83 proved cases. JAMA 133:147, 1947

Bruce KW, Royer RQ: Multiple myelomas occurring in jaws. Oral Surg 6:729, 1953

Cranin AM, Gross ER: Severe oral and perioral amyloidosis as primary complication of multiple myeloma. Oral Surg 23:153, 1967

Flick WG, Lawrence FR: Oral amyloidosis as initial symptom of multiple myeloma. Oral Surg 49:18–20, 1980

Gross SD, Roth NA, Koudelka BM: Multiple myeloma presenting as a hemorrhagic diathesis. J Oral Maxillofac Surg 41:125, 1983

Kraut RA, Buhler JE, LaRue JR, Acevado A: Amyloidosis associated with multiple myeloma. Oral Surg 43:63, 1977

Smith DB: Multiple myeloma involving the jaws. Oral Surg 10:910, 1957

Infectious Mononucleosis

McCarthy JT, Hoagland RJ: Cutaneous manifestation of infectious mononucleosis. JAMA 187:153, 1964

Niederman JC et al: Infectious mononucleosis: clinical manifestations in relation to EB virus antibodies. JAMA 203:205, 1968

Red Cell Disorders

Alexander WN, Bechtold WA: Alpha thalassemia minor trait accompanied by clinical oral signs. Oral Surg 43:892, 1977

Beutler E: Genetic disorders of human red blood cells. JAMA 233:1184, 1975

Caffey J: Cooley's anemia. Am J Roentgenol 78:381, 1957

Cahn LR: The Plummer-Vinson syndrome facies: an oral pre-cancerous sign. Arch Clin Oral Pathol 2:308, 1938

Friedlander AH et al: Mental nerve neuropathy: a complication of sickle cell crisis. Oral Surg 49:15, 1980

Goldsby JW, Staats OJ: Nuclear changes of intraoral exfoliated cells of six patients with sickle-cell disease. Oral Surg 16:1042, 1963

Greenberg MS: Clinical and histologic changes of the oral mucosa in pernicious anemia. Oral Surg 52:38, 1981

Halstead CL: Oral manifestations of hemoglobinopathies. J Oral Surg 30:615, 1970

Hays GL: Nuclear characteristic of buccal mucosa cells in sickle cell anemia. Oral Surg 43:554, 1977

Kirson LE, Tomaro AJ: Mental nerve paresthesia secondary to sickle cell anemia. Oral Surg 48:509, 1979

Lasser SD et al: Dental management of patients undergoing bone marrow transplantation for aplastic anemia. Oral Surg 43:181, 1977

Mittleman G et al: Alveolar bone changes in sickle cell anemia. J Periodontol 32:74, 1961

Moore CV: The importance of nutritional factors in the pathogenesis of iron-deficiency anemia. Am J Clin Nutr 3:3, 1955

Moore CV, Dubach R: Metabolism and requirements of iron in the human. JAMA 162:197, 1956

Novak AJ: The oral manifestations of erythroblastic anemia. Am J Orthodont 30:542, 1944

Prowler JR, Smith EW: Dental bone changes occurring in sickle-cell disease and abnormal hemoglobin traits. Radiology 65:762, 1955

Robinson IB, Sarnat BG: Roentgen studies of the maxillae, and mandible in sickle-cell anemia. Radiology 58:517, 1952

Sanger RG et al: Differential diagnosis of some simple osseous lesions associated with sickle cell anemia. Oral Surg 43:538, 1977

Thomas ED: Bone marrow transplantation. JAMA 249:2528, 1983

23

Bleeding and Clotting Disorders

MALCOLM A. LYNCH

Hemorrhage is one of the most common manifestations of disease in the oral cavity and is of vital concern to every dental practitioner. It is also one of the most dramatic and powerful stimuli to motivate the patient to seek medical or dental attention. Amounts varying from profuse postsurgical or post-traumatic bleeding to minimal quantities collected on a pillow during the night from blood-stained saliva may bring the patient scurrying to the office door or prompt a hysterical phone call to the dentist. Whatever the etiology of the bleeding, the dentist should be able to reassure the patient while he systematically assesses the amount of blood lost, decides whether emergency replacement is indicated, and ascertains the cause of the loss and the proper long-term therapy.

ASSESSING BLOOD LOSS

The amount of blood lost by a patient is often difficult to assess because many patients overreact emotionally to even small amounts of blood. If on examination of the oral cavity, profuse or brisk hemorrhage is occurring, assessment is easy; however, if the patient presents a collection of blood-tinged saliva, a blood-stained pillowcase, or a histrionic description of blood loss, it is difficult to evaluate how much bleeding has actually occurred. If bleeding is reasonably slow and the patient has been able to maintain proper fluid intake, a measurement of the hemoglobin or hematocrit should give a rough idea of the amount of blood loss. This is especially helpful if the normal values for *that particular patient* are known (*e.g.*, preoperative hemoglobin or hematocrit in surgical cases). In *acute* bleeding, the hemoglobin or hematocrit may not give an accurate assessment of the oxygen-carrying capacity of the blood inasmuch as blood volume may not have yet been totally replaced at the expense of the extravascular fluid volume. The hemoglobin and hematocrit levels would not decrease until this migration of extravascular fluid into the vascular space has occurred, thereby diluting the hemoglobin and hematocrit concentrations.

In a hospital situation where time permits, measurement of the total red cell mass using radioactive chromium tagging of the red cells will give the most accurate assessment of total body red cell hemoglobin. In an acute situation and in a location where sophisticated radioactive studies are not available (as in a dentist's or a physician's office), a far simpler and more rapid method of measuring decrease in the blood volume is the *positional determination of the pulse and blood pressure*. The patient should be placed in the supine position for a few minutes and the pulse rate and the blood pressure obtained. Then the patient should be changed to the sitting position and within 45 seconds, the pulse rate and blood pressure retaken. If there has been a significant decrease in blood volume, the pulse rate will *increase* by at least 20, and the blood pressure will *decrease* by 20 or more mm Hg. If such a situation occurs in a patient with a history of significant blood loss, blood volume replacement therapy should be instituted as soon as possible without awaiting the results of more sophisticated laboratory studies.

CAUSES OF BLEEDING IN THE ORAL CAVITY

Bleeding into the oral cavity may be classified, on the basis of etiology, into the following categories:

HEMORRHAGE DUE TO LOCAL CAUSE

- Infection
  Fusospirochetal infection
  Primary herpes simplex infection
- Local irritants
  Malposed teeth
  Calculus accretions
  Prosthetic appliances
- Postsurgical or post-traumatic
- Rupture of blood-containing bullae caused by local trauma (*e.g.*, cheek biting)
- Congenital malformation
  Hemangiomata
  Hereditary hemorrhagic telangiectasia

HEMORRHAGE DUE TO CLOTTING FACTOR DEFICIENCIES OR CLOTTING FACTOR DYSFUNCTION

- Deficiencies
  Hereditary
    Hemophilia A
    Hemophilia B

Von Willebrand's disease
Hemorrhage Due to Other Clotting Factor Deficiencies
Iatrogenic
  Anticoagulant therapy
  Therapy with drugs other than anticoagulants
Liver disease
  Factor II, VII, IX, and X deficiencies
• Dysfunction
Multiple myeloma
Systemic lupus erythematosus
Macroglobulinemia

HEMORRHAGE DUE TO PLATELET DEFICIENCY, EXCESS, OR DYSFUNCTION

• Deficiency
Idiopathic thrombocytopenic purpura
Secondary thrombocytopenic purpura
Incompatible transfusion reaction
Leukemia
Multiple myeloma
Systemic lupus erythematosus
Aplastic anemia
Drug or chemical allergy
Cytotoxic drug therapy
Hypersplenism
Diffuse intravascular coagulation (usually obstetric complication)
• Excess
Thrombocytosis
• Dysfunction
Defective Adherence
  Von Willebrand's disease
  Bernard-Soulier syndrome
Defective platelet release reaction
  Storage pool disease
  Drugs (aspirin, phenylbutazone, indomethacin)
Defective aggregation
  Thrombasthenia
Other defects of uncertain nature
  Uremia
  Cryoglobulinemia
  Macroglobulinemia
  Liver disease

HEMORRHAGE DUE TO SYSTEMIC DISEASES OTHER THAN THOSE INVOLVING THE BLOOD OR BLOOD-FORMING ORGANS

• Septic embolization in bacterial endocarditis
• Meningococcemia

• Viral infections
• Scurvy (dentulous patients only)
• Rupture of blood-containing bullae (of systemic origin)
Erythema multiforme
Pemphigus
Pemphigoid
• Allergy

Hemorrhage Due to Local Cause

Hemorrhage due to local cause is probably the most common type of bleeding the dentist will encounter. The dentist should keep in mind that local causes may be a contributing factor in bleeding of systemic etiology and should, therefore, be prepared to search more thoroughly for such a systemic cause if the bleeding does not respond to local therapy, is disproportionate to the degree of local disease, or if there is a strong personal or family history of bleeding.

Marginal gingivitis caused by calculus deposits or debris on the tooth surfaces, rough and badly broken down teeth, or faulty restorations is likely to bleed on the slightest provocation. Bleeding and a blood-stained toothbrush are good evidence of the hyperemic gingiva. Minimal bleeding in the absence of marginal gingivitis may sometimes be seen coming from the periodontal space in the case of occlusal traumatism or teeth undergoing rapid orthodontic movement. This is usually noted by the patient only during toothbrushing.

Probably the most common cause of bleeding when brushing the teeth or a blood-stained pillow at night is a fusospirochetal infection. The bleeding takes place from the necrotic tissue on the surface of the cratered interdental papilla. The bleeding is usually minimal but is often the first symptom noticed by a patient with an incipient fusospirochetal infection.

Therapy for any of the above local causes of oral hemorrhage consists of removal of the local irritating factors. In the case of a fusospirochetal infection, hydrogen peroxide mouthrinses aid in destroying the organisms and by local foaming action, also act as a debriding agent. In rare cases in which patients do not respond to either hydrogen peroxide or local debridement, the dentist must resort to antibiotic therapy (usually penicillin). Fusospirochetal infections are discussed in more detail in Chapter 5.

The hemorrhage associated with a primary herpes simplex infection results from the tender, boggy, hyperemic gingivae associated with the viral infection. The amount of hemorrhage is minimal, and the patient zealously guards against trauma to the gingiva that would incite hemorrhage because of the exquisite tenderness of the gingiva. There is no specific treatment for the hemorrhage, which will cease with the resolution of the infectious process within 7 to 14 days.

Postsurgical or posttraumatic bleeding may be quite profuse. It is assumed that a dentist will have taken a thorough history before embarking on procedures involving the loss of blood. The patient who bleeds abnormally for the *first* time despite *prior* extensive oral surgical procedures is almost certainly doing so because of local factors, or more rarely, acquired hemorrhagic diathesis, rather than an inherited clotting disorder. Often, simple compression of the buccal and lingual plates of bone contiguous to the alveolar socket will suffice to stop hemorrhage. Sometimes it may be necessary to debride the socket of foreign material, necrotic bone, or an "infected" clot and allow another clot to form. Application of firm pressure over the occlusal surface of the alveolus with a gauze pad will usually stop capillary oozing. If local measures are ineffective in stopping postsurgical bleeding, the patient must be investigated thoroughly for platelet or clotting factor deficiencies.

Blood-filled bullae are sometimes seen on oral examination; these may be caused by cheek biting or more ominously, by pemphigus, pemphigoid, or erythema multiforme. (The last three diseases are classified under rupture of blood-containing bullae of systemic origin. When the bullous lesion bursts, blood is released into the mouth, but with the exception of erythema multiforme, further bleeding is distinctly unusual. Except with erythema multiforme, the patient is often unaware either of the presence of the bullae or of the bleeding when they rupture.

Congenital malformations may also be a source of oral bleeding of local cause. These include hereditary hemorrhagic telangiectasia and hemangiomata.

Hereditary Hemorrhagic Telangiectasia

Hereditary hemorrhagic telangiectasia, although relatively rare, should be recognized by every dentist who comes in contact with a case. This condition was first described by Osler in 1901, and it frequently bears his name (Osler–Rendu–Weber syndrome). It is transmitted as a nonsex-linked, simple dominant mendelian characteristic. Bird and associates studied a large family in which 32 of 170 members were affected. There was no genetic linkage between hereditary hemorrhagic telangiectasia and any specific blood group.

This disease is characterized by multiple localized angiomata or telangiectases on the skin, particularly in the circumoral region. The skin of the cheeks, the nasal orifices, and the ears may present the characteristic lesions. Oral mucosal involvement is estimated to occur in 60% of cases with the lips and tongue being most frequently affected (see Fig. 23-1). The lesions may be present in childhood but more often appear in puberty and become progressively worse with increasing age. They often give rise to profuse hemorrhage, either spontaneously or as a result of trauma. This hemorrhage is most likely to occur spontaneously or with slight provocation, such as an episode of epistaxis. The oral lesions do not often bleed, but the bleeding may occur without any known or apparent injury or irritation.

Severe oral hemorrhage may be experienced several times a day for weeks. At times, there will be a gush of blood when the involved areas are simply touched with cotton. The skin lesions virtually never bleed. Severe bleeding may occur from the mucosa of the gastrointestinal tract, which is very difficult to control because of the multiplicity of bleeding sources and difficulty of localization. Bleeding is not associated with any derangement of laboratory tests of the hemostatic mechanism.

The typical lesion is a cherry-red to purplish macule or small papule that resembles a crushed spider. Raised vascular nodules may also occur. The lesions blanch on pressure and regain their color when the pressure is removed. The telangiectatic areas are nonpulsating, although when there is hemor-

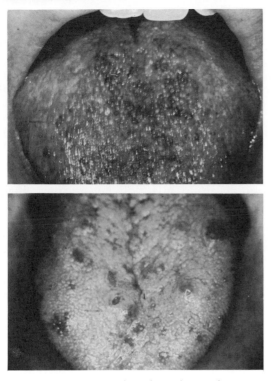

Fig. 23-1 Oral lesions in hereditary hemorrhagic telangiectasia.

rhage from the oral lesions, it is usually profuse and appears as if a small artery had been severed. As the affected individual grows older, the bleeding episodes tend to increase in frequency and intensity. Most of these patients, as might be expected, will have a low hemoglobin as a manifestation of the iron-deficiency anemia caused by the hemorrhage.

This disease can be diagnosed on the basis of the familial history and the presence of multiple angiomata of the skin and the mucosa, which have a tendency to profuse and recurrent hemorrhage. One may encounter difficulty in differentiating angiomata from petechiae and ecchymoses. Pressure with the tip of a moderately sharp lead pencil or a glass slide will blanch the angiomata. Petechiae will be unaffected by the pressure.

Dental Considerations. Other than spontaneous hemorrhage in the oral cavity, which is relatively rare, hemorrhage may be encountered during dental treatment that en-

croaches on the telangiectatic lesion. Prostheses that impinge on telangiectatic areas may also incite irritation or hemorrhage. For prophylaxis of bleeding, the use of a sclerosing agent such as morrhuate sodium or sodium tetradecyl sulfate injected into a lesion is useful. Electrocautery is also useful when applied prophylactically to lesions likely to cause bleeding. The usual procedures for the control of active hemorrhage can be used during an acute bleeding episode. Electrocoagulation is particularly effective in controlling the oral or nasal hemorrhages (where accessible), although chemical coagulation with 50% trichloroacetic acid can also be used.

Hemangiomata

One final local cause of oral hemorrhage is hemangiomata. These are congenital malformations and unlike the lesions of hereditary hemorrhagic telangiectasia, are usually larger (up to 1 cm in diameter) and tend to decrease in size at puberty. Larger malformations may persist through adult life. Histologically, hemangiomata may be capillary or cavernous in character, but from a therapeutic standpoint this is not important. They may vary in size, being as unobtrusive as macules or as predominant as a pedunculated lesion. As might be expected, the macular lesions are less prone to hemorrhage. They may occur anywhere in the oral cavity—lips, gingiva, tongue (see Fig. 23-2), buccal mucosa, or within the jawbones. When lesions are pres-

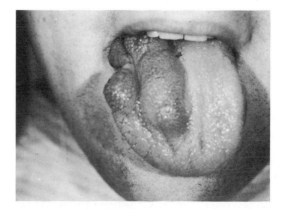

Fig. 23-2 Large hemangioma affecting the tongue and side of the face.

ent within the jawbones, the patient may present with mobile teeth, bleeding from the gingival crevice, and expansion of the cortex of the jawbone in the area of involvement. Diagnosis is by routine and angiographic radiography.

Therapy can entail the use of sclerosing agents such as sodium tetradecyl or morrhuate sodium, injected directly into the lesion. This is especially effective with the larger lesions. Complete surgical excision is also possible, but it is often difficult to assess the size of the lesion preoperatively, and profuse hemorrhage during the operation may be encountered with deep, extensive lesions. Preoperative embolization of the major afferent vessels, which have been identified by angiography as supplying central hemangiomas of the jawbone, frequently reduces hemorrhage at the time of surgery. Various materials have been used: embolizing agents including fragment of muscles, silicone pellets, Gelfoam pellets, and lead pellets. Unless the lesion is pedunculated and the size therefore easily ascertainable, surgery should be performed in a hospital with typed and crossmatched blood ready for the patient in case of need. Radiation has been used effectively, but its use is on the decline, as is generally the use of therapeutic radiation for nonneoplastic lesions.

Hemorrhage Due to Clotting Factor Deficiencies or Dysfunctions

The normal clotting mechanism can be seen in Figure 23-3. Those factors involved with release of substances from injured tissue are tissue factors or tissue thromboplastin and belong to the *extrinsic system;* the *intrinsic system* requires factors present in the plasma. In addition, vascular factors such as blood vessel contractility and tissue tonus are important in old age, when there may be loss of tissue tone. The extrinsic system, with the aid of vascular factors, can cause clotting with minor trauma even without activation of the intrinsic system. This explains why hemophiliacs, who have a deficiency in one of the intrinsic factors, do not often have trouble with hemorrhage from minor scratches on the skin or toothbrush abrasion of the gingiva. Patients with intrinsic factor deficiency

will often be able to form an initial clot when injury occurs because of release of tissue thromboplastin. Later on, if the clot is disturbed without further tissue injury, profuse bleeding may occur. Hemophiliacs usually have a normal bleeding time but may resume bleeding at the site of the test several hours afterward.

Hemophilia is now a term applied to a group of genetically determined bleeding disorders. In evaluating reports in the literature of the bleeding diatheses, one must keep in mind certain historical perspectives. Before 1900, "hemophilia" probably referred to any sort of bleeding diathesis, and only as late as 1952 was it realized that there was a difference between hemophilia A (factor VIII coagulant activity deficiency) and hemophilia B (factor IX deficiency). The relationship between hemophilia A and a closely related factor deficiency, von Willebrand's disease, was not clearly delineated until the late 1970s. Patients manifesting oral bleeding caused by hereditary clotting deficiencies may have a family history of such bleeding, although some of these heritable deficiencies often arise as mutations.

Laboratory Diagnosis

Screening of patients with suspected bleeding disorders can be accomplished by a relatively small number of laboratory tests without inordinate expense to the patient. These tests include the prothrombin time, the partial thromboplastin time, the platelet count (direct method), and the Ivy bleeding time. In instances in which disseminated intravascular coagulation or deficient fibrinogen is suspected, a blood fibrinogen level should also be assayed. The prothrombin test is a reasonably accurate screener of the extrinsic pathway to coagulation and the partial thromboplastin time of the intrinsic pathway. The platelet count detects those causes of bleeding due to thrombocytopenia or thrombocytosis, and the bleeding time is particularly useful in detecting diseases caused by capillary abnormalities or in detecting abnormalities in platelet function as in von Willebrand's disease.

Good clinical judgment should prevail in ordering any of the above screening tests,

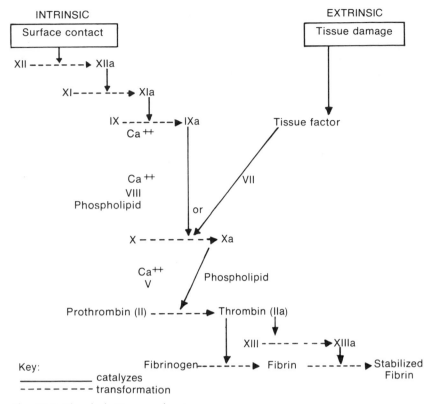

Fig. 23-3 Blood-clotting mechanism.

and testing should probably be limited to patients in whom it is reasonable to suspect that a bleeding diathesis may exist. Eisenberg and colleagues studied the use of the prothrombin and partial thromboplastin times as presurgical screening tests and concluded that based on the history or physical examination, the selective use of the presurgical screening test was justified in patients in whom a bleeding disorder was suspected. On the other hand, the use of these routine presurgical screening tests in patients without suspected bleeding disorders was of little or no value and did not justify the expense involved.

If any of the above screening tests are abnormal, more sophisticated (and expensive) tests are usually necessary to determine exactly which factor is missing in the clotting mechanism. Referral to a hematologist specializing in coagulation disorders should be considered in all patients with a strong history suggestive of a bleeding diathesis even though the above screening tests are normal. Some of these patients may have a rare co-

agulation disorder requiring a very sophisticated evaluation beyond the scope of most medical or dental practitioners. The reader is also referred to Chapter 3 for further discussion of laboratory testing and the clotting mechanism.

Hemophilia A

The largest number of *known* patients with a severe heritable clotting factor deficiency are patients with hemophilia A (factor VIII co-agulant factor deficiency; AHG deficiency). Hemophilia A occurs ten times more commonly than the next known clotting factor deficiency, hemophilia B (factor IX, PTC, Christmas factor deficiency), and 200 to 300 times more commonly than the other known clotting factor deficiencies (see Table 23-1). Hemophilia A (true hemophilia) occurs predominantly in males (less than a half-dozen females have been documented) and is inherited as a sex-linked recessive trait carried on the X chromosome. There is usually a

Table 23-1. Incidence of Factor Deficiencies

Factor	Probable Inheritance	Incidence per Million of Population of Congenital Defect
I	Autosomal recessive	0.5
II	Autosomal recessive	0.5
III	and	
IV	No deficiency	
V	Autosomal recessive	0.5
VII	Autosomal recessive*	0.5
VIII/c**	Sex-linked recessive	60–80
VIII/VWF**	Autosomal dominant	5–10
IX	Sex-linked recessive*	15–20
X	Autosomal recessive*	<0.5
XI	Autosomal dominant	<1.0
XII	Autosomal recessive	<1.0
XIII	Autosomal recessive	<0.5

* Most clinical deficiencies of factors II, VII, IX, and X are caused by liver disease, vitamin K deficiency, or coumarin anticoagulants.
** VIII/c is classic hemophilia A; VIII/VWF is von Willebrand's disease.

family history, although 25% of cases are said to arise as spontaneous mutations. Spontaneous hemorrhage in moderate and severe hemophilia usually takes the form of hemarthrosis into the larger joints (hip, knee, ankle). Spontaneous *oral* hemorrhage is more likely to occur for the first time in *mild* hemophilia. A study by Sonis and Musselman of 132 patients with hemophilia A found that 13.6% of the patients first presented with an oral bleeding episode, and the majority of these were patients with mild hemophilia. The most common site was the lip frenum with the tongue being a much less frequent second site. Nine percent of spontaneous bleeding episodes requiring infusion therapy were in the oral cavity. Patients with hemophilia A bleed excessively with oral trauma such as a tongue laceration or after tooth extraction.

Hemophiliacs may be classified as mild (less than 4% AHG); moderate (1% to 3% AHG); moderate to severe (0.0% to 0.9% AHG); and severe (0% AHG); from 50% to 150% is normal AHG. These are merely percentages, and quantitation of the actual normal AHG concentration shows it to be less than 1 mg/dl.

Results of laboratory tests to measure clotting (for techniques, see Chap. 3) are as follows: the bleeding time and tourniquet test are normal; the clotting time (not a particularly useful test) is abnormal only in those patients with less than 2% AHG; prothrombin time is normal and the prothrombin consumption abnormal, with less than 10% AHG. The thromboplastin generation time was the standard diagnostic test for many years. Because of the difficulty of performance and reproducibility of the results of this test other than in the hands of special laboratory technicians, it is being replaced by the partial thromboplastin time. At present, this rapid, simple test is the procedure of choice for diagnosis of hemophilia A and is prolonged in patients with AHG levels of less than 20%.

Because the hemophilia gene is no longer necessarily lethal at a very young age, more hemophiliacs are reproducing, and this increases the need for carrier detection. In the past, most carriers went undetected, but in recent years it has become possible to identify approximately 90% of women whose male off-spring are at risk for hemophilia A. The enabling tool is the ratio of factor VIII activity (measured in a clotting test) to the amount of factor-VIII-related antigen (a protein in plasma that can be measured by immunologic assays).

Since 1940 it has been known that there is also an acquired factor VIII deficiency caused by a circulating inhibitor of factor VIII. Clinically, the disease is similar to inherited factor VIII deficiency. The cause of those cases that arise *de novo* is not known, but inhibitors also develop in true hemophiliacs who secondarily develop factor VIII inhibitors in their blood after receiving many transfusions. The presence of inhibitors to factor VIII in a patient's blood may be demonstrated by adding a purified, standardized preparation of AHG to the patient's blood and then assaying for factor VIII concentration. If an inhibitor is present, it may be very difficult to increase the AHG concentration in a patient's blood before surgery by giving AHG concentrates.

Treatment of patients with hemophilia A will be discussed after the section on hemophilia B because in many aspects, dental care of these patients is quite similar.

Hemophilia B

Hemophilia B is caused by a deficiency in clotting factor IX. It is also known as PTC (plasma thromboplastin component) deficiency or Christmas disease after the surname of one of the first families in which the disease was recognized. The clinical manifestations are identified with those of hemophilia A, and it is inherited in the same manner— as a sex-linked recessive trait carried on the X chromosome. Several cases in females have been reported. Spontaneous mutations arise in about 15% of cases (25% in hemophilia A). The proportion of patients who have severe hemorrhagic tendencies is far greater in factor VIII than in factor IX deficiency. This does not mean that hemophilia B is a milder disease but only that fewer afflicted patients have virtually complete lack of the deficient factor. PTC deficiency has been reported to be from about one tenth to one fourth as common as hemophilia A deficiency. In the laboratory, hemophilia A may be differentiated from hemophilia B by a modification of the prothrombin consumption time or the partial thromboplastin time.

Factor IX differs from factor VIII in that factor VIII has poor stability on being stored in plasma, whereas factor IX is relatively stable; factor VIII is not present in serum, whereas factor IX is; vitamin K deficiency will not affect the plasma levels of factor VIII but will reduce levels of factor IX, and correspondingly, anticoagulant therapy with dicumarol will reduce factor IX levels but not factor VIII levels.

Dental Treatment of Patients with Hemophilia A or B

Endodontic Therapy. Although surgical techniques are generally not advisable in hemophiliacs, common endodontic techniques are quite acceptable provided that care is taken not to extend beyond the apex of the tooth. Hemorrhage into the canal can usually be controlled with 1:1000 aqueous epinephrine on an endodontic paper point. Pulpectomies in deciduous teeth are not associated with undue hemorrhage.

Prosthodontic Therapy. Hemophiliac patients tolerate full dentures very well. Partial dentures are also well tolerated as long as the patient maintains meticulous oral hygiene, because clasps can trap food debris, resulting in gingivitis and subsequent hemorrhage.

Periodontic Therapy. Conservative periodontic treatment is generally more desirable than gingival and osseous surgery because of the hospitalization and extensive amount of replacement factor therapy necessary with surgery.

Anesthesia. Local anesthesia is contraindicated in the severe hemophiliac without prior replacement factor therapy. Block local anesthesia is particularly pernicious inasmuch as it can lead to bleeding in the tissue planes, formation of a hematoma, and obstruction of the airway. Nitrous oxide anesthesia by mask is quite useful in these individuals. General anesthesia with intubation is not indicated because of the great danger of laryngeal bleeding from intubation.

Restorative Therapy. Restorative procedures may be carried out in the hemophiliac patient as in normal patients, but the rubber dam must be used to prevent trauma to the gingiva and other oral soft tissues. The dam is particularly effective in preventing laceration of the tongue. When use of the rubber dam is not practical, an epinephrine-impregnated hemostatic cord placed in the gingival sulcus before preparation of the crown or inlay margin is also helpful in preventing hemorrhage.

Oral Surgical Procedures. Surgical treatment of the patient with hemophilia should be a concerted effort on the part of the dentist and the physician (usually a hematologist) responsible for the medical management of the patient's hemophilia and should be done in a hospital.

Local Hemostatic Agents. Lucas reported good results with the use of oxidized cellulose saturated with bovine thrombin-$NaHCO_3$ solution. After oral surgical procedures, the solution is placed in each *individual* root socket, which has been previously cleaned and dried with sterile gauze. Even the smallest amount of fibrin or partially clotted blood will interfere with the hemostatic activity of locally applied thrombin. After packing, the tooth socket must be protected by mechanical devices to prevent disturbance of the clot, which would lead to further bleeding. In patients treated locally who developed secondary bleeding, Lucas found that removal of the clot and repacking with oxidized cellulose-thrombin-$NaHCO_3$ was sufficient to stop the hemorrhage in most cases.

Many workers maintain that hemophiliacs cannot be treated with local measures alone. Lucas attributes their lack of success to improper attention to detail (careful packing of the socket) and indeed has reported success in some of his hemophiliac patients treated *only* with local measures. The degree of success partially depends on the severity of the hemophilia (*i.e*, factor VIII or IX level).

Mechanical Splints. There is almost universal agreement that once a clot forms in a hemophiliac, it must be zealously protected against dislodgment, which would lead to further profuse bleeding. The splint must be constructed so that it will guard the clot without applying undue pressure. When pressure is applied to a clot in a hemophiliac, whether with a mechanical splint or gauze pad, it will not arrest bleeding; in fact, it will serve only to prevent the blood from escaping by way of the normal route at the top of the socket and lead to intratissue hemorrhage and hematoma formation. This can be life-threatening in the fascial planes of the neck by closing off the airway. Splints must be used in *conjunction* with local or systemic therapy to induce clotting.

Sutures. The use of sutures is controversial and probably depends on the individual case. On the one hand, approximation of the tissue with sutures tends to aid in protection of the clot. On the other hand, sutures tend to move slightly with the actions of the tongue and buccinator muscle, and bleeding often occurs at the suture site. In some areas (*e.g.,* lacerated tongue), suture use is practically unavoidable. When used, sutures should be of the smallest size practicable, placed with an atraumatic needle, and in number, only the minimum necessary to provide clot protection and tissue approximation. Sutures must be used in conjunction with local or systemic coagulation therapy.

Factor VIII or IX Replacements or EACA. Factor VIII (AHG) is unstable, so plasma must be used soon after the blood is taken from a patient or cold centrifuged or fresh frozen. Cryoprecipitate or lyophilized concentrates are the most common vehicles in use today for raising AHG levels in hemophiliacs before surgical procedures. Fresh plasma may be used, but it has several disadvantages. It can transmit hepatitis. It is highly antigenic because it contains all blood proteins except those in the red cells. In patients needing a great deal of AHG (*i.e.,* those with inhibitors to AHG in their blood), problems of hypervolemia and congestive heart failure occur. For these reasons, cryoprecipitate or lyophilized concentrates of AHG have been made from fresh plasma.

Probably the easiest to make of the concentrates is a cryoprecipitate of AHG. It can be made by any blood bank by cooling fresh plasma until a white precipitate forms (this precipitate is relatively pure AHG), and the blood bank can then use the plasma in other patients (not hemophiliacs, of course), which keeps the cost low. The only real disadvantages of the cryoprecipitate are the lack of assured potency (in normal individuals AHG ranges from 50% to 150%) and the fact that it must be stored in a freezer. The amount of AHG contained in a unit of plasma (300 ml) can be administered as a cryoprecipitate in 15 ml after thawing and resuspension in normal saline.

Glycine precipitates of AHG are now commercially available. Although more expensive than cryoprecipitates, they have the advantage of needing only refrigeration for storage and of being assayed and of standardized potency. Because of higher purification, there is less chance of an untoward allergic reaction and of transmitting hepatitis. The high-potency concentrates are particularly useful in treating patients with AHG inhibitors who may have enough inhibitor present to require more than 150 units of fresh plasma to gain therapeutic (50%) AHG levels—a clearly impossible feat.

Factor IX (PTC) is relatively stable and unlike AHG, is present in both plasma and serum. Compared with patients with AHG deficiency, who may have inhibitors to AHG in their blood and thereby need enormous quantities of AHG supplementation, patients with PTC deficiency usually do not need such large amounts of PTC, and serum or plasma suffices in most cases to prepare the patients preoperatively and treat them postoperatively. Another reason for the lesser requirement of PTC supplementation is that patients with PTC deficiency usually have higher initial levels of PTC than patients with hemophilia A have of AHG.

Because PTC deficiency is also rarer than AHG deficiency, there has been less impetus for the commercial development of PTC concentrates. Nonetheless, chromatographic DEAE-Sephadex absorbed prothrombin complexes (Konyne, Proplex, Profilate) have been developed. The concentration of factor IX in these preparations is increased considerably over plasma, and in addition they contain factors II, VII, and X. They are also useful in treatment of cases of hypothrombinemia induced by liver disease or bishydroxycoumarin therapy. There is an extraordinarily high risk of acquiring viral hepatitis from the use of these products. It is documented to be as high as 50% of patients in some studies. Fortunately, almost all patients with hemophilia B resulting from multiple exposures to blood products containing the virus will have acquired immunity and will be at a relatively low risk.

Epsilon-aminocaproic acid (EACA) has antifibrinolytic properties and thus acts as a clot stabilizer. When used in conjunction with appropriate factor replacement therapy, it appears to reduce the need for a high circulating level of infused factor VIII or IX and considerably reduces the cost.

Webster and co-workers concluded that dental surgery can be accomplished safely in even the most severe hemophiliac when the deficient factor is replaced by infusion. Both continuous and intermittent infusion therapy provide maximal hemostasis for major surgical procedures. Very minor oral surgical procedures and other less traumatic surgical procedures such as tooth extraction may be completed with a single dose of factor VIII or IX concentrate and EACA. In the severe hemophiliac, it appears that EACA alone is not sufficient to provide adequate hemostasis.

Von Willebrand's Disease

Von Willebrand's disease is the most common of the hereditary clotting disorders, but it has only recently begun to be recognized because of the development of newer and more definitive diagnostic techniques. With the advent of these newer tests for diagnosis, the discovery of new cases, and a more thorough understanding of the mechanisms involved in this disease, it is likely that it will be found to be the *most common hereditable cause of spontaneous intraoral hemorrhage*. Unlike hemophilia A and B, the clinical manifestations are usually mild; fatal hemorrhage almost never occurs and hemarthroses are rare.

In this disease there are at least two demonstrable defects. Platelet adhesiveness to the subendothelial collagen of the disrupted capillary wall is reduced (the probable explanation for a prolonged bleeding time), and, as in classic hemophilia A, factor VIII levels are low—usually in the range of 5% to 15%.

The complex molecule known collectively as factor VIII is actually a macromolecular protein composed of at least two molecular portions responsible for several biological activities. A smaller molecular portion appears to be associated with classical factor VIII coagulant activity, whereas the larger molecular portion is associated with von Willebrand factor activity. In von Willebrand's disease there is a quantitative and qualitative deficiency in this portion of the factor VIII molecule. Von Willebrand factor activity is responsible for platelet adhesion to subendothelium, regulates the plasma levels of factor VIII coagulant activity and thereby influences normal hemostasis. Although a prolonged bleeding time is characteristic of von Willebrand's disease, it may also be prolonged in other diseases, and more specific laboratory tests are available to identify von Willebrand factor deficiency in plasma. Results of two of these tests are abnormally decreased platelet retention to glass beads in von Willebrand's disease, and failure of ristocetin to induce platelet aggregation in patients with von Willebrand's disease as it does in normal patients.

Transmission is by a dominant autosomal gene, and it occurs with equal frequency in both sexes. Menorrhagia, epistaxis (75% of children with the disease), and gingival bleeding often occur. Hemarthroses are uncommon as are petechiae. Bleeding tendencies usually appear early in childhood and decrease in middle and old age.

Diagnosis is made in a patient with a family history of bleeding in *either* parent, gingival bleeding or epistaxis and a prolonged bleeding time (not often seen in hemophilia A or B), low AHG levels, abnormal platelet retention to glass beads, and decreased platelet aggregation with ristocetin as described above. The platelet count, clotting time, and prothrombin consumption are normal. Quick has described an aspirin tolerance test that appears to be positive in patients with von Willebrand's disease or thrombocytopathia. The bleeding time is determined 2 hours before the patient is given 10 gr of aspirin (5 gr for children); 2 hours later the bleeding time is again determined. In von Willebrand's disease the time is significantly prolonged: three times normal or greater after aspirin administration.

Dental Treatment. Patients with von Willebrand's disease should not be given aspirin because of the prolongation of the bleeding time that may occur. Local attention to meticulous details during surgical, periodontal, or restorative procedures usually suffices to prevent bleeding. In patients who tend to bleed profusely, hospitalization may be necessary. Transfusion with factor VIII cryoprecipitate preoperatively is usually adequate to control hemorrhage.

Hemorrhage Due to Other Clotting Factor Deficiencies

As can be seen in Table 23-1, the incidence of hereditary clotting factor deficiencies other than hemophilia A and B or von Willebrand's disease is quite low. As might be expected, bleeding from these disorders while they can occur are quite rare and not likely to be encountered in the average dental practice. A case was reported by Evian and co-authors in which a patient with no prior history of bleeding experienced profuse hemorrhage subsequent to periodontal surgery. Evaluation of the patient indicated that there was a previously undiagnosed factor XI deficiency. This case illustrates that patients who bleed unduly and unexpectedly subsequent to dental procedures should be referred to a hematologist for a coagulation evaluation.

Hemorrhage of Iatrogenic Cause

Anticoagulation Therapy

Common reasons or patients to be placed on anticoagulant therapy are an acute myocardial infarction, a cerebrovascular accident (stroke) caused by embolism or thrombosis, or an episode of pulmonary embolism—presumably originating from the veins in the iliac region or lower extremities. Most patients who are on anticoagulant therapy are warned by their physician to consult with him before any dental or surgical procedures. Nonetheless, the dentist should always question the patient as to the use of anticoagulants.

Two types of anticoagulants are used: heparin and the bishydroxycoumarin derivatives, which are used much more commonly than the heparin in ambulatory patients likely to be seen in the average dental office.

Because it must be given by injection, heparin is usually used only on hospitalized patients. It acts primarily by preventing thrombin formation, although in large doses it also inhibits platelet aggregation. When given subcutaneously, the duration of action is about 6 hours. The degree of anticoagulation is determined by performing Lee White clotting times, partial thromboplastin times, or activated partial thromboplastin times on the patient's blood. The usual therapeutic level is a time two to three times normal using any of the above tests of clotting functions. After dental procedures causing hemorrhage, the patient may usually be managed with topical thrombin. If necessary, the level of anticoagulation may be decreased rapidly (since the duration of action of heparin is only 6 hours) by reducing the heparin dosage the patient is receiving. This should be done by the patient's physician on the dentist's request. In an emergency situation in which profuse hemorrhage is present, the action of heparin may be reversed within a matter of minutes by the administration of intravenous protamine.

The bishydroxycoumarin derivatives are by far the safest and most widely used anticoagulants in medical practice today. They are given orally, usually as a single daily dose in the late afternoon. They act as vitamin K antagonists and depress the production of four clotting factors in the liver: factors II, VII, IX, and X. The degree of anticoagulation is determined by the Quick one-stage prothrombin time, and most patients are maintained at a therapeutic level of two to two and one half times the control level in seconds. Vitamin K antagonizes the action of these drugs, and their action is potentiated by salicylates and broad-spectrum antibiotics (which suppress the normal intestinal flora necessary for vitamin K synthesis). *Patients taking these drugs may occasionally be given salicylates for the relief of pain, but not in frequent or prolonged dosage.* Acetaminophen, which is often used as a substitute analgesic for aspirin, has also been demonstrated to potentiate the effects of therapeutic anticoagulants.

When dental procedures that might cause excessive hemorrhage are contemplated, the patient should be hospitalized (see Fig. 23-4). Many oral surgeons feel that these pa-

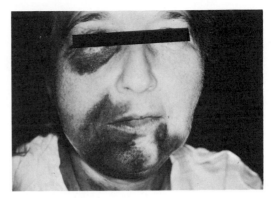

Fig. 23-4 Extensive ecchymosis that followed extraction of several molar teeth in a patient receiving dicumarol therapy.

tients can be treated without any reduction of the anticoagulant drug, provided that they are watched closely postoperatively and that topical thrombin is available. Although the action of the bishydroxycoumarin derivatives may be reversed by giving intramuscular vitamin K_1, it takes about 12 to 24 hours for this reversal to take place. In an emergency situation, patients have been given plasma transfusions to restore the missing factors. A concentrate is now available that will restore all four missing factors without the danger of hypervolemia, as is the case with plasma. This concentrate is discussed in the section on therapy of hereditary factor IX deficiency (Christmas disease).

Therapy with Drugs Other than Anticoagulants

On occasion therapy with drugs that do not generally have an anticoagulant effect may cause bleeding owing to effects on platelets such as aspirin or on the clotting factors themselves, or for unknown reasons. Hassell reported a case in which valproic acid, an antiepileptic drug, was shown to have an association between defective blood clotting and spontaneous hemorrhage. The exact mechanism in which valproic acid acted on hemostasis was unknown.

Hemorrhage Due to Liver Disease

Liver disease such as cirrhosis or hepatitis rarely causes oral hemorrhage until near terminal stages are reached. The mechanism is similar to that in iatrogenic anticoagulation therapy (suppression of formation of the clotting factors II, VII, IX, and X) and may be caused by two mechanisms because both an intact hepatic cell and vitamin K available to that cell are necessary for formation of the four clotting factors. In the case of hepatocellular diseases, suppression is directly caused by derangement of hepatic cell function. In the case of obstructive liver disease, another mechanism operates. Vitamin K is a fat-soluble vitamin, and the lack of intestinal bile, which is necessary for the emulsification of fats for digestion, inhibits vitamin K absorption. The formation of the four clotting factors is thereby inhibited because of the inavailability of vitamin K to the hepatic cell.

Dental treatment in these patients should be deferred until the patient's condition has improved. If emergency oral surgery is necessary, topical thrombin is of inestimable value. The concentrates discussed under hereditary factor IX deficiency are also available when it is absolutely necessary, but unlike hemophilia B patients, these patients will not likely have immunity to hepatitis, and the high (50%) risk of hepatitis with infusion of the concentrates must be weighed against the possible benefit.

Bleeding Due to Macroglobulinemia, Multiple Myeloma, and Systemic Lupus Erythematosus

Macroglobulinemia (*e.g.*, Waldenström's macroglobulinemia), multiple myeloma, and systemic lupus erythematosus are diseases in which abnormal serum proteins are produced. Oronasal bleeding is seen often—up to 80% of cases of macroglobulinemia—and is often the first manifestation of this disease. Bleeding occurs both as frank hemorrhage and as ecchymoses on the oral mucosa. The formation of complexes between the abnormal immunoglobulin M macroglobulins and clotting factors, thereby inactivating the clotting factors, is thought to cause the oral bleeding.

Oral bleeding is seen less commonly in multiple myeloma than in macroglobulinemia, and the bleeding may be caused by a similar inactivation of clotting factors. It may also be caused by thrombocytopenia secondary to plasma cell proliferation in the bone marrow. Multiple myeloma is discussed more fully in Chapter 22, Hematologic Diseases.

The abnormal serum proteins in systemic lupus erythematosus do not often cause oral bleeding, but the mechanism involving abnormal serum proteins would be operative in those rare instances in which it does occur.

Hemorrhage Due to Platelet Deficiency or Excess

Diseases of the platelets may be classified into three major categories as follows:

1. Thrombocytopenias—a decreased number of circulating platelets
2. Thrombocytosis—an increased number of circulating platelets
3. Platelet dysfunction—normal numbers of platelets that fail to function normally

Oral Manifestations. Because oral manifestations of all of the platelet disorders are similar, they will be discussed before consideration of each separate category.

The oral manifestations usually begin as petechiae-extravasated blood into the intercellular spaces visible just beneath the oral mucosa (see Figs. 23-5 and 23-6). Petechiae are reddish spots less than a pinhead in diameter that often first appear near the junction of the hard and soft palates. These spots do not blanch on pressure in contrast with the lesions of hereditary hemorrhagic telangiectasia, and this aids in differentiating petchiae or ecchymotic spots from vascular

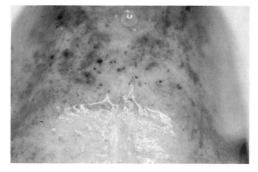

Fig. 23-5 Petechial hemorrhages on the palate under a full denture in a 44-year-old woman with idiopathic thrombocytopenic purpura. (From Dr. Burton Goldstein)

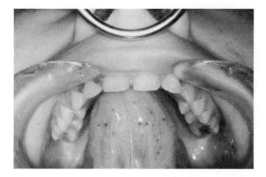

Fig. 23-6 Petechial hemorrhages of the oral mucosa.

anomalies. When the hemorrhage progresses and spreads along the tissue planes ecchymoses develop. Ecchymoses differ from petechiae only in extent, being larger than a pinhead.

With further development of the platelet disorder, frank hemorrhage into the oral cavity begins. At first this hemorrhage is seen at sites of minor trauma (*e.g.*, toothbrushing), but it may eventually occur spontaneously without known provocation. No local irritants are required to produce frank hemorrhage and even ecchymoses when the platelet count falls below 10,000/mm³. With very low platelet counts (less than 5,000), profuse hemorrhage usually occurs into the gingival papillae, enlarging them two to three times normal size and making them an ominous dark red color (see Fig. 22-26). Capillary oozing from the entire marginal gingiva is not unusual, and spontaneous pulpal hemorrhage has been observed. The decomposing blood in the gingival sulcus and the interdental areas produces a fetid odor and forms a favorable medium for microbial growth. When there is necrosis of tissue due to profuse intercellular hemorrhage, a fusospirochetal infection may be superimposed.

Diagnosis. Diagnosis of a platelet disorder may be suspected when petechiae, ecchymoses, or unexplainable bleeding occurs in the mouth and when a smear of the peripheral blood shows few or no platelets, too many platelets, or platelets exhibiting abnormal morphology. More definitive diagnosis depends on the actual platelet count, which is decreased in thrombocytopenia and increased in thrombocytosis. In disorders of

platelet function, the platelet count may be normal, but laboratory tests of platelet function such as clot retraction; platelet adhesiveness in glass bead column; platelet aggregation tests using ADP, ristocetin, connective tissue, and epinephrine; and platelet factor 3 release will be abnormal. The clinical test of bleeding time may be abnormal in both qualitative and quantitative disorders (see Chap. 3 for details of these tests).

Thrombocytopenia

Thrombocytopenia is a decrease in the number of circulating platelets. Depending on the technique, the number of platelets normally found in a cubic millimeter of blood is 150,000 to 500,000. Bleeding manifestations do not usually occur until the count has fallen to less than 60,000/mm³. Thrombocytopenia may be subdivided into two broad categories: in one the cause is unknown, idiopathic thrombocytopenic purpura; and in the other the cause is known, secondary thrombocytopenia.

Idiopathic thrombocytopenic purpura (ITP) may be the result of two mechanisms: decreased production of platelets, increased destruction of platelets, or both. Increased destruction of platelets has been demonstrated to be present in most patients with ITP, and it is thought to be on an autoimmune basis. No exogenous antigen is necessary to induce this autoimmunity. Many of these patients respond well to corticosteroid therapy. Other patients with increased platelet destruction have been found to have splenomegaly, suggesting that stasis of blood in the spleen may account in part for the destruction. Many of these patients respond to splenectomy. ITP is most common in postmenopausal women and in children. The most common causes of secondary thrombocytopenia are seen below.

DRUGS

1. Myelosuppressive agents used in therapy of neoplastic disease; these drugs when used in sufficient dosage cause thrombocytopenia in *all* patients.
2. Drugs causing thrombocytopenia as a side-effect on an individual patient-sensitivity basis, usually by inducing autoimmunity; those drugs that might be used

by the dentist and have been most frequently implicated are sedatives (barbiturates), analgesics (phenylbutazone, salicylates), antihistamines (diphenhydramine hydrochloride), and tranquilizers (meprobamate and diazepam). Although not often used in dental therapy, the sulfonamides, quinine, quinidine, and the oral diuretics are most commonly implicated.

DISEASES

1. Infectious—viral, bacterial
2. Metabolic—uremia, megaloblastic anemias
3. Neoplastic—carcinoma, leukemia, sarcoma, lymphoma, Hodgkin's disease
4. Bone marrow replacement or destruction other than neoplastic—myelofibrosis, radiation therapy
5. Systemic lupus erythematosus

Although the etiologic mechanisms affect the platelets in the same way as in ITP (*i.e.,* decreased production or increased destruction), in the case of secondary thrombocytopenia the cause is demonstrable. From the clinical standpoint, it can be said that a case of thrombocytopenia in which a cause is demonstrated is properly classified as secondary thrombocytopenia. This form of thrombocytopenia is more common in adults.

Treatment. Systemic treatment involves eliminating the cause when known and may consist of corticosteroids, splenectomy, and platelet transfusions.

Corticosteroids may decrease bleeding in patients with ITP or those with autoimmune, drug-induced thrombocytopenia. Steroids reduce bleeding even without producing a demonstrable rise in the platelet count. Splenectomy is sometimes useful in patients who have megakaryocytes in the bone marrow (*i.e.,* in those patients in whom the thrombocytopenia is caused by increased destruction rather than decreased production of platelets). Although it is not the treatment of choice, it is often used when corticosteroids fail. Platelet transfusions are useful in treating secondary thrombocytopenia but have little or no effect on patients with ITP. They

must be given every 3 to 4 days at first (the life-span of the platelet is 9 to 10 days), but with the frequent use of transfusions, antibodies develop, and the transfusions are less effective. It is usually sufficient to raise the platelet count to 20,000/mm^3.

Oral Treatment. The spontaneous gingival hemorrhages can often be controlled by the local use of hemostatics of the noncaustic type, such as fibrin foam, Gelfoam, or absorbable cellulose with thrombin. At times a 1.5% strength hydrogen peroxide mouthwash (1:1 dilution U.S.P. H$_2$O$_2$) will stop the gingival oozing, but at other times all measures are ineffective in controlling it. The diet should be soft or semisolid in order to minimize the trauma to the gums.

Do not attempt elective dental procedures when purpuric symptoms are present. Patients with secondary thrombocytopenia requiring emergency dental procedures that involve significant hemorrhage should be hospitalized and treated with the cooperation of the patient's physician. The platelet count should be at least 30,000/mm^3 before the dental procedure, and subsequent to the dental treatment the patient should be observed for further bleeding for several days. Give additional platelet transfusions if necessary. Meticulously observe local measures in order to keep the dental procedure as atraumatic as possible.

Thrombocytosis

Thrombocytosis is a rare disorder in which the level of platelets in the blood rises to greater than 1,000,000/mm^3. Although there is an excess of platelets, mucocutaneous petechiae, ecchymoses, and bleeding, as well as thrombotic lesions, are frequently seen throughout the body. The cause of the increase in platelets may be unknown (essential thrombocytosis, thrombocythemia hemorrhagica), transiently caused by a fracture of one of the long bones (*e.g,* femur) or profuse hemorrhage, or it may accompany malignant disease (*e.g.,* lung cancer, polycythemia vera, chronic granulocytic leukemia, or myelofibrosis). The thrombocytosis may be the first sign of a leukemia and may be present for several years before abnormalities of the white cells become manifest. Diagnosis is made by the platelet count. Systemic treatment consists acutely, of platelet pheresis and chronically, of myelosuppression using agents such as busulfan, melphalan, and radioactive phosphorus for bone marrow suppression.

Dental Considerations. Dental treatment of thrombocytosis should be conservative, and elective treatment should be deferred. If gingivitis or periodontal disease provides local stimuli for bleeding, cautiously and lightly scale one quadrant of the teeth at a time with the generous use of hydrogen peroxide or local hemostatic agents to stop bleeding as it occurs. If extractions are absolutely necessary, packing of the socket with an absorbable material such as Gelfoam will usually suffice to stop the hemorrhage. Frequently and carefully observe the patient for bleeding for at least 2 days postoperatively.

Hemorrhage Due to Platelet Dysfunction

In order to understand the various ways in which platelet dysfunction is involved in hemorrhage, it is necessary to understand how platelets function in the clotting mechanism. In the first step platelets adhere to the subendothelial collagen of the damaged vascular wall. This *adherence* is mediated in part by Von Willebrand's factor (see discussion in previous section). The next step after adherence of platelets is the *release* reaction in which adenosine diphosphate (ADP) is released and acts as a primary platelet aggregating agent. The release reaction is mediated by thrombin, which is generated either through the extrinsic or intrinsic clotting system as well as by an intraplatelet enzyme. The release reaction eventually forms prostaglandins and thromboxanes. Aspirin inhibits the latter action, and its interference with the clotting mechanism is responsible at least in part for this inhibitory effect. The ADP released in the release reaction acts as a primary platelet aggregating agent, thus leading to the next step of platelet action in which platelets *aggregate* at the site of injury providing a plug causing initial hemostasis. Platelet dysfunction may thus occur because of de-

fects in adherence, defects in the release, or defects in aggregation.

Defects in Adherence

Bernard–Soulier Syndrome. In this disease, transmitted as an autosomal dominant defect with variable penetration, the bleeding time is prolonged and aggregation with ristocetin is defective. It is theorized that a membrane receptor on the platelet is absent in this syndrome and accounts for the bleeding problems. The only known treatment is to use platelet transfusion during acute bleeding episodes.

von Willebrand's Disease. This disease is not felt to be a primary platelet disorder but rather a defect of the Von Willebrand's portion of the factor VIII molecule, which is necessary for platelet adherence. Treatment is discussed in the section on Von Willebrand's Disease.

Defects in Release

A number of drugs have been implicated in inhibiting the platelet release reaction. Among these are aspirin and other nonsteroidal anti-inflammatory agents such as phenylbutazone and indomethacin. Diagnosis is made by noting the abnormalities produced in the bleeding time and tests of platelet aggregation subsequent to the afflicted patient's ingestion of these agents. The dentist should avoid administering drugs that contribute to bleeding in these patients.

Some patients appear to have a primary defect in the platelet-release reaction of unknown cause but not apparently mediated by drugs.

Defects in Aggregation

Perhaps the prototype of defective aggregation is Glanzmann's disease or thrombasthenia. It was first described in 1918 as an inability of a patient's platelets to cause clot reaction, but it has since been learned that the defect is actually an aggregation of the platelets most likely caused by a defect in the platelet membrane.

Oral Manifestations

Oral manifestations of platelet dysfunction are similar to those of the other platelet disorders: spontaneous petechiae, ecchymoses and bleeding, and inordinate bleeding after minor oral trauma.

Diagnosis

Diagnosis of platelet dysfunction consists of platelet count (normal), platelet morphology (platelets may sometimes be abnormally large), and tests of platelet function including clot retraction (abnormal); decreased platelet adhesiveness in glass bead columns; defective platelet factor 3 release; platelet aggregation tests using ADP, ristocetin, connective tissue, and epinephrine; and prothrombin consumption (abnormally low).

Treatment

Dental. Use hemostatics locally in the oral cavity to control capillary bleeding. (Perkin and colleagues recently reported two cases of Glanzmann's thrombasthenia in which extractions were performed using microfibrillar bovine collagen and epsilon-aminocaproic acid to control postoperative hemorrhage. Results were excellent, and this method of treatment was suggested as a good therapeutic modality in these disorders.) Keep dental procedures as atraumatic as possible. Hospitalize patients with Glanzmann's hereditary thrombasthenia for dental procedures which are likely to cause appreciable bleeding (*e.g.*, tooth extraction, gingivectomy, deep periodontal scaling). Because clinical manifestations of the disease may be mild to severe in expression, the necessity of hospitalization and transfusion before restorative dental treatment must be evaluated for each patient. Because aspirin may aggravate the hemorrhage, choose other analgesics.

Systemic. Treatment to control bleeding episodes consists of transfusions of fresh platelet-rich plasma collected in a plastic bag. These transfusions should be kept to a minimum and used only when absolutely necessary inasmuch as patients tend to develop isoantibodies to platelet antigen. Sugar re-cently reported a case in which dental extractions in a patient with thrombasthenia were complicated by bleeding caused by the development of isoantibodies to donor platelets.

Systemic therapy in acquired thrombasthenia is often ineffective; therefore, confine dental treatment to what is absolutely necessary, and choose the treatment that would cause the least possible hemorrhage. When the local oral condition provides the stimulus for the hemorrhage, conservative scaling is indicated. Although scaling may produce profuse hemorrhage at the time, it is better than allowing the patient to bleed chronically from the gingiva over a period of many weeks. The life expectancy in these diseases when they are severe enough to cause spontaneous oral hemorrhage is not good, and specific temporary dental treatment to make the patient as comfortable as possible must be suggested to the physician responsible for the care of the patient.

Hemorrhage Due to Systemic Diseases Other Than Those Involving the Oral Cavity

Oral hemorrhagic manifestations of systemic disorders other than those involving the blood and blood-forming organs directly are relatively rare. In both bacterial endocarditis and meningococcemia, petechiae may be seen anywhere on the oral mucosa. These petechiae are not caused by platelet deficiency or dysfunction but rather by bacterial emboli that destroy the capillary wall, allowing erythrocytes to escape into the tissues surrounding the vessel. Like petechiae from any cause, these do not blanch on pressure. Sometimes the petechiae arising from bacterial endocarditis may have a small white spot in the center.

Pharyngitis caused by viral or streptococcal infections may produce petechiae in the soft palate as an extension of the pharyngeal disease, presumably by the same mechanism as that in endocarditis—small breaks in the capillary wall induced by the infectious agent.

The oral manifestations of scurvy are well-known and are extremely rare in these days of self-prescribed vitamin therapy. Unlike the perifollicular cutaneous lesions seen in *all* adults with serious vitamin C deficiency, the oral lesions are not present in edentulous patients. The gingivae become engorged with blood, are boggy, and bleed quite easily. The teeth eventually become loose and if the deficiency progresses, will be exfoliated. It has been shown that at least 6 months of vitamin C deficiency are necessary for oral manifestations to develop.

Patients may appear to be bleeding from the mouth from diseases such as erythema multiforme, pemphigus, and pemphigoid when bullae that contain blood rupture discharging blood into the oral cavity. These diseases are discussed in detail in Chapter 5.

In allergies, patients have been reported to have petechial lesions on the skin and on the mucosa, presumably caused by a localized vasculitis allowing blood to leak through the capillary wall.

BIBLIOGRAPHY

Baehner RL, Strauss HS: Hemophilia in the first year of life. N Engl J Med 275:524, 1966

Bayard ED et al: Macroglobulinemia, its recognition and treatment. JAMA 193:724, 1965

Brinkhous KM (ed): Handbook of Hemophilia, pp 767–853. Amsterdam, Excepta Medica, 1975

Brockway WJ, Fass DN: The nature of the interaction between ristocetin-Willebrand factor VIII coagulant activity molecule. J Lab Clin Med 89:1925, 1977

Eisenberg JM et al: Prothrombin and partial thromboplastin times as preoperative screening tests. Arch Surg 117:48, 1982

Evian CI et al: Complications of severe bleeding in a patient with undiagnosed factor XI deficiency. Oral Surg 52:12, 1981

Hassel TM et al: Valproic acid: A new antiepileptic drug with potential side effects of dental concern. J Am Dent Assoc 99:983, 1979

Hattler AB, Summers RB: Hereditary hemorrhagic telangiectasia: Report of a case and clinical considerations. J Am Dent Assoc 103:421, 1981

Kushlan SD: Gastro-intestinal bleeding in hereditary hemorrhage telangiectasia. Gastroenterology 7:199, 1946

Lucas ON, Albert TW: Epsilon aminocaproic acid in hemophiliacs undergoing dental extractions: A concise review. Oral Surg 51:115, 1981

Merril A, Peterson LJ: Gingival hemorrhage secondary to uremia. Oral Surg 29:530, 1970

Osler W: On a family form of recurring epistaxis associated with multiple telangiectases of the skin and mucous membrane. Bull Johns Hopkins Hosp 12:333, 1901

Perkin RF et al: Glanzmann's thrombasthenia. Oral Surg 47:36, 1979

Sadowsky D et al: Central hemangioma of the mandible. Oral Surg 52:472, 1981

San Miguel JG, Castillo R: Investigation of uremic thrombopathy. Acta Haematol 40:113, 1968

Sonis AL, Musselman RJ: Oral bleeding in classic hemophilia. Oral Surg 53:363, 1982

Sugar AW: The management of dental extractions in cases of thrombasthenia complicated by the development of isoantiobodies to donor platelets. Oral Surg 48:116, 1979

Weiss HJ et al: Effect of salicylates on hemostatic properties of platelets of man. J Clin Invest 47:2169, 1968

Weiss HJ et al: Pseudo-von Willebrand's disease. N Engl J Med 306:326, 1982

Wilson WB: Emergency management of unexpected defects of hemostatic function in surgical patients. JAMA 201:123, 1967

24

Immunologic Diseases

MARTIN S. GREENBERG

GENERAL PRINCIPLES

The science of immunology, once a small branch of microbiology, has grown into one of the principal sciences dealing with human disease. One need only glance at the number of texts, journals, and papers published each year on the subject to realize the extensive investigation now being carried out in the field.

Concepts of disease are changing because of knowledge gained in immunologic research. A competent clinician should understand the basic concepts of modern immunology and how it relates to disease. Much of the current research dealing with dental caries, periodontal disease and oral ulcers uses the techniques of immunology to investigate the etiology and treatment of these diseases. In this chapter pertinent basic principles of clinical immunology will be reviewed, diseases that involve the immune system will be discussed, and the relationship of these diseases to oral mucosal disease will be highlighted.

The function of the immune system is to distinguish self from nonself and eliminate potentially destructive foreign substances from the body. This function has direct clinical application in the fields of infectious and neoplastic diseases and in transplant immunology. Current concepts of human immunology support the theory that the cells responsible for the immune response are derived from an undifferentiated stem cell precursor that originates in the bone marrow. These stem cells differentiate into two distinct populations of lymphocytes that form the two components of the immune system. One population of lymphoid stem cells contacts the thymus and forms the thymus-dependent or the T-cell system. Other cells contact the human equivalent of the bursa of Fabricius of birds, possibly the intestinal lymphoid tissue of Peyer's patches or the appendix, to differentiate into the bursa or B-cell system.

The T-cell system is responsible for cell-mediated immunity, which serves as the body's primary defense against viruses and fungi. The T-cell system is also responsible for delayed hypersensitivity reactions and graft rejection and helps to regulate the B-cell system. T lymphocytes perform many of their functions by releasing mediators: cytotoxic mediators destroy grafts and tumor cells, while migration inhibition factor (MIF) attracts phagocytic macrophages to the site of bacterial infection. T cells populate the paracortical areas of lymph nodes and the white pulp of the spleen, and constitute 60% to 80% of lymphocytes in the peripheral blood.

The B cells populate the follicles around germinal centers of lymph nodes, spleen, and tonsils. B lymphocytes have immunoglobulin receptors on their surface. When these receptors combine with antigen, they differentiate into plasma cells and produce antibody. Antibodies are the body's primary defense against bacterial infection. Five major classes of antibodies or immunoglobulins (Ig) are now recognized: IgM, IgG, IgA, IgD, and IgE. Each of these immunoglobulins has different chemical as well as distinct biological properties.

IgM antibodies are macromolecules composed of five antibody monomers and are produced chiefly in the body's primary response to a foreign antigen. IgG constitutes 75% of the serum immunoglobulins, is the major component of the secondary antibody response, and is also the immunoglobulin that crosses the placenta, giving protection to the newborn. Four subgroups of IgG have been identified. IgA antibodies are found in blood in small amounts, but secretory IgA is the main antibody found in external secretions such as saliva, tears, and bile. Levels of secretory IgA in saliva may have an important role in protecting oral tissues against disease by preventing microorganisms from attaching to the mucosa. Dysfunction of the IgA system may help explain certain oral diseases, and in the future, induction of specific salivary secretory IgA antibodies may protect patients from dental caries and periodontal disease. Both IgD and IgE are found in normal human serum in low quantities. IgD acts as a receptor for antigen on B lymphocytes; IgE binds to mast cells triggering the release of histamine during allergic reactions, such as anaphylaxis, hay fever, and asthma.

The immune reaction is being actively investigated as a cause or contributing factor in a variety of diseases ranging from periodontal disease to cancer. The immune nature of the clinical signs noted in an allergic reaction is well accepted, but the relationship of the immune response to other diseases remains controversial. Particularly debated is the topic of autoimmune disease, where it is theorized that antibodies produced against the individual's own tissues cause damage. Strong evidence exists that autoantibodies play a significant role in the pathogenesis of pemphigus and Hashimoto's thyroiditis. The evidence is cloudier in other diseases because normal individuals may produce autoantibodies without apparent disease.

Immune complex disease is another subdivision of immunologic disorders. In these diseases antibody-antigen complexes combine with complement to cause a nonspecific vasculitis and nephritis. Systemic lupus erythematosus, glomerulonephritis, and Behcet's syndrome are examples of immune complex disorders.

Antibodies may also cause disease by blocking the receptor sites, preventing chemical agents that normally attach there from functioning. Myasthenia gravis and insulin-resistant diabetes are caused by receptor sites blocked by antibody.

PRIMARY IMMUNE DEFICIENCIES

Primary immune deficiencies are hereditary abnormalities characterized by an inborn defect of the immune system. These diseases may solely involve the B-cell system with a resultant deficiency of humoral antibodies, or solely the T-cell system with a deficiency of cellular immunity. There are also combined deficiencies that affect both the B- and T-cell systems and others with associated findings that make them difficult to classify. Five illustrative primary immune deficiencies are discussed below. Oral manifestations of these deficiencies are discussed together at the end of the section.

Sex-Linked Agammaglobulinemia

This hereditary disease (Bruton's agammaglobulinemia) of male children is caused by a defect in B-cell function; T-cell function remains intact. As a result these patients lack the ability to synthesize all classes of antibody including the secretory immunoglobulins, making them considerably more susceptible to bacterial infection. The symptoms begin at 6 months of age when transplacentally acquired maternal antibodies have been metabolized. The patients experience severe recurrent bacterial infections of the lungs, meninges, skin, and sinuses. The most common organisms involved in these infections are pneumococci, streptococci, staphylococci, and Hemophilus influenzae. The patient's ability to combat most viral and fungal infection is normal because of the intact T-cell system. Examination of these patients will reveal hypoplasia of the lymph nodes, tonsils, and adenoids. Biopsy of lymphoid tissue reveal a lack of germinal centers and plasma cells.

Patients with agammaglobulinemia have an increased incidence of rheumatoid arthritis, dermatomyositis, lymphoma, and leukemia.

Primary Adult Immunoglobulin Deficiencies

This group of disorders is characterized by an abnormality of the B-cell or humoral antibody system that does not become clinically apparent until adulthood. Usually only one or two Ig classes are deficient. This selective deficiency accounts for the relatively asymptomatic nature of the disease throughout childhood. There is evidence that patients with deficiencies of one immunoglobulin will compensate with increased production of others. For this reason selective immunoglobulin deficiencies have been difficult to detect. Routine serum protein electrophoresis appears normal, and selective tests, described below, must be used in diagnosis.

The primary adult deficiencies rarely become apparent until the third decade of life. The most common symptoms include recurrent gram-positive bacterial infections, especially of the upper and lower respiratory tract. The infections are severe in patients who lack all classes of immunoglobulins and moderate to mild in patients with selective immunoglobulin deficiency. Hill studied 176 patients with immunoglobulin deficiency in the United Kingdom; one half of the patients had respiratory tract infections. Other organ systems commonly involved were the joints, gastrointestinal tract, and skin. Chronic compensatory hyperplasia of the lymphoid tissue has also been noted by others, causing these disorders to be confused with lymphomas.

The most common selective Ig deficiency is that involving decreased levels of serum and secretory IgA. Population studies have demonstrated IgA deficiencies in one of every 500 to 1,000 adults. A majority of these patients are apparently normal, having no specific clinical symptoms related to the deficiency and no obvious susceptibility to infection. These patients having clinical disease have been reported to have chronic sinusitis, chronic pulmonary infection, malabsorption syndromes similar to sprue, and oral ulcers (see Fig. 24-1). Adults, like children with B-cell deficiencies, also have an increased incidence of collagen vascular disease such as systemic lupus erythematosus and rheumatoid arthritis. The reason for this is not clear, but some have speculated that in the normal patient secretory IgA blocks antigens that cause autoimmune diseases in immunodeficient patients.

Thymic Hypoplasia

The two classic T-lymphocyte deficiency disorders are DiGeorge's syndrome and Nezelof's syndrome. These patients have normal levels of serum immunoglobulins but a lack of cell-mediated immunity. The syndrome as described by DiGeorge originates with faulty development of the third and fourth pharyngeal pouches, producing abnormalities of both the thymus and the parathyroid glands. The lack of parathyroid hormone will lead to hypocalcemia and tetany, and the lack of normal thymus function causes an absent T-lymphocyte response. DiGeorge's syndrome was important in the development of the concept of separate immune systems for humoral and cellular hypersensitivity because hypoplasia of the thymus produced impairment of only cellular immunity. Partial DiGeorge's syndrome exists with partial aplasia of the thymus and parathyroids. Nezelof's syndrome, a hereditary disorder, is characterized by hypoplasia of the thymus, a decrease in the delayed-type hypersensitivity reaction, and normal immunoglobulin levels.

During the first few months of life, the T-cell abnormality becomes apparent in children with both syndromes because of the increased susceptibility to infections with viruses and fungi. Infections with *Candida albicans* are especially prominent (see Fig. 24-2). Most patients have normal leukocyte function and normal humoral immunity but almost a total lack of cellular immunity. Cleveland and associates as well as August and co-workers have treated patients with thymic hypoplasia by transplanting fragments of fetal thymus into the rectus abdominis muscle. This therapy has been successful in restoring cellular immunity in some patients.

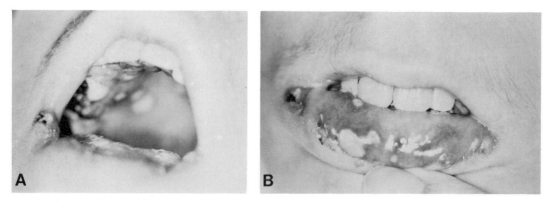

Fig. 24-1 Oral ulcers in a 32-year-old female with hypogammaglobulinemia. The ulcers are of 3 days' duration and were accompanied by a skin rash of the legs. (Courtesy Dr. David Reiter)

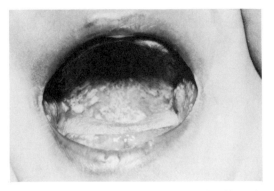

Fig. 24-2 Oral candidiasis in a 5-month-old male with severe combined immunodeficiency. (Courtesy Dr. Mary Ann South)

Severe Combined Immunodeficiency

This genetic disease (Swiss-type agammaglobulinemia) can be inherited as either a sex-linked or an autosomal-recessive trait. It is theorized that in some cases the basic defect involves the lymphoid stem cell with a resultant deficiency of both B-cell and T-cell function. Other cases, particularly in the autosomal-recessive form, are related to a deficiency of the enzyme adenosine deaminase. The patients have low peripheral lymphocyte counts, severe deficiency of immunoglobulins, and complete lack of cellular immunity. Symptoms of this disease begin in the first few weeks of life and include bacterial, viral, and fungal infections; localized or systemic candidiasis is common. The patient dies of overwhelming infection during the first year of life unless a histocompatible relative is found for a bone marrow transplant.

Immunodeficiency with Ataxia Telangiectasia

This immune disorder is inherited as an autosomal recessive trait. The cardinal signs of this disease include the following:

1. Combined T-cell and B-cell deficiency causes both an abnormal cellular response as well as a deficiency of immunoglobulins. The majority of these patients have a deficiency of secretory and serum IgA with elevated levels of IgM. Severe pulmonary infection occurs in 85% of cases and is a common cause of death.

2. Progressive neurologic disease originates from severe degenerative changes in the cerebellum leading to cerebellar ataxia. This sign becomes apparent when the child begins to walk.
3. Telangiectasias of the skin and eyes become apparent at about 3 years of age. The lesions become progressively more extensive with age and mainly occur on conjunctiva, ears, and malar eminences.
4. Gonadal dysgenesis.
5. Increased incidence of malignancies of the lymphoreticular system.

Oral Manifestations

Patients with T-lymphocyte abnormalities have more oral disease than do patients with B-lymphocyte disorders because T-lymphocyte abnormalities lead to chronic fungal and viral infections, which are more likely to occur on the oral mucosa than are the bacterial infections seen in B-lymphocyte deficiencies.

A consistent oral sign noted in patients with T-cell diseases such as thymic hypoplasia or ataxia telangiectasia is chronic oral candidiasis (see Fig. 24-3). Lehner studied 15 patients with chronic oral candidiasis, and each one had an impaired cellular immune response. Lawlor reported on six patients with decreased cellular immune deficiency; five of the six patients had severe chronic oral candidiasis.

Herpes simplex virus infections are also common in patients with T-cell disease. The infections may be localized to the mouth but frequently become disseminated and are potentially lethal.

Other oral signs seen with T-cell deficiencies include the skin and mucosal telangiectases of ataxia telangiectasia. Boder and Sedgwick reported on eight patients with this disease; two of the patients had extensive telangiectasis of the hard and soft palates, and one had severe malocclusion caused by micrognathia. Oral signs were not noted in the other six patients. Congenital defects of the mouth and jaws have also been seen in patients with thymic hypoplasia and include cleft palate, micrognathia, bifid uvula, and short philtrum of the upper lip.

The major sign in patients with B-cell abnormalities is recurrent bacterial infections.

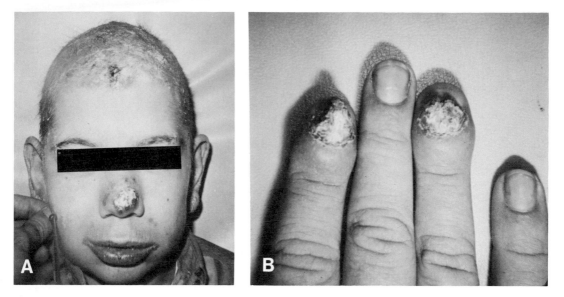

Fig. 24-3 Mucocutaneous candidiasis in a 12-year-old male with immunodeficiency. (Courtesy Dr. Mary Ann South)

These infections frequently involve the respiratory tract. The most common of these infections that comes to the attention of dentists is chronic maxillary sinusitis.

The weight of evidence indicates that patients with primary immunoglobulin deficiencies do *not* have an increase in dental caries or periodontal disease. Robertson and co-workers studied 23 patients with primary immune deficiency and control subjects and found no increase in either dental caries or periodontal disease. In a follow-up study, Robertson found a decrease in gingival inflammation, periodontal breakdown, and dental caries when compared to a group of controls. Brown and colleagues also found a decrease in caries rate among patients with primary immunoglobulin deficiency and found minimal differences in the microbial flora of the supragingival plaque.*

Although oral ulceration has been occasionally described in patients with primary immune deficiency it is not a characteristic finding. Neutropenia and neutrophil dysfunction syndromes commonly cause oral ulcers; immunoglobulin deficiencies do not.

Factors other than primary immune defi-

ciency may cause candidiasis and maxillary sinusitis, but patients with these infections who are not successfully treated by antibiotic or antifungal therapy or who have a history of other recurring infections should have immune deficiency ruled out. This should be done with a careful history, including past episodes of pneumonia, recurrent otitis media, autoimmune disease, severe asthma, malabsorption syndrome, or pyoderma. Laboratory studies should be performed when the history suggests immune deficiency. The dentist may order preliminary laboratory studies himself or refer the patient to a clinical immunologist. Laboratory studies to rule out B-lymphocyte function should include quantitation of the major immunoglobulins. In questionable cases the clinical immunologist will test the patient's ability to synthesize specific antibody after immunization with standard antigens.

Screening patients for T-lymphocyte function must be performed by a clinician used to dealing with the tests. Cellular function is tested by skin testing for commonly occurring antigens including purified protein derivative of tuberculin (PPD), *Candida,* and *Trichophyton.* Negative reactions to these antigens suggest a defect of cellular (T-cell) immunity. Laboratory studies used to check

* Legler and associates described an increased rate of caries in patients with a selective IgA deficiency.

T-cell activity include blast cell transformation and inhibition of macrophage migration.

Dental Management

Dental treatment for patients with primary immune deficiency must minimize the chances of local infection or septicemia. Although the risk of spreading oral candidiasis by dental treatment is not known, a patient with decreased T-cell function and oral candidiasis should be treated with antifungal therapy prior to dental treatment in order to minimize the risk of systemic fungal infection.

Patients with symptomatic B-cell abnormalities are usually given continuous therapy with concentrated human gamma globulin. Prior to instituting dental treatment, the gamma globulin level should be checked to ensure that it is at least 200 mg/dl. When oral surgery is necessary, an extra dose of gamma globulin should be administered the day before surgery in a dosage usually between 100 mg and 200 mg/kg of body weight. This dose should be given intramuscularly and not intravenously to minimize the risk of severe transfusion reactions.

Unusual transfusion reactions occur frequently in patients with primary immune deficiency, and this must be taken into account when using blood replacement therapy. Patients with B-cell deficiency resulting in the absence of particular immunoglobulins may experience severe transfusion reactions when receiving blood from a patient who has normal immunoglobulin levels. The immunoglobulin acts as a foreign protein and causes an allergic response. For this reason the patient with selective IgA deficiency must be given IgA-depleted blood.

Another problem in administering a transfusion to a patient with primary immune deficiency is the development of graft-versus-host disease. The immunocompetent cells in the transfused blood will react against the tissues of the immunodeficient recipient. Only fresh blood in which the immunocompetent lymphocytes have been destroyed can be used. This can be accomplished by saturating the blood with oxygen and radiating with 1,000 rad. Huggins recommends processing the blood in a cytoagglomerator and

freezing in glycerol at $-60°$ C to make it safe; while Fudenberg and colleagues recommend repeated freezing and thawing.

Dental infections in patients with primary immune deficiencies must be treated vigorously. A culture for bacteria and fungi and sensitivity should be taken prior to instituting antibiotic therapy. Few dentists do this routinely for normal patients with abscesses, but it is particularly important for immunodeficient patients because these patients get unusual infections with fungi and gram-negative bacteria.

SECONDARY IMMUNE DEFICIENCIES

Secondary immune deficiencies can be caused by immunosuppressive drug therapy, malignancy or granulomatous disease of the lymphoid system, and protein-depleting disorders. Specific diseases that result in secondary immune deficiency include leukemia, Hodgkin's disease, non-Hodgkin's lymphoma, nephrotic syndrome, multiple myeloma, sarcoidosis, and Waldenström's macroglobulinemia. The above disorders are discussed in detail in other chapters of this text. This section confines itself to a discussion of the immunologic aspects of the diseases.

Leukemia

Infection is the major cause of death in patients with leukemia, and it poses a major clinical management problem. A majority of these infections are caused by microorganisms that rarely cause fatal illness in normal individuals (e.g., gram-negative bacilli, fungi, and herpes viruses; see Fig. 24-4).

Infections in patients with acute leukemia are caused by a severe decrease in mature, functioning granulocytes. The function of the B and T lymphocytes appears to be intact until cytotoxic chemotherapy is initiated. Studies of neutrophils from patients with acute leukemia show both an impaired ability to migrate and diminished bactericidal and chemotactic functions.

Chronic lymphatic leukemia involves the B lymphocytes in most cases, affecting the hu-

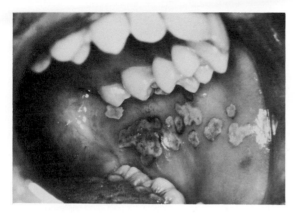

Fig. 24-4 A patient taking chemotherapy for leukemia who developed extensive recurrent herpes simplex lesions of the buccal mucosa and palate.

moral antibody response and resulting in hypogammaglobulinemia. A few cases of chronic lymphatic leukemia involving T lymphocytes have been reported, but these are rare. Shaw studied 42 patients with chronic lymphatic leukemia; 52% developed bacterial infections—most frequently involving the respiratory tract. This is similar to the type of infection observed in patients with primary B-lymphocyte disorders.

Patients with chronic myelocytic leukemia have a lower incidence of infection, consistent with laboratory studies that show a good antibody response in these patients.

Hodgkin's Disease

Patients with Hodgkin's disease have a loss of T-lymphocyte function that worsens as the disease progresses. The radiotherapy and chemotherapy used to treat the disease further suppress normal immune function.

Studies of patients with advanced Hodgkin's disease reveal changes consistent with the deficient T-cell response, including unresponsiveness to skin tests with previously encountered antigens and prolonged skin graft survival time. *In vitro* studies of lymphocytes from patients with Hodgkin's disease show an abnormal response to antigens. The major clinical infections seen in patients with Hodgkin's disease are fungal, viral, and protozoal. The most common fungal infections are *Cryptococcus*, *Candida albicans*, actinomycetes, and histoplasmosis. The viral in-

fections are herpes simplex, varicella zoster, and cytomegalovirus. The protozoal infections include *Pneumocystis carinii* and toxoplasmosis. Chemotherapy and radiotherapy may suppress neutrophil and antibody function for years, increasing the patient's susceptibility to bacterial infection.

Non-Hodgkin's Lymphomas

The immune response of patients with non-Hodgkin's lymphoma has not been studied as extensively as the response in Hodgkin's disease. Some patients with non-Hodgkin's lymphoma have deficiency of the B-cell or T-cell system caused by the disease itself or by chemotherapy. This deficiency becomes more severe late in the course of the disease. Lymphoma patients have an increased rate of infections with bacteria, viruses, and fungi.

Nephrotic Syndrome

Patients with nephrotic syndrome lose large amounts of serum protein through the destroyed or damaged glomeruli, causing a secondary hypogammaglobulinemia. Bacterial infections secondary to the hypogammaglobulinemia have been described as a cause of death in children with nephrotic syndrome. The common sites of infection seen in these patients are the oropharynx, skin, and lungs. Prophylactic use of gamma globulin and antibiotics has decreased the incidence of infection dramatically.

Multiple Myeloma

Multiple myeloma is a malignancy of plasma cells, the cells primarily responsible for the humoral antibody response. These defective plasma cells produce large quantities of myeloma proteins instead of the normal immunoglobulins. The myeloma proteins offer no protection against infection, and repeated bouts of bacterial infection, particularly pneumococcal pneumonia, are common. Bone marrow suppression by malignant plasma cells and chemotherapy further increases the patient's susceptibility to infection. A viral infection that occurs with increased frequency in multiple myeloma patients is varicella zoster infection, which may occur as localized herpes zoster or generalized varicella.

Sarcoidosis

Sarcoidosis is a systemic granulomatous disease of unknown etiology that most commonly involves the lungs, lymph nodes, mucocutaneous surfaces, eyes, and salivary glands. Patients with sarcoidosis show decreased T-cell mediated response as has been demonstrated by a decreased response to skin test antigens, diminished transplantation immunity, and *in vitro* testing of lymphocytes. The humoral antibody response in patients with sarcoidosis is unimpaired. Although the cellular immune response is defective, it is not as depressed as in patients with primary T-cell deficiencies or in Hodgkin's disease, and sarcoidosis patients do not appear to be more susceptible to viral or fungal infection.

Acquired Immune Deficiency Syndrome

In 1981, a previously little known acquired immune deficiency syndome (AIDS) was reported by groups from several medical centers (see also Chapter 28). AIDS is associated with a high incidence of Kaposi's sarcoma and opportunistic infections. The etiology of AIDS is unknown, but the epidemiology suggests an infectious agent spread by sexual contact or intravenous drug use. Most initial cases were reported in homosexual males and Haitians, but recently cases have been detected in heterosexuals with multiple sexual contacts and a history of intravenous drug abuse, hemophiliacs, and children living with high-risk patients. The majority of cases have been from New York, California, Florida, New Jersey, and Texas.

The immune defect affects the function of the T lymphocytes (cellular immunity), and many of the patients are anergic to routine skin tests. They also demonstrate an absolute lymphopenia and a significant decrease in helper T-cells with an increase in suppressor T-cells. B lymphocytes, antibody levels, and complement levels appear to be normal. A major clinical finding is the high incidence of Kaposi's sarcoma, a rare malignancy usually occurring in Jewish or Italian men over 50.

AIDS patients have Kaposi's sarcoma at a younger age, and it disseminates rapidly. The lesions of Kaposi's sarcoma occur on any skin or mucosal surface and start as reddish to brown macules or papules measuring 1 cm to 2 cm in diameter that enlarge to form dark plaques and nodules. Gastrointestinal lesions are common.

AIDS patients, like other immunocompromised patients, are susceptible to infection with opportunistic microorganisms. Particularly prevalent is pneumonia with *Pneumocystis carinii*, a protozoan. Many of the AIDS cases have been detected because of infection with this unusual organism. The patients also have an increased susceptibility to infection with fungi and viruses of the herpes group. AIDS patients often have many months of nonspecific complaints such as fever, malaise, and weight loss before the diagnosis is made. Examination at this early stage reveals nontender, enlarged lymph nodes and splenomegaly with no apparent cause.

Oral lesions of Kaposi's sarcoma have been described in AIDS patients. The lesions are red to brown macules, papules, or nodules. Friedman–Kein and associates described a palatal lesion of Kaposi's sarcoma in an AIDS patient, and Kaposi's sarcoma lesions have also been described on the gingiva, soft palate, and tongue. Other reported oral lesions include infections often seen in patients with a T-lymphocyte disorder, particularly chronic candidiasis and recurrent herpes infections.

A major role of dentists at this initial state of knowledge regarding AIDS is in early detection. Patients with oral lesions of Kaposi's sarcoma, chronic oral candidiasis, or other infections associated with T-cell abnormalities should have AIDS included in the differential diagnosis. Suspicion of AIDS should increase if the patient is homosexual, an intravenous drug abuser, a hemophiliac, or has a history of multiple sexual contacts. Because this disease has recently been identified, it is possible that the epidemiologic picture may change over the next few years as contacts increase. The risk of dental treatment is unknown, but it would be wise for dentists treating patients with AIDS to take precautions similar to those used for patients who are carriers of hepatitis B.

Immunosuppressive Drug Therapy

Corticosteroids are administered alone or in combination with cytotoxic drugs for their immunosuppressive, anti-inflammatory, and antineoplastic actions. These effects of corticosteroids result from the decrease of lymphocytes in the peripheral blood as well as the drug actions in interfering with the normal functioning of lymphocytes and neutrophils.

A widely studied group of immunosuppressed patients are those taking azathioprine (Imuran) and corticosteroids (usually prednisone) to prevent graft rejection after renal transplantation. Azathioprine, an analogue of 6-mercaptopurine, is the major drug used to prevent rejection of renal homografts and is a potent inhibitor of both cellular and humoral immunity. Prednisone, a commonly used corticosteroid, is customarily given as an adjunct to azathioprine for long-term immunosuppressive therapy. Prednisone is also given in extremely high doses (200 to 1,000 mg per day) during episodes of graft rejection. A frequent complication in patients immunosuppressed with these two drugs is infection. A majority of these infections are caused by microorganisms that are of little pathologic significance in the normal individual, but often cause fatal infection in the patient taking immunosuppressive drugs. Tapia and co-workers studied 16 patients who died after renal transplantation, 69% of deaths being caused by infection.

Eickhoff studied 224 renal transplant recipients and found infectious complications in 80%. The results of these studies and others show that the most common infections occurring in patients on immunosuppressive drug therapy are caused by gram-negative bacteria such as *Klebsiella*, *Pseudomonas*, and *Bacteroides*; fungal infections with *Candida*, *Aspergillus*, and *Cryptococcus*; nocardial and viral infections, especially with herpes simplex, varicella zoster, and cytomegalovirus.

Oral and Dental Implications

The major clinical problem in the management of patients with secondary immune deficiency is the prevention and treatment of infection. This is particularly important when severe neutropenia or neutrophil dysfunction is a component of the clinical status, increasing the patient's susceptibility to bacterial infection. The patient with acute leukemia taking chemotherapy is at risk of severe life-threatening infection originating from the oral flora. Potential sources of oral infection such as pulpal or periodontal disease should be eliminated before chemotherapy (see Acute Leukemia, Chap. 22).

Patients taking immunosuppressive drug therapy to prevent rejection of transplanted organs are also susceptible to oral infection. The risk of infection is highest just after transplantation or during a rejection crisis when huge doses of corticosteroids are administered. During long-term maintenance therapy when the dose of drugs is lower, the risk of infection decreases, but the incidence of viral and fungal infection remains significant and may be lethal. Oral lesions commonly seen are oral candidiasis and herpes simplex infections. The dentist must also be aware of the incidence of severe chronic fungal infections that can be manifest as oral ulcers such as mucormycosis or histoplasmosis. Chronic oral ulcers should be biopsied when these infections are suspected so that early diagnosis will lead to prompt successful treatment. Chronic herpes simplex infections of the oral mucosa can develop (Fig. 24-5) that

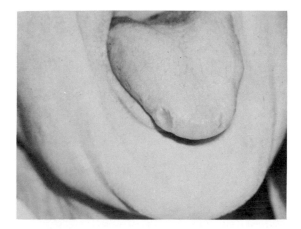

Fig. 24-5 Chronic herpes simplex infection involving the tongue in a patient taking high doses of corticosteroids. These lesions were 4 weeks old and did not resolve until topical antiherpes medication (Acyclovir) was used.

may lead to disseminated infection (see section on chronic ulcers, Chap. 5).

Tyldesley and associates described superficial mucosal bacterial lesions occurring in transplant patients during high-dose corticosteroid therapy. The lesions resembled candidiasis but did not respond to antifungal therapy. Greenberg and Cohen studied the incidence of oral infections over 10 months in 27 renal transplant patients who were taking maintenance doses of immunosuppressive drugs. Oral infections occurred as frequently as pulmonary or urinary tract infections. The acute dental infections that developed remained localized and resolved after routine oral treatment and antibiotics. Although *Klebsiella* and *Pseudomonas* were cultured from the oral cavity of several patients, the predominant organism cultured from the acute dental abscesses was alpha-*Streptococcus*. Reyna and co-workers studied the incidence of head and neck infections in 128 renal transplant recipients; 14 developed head and neck infections including five cases of sinusitis, three dental abscesses, one Ludwig's angina, and one parotitis. The dental infections did not become generalized and resolved with routine extraction and antibiotics.

Although most dental infections reported to date in renal transplant patients have occurred with gram-positive cocci, the dentist must remember that infections with gram-negative bacilli are common in all hospitalized immunosuppressed patients. All infections should be cultured. The gingival area to be treated should be prepared preoperatively with povidone-iodine solution to decrease the risk of bacteremia following extraction, periodontal curettage, or other dental procedures. Periodontal disease in patients taking immunosuppressive drugs has been studied by several groups of investigators. The patients have less gingival response to local irritants, but there is no evidence of an increase in periodontal disease. Some preliminary reports suggest a decrease in periodontal disease among immunosuppressed patients.

If practicing in hospitals where immunosuppressive drugs are administered, the dentist should set up close liaison with departments administering the drugs. Each patient should be seen by the dental department prior to the institution of immunosuppressive drug therapy. Clinical and radiographic examination of the mouth, jaws, and maxillary sinuses should be carried out. When possible, treat or remove teeth involved with pulpal or periodontal disease if they are a potential source of infection prior to drug therapy.

THE CONNECTIVE TISSUE DISEASES

Connective tissue diseases are customarily grouped together under titles such as collagen disease, collagen vascular disease, hyperimmune disease, or autoimmune disease. They include systemic lupus erythematosus, rheumatoid arthritis, scleroderma (progressive systemic sclerosis), dermatomyositis, and polyarteritis nodosa. Rheumatic fever is also sometimes classified with these disorders.

The term autoimmune has been used to describe this group of diseases because autoantibodies that react with normal tissue *in vitro* have been detected in significant quantities. Use of the term *autoimmune* appears justified when it is used to describe pemphigus or Hashimoto's thyroiditis, diseases in which autoantibodies appear to cause direct, specific damage to tissues. In connective tissue diseases the term *immune complex* more accurately describes the source of most of the tissue damage, although autoantibodies appear to cause some hematologic changes. In immune complex disease, a nonspecific inflammatory response results from the accumulation of antibody-antigen complexes rather than specific destruction by antibody. Serum sickness, a generalized allergic reaction, is a classic example of a self-limiting disease caused by circulating immune complexes.

Among the connective tissue diseases, immune complexes have been closely related to disease activity in systemic lupus erythematosus and rheumatoid arthritis. In lupus, the immune complexes consist of nucleic acid combined with antibody, while in rheumatoid arthritis the immune complexes consist of a combination of immunoglobulins. When immune complexes form they activate the complement system, which attracts neutrophils and macrophages. Vasculitis and tissue damage result when immune complexes are present in sufficient quantity.

The stimulus that causes formation of the abnormal antibodies triggering the immune complexes is unknown, but some investigators believe that viruses or other microorganisms trigger the reaction.

Lupus Erythematosus

Systemic lupus erythematosus (SLE) is a disease characterized by the presence of abnormal serum antibodies and immune complexes. The disease can affect any organ system and therefore has a variety of clinical manifestations. Although the disease may affect both children and older individuals, the peak incidence is the 20- to 40-year-old age range. SLE occurs ten times more frequently in females and has a higher incidence among blacks. It is rare among Orientals.

The abnormal antibodies occur in all autoimmune diseases, but the amount is significantly higher in SLE. The autoantibodies of SLE may be directed against nucleoprotein, erythrocytes, leukocytes, platelets, coagulation factors and liver, kidney, or heart tissue. A false-positive serologic test for syphilis (STS) is also common and should make the clinician suspicious of the possibility of SLE.

Etiology. The specific etiology of SLE is not known with certainty, but several factors play a significant role.

1. Endocrine. A hormonal component to SLE is suggested by its high incidence in women of child-bearing years, the many reports of remission during pregnancy, and the finding of increased estrogen levels in SLE patients.
2. Genetic. Relatives of SLE patients have higher incidences of autoantibodies and immune deficiency. This tendency is greater among identical twins.
3. Biochemical. The theory of biochemical defects is supported by the finding of increased excretion of metabolic products particularly tyrosine and phenylalanine in certain SLE patients.
4. Viral. Viral-like particles to RNA viruses have been detected in tissues of SLE patients.
5. Immune. Immune complexes consisting chiefly of nucleic acid and antibody account for the majority of the tissue damage seen in SLE patients. Patients with increased circulating immune complexes have more severe disease, particularly of the kidney. Immune complexes also account for tissue damage in the central nervous system, skin, and lung.

Autoantibodies are a cause of the hemolytic anemia and thrombocytopenia seen in SLE patients. The formation of autoantibodies is thought to be related to decreased functioning of suppressor T-lymphocytes. A unified theory that accounts for many of the findings described above has been developed. In this theory, many factors acting together result in SLE. An individual with a genetic predisposition develops a chronic viral infection that releases nucleic acid antigens. Sunburn or damage from chemicals may also contribute to antigen release. Lack of normal suppressor T-lymphocyte function leads to the formation of autoantibodies and immune complexes; widespread tissue damage results.

Clinical Manifestations. SLE is a disease with multiorgan involvement. One patient may present with dermatitis and kidney disease; another presents with arthritis, anemia, and pleurisy. Thus, whenever a patient demonstrates signs and symptoms of multiorgan involvement, SLE should be considered in the differential diagnosis, especially in a female in the 20- to 40-year-old age range.

Lupus erythematosus confined to the skin and mucosa is called *discoid lupus erythematosus* (DLE). Approximately 10% to 20% of patients with DLE develop systemic manifestations later in the course of the disease and it is likely that SLE and DLE are variants of the same disease process. The skin lesions of DLE begin as erythematous scaling lesions with sharp borders that slowly expand and form telangiectases (see Fig. 24-6). An important clinical feature of DLE is follicular plugging. This can be observed when the scale is removed and it extends down into the skin follicles. The malar or so-called "but-

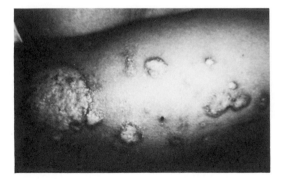

Fig. 24-6 Skin lesions in a patient with systemic lupus erythematosus. (Courtesy Dr. George Ehrlich)

terfly rash'' is common, but does not always occur and is not pathognomonic for DLE inasmuch as it is also seen in other dermatologic diseases such as seborrheic dermatitis (see Fig. 24-7).

The skin lesions of SLE differ from those of DLE as follows:

1. There are signs of acute inflammation, especially diffuse edema.
2. The lesions tend to be bilateral in SLE and also more widespread.

Other skin manifestations are Raynaud's phenomenon of the fingers and toes and skin ulcers secondary to vasculitis. The other clinical manifestations of SLE include arthritis, which can be migratory as in rheumatic fever. Deforming arthritis is uncommon in SLE. Muscle atrophy, pericarditis, pulmonary infiltrates, convulsions, and psychosis also may occur. Kidney involvement in the form of glomerular destruction is seen in approximately 50% of patients, and the severity of kidney disease is often a good indication of the prognosis. The glomerulonephritis results from the deposition of complement and immune complexes in the basement membrane of the glomerulus. Nephrotic syndrome results from massive destruction and is a common cause of death in SLE. Central nervous system involvement is a poor prognostic sign.

The important findings on routine laboratory tests include thrombocytopenia, which may occasionally be severe enough to cause purpura, increased levels of globulins, and a biological false-positive STS (serological test for syphilis). This may be the first laboratory sign of SLE.

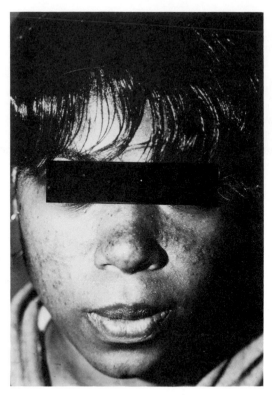

Fig. 24-7 "Butterfly" rash in patient with systemic lupus erythematosus. (Courtesy Dr. Robert Arm)

Diagnosis. The most important diagnostic laboratory test for SLE is the detection of antinuclear antibody (ANA) in the serum. This test is positive in 99% of patients with SLE. The clinician should remember that the ANA is also positive in a minority of patients with scleroderma or rheumatoid arthritis, so the diagnosis must made on the total clinical picture, not on a single laboratory test.

Levels of complement are decreased in patients with active SLE, and 80% will have a positive LE cell phenomenon sometime during the course of the disease. This LE cell test is obtained *in vitro* by observing leukocytes phagocytizing particles of other leukocytes. The LE test has been replaced by sophisticated ANA tests.

Oral Manifestations. Oral manifestations of LE were first described by Bazin in 1861. The first report in the American dental literature

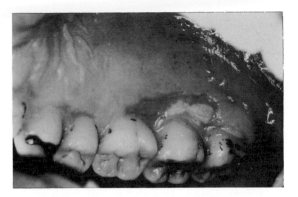

Fig. 24-8 A chronic palatal lesion was initial sign in this patient with systemic lupus erythematosus.

was by the dermatologist Monash in 1931. Monash examined 22 patients with LE; 50% had oral lesions. The most common sites for the lesions were the buccal mucosa, lips, and palate. Other authors noted that 10% to 25% of LE patients had oral involvement. The most common sites were the buccal mucosa, lip, palate (Fig. 24-8), and alveolar ridges. A recent study of this was performed by Schiodt and colleagues.

Andreasen described the oral lesions present in 16 patients with LE. The lip lesions consisted of a central atrophic area with small white dots surrounded by a keratinized border composed of small radiating white striae. There was occasional ulceration of the central area (Fig. 24-9). The intraoral lesions were somewhat different because of the relatively thin epithelium and secondary infection from oral flora. The intraoral lesions were composed of a central, depressed, red atrophic area surrounded by a 2- to 4-mm elevated keratotic zone that dissolved into small white lines.

Andreasen noted more ulceration, edema, and petechiae in SLE patients than in DLE patients; other authors noted similar lesions. Patients with acute SLE frequently have nonspecific oral ulcers (Fig. 24-9). Oral lesions usually accompany extensive skin lesions, but patients with oral lesions as the initial sign have been reported, and initial involvement of the gingiva has also been described.

The oral lesions of LE are sometimes confused with the lesions of lichen planus, and biopsy alone will often not distinguish between the two diseases. Direct immunoflu-orescent demonstration of immunoglobulin and complement deposits in biopsy specimens can be used to help distinguish LE from lichen planus. LE lesions characteristically have a band of immunoglobulines and complement along the dermal-epidermal junvtion while lichen planus lesions show fluorescent ovoid bodies.

Schiodt and associates studied biopsy specimens from oral lesions of patients with LE, lichen planus, and leukoplakia. They found that immunofluorescent staining for immunoglobulins was an excellent means of distinguishing the oral lesions of LE from lichen planus or leukoplakia. Immunoglobulin deposits were detected in 100% of oral lesions of SLE and 73% of DLE, while those deposits were rare in lichen planus or leukoplakia.

There appears to be a small number of cases where DLE and lichen planus overlap. Romero and colleagues reported 11 cases, two with oral lesions suggestive of both LE and lichen planus, clinically and histologically. Direct immunofluorescent staining for immunoglobulins also could not distinguish between the two diseases.

A careful review of systems is necessary to determine whether symptoms of multiorgan involvement exist. Especially pertinent are symptoms of kidney, joint, skin, and central nervous system disease. An ANA test should be ordered along with a routine complete blood count and an erythrocyte sedimentation rate (ESR) when SLE is suspected after clinical evaluation. A patient with oral lesions

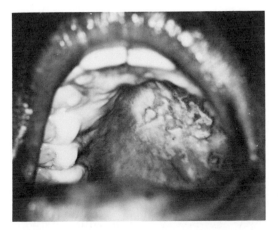

Fig. 24-9 Palatal ulcers in a patient with SLE. (Courtesy Dr. Robert Arm)

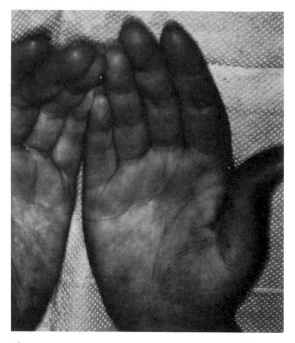

Fig. 24-10 Lesions of the palms in a patient with systemic lupus erythematosus.

and negative laboratory tests may have to be followed carefully for months or even years before the final diagnosis of either DLE or SLE can be made.

Dental Considerations. Although the diagnosis of oral lesions of LE is often emphasized, treatment for a patient with SLE is a much more common problem for the dental practitioner. Because SLE can be a widespread disease affecting many organ systems, the dental management of an SLE patient requires a good understanding of general medicine. The more common problems seen in SLE patients are as follows:

1. Thrombocytopenia may sometimes be severe. Have the results of a recent platelet count before undertaking oral surgery.
2. Bacterial Endocarditis. Libman–Sacks vegetations under the mitral valve leaflets may occur in patients with SLE. These vegetations rarely affect function but can lead to bacterial endocarditis. Give patients with SLE and heart murmurs antibiotic prophylaxis before dental treatment likely to cause a bacteremia.

3. Exacerbation by Drug Therapy. Drugs that have been related to these exacerbations include penicillin and sulfonamides. Avoid using these drugs whenever possible; use all drugs with caution.
4. Exacerbation by Surgery. This has occurred in SLE patients. Avoid all elective surgery, including elective dental procedures.
5. Susceptibility to Shock and Infection. Patients with SLE may be taking adrenal suppressive doses of corticosteroids or cytotoxic drugs, and these patients may be susceptible to shock and infection (see section on immunosuppressive drugs).

Scleroderma

Scleroderma is a disease that involves connective tissue and blood vessels, leading to fibrosis. This causes a clinical picture characterized by hardening and tightening of the skin. There is a localized skin disease, morphea, which may be deforming but not life-threatening, and a diffuse disease, progressive systemic sclerosis (PSS), in which skin as well as internal organs are involved.

Localized scleroderma begins with violaceous patches on the skin. These lesions enlarge, become indurated, and eventually lose hair and the ability to sweat. Later in the course of the localized disease the lesion "burns out" and appears as a hypo- or hyperpigmented area depressed below the level of the skin. These lesions may appear at any age and are of little clinical consequence unless they become extensive or involve the visible skin surface. A linear form of the localized disease may develop during childhood and usually involves the arms, legs, or head. This form of the disease develops as a thin band of sclerosis that may run the entire length of an extremity involving underlying muscle, bones, and joints. Linear localized scleroderma of the head and face is called *en coup de sabre* and may result in hemiatrophy of the face. Scleroderma localized to the hands is called *acrosclerosis*.

PSS is a systemic disease categorized with other connective tissue diseases such as SLE, rheumatoid arthritis, and dermatomyositis. This categorization has resulted from the many patients with overlap syndromes that

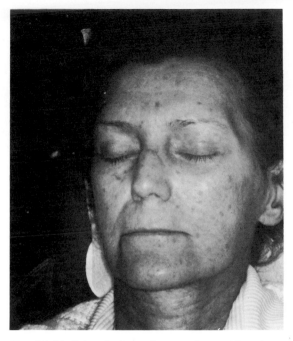

Fig. 24-11 Telangiectases in a patient with scleroderma.

combine PSS with rheumatoid arthritis or SLE. Other indications of immunologic abnormality in PSS include increased levels of plasma gamma globulins, especially the IgG fraction, the large collection of lymphocytes and plasma cells seen in histologic sections of early lesions, increased positive latex fixation reactions, the presence of antinuclear serum antibodies, and positive LE cell reactions. PSS affects women twice as frequently as men and also occurs in high frequency in occupations such as coal mining where there is a high incidence of silicosis.

The initial sign of PSS is frequently Raynaud's phenomenon, a paroxysmal vasospasm of the fingers. This is followed by early skin changes starting with pitting edema, often involving the extremities and face. In several months the edema is replaced by a tightening and hardening of the skin, which results in difficulty in movement of the affected parts. Hyperpigmentation, telangiectases (see Fig. 24-11), and subcutaneous calcifications may also occur leading to deformity and severe cosmetic problems.

Involvement of internal organs may cause dilation of the esophagus, fibrosis of the in-

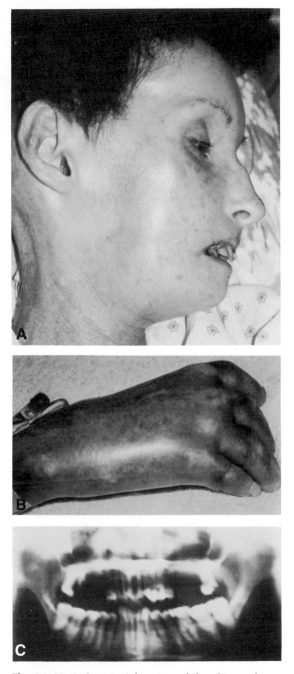

Fig. 24-12 *A,* Severe tightening of the skin and narrowing of the oral aperture in a patient with scleroderma. *B,* Extensive involvement of fingers and hand in the same patient causing lack of mobility and resorption of phalanges. *C,* The severe tightening of the face caused resorption of the body, angle, and inferior border of the mandible.

testine, pulmonary destruction, fibrosis of the myocardium, arthritis, and renal damage. Remissions may occur, or PSS may cause death from renal disease, heart failure, or severe intestinal malabsorption.

A variant of scleroderma is called *CREST syndrome*, which stands for *c*alcinosis, *R*aynaud's phenomenon, *e*sophageal involvement, *s*clerodactyly, and *t*elangiectasia.

Oral Findings. The clinical signs of scleroderma of the mouth and jaws is consistent with findings elsewhere in the body. The lips become rigid, and the oral aperture narrows considerably. Skin folds are lost around the mouth, giving a masklike appearance to the face. The tongue can also become hard and rigid, making speaking and swallowing difficult. Involvement of the esophagus causes dysphagia. When the soft tissues around the temporomandibular joint are affected, they restrict movement of the mandible, causing a pseudoankylosis (Fig. 24-13).

The linear form of localized scleroderma may involve the face as well as underlying bone. Looby and Burket reported a case in which the alveolar process was involved, preventing the eruption of a permanent central incisor. Dental radiographic findings have been reported and widely described. These classical findings include uniform thickening of the periodontal membrane, especially around posterior teeth. It should be emphasized that these findings are not common. Stafne and Austin found increased width in the periodontal membranes of nine of 127 (7%) cases of PSS. Green observed widening in one of three cases (see Fig. 24-14). Other characteristic radiographic findings include calcinosis of the soft tissues around the jaws. The areas of calcinosis will show up on dental films and may be misinterpreted as radiographic intrabony lesions. A thorough clinical examination will demonstrate that the calcifications are present in the soft tissue.

When the facial tissues and muscles of mastication are extensively involved the pressure exerted will cause resorption of the mandible. This resorption is particularly apparent at the angle of the mandible at the attachment of the masseter muscle. The coronoid process or the condyle may also be damaged by the continual pressure.

Dental Management. The most common problem with dental treatment of scleroderma patients is the physical one caused by the narrowing of the oral aperture and rigidity of the tongue. Procedures such as molar endodontics, prosthetics, or restorative pro-

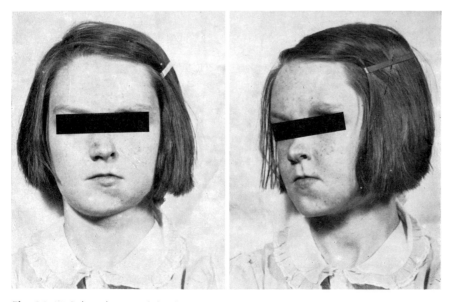

Fig. 24-13 Scleroderma of the face (*coup de sabre* form) that follows the terminal distribution of the fifth nerve. (Looby JP, Burket LW: Am J Orthod 28:493)

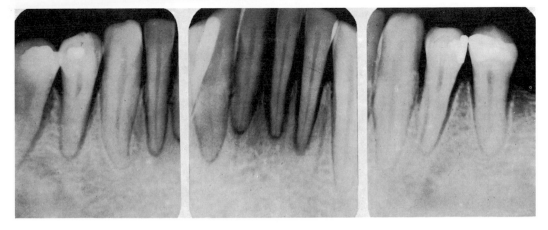

Fig. 24-14 Thickening of periodontal membrane in patient with scleroderma.

cedures in the posterior portions of the mouth become difficult, and at times the dental treatment plan may have to be changed because of the physical problem of access. Sanders and associates reported a case of severe microstomia secondary to an overlap syndrome of scleroderma and dermatomyositis. They increased the oral opening using a bilateral commisurotomy. The procedure was successful and the patient was able to wear dentures.

When treating a patient with scleroderma, determine whether he has the localized or diffuse form of the disease. If PSS is present, consider the extent of the heart, lung, or kidney involvement, and treat the patient as for renal or myocardial failure.

Patients with extensive resorption of the angle of the mandible are at risk for developing pathologic fractures from minor trauma including dental extractions.

Dermatomyositis

Dermatomyositis (polymyositis) is an inflammatory degenerative disease characterized by skin lesions and progressive muscle atrophy. When the disease affects only muscles it is called *polymyositis*. The disease occurs most frequently during early adolescence and between the fourth and sixth decades of life.

The etiology of dermatomyositis is unknown, but it is classified with the connective tissue diseases because of many overlapping clinical features and the fact that dermatomyositis is seen together with either scleroderma, SLE, rheumatoid arthritis, or Sjögren's syndrome. As in the other connective tissue diseases, immunologic abnormalities have been noted. The tissue damage seen is consistent with a T-lymphocyte (cell-mediated) reaction.

Symptoms usually begin with a symmetrical, painless weakness of proximal muscles of the arms, legs, and trunk. The weakness is progressive and characteristically spreads to the face, neck, larynx, pharynx, and heart. Muscle involvement may become severe enough to confine the patient to bed or cause death owing to failure of the respiratory muscles.

The typical skin lesions include a "heliotrope" (lilac-colored) change around the face and fingers. The facial changes may take on the butterfly distribution associated with SLE. Other skin changes are nonspecific diffuse erythema, erythematous plaques, macules, papules, and telangiectasis. Diagnosis from skin lesions alone is rarely possible.

Other clinical features include Raynaud's phenomenon, arthritis, cardiac failure, and renal damage. Laboratory reports will show evidence of muscle destruction with elevated levels of serum glutamic-oxaloacetic transaminase (SGOT), lactate dehydrogenase (LDH), serum glutamic-pyruvic transaminase (SGPT) and creatine phosphokinase (CPK). Ten percent of adults with dermatomyositis have concomitant carcinoma.

Diagnosis. Diagnosis is based on the clinical findings of muscle weakness and skin lesions, elevated "muscle" enzymes, positive findings on muscle biopsy, and electromyographic (EMG) changes. The best available treatment is systemic corticosteroids.

Oral Features. The most common clinical manifestations of dermatomyositis around the mouth and jaws include weakness of the pharyngeal and palatal muscles, causing difficulty in swallowing (dysphagia), and nasal speech (dystonia). The muscles of mastication and facial muscles may also be involved, causing difficulty in chewing. Involvement of the oral mucosa has been described, but the lesions are not diagnostic. Lesions seen include shallow ulcers, erythematous patches, and telangiectases. Calcinosis of the soft tissues is seen, especially in children. These calcified nodules may appear in the face and show up on dental x-rays, leading to misinterpretation. The tongue may also become rigid owing to severe calcinosis.

Sanger and Kirby reported a case of dermatomyositis with generalized calcinosis. Dental radiographs showed severe calcification and obliteration of the pulp chambers of deciduous and permanent dentitions, and there was also purplish black intrinsic staining of the teeth.

Dental Management. The medical management of dermatomyositis involves high doses of systemic corticosteroids. Precautions necessary for dental treatment of patients on high steroid dosage were reviewed earlier in this chapter. Some medical centers are also using antimetabolites and immunosuppressive drugs to manage these patients. This practice causes an increased risk of infection after dental and oral surgery.

Rheumatoid Arthritis

Rheumatoid arthritis (RA) is a generalized inflammatory disease of unknown etiology that occurs most frequently in temperate climates and has its highest incidence in women from 20 to 50 years of age. Unlike degenerative joint disease (osteoarthritis), which is localized to the joints in middle age and elderly individuals, rheumatoid arthritis affects all age groups and may affect muscles, blood, the lymphatic system, heart, and lungs. Although this disease is called arthritis, there are frequent extra-articular manifestations.

The pathogenesis of the rheumatoid arthritis is unknown, but many theories have been advanced to explain this disease, which affects three out of 100 adults in the United States.

Genetic. A hereditary predisposition has support in statistical studies in population groups and identical twins, but none of these studies suggests anything but a weak genetic influence.

Infectious. Many experiments have been performed to isolate microorganisms from affected joints; these efforts have proved largely unsuccessful. The most recent reports include isolation of mycoplasma, but this study has not been confirmed.

The theory of "focal infection" has been discredited, although some still believe that areas of low-grade chronic infection may cause exacerbation of already existing disease. According to the *Primer on Rheumatic Disease,*

> No one now believes that the removal of an infected focus will alter the course of rheumatoid arthritis and extraction of teeth, tonsils, gall bladders and pelvic organs is to be condemned unless they are to be removed for their own sake.

Psychosomatic. Studies have been performed relating emotional trauma, anxiety, and environmental strain to the onset of rheumatoid arthritis. Others have noted stress as a cause of exacerbations, but this observation will need further study with large populations. It has also been difficult to separate the reaction to the disease from personality traits present before the onset of the disease.

Immunologic. The majority of the present investigation involves the immune system as a cause of the disease. There is no doubt that the inflammatory response causing joint and other injury is immune in nature. The initiating factor of this immune response is unknown. The evidence of immune features of this disease include the following:

1. The presence of rheumatoid factors in the serum and synovial fluid of affected patients. Rheumatoid factors are antigammaglobulin antibodies that form soluble complexes. They are measured in the serum of patients suspected of RA by coating latex particles with IgG and testing the agglutinating properties of the patient's serum.
2. Extensive collections of plasma cells and lymphocytes on histologic examination of affected tissues.
3. Decreased complement levels demonstrated in the synovial fluid of affected patients. This suggests complement utilization during hypersensitivity reactions.
4. The overlap of RA with SLE and other diseases suspected of an immune pathogenesis.

Clinical Manifestations. The major early involvement in RA includes a symmetrical polyarthritis characterized by a complaint of stiffness and a finding of spindle-shaped swelling of the involved joints. The proximal interphalangeal (PIP) joints of the fingers and metacarpophalangeal joints (MCP) of the hands are most commonly involved (Fig. 24-15) with the wrists, elbows, knees, and ankles also frequently affected (Fig. 24-17). All joints may be involved in some patients, including the temporomandibular joint and the cricoarytenoid joints of the larynx. The joints affected with RA become red, swollen, and warm to the touch. Muscle atrophy around the affected joints is common.

Extracapsular manifestations include subcutaneous nodules especially over pressure points in 20% to 25% of patients (Fig. 24-16), enlargement of the lymph nodes and spleen, chronic skin ulcers from a diffuse arteritis, pleural effusion, and pulmonary fibrosis. Rheumatoid granulomas may affect the heart, eye, or brain.

Some patients may have a short course of nondisabling disease, whereas others have an unrelenting downhill course of crippling and severe disability. A fluctuating course of

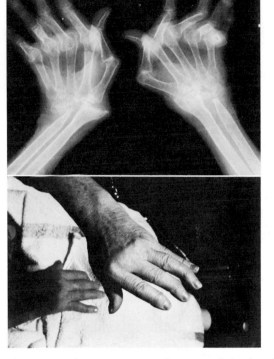

Fig. 24-15 Characteristic involvement of the hands in a patient with rheumatoid arthritis. (Courtesy Dr. George Ehrlich)

remissions and exacerbations is seen in many patients and this unpredictable course makes choice of therapeutic regimens difficult.

Laboratory findings include positive rheumatoid factor, elevated erythrocyte sedimentation rate, and a normochromic, normocytic anemia.

Several variations of RA exist. Felty's syndrome comprises fewer than 5% of the total cases. In addition to the usual manifestations of RA, these patients also have splenomegaly and leukopenia, with the neutrophils showing the greatest decrease. In severe cases recurrent bacterial infection is a common cause of death.

Another variant is juvenile RA (Still's disease), which is thought by some rheumatologists to be a separate disease and not a simple variation of adult RA. Systemic extraarticular symptoms are prominent including fever, lymphadenopathy, hepatosplenomegaly, carditis, and rash. Visual impairment secondary to iridocyclitis (inflammation of the iris and ciliary body) may also occur. In 50% of patients growth and sexual maturation are delayed during active stages of the disease.

Sjögren's syndrome, in which rheumatoid arthritis is associated with salivary gland and lacrimal involvement, is also extensively studied. Details of this syndrome are discussed in Chapter 12.

Oral Signs. The sign of RA of interest to clinicians who treat the oral facial region is involvement of the temporomandibular joint (TMJ). Joint disease can range from mild symptoms of crepitus and stiffness to ankylosis of the joint requiring condylectomy (Fig. 24-18). Patients with juvenile RA may get severe micrognathia secondary to TMJ disease with involvement of growth centers.

The percentage of patients with RA exhibiting TMJ disease has been studied, but there is a large discrepancy in results. Lamont–Havers estimated that only 5% of RA patients had TMJ disease. Bayles and Russell stated that 51% had TMJ disease. Franks studied 100 patients and placed TMJ disease at 53%. This large discrepancy is probably caused by the use of different criteria by the investigators to define TMJ disease.

Crum studied 53 male patients with a diagnosis of RA; 43% had TMJ complaints during the course of the disease, but only one had residual joint damage.

In a recent controlled study of 100 patients with severe RA, Chalmers and Blair included a detailed clinical examination of the TMJ and mouth as well as radiographic examination

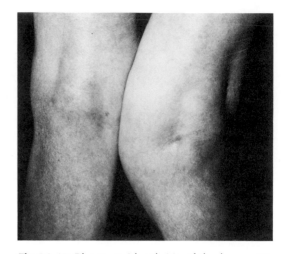

Fig 24-17 Rheumatoid arthritis of the knees. (Courtesy Dr. George Ehrlich)

using circular tomography. Some clinical abnormality occurred in 71% of RA patients with radiographic abnormalities evident in 79%. The most prominent clinical symptoms included stiffness, crepitus, limitation of opening, tenderness on biting, and decreased mobility. Radiographic abnormalities included erosion and flattening of the condyle and marginal proliferations.

It appears that the bulk of the evidence supports the concept that a majority of RA patients will have transient TMJ disease during the course of their disease. Severe permanently disabling TMJ disease requiring special therapy or surgery is present in only a small percentage of patients. Therapy of TMJ disease in RA is discussed in Chapter 12.

Dental Management. Before initiating dental therapy on an RA patient, consult the physician to determine whether hematologic involvement is a component of the disease, and take a careful drug history. Many patients take aspirin at doses approaching 5 grams per day. Acetylsalicylic acid may affect platelet function, causing a prolongation of the bleeding time and hemorrhage after surgery. Perform a bleeding time before oral surgery on all patients on high dosages of aspirin.

Intramuscular doses of gold salts are used in patients refractory to other forms of treatment. Side-effects to this therapy are common and include stomatitis, blood dyscra-

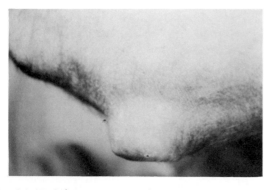

Fig. 24-16 Subcutaneous nodules of the arm in a patient with rheumatoid arthritis. (Courtesy Dr. George Ehrlich)

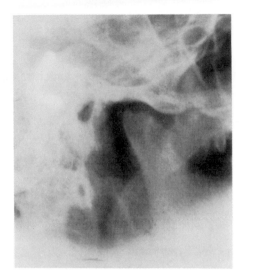

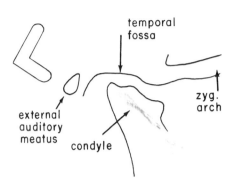

Fig. 24-18 Rheumatoid arthritis and evidence of flattening of condylar articular surface with deepening radiolucency. Note the lack of depth of temporal bone fossa.

sias, and nephrotic syndrome. Have total and differential white blood cell counts done on patients taking gold who develop oral ulcers to rule out the possibility of neutropenia as a cause of the ulcers. Before undertaking dental therapy, get recent results of a hematology report including a platelet count as well as a urinalysis.

Phenylbutazone (Butazolidin) and indomethacin are used extensively by some rheumatologists to suppress joint inflammation. Because these drugs may also cause blood dyscrasias, a complete blood count must be performed before dental treatment. In many cases new blood studies are not necessary because the physician managing the patient may have recent results. Long-term systemic corticosteroids are not used as frequently as in the past to manage RA. Some medical centers are now using a combination of corticosteroids and immunosuppressive agents.

ALLERGY

The modern dentist uses a wide variety of drugs to treat his patients including antibiotics, hypnotics, and anesthetics. All practitioners who use these medications must know how to cope with reactions secondary to their use. In the following section acute allergic reactions and their management will be discussed. Stomatitis associated with allergy is discussed in Chapter 6.

Acute allergic reactions are caused by an immediate type hypersensitivity reaction. A good model for understanding this mechanism is anaphylaxis. A patient, previously exposed to a drug or other antigen has antibody, primarily IgE, fixed to basophils and mast cells. When the antigen in the form of a drug, food, or airborne substance is reintroduced into the body it will react with the fixed antibody, bind complement, and open mast cells, releasing active mediators such as histamine and slow-reacting substance of anaphylaxis (SRS-A). These substances cause vasodilation and increased capillary premeability resulting in fluid and leukocytes leaving the blood vessels and accumulating in the tissues forming areas of edema. Constriction of bronchial smooth muscle also may result when IgE is bound in the pulmonary region. The anaphylactic reaction may be localized and lead to urticaria and angioneurotic edema, or a generalized reaction may result, causing anaphylactic shock.

Localized Anaphylaxis

When a localized anaphylactic reaction involves superficial blood vessels, urticaria results. Urticaria (hives) begins with pruritus in the area of release of histamine and other active substances. Wheals (welts) then appear on the skin as an area of localized edema on an erythematous base. These lesions can occur anywhere on the skin or mucous membranes. Urticaria of the lips and oral mucosa occur most frequently after food ingestion by an allergic individual. Common allergies are to chocolate, nuts, shellfish, and tomatoes. Drugs such as penicillin and aspirin may cause urticaria, and cold, heat, or pressure may cause the reaction in susceptible individuals.

Angioneurotic edema (angioedema) occurs when blood vessels deeper in the subcutaneous tissues are affected, producing a large diffuse area of subcutaneous swelling under normal overlying skin. This reaction may be caused by contact with an allergen but a significant number of cases are idiopathic. A recurrent form is inherited as an autosomal dominant trait. Hereditary angioneurotic edema is fatal in approximately one quarter of cases because of the severe laryngeal edema. The mechanism of the hereditary form of the disease has been shown to be a deficiency of an alpha-2 globulin, which normally acts as an inhibitor of the first component of complement and kallikrein.

Angioedema commonly occurs on the lips, tongue, and around the eyes (Figs. 24-19 and 24-20). It is a temporarily disfiguring but not serious disorder unless the posterior portion of the tongue or larynx compromises respiration. The patient in respiratory distress should be treated immediately with 0.5 ml epinephrine 1:1000 subcutaneously or 0.2 ml injected slowly, intravenously. When the immediate danger has passed, 50 mg of diphen-

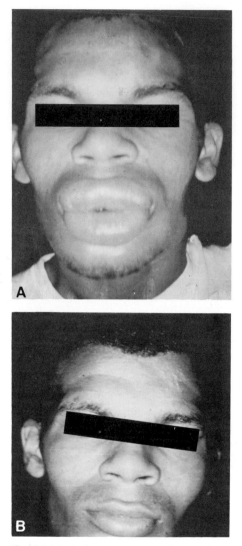

Fig. 24-20 *A,* Angioneurotic edema of allergic reaction to penicillin administered intramuscularly. *B,* Same patient 48 hours later following therapy with epinephrine and antihistaminic agents.

hydramine hydrochloride (Benadryl) should be given four times a day until the swelling diminishes.

Serum Sickness

Serum sickness is named for its frequent occurrence after administration of foreign serum, which before antibiotics, was given for the treatment of infectious diseases. The reaction is less common now but still occurs from tetanus antitoxin, rabies antiserum, and

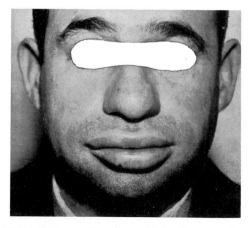

Fig. 24-19 Angioneurotic edema of the lips and the eyes. (Haden: Allergy in Clinical Practice. Philadelphia, JB Lippincott)

drugs that combine with body proteins to form allergens. Penicillin is a drug commonly prescribed by dentists that may cause serum sickness.

The pathogenesis of serum sickness differs from anaphylaxis. Antibody forms immune complexes in blood vessels with administered antigens. The complexes fix complement, which attracts leukocytes to the area causing direct tissue injury.

Serum sickness and vasculitis usually begin 7 to 10 days after administration of the allergen, but in some cases it may be as short as 3 days or as long as 1 month until symptoms appear. Unlike other allergic diseases, serum sickness may occur during the initial administration of the drug.

Major symptoms consist of fever, swellings, lymphadenopathy, joint and muscle pains, and rash. Less common manifestations include peripheral neuritis, kidney disease, and myocardial ischemia. Serum sickness is usually self-limiting with spontaneous recovery in 1 to 3 weeks. Treatment is symptomatic with aspirin given for arthralgia and antihistamines for the skin rash. Severe cases should be treated with a short course of systemic corticosteroids, which significantly shorten the course of the disease. Although this reaction is rare, the dentist prescribing penicillin should be aware of the possibility of its occurring even weeks after use of the drug.

Generalized Anaphylaxis

Generalized anaphylaxis is an allergic emergency. There is often no time to call consultants.

The mechanism of generalized anaphylaxis is the reaction of IgE antibodies with an allergen causing the release of histamine, bradykinin, and SRS-A (slow-reacting substance of anaphylaxis). These chemical mediators cause contraction of smooth muscles of the respiratory and intestinal tracts as well as increased vascular permeability.

The following factors increase the risk to anaphylaxis:

1. History of allergy to other drugs or food
2. History of asthma
3. Family history of allergy
4. Parenteral administration of the drug

5. Administration of high-risk allergens such as penicillin

Anaphylactic reactions may occur within seconds of drug administration or occur 30 to 40 minutes later, thus leading to confusion in diagnosis. The symptoms of generalized anaphylaxis should be known so that prompt treatment may be initiated and psychic or toxic reactions are not confused with true allergy. For example, patients have been diagnosed as allergic to local anesthetics when a psychic reaction to an injection occurred. This erroneous diagnosis makes future dental management difficult.

The generalized anaphylactic reaction may involve four systems: cardiovascular, intestinal, respiratory, and skin. The first signs often occur on the skin and are similar to those seen in localized anaphylaxis including urticaria, angioedema, erythema, and pruritus. Pulmonary symptoms include dyspnea, wheezing, and asthma. Gastrointestinal tract disease (*e.g.,* vomiting, cramps, and diarrhea) often follows skin symptoms. If these are untreated, symptoms of hypotension appear that result from the loss of intravascular fluid. If untreated this leads to shock. Patients with generalized anaphylactic reactions may die from respiratory failure, hypotensive shock, or laryngeal edema.

The most important treatment for generalized anaphylaxis is administration of epinephrine. All clinicians who administer drugs should have a vial of aqueous epinephrine at a 1:1000 dilution and sterile syringe easily accessible. Administer 0.5 ml of epinephrine intramuscularly or subcutaneously in an adult; use smaller doses from 0.1 ml to 0.3 ml for children, depending on their size. If the allergen was administered in an extremity, place a tourniquet above the injection site to minimize further absorption into the blood. The absorption can be further reduced by injecting 0.3 ml of 1:1000 epinephrine directly into the injection site. Remove the tourniquet every 10 minutes.

Epinephrine will usually reverse all severe signs of generalized anaphylaxis. If improvement is not observed in 10 minutes, readminister epinephrine. If the patient continues to deteriorate, take the following steps:

1. For bronchospasm, slowly inject aminophylline 250 mg intravenously over a pe-

riod of 10 minutes. Too rapid administration can lead to fatal cardiac arrhythmias. Do not give aminophylline if hypotensive shock is a part of the clinical picture. Inhalation sympathomimetics may also be used to treat bronchospasm, and oxygen should be given to prevent or manage hypoxia.

2. For laryngeal edema, establish an airway. This may necessitate endotracheal intubation; in some cases, a cricothyroidotomy may be necessary.

BIBLIOGRAPHY

Primary Immune Deficiencies

Ammann AJ, Hong R: Selective IgA deficiency: Presentation of 30 cases and a review of the literature. Medicine 50:223, 1971

August CS et al: Implantation of a foetal thymus, restoring immunological competence in a patient with thymic aplasia (DiGeorge's syndrome). Lancet 2:1210, 1968

Bachmann R: Studies on serum gamma A globulin level. 3. The frequency of agammaglobulinemia. Scand J Clin Lab Invest 17:316, 1965

Barrickman RW, Callerame ML, Condemi JJ: Gingivitis in hypogammaglobulinemia. J Periodontol 44:171, 1973

Boder E, Sedgwick RP: Ataxia telangiectasia. A familial syndrome of progressive cerebellar ataxia, oculocutaneous telangiectasia and frequent pulmonary infection. Pediatrics 21:526, 1958

Brown LR et al: Comparison of the plaque microflora in immunodeficient and immunocompetent dental patients. J Dent Res 23:44, 1979

Bruton OC: Agammaglobulinemia. Pediatrics 9:722, 1952

Claman NH et al: Isolated severe gamma A deficiency. J Lab Clin Med 75:307, 1970

Cleveland WW et al: Foetal thymic transplant in a case of DiGeorge's syndrome. Lancet 2:1211, 1968

Collins JR, Ellis DS: Agammaglobulinemia, malabsorption and rheumatoidlike arthritis. Am J Med 39:476, 1965

Crabbé PA, Heremans JF: Selective IgA deficiency with steatorrhea, a new syndrome. Am J Med 42:319, 1967

Della BG et al: Congenital alymphoplasmacytic agammaglobulinemia with thymic dysplasia. JAMA 194:507, 1965

DiGeorge AM: Congenital absence of the thymus and its immunologic consequences: Concurrence with congenital hypoparathyroidism. Birth Defects: Original Article Series, 4(1):116, 1968

Fudenberg H et al: Primary immunodeficiencies: report of a World Health Organization Committee. Pediatrics 47:927, 1971

Fudenberg HH, Spitler LE, Levin AS: Treatment of immune deficiency. Am J Pathol 69:529, 1972

Gatti RA, Good RA: The immunologic deficiency diseases. Med Clin North Am 54:281, 1970

Hill LE: Clinical features of hypogammaglobulinemia in the United Kingdom. H. M. Stationery Office, London, M.R.L. Special Report Series, No 310, 1971

Kirkpatrick CH, Ruth WE: Chronic pulmonary disease and immunologic deficiency. Am J Med 41:427, 1966

Kretschmer R et al: Congenital aplasia of the thymus gland (DiGeorge's syndrome). N Engl J Med 279:1295, 1968

Lawlor GJ et al: The syndrome of cellular immunodeficiency with immunoglobulins. J Pediatr 84:183, 1974

Legler DW et al: Immunodeficiency disease and implications for dental treatment. J Am Dent Assoc 105:803, 1982

Lehner T, Wilton JMA, Ivanyl L: Immunodeficiencies in chronic mucocutaneous candidiasis. Immunology 22:775, 1971

Mawhinney H et al: Selective IgA deficiency. Lancet 2:546, 1972

Medical Staff Conference, Univ. of Calif. San Francisco: Immunoglobulin deficiency disorders. West J Med 120:471, 1974

Moore EC, Meywissen HJ: Immunologic deficiency disease. New York State J Med 73:2437, 1973

Peterson RDA, Cooper MD, Good RA: The pathogenesis of immunologic deficiency diseases. Am J Med 38:579, 1965

Robertson PB et al: Periodontal status of patients with abnormalities of the immune system. J Periodont Res 13:37, 1978

Robertson PB et al: Periodontal status of patients with abnormalities of the immune system II. Observations over a two year period. J Periodontol 51:70, 1980

Schaller J, Davis SC, Wedgwood RJ: Failure of development of the thymus, lymphopenia, hypogammaglobulinemia. An atypical case. Am J Med 41:462, 1966

Seward MH: Oral manifestations of hypogammaglobulinemia in a young child. Br J Oral Surg 11:246, 1974

Vyas GN, Perkins HA, Fudenberg HH: Anaphylactoid transfusion reactions associated with anti IgA. Lancet 2:312, 1968

Webster ADB: Immune deficiency in the adult. Br J Clin Pract 26:323, 1972

Secondary Immune Deficiencies

Aisenberg AC: Manifestations of immunological unresponsiveness in Hodgkin's disease. Cancer Res 26:1152, 1966

Anderson RJ et al: Infectious risk factors in the immunosuppressed host. Am J Med 54:453, 1973

Bach MC et al: Influence of rejection therapy on fungal and nocardial infections in renal transplant recipients. Lancet 1:180, 1973

Craig JM, Facher S: The development of disseminated visceral mycosis during therapy for acute leukemia. Am J Pathol 29:601, 1953

Eickhoff TC: Infectious complications in renal transplant recipients. Trans Proc 5:1233, 1973

Erlichman MC, Trieger N: Aspergillus infection in a patient receiving immunosuppressive drugs. Oral Surg 36:978, 1978

Friedman–Kein AE et al: Disseminated Kaposi's sarcoma in homosexual men. Ann Intern Med 96:693, 1982

Greenberg MS, Cohen SG: Oral infection in immunosuppressed renal transplant patients. Oral Surg 43:879, 1977

Greenberg MS, Cohen SG, McKitrick J, Cassileth P: The oral flora as a source of septicemia in patients with leukemia. Oral Surg 53:32, 1982

Hirschberg N: Phagocytic activity in leukemia. Am J Med Sci 197:706, 1939

Holm G, Perlmann P, Johansson B: Impaired phytohaemagglutinin-induced cytotoxicity in vitro of lymphocytes from patients with Hodgkin's disease or chronic lymphocytic leukemia. Clin Exp Immunol 2:351, 1967

Keyes JD et al: Fungal diseases in a general hospital. Study of 88 cases. Am J Clin Pathol 26:1235, 1956

Larson DL, Tomlinson LJ: Quantitative antibody studies in man; III. Antibody response in leukemia and other malignant lymphomata. J Clin Invest 32:317, 1953

Lopez C et al: Role of virus infections in immunosuppressed renal transplant patients. Trans Proc 5:803, 1973

McGowan DA, Gorman JM, Otridge BW: Intensive dental care in adult acute leukemia. Dent Pract 20:239, 1970

Miller DG: Patterns of immunological deficiency in lymphoma and leukemias. Ann Intern Med 57:703, 1962

Miller DG, Karnofsky DA: Immunologic factors and resistance to infection in chronic lymphocytic leukemia. Am J Med 31:748, 1961

Oshrain HI, Mender S, Mandel ID: Periodontal status of patients with reduce immunocapacity. J Periodontol 50:185, 1979

Reyna J et al: Head and neck infection after renal transplantation. JAMA 247:3337, 1982

Rifkind, D et al: Systemic fungal infections complicating renal transplantation and immunosuppressive therapy. Am J Med 43:28, 1967

Schuller PD, Freedman HL, Lewis PW: Periodontal status of renal transplant patients receiving immunosuppressive therapy. J Periodontol 44:167, 1973

Scopp IW, Orvieto LD: Gingival degerming by povidone-iodine irrigation: Bacteremia reduction in extraction procedures. J Am Dent Assoc 83:1294, 1971

Shier WW et al: Hodgkin's disease and immunity. Am J Med 20:94, 1956

Tapia HR et al: Causes of death after renal transplantation. Arch Intern Med 131:204, 1973

Tyldesley WR, Rotter E, Sells RA: Oral lesions in renal transplant patients. J Oral Pathol 8:53, 1979

Ulfmann JE et al: The clinical implications of hypogammaglobulinemia in patients with chronic lymphocytic leukemia and lymphosarcoma. Ann Intern Med 51:501, 1959

Wilson JD, Nossal GJV: Identification of human T and B lymphocytes in normal peripheral blood and in chronic lymphocytic leukemia. Lancet 2:788, 1971

The Connective Tissue Diseases

Andreasen JO, Poulsen HE: Oral discoid and systemic lupus erythematosus. I. Clinical investigation. Acta Odontol Scand 22:295, 1964

Andreasen JO: Oral manifestations in discoid and systemic lupus erythematosus II. Histologic investigation. Acta Odontol Scand 22:389, 1964

Archard HO, Roebuck NF, Stanley HR, Jr: Oral manifestations of chronic discoid lupus erythematosus. Oral Surg 16:696, 1963

Arnold HL, Tilden IL: Fatal scleroderma with L.E. phenomenon, report of a case. Arch Dermatol 76:427, 1957

Bardawil WA et al: Disseminated lupus erythematosus, scleroderma, and dermatomyositis as manifestations of sensitization to DNA-protein, I. An immunohistochemical approach. Am J Pathol 34:607, 1958

Barnett AV: Lupus erythematosus. Aust Dent J 6:40, 1961

Bartholomew LE: Characterization of mycoplasma strains and antibody studies from patients with rheumatoid arthritis. Ann NY Acad Sci 143:522, 1967

Bassett ER, Kutscher AH: Acute disseminated lupus erythematosus of oral mucosa. J Clin Stomatol Conf 4:10, 1963

Bayles TB, Russell LA: Temporomandibular joint in rheumatoid arthritis. JAMA 116:2842, 1941

Blackwood HJJ: Arthritis of the mandibular joint. Br Dent J 115:317, 1963

Caplan HI, Benny RA: Total osteolysis of the mandibular condyle in progressive systemic sclerosis. Oral Surg 46:362, 1978

Chalmers IM, Blair GS: Rheumatoid arthritis of the temporomandibular joint. Q J Med 42:369, 1973

Cooke BED: Chronic lupus erythematosus with oral manifestations. Proc R Soc Med 46:872, 1953

Crum RJ, Loiselle RJ: Incidence of temporomandibular joint symptoms in male patients with rheumatoid arthritis. J Am Dent Assoc 81:129, 1970

Dawkins RL, Mastaglia FL: Cell-mediated cytotoxicity to muscle in polymyositis. N Engl J Med 288:434, 1973

Editorial: Scleroderma or sclerodermas. Br Med J 4:249, 1973

Edwards MB, Gayford JJ: Oral lupus erythematosus, three cases demonstrating three variants. Oral Surg 31:332, 1971

Estes D, Christian CL: The natural history of systemic lupus erythematosus by prospective analysis. Medicine 50:85, 1971

Franks AST: Temporomandibular joint in adult rheumatoid arthritis: A comparative evaluation of 100 cases. Ann Rheum Dis 28:139, 1969

Gores RJ: Dental features of acrosclerosis and scleroderma. J Am Dent Assoc 54:755, 1957

Green D: Scleroderma and its oral manifestations. Oral Surg 15:1313, 1962

Greenberger NJ et al: Intestinal atony in progressive systemic sclerosis (scleroderma). Am J Med 45:301, 1968

Harvey AM et al: Systemic lupus erythematosus, review of the literature and clinical analysis of 138 cases. Medicine 33:291, 1959

Herschfus L: Lupus erythematosus. J Oral Med 27:12, 1972

Herschfus L: The significance of lupus erythematosus in oral medicine. J Michigan State Dent Assoc 54:248, 1972

Jansson E, Vainio U, Tuuri S: Cultivation of a mycoplasma from the bone marrow in systemic lupus erythematosus disseminatus. Acta Rheumatol Scand 17:223, 1971

Kellgren JH, Ball J: Clinical significance of the rheumatoid serum factor. Br Med J 1:523, 1959

Lamont–Havers RW: Arthritis of the temporomandibular joint. Dent Clin North Am November 1966, 621

Lever WF: Histopathology of Skin, 5th ed. Philadelphia, JB Lippincott, 1975

Lite T: Gingival manifestations of lupus erythematosus. J Periodontol 24:119, 1953

Looby JP, Burket LW: Scleroderma of the face with involvement of the alveolar process. Am J Orthod 28:493, 1942

Martis CS, Karakasis DT: Ankylosis of the temporomandibular joint caused by Still's disease. Oral Surg 35:462, 1973

Michanowicz A: Arrested diffuse scleroderma. Oral Surg 15:1325, 1962

Monash S: Oral lesions of lupus erythematosus. Dent Cosmos 73:511, 1931

Nishimura N et al: Phenylalanine and tyrosine in collagen diseases: Urinary excretion of general intermediary metabolites in tyrosine in patients with collagen disease and liver disease. Arch Dermatol 83:644, 1961

Rodnan GP: A review of recent observations and current theories on the etiology and pathogenesis of progressive systemic sclerosis (diffuse scleroderma). J Chronic Dis 16:929, 1963

Rodnan GP, McEwen C, Wallace SL: Polymyositis and dermatomyositis. JAMA 5 (Suppl):55, 1973

Romero RW, Nesbitt LT, Reed RJ: Unusual variant of lupus erythematosus or lichen planus. Arch Dermatol 113:741, 1977

Rosenthal IH: Generalized scleroderma, hidebound disease, its relation to the oral cavity with case history and dental restoration. Oral Surg 1:1019, 1948

Samuelson SJ, Friedlander AH, Swerdloff M: Systemic lupus erythematosus. J Am Dent Assoc 100:553, 1980

Sanders B, McKelvey B, Cruickshank G: Correction of microstomia secondary to sclerodermatomyositis. Oral Surg 35:57, 1977

Sanger RG, Kirby JW: The oral and facial manifestations of dermatomyositis with calcinosis. Oral Surg 35:476, 1973

Schiodt M, Halberg P, Hentzer B: A clinical study of 32 patients with oral discoid lupus erythematosus. Int J Oral Surg 7:85, 1978

Schiodt M et al: Deposits of immunoglobulins, complement, and fibrinogen in oral lupus erythematosus, lichen planus and leukoplakia. Oral Surg 51:603, 1981

Seifert MH, Steigerwald JC, Cleff MM: Bone resorption of the mandible in progressive systemic sclerosis. Arthritis Rheum 18:507, 1975

Sharp JT: Mycoplasmas and arthritis. Arthritis Rheum 13:263, 1970

Smith DB: Scleroderma: Its oral manifestations. Oral Surg 11:865, 1958

Stafne EC, Austin LT: A characteristic dental finding in acrosclerosis and diffuse scleroderma. Am J Orthod 30:25, 1944

Sugarman MM: Lupus erythematosus. Oral Surg 6:836, 1953

Sugarman MM, Stillerman HB: Systemic lupus erythematosus: a seven year case report. J Periodontol 31:47, 1960

Tuffanelli DL, Dubois EL: Cutaneous manifestations of systemic lupus erythematosus. Arch Dermatol 90:377, 1964

VanBelois HJ, Sugg WE: Calcinosis universalis lesions in scleroderma. Oral Surg 46:329, 1978

Vaughan JH: Infectious and immunological consideration: In Hollander JL, McCarthy DJ (eds): Rheumatic Diseases, Arthritis and Allied Conditions, 8th ed. Philadelphia, Lea & Febiger, 1972

Wade GW: Scleroderma. Dent Progr 3:236, 1963

Weiner SN, Wolf M: Changes in the mandible in scleroderma. Oral Surg 51:329, 1981

Weisman RA, Calcateria TC: Head and neck manifestations of scleroderma. Ann Otorhinolaryngol 87:332, 1978

Whitaker, JN, Engel WK: Vascular deposits of immunoglobulin and complement in inflammatory myopathy. N Engl J Med 286:333, 1972

White SC et al: Oral radiographic changes in patients with progressive systemic sclerosis (scleroderma). JAMA 94:1178, 1977

Witebesky E: Historical roots of present concepts of immunopathology. In Graber P, Muocher PA (eds): Immunopathology (First International Symposium) Basel, Schwaber, 1959

Zampelli M et al: Rheumatoid arthritis of the temporomandibular joint: Case report. J Periodontol 45:26, 1974

25

Endocrine Disease and Dysfunction

MARK B. SNYDER

The endocrine system is a network of anatomically distinct structures located throughout the body. These glands secrete chemical substances called *hormones* that act at locations remote from their source of production and release into the bloodstream. Hormones control the body's vegetative and adaptive functions and maintain both an internal and external environmental "steady state." This homeostasis is achieved by a complex system of feedback control mechanisms linked in part to the autonomic nervous system.

The widely distributed signs and symptoms of endocrine diseases stem from the fact that hormones are secreted either directly or indirectly into the circulatory system.

NONSPECIFIC PHYSICAL FINDINGS SUGGESTIVE OF ENDOCRINE DYSFUNCTION

- Retarded or excessive growth pattern
- Obesity
- Hyperpigmentation of skin
- Cachexia
- Muscle weakness
- Hirsutism
- Anorexia or increase in appetite
- Polyuria and polydipsia
- Precocious puberty
- Menstrual abnormalities
- Arthralgia
- Kidney stones
- Tetany
- Behavioral changes
- Pathologic fractures

Endocrine dysfunction, in fact, is best regarded in terms of hyperfunction or hypofunction of endocrine tissues or failure of target organs to appropriately respond to hormones. These functional abnormalities are most commonly caused by acute or chronic pathosis such as tumors, infections, or degenerative changes affecting the endocrine glands. In addition, agents prescribed for the control or treatment of a wide variety of systemic diseases can also cause endocrinopathies.

This chapter presents the salient features of endocrine disorders of particular relevance to the dentist. The primary goals of this chapter are to give the dentist sufficient information with which to suspect an endocrinopathy, to describe the clinical and radiographic oral manifestations of the various endocrine diseases (Table 25-1), and to discuss special

Table 25-1. Dental and Oral Findings Associated with Endocrine Dysfunction

TYPE OF ABNORMALITY	MANIFESTATIONS
Soft tissue abnormalities	Macroglossia Abnormal pigmentation of skin and mucosa Neck masses (goiters, adenomas, carcinomas) Salivary gland dysfunction (xerostomia) Ectopic glandular tissue (lingual thyroid gland)
Radiographic abnormalities	Loss of lamina dura Delayed root formation (root blunting) Enlargement of paranasal sinuses Abnormal calcifications Osteolytic lesions (giant cell tumors) Osteoporosis Altered trabecular pattern (ground glass appearance)
Jaw and tooth abnormalities	Disproportionate jaw growth (prognathism, micrognathia) Malocclusion Tooth spacing and flaring Retarded or accelerated eruption pattern (primary and adult dentition) Defects in enamel and dentin formation

dental management considerations in patients with suspected or proven endocrine dysfunction.

DISEASES OF THE PITUITARY GLAND

Anatomy and Physiology

The pituitary gland sits within the sella turcica and is composed of functionally and anatomically distinct anterior (adenohypophysis) and posterior (neurohypophysis) lobes. The secretory activity of the pituitary is modulated by the hypothalamus through a series of complex feedback loop interactions whereby specific releasing hormones elaborated in the hypothalamus are transported to the pituitary, which in turn generates hormones directed at target organs. For example, pituitary release of adrenocorticotropin (ACTH) stimulates production of cortisol by the adrenal glands. Once physiologic blood levels of cortisol are reached, negative feedback to the pituitary and hypothalamus inhibits further release of ACTH (Fig. 25-1).

The pituitary gland governs and coordinates the varied activities of all the endocrine glands. Seven hormones are produced by the adenohypophysis:

1. Adrenocorticotropin (ACTH)
2. Growth hormone (GH)
3. Follicle-stimulating hormone (FSH)
4. Luteinizing hormone (LH) and interstitial-stimulating hormone (ICSH) acting on the corpus luteum of the ovaries or on the interstitial cells of the testes
5. Thyroid-stimulating hormone (TSH), acting on the thyroid gland
6. Lactogenic hormone (prolactin, LTH), acting on the mammary glands
7. Melanocyte-stimulating hormone (MSH)

Hormones elaborated by the neurohypophysis include the following:

1. Antidiuretic hormone (ADH), which regulates the flow of water through the kidneys, stimulates intestinal musculature, and produces contraction of peripheral blood vessels
2. Oxytocin, which induces contraction of the uterine musculature and milk ejection

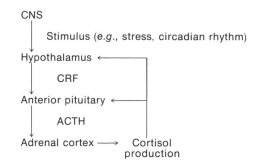

Fig. 25-1 Diagram of hypothalamic–pituitary–adrenal axis. Secretion of ACTH by the anterior pituitary stimulates the release of cortisol in the adrenal cortex. The circulating levels of cortisol control ACTH release by a negative feedback mechanism such that high levels of glucocorticoid inhibit and low levels stimulate ACTH release. Hypothalamic secretion of corticotropin-releasing factor (CRF) is also regulated by cortisol levels and by stimuli mediated by the central nervous system (CNS).

Synthesis and secretion of anterior pituitary hormones is controlled by short-chain polypeptides called *releasing factors*, which are produced in the hypothalamus and are transported to the pituitary by the hypophyseal portal veins. Posterior pituitary hormones are produced in the hypothalamus and are transported from axons of the neurohypophyseal tract to the nerve endings in the posterior pituitary where they are released in response to specific stimuli. Diseases causing hyperfunction or hypofunction of the pituitary gland of relevance to the dentist are discussed below.

Hypopituitarism

Pathologic changes can result from a variety of pituitary gland malfunctions. When single or multiple pituitary hormones are not produced in normal amounts, hypopituitarism results; total absence of all pituitary secretions is known as *panhypopituitarism* (Simmonds' disease). The nature of the clinical manifestations of pituitary hypofunction depends on which target organs or tissues are affected. For example, Kallmann's syndrome is characterized by deficiency of gonadotropin-releasing hormone; therefore, insufficient amounts of LH and FSH are produced. The signs and symptoms associated with this are decreased spermatogenesis and inadequate production of testosterone in males and failure of ovulation and ovarian production of estrogen in females.

Hypopituitarism can result from space-occupying lesions involving the sella turcica. Examples include craniopharyngiomas, chromophobe or acidophil adenomas of the pituitary, metastatic carcinomas, sarcoidosis, and histiocytosis. *Sheehan's syndrome* is a form of hypopituitarism caused by infarction of the pituitary associated with postpartum hemorrhage.

Signs and Symptoms. Growth hormone (GH) does not act on a single target organ but has a more general metabolic effect. Deficiency of GH produces a very different clinical picture in children than in adults. In children, pituitary insufficiency leads to *pituitary dwarfism* (Fig. 25-2). The cause is usually a craniopharyngioma, or the disorder is idiopathic. Clinically, the hallmark of this condition is growth retardation; as a general rule, growth is retarded to a greater degree than is bone development, and dental development is least affected. Most patients have normal birth length and weight and growth retardation is often not noticed until the second or third year. Signs of hypothyroidism are not a prominent feature of this condition. Hypoglycemia may occur because of GH deficiency and lack of cortisol. The presence of diabetes insipidus associated with deficient secretion of vasopressin is suggestive of pituitary dysfunction. Lack of gonadotropins also delays the onset of puberty. It is important to note that patients with hypopituitarism, despite retarded growth, have normal body proportions. This is a contrast to patients with primary hypothyroidism who have infantile proportions. In adults, hypopituitarism is usually secondary to tumors or infiltrative diseases involving the pituitary gland. Some examples include Frölich's syndrome (adiposogenital dystrophy), Sheehan's syndrome, and Simmonds' disease. Clinical symptoms vary according to the location of the primary lesion and according to which pituitary hormones are affected.

Oral Changes. No dental anomaly is pathognomonic for a particular endocrine disorder and many of the symptoms of pituitary dwarfism are also seen in other forms of growth retardation. In hypopituitarism, both facial and dental development are slowed. Facial height is affected because the mandible is underdeveloped owing to lack of condylar growth and a short ramus, and this can lead to severe malocclusion and crowding of the teeth. The eruption pattern of the teeth is likewise delayed, and there may be overretention of primary teeth and incomplete apexification of the permanent dentition.

Treatment. Pituitary dwarfism is successfully treated by the use of GH prepared from human pituitary glands. If therapy is instituted early enough, normal growth and development will occur. Hypopituitarism caused by tumors may require surgery or radiotherapy. Deficiencies in end-organ hormones (*e.g.* cortisol, thyroxine) are corrected by hormone replacement therapy when appropriate.

Hyperpituitarism

Excessive secretion of GH caused by a pituitary adenoma produces *gigantism* in children and *acromegaly* in adults.

Signs and Symptoms. Hypersecretion of GH before the closure of epiphyses leads to an increase in bone length and width in a proportional manner. The term *pituitary gigantism* is used to describe individuals who achieve monstrous size because of tumors of the pituitary gland. After closure of epiphyses, excessive GH leads to periosteal overgrowth and cortical thickening. Bone overgrowth and thickening of the soft tissues cause a characteristic coarsening of facial features termed *acromegaly* (Fig. 25-3). It is common for the hands and fingers to enlarge to a point at which jewelry no longer fits properly. Increase in the size of the calvarium may change the hat size. Other changes include erosion of articular surfaces and symptoms such as arthralgias, headache, visual problems, and the carpal tunnel syndrome. In addition to GH excess, pituitary tumors may also induce deficiencies of other pituitary hormones causing signs of hypogonadism including decreased libido and menstrual problems in women.

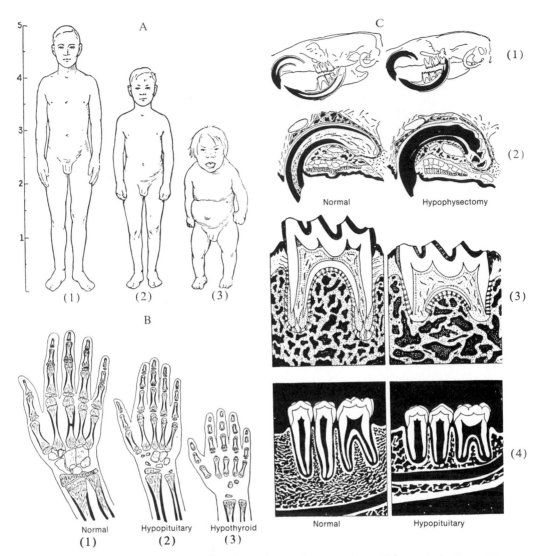

Fig. 25-2 *A,* Composite drawings of male patients: (1) normality, (2) hypopituitarism, (3) congenital untreated hypothyroidism (cretinism). The smaller size but symmetric proportions are noted in (2) and the dysplasia in (3). (Composite drawings of figures in Wolf's *Endocrinology,* Zondek's *Diseases of the Endocrine Glands,* and photographs supplied by I.P. Bronstein.) In (1) the chronological age is 13 years; statural age, 12 years; height, 5 ft. In (2) the chronological age is 13 years; statural age, 8 years; height, 4 ft. 2 in. In (3) the chronological age is 13 years; statural age, 24 years; height, 3 ft. 1 in.

B, Composite tracings of handplates taken of patients and similar to those shown in *A:* (1) normality; (2) hypopituitarism; (3) congenital untreated hypothyroidism (cretinism). In (1) the chronological age is 16 years; carpal age, 16 years. In (2) the chronological age is 16 years; carpal age, 7 years. In (3) the chronological age is 16 years; carpal age, 2 years.

C, Effect of deficiency in secretion of growth hormone from anterior pituitary. (1) Drawings of lateral radiograms of skulls of albino rats. (2) Enlarged drawing of rat incisors in sagittal section. (3) Enlarged drawing of rat molars in mesiodistal section. The albino rats from which these sections and drawings were made were 300 days old at the time they were killed, but the ones on the right were hypophysectomized at 40 days. (4) Drawing from intraoral radiograms from normal and hypopituitary males aged 16 years. The effect of hypopituitarism upon growth of bone and eruption of the teeth is to be noted. (Schour I, Massler M: JADA, 30:595)

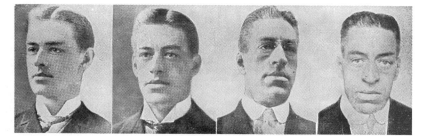

Fig. 25-3 A case of acromegaly. (*Left to right*) The patient at 24 years of age before the onset of the malady; at 29 years of age at the time of onset; at 37 years of age; and at 42 years of age when outspoken acromegalic changes are evident. (Cushing N: The Pituitary Body and Its Disorders. Philadelphia, JB Lippincott)

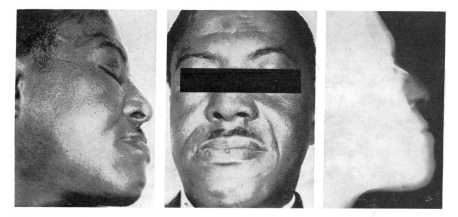

Fig. 25-4 Acromegalic features showing the abnormal development of the mandible. (*Left*) profile of patient; (*center*) front view; (*right*) profile radiogram.

Oral Changes. The most striking change in the dental structures is overgrowth of the mandible leading to prognathism (so-called lantern jaw; Fig. 25-4). Accelerated dental development including eruption of the teeth is apparent clinically and radiographically. Radiographs show marked thickening of the cranium and the cortical plates of the mandible and often show sinus enlargement. Periosteal calcification may be seen at muscle and tendon insertions.

Characteristically, the lips and nose are greatly enlarged in acromegaly (Fig. 25-5). The mandible may reach extraordinary proportions creating a major discrepancy between the upper and lower jaws and a pronounced class III malocclusion. The palatal vault is usually flattened. The tongue increases in size and may show crenations on its lateral borders. There is usually tremendous flaring of the dental arches, and fanning out and spacing of the teeth is common. In the edentulous patient, enlargement of the alveolus may prevent the comfortable fit of complete dentures. When this occurs the dentist should suspect the possibility of underlying endocrine disease as a source of the problem.

Diagnosis. Diagnosis can be made from the characteristic clinical findings. Radiographs of the skull reveal cortical thickening, frontal sinus enlargement, and erosion of the sella turcica. GH concentrations can be measured by radioimmunoassay techniques.

Treatment. Treatment of hyperpituitarism depends on the nature and location of the

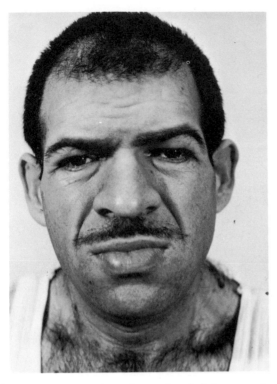

Fig. 25-5 Acromegaly and associated diabetes mellitus. This 36-year-old man's maximum serum growth hormone (GH) level was 160 ng/ml (normal, under 5). His GH did not respond to stimulation with insulin-induced hypoglycemia or arginine; thus the pituitary adenoma was secreting maximally, and GH production by remainder of the gland was suppressed by tumor. In the normal individual, GH level falls when blood sugar level rises. In this man, as in all "active" acromegalics, the GH level did not fall during a glucose tolerance test, an indication that the tumor is relatively autonomous. (Ezrin C, Godden JO, Volpé R: Systematic Endocrinology, 2nd ed, p 67. New York, Harper & Row, 1979)

lesion. Both surgery and radiotherapy are used effectively to irradicate functional tumors. A possible complication of treatment is the development of panhypopituitarism.

THYROID DISEASES

Anatomy and Physiology

The normal thyroid gland is a midline, butterfly-shaped organ, consisting of two lobes on either side of the trachea at the level of the cricoid cartilage connected by an isthmus. A pyramidal lobe also extends from the isthmus in over one third of the population. The gland is bordered laterally by the carotid sheath and sternocleidomastoid and anteriorly by the infrahyoid musculature.

Embryologically, the thyroid gland develops as a downgrowth from portions of the fourth pharyngeal pouches and the ultimobrachial body. The anlage of the median lobe arises at the base of the tongue (foramen cecum), and as downgrowth occurs, the thyroglossal duct maintains continuity between the lingual and pharyngeal areas. By the sixth week *in utero*, this structure usually is obliterated; however, epithelial remnants may persist anywhere along the path of descent of the thyroid anlage leading to *thyroglossal duct cysts*. The vast majority of these cysts (80%) occur in the midline and move superiorly with swallowing or protrusion of the tongue.

Another rare developmental condition caused by incomplete descent of the gland is known as *lingual thyroid gland*. In this condition, the thyroid gland may persist as a raised, purplish mass, usually located at the base of the tongue. This is of clinical significance because it may represent the only functional thyroid tissue in the body. Radioisotope studies and biopsy are used to establish the diagnosis when ectopic thyroid tissue is suspected and to rule out neoplastic disease.

Synthesis of thyroxine (T_4) and triiodothyronine (T_3) occurs in the thyroid and depends on the presence of iodine. Synthesis and secretion of thyroid hormones is controlled by thyroid-stimulating hormone (TSH) produced in the anterior pituitary gland. TSH, in turn is regulated by thyrotropin-releasing hormone TRH), which is elaborated by the hypothalamus and transported to the pituitary. A negative feedback loop works as follows: when thyroid hormone levels are depleted in the tissues, TSH synthesis is stimulated in the pituitary, which acts on the thyroid causing production and release of T_3 and T_4 until adequate serum levels of hormone are achieved. Conversely, excess T_3 and T_4 concentrations in the blood act to inhibit further pituitary TSH secretion (Fig. 25-6). This mechanism effectively maintains normal levels of circulating thyroid hormone.

The thyroid hormones are essential for nor-

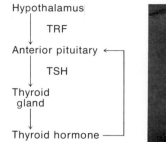

Hypothalamus

| TRF

Anterior pituitary ←

| TSH

Thyroid gland

|

Thyroid hormone ──

Fig. 25-6 Regulation of thyroid hormone secretion. Classic negative feedback system showing inhibition of thyroid-stimulating hormone (TSH) secretion by circulating thyroid hormone levels. This inhibition antagonizes the stimulating effect of the thyroid-releasing factor (TRF) from the hypothalamus.

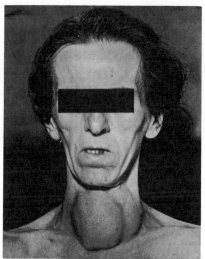

Fig. 25-7 Toxic goiter. A patient with a large nodular goiter who was suffering from severe hyperthyroidism. Note the absence of exophthalmos. (Courtesy Dr. George Crile and Surg Gynecol Obstet)

mal growth and maturation and are known to affect oxygen consumption and protein synthesis throughout the body; therefore, thyroid disease can be characterized by severe metabolic derangements associated with overproduction of hormone or insufficient hormone production. Furthermore, enlargement of the gland caused by dietary deficiency of iodine or neoplastic disease can produce alarming anatomic abnormalities (Fig. 25-7).

Hyperthyroidism and Graves' Disease*

In hyperthyroidism or thyrotoxicosis, thyroid hormone is produced in excess. This may be caused by ectopic thyroid tissue, Graves' disease, multinodular goiter, thyroid adenomas, or pituitary dysfunction.

TYPES OF HYPERTHYROIDISM

- Graves' disease
- Toxic nodular goiter (toxic adenoma) or toxic multinodular goiter
- The hyperthyroid phase of subacute thyroiditis (this may be painless)
- Hyperthyroidism associated with acromegaly
- Hyperthyroidism caused by HCG produced by choriocarcinoma
- Hyperthyroidism in thyroid carcinoma

* From Ezrin C, Godden JO, Volpe R, Wilson R: Systematic Endocrinology, 2nd ed, p 208. New York, Harper & Row, 1979

caused by a toxic carcinomatous nodule or excess thyroxine from widespread metastases (the tissue is not hyperfunctioning, but the total mass is very large)
- Hyperthyroxinemia caused by excessive administration of thyroid hormone
- Hyperthyroidism caused by excess pituitary TSH
- Hyperthyroidism caused by an autonomous struma ovarii
- Iodide-induced hyperthyroidism (Iod–Base dow's disease)
- Hyperthyroidism related to polyostotic fibrous dysplasia

Graves' disease (toxic diffuse goiter; Fig. 25-8) is the most common form of hyperthyroidism, usually affecting middle-aged women and characterized by a syndrome of nodular thyroid enlargement, exophthalmos, and pretibial myxedema (Fig. 25-9). The etiology of the hyperthyroidism may be related to severe emotional trauma or infection, but recent evidence suggests an immunologic basis. In fact, a significant percentage of patients with Graves' disease have a circulating thyroid stimulator in their serum known as *long-acting thyroid stimulator* (LATS), which has the characteristics of an antibody.

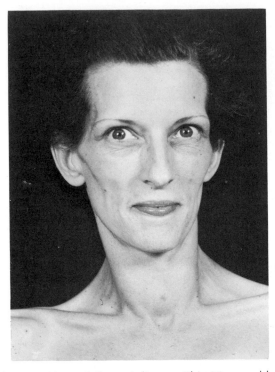

Fig. 25-8 Signs of Graves' disease. This 35-year-old woman shows obvious weight loss, diffuse goiter, widened palpebral fissure, and some puffiness of her upper lids. (Ezrin C, Godden JO, Volpé R: Systematic Endocrinology, 2nd ed, p 106. New York, Harper & Row, 1979)

Signs and Symptoms. A group of classic signs and symptoms is common to all forms of hyperthyroidism (Table 25-2). In Graves' disease, exophthalmos is produced by excessive retro-orbital tissue and lymphocytic infiltration of the ocular muscles, producing vision problems (Figs. 25-10 and 25-11). Patients with Graves' disease may also exhibit *pretibial myxedema,* characterized by a nonpitting mucinous infiltration of the tissues.

Untreated thyrotoxicosis can lead to a rare and life-threatening condition known as *thyroid storm.* This condition may be precipitated by infection, trauma, or dental surgery under local anesthesia with epinephrine. It is characterized by rapid onset of muscle weakness, fatigue, fever, nausea, vomiting, and abdominal pain. Profuse sweating, marked tachycardia, congestive heart failure, and cardiac arrythmias also develop. The patient may be-

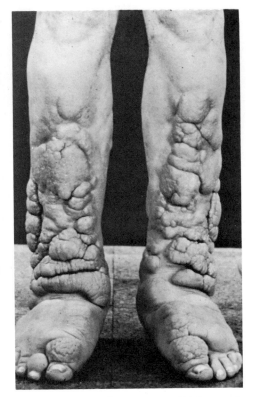

Fig. 25-9 Unusually severe pretibial myxedema. Mucopolysaccharide has gathered in locules, giving the appearance of elephantiasis. This patient had had hyperthyroidism 18 years before and had moderate pretibial myxedema at that time. He was treated with radioactive iodine and became euthyroid; however, over the years his pretibial myxedema slowly increased. He also has moderate exophthalmos and clubbed fingers. The titer of plasma LATS was very high. (Ezrin C, Godden JO, Volpé R: Systematic Endocrinology, 2nd ed, p 107. New York, Harper & Row, 1979)

come psychotic or comatose. Profound hypotension eventually develops and can cause death. Emergency treatment of thyroid storm consists of large doses of propylthiouracil, propranolol, potassium iodide, hydrocortisone, and intravenous fluids.

Oral Changes. No pathognomonic oral signs and symptoms are associated with hyperthyroidism. Although occasional reports appear in the literature describing unusual dental changes in these patients, there is no causal relationship between a hyperactive thyroid

Table 25-2. Signs and Symptoms of Hyperthyroidism (Thyrotoxicosis)

SIGNS	SYMPTOMS
Thyroid enlargement	Nervousness
Tachycardia	Increased sweating
Widened pulse pressure	Hypersensitivity to heat
Warm, moist skin	Palpitations
	Increased appetite
Tremor	Fatigue
Eye signs	Insomnia
Atrial fibrillation	Muscle weakness

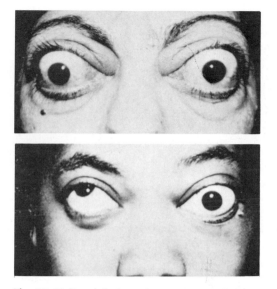

Fig. 25-10 Exophthalmos in a patient with hyperthyroidism. (Haddad HM: JAMA 199:559)

gland and altered susceptibility to dental caries or periodontal disease. Growth and development of the jaws and eruption pattern of the teeth are likewise unaffected.

Diagnosis. Diagnosis begins with the history and physical examination. In patients with hyperthyroidism resulting from Grave's disease, the classic signs and symptoms are usually characteristic enough to make the diagnosis. In other patients laboratory studies become important. Serum levels of T_3 and T_4 are elevated, and the most useful tests are the serum thyroxine or free-thyroxine index, serum T_3, and thyroidal radioactive iodine uptake (RAIU; see Chapter 3).

Treatment. Treatment for hyperthyroidism in young patients is antithyroid drugs such as propylthiouracil or methimazole (Tapazole), which interfere with the synthesis of thyroxine and can be supplemented with the use of propranolol, a beta-adrenergic blocking agent. In a significant percentage of patients, remission occurs within 1 year and if thyroid laboratory studies return to normal, patients are weaned from drug therapy to evaluate thyroid function. In patients who do not experience a prolonged remission from antithyroid drugs, surgery may be necessary. Radioisotope therapy is also effectively used in many cases. In older patients with large goiters who are unresponsive to drug therapy or radioactive iodine treatment, surgery is a common mode of therapy. Hypothyroidism is the most common side-effect following

radioisotope therapy or surgery and sometimes requires hormone replacement to stabilize the patient.

Dental Considerations. The primary consideration in the treatment of the dental patient with a history of hyperthyroidism relates to an evaluation of the current thyroid status. Euthyroid patients whose hyperthyroidism is controlled can be managed uneventfully; however, patients with active disease have an increased likelihood of cardiovascular complications that could precipitate a life-threatening episode in the dental chair. Specifically, the use of epinephrine with local anesthetics or in gingival retraction cord is strictly contraindicated in these patients until thyroid hormone levels are brought under control. Emergency dental problems in uncontrolled hyperthyroid patients should be managed in consultation with a physician to avoid untoward reactions.

Hypothyroidism and Myxedema

Hypothyroidism is a condition caused by a deficiency of thyroid hormone. It is characterized by an insidious and progressive slowdown of body metabolic functions. Initially, the patient may be asymptomatic; however,

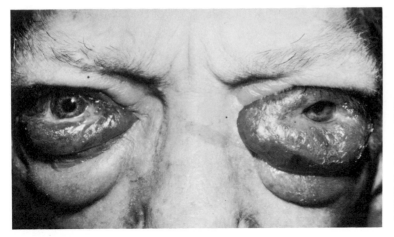

Fig. 25-11 Ocular manifestations in Graves' disease. This man has advanced ophthalmopathy ("malignant exophthalmos"). His severe conjunctival edema obscures the moderate exophthalmos. (Ezrin C, Godden JO, Volpé R: Systematic Endocrinology, 2nd ed, p 108. New York, Harper & Row, 1979)

as hormone depletion persists the signs and symptoms of hypothyroidism become clinically apparent.

SYMPTOMS OF HYPOTHYROIDISM

- Fatigue; muscle weakness
- Coarse, dry skin
- Edema of extremities
- Cold intolerance
- Hoarseness
- Slight weight gain with loss of appetite
- Paresthesias; arthralgias
- Muscle cramps
- Constipation

In the most advanced form of the disease, *myxedema*, the skin is infiltrated by a mucoprotein and mucopolysaccharides, resulting in a puffy, edematous appearance. The signs of hypothyroidism are related to deposition of these mucopolysaccharides; for example, deposition in the cardiac tissues may cause several problems including cardiomyopathy and pleural and pericardial effusions.

The etiology of hypothyroidism is multifactorial. The disease is most commonly (over 95% of cases) caused by thyroid gland malfunction (primary hypothyroidism) owing to iatrogenic causes as in patients with Graves' disease, following the administration of radioisotope therapy, or after subtotal thyroidectomy. It may also be a feature of Hashimoto's thyroiditis (see Thyroiditis). Less frequently, the condition is associated with

pituitary TSH deficiency or hypothalamic deficiency of thyrotropin-releasing hormone (secondary hypothyroidism). Hypothyroidism is also observed in patients with congenital metabolic defects of thyroid hormone production or endemic iodine deficiency.

Hypothyroidism in Children (Cretinism)

Cretinism is encountered in infants and young children and results from a lack of thyroid hormone during the fetal or perinatal period (Fig. 25-12). It is the most common preventable cause of mental retardation. Cretinism can be caused by failure of the thyroid gland to develop normally, by iodine deficiency in regions of endemic goiter, or by inborn errors of thyroid hormone synthesis. Early recognition of hypothyroidism, particularly in infants, is essential to prevent permanent brain damage.

Signs and Symptoms. Cretinism results from an aplastic thyroid gland or a gland replaced by fibrous scar tissue and lymphocytes. Clinically, cretins show generalized evidence of retarded growth and development manifesting as delayed ossification of bones, epiphyseal dysgenesis, cerebal hypoplasia, and jaw and tooth anomalies (Fig. 25-13). The skin is thick, dry, and wrinkled. There is macroglossia, thickening of the lips, open bite, and persistent drooling. The face is broad, and the nose is short and flattened. Mental retardation may accompany the characteristic un-

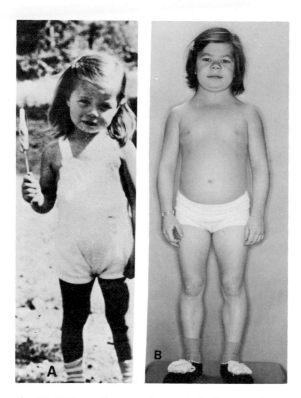

Fig. 25-12 Juvenile myxedema. *A*, At 2 years of age, this girl shows no signs of cretinism. Growth and physical appearances were normal up to 7 years of age. School progress was not affected by her hypothyroidism. *B*, The same girl at 13 years after she developed juvenile myxedema. (Ezrin C, Godden JO, Volpé R: Systematic Endocrinology, 2nd ed, p 537. New York, Harper & Row, 1979)

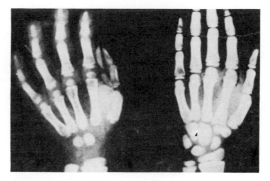

Fig. 25-13 Significant among the body processes affected by thyroid hormone deficiency is delayed ossification in children. Compare the wrist radiogram of a 5-year-old hypothyroid patient (*left*) with that of a normal child (*right*). (Starr P: JAMA 165:1311)

derdevelopment of body structures, and as the aging process continues, cretins remain dwarfed.

Oral Changes. The retardation of growth and development associated with the hypothyroid state has profound manifestations in the head, neck, and oral regions. In *athyreotic cretinism,* there is dysgenesis of the thyroid gland *in utero* that interferes with normal development of the cranium, facial bones, jaws, and the primordia of the teeth. The newborn athyreotic infant typically has massive macroglossia. Osseous development is retarded, and the growth of the cranial vault is slowed. The face develops with coarse features, and the bridge of the nose is broad and flat. The lips are puffy, thickened and pro-

truding. Jaw development is markedly retarded and impaired. Retarded condylar growth leads to a characteristic micrognathia and open bite relationship. The dental age is likewise affected, lagging behind the chronologic age; this is manifested by retarded eruption of the primary dentition and delayed exfoliation of these teeth. Eruption of the permanent dentition is also retarded (Fig. 25-14). In some cases, there is also delayed apexification of the adult dentition, which may be caused by abnormal deposition of mucoproteins in and around the developing tooth buds. A high incidence (80%) of enamel hypoplasia has been reported in the primary and secondary dentition in some series of patients. Abnormalities of dentin formation may also occur leading to enlarged pulp chambers. It is interesting to note that these tooth abnormalities may be of diagnostic significance in pinpointing the time of onset of the hypothyroidism.

In the adult patient with myxedema, similar metabolic and structural derangements occur as described for infants and children. The extent to which the facial and dental structures are affected depends on the age at which the thyroid hormone deficiency occurs.

Diagnosis. Cretinism is often suspected at birth; however, the typical physical appearance and behavioral changes may not become apparent until the third to sixth month of life. Early diagnosis may therefore be predicated

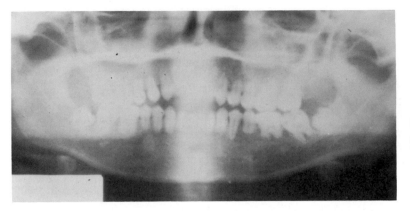

Fig. 25-14 Panoramic radiograph of an adult patient with hypothyroidism. Note blunted roots, enlarged pulps, alterations in trabecular bone pattern, and anterior open bite.

on a screening heel-stick serum T_4 determination in the perinatal period. In infants with values less than 7 μg/dl, repeat T_4 and serum TSH tests are used to confirm the diagnosis. It is also important to determine whether the cause of the hypothyroidism is primary (*i.e.,* associated with decreased function of the thyroid gland or secondary, involving the hypothalamic–pituitary axis). The diagnosis of primary hypothyroidism is made if the serum TSH level is elevated. In pituitary or hypothalamic hypothyroidism, serum TSH levels are normal to slightly decreased. Cretinism must be differentiated from Down's syndrome (mongolism), a genetic defect that has different physical findings and where the thyroid function studies are usually normal.

Treatment. Cretinism is treated with thyroid hormone replacement therapy. If discovered and treated early, a normal growth pattern will result with minimal retardation of mental capacity.

Myxedema

Myxedema results from thyroid hormone deficiency in adults and is usually seen following radioisotope therapy or thyroid surgery. Secondary hypothyroidism may be caused by a malfunction of the pituitary gland or hypothalamus.

Signs and Symptoms. Hypothyroid patients are lethargic and overweight. Typical changes include facial puffiness, watery eyes, brittle hair, and patchy alopecia (Fig. 25-15). The skin is thickened and dry, and there is a diminution of sweating. Marked edema of the face and extremities occurs. The tongue is enlarged and thick. In approximately 12% of patients there is a concurrent pernicious anemia that may cause lingual depapillation. Lassitude, drowsiness, sensitivity to cold, and constipation are frequently observed. In females, there are menstrual complaints. Neurologic signs include deafness, paresthesias, and coordination problems. The heart may be enlarged. and the pulse rate is usually slow. Characteristically, there is slow relaxation time of the Achilles tendon reflex.

Diagnosis. Diagnosis of myxedema is based on recognition of the characteristic signs and symptoms of the disease and is confirmed by laboratory studies. Serum thyroxine (T_4) levels were used in the past to detect hypothyroidism, but a more sensitive radioimmunoassay for serum TSH has improved diagnosis. With this test a greater than twofold increase in serum TSH is regarded as the initial indication of primary hypothyroidism. When a clinically hypothyroid patient presents with normal serum TSH and T_3-resin uptake but a low serum T_4, further studies must be done to determine whether the symptoms are caused by pituitary or hypothalamic failure. The TRH stimulation test is used for this purpose. Hypothyroidism secondary to pituitary dysfunction shows no TSH elevation with TRH injection,whereas a definite rise is seen when the cause is hypothalamic failure.

Treatment. Sodium levothyroxin is the recommended medication to replace deficient thyroid hormone; dessicated thyroid is no longer widely used because it is poorly stan-

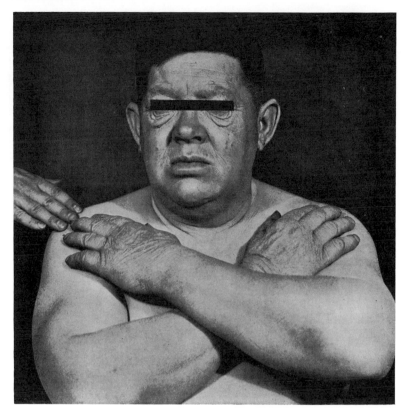

Fig. 25-15 Myxedema. Note the typical facial expression and the shape of the fingers in a man, 52 years of age, suffering from myxedema. (Grollman A: Essentials of Endocrinology. Philadelphia, JB Lippincott)

dardized. The prognosis for hypothyroid patients is excellent; however, treatment must be continued indefinitely.

Dental Considerations. The dentist must be aware that alterations in metabolism in hypothyroidism may be associated with impaired healing following routine oral surgical or periodontal procedures. These patients may also exhibit untoward reactions to dental anesthetics or analgesic compounds; therefore, elective dental treatment should be postponed until hypothyroid patients are properly treated from a medical standpoint and potential underlying cardiac, neurologic, and metabolic abnormalities are investigated and controlled.

Hashimoto's Thyroiditis

This chronic, autoimmune disorder is characterized by diffuse lymphocytic infiltration of the thyroid parenchyma and deposition of fibrous scar tissue progressing to goiterous changes and thyroid hormone deficiencies.

In this condition, antibodies are produced that react with thyroglobulins, producing hypothyroidism in about one third of the cases.

Hashimoto's thyroiditis is associated with other suspected autoimmune diseases such as pernicious anemia, idiopathic adrenal insufficiency, rheumatoid arthritis, Sjögren's syndrome, ulcerative colitis, systemic lupus erythematosus, and hemolytic anemia. The disease is seen most frequently in females and is more common in the 30- to 50-year-old age group. The serum thyroxin concentration may be decreased in these patients. Diagnosis of Hashimoto's thyroiditis is established by needle biopsy of the gland or by demonstrating circulating antithyroid antibodies. The test of choice is the tanned RBC agglutination test of antibodies to thyroglobulin.

Recently, another form of thyroiditis known as *lymphocytic* or *silent thyroiditis* has been identified as causing hypothyroidism. Unlike Hashimoto's thyroiditis, this condition usually resolves spontaneously within 1 year. It is usually seen in postpartum women, and there are no circulating antithyroid antibodies detected.

Thyroid Neoplasms

Thyroid neoplasms are classified as benign adenomas (nontoxic nodular goiters) and malignant tumors (papillary, follicular, medullary, or anaplastic carcinomas). *Adenomas* most frequently present as solitary thyroid nodules and consist of a well-encapsulated new growth of glandular structures. They are usually asymptomatic but may cause hoarseness, pain, or dysphagia. The majority of these nodules are found in otherwise healthy individuals: therefore, the primary role of the dentist is to detect such nodules during routine head and neck examination and to refer patients with suspicious findings to a physician.

Benign adenomas must be differentiated from malignancies. Thyroid nodules in patients under 30 years and in males are cause for the most concern. On the other hand, those detected in women over 40 are most likely to be benign. A history of prior radiation therapy to the thyroid region should also increase the clinician's index of suspicion because in 30% of thyroid malignancies there is a prior history of radiotherapy. As a matter of routine course, all isolated thyroid nodules in younger patients (especially males), should be biopsied to rule out carcinoma.

Malignant thyroid tumors generally present as a mass in the neck that may extend by local invasion or metastasis to regional lymph nodes. The enlarged area is hard, irregularly shaped, and usually fixed to adjacent structures. Papillary carcinomas account for 50% to 80% of thyroid malignancies. A less common form of medullary thyroid carcinoma is a feature of the *multiple endocrine neoplasia syndrome*. Other features of this rare syndrome include mucosal neuromas involving the tongue, intestinal ganglioneuromas and pheochromocytomas.

DISEASES OF THE ADRENAL GLAND

Anatomy and Physiology

The adrenals are triangular-shaped structures that sit on the superior poles of the kidneys. They produce and secrete a number of compounds that are essential for maintenance of life and adaptation to stress. Each gland is divided anatomically and functionally into a medulla and a cortex.

Adrenal Medulla

The adrenal medulla arises from ectodermal tissues and functions as a part of the sympathetic nervous system. The medulla manufactures and secretes two catecholamines, epinephrine and norepinephrine, which have similar actions. Epinephrine supports blood pressure by increasing heart rate while norepinephrine increases peripheral resistance by its vasoconstrictor effects. Epinephrine also increases oxygen consumption by the tissues and glucose release by the liver. Gastrointestinal motility is slowed by both substances.

Epinephrine and norepinephrine also exert important metabolic effects by promoting lipolysis, increasing blood sugar levels by stimulating glycogenolysis, elevating body temperature, and increasing basal metabolic rate. Perhaps the most important action occurs during emergency situations when these compounds aid the body in adapting to stress. This has potential importance in the dental setting because release of endogenous epinephrine during stressful dental procedures can produce significant changes in blood pressure and pulse rates.

Adrenal Medullary Disease

Pheochromocytoma

This catecholamine-producing tumor arises from the chromaffin cells of the adrenal medulla or from the extradrenal tissues of the sympathetic nervous system (paragangliomas). The major clinical symptom associated with this tumor is paroxysmal hypertension. It is of interest to the dentist because reports have appeared in the literature describing patients with a distinct symptom complex characterized by endocrine neoplasms (pheochromocytoma and medullary carcinoma of the thyroid gland) and multiple mucosal neuromas involving the lips, tongue, larynx, and eyelids. This condition is referred to as the multiple mucosal nervous system or *Sipple's syndrome* and is inherited as an autosomal dominant trait.

Adrenal Cortex

The adrenal cortex secretes three major classes of hormones: the glucocorticoid *cortisol*, which affects the inflammatory process and carbohydrate and protein metabolism; the mineralocorticoid *aldosterone*, which affects water and electrolyte balance; and the sex hormones *testosterone*, *estrogen*, and *progesterone*.

The synthesis and secretion of the glucocorticoids and to a lesser extent sex hormones, is regulated by the pituitary-adrenal axis. For the normal individual the daily secretion of cortisol is kept within physiologic limits by a finely tuned negative feedback system. The secretion of cortisol is characterized by a *diurnal rhythm* whereby peak blood levels are attained in the early morning and taper off in the late afternoon and early evening. In response to the circadian rhythm of cortisol production and secretion and various noxious stimuli such as surgical trauma, the hypothalamus produces corticotropin-releasing factor (CRF), which stimulates secretion of adrenocorticotropic hormone (ACTH) by the anterior pituitary; ACTH, in turn, promotes the synthesis and secretion of cortisol in the adrenal cortex. This negative feedback system works in such a way that rising plasma levels of cortisol render the pituitary unresponsive to CRF, thereby decreasing ACTH output so that cortisol levels are kept within normal limits.

The glucocorticoids have a wide range of physiologic actions that affect carbohydrate, fat, and protein metabolism. They increase serum glucose levels through gluconeogenesis in the liver and promote mineral, protein, and nucleic acid catabolism; they also influence lipolysis and distribution of adipose tissue in the body. In addition, the glucocorticoids are used therapeutically to suppress or modify the immune and inflammatory responses. The synthesis and secretion of the mineralocorticoids is regulated by the renin-angiotensin system in the kidneys. Aldosterone maintains fluid and electrolyte balance by controlling sodium and potassium levels and by monitoring renal tubular function.

Diseases of the Adrenal Cortex

Addison's Disease

The majority of cases of Addison's disease *(primary adrenocortical insufficiency)* are caused by idiopathic destruction of the adrenal cortex, thought to be on a autoimmune basis. The remainder of the cases are caused by granulomatous infiltration of the cortex by tuberculosis, amyloidosis, inflammatory necrosis, or neoplastic disease of the gland. The disease affects all age groups and both sexes equally.

Signs and Symptoms. The signs and symptoms of primary adrenal insufficiency all relate to deprivation of aldosterone and cortisol. In Addison's disease, sodium excretion is increased and potassium excretion is decreased, resulting in high blood levels of potassium and low concentrations of sodium and chloride. This electrolyte imbalance produces increased diuresis with dehydration, decreased fluid volume, hypotension, and potential circulatory collapse.

Deficiency in cortisol adds to the problem of hypotension and causes disturbances in carbohydrate, protein, and fat metabolism. Decreased cortisol levels interfere with the manufacture of carbohydrates from protein, causing hypoglycemia and diminished glycogen storage in the liver. Neuromuscular function is inhibited, producing muscle weakness. There is also a reduced resistance to infection, trauma, and stress. In addition, cardiac output is adversely affected resulting in possible circulatory failure. Finally, low blood levels of cortisol increase pituitary ACTH output and increase release of melanocyte-stimulating hormone (MSH), which accounts for the hyperpigmentation of skin and mucous membranes with Addison's disease.

Addison's disease often occurs in association with other diseases including diabetes mellitus and thyroid and parathyroid dysfunction. The most common clinical manifestations are generalized weakness, fatigue, hypotension, and abnormal pigmentation. *Increased pigmentation* may take the form of diffuse tanning, black freckles on the skin of the face and extremities, areas of vitiligo, and bluish-black discoloration of the areolas and mucous membranes of the lips, mouth, rectum, and vagina. Weight loss, dehydration, anorexia, vomiting, and nausea are also common complaints.

Oral Changes. Pigmentation of the skin of the face and mucosa is an early and characteristic sign of Addison's disease. The pigmented areas are blueish-black in color and most commonly involve the mucosa of the cheeks. The gingiva, palate, tongue, and lips can be likewise affected (Fig. 25-16). It is important to differentiate the lesions from hyperpigmentation associated with *Peutz–Jeghers syndrome* and neurofibromatosis. In these latter disorders, steroid replacement therapy of course does not result in a reversal of the changes.

Diagnosis. Laboratory studies reveal a low serum sodium level, high serum potassium levels, and an elevated blood urea nitrogen

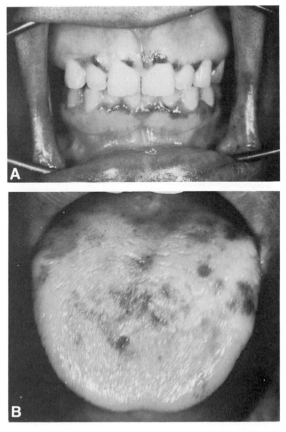

Fig. 25-16 Oral pigmentation in a patient with Addison's disease. *A,* Involvement of attached gingiva. *B,* Hyperpigmented areas on dorsum of tongue.

(BUN). These findings in conjunction with the characteristic clinical picture suggest the possibility of Addison's disease. The diagnosis is confirmed by the failure of administered synthetic ACTH to produce an appropriate rise in blood cortisol levels; demonstrating low cortisol levels in the presence of high serum ACTH levels provides additional confirmation.

Treatment. Therapy of primary adrenal insufficiency consists in replacement of the glucocorticoid in a dose approximating normal daily requirements. The dose is divided such that larger amounts are given in the early morning hours and less in the late afternoon. Supplemental mineralocorticoids may also be required. Because Addison's disease prevents the stress-related release of cortisol that occurs in normal individuals, additional steroids may have to be given during stressful situations such as surgery, trauma, and dental treatment. Secondary adrenal insufficiency resulting from failure of the pituitary gland to produce physiologic amounts of ACTH will also cause symptoms of glucocortical deficiency. In this situation patients are also treated with corticosteroid replacement therapy.

Cushing's Syndrome

Hypersecretion of one or more of the hormones produced by the adrenal cortex (adrenocortical hyperfunction) causes distinct clinical syndromes. When androgens are produced in excess the result is adrenal virilism; *aldosteronism* is caused by hypersecretion of aldosterone; Cushing's syndrome is seen when excess quantities of glucocorticoids are produced.

BIOLOGIC EFFECTS OF HYDROCORTISONE OVERPRODUCTION*

- Protein metabolism
  Thinning of skin
  Reddish striae
  Loss of bone matrix and demineralization
  Poor wound healing

* From Ezrin C, Godden JO, Volpe R, Wilson R: Systemic Endocrinology, 2nd ed, p 103. New York, Harper & Row, 1979

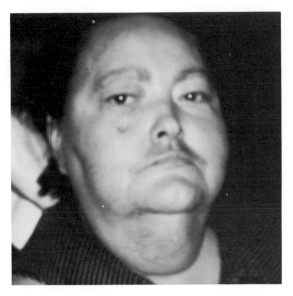

Fig. 25-17 Moon facies in a patient with Cushing's syndrome.

Muscle wasting and weakness
Capillary fragility and bruising
Impaired growth (children)
• Carbohydrate metabolism
Abnormal glucose tolerance curve
Overt diabetes mellitus
• Lipid metabolism
Centripetal fat distribution
Moon facies
• Electrolyte balance
Sodium retention, potassium loss
Hypertension
Hypervolemia
• Hematopoietic effects
Eosinopenia, lymphopenia
Polymorphonuclear leukocytosis
Erythrocytosis
• General effects
Hypercalciuria and renal calculi
Gastric ulceration
Psychosis
Impaired immunologic tolerance

These syndromes may be the result of congenital or acquired hyperplasia of the gland. Adenomas and adenocarcinomas also cause adrenocortical hyperfunction. The features of Cushing's syndrome are discussed here because the most common cause of signs and symptoms adrenocortical hyperfunction is exogenous administration of corticosteroids.

It is therefore important that the dentist recognize these changes as an indication that a patient may be taking supraphysiologic doses of corticosteroids for the management of a serious medical problem.

Signs and Symptoms. The classic syndrome includes a rounded moon facies with a plethoric appearance (Fig. 25-17). There is truncal obesity with prominent supraclavicular and dorsal cervical fat pads giving rise to the characteristic "buffalo hump" appearance (Fig. 25-18). The distal extremities are usually thin. Signs of muscle weakness and wasting are usually present. The skin is atrophic, and there is poor wound healing, easy bruising, and osteoporosis. Purple straie (stretch marks) commonly appear on the abdomen. Increased production of androgens, if present, may lead to hypertrichosis and abnormal distribution of facial hair in women.

Oral Changes. There are no pathognomonic changes involving the oral structures with adrenocortical hyperfunction. In children growth and development including skeletal and dental age may be retarded. In some instances there may be osteoporosis of the jaws.

The dentist should be suspicious of any patient with cushingoid changes and should make specific enquiries about a past history of adrenal or pituitary gland disease and possible corticosteroid therapy.

Treatment. Treatment of adrenocortical hyperfunction is based on correction of the underlying physiologic abnormality. If a lesion in the pituitary gland is the cause, therapy usually consists of a combination of surgery and irradiation. Tumors involving the adrenal cortex are removed surgically and often require post-operative administration of corticosteroids to maintain normal glucocorticoid levels.

Corticosteroid Therapy

Over the past 20 years, corticosteroids have been used with increasing frequency to treat many acute and chronic systemic diseases. Corticosteroids are used locally to treat skin rashes and inflammation and systemically to control severe ulcerative bullous disorders such as pemphigus vulgaris and erythema

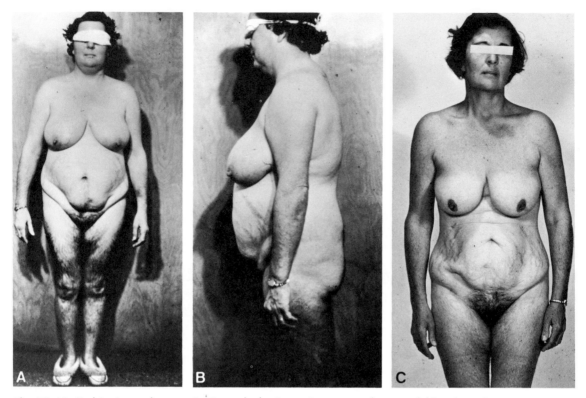

Fig. 25-18 Cushing's syndrome. *A,* Truncal obesity, striae, moon face, and hirsutism. *B,* Lateral view of same patient shows obvious buffalo hump, and lateral abdominal striae are more clearly seen than in front view. *C,* Same patient is shown following cure of Cushing's syndrome by removal of both adrenals, which were hyperplastic. Note regression of obesity and moon face and increase in pigmentation, particularly of the areolae. This pigmentation is probably caused by a pituitary oversecretion of ACTH. (Ezrin C, Godden JO, Volpé R: Systematic Endocrinology, 2nd ed, p 208. New York, Harper & Row, 1979)

multiforme. Long-term corticosteroid therapy is used in the treatment of ulcerative colitis, regional enteritis, and collagen diseases. The corticosteroids are also widely used as adjuncts in the treatment of malignancy and in the management of organ transplant patients requiring immunosuppression to prevent rejection and graft-versus-host disease.

Exogenous administration of corticosteroids has the potential side-effect of causing suppression of normal adrenal function. The major determining factors that must be considered in evaluating the degree of adrenal suppression are the anti-inflammatory potency of the drug (as compared to hydrocortisone), the dosage, and the duration of therapy (see Table 25-3). Dosages above 20 mg

hydrocortisone or its equivalent for 5 days or longer may cause adrenal suppression and prevent the physiologic release of glucocorticoid required to adapt to acute stress. It can take up to 1 year following cessation of corticosteroid therapy before the hypothalamic–pituitary–adrenal axis recovers and normal production of cortisol is resumed by the body.

Dental Considerations. Although there is some evidence that prolonged use of topical steroid preparations can result in a degree of adrenal suppression, the dentist should be most concerned with patients undergoing long-term steroid therapy above physiologic levels. In general, short-term high-dose therapy, alternate day therapy, and topical ad-

Table 25-3. Relative Potencies of Corticosteroid Drugs

Steroid	Glucocorticoid (Anti-Inflammatory) Activity	Equivalent Dose (mg)
Hydrocortisone (cortisol)	1	20
Cortisone	0.8	25
Prednisone	4	5
Prednisolone	4	5
Methylprednisolone	5	5
Triamcinolone	5	4
Dexamethasone	25	0.75

ministration produce minimal adrenal side-effects and little in the way of adrenal suppression.

In patients receiving long-term therapeutic doses of corticosteroids, the dentist should look for Cushingoid symptoms, osteoporotic changes in the jaws, and degenerative changes in the periodontal ligaments. Suppressed patients may show any of the following signs when placed in stressful situations: hypotension, fatigue, anorexia, postural dizziness, nausea, vomiting, glucose intolerance, and arthralgia. These symptoms may herald an adrenal crisis characterized by cardiovascular collapse. In such cases. the dentist must be prepared to administer emergency care in the form of hydrocortisone succinate or phosphate, 100 mg to 200 mg intravenously. In addition, measures must be taken to support blood pressure and fluid volume and to maintain normal electrolyte balance.

The following recommendations are guidelines for the dental management of patients taking corticosteroids in doses above physiologic levels for more than 5 days. When a question exists regarding the level of adrenal suppression, it is prudent to consult with the patient's physician in determining what changes, if any, should be made in the dosage prior to operative procedures. *No increase* in corticosteroid medication is required in the suppressed patient undergoing *minor dental procedures with minimal stress.* Examples of these procedures include routine periodontal probing, alloy restorations, minor biopsies, denture and orthodontic adjustments or scaling, and prophylaxis.

For *moderately stressful* dental procedures in the suppressed patient, the normal daily dosage should be *doubled* approximately 8 hours before the procedure. Dental manipulations in this category include procedures generally performed under local anesthesia that take less than 1 hour, such as third-molar impactions, multiple extractions, incision and drainage of dental infections, extensive restorative dentistry, or periodontal surgery. Procedures taking *longer periods* of time may require the preoperative dose to be *tripled.* The dosage should be tapered back to the normal regimen during the postoperative period in a manner that parallels the cessation of pain, fear, fever, and other symptoms of stress. In most cases this means that the patient is returned to his normal oral dosage by the second or third postoperative day.

For *major dental surgery* under general anesthesia such as orthognathic surgery, management of acute facial trauma, or treatment of severe oral infections, parenteral administration of corticosteroids is mandatory. This usually consists of an intramuscular injection of 100 mg of cortisone acetate 8 hours before the procedure, followed by intravenous infusion of hydrocortisone or its equivalent during the procedure so that the total 24-hour dose approximates 300 mg cortisol. Alternatively, sodium dexamethasone (Decadron), 6 mg, is given intravenously 2 to 3 hours before the procedure and supplemented with 4 mg every 8 hours for 24 hours. The dosage is then tapered during the postoperative period usually by halving the dose each day until the normal replacement dosage is reached.

Patients taking long-term high-dose corticosteroid therapy may have an increased risk of infection owing to inhibition of the inflammatory response. Although antibiotics are not recommended on a routine basis, particularly traumatic dental procedures or severe infections may require the concurrent use of appropriate antibiotics. Consultation with a qualified physician or endocrinologist is recommended when extensive dental treatment is contemplated for a patient suspected of having persistent adrenal suppression. In communicating with the physician, the dentist must indicate the nature of the dental treatment planned and the duration of such treatment. If there is doubt regarding the degree of suppression, the physician can determine this by using the ACTH stimulator test preoperatively.

Therapeutic Use of Corticosteroids for Oral Disease

Corticosteroid preparations can be a useful treatment in the management of acute and chronic ulcerative stomatitis that is unresponsive to other forms of therapy. In patients with recurrent aphthous stomatitis, 0.1% topical triamcinolone acetomide in an emollient dental paste (Kenalog in Orabase) can be applied three to four times daily to the affected areas. For the best results, the patient should be instructed to first dry the area surrounding the ulcer before applying a thin coating of the paste with a cotton swab. This approach is most effective when the ulcers being treated are inside the lower lip or in other accessible parts of the mouth. It is more difficult to retain the medication on ulcers involving the tongue or posterior buccal mucosa, and therefore, the results of this form of therapy are less successful.

In patients with diffuse ulceration of the oral mucous membranes, short-term systemic steroids have proven useful. For example, in patients with erythema multiforme, bullous pemphigoid, or benign mucous membrane pemphigoid, a short course of prednisone can be given in situations where there are no contraindications for

the use of corticosteroids. This, of course, requires a thorough grasp of the past medical history of the patient and an awareness of the possible complications of steroid therapy, such as hyperglycemia, electrolyte imbalance, peptic ulcer, or reactivation of tuberculosis. The usual course of treatment in these patients is 25 mg to 40 mg prednisone (or the equivalent) daily in divided doses for a period of 3 to 4 days. The dosage should be reduced and the patient tapered off the medication over a 2-week period depending on the extent of the ulceration and response to therapy. Patients requiring more than 2 weeks of this regimen are best placed on alternate-day treatment to minimize the possibility of adrenal suppression. Treatment of pemphigus and other severe mucocutaneous disorders require high-dose corticosteroid therapy, usually in the range of 100 mg prednisone per day initially. In these cases, hospitalization of the patient is often required, and the treatment program should be the responsibility of a dermatologist or physician.

DISEASE OF THE PARATHYROID GLANDS

Anatomy and Physiology

The parathyroid glands are usually four in number and are located on the posterior aspect of the thyroid gland. They secrete parathyroid hormone (parathormone, PTH) a polypeptide that plays an important role in calcium and phosphorous metabolism.

Any discussion of disease of the parathyroid glands is predicated on a thorough understanding of calcium metabolism. Calcium is an important constituent of biologic membranes, and it exerts an influence on membrane permeability and excitability. Calcium also plays an essential role in the contraction of all types of muscle and in the release of parathyroid hormone.

The total calcium content of a normal adult male is 1000 g to 1100 g; 99% of this amount is in the bones and teeth. Normal serum calcium levels range between 8.8 mg/100 ml and 10.4 mg/100 ml; the upper limit of normal for total serum calcium is slightly lower in women than in men. Normal serum calcium values in children are slightly higher than in adults. Approximately 40% of the total blood calcium is bound to serum proteins—chiefly albumin. The remaining nonprotein bound calcium is ultrafilterable and consists of ionized calcium and calcium complexed with phosphate and citrate. The ionized calcium is the fraction that affects biologic processes and must be kept normal by the parathyroids and other homeostatic mechanisms.

Maintenance of normal blood calcium levels depends on dietary intake of calcium, gastrointestinal absorption of calcium, and renal calcium excretion. The bone calcium reservoir serves as the major factor in preserving a constant blood calcium concentration. The level of ionic calcium in the blood influences parathyroid activity by a negative feedback mechanism as follows: when the blood calcium drops below normal, secretion of PTH increases; and when blood calcium exceeds normal, secretion ceases.

Dietary calcium is absorbed in the small intestine and is vitamin-D dependent. Absorption of calcium is inversely related to dietary intake of calcium. PTH produced by the parathyroid glands promotes renal formation of the active metabolite of vitamin D (1, 25-dihydroxycholecalferol), which increases calcium absorption from the gastrointestinal tract.

PTH and vitamin D are the principal mediators of calcium and phosphate homeostasis. The most important actions of PTH are increasing the rate of bone resorption by mobilization of Ca and P from bone, increasing renal tubular reabsorption of Ca, increasing intestinal absorption of Ca, and decreasing renal tubular reabsorption of phosphate. These actions account for the majority of the important clinical manifestations of hyperparathyroidism and hypoparathyroidism. PTH maintains normal blood levels of calcium by its action on three target organs: bone, gastrointestinal tract, and kidney. The most important action of PTH is the stimulation of bone resorption, which liberates calcium and phosphorus into the extracellular fluids. PTH appears to promote osteoclastic osteolysis and activates adenyl cyclase in bone and kidney leading to the formation of cyclic adenosine monophosphate (cAMP). The hormone *calcitonin*, which is probably produced in the thyroid gland, has an antagonistic action to PTH. It reduces calcium levels by direct inhibition of bone resorption. This hormone is useful in the management of Paget's disease of bone.

Hypoparathyroidism

Hypoparathyroidism is caused by a deficiency in parathyroid hormone production; it is characterized by metabolic disturbances leading to hypocalcemia and increased neuromuscular excitability. The four types of hypoparathyroidism are DiGeorge's syndrome, postoperative hypoparathyroidism, idiopathic hypoparathyroidism, and pseudohypoparathyroidism.

DiGeorge's Syndrome

This symptom complex consists of congenital absence of the parathyroid glands and thyroid, aortic arch anomalies, and congenital heart defects. It is caused by an error in formation of the third and fourth pharyngeal pouches. Thymic aplasia results in severe immune deficiencies that may not be consistent with life.

Postoperative Hypoparathyroidism

This form of hypoparathyroidism occurs when the parathyroid glands are inadvertently removed or injured during thyroid surgery, the most common cause of hypoparathyroidism. The clinical symptoms parallel those of idiopathic hypoparathyroidism (see below), and their severity depends on whether the parathyroid glands are partially or totally removed.

Idiopathic Hypoparathyroidism

This rare form of hypoparathyroidism has an unknown etiology. It is sometimes considered to be congenital; in other cases, it does not occur until later in childhood or adolescence.

Signs and Symptoms of Hypoparathyroidism. The important signs and symptoms relate to *hypocalcemia;* therefore, clinical manifestations are primarily neurologic. *Tetany* is a characteristic, as are paresthesias of the lips, tongue, fingers, and feet and myalgia and spasm of the facial musculature. The neuromuscular instability associated with hypocalcemia can be provoked by tapping the facial nerve, which produces twitching of the facial muscles (Chvostek's sign). Another useful test is *Trousseau's sign* (carpopedal spasm; Fig. 25-19), which occurs when blood supply to the hand is reduced by application of a blood pressure cuff above the systolic pressure. Other symptoms include muscle weakness, cramps, heart palpitations, and bizarre behavior patterns. Abnormalities of hair, skin, nails, and teeth are common findings. The skin is coarse, scaly, and dry, and the nail beds are deformed; hair is thin and alopecia may be present.

Oral Changes. The dental changes in hypoparathyroidism are helpful in pinpointing a diagnosis. The dental age is usually delayed in relation to the chronologic age. If the disease occurs while the primary and permanent teeth are calcifying the result is enamel hypoplasia and abnormal dentin formation. Specifically, bands of enamel hypoplasia and pits and grooves are observed, and these correspond to the onset of the endocrinopathy. Dentin is layed down in an irregular fashion and is observable in histologic sections. Incomplete root formation and premature narrowing of the apices are commonly observed.

A rare syndrome of idiopathic hypoparathyroidism, candidiasis, Addison's disease, and enamel hypoplasia has been described by some authors. This congenital disorder appears to be inherited as an autosomal recessive trait. In the case reported by Greenberg and associates, severe mucocutaneous candidiasis including oral involvement that was refractory to treatment and enamel hypoplasia led to a presumptive diagnosis of idiopathic hypoparathyroidism many years before chemical abnormalities became apparent.

Diagnosis. Laboratory findings are useful in establishing the diagnosis. The serum calcium is decreased and usually below 7 mg/dl when tetany is present. Serum phosphorous is correspondingly elevated, and the alkaline phosphatase level is normal. Urinary calcium is low or absent.

Treatment. Hypoparathyroidism is treated by supplemental calcium and vitamin D, depending on the severity of the hypocalcemia and the nature of the associated signs and symptoms. There are at present no therapeutic parathormone preparations available.

Pseudohypoparathyroidism

This rare genetic disorder is transmitted as an X-linked dominant trait in which the parathyroid glands are normal and there is no deficiency of PTH. Instead, a defect exists in the target organs (bone and kidney), which are unresponsive to the action of PTH.

These patients are typically small and have short metacarpal and metatarsal bones; mental retardation is common. Plasma levels of PTH are often increased, and the bone may show evidence of osteitis fibrosa cystica.

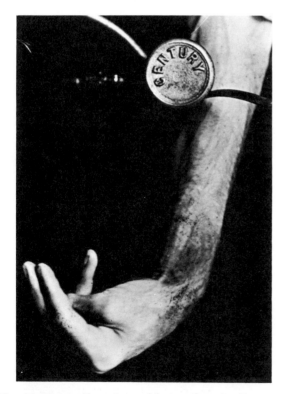

Fig. 25-19 Manifestations of hypocalcemia. Trousseau's sign in a patient with hypoparathyroid tetany. (Ezrin C, Godden JO, Volpé R: Systematic Endocrinology, 2nd ed, p 151. New York, Harper & Row, 1979)

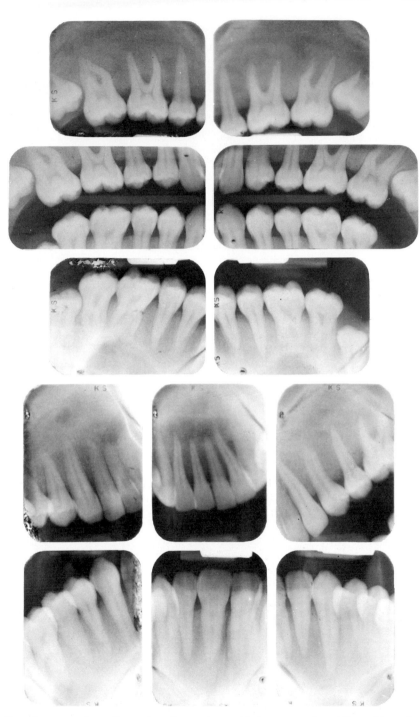

Fig. 25-20 Complete mouth radiographs of a patient with hyperparathyroidism. Note the altered trabecular pattern with "ground glass" appearance and loss of lamina dura. Also present are radiolucent areas in the lower incisor region suggestive of "brown tumors."

Hyperparathyroidism

A rare generalized disorder resulting from hypersecretion of PTH, hyperparathyroidism is characterized by hypercalcemia, hypophosphatemia, and abnormal bone metabolism. In the majority of cases the cause is an adenoma of one of the parathyroid glands. The disease is most frequently seen in the 20- to 50-year-old age group, and females are more frequently affected.

Signs and Symptoms. Signs and symptoms are primarily referable to the bones, kidneys, and gastrointestinal tract. Approximately 30% of patients exhibit *osteitis fibrosis cystica,* in which increased osteoclastic activity causes osteoporotic changes, fibrous degeneration, and cyst formation. Skeletal complaints include bone pain and pathologic fractures. Renal calculi are formed in over half of the patients, and hematuria, back pain, urinary tract infection, and hypertension are common. Gastrointestinal difficulties such as anorexia, nausea, vomiting, and crampy pain may be present; in over 20% of patients peptic ulcers develop. Hypocalcemia in these patients is associated with muscle weakness, fatigue, weight loss, cardiac irregularities, insomnia, headaches, and polyuria.

Oral Changes. Radiographic changes in hyperparathyroidism are characteristic enough to assist in the diagnosis. The skull may have an even ground glass, "moth-eaten," or "salt and pepper" appearance. Calcification of the basal ganglia is sometimes seen. The trabecular pattern of the alveolus and mandible is indistinct, and loss of lamina dura is regarded by some to be pathognomonic of hyperparathyroidism (Figs. 25-20 and 25-21). Cystic lesions involving the jaws and gingiva are seen in over 10% of cases. Central and peripheral lesions known as *brown tumors* occur, having the same histologic features as giant cell reparative granulomas (Fig. 25-22).

This disease should be considered by the dentist whenever single or multiple radiolucencies of the jaws are observed radiographically. Although cystic changes usually develop late in the course of the disease, jaw or soft tissue lesions may be the first mani-

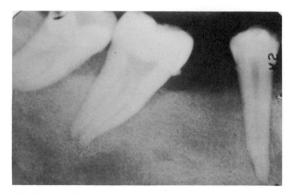

Fig. 25-21 Periapical radiograph of a patient with hyperparathyroidism. Note ground glass trabecular pattern and loss of lamina dura.

festation of hyperparathyroidism. A history of recurrent osseous or soft tissue lesions is highly suspicious of this endocrinopathy and mandates both histopathologic examination of tissue and laboratory investigation.

The oral findings must be differentiated from Paget's disease, polyostotic fibrous dysplasia, multiple myeloma, ameloblastoma, and osteomalacia. In Paget's disease, calcium metabolism is normal and bone formation usually exceeds bone resorption, resulting in an elevated blood alkaline phosphate. In osteomalacia, blood calcium and phosphorous levels are decreased. In fibrous dysplasia, osseous changes are frequently localized, and there is no loss of lamina dura.

Biopsy studies may be required to differentiate hyperparathyroidism from multiple myeloma and fibrous dysplasia. In multiple myeloma the skull is often involved, Bence–Jones protein can be demonstrated in the urine, and there are characteristic serum protein abnormalities on electrophoresis.

Diagnosis. Laboratory studies reveal elevated blood calcium and decreased blood phosphorous levels. Alkaline phosphatase levels are also increased when there is significant osteolytic activity. Urinary excretion of calcium is elevated in some patients, and urinary phosphorous excretion is usually elevated. An increase in circulating PTH can be demonstrated by radioisotope studies. Radiographic findings may aid in the diagnosis (Fig. 25-23).

PREGNANCY

Pregnancy causes physiologic changes throughout the body that are of relevance to the dentist. For example, alterations in the level of circulating female sex hormones have been implicated in modifying the response of the oral soft tissues (periodontium) to local irritants. In addition, the hemodynamic and metabolic changes caused by pregnancy may require special dental treatment planning considerations for the protection of the expectant mother and the developing fetus.

Medical Aspects

The normal pregnancy lasts for 40 weeks. During pregnancy, there is a marked increase in cardiac output (30% to 50%); blood volume increases to help sustain the fetus, and the

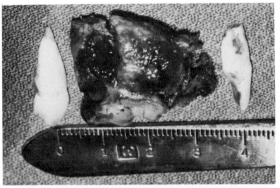

plasma volume may increase by as much as 50%. Other important physiologic changes of concern to the dentist include mild hypotension, dyspnea on exertion, fatigability, and an increased requirement for iron. The additional burden placed on the maternal cardiovascular system may result in an increased heart rate and the detection of functional murmurs. Cardiomyopathies may also become apparent during pregnancy.

The endocrine changes in pregnancy consist of increased production of female sex hormones and glucocorticoids. In addition, trophic hormones are manufactured by the placenta. Circulating levels of estrogen and progesterone steadily increase during the first and second trimesters of pregnancy and generally peak at the start of the third trimester.

During the first trimester of gestation, *organogenesis* occurs and all the major organ systems of the fetus are formed. It is at this time that the fetus is most susceptible to injury and that the vast majority of spontaneous abortions occur. The second and third trimesters are devoted to further growth and maturation of the fetus.

Oral Changes

The term *pregnancy gingivitis* has been coined to describe the clinical picture of localized

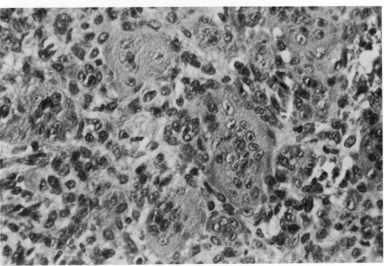

Fig. 25-22 Histologic appearance of a brown tumor showing multinucleate giant cells.

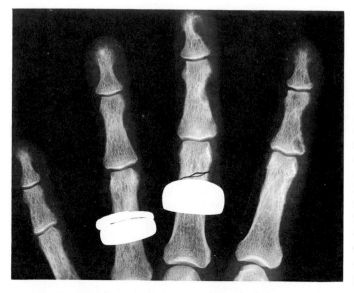

Fig. 25-23 Subperiosteal resorption in hyperparathyroidism. Such resorption is pathognomonic. The frayed, irregular periosteal surface of the bone is particularly marked on radial aspect of middle phalanx of second finger. Punched-out lesions seen at the base of this phalanx and in terminal phalanx of third finger are caused either by cyst formation or osteoclastomas. The cortices of all phalanges are abnormally thin. (Ezrin C, Godden JO, Volpé R: Systematic Endocrinology, 2nd ed, p 166. New York, Harper & Row, 1979)

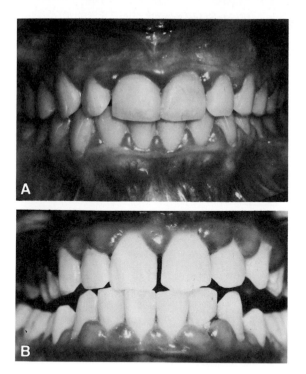

Fig. 25-24 Gingival changes in pregnancy. *A,* Gingival inflammation in anterior region of mouth. *B,* Marked gingival enlargement and hyperemia during the second trimester. Both patients had poor oral hygiene with abundant plaque and calculus deposits. There was a favorable response to scaling, root planing, and plaque control measures.

and diffuse gingival inflammation that occurs in many pregnant patients. There is increased vascularity of the gingiva in this condition, and edema, redness, and bleeding of the tissues are prominent features (Fig. 25-24); "pregnancy tumors" having the same histopathologic appearance as pyogenic granulomas are also occasional findings (Fig. 25-25). These are exuberant growths of granulation tissue that develop in the interdental papilla region. The lesions may regress following birth; however, surgical excision is usually warranted (Fig. 25-26).

During pregnancy, the amount of gingival exudate appears to correlate with the severity of gingival inflammation and with circulating levels of estrogens and progesterones. The role of microbial plaque and calculus as etiologic agents in the pathogenesis of gingivitis in pregnant women has been studied by Löe and Cohen, and associates. These investigations suggest that pregnancy gingivitis represents an exaggerated response to the same local factors that are associated with marginal gingivitis. Presumably, the increased levels of female sex hormones during pregnancy are responsible for the altered gingival response. This theory is supported by the fact that gingival inflammation tends to lessen in severity postpartum and that meticulous plaque con-

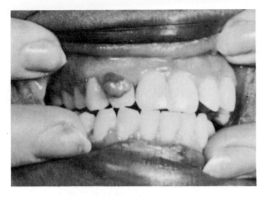

Fig. 25-25 Pregnancy tumor that remained after parturition 6 months previously. The lesions was removed surgically.

trol during pregnancy tends to minimize gingival inflammation during the gestational period.

Dental Treatment

Treatment of the pregnant patient must be structured in a manner that affords maximum protection to both the mother and the developing fetus. The following recommendations should be regarded as general guidelines that may be modified based on the patient's medical or dental status or by communication with the patient's physician.

Patient Education. The importance of good oral hygiene during pregnancy should be stressed with the patient. Scaling and prophylaxis should be performed as often as is necessary to control local etiologic factors and reduce gingival inflammation. Proper methods of toothbrushing and flossing should be taught, monitored, and reinforced during the course of the pregnancy. It is important to explain to the patient the need for good plaque control in view of the relationship between local irritants, hormonal changes, and gingival disease during pregnancy.

Timing of Dental Treatment *Emergency dental treatment* can safely be administered at any time during pregnancy, however, it may be necessary to consult with the patient's physician regarding unusual or especially stressful dental procedures. The *second trimester* is

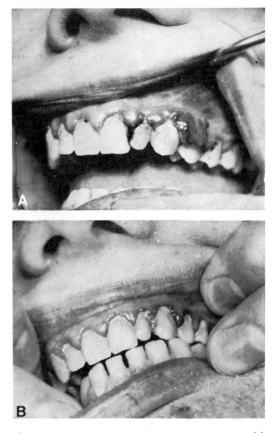

Fig. 25-26 *A,* Pregnancy tumor in a 21-year-old patient who was 7 months pregnant. The growth in the left canine and the premolar region bled easily. *B,* Same patient 2 months after delivery, showing regression of gingival hypertrophy and pregnancy tumor without treatment. (Courtesy Dr. John P. Looby, Philadelphia, PA)

the *safest* period during which to perform routine dental care. In general, dental treatment should be limited to palliative care, and electrive therapy should be postponed until after birth. Specifically, stressful procedures such as periodontal surgery, impactions, and extensive restorative dentistry should be avoided during pregnancy.

Radiographs are not contraindicated during pregnancy, but the practitioner should use good clinical judgement and limit the number of x-rays taken. A lead apron, of course, must be used to shield the fetus and gonads. Many drugs cross the placental barrier, therefore, there is potential risk of injury to the fetus. If possible, avoid the use of any drugs during the pregnancy. It is well known that the administration of tetracyclines during the last trimester will cause permanent discoloration of the teeth and enamel hypoplasia; therefore, they should not be prescribed unless other antibiotics are contraindicated.

MENOPAUSE

Medical and Dental Considerations

Medical aspects. Menopause begins when menstrual function ceases. It represents a decline in ovarian function and usually occurs between ages 40 and 55. Artificial menopause will occur if the ovaries are removed or receive irradiation therapy.

Signs and symptoms. There are numerous symptoms associated with menopause, and when symptoms develop, they are usually caused by deficiency of estrogen. Any of the following symptoms may be associated with menopause: irritability, hot flashes, depression, paresthesias, insomnia, nervousness, or menstrual disturbances. During the advanced stages of menopause, osteoporosis, resulting in back or joint pain, may occur.

Oral Changes. The hormonal changes associated with menopause may cause oral symptoms. Complaints of burning mouth and tongue, taste abnormalities, and dryness of the mucous membranes are not uncommon. Patients occasionally present with *desquamative gingivitis* (Fig. 25-27). In this condition, there is atrophy and ulceration of the gingival tissues that can produce extreme gingival pain and bleeding. Although the etiology of this form of gingivitis may be deficiency in femal sex hormones, it is important to rule out erosive lichen planus, mucous membrane pemphigoid, and other dermatologic conditions that are possible sources of the problem; therefore, biopsy is usually indicated to establish a definitive diagnosis before instituting treatment.

Treatment. Treatment consists of estrogen replacement therapy and depends on the ex-

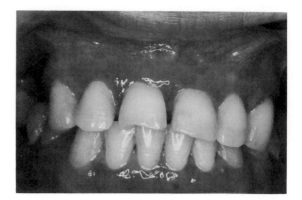

Fig. 25-27 Desquamative gingivitis. Biopsy of the lesions revealed histologic changes suggestive of erosive lichen planus.

tent and severity of symptoms. If the desquamative gingivitis is determined to be an oral manifestation of a skin disease, topical or systemic corticosteroid therapy may be indicated.

BIBLIOGRAPHY

Bahn SL: Glucocorticosteriods in dentistry. J Am Dent Assoc 105:476–481, 1982

Brown AE et al: Oral ulceration associated with hypothyroidism—Report of a case. Oral Surg 46:216–219, 1978

Brown J, Solomon D et al: Autoimmune thyroid disease-Graves' and Hashimoto's. Ann Intern Med 88:379–39l, 1978

Braverman LE: Update on tests and treatment for thyroid disease. Modern Med pp. 58-81, May 1982

Burch WM Jr, Francis AN: Using adrenal steroids in endocrine disease. J Clin Therapeutics 12:89–104, 1982

Cawson RA, James J: Adrenal crisis in dental patients having systemic corticosteroids. Br J Oral Surg 10:305–309, 1973

Cohen DW et al: A longitudinal investigation of the periodontal changes during pregnancy. J Periodontal 40:563–570, 1969

Cohen DW et al: A longitudinal investigation of the periodontal changes during pregnancy and 15 months post partum II. J Periodontal 42:653, 1971

Council on Dental Therapeutics: Accepted Dental Therapeutics, 37th ed, pp 227–230. Chicago, American Dental Association, 1977

Edler RJ: Dental and skeletal ages in hypopituitary patients. J Dent Res 56:1145–1153, 1977

Ellyin F, Singh SP: Cushing's disease, A review of pathogenesis, diagnostic methods and treatment. Postgrad Med 70:131–143, 1981

Fletcher PD et Al: Oral manifestations of secondary hyperparathyroidism related to long term hemodialysis therapy. Oral Surg 43:218–226, 1977

Frensilli J et al: Dental changes of idiopathic hypoparathyroidism. J Oral Surg 29:727–731, 1971

Garfunkel AA et al: Familial hypoparathyroidism, candidiasis, and mental retardation—A histopathological study of dental structure. J Oral Med 34(1):13-17, 1979

Hanson LI et al: Affect of thyroxine and growth hormone on dentin production in maxillary incisors in rats. Scand J Dent Res 86:169–173, 1978

Kosowitz J, Rzymski K: Abnormalities of tooth development in pituitary dwarfism. Oral Surg 44:853–863, 1977

Ledbetter CA: Osteitis fibrosa cystica secondary to parathyroid adenoma with normocalcemia. J Arkansas Med Soc 78:331–335, 1982

Löe H : Periodontal changes in pregnancy. J Periodontal 36:37–47, 1965

Meuller WA et al: Management of a hyperthyroid dental patient utilizing general anesthetic. Pediatr Dent 3:20l–203, 1981

Miller RL et al: The ultrastructure of oral neuromas, multiple mucosal neuromas, pheochromocytoma, medullary carcinoma syndrome. J Oral Pathol 6:253–263, 1977

Myllärniemi S et al: Oral findings in autoimmunepolyendocrinopathy-candidosis syndrome (APECS) and other forms of hypoparathyroidism. Oral Surg 45:721–729, 1978

Myllärniemi S: Dental maturity in hypopituitarism and dental response to substitution treatment. Scand J Dent Res 86:307–312, 1978

Pisanty S et al: Familial hypoparathyroidism with candidiasis and mental retardation. Oral Surg 44: 374–383, 1977

Picoides AM: Pharmacology and therapeutic use of vitamin D and its analogues. Drugs 27:241–256, 1981

Rosen IB et al: Fibrosseous tumors of the facial skeleton in association with primary hyperparathyroidism endocrine syndrome or coincidence? Am J Surg 142:494–498, 1981

Rosenberg E, Guralnick W: Hyperparathyroidism: A review of 220 proved cases with special emphasis on findings in the jaws. Oral Surg 15 (suppl.2):84–92, 1962

Schaffer TC, Dishart PW: Hypothyroidism: Outpatient management. Fam Pract Recert 4:23–43, 1982

Scopp IW: Dentistry for the patient on steroids: Steroids in medicine and dentistry. NY J Dent 49:179–182, 1979

Sheikh MM et al: Brown tumors of the jaw. Alex Dent J 2:173–193, 1977

Silverman S et al: Dental aspects of hyperparathyroidism. Oral Surg 26:184–189, 1968

Smith MJ et al: Subacute thyroiditis as a cause of facial pain. Oral Surg 43:59–62, 1977

Spiegel RJ et al: Adrenal suppression after short term corticosteroid therapy. Lancet 630–633, March 24, 1979

Streck WF, Lockwood DH: Pituitary adrenal recovery following short term suppression with corticosteroids. Am J Med 66:910–913, 1979

Terezhalmy GI et al: Initial incidence of primary hyperthyroidism presenting in the mouth: A case report. J Oral Med 33:4–8, 1978

Wells SA Jr: Primary hyperparathyroidism. Curr Probl Surg 17:398–463, 1980

Zack B: Hypothyroidism in children. Postgrad Med 70:177–184, 1981

26

Diabetes

MALCOLM A. LYNCH

Diabetes mellitus, one of the more prevalent diseases common to man is estimated to occur in the diagnosed form in about 2% of the population with at least another 2 percent who are undiagnosed. In the United States at the present time, an estimated 12 million people are presently or will be affected by diabetes. Consequently, virtually every practicing dentist will treat diabetic patients.

Diabetes may be described as a chronic disease of carbohydrate metabolism caused by a relative or absolute deficiency of insulin and characterized by hyperglycemia. It is accompanied by blood vessel disease consisting of microangiopathy, manifested by a thickening of the basement membrane in the smaller blood vessels, and atherosclerosis caused by increased serum levels of cholesterol and tryglycerides.

Diabetes has been classified by the National Diabetes Data Group.

CLASSIFICATION OF DIABETES AND OTHER CATEGORIES OF GLUCOSE INTOLERANCE

- Idiopathic diabetes mellitus
  Insulin-dependent type (type I)
  Noninsulin-dependent type (type II)
    Nonobese
    Obese
- Impaired glucose tolerance
- Gestational diabetes
- Previous abnormality of glucose tolerance
- Potential abnormality of glucose tolerance
- Glucose intolerance associated with certain conditions

Idiopathic diabetes mellitus, which comprises the vast majority of cases, is subdivided into two genetically and clinically distinct types. Insulin-dependent diabetes mellitus (type I) and noninsulin-dependent diabetes mellitus (type II). Studies have shown that microvascular complications of diabetes are largely confined to persons with fasting plasma glucose values higher than 140 mg/dl and to persons who have a sustained elevation of the plasma glucose level greater than 200 mg/dl 2 hours after an oral challenge of 75 g of glucose. Only individuals with plasma glucose above these levels may be

considered to be diabetic, and there are some exceptions to this as described below under other classifications of impaired glucose tolerance.

It is no longer considered accurate to diagnose individuals as being diabetic who exhibit fasting plasma glucose levels greater than normal (> 100 mg/dl) but less than those described above. These individuals are referred to as having *impaired glucose tolerance,* and it has been found that they either remain in this state of impaired glucose tolerance for years or return to normal tolerance without developing the microvascular complications of diabetes. *Gestational diabetes* is a temporary form of glucose intolerance that occurs during pregnancy. The classification *previous abnormalities of glucose tolerance* refers to individuals who have previously experienced transient episodes of hyperglycemia but who presently do not exhibit glucose intolerance according to the plasma glucose parameters described above.

Potential abnormalities of glucose tolerance refers to individuals who are not diabetic but who are at substantially higher risk than the general population to develop diabetes. These include individuals with islet cell antibodies and those who are genetically predisposed. Finally, a small number of cases of *glucose intolerance* are *associated with certain diseases or conditions* including patients on drugs known to have a hyperglycemic effect and diseases such as hemochromatosis, carcinoma of the pancreas, acromegaly, Cushing's disease, hyperthyroidism, and in patients who have had their pancreas removed.

IDIOPATHIC DIABETES MELLITUS

By definition the etiology of idiopathic diabetes mellitus is unknown; however, there are definite demonstrable genetic and environmental influences that determine whether a person will develop the disease. Insulin-dependent diabetes has been associated with particular human leukocytic antigens (HLA). Environmental factors appear to determine whether this form of the disease will be expressed clinically. For example, seasonal variations in manifestations of the disease have coincided with attacks of rubella and mumps, and elevated antibody titers of these viruses have been shown in some insulin-dependent diabetic patients. Experimentally, coxsackievirus B4 was isolated from the pancreas of a young person who died from insulin-dependent diabetes, and this virus was shown to produce diabetes in animals. Siblings of insulin-dependent diabetics, especially those with identical HLA haplotypes are at increased risk for developing diabetes.

Noninsulin-dependent diabetes has not been associated with any particular HLA; however, genetic factors certainly play a part as evidenced by the fact that concordance between identical twins for noninsulin-dependent diabetes approaches 100% Siblings, parents, and offspring of insulin-dependent diabetics are at an increased risk of developing the disease. A mild form of insulin-independent diabetes mellitus with onset at an early age has been shown to be inherited by autosomal dominance. Obesity has also been shown to play an important role in the development of insulin-independent diabetes as has belonging to a racial or ethnic group with a high prevalence of the disease.

Insulin-Dependent

This type of diabetes mellitus also known as type I comprises 10% to 20% of all patients with diabetes. The disease may come on at any age although its time of onset is usually before age 25. Onset is usually abrupt, and patients are prone to develop ketoacidosis. Difficulty of control is the hallmark of this disease with abrupt shifts in the blood sugar level from hypoglycemia to hyperglycemia with small doses of insulin. Plasma insulin is nearly or virtually absent, and there is total destruction of pancreatic beta cells. Islet cell antibodies are frequently present at diagnosis. Cellular receptors for insulin are usually unimpaired, and there may even be a physiological increase in the number of insulin receptor sites. These patients must be treated by insulin.

Insulin-Independent

This type of diabetes also known as type II comprises 80% to 90% of patients with idiopathic diabetes mellitus. Circulating plasma insulin levels are generally normal or slightly increased, and a few patients in this category have markedly increased plasma insulin levels. There are a decreased number of cellular receptor sites for insulin, and some receptor sites have been shown to be inactivated by autoantibodies especially in those patients with markedly increased plasma insulin levels. Most of these patients are obese at the onset of the disease, although they may lose weight as symptoms develop. The onset is quite gradual, and the disease may be discovered accidentally when the patient has a blood sugar test done for another reason such as admission to a hospital or routine screening of the population for hyperglycemia such as during Diabetes Week. These patients are not usually prone to ketoacidosis. Treatment is by weight reduction, insulin, or drugs that increase cellular receptor sites.

PATHOPHYSIOLOGY

Decreased resistance to infection is seen in patients with uncontrolled diabetes but not in those who have normal blood glucose levels. In hyperglycemia, phagocytosis by granulocytes is decreased, and in the presence of ketosis, mobility of granulocytes is decreased. After several years of hyperglycemia the capillary basement membrane thickens, hampering both granulocyte mobilization and the transport of oxygen and nutrients.

CLINICAL MANIFESTATIONS

The clinical manifestations of diabetes mellitus are protean and include visual difficulties secondary to involvement of the retina (seen in 90% of all diabetics who have had their disease more than 20 years), skin infections especially furuncles (boils), generalized itching, vaginal pruritus, renal disease that often is terminal, and neurologic manifestations characterized by a peripheral neuropathy, which are estimated to eventually occur in 90% of patients with diabetes. This neuropathy also contributes to bladder infection in that the patient is unable to completely empty the urinary bladder thus leading to chronic residual urine that is susceptible to infection.

Lower extremity lesions often occur. These are caused by atherosclerosis, the development of which is accelerated in the diabetic patient, and by the impairment of the microcirculation. Lower extremity infection is exacerbated by the diabetic neuropathy in which the patient is unable to appreciate small lesions of the skin, allowing pathogenic organisms to perforate and initiate infection.

In addition to the above, the patient may develop ketoacidosis (see below), which may proceed to coma. In uncontrolled diabetes, the patient exhibits polyuria caused by spilling of glucose into the urine, polydipsia (increased thirst) caused by dehydration, and polyphagia (increased appetite and eating) caused by starvation of the cells secondary to their inability to absorb glucose.

While many patients can survive with chronically elevated blood sugar levels, it has become increasingly evident in recent years that chronic close control of blood glucose levels is important in preventing the microvascular complications of the disease. Acutely, one overriding reason for controlling the blood sugar level is to prevent the development of ketoacidosis. Ketoacidosis is produced by an alternate pathway of metabolism of fatty acids in the liver leading to an accumulation of ketone bodies (acetoacetic acid, beta-hydroxybuteric acid, and acetone) in the blood. These in turn lead to a lowering of the blood pH, which is ameliorated by the blood buffer systems. When the buffer systems are exhausted, the blood pH goes below a range compatible with life. The buffer system involved most closely with the protection of the blood pH is the bicarbonate system. For this reason the severity of the ketoacidosis can often be measured by measuring the decrease in the blood bicarbonate level. Alternatively, direct measurements of serum pH may also be used. The characteristic finding in the blood of ketoacidosis is a lowered pH, a lowered bicarbonate level, and hyperglycemia. There is also acetone and glucose in the urine as measured by the usual techniques.

Diabetic Coma

Diabetic coma is an ambiguous term inasmuch as it is used to refer to the state of unconsciousness that results from either hyperglycemia and ketoacidosis or at the other end of the spectrum, hypoglycemia. When using the term one should be careful to orient thinking and terminology so that there is no confusion between the two. The two comas can usually be differentiated on the basis of a history if the patient is coherent enough to give one, or if he is accompanied by someone who can give an adequate history. In cases of doubt, 50 ml of 50% glucose solution should be given intravenously or alternatively 1 to 2 mg glucagon administered subcutaneously or intramuscularly. The dosage of glucagon may be repeated in 15 minutes. The above treatments will alleviate hypoglycemia but not appreciably worsen hyperglycemia.

Factors leading to coma secondary to hypoglycemia are those of decreased food intake, increased insulin administration, or increased exercise. The period of onset can vary from a few hours in the case of a patient taking a short-acting insulin to many hours in a patient taking a long-acting insulin. The urine is usually negative for both glucose and acetone, and the blood sugar is less than 40 mg/dl. Symptoms preceding the onset of coma are anxiousness, sweating, hunger, headache, diplopia, convulsions, and palpitations.

On the other hand, coma secondary to hyperglycemic ketoacidosis usually takes days to develop and is associated with the following:

1. Infection, the most common cause, may be respiratory, genitourinary, gastrointestinal, of the skin, in the oral cavity (which may be asymptomatic), or anywhere else in the body
2. Dehydration
3. Exogenous steroid administration
4. Gastrointestinal upsets, along with nausea, vomiting and diarrhea
5. Emotional upsets
6. Failure to take insulin in prescribed dosage or to follow the proper diet

The biochemical values are as noted earlier. Symptomatology is that of polyuria, polyphagia, polydipsia, anorexia, nausea, vomiting, weakness, and drowsiness gradually increasing to coma.

DIAGNOSIS OF DIABETES

Presently accepted criteria for diagnosis of diabetes are, in adults, 1. unequivocal elevation of plasma glucose concentration (greater than 140 mg/dl) *together with* the classical symptoms of diabetes, or 2. elevated fasting plasma glucose concentration (greater than 140 mg/dl) on more than one occasion, or 3. elevated plasma glucose concentration (greater than 200 mg/dl) 2 hours after a 75-g oral glucose challenge on more than one occasion. Diagnosis of diabetes in children requires either 1 or 2 described above, *and* 3.

Urine Sugars

Urine sugars are often misused in the diagnosis of diabetes and are both insensitive and nonspecific. False positives can result from the hereditary familial condition renal glucosuria, in which the patient has a lowered renal threshold for glucose and spills it into the urine, although the blood glucose level is normal. If the test for urinary glucose is not a glucose oxidase test and therefore not specific for glucose, the presence of other reducing sugars in the urine such as lactose in lactating mothers may also give a false-positive result. False negatives can occur in early diabetes when the patient has only transient glucosuria, which when diluted with normal urine gives a negative test or conversely, with advanced diabetic nephropathy wherein the renal threshold for glucose is markedly elevated.

Blood Glucose

There is controversy as to whether a blood test for glucose should be performed in the fasting state or in the postprandial state. Either should suffice providing the diagnostic criteria described previously are met. The fasting plasma glucose is a more specific test in that patients who have significantly elevated fasting plasma glucose levels with no other cause almost always turn out to be diabetic; however, to meet diagnostic criteria, an elevation of plasma glucose greater than 140mg/dl must be demonstrated on more than one occasion. On the other hand, a 2-hour postprandial determination of the plasma glucose is a more sensitive test, because some diabetics who have normal fasting glucose levels early in this disease will exhibit hyperglycemia only when challenged with an oral glucose load.

Glucose Tolerance Test

An oral glucose tolerance test may be indicated when a patient's signs and symptoms are suggestive of diabetes, but the fasting plasma glucose cannot be demonstrated to be greater than 140 mg/dl on *more* than one occasion. It is *not* necessary when the fasting blood glucose concentration is greater than 140 mg/dl on more than one occasion. When indicated, the test should be performed in the morning after at least 3 days of unrestricted diet containing the usual amount of carbohydrates and normal physical activity. The patient should fast for 10 to 16 hours before the test is performed. A standardized oral 75-g dose of glucose is given, and the plasma glucose is measured at the beginning and at 30-minute intervals for up to 2 hours. The test is interpreted as positive if the 2-hour level and any other sample taken between time 0 and 2 hours is equal to or greater than 200 mg/dl.

Hemoglobin A_{1c} Levels

Hemoglobin A_{1c} is a postsynthesis modification of the hemoglobin molecule produced by an addition of a glucose molecule to the N-terminus of the beta chain of hemoglobin A. It is synthesized at a constant rate throughout the life span of the red cell. The rate of synthesization is proportional to the blood glucose level. Because the life span of the red cell is about 120 days, the level of hemoglobin A_{1c} is a useful index of control of hyperglycemia and blood glucose levels during the 2 to 3 months immediately prior to the measurement. Normal level is 5.5% and in diabetics generally runs higher, averaging 7% to 10%. The clinical usefulness of measurement of hemoglobin A_{1c} lies in diagnosis of diabetes and monitoring of control. It is particularly useful in the latter instance in that it gives a long-term, chronic measurement of blood glucose levels. In this respect it also looks promising as a research tool.

Hemoglobin A_{1c} levels have also been found to be useful in differentiating the hyperglycemia that often occurs after an acute myocardial infarction from that associated with diabetes. In the former, the levels of hemoglobin A_{1c} are not elevated while in the latter (diabetes) they are.

TREATMENT OF DIABETES

Medical control of diabetes mellitus depends on striking a balance between dietary intake and absorption, glucose transport from the exterior to the interior of the cell as mediated by insulin, or oral hypoglycemic agents and glucose utilization as determined by body needs of basal metabolism plus level of activity.

The mainstay of diabetic treatment is in reasonably rigid control of the diet and thereby the blood glucose levels. In many insulin-independent diabetics, the disease can be controlled by weight loss and diet alone without the use of any medication. Total calories taken in must be balanced with activity and body weight; in contrast to what was formerly thought, the precise breakdown of food between carbohydrate, fat, and protein is not terribly important, and rigid carbohydrate restriction is no longer thought necessary. A reasonably balanced diet will suffice as long as caloric content is controlled.

Diabetics should be warned about the blood glucose-lowering effects of alcohol and urged to temper use of this drug. Alcohol interferes with hepatic glyconeogenesis and induces hypoglycemia whenever glyconeogenesis is required to maintain normal glucose levels as in instances of insulin overdosage, inadequate oral intake, or markedly increased exercise. Any or all of these could lead to serious hypoglycemia unless compensated for by mechanisms such as hepatic glyconeogenesis.

If dietary management is not sufficient to control the blood glucose level, hypoglycemic drugs must be used. These consist of either insulin or an oral hypoglycemic agent, one of the sulfonylurea drugs. Sufonylurea drugs act primarily by stimulating the release of insulin from the pancreas, but they also act by decreasing gluconeogenesis and by increasing sensitivity of cell receptor sites for insulin. Newer sulfonylurea drugs are being developed that in addition to the above actions will also stimulate an increase in number of cellular receptor sites for insulin. Sulfonylurea drugs presently available include tolbutamide, chlorpropamide, acetohexamide, and tolazamide. The oral agents should not be used during pregnancy and should be used only in certain rare situations with insulin-dependent diabetes in conjunction with insulin. They are usually not effective in patients who require more than 40 units of insulin a day.

Patients whose diabetes cannot be controlled by diet alone and in whom use of oral agents is considered injudicious, must be given insulin. Insulin can be given by injection only. The types of insulin vary according to the speed of onset and duration of action: crystalline (regular) insulin is the fastest acting, and other types of insulin are combinations with crystalline to increase the molecular size and prolong the duration of action. Table 26-1 shows examples of various kinds of insulin available. The usual concentration is 100 units per cubic centimeter "U-100" insulin. Insulin syringes are calibrated to deliver the desired amount of insulin by units. Dosage of insulin must be adjusted for each patient and balanced against diet and excercise. When the patient's blood glucose is at approximately normal levels, the insulin dosage is considered to be adjusted.

For years it was thought optimum that the patient should take insulin only once a day in order to achieve control. It has now become apparent that close control of blood glucose levels is important in order to prevent microvascular complications. Periodic measurement of blood glucose levels during the day with supplemental insulin as needed represents optimum therapy. Patients may now measure their blood glucose levels at home using chemically impregnated strips (see chapter on Laboratory Diagnosis) and reading the color reaction to determine the glucose level either visually or through use of the electronic reflectance meter.

A promising development on the horizon is the use of insulin pumps. One type of

Table 26-1. Insulin Preparations

	HOURS AFTER SUBCUTANEOUS INJECTION FOR:		
TYPE	ONSET OF ACTION	MAXIMUM ACTION	DURATION OF ACTION
Crystalline (regular)	¼	4–6	6–8
NPH	1–3	8–12	18–24
PZI	4–8	15–20	24–36
Lente	1–3	8–12	18–30
Semilente	1	4–6	8–14
Ultralente	6–8	16–18	36

pump, the open loop, provides a previously determined, preprogrammed insulin dose usually by subcutaneously implanted catheters continuously throughout the day. The patient can deliver supplemental doses before each meal and after periodic measurement of blood glucose levels as described in the preceding paragraph. A more sophisticated implanted device, the closed-loop pump, automatically detects the level of glucose in the blood of diabetic patients and delivers an appropriate amount of insulin on a continuous basis similar to normal pancreatic function. Both types of pumps appear promising, and once the difficulties inherent in their development (such as malfunction and body rejection of the implanted materials) are solved, very close controls of blood glucose levels should be possible. Studies are also ongoing in attempts to develop pancreatic beta cell transplantation. A number of problems in this area include those of immunologic rejection and the source of donor beta cells.

The third factor (other than dietary intake and glucose transport into the cell, as mediated by insulin or oral hypoglycemic agents) to be considered in the treatment of diabetes is exercise. If the exercise level during a 24-hour period varies considerably, consideration must be given to supplementing increased exercise with increased intake of glucose and decreasing glucose intake and exogenous insulin during periods of decreased activity. Because active muscle can take up blood glucose by a process *not* related to insulin, the diabetic must decrease insulin and increase glucose intake during exercise. Insulin should not be injected directly into a muscle before or during exercise because in-

creased insulin absorption by muscle tissue can increase glucose entry into the cells with resultant lowering of blood glucose levels and onset of hypoglycemic symptoms.

Great advances have been made in the treatment of eye disease secondary to diabetes. Laser photocoagulation is very effective in halting the progress of proliferative retinopathy, and hemorrhage into the vitreous body, which can result in blindness, can be treated by surgical vitrectomy.

ORAL MANIFESTATIONS

No specific oral lesions are associated with or are pathognomonic of diabetes; however, numerous investigators both in studies of experimental animals and in some carefully controlled human studies have indicated an increased incidence of gingivitis and periodontal disease in diabetic patients. Studies by Cianciola and colleagues demonstrated that insulin-dependent diabetic patients had a higher prevalence of severe gingivitis and periodontitis than did normal controls. Periodontal disease showed a stronger relationship to chronologic age than to the duration of the diabetes. Diabetics and controls had comparable amounts of supragingival dental plaque, apparently negating this as a factor accounting for the higher prevalence of periodontal disease in the diabetic patient.

Reports indicating an increased likelihood of oral candidiasis in diabetes have not been confirmed by other investigators. One of the most perplexing problems to the dentist (and to the patient) is an oral manifestation of the peripheral neuropathy that presents as a burning tongue. Although not all patients with a burning tongue have diabetes, it is *sine qua non* that all patients presenting with this symptom have diabetes excluded as the cause of the disease.

DENTAL MANAGEMENT OF THE PATIENT WITH DIABETES MELLITUS

Diagnosis

Diabetic patients will be either known diabetics, who are under a physician's care and report this to their dentist, or alternatively may be suspected to be diabetic on the basis of the health questionnaire. Symptoms that should lead a dentist to suspect diabetes were discussed earlier in the chapter. Remember that insulin-dependent diabetics rarely have insidious onset of their disease, and undiagnosed diabetes in this age group (under 25 years) usually have striking symptoms of short duration. On the other hand, insulin-independent diabetics will have insidious onset of their disease and may not be aware of it until the symptoms are elicited by a carefully administered and accurately interpreted health questionnaire.

If diabetes is suspected solely on the basis of polyuria, tests for glucosuria should be sufficient to include or exclude glucosuria as a cause of this symptom, although a single negative urine test is not sufficient to exclude glucosuria. A single test for hyperglycemia is best made in the dental office about 2 hours after a heavy meal. Although biochemical laboratory evaluation of the blood sugar level is more accurate than a finger prick Dextrostix test, the latter is reasonably accurate to test hyperglycemia of sufficient magnitude to be of dental importance and can be performed easily in the dental office (see the chapter on Laboratory Diagnosis for details of performing this test).

If diabetes is still suspected even though there is no glucosuria and normal fasting or 2-hour postprandial blood glucose levels, it is usually because of either rampant caries or far advanced periodontal disease disproportionate to the patient's age or state of oral hygiene. In this event, a glucose tolerance test may be ordered, but search for diabetes in such patients is seldom fruitful, and there is only a questionable relationship to the patient's dental disease even when transitory abnormalities of glucose metabolism are discovered. Although either a dentist or physician may order a glucose tolerance test, it is often best for convenience, for good medical-dental relations, and for possible further medical management to refer the patient to his physician to determine whether he feels that the glucose tolerance test is justified on the basis of symptomatology elicited.

Assessment of Severity of Diabetes

A questionnaire for diabetics is often helpful in assessing the severity of the disease and propensity toward ketoacidosis or hypoglycemia in order to aid in dental management. The pertinent data are as follows:

1. Physician supervising diabetes (name and address)_____
2. Diabetes discovered at age _____
3. Are you on a special diet? _____
4. Do you take oral antidiabetic medication or insulin? _____
5. If you take insulin, how long have you taken the present dose of insulin? _____ How much insulin is taken daily? (give type of insulin and number of units)____
6. How many times have you been in a hospital because of your diabetes? _____
7. When was your most recent hospitalization for diabetes? _____
8. How often have you been in insulin shock? _____times. Date of last time _____.
9. How often do you see your physician in regard to your diabetes? _____Date last visit _____.
10. Do you check your urine or blood for glucose? _____If so, which, and how often? _____What test do you use? _____Results of last three times tested? _____
11. Do you test your urine for acetone? ____ If so, how often? _____.

An insulin-dependent diabetic is usually more likely to develop hypoglycemia or hyperglycemia than an insulin-independent diabetic. Diabetic patients who are controlled on diet alone or who are controlled with oral agents alone are usually more stable. Ketoacidosis is unlikely to develop in such patients except with the most severe infections. The higher the insulin dosage, the more difficult the patient may be to control. Frequent changes in insulin dosage (except in a growing child) are an indicator of instability of control as are the number of hospitalizations and the number of times in hypoglycemic (insulin) shock. Diabetics who give a history of instability of control of their diabetes, who do not see their physician regularly, or do not check glucose levels in blood or urine regularly should be regarded with suspicion and checked several times for glucosuria. Check with the patient's physician if the patient reports (or you find) persistent 3+ or 4+ glucosuria.

For routine elective dental treatment, be sure that the patient takes his usual insulin dose on the day of dental treatment and that he eats his prescribed usual diet on the day of the procedure. If the patient is on a diet that prescribes the number of calories and carbohydrate-fat-protein ratios, be sure that he can *mechanically* ingest it before and after dental treatment. If dental treatment is such that the patient cannot masticate properly (*e.g.*, full mouth extractions or extensive periodontal surgery), he must have a diet substitute equal in caloric content and carbohydrate-fat-protein ratios but that is soft or liquid. Often the patient will be able to puree his usual diet in a blender or other food processor until he is able to masticate it properly.

If the patient is a brittle diabetic, his urine should be tested for glucosuria and acetone at least on the day of the procedure and perhaps several days afterward depending on the nature of the dental treatment. Promptly refer the patient to the physician if persistent glucosuria or acetonuria develop. With very unstable diabetics it is best to consult with the patient's physician before dental treatment and discuss the intended dental treatment and proposed procedure for following the course of the patient's diabetes during the course of the dental treatment. This is done so that if unanticipated complications develop, the physician will be able to work with the dentist more readily and have better understanding and control of the situation. Some dentists use antibiotic premedication routinely in diabetics, but there is no good experimental evidence that this is useful or effective in preventing infection. The foregoing statement does not apply to the treatment of established infections.

Emergency Dental Treatment in Patients with Infections or Traumatic Injuries

The patient's diet should be controlled according to his ability to eat it (see preceding section). If the patient is hospitalized, diet control may be done in conjunction with the physician responsible for the care of the diabetes. In patients with severe infections, ketoacidosis is likely to develop. Such patients should be watched very carefully with frequent urine checks for glucosuria and acetonuria. If the patient is going into ketoacidosis, consult his physician and manage dental and diabetic therapy on a cooperative basis. Use antibiotic therapy in patients with established infections and in patients in whom infection is likely to develop (regardless of whether the patient is diabetic) such as in severely contaminated wounds. Also use antibiotic therapy prophylactically in patients with acetonuria. Neutrophilic function in ketoacidotic blood is known to be seriously impaired.

BIBLIOGRAPHY

Bierman EL et al: Principles of nutrition and dietary recommendations in patients with diabetes mellitus. J Diabetes 20:633, 1971

Cianciola LJ et al: Prevalence of periodontal disease in insulin-dependent diabetes mellitus (juvenile diabetes). J Am Dent Assoc. 104:653, 1982

Cohen DW et al: Diabetes mellitus in periodontal disease: 2-year longitudinal observations. Part l. J Periodontal 41:709, 1970

Cohen MM: Clinical studies of dental caries susceptibility in young diabetics. J Am Dent Assoc 34:239, 1947

Crosby B, Allison F: Phagocytic and bactericidal capacity of polymorphonuclear leukocytes recovered from venous blood of human beings. Proc Soc Exp Biol Med 123:660, 1966

Fajans SS: What is diabetes? Definition, diagnosis, and course. Med Clin North Am 55:793, 1971

Goldmer MG, Knatterud GL, Prout TE: Effects of hypoglycemic agents on vascular complications in patients with adult onset diabetes. JAMA 218:1400, 1971

Howard EE, Marlette RH: The rationale of management in oral surgery procedures in diabetics. Oral Surg 9:1032, 1956

National Diabetes Data Group: Classification and diagnosis of diabetes mellitus and other categories of glucose intolerance. Diabetes 28:1039, 1979

Newmark SR, Himathongkam T, Shane SM: Hyperglycemic and hypoglycemic crises. JAMA 231:185, 1975

New Standards for Classification and Diagnosis of Diabetes. JAMA 243:2296, 1980

Niejaklik DC, Dube AH, Adamko SM: Glucose measurements and clinical correlations. JAMA 224:1734, 1973

Peters V: Candida albicans in the oral cavities of diabetics. J Dent Res 45:771, 1966

Report of the committee for the assessment of biometric aspects of controlled trials of hypoglycemic agents. JAMA 231:583, 1975

Robinson SC et al: Relationship of pregnancy, vaginal candidiasis and glucose metabolism. Can Med Assoc J 96:583, 1967

Salans LB: Diabetes mellitus—a disease that is coming into focus. JAMA 247:590, 1982

Schade DS, Eaton RP: Prevention of diabetic ketoacidosis. JAMA, 242:2455, 1979

Soler NG, Franks: Value of glycosolated hemoglobin measurements after acute myocardial infarction. JAMA 246:1690, 1981

Waxler SH, Leef MR, Craig LS: Errors inheritant in use of abbreviated screening procedures for diabetes mellitus. Geriatrics 26:98, 1971

Williams RC, Mahan CJ: Periodontal disease and diabetes in young adults. JAMA 172:776, 1960

27

Neuromuscular Diseases

MARTIN S. GREENBERG

Cerebrovascular Disease
Epilepsy
Multiple Sclerosis
Parkinson's Disease
Myasthenia Gravis
Muscular Dystrophy

In this chapter diseases affecting the nerves, muscles, and neuromuscular junction are discussed. This is an extensive topic, but the diseases discussed here include only those that affect the orofacial region or have a significant effect on dental management. Polymyositis, a disorder that could have been included in this chapter, is discussed with the immune diseases in Chapter 24.

CEREBROVASCULAR DISEASE

Cerebrovascular disease is the most common neurologic disorder of adults in the United States, and all dentists will treat patients with sequelae of this disorder. In order to manage these patients safely, it is important to understand the basic principles of the disease. This knowledge gives a rational approach to managing these patients in the dental office.

Cerebrovascular disease includes all disorders that damage the blood vessels supplying the brain, thus producing neurologic damage. The end result of the blood vessel damage is an acute episode referred to as a *cerebrovascular accident* (CVA) or stroke. Eighty percent of CVAs are caused by infarction; hemorrhage accounts for the other 20%.

The most common cause of infarction in the brain is atherosclerosis. Atheromatous plaques develop in artery walls; the plaque ulcerates causing a thrombus (or blood clot), which may eventually stop the flow of blood to the portion of the brain supplied by that artery and lead to acute infarction of brain tissue. Sites that commonly develop atheromatous plaques are the branching portions of the arterial system such as the internal carotid artery where it branches from the common carotid artery. Thrombi also commonly form in the vertebral, basilar, and middle cerebral arteries. Occlusion of each of these arteries causes a characteristic syndrome, of which the signs depend on the portion of the brain in which there is an infarction. Diabetes and hypertension are predisposing factors to thrombus formation, and patients with these disorders have an increased susceptibility to CVA.

Emboli may also cause occlusion of a cerebral vessel. An embolism is a blockage of a blood vessel by a blood clot, bacterial mass or other material that originates in another part of the body. Whereas a thrombus builds up slowly in the affected vessel, the embolus builds up elsewhere, breaks off, and suddenly occludes a vessel at another site. The majority of emboli that affect the brain break away from a thrombus that has formed in the left side of the heart. Most emboli that form elsewhere in the body, such as in thrombophlebitis in the legs, will lodge in the lungs. Emboli from the heart result from thrombus formation at the site of an acute myocardial infarction, chronic atrial fibrillation, or rheumatic heart disease. Septic emboli may result from bacterial endocarditis.

Other causes of ischemia and infarction of the brain include decreased blood flow secondary to sudden severe hypotension, acute hypertension that causes a spasm of cerebral vessels, arthritis caused by collagen diseases, polycythemia, sickle-cell anemia, and cavernous sinus thrombosis.

Hemorrhage of an intracranial vessel may also cause a CVA. The two most common causes of hemorrhage are hypertension and rupture of a saccular (berry) aneurysm. Less common causes of brain hemorrhage include trauma, bleeding, and clotting disorders, and ruptured angiomata.

Clinical Manifestations

The initial sign of thrombosis in the brain may be a CVA, but in many cases CVA from a thrombus is preceded by transient ischemic attacks (TIA). These reversible strokes may occur weeks to years before a true CVA, and they often indicate an impending stroke from thrombus formation. The frequency of TIAs varies, but each event lasts only a few minutes. A RIND (reversible ischemic neurologic disability) causes a neurologic deficit that lasts several days. Some patients may experience only one or two TIAs prior to a CVA; others may have several per day for months. During the attack, which usually lasts from several seconds to 10 minutes, a wide variety of neurologic signs and symptoms can appear depending on the site of the developing thrombus. Common clinical signs include unilateral weakness of the extremities, face, tongue, and palate; dysphagia, paresthesia; diplopia; and dizziness. *Many patients experi-*

encing TIAs will be taking anticoagulants to help prevent infarction. CVA caused by a thrombus often evolves slowly and may take hours or even days for the full neurologic picture to develop. This clinical picture commonly includes hemiplegia, aphasia, and cranial nerve defects including involvement of nerves V, VII, IX, and X.

Signs and symptoms of a CVA caused by an embolus come on suddenly. It is not preceded by TIAs, and the CVA itself does not evolve slowly because the clot originates elsewhere and suddenly blocks a cerebral vessel. Although the neurologic manifestations are similar, CVA caused by a thrombus may take hours to develop, and neurologic damage is progressive; the signs and symptoms of an embolus are swift and sudden.

Hemorrhage, the third cause of CVA, is commonly a result of either a rupture of a saccular (berry) aneurysm at the circle of Willis, a rupture of an intracerebral arteriovenous malformation, or rupture of a cerebral vessel caused by hypertension. Bleeding and clotting disorders and neoplasms of the brain may also cause intracranial hemorrhage. The signs and symptoms of a CVA caused by hemorrhage are sudden and often accompanied by a severe headache. Vomiting, nuchal rigidity, and seizures more commonly accompany hemorrhage than infarction, and localizing neurologic signs are less common.

Dental Considerations

The responsibility of the dentist in the field of cerebrovascular disease falls into two categories: minimizing the risk of CVA for dental patients and adequate dental care for post-CVA patients.

The dentist must realize that most of the factors that cause strokes are beyond his control. There are no "five steps" that will guarantee a stroke-free patient. Years of atherosclerosis or a weakened blood vessel at the circle of Willis cannot be reversed by medication; therefore, the dentist must settle for minimizing the risk to his patients. A patient cannot remain in severe pain or with an acute infection because of a risk of stroke.

To reduce CVA in dental patients, begin with a history that includes questions identifying patients with an increased risk. Included in this group are patients with history of CVA, diabetes, or hypertension and women taking oral contraceptives. In the history also include questions in the review of systems of intermittent neurologic signs of paresthesia, weakness, aphasia, visual changes, syncope, diplopia, or dysarthria. These latter questions are important in recognizing patients who have experienced TIAs or RIND. If a patient experiencing TIAs or RIND is not under a physician's care, refer him for evaluation before performing any dental treatment other than minimal emergency care. The physician may be able to reduce the risk of stroke by controlling hypertension, treating heart disease, and using platelet antiaggregants such as aspirin. The risk of stroke is also diminished by taking blood pressure in the dental office on all adult patients and referring hypertensive patients to a physician for evaluation and management.

Dental treatment may, of course, still be necessary for a patient with a high risk of CVA. Prolonged elective procedures are contraindicated, but do not ignore conservative control of dental caries and periodontal disease. Management of acute infection or severe pain that results from neglect may be more of a risk than routine care. Patients taking anticoagulants prophylactically to prevent emboli or thrombus formation, should *not* be removed from the drug for routine dental procedures.

Patients who have a high risk of CVA may be lightly sedated prior to treatment, but heavy sedation of patients with severe atherosclerosis is contraindicated because hypotension can lead to cerebral ischemia when large atheromas are present in vessels leading to the brain.

Take the blood pressure at the beginning of each dental appointment for all patients who have been previously identified as hypertensive. Have blood pressure readings listed on the patient's record. If the blood pressure remains elevated even after medical consultation, ask the physician to determine whether the blood pressure is controlled as closely as possible. In some patients pressure is elevated because they are not following their prescribed regimen; others cannot be adequately controlled with medications available. The risk of CVA can be reduced by establishing that each patient is under the best possible control at the beginning of each visit.

Be aware that osteoarthritis of the cervical spine may cause cerebral ischemia by pressing on cerebral arteries when the patient turns his head. Study of atherosclerotic changes in the lingual artery to predict changes in intracranial vessels has been considered. One noninvasive technique is use of Doppler ultrasound. Myers and co-workers demonstrated changes in lingual artery dynamics of CVA patients using this technique.

Many dentists tend to avoid the oral care of the post-CVA patient, although a majority of the patients may be managed with a minimal change in routine. Methods of coping with dental prosthetic problems that develop in patients with facial nerve weakness or paralysis are described by Salley as well as by Zafron and Zayon. Cheek biting or food collecting in the buccal sulcus on the affected side are reduced by adding a large buccal flange to a lower denture, which fills the buccal sulcus and holds the cheek away from the occlusal surfaces of the teeth. Salley has also described a palatal training appliance that is used to reduce speech and swallowing difficulties present in patients with palatal paralysis.

Poor oral hygiene is common among post-CVA patients because of the mental depression that is frequently seen in many chronically debilitated patients, as well as the physical inability to brush the teeth because of the paralysis. Combine ingenuity and compassion in motivating CVA patients to maintain a healthy mouth; in instances of severe disability, the cooperation of the family is necessary.

Disabled patients who cannot transfer to a dental chair will need specialized dental facilities. Anderson has described an apparatus that can be used to adapt a wheelchair into a dental chair.

EPILEPSY

Epilepsy is caused by intermittent abnormal electrical discharges in the brain. These abnormal discharges may cause episodes of sensory and motor abnormalities as well as loss of consciousness. Epileptics are categorized as follows: 75% are idiopathic having no known organic brain lesion, 25% are secondary to diseases known to affect the brain such as trauma, anoxia, and meningitis, encephalitis, or tumors.

The incidence of epilepsy is estimated at 0.5% of the population. Onset is most frequent during infancy and puberty. Epilepsy developing later in life is more commonly associated with known organic brain disease.

Clinical Manifestations

Epilepsy is generally categorized according to the type of seizure the patient experiences. The four major types of seizures are petit mal, grand mal, Jacksonian, and psychomotor. Approximately 25% of epileptics experience more than one type of seizure.

Grand Mal. The most common type of seizure is grand mal, with 90% of epileptics experiencing it alone or in combination with another type of seizure. A grand mal seizure characteristically begins with an aura. The characteristics of the aura depend on which portion of the brain is the focus of the abnormal electrical discharge. The aura may be experienced as epigastric discomfort, an emotion, or hallucination of hearing, vision, or smell. The aura is followed in seconds to minutes by unconsciousness, a cry, and tonic muscle spasms; this rigid phase lasts about 30 seconds. During this period the patient does not breathe because of the spasm of the respiratory muscles, and he becomes cyanotic. The tonic phase is followed by a clonic phase composed of convulsive jerky movements, incontinence, and tongue biting (see Fig. 27-1). The patient may injure himself seriously if he is near hard or sharp objects. A postictal state characterized by headache, confusion, lethargy, occasional temporary neurologic deficit, and deep sleep usually follows a grand mal seizure.

The number, severity, and duration of grand mal seizures vary considerably from one patient to another. A severe form of the disorder, status epilepticus, occurs when a series of seizures follow each other before the patient is able to regain consciousness.

Petit Mal. Petit mal is the second most common type of seizure and occurs without an aura and with little or no clonic or tonic movements. They are present almost exclu-

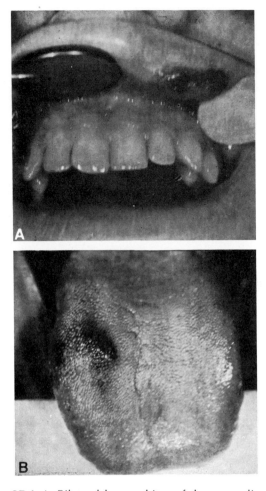

Fig. 27-1 *A,* Bilateral human bites of the upper lip that were received during an epileptic convulsion. *B,* Traumatic injury (bite) to tongue that occurred during an epileptic seizure.

sively in children and frequently disappear during the second decade of life. A single seizure lasts just seconds. The patient loses consciousness and appears to stare into space. He will continue normal activity immediately after the seizure is over. Petit mal seizures may occur several times each day and in severe cases may interfere with school and social activities.

Psychomotor. The seizures are preceded by an aura that is often a hallucination or a feeling of *déjà vu.* During the seizure the patient exhibits purposeless movements and bizarre behavior. Patients may wander about aim-

lessly, undress, or exhibit violent behavior during a seizure.

Jacksonian. This form of epilepsy accompanies known organic brain disease. The seizure begins with clonic movements of a distal portion of an extremity or the face. Initial movements of the seizure involving toes or fingers are common. The convulsive movements spread up the affected limb, becoming generalized and causing loss of consciousness.

Treatment of Seizures

All forms of epilepsy are managed by anticonvulsive drug therapy. The drug of choice for the management of grand mal, psychomotor, or Jacksonian seizures is phenytoin (Dilantin), often in combination with phenobarbital. When these drugs do not give the desired results, primidone (Mysoline) is used. In patients with seizures resistant to the above drugs, mephenytoin (Mesantoin) is prescribed. Patients taking mephenytoin may experience serious side-effects including neutropenia, agranulocytosis, and thrombocytopenia. Dermatitis and stomatitis have also been reported, including severe erythema multiforme reactions. Mephenytoin is used only in patients who do not improve using the other less toxic drugs. Tegretol and sodium valproate are also being used with increased frequency.

The drug of choice for petit mal seizures is ethosuximide (Zarontin) because of the few side-effects associated with it. Other drugs used are trimethadione (Tridione), paramethadione (Paradione), and acetazolamide (Diamox); the latter three drugs may cause blood dycrasias.

Dental Considerations

Patients taking anticonvulsant drugs are subject to gingival hyperplasia (see Fig. 27-2). This hyperplasia is usually associated with phenytoin, but cases have been reported of gingival changes in patients taking primidone. The etiology of the gingival hyperplasia has been studied, and workers have related it to levels of drug in the gingival tissues and the effect of the drug on gingival mast cells. Hall observed increased mast cells in the gingivae of patients with phenytoin gin-

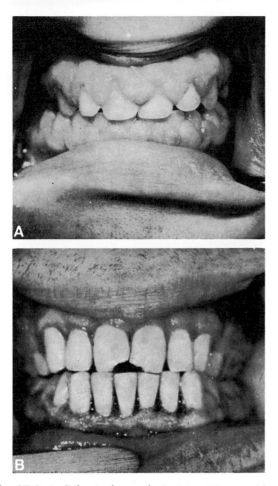

Fig. 27-2 *A,* Dilantin hyperplasia in a 17-year-old girl. The enlarged tissues are light pink in color and fibrous, and they show no evidence of edema, inflammation, or ulceration. *B,* Patient with Dilantin hyperplasia following electrocautery of the enlarged gingival tissues. The excess maxillary gingival tissue had been removed 10 days previously. The excess mandibular gingival tissue had just been removed. Fractures of the mesioincisal angles of the maxillary first incisors occurred during a seizure.

gival hyperplasia. Angelopoulos also suspects the role of mast cells. He believes that chemical mediators from the mast cells (heparin, histamine, hyaluronic acid) cause increased connective tissue to be produced by fibroblasts. Most workers now agree that local inflammatory factors also play an important role in the etiology of phenytoin hyperplasia. Hall studied 20 patients taking phenytoin who received a dental prophylaxis and oral hygiene instruction; none of the patients developed gingival hyperplasia. Nuki studied cats taking phenytoin and noted that gingival hyperplasia developed only when local inflammatory factors were present.

Clinically, phenytoin hyperplasia starts in the interdental papillae and occurs only where teeth are present. The papillae enlarge buccally and lingually. The enlarged areas are firm, pink, and covered with normal mucosa. The severity of the hyperplasia varies. In some patients the enlarged gingivae may involve just one or two papillae; in other cases the crowns of the teeth are completely covered with hyperplastic tissue. The best treatment of phenytoin hyperplasia begins with prevention. Little doubt remains that careful oral hygiene can prevent or at least minimize the gingival enlargement. Soon after being placed on anticonvulsant therapy, each patient should be referred to a dentist for oral hygiene instruction and gingival curettage. Patients who have not been properly managed and develop gross gingival enlargement will require gingivectomy. Curettage and careful attention to oral hygiene must follow the surgery, or the hyperplastic tissue will return.

It is known that side-effects other than gingival hyperplasia also occur in patients taking phenytoin. This includes megaloblastic anemia, hirsutism, and lymphadenopathy. Connective tissue and bone changes have also been reported, including osteomalacia, thickening of the heel pad and of the calvarium, and coarse facies. Harris and Goldhaber studied 112 adult epileptics on prolonged phenytoin therapy; they found root abnormalities in 14. These two workers hypothesized that phenytoin blocks the effect of parathyroid hormone on bone, inducing a type of pseudohypoparathyroidism with resulting bone and root changes. Routine dental treatment for well-controlled epileptics may be performed with no change in normal treatment. There is no reason to increase the dose of anticonvulsant therapy prior to dental treatment, and routine use of sedation is not indicated.

MULTIPLE SCLEROSIS

Multiple sclerosis (MS) is a chronic neurologic disease caused by demyelination of the axon sheath of the brain and spinal cord.

There is increasing evidence that the demyelination is caused by a virus. Some investigators believe that the viral infection is acquired in childhood but does not become clinically apparent until adult life. Other theories focus on an immunologic cause.

The average age of onset is during the fourth decade of life, the disease occurs more frequently in females. In the northern hemisphere, the number of cases increases the farther one goes above the equator. For instance in Europe, the incidence is much higher in Scandinavia than in Italy, and in North America the incidence is higher in Nova Scotia than in Louisiana.

Clinical Manifestations

The clinical signs and symptoms of MS depend on the site of the demyelinating lesion. The lesions may occur almost anywhere in the central nervous system, but they have a predilection for certain areas. A common initial sign of the disease is loss of vision caused by demyelinating lesions of the second cranial nerve. The loss of vision occurs over a period of days to weeks. Another ophthalmic sign is diplopia caused by involvement of the third, fourth, or sixth cranial nerve.

Weakness or paresthesia of the extremities, with increase of the deep tendon reflexes, is another common early finding in MS. Other common signs of the disease include bladder dysfunction, euphoria, ataxia, vertigo, and incoordination.

Most cases of MS are chronic and are characterized by exacerbations and remissions over a period of many years. During acute episodes, severe neurologic involvement is evident. This slowly disappears, but after each episode some permanent neurologic involvement remains. The extent and severity of the permanent involvement varies considerably from patient to patient. In mild cases little permanent effect is noted, and patients may have a normal life span. In severe acute cases a patient may be totally paralyzed within months. Millar studied severe cases of MS finding that the average duration of the disease was 20 years. He found minimal disability for the first 7 years, deterioration for the second 7 years, and a confinement to a chair and bed during the last 6 to 7 years.

Death is most frequently caused by urinary tract and pulmonary infections.

The diagnosis of MS is clinical and is based on the age of the patient, neurologic signs that cannot be explained by a single lesion, the progressive nature of the disease, and a history of exacerbations and remissions.

There are no definitive laboratory tests for MS, but the presence of increased immunoglobulins in the cerebral fluid without infection is considered strong evidence for the diagnosis. A CT scan is used to rule out tumors and show multiple brain abnormalities.

Treatment

There is no definitive treatment for MS. Some investigators consider adrenocorticotropin (ACTH) helpful during acute exacerbations, but long-term use of the drug does not alter the course of the disease. Use of corticosteroids has also been tried but with less success.

Dental Considerations

In some MS patients the trigeminal nerve is involved in the disease, and there may be paresthesia or anesthesia of any or all of the three divisions. Approximately 2% of MS patients develop trigeminal neuralgialike pain that is severe and lancinating, but there is no trigger zone. In time the pain becomes less severe but more continuous. The dentist should include MS in the differential diagnosis of facial or oral pain and numbness, especially when these symptoms are seen in young adults. Unnecessary extractions, surgery, and endodontic therapy have been performed when the true etiology of the symptoms is not dental but neurologic.

When a patient presents with orofacial pain or numbness with no local cause, take a careful review of systems, emphasizing a recent history of blurred vision, diplopia, and weakness or paresthesia of the extremities. Carefully examine the trigeminal nerve, checking the response of the nerve to sharp, dull, hot, and cold stimuli as well as to vibration. Also evaluate the other cranial nerves. If this screening history and examination is suggestive of a central nervous system lesion, refer the patient to a neurologist for final evaluation.

Severe facial pain secondary to MS have been treated successfully with carbamazepine (Tegretol). Patients who take this medication should have monthly hematologic evaluations because bone marrow suppression may result in some patients. Phenytoin has also been used with success. When medication proves inadequate, surgical sectioning of the nerve or alcohol injection has been helpful.

PARKINSON'S DISEASE

Parkinson's disease is a major cause of chronic disability in patients over 50 years of age. The best evidence available to date indicates that parkinsonism is caused by a depletion of the neurotransmitters, dopamine, and norepinephrine in the basal ganglia. Most cases are idiopathic, but some are caused by encephalitis, trauma, carbon monoxide intoxication, atherosclerosis, metal poisoning, or brain tumor. A form of drug-induced parkinsonism is caused by a reaction to phenothiazine derivatives. This latter form of the disease is caused by a drug-induced reduction of dopamine in the brain and disappears when use of the drug is stopped.

Clinical Manifestations

The three major clinical features of Parkinson's disease are rigidity, tremor, and akinesia (slowness in the initiation of movements). The onset of the disease is insidious. Mild stiffness of the muscles of the extremities and tremor of the hands are frequent early signs. The typical hand tremor is often called a *pill-rolling movement* and is caused by the movement of the thumb and fingers rubbing against one another. The stiffness slowly progresses until significant disability is noted by the patient. Walking becomes more difficult, and the patient develops a slow shuffling gait in a stooped position because of the inability to stand straight. Speech becomes slow owing to lack of muscle control (dysarthria), and as the disease progresses there is a decrease in all voluntary movements and an increase in tremor, which is prominent at rest. In

some patients the tremor may remain confined to the hands, but in others the arms and trunk may also be involved.

Akinesia is an important characteristic of the disease. Patients notice an inability to coordinate two movements. For example, a normal individual will be able to get out of a chair and begin walking across a room all in one motion. A patient with parkinsonism completes one motion before initiating another. Motions also tend to be jerky (cogwheel motion).

Treatment

Levodopa can cause dramatic reversal of the symptoms of Parkinson's disease and is the mainstay of treatment. Side-effects of levodopa such as nausea and vomiting can be minimized by taking a peripheral dopa decarboxylase inhibitor. Sinemet is a commonly used medication that contains both levodopa and the peripheral inhibitor. Mild forms of Parkinson's can be managed by anticholinergic drugs such as trihexyphenidyl (Artane), benztropine mesylate (Cogentin), or ethopropazine (Parsidol).

Oral Manifestations

Many signs of Parkinson's disease are found in the head and neck region. Rigidity of the facial muscles is common. This loss of flexibility gives the patient an expressionless or masklike face. The muscle rigidity also causes difficulty swallowing, resulting in drooling. Tremor of the tongue and mandible is also common, making speech and eating difficult for the patient and dental procedures difficult for the dentist. Sacks reported a case of Parkinson's disease with jaw tremors severe enough to cause repeated dislocation of the mandible.

Because levodopa has been used extensively in the management of Parkinson's disease, many of the oral signs seen are not related to the disease but to the drug. Abnormal involuntary movements of a choreic or athetoid nature may follow levodopa therapy and may be severe around the mouth. Patients exhibit purposeless chewing, grinding, and sucking movements that may be quite bizarre. The patient may thrust or shake his tongue and chew or suck vigorously when there is nothing in his mouth.

Sacks and associates studied 60 patients taking levodopa and noted abnormal oral movements in a majority of them. Some of the movements were forceful enough to cause flaring of the teeth and breaking of prostheses. Walter studied movement of teeth in a patient with involuntary oral movements from levodopa therapy. He treated this problem by the fabrication of a prosthesis adapted to the occlusal surfaces of the teeth. Night guards and other devices used to hold the teeth in place may also be helpful in some patients.

Dental Considerations

Because anxiety causes an increase in the tremors, sedation before dental treatment is helpful in minimizing them. Because the tremor is increased at rest, request the patient to concentrate on placing his tongue or jaw in a certain position that will help decrease tremors around the mouth, making dental treatment easier to perform.

MYASTHENIA GRAVIS

Myasthenia gravis (MG) is a disease characterized by easy fatigability of striated muscle secondary to a disorder at the neuromuscular junction. Acetylcholine normally transmits the impulse from nerve to muscle at the neuromuscular junction, and cholinesterase hydrolyzes acetylcholine. In patients with MG, autoantibodies are present that combine with the acetylcholine receptor sites at the neuromuscular junction, preventing proper transmission of nerve impulses to the muscle. The etiology of the autoantibodies is unknown, but other findings linking MG to autoimmunity include the incidence of thymoma in MG patients, the improvement of symptoms after thymectomy, the association of MG with other diseases involving abnormal immune phenomena such as pemphigus, pemphigoid, systemic lupus erythematosus, and rheumatoid arthritis. The disease occurs more frequently in women than in men particularly during the third and fourth decades of life.

Clinical Manifestations

The chief complaint of patients with MG is muscle weakness following exercise. The initial signs of this disease commonly occur in areas innervated by the cranial nerves, frequently the eye muscles. Thus, intermittent diplopia caused by weakness of the extraocular muscles or ptosis caused by weakness of the lid are common early signs of MG. In some patients the disease remains confined to the eye muscles, but in most cases it progresses to other cranial nerves as well as to the shoulders and limbs. MG follows an unpredictable course, and exacerbations and remissions occur frequently. In severe, advanced cases, respiratory difficulty arises.

The diagnosis is made on the basis of a history of intermittent muscle weakness. Inability to continue to blink the eyes voluntarily is highly suggestive of MG. The clinical diagnosis can be confirmed by dramatic improvement of the symptoms with the administration of parenteral neostigmine or the shorter-acting drug edrophonium chloride (Tensilon). Neostigmine antagonizes the effect of cholinesterase on acetylcholine, allowing for increased levels of this chemical at the neuromuscular junction.

Treatment

Symptoms of MG can be controlled by the use of anticholinesterases such as neostigmine (Prostigmin) or pyridostigmine bromide (Mestinon). In patients with more severe disease, remission may be obtained by thymectomy. In other cases, long-term corticosteroids and immunosuppressive drugs are necessary. Plasmapheresis has been of temporary value in patients with severe exacerbations of MG.

Oral Manifestations

Oral and facial signs are an important component of the clinical picture of MG. The facial muscles are commonly involved, giving the patient an immobile, expressionless appearance. This has led to the incorrect diagnosis of psychiatric disease in MG patients. Difficulty in chewing is another prominent symptom; patients whose muscles of mastication have been involved will be unable to finish chewing a bolus of food because of the easy fatigability of the muscles. It is essential to be aware that this may be an early sign of disease. The patient's masticatory muscles may become so tired that the mouth remains open following eating. An important indication of MG is a patient who must hold his jaws closed with his hand.

Weakness of the tongue and palatal muscles are also frequent clinical signs. Mason reported a case in which fluid entering the nose after drinking was the first sign of MG. This same patient also experienced fatigue of the masticatory muscles, requiring rest during chewing. When examining a patient with recent onset of difficulty in chewing or swallowing, be sure that MG is part of the differential diagnosis. Ask questions concerning diplopia, ptosis, or weakness of other muscles. If MG is suspected, refer the patient for further evaluation by a neurologist and for testing with cholinergic drugs.

Dental Considerations

When treating known MG patients, the dentist must be aware that a respiratory crisis may develop from the disease itself or from overmedication. If a patient is at risk for developing a respiratory crisis, dental treatment should be performed in a hospital where endotracheal intubation can be performed. The airway must be kept clear because aspiration may occur in patients whose swallowing muscles are involved. Adequate suction and use of a rubber dam is an aid in these cases.

The dentist should avoid prescribing drugs that may affect the neuromuscular junction, such as narcotics, tranquilizers, and barbiturates. Certain antibiotics including tetracycline, streptomycin, sulfonamides, and clindamycin may reduce neuromuscular activity and should be avoided.

MUSCULAR DYSTROPHY

Muscular dystrophy (MD) is a genetic disease characterized by muscle atrophy that causes severe progressive weakness. The primary biochemical defect has not been identified, but evidence is accumulating that implicates an enzymatic dysfunction at the muscle surface membrane.

Clinical Manifestations

MD is generally classified according to a combination of the mode of genetic transmission and clinical manifestations. Using these criteria, four major types of MD are as follows.

Duchenne's Pseudohypertrophic Dystrophy. Most cases of Duchenne's are inherited as a sex-linked recessive trait and are therefore seen only in males. There is a milder form of the disease inherited as an autosomal recessive trait, but this form is rare. Clinical manifestations begin during the first 3 years of life. Early signs begin as difficulty in walking, frequent falling, and inability to run. Symptoms progress as muscles continue to atrophy. Initially the atrophy is marked, although muscles may appear even larger than normal, primarily because of the fat deposition in the muscles.

At the end of the first decade of life, the child will be unable to walk and will be bedridden. Respiratory muscles will begin to be affected, and most patients are dead by 20 years of age. The muscles of the pelvis and femoral region are most severely affected by the Duchenne form of MD, but the muscles of the face, head, and neck are not involved. Elevation of the enzyme creatinine phosphokinase in serum is elevated in affected males as well as in femal carriers.

Facioscapulohumeral Dystrophy. This form of MD is inherited as an autosomal dominant trait and will affect both males and females. Symptoms do not usually begin until the second decade of life. It is not as universally devastating as the Duchenne form of MD, and some patients may live a normal life span with minimal physical disability. The muscles of the face and pectoral girdle are most severely involved, and characteristically these patients exhibit weakness of the arms, winging of the scapulae, and weakness of the muscles of the eyes and mouth.

Limb Girdle Dystrophy of Erb. This is inherited as an autosomal recessive trait. It affects both sexes and has its onset in the second and third decades of life. The weakness starts in either the shoulders or the pelvis, but will eventually spread to both. This is characteristically a slowly progressing form of MD. Facial muscles are not involved.

Myotonic Dystrophy. This form of the disease has its onset during adult life and is inherited as an autosomal dominant trait. The most severe involvement occurs in the muscles of the head and neck as well as the distal extremities. Myotonia is the persistence of contraction of muscles, and in this form of MD the patient is unable to relax his muscle after contraction. This can be best observed in the forearm, thumb, and tongue. Wasting of muscles and subsequent weakness are as prominent as in other forms of MD . Involvement of the facial muscles and hands is especially striking. Myotonic dystrophy is also associated with testicular atrophy, frontal baldness and cataracts.

Treatment

All forms of MD are incurable, and no satisfactory method of retarding the muscle atrophy exists. Physical therapy may help prolong use of specific muscle groups, but the ultimate outcome in severe forms of the disease is grave.

Oral Manifestations

Oral and facial signs are prominent in the facioscapulohumeral and myotonic forms of MD. Patients with the myotonic-type disease develop severe atrophy of the sternomastoid muscles with a resultant difficulty in the ability to turn the head. The muscles of facial expression and mastication are also commonly affected, such that the patient has difficulty chewing or pursing his lips. The tongue in the myotonic form of disease can be forced into continuous contraction by placing a tongue blade under the tongue and striking the blade with a percussion hammer. Weakness of the facial muscles and enlargement of the tongue caused by fatty deposits has been noted by several authors.

Dental Considerations

Occlusal abnormalities have been reported in MD. This is thought to result from the lack of proper muscle tension to keep the teeth properly aligned in the dental arch. If the tongue is enlarged and the facial muscles are weak, the teeth will be pushed out. Thayer reported severe open bite and the development of diastemata in patients with MD. White measured the force of the facial muscles and tongue with a pressure gauge and found a 50% reduction in cheek muscle efficiency, but only a 10% reduction in efficiency of tongue muscles. This would account for the tendency of the teeth to be pushed outward. Friedman and colleagues reported a case of an MD patient with a constricted dental arch.

Brown and Losch studied five children with MD; all five had deformities of the dental arch, and four of the five had macroglossia. Proffit as well as Ardran reported anterior open bite in patients with MD. Temporomandibular joint dysfunction has also been described in MD patients. Gold studied 15 patients with myotonic dystrophy; three had significant joint disability, three others had minor symptoms. The major symptoms included frequent dislocations, inability to chew, and locking and clicking of the jaws.

BIBLIOGRAPHY

Cerebrovascular Diseases

Anderson CF: Modified dental chair for patients in wheelchairs. J Am Dent Assoc 74:1250, 1967

Fisher CM, Mohr JP, Adams RD: Cerebrovascular diseases. In Harrison's Principles of Internal Medicine, 6th ed. New York, McGraw-Hill, 1970

McCarthy FM: Cardiovascular and other medical emergencies in the dental office. Dent Clin North Am p 711, November, 1965

McDowell FH: Cerebrovascular diseases. In Beeson PB, McDermott W (eds): Textbook of Medicine, 14th ed. Philadelphia, WB Saunders, 1975

Myers DE, Davis S, Barker JN: Evaluation of lingual artery hemodynamics in stroke patients using Doppler ultrasound. Oral Surg 51:252, 1981

Selley WG: Dental help for stroke patients. Br Dent J 143:409, 1977

Zafran JN, Zayon GM: Prosthodontics and the stoke patient. J Am Den Assoc 74:1250, 1967

Epilepsy

Angelopoulos AP: Diphenylhydantoin gingival hyperplasia—A clinicopathological review 1. Incidence, clinical features, histopathology. J Can Dent Assoc 41:103, 1975

Angelopoulos AP: A clinicopathological review, diphenylhydantoin gingival hyperplasia 2. Aetiology, pathogenesis, differential diagnosis, and treatment. J Can Dent Assoc 41:275, 1975

Angelopoulos AP, Goaz PW: Incidence of diphenylhydantoin gingival hyperplasia. Oral Surg 34:898, 1972

Conard GJ et al: Levels of 5,5-diphenylhydantoin and its major metabolite in human serum, saliva and hyperplastic gingiva. J Dent Res 53:1323, 1974

Dent CE et al: Osteomalacia with long term anticonvulsant therapy in epilepsy. Br M J 4:69, 1970

Dreyer WP, Thomas CJ: Diphenylhydantoinate induced hyperplasia of the masticatory mucosa in an edentulous epileptic patient. Oral Surg 45:70l, 1978

Evans DEN: Anaesthesia and the epileptic patient—A review. Anesthesia 30:34, 1975

Hall WB: Dilantin hyperplasia: a preventable lesion. J Periodont Res 4:36, 1969

Harris M, Goldhaber P: Root abnormalities in epileptics and the inhibition of parathyroid hormone induced bone resorption by diphenylhydantoin in tissue culture. Arch Oral Biol 19:981, 1974

Hawkins CF, Meynell MJ: Megaloblastic anaemia due to phenylhydantoin sodium. Lancet 2:737, 1954

Katten KR: Calvarial thickening after dilantin medication. Am J Roentgenol Radium Ther Nucl Med 110:102, 1970

Katten KR: Thickening of the heel pad associated with long term dilantin therapy. Am J Roentgenol Radium Ther Nucl Med 124:52, 1975

Lefebrose EB et al: Coarse facies, calvarial thickening and hypophosphatasia associated with long term anticonvulsant therapy. N Engl J Med 286:1301, 1972

Nuki K, Cooper SH: The role of inflammation in the pathogenesis of gingival enlargement during the administration of diphenylhydantoin sodium in cats. J Periodontol Res 7:102, 1972

Panuska HJ et al: The effect of anticonvulsant drugs upon the gingiva—A series of analyses of 1048 patients. J Periodontol 32:15, 1961

Reynolds NC, Kirkham DB: Therapeutic alternatives in phenyltoin-induced gingival hyperplasia. J Periodontol 51:516, 1980

Stein GM, Lewis H: Oral changes in a folic acid deficient patient precipitated by anticonvulsant drug therapy. J Periodontol 44:645, 1973

Multiple Sclerosis

Friedlander AH, Zeff S: Atypical trigeminal neuralgia in patient with multiple sclerosis. J Oral Surg 32:30l, 1974

Millar JHD, Allison RS: Multiple sclerosis—A disease acquired in childhood. Springfield, IL, Charles C Thomas, 1971

Miller J et al: Multiple sclerosis: Trials of maintenance treatment with prednisone and soluble aspirin. Lancent 1:27, 1961

Rose AS et al: Cooperative study in the evaluation of therapy in multiple sclerosis, ACTH vs placebo in acute exacerbations. Neurology 18:1, 1968

Tweedle JA, Morrissey JB, Rankow RM: Mistaken TMJ Pathology in unrecognized multiple sclerosis: Report of a case. J Oral Surg 28:785, 1970

Parkinson's Disease

Merrill RG: Habitual subluxation and recurrent dislocation in a patient with Parkinson's disease. J Oral Surg 26:473, 1968

Sacks OW et al: Abnormal mouth—Movements and oral damage associated with L-DOPA treatment. Ann Dent 29:130, 1970

Walter DC, Barbeau A: Parkinson's disease—the effect of levodopa therapy on the dentition—report of a case. J Am Dent Assoc 85:133, 1972

Myasthenia Gravis

Bottomley WK, Terezhalmy GT: Management of patients with myasthenia gravis who require maxillary dentures. J Prosthet Dent 38:609, 1977

Gallager DM, Erickson KL, Genkins G: Current concepts in the surgical treatment of patients with myasthenia gravis. J Oral Surg 39:30, 1981

Goldstein G: The thymus and neuromuscular function. Lancet 2:119, 1968

Havard CWH: Progress in myasthenia gravis. Br Med J 3:437, 1973

Mason DK: Oral aspects of myasthenia gravis. Dent Pract 15:23, 1964

Perlo VP et al: Myasthenia gravis: Evaluation of treatment in 1,355 patients. Neurology 16:43l, 1966

Steinhauser EW, Lines PA: Correction of severe open-bite associated with muscular disease. Oral Surg 39:509, 1975

Muscular Dystrophy

Ardran GM, Hamilton A, Kemp FH: Enlargement of the tongue and changes in the jaws with muscular dystrophy. Clin Radiol 24:359, 1973

Brown JC, Losch PK: Dental occlusion in patients with muscular dystrophy. Am J Orthodont 25:1040, 1939

Duborowitz M: Progressive muscular dystrophy in childhood. M.D. Thesis. University of Capetown, 1960

Friedman RD, Joe J, Bodak GLZ: Myotonic dystrophy: Report of a case. Oral Surg 50:229, 1980

Gold GN: Temporomandibular joint dysfunction in myotonic dystrophy. Neurology 16:212, 1966

Greene HJ, Doyles BL: Alleviating respiratory problems in a muscular dystrophy patient. J Prosthet Dent 20:565, 1968

Proffit WR, Gamble JW, Christiansen RL: Generalized muscular weakness with severe anterior open-bite. Am J Orthodont 54:104, 1968

Thayer HH, Crenshaw J: Oral manifestations of myotonic muscular dystrophy: Report of a case. J Am Dent Assoc 72:1405, 1966

Weitzner S: Pathosis of the tongue in oculopharyngeal muscular dystrophy. Oral Surg 28:613, 1969

White RA, Sackler AM: Effect of progressive muscular dystrophy on occlusion. J Am Dent Assoc 49:449, 1954

28

Sexually Transmitted Diseases

VERNON J. BRIGHTMAN

865

INTRODUCTION

The extended contact and friction between skin and mucosal surfaces, and the transfer of oral and genital secretions that can occur during sexual intercourse provide many opportunities for transmission of infectious material. Fastidious microorganisms that would not survive less direct methods of transmission (*e.g.*, *Neisseria gonorrhoeae*, *Treponema pallidum*, herpes simplex), and those microorganisms commonly acquired by other routes (*e.g.*, hepatitis B, *Candida*, warts and some viral upper respiratory and gastrointestinal infectious agents) are known to be transmitted in this way. The term *sexually transmitted disease** (STD) is currently used to describe those infections acquired almost exclusively through sexual intercourse, and those for which sexual transmission is frequent enough to be considered a public health problem. The list of sexually transmitted diseases currently includes those traditionally described as venereal diseases (syphilis, gonorrhea, chancroid, lymphogranuloma venereum and granuloma inguinale), as well as those that have only more recently been included in literature on sexually transmitted disease because of improved methods of culturing and identification (*e.g.* hepatitis B, herpes simplex type 2, *Chlamydia* and mycoplasma). The term *venereal disease (VD)* has largely disappeared from both the lay press and scientific literature, partly because of intentional efforts to separate sexually acquired infections from any pejorative or illicit connotation that might inhibit discussion of these diseases by patients, clinicians and teachers. The term VD is also used less frequently because the more comprehensive term, sexually transmitted disease (STD), better describes the broad range of the current epidemiologic picture of sexually acquired infections.*

Sexually transmitted infections are of professional concern to the dentist because of their oral manifestations, and because inadvertent contact between the dentist's fingers and organisms present in a patient's blood and saliva could conceivably lead to *nonvenereal infection of the dentist*, where the organisms could enter his tissues by percutaneous or mucosal routes. Of particular dental interest are those sexually transmitted diseases in which the oropharynx is colonized by the infectious agent, either with or without development of obvious oral lesions, and those in which the infectious agent is found in mixed saliva as a consequence of the bacteremia or viremia accompanying the infection. The hazard to the dentist from this source varies considerably depending on the sexually transmitted disease itself, the stage of the infection, and the nature of the contact (*e.g.* percutaneous inoculation by a contaminated sharp instrument, versus contamination of an intact skin surface). There is no doubt that hepatitis B and herpes simplex, for example, can be transmitted in this way from an infectious agent in the patient's saliva.

Until recently, literature dealing with nonvenereal transmission in the dental office, of organisms commonly associated with sexually transmitted disease was limited to a number of 1930's publications concerned with inadvertent syphilitic infections of the hands acquired through professional activities (referred to as syphilis innocentum or insontium). With the appearance of more effective treatments for syphilis in the 1940's, these non-venereally acquired infections almost disappeared, although screening for syphilis by questionnaire and laboratory tests was maintained in many dental clinics and innocently acquired venereal disease was still perceived as a hazard for the careless oral diagnostician. In the last 20 years, changes in the observed patterns of sexually transmitted diseases have given rise to a resurgence of interest in non-venereal transmission of these infections. Experts now have a better appreciation of actual hazards than they did in the decades preceding 1960. Two factors have contributed to this new interest: a widely publicized epidemic of sexually transmitted disease and the recognition that several different sexually transmitted diseases, including syphilis, may be associated with a carrier state, during which time the infectious agents of these diseases are present in the oropharynx. The dentist now has good rea-

* Since a number of sexually transmitted diseases may also be transmitted by non-venereal contact, the term *sexually transmissible disease* is a more accurate name for the diseases included under the designation STD, and is gradually appearing in the literature.

son to be interested in gonorrhea, hepatitis B and herpes, as well as syphilis. There is now good justification for including questions about these diseases in the medical questionnaires and health evaluations that the dentist routinely completes on all patients, since oropharyngeal involvement may occur in all of these infections.

This chapter begins with a section describing the current epidemiologic patterns of sexually transmitted diseases, the ranges of sexually transmitted infections and the epidemic natures of certain of these infections at this time. The pathologic and clinical features of each of these infections are briefly summarized in the following section as a necessary background for understanding their oral manifestations and associated infectious hazards. The remainder of the chapter deals specifically with the oral lesions and management of the sexually transmitted diseases with well-established oropharyngeal involvement (gonorrhea, condyloma acuminatum, herpes simplex, molluscum contagiosum, syphilis and hepatitis B, the acquired immune deficiency syndrome, and lymphogranuloma venereum), and concludes with a consideration of the hazards to the dentist who may be providing dental care for patients with particular sexually transmitted diseases. Diseases caused by several of the agents associated with sexually transmitted diseases, but which are also commonly transmitted nonvenereally, are described in detail elsewhere in this textbook (*e.g.* hepatitis B in Chapter 20, herpes simplex in Chapter 5, candidiasis in Chapter 6, and warts and molluscum contagiosum in Chapter 8). Discussion of these particular infections in this chapter is therefore restricted to topics associated with their sexual transmission and their specific hazards during dental treatment.

EPIDEMIOLOGIC FEATURES OF THE SEXUALLY TRANSMITTED DISEASES

Frequency of the More Common Sexually Transmitted Diseases

As a result of changes in the methods used to identify and report sexually transmitted disease, accurate figures allowing for a comparison of the prevalence of different types of sexually transmitted diseases over several decades are not generally available. It is also acknowledged that the dismantling of the system of venereal disease clinics and laboratories, which occurred in the United States in the years following the introduction of penicillin owing to a reduction in federal support for treatment of diseases commonly believed to be "wiped out," led to serious gaps in the United States' statistics on the prevalence of sexually transmitted diseases. Data from England, where over 90% of all new known cases of sexually transmitted disease have been treated in a coordinated system of clinics throughout the country for over 40 years; and from Scandinavia, where STD testing is done in centralized laboratories, are usually accepted as more accurate. Using data from these sources, the comparative frequency of the more common sexually transmitted diseases is illustrated in Table 28-1.

Non-specific genital infection (non-gonococcal urethritis, NGU), which heads the list in Table 28-1 as the most common sexually transmitted disease reported in England, is not a reportable condition in the United States, but is believed to be this country's and other western countries' most common sexually transmitted disease. The frequency of gonorrhea approaches that of non-specific genital infection. At a rate of 200 million new cases reported annually in the world (208, and 124 cases per 100,000 population in England and the United States, respectively), gonorrhea is currently considered to be the most important sexually transmitted disease, and a disease of epidemic proportions. The rates for genital candidiasis, trichomoniasis, and venereal warts are less than, but of a similar order of magnitude to, the rate for gonorrhea. Like non-specific genital infection, genital candidiasis and trichomoniasis have no recognized venereally acquired oropharyngeal component. Genital warts, which, by contrast, are difficult to distinguish biologically from skin, lip and oropharyngeal warts (except for the more obvious venereal etiology and usually more florid appearance of genital warts on the genital area) are approximately one half as frequent as gonorrhea. Genital herpes, pubic lice ("crabs"), and syphilis constitute the next most prevalent group, with frequencies only one-ninth

Table 28-1. Relative Frequency of the Sexually Transmitted Diseases. Reported Cases in England in 1972 and 1978.*

SEXUALLY TRANSMITTED DISEASE	NUMBER OF REPORTED CASES	
	1972[†]	1978[‡]
Non-specific genital infection	76,916	97,062
Gonorrhea	53,439	57,501
Candidiasis	29,844	38,465
Trichomoniasis	19,100	19,943
Genital warts	15,820	23,332
Genital herpes	4,380	7,992
Pediculosis pubis	4,099	6,206
Syphilis	2,965	6,084
Scabies	2,771	2,237
Other treponemal diseases	853	1,140
Molluscum contagiosum	634	933
Lymphogranuloma venereum	59	27
Chancroid	49	49
Granuloma inguinale	5	14

* Population of England in 1972 and 1978 was approximately 46 million people. Patients who were treated in general or in private practices or in antenatal and gynecology clinics are not included in the figures in this table.

[†] (Data from Catterall RD: The situation of gonococcal and non-gonococcal infections in the United Kingdom. In Danielsson D, *et al* (eds) Genital Infections and Their Complications, Proc Wellcome Fdn. Sympos. Stockholm, Sweden Oct 9-11, 1974; Almquist and Wiskell Pubs. Stockholm, Sweden 1975).

[‡] (Data from Sexually Transmitted Diseases. Extract from the Annual Report of the Chief Medical Officer of the Dept. Health & Social Services for the year 1978. Br J Ven Dis 56:178, 1980) (Courtesy Almquist and Wiskell, Int Pubs. Stockholm, Sweden; and Br Med Assoc, London)

to one-sixteenth of those for gonorrhea and non-specific genital infections. Other miscellaneous infections, including the three classic "minor" venereal diseases—chancroid, lymphogranuloma venereum, and granuloma inguinale, other treponemal diseases (yaws), and two superficial dermatologic infections—scabies and molluscum contagiosum, complete the list, but with rather low frequencies. The great difference in the frequency for gonorrhea and syphilis should be noted: syphilis is approximately one-tenth as frequent as gonorrhea and now a relatively rare disease except in urban populations. A number of other sexually transmitted diseases are also more prevalent than syphilis.

Hepatitis B has been considered a sexually transmitted disease only in recent years, and statistics describing the proportion of cases that are sexually acquired as opposed to those acquired from parenteral drug abuse, or associated with administration of contaminated blood products or renal dialysis, are

not generally available. Hepatitis B infection, like genital herpes, gonorrhea, syphilis and the recently described aquired immune deficiency syndrome has been described as a prevalent sexually transmitted disease among male homosexuals. Each of these infections is also sexually transmitted by heterosexuals, and the correlation between sexual behavior and hepatitis B (as well as other sexually transmitted diseases) is more accurately an illustration of frequency, number and promiscuity of sexual partners rather than sexual preference. Even so, studies of sexually transmitted disease in male homosexuals have recently added an even broader range of sexually acquired infections (*e.g.*, enteric microorganisms such as *Cryptosporidium*, *Isospora*, *Giardia*, and *Entamoeba*, and *Shigella*) to the list of sexually transmitted diseases. As a result, sexually transmitted diseases in male homosexual communities have received considerable attention in the literature over the last decade.

Gonorrhea, genital herpes, hepatitis B and the acquired immune deficiency syndrome, which is largely confined to male homosexuals and one or two other special high-risk groups, are currently considered to be the most serious problems that a promiscuous individual can acquire, based upon either the frequency of the infection, or the severity of its complications. Gonorrhea and genital herpes pose threats to the individual's reproductive system, threats of morbidity from systemic spread of the infection in gonorrhea, acute pain, discomfort, limitation of sexual activity (in the case of genital herpes), and the risk of transmission of infection to the newborn child. Antibiotic treatment is now available for both gonorrhea and primary genital herpes but, in the former disease, may fail to eradicate chronic infection. Hepatitis B infection is associated with a 10% to 12% mortality rate in the United States, and a proportion of infected individuals may become chronic carriers. While a vaccine for prevention of hepatitis B is now available, there is still no practical way of curing the chronic carrier. The acquired immune deficiency syndrome has an even higher mortality rate and has, as yet, no identified etiologic agent.

The Sexually Transmitted Disease Epidemic

The diminishing importance of syphilis in relation to gonorrhea over the last 40 years is well illustrated in Figure 28-1, which shows the changes in annual rates for syphilis and gonorrhea over this period. This graph also provides the basis for recognizing an epidemic of gonorrhea commencing in the early 1960's and far surpassing the previous epidemic of the Second World War. This epidemic has been well publicized in both lay and professional literature, and supporting data are available from England and Scandinavia as well. A similiar increase in cases has probably also occurred worldwide. An increase in the number of cases of gonorrhea is the most prominent feature of this epidemic, but an increased prevalence of newer sexually transmitted diseases, such as genital herpes (quoted for females by one author as one case for every three cases of gonorrhea)

and hepatitis B, has also contributed significantly to the extent of the problem. Other features of the epidemic are the increased number of cases in the younger age group (50% under 24 years of age in 1956, 70% in 1974); proportionately higher prevalence rates in urban areas, which account for over 50% of cases; and the recognition of extremely high prevalence rates among special groups, such as male homosexual communities.

While the reality of this epidemic is not to be doubted, several factors have contributed to its apparent magnitude in the United States. Based on a belief that sexually transmitted diseases, and gonorrhea in particular, had been conquered by penicillin, special "VD" treatment facilities were discontinued, and case reporting in the United States fell off. By the late 1950's the number of reported cases and rates dropped to an all-time low, no doubt contributing to the steepness of the curve in the 1960's and 1970's when better surveillance methods were reinstituted. In the 1970's, a program of screening cultures for gonorrhea in asymptomatic females was introduced that also produced an increase in the number of reported cases, particularly for women attending clinics. Other factors that potentially may have affected the prevalence of gonorrhea and other sexually transmitted diseases, and contributed to the current epidemic are: development of antibiotic-resistant strains of $N. gonorrhoeae$, sexual promiscuity and changing methods of contraception, emergence of homosexual communities in urban areas, and a more casual attitude to sexually transmitted diseases in an era when effective antibiotic therapy of the traditional venereal diseases is readily available.

With few exceptions, this epidemic continues. The total number of reported cases of gonorrhea in the United States has stabilized at about a million cases annually since 1976, and a decrease in the number of cases of gonorrhea has been observed in Scandinavia since the middle 1970's. This decrease has been tentatively associated with more widespread use of condoms following a campaign that included attractive packaging and sales promotion of these products, as well as education of the public about their value in sex-

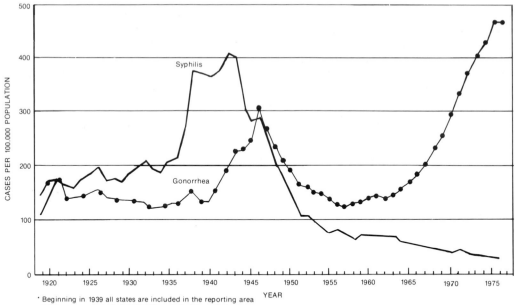

* Beginning in 1939 all states are included in the reporting area
(Military cases included 1919-1940 excluded thereafter)
** 1919-1940 Fiscal years. Twelve month period ending June 30 of year specified 1919-1940
1941-1976 calendar years

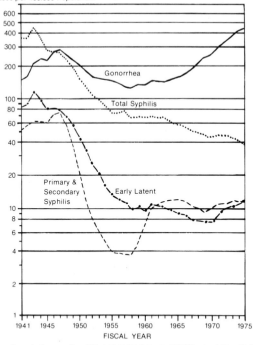

Reported cases of syphilis and gonorrhea per 100.000 population: United States. fiscal years 1941-1975.

Fig.28-1 (A & B) (A) Annual reported cases of gonorrhea and all stages of syphilis in the United States between 1919 and 1976, per 100,000 population. (From Fuerst R: Frobischer and Fuerst's Microbiology in Health and Disease, 14th ed, Philadelphia, W.B. Saunders, 1978. Reprinted from Morb Mort Wkly Rep 1975 Annual Supplement) (B) Annual reported cases of gonorrhea and syphilis (total and by stages) in the United States between 1941 and 1975, per 100,000 population. (From Arthes FG: Some aspects of the epidemiology of venereal diseases. In Castelazo-Ayala L and MacGregor C (eds): Gynecology and Obstetrics, Proc VIII World Congress of Gynecology and Obstetrics, Mexico City, 1976. Courtesy of Excerpta Med., Amsterdam, 1977)

ual hygiene. It is stated that such educational programs have been less effective in the United States, although it is interesting to speculate whether more prominent and attractive marketing of condoms as contraceptives, which has occurred in the United States in recent years, may have a similar effect.

The introduction in the United States of oral contraceptives and intrauterine devices (IUD's) in the early 1960's displaced the use of the condom and diaphragm (use of these methods dropped from a quoted figure of 64% in 1955 to 16% or less in 1970) and paralleled the increase in the number of cases of venereal disease. Increased promiscuity is often blamed on the availability of oral contraceptives and intercourse between unmarried partners is believed to have increased significantly for both men and women in the last two decades. No clear association between use of oral contraceptives or promiscuity (as defined by the number of sex partners per unit time) in the general population and the risk of acquiring one of the major sexually transmitted diseases (gonorrhea) has been found. Other factors, such as the increased urban population, and the ease of travelling, both of which favor the growth of special groups with high prevalence rates, are probably also important determinants of the epidemic.

High Risk Groups, Recidivisim and Multiple Sexually Transmitted Infections

The concept, *high risk group* has always been an important aspect of the epidemiology of sexually transmitted disease whether it was the prostitute, seaman, military personnel, commercial traveler, traveling entertainer, or conference attendee who was so identified. Recognition of a patient as a member of a "high risk group" is an important item in a diagnostic evaluation for suspected sexually transmitted disease and will be stressed again in the section dealing with oropharyngeal infection.

In recent years, with increased public awareness of homosexuality, and the development of "gay" communities, various sex-

ually transmitted diseases have been shown to be particularly prevalent among male homosexuals, and they currently constitute the most discussed "high risk group"in the sexually transmitted disease literature. Gonorrhea, primary and secondary syphilis, hepatitis B, genital herpes, genital warts and the acquired immune deficiency syndrome have been identified as special problems in this high risk group, based not only on the percentage of patients seeking treatment for sexually transmitted disease (who give a history of homosexual practices), but also on the frequency of both symptomatic and asymptomatic sexually transmitted disease among the users of "gay" establishments.

The basic factors leading to inclusion in a high risk group are reported to be multiple sex contacts, inability to discriminate in the choice of sex partners, failure to take precautions, and the frequency of repetition of the contact that carries the risk of infection. *Recidivism,* or repeated infection, is an important feature of "high risk groups" and many studies of this phenomenon emphasize that treatment of an episode of sexually transmitted infection in a promiscuous individual is no guarantee that repeated episodes will not occur. One study in the United States demonstrated that gonorrhea occurred more than once in 23% of patients treated for sexually transmitted disease, and that "recidivists" accounted for 48% of all cases of gonorrhea reported. Infection with one sexually transmitted disease also does not preclude coexisting or subsequent infection with other sexually transmitted disease agents, and numerous case reports describe patients whose second sexually transmitted disease would have been missed if a specific search had not been made for it, despite the prominence of clinical findings suggesting an alternate diagnosis.

High risk groups have also been identified for hepatitis B infections and for the acquired immune deficiency syndrome, and are used in determining which groups of patients should be screened more carefully for markers of hepatitis B infection in the one case, and as supporting data for a diagnosis of the acquired immune deficiency syndrome in the other.

PATHOLOGIC AND CLINICAL FEATURES OF THE SEXUALLY TRANSMITTED DISEASES

A list of the sexually transmitted diseases discussed in this section and their associated etiologic agents is provided in Table 28-2.

Nonspecific Urethritis

Nonspecific urethritis (NSU) describes a somewhat imprecise group of infections manifesting themselves as genital discharges in both sexes, from which gonorrhea, candidiasis, trichomoniasis, and some other more recently identifiable causes have been excluded. This group of infections is also referred to as non-gonococcal urethritis (NGU) or non-specific genital infection. Pathologically, it includes non-specific infections of the urethra (including Reiter's syndrome), rectum, vagina and/or uterine cervix. With the availability of routine laboratory isolation and sero-diagnostic procedures for certain groups of fastidious microorganisms found in the urogenital tract, an increasing number of

Table 28-2. Etiologic Agents of the More Common Sexually Transmitted Diseases

DISEASE	ETIOLOGIC AGENT(S)
Non-specific urethritis (non-gonococcal urethritis, post-gonococcal urethritis, non-specific genital infection, Reiter's syndrome)	*Ureaplasma urealyticum* (= T strain *Mycoplasma*) *Chlamydia trachomatis*
Gonorrhea	*Neisseria gonorrhoeae*
Genital candidiasis	*Candida* (*Monilia*) sp.
Genital warts (condyloma acuminatum)	Papilloma (warts) virus
Oropharyngeal herpes simplex Genital herpes simplex	Herpes simplex virus types 1 & 2
Pediculosis pubis Scabies Molluscum contagiosum	*Phthirus pubis* *Acarus* (*Sarcoptes*) *scabiei* Virus of molluscum contagiosum
Acquired & congenital syphilis Yaws Pinta Endemic syphilis (bejel)	*Treponema pallidum* "*Treponema pertenue*"* "*Treponema carateum*"* *Treponema pallidum*
Hepatitis B Cytomegalic inclusion body disease Infectious mononucleosis & other EB virus infections	Hepatitis B virus Cytomegalovirus Epstein-Barr (EB) virus
The acquired immune deficiency syndrome[†]	(?) Retrovirus (HTLV)
Granuloma inguinale Lymphogranuloma venereum Chancroid	*Donovania granulomatis* *Chlamydia* (LGV strain) *Hemophilus ducreyi*

* Microbiologically indistinguishable from *T. pallidum*. Yaws, pinta and bejel are transmitted non-venereally.

[†] Opportunistic infections with a variety of bacterial, fungal, protozoal, and viral agents are a prominent feature of this syndrome. Proof of an infectious etiology and specific identification of a causative agent are both lacking at this time.

cases of non-specific urethritis have been shown to be associated with either *Ureaplasma urealyticum* (previously referred to as T-strain or tiny *Mycoplasma* of the urogenital tract, see Figure 28-2) or *Chlamydia trachomatis* (also referred to as the TRIC or trachoma-inclusion conjunctivitis agents).

Non-specific urethritis occurs more commonly than gonorrhea and affects males and females equally. Gonorrhea and non-specific urethritis may be acquired simultaneously, with the latter infection not being recognized until after penicillin treatment has freed the urogenital discharge of *Neisseria*. *Chlamydia* and *Mycoplasma sp.* are resistant to penicillin and tetracycline respectively, and account for many of the infections previously described as postgonococcal urethritis. Tetracycline-responsive *Chlamydia trachomatis* is said to be responsible for 30% to 60% of cases of non-specific urethritis, and *Ureaplasma urealyticum* for 10% to 30%. The majority of cases of non-specific urethritis and proctitis are cured by one week of treatment with adequate doses of tetracycline hydrochloride, although patients with *Chlamydia*-negative, non-specific urethritis have a high relapse rate that requires additional and usually different antibiotic treatment. Eradication of non-specific vaginitis and cervicitis may require systemic as well as local antibiotic therapy.

Fewer than 1% of patients with non-specific urethritis develop symptoms of *Reiter's syndrome,* characterized by arthritis, sacroiliitis, conjunctivitis, balanitis (redness of the gland penis) and thickened skin on the soles of the hands and feet (keratitis blenorrhagica). A markedly raised erythrocyte sedimentation rate is common, and less frequently there may also be electrocardiographic abnormalities and oral ulcerations and psoriasiform lesions (geographic tongue-like lesions or circinate stomatitis). Reiter's syndrome must be distinguished from gonococcal arthritis and disseminated gonococcal dermatitis syndrome *(q.v.),* in which oral lesions are uncommon. While negative cultures for *N. gonorrhoeae* will rule out the possibility of gonococcal infection, there is no specific test for Reiter's syndrome, except perhaps for the presence of the HLA type 127 tissue antigen. Reiter's syndrome appears to occur almost exclusively in patients with this particular inherited tissue antigen. The so-called Reiter's treponeme, a laboratory strain of spirochetes that was used in the Reiter-protein-complement-fixation test (RPCF) for syphilis, is unrelated to Reiter's syndrome and the RPCF test is of no diagnostic value in this condition.

While other strains of *Mycoplasma* and bacterial L-forms (amorphous bacterial species without cell walls produced by treatment with penicillin, and which may be difficult at times to distinguish from *Mycoplasma*) constitute part of the normal oral bacterial flora (see Figure 28-2), there is no convincing evidence that these organisms, or *Ureaplasma* and *Chlamydia,* are associated with oral infection or oral lesions. The contention that recurrent aphthous ulcers are due to L-forms of *Streptococcus sanguis* still lacks adequate proof, and evidence previously presented to support this belief can equally well be interpreted as contamination of the oral ulcers by the normal oral flora. The etiology of oral ulcers and oral psoriasiform lesions in Reiter's syndrome is also unexplained. Specific therapy, other than the administration of antibiotics and nonsteroidal antirheumatic drugs prescribed for the systemic symptoms, and topical oral analgesics for relief of ulcer pain, is not available.

There is no known infectious hazard associated with the oropharyngeal secretions of patients with Reiter's syndrome, whether oral lesions are present or not. Antibiotic treatment provided for the systemic component of Reiter's syndrome should also usually eliminate concern about other concomitant sexually transmitted infections.

Gonorrhea (see Fig. 28-3)

Gonorrhea is an almost exclusively sexually transmitted infection caused by a gram-negative intracellularly located diplococcus, *Neisseria gonorrhoeae.* [Transmission of the infectious agent to infants born of mothers with gonococcal infection may occasionally result in inflammation of the ocular conjunctiva *(ophthalmia neonatorum)* or more rarely disseminated infection with septicemia. The prevalence of ophthalmia neonatorum is now extremely low owing to the standard practice of instilling 1% silver nitrate or an antibiotic

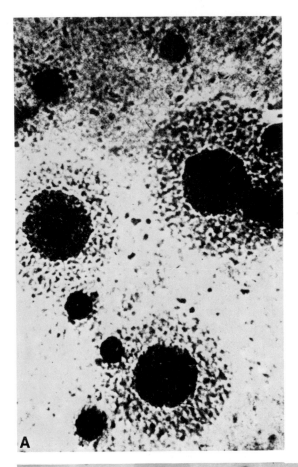

Fig. 28-2 (A & B) *Mycoplasma* appears on artificial media. (A) Colonies of *M. hominis* (large 'fried eggs') and T-strain *Mycoplasma* (small dark urease positive colonies), also referred to as *Ureaplasma urealyticum,* are isolated from the human urogenital tract. (A) shows a significantly higher magnification than (B). (From Mårdh PA In Danielsson D et al (eds): Genital Infections and Their Complications. Proceeding of the Wellcome Foundation Symposium, Stockholm, Oct. 9-11, 1974. Courtesy of the Wellcome Foundation, Ltd. Sweden) (B) Colonies of *Mycoplasma* species from filtered human saliva are isolated on an antibiotic free medium. No pathogenic role has been identified for oral *Mycoplasma*. (From Brightman VJ et al: Isolation of oral PPLO in the absence of known cell-wall inhibitors (abstr 130:68). Proc. Int. Assoc. Dent. Res. 45th Annual Meeting, Washington, DC, 1967)

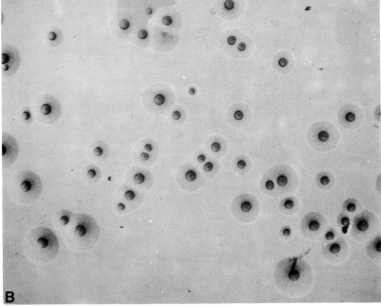

Fig. 28-3 Reported cases of gonorrhea epidemic in the United States between 1965 and 1978. (From Wiesner PJ and Thompson SE: Gonococcal diseases. Disease-a-Month 26:7, 1980; Courtesy Year Book Medical Publs Inc., Chicago, IL 60601)

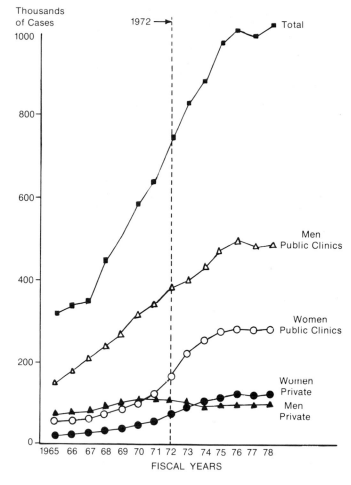

solution into the eyes of the neonate in the delivery room.]

In the adult, the most important primary sites of infection are the urethra, rectum and oropharynx, in each case owing to the direct involvement of the particular mucous membrane in sexual contact. Infection may be uncomplicated, in which case the microorganisms are restricted to the lower urogenital tract or other involved mucous membrane, or complicated by local spread within the urogenital tract, pelvic inflammatory disease in the female, or systemic involvement (pustular or hemorrhagic skin rashes, arthritis, iritis, and rarely septicemia with gonococcal endocarditis and meningitis).

The classic presenting symptom of gonorrhea is a profuse purulent urethral discharge, but urethral, rectal and oropharyngeal infections are often asymptomatic at the time they are recognized, and a diagnosis can only be made by means of a stained smear (for a presumptive diagnosis only, in the case of urogenital and rectal, but *not* oropharyngeal infections) or a culture inoculated directly from the particular mucous membrane involved. Asymptomatic infection is considered to be more common in females than in males. There is still no satisfactory blood test for diagnosing gonorrhea despite extensive recent work on development of a serologic test based on the small external antigenic protein threads (pili) on the gonococcus, which apparently secures its attachment to the columnar epithelium of the urogenital tract and oropharynx.

Owing to the frequency with which more than one sexually transmitted disease is acquired simultaneously, it is customary to test patients with confirmed gonorrhea for evidence of other infections, such as syphilis, hepatitis B, trichomoniasis, and even herpes simplex (in the female), when facilities are available.

Complications of Infection in the Adult

The *symptoms of uncomplicated gonorrhea* may on occasion subside with time and with inadequate antibiotic treatment, but unfortunately the symptoms will recur or the disease will pass to a *complicated state.* Persistent gonococcal infection of the urogenital tract may lead to inflammation of the periurethral glands (painful perineal swelling or Cooper's abscess), urethral stricture (difficulty passing water), prostatitis (urinary frequency, dysuria, chills, and pain on defecation), and epididymitis (painful swollen testicle) in the male, and in the female, to periurethral inflammation (painful vulvar swelling, Bartholin's abscess), salpingitis, or pelvic inflammatory disease (lower abdominal pain, metrorrhagia, and pelvic tenderness on vaginal or rectal examination), fever and headache. Pelvic inflammatory disease (PID) due to gonorrhea is characterized by blocking, dilation, abscess formation, fibrosis in the fallopian tubes, and an increased frequency of ectopic pregnancies and sterility. Pelvic inflammatory disease may also be caused by non-venereal causes such as displaced intrauterine contraceptive devices, septic abortions, childbirth (puerperal) infections, hematogenous infections (such as tuberculosis), or other sexually transmitted agents such as *Chlamydia.*

Disseminated Systemic Infection

Disseminated systemic infection with N. gonorrhoeae (gonococcal arthritis/dermatitis syndrome) is manifested by gonococcemia (positive blood cultures) and septic arthritis with or without a characteristic rash (see Fig. 28-4). This is a less common complication, but

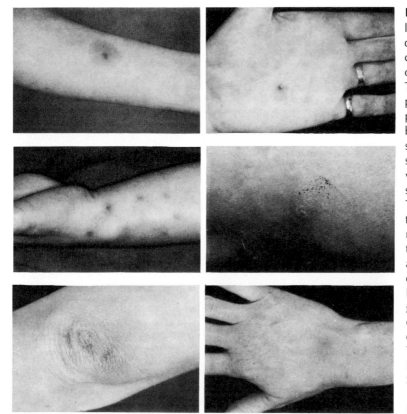

Fig. 28-4 Various types of skin lesions are seen in patients with disseminated gonococcal septicemia (known as the septic gonococcal dermatitis syndrome). These lesions are usually multiple and can be located on any part of the body, but have not been observed intraorally. Lesions are either macular or vesicular and may develop into vesiculopustules similar to those seen in varicella-virus infections. The latter, however, can be distinguished by culture techniques, the Tzanck smear, and the fact that lesions of varicella are often seen on keratinized oral mucosa. (From Barr J and Danielsson D: Disseminated gonococcal infections (gonococcal septicemia) in Danielsson D et al (eds): Genital Infections & Their Complications, Proceeding of the Wellcome Foundation Symposium, Stockholm, Oct. 9-11, 1974; courtesy Wellcome Foundation Ltd., Sweden)

serves to remind the clinician that acute arthritis with a limited vesicular, pustular or hemorrhagic skin rash (usually no more than 8 to 10 vesiculae or pustules that progress to hemorrhagic spots on the dorsum of the elbows and wrists) in a sexually active individual requires laboratory study for evidence of genital, rectal, or oropharyngeal–gonococcal infection.

Oropharyngeal Gonorrhea

Controversy continues as to whether or not specific clinical signs and symptoms are associated with oropharyngeal gonococcal infection (see discussion under section dealing with oral manifestations of gonorrhea). However, oropharyngeal infection, like urogenital infection, may be associated with systemic involvement. Complaints of sore throat and clinical signs of tonsillitis in a patient exposed to gonorrhea are therefore indications for submission of a special throat culture for *N. gonorrhoeae*, especially if a routine throat culture (β-Hemolytic *Streptococcus* screen) has failed to reveal a pathogen. In most cases, oropharyngeal gonococcal infection coexists with urogenital gonorrhea, but cases have been reported in which oropharyngeal infection alone was associated with the gonococcal arthritis/dermatitis syndrome.

Treatment

For many years, gonorrhea was treated like syphilis by intramuscular aqueous procaine penicillin G. With the recognition of penicillinase-producing strains of *N. gonorrhoeae* and their introduction to the United States during the Vietnam War, with the knowledge that gonorrhea is often acquired along with other sexually transmitted infections, and with the importance of eradicating the infection and not allowing chronic subclinical infection to persist, revised recommendations for antibiotic treatment of gonorrhea have been published on several occasions over the last decade. The recommendations issued by the United States Public Health Service Centers for Disease Control in 1982 for the treatment of uncomplicated urogenital gonorrhea are: one time oral administration of 3.5 g ampicillin with 1 g of probenecid; *or* one time administration of 3 g amoxicillin with 1 g probenecid; *or* oral administration of 2 g/day tetracycline hydrochloride, or other tetracycline, for seven days; *or* intramuscular injection of 4.8 million units of aqueous penicillin G at two sites at one visit, preceded by 1 g probenecid orally; *or* amoxicillin or ampicillin as above, followed by tetracycline hydrochloride 2 g daily for one week. Intramuscular injection of penicillin G is preferred over oral administration where patient compliance is uncertain, and tetracycline hydrochloride or intramuscular penicillin in larger doses is recommended for treatment of oropharyngeal gonococcal infections, which should be considered more resistant to systemic ampicillin and spectinomycin therapy than uncomplicated urogenital infections. Patients who are allergic to penicillin or probenecid are treated with tetracyclines or doxycycline. Intramuscular spectinomycin hydrochloride was introduced for treatment of penicillinase-producing strains of *N. gonorrhoeae* and may be also used for patients with gonorrhea who are allergic to tetracycline or penicillin. Cefoxitin sodium with probenecid and trimethoprim-sulfamethoxazole are also used for this purpose.

Treatment of gonorrhea by any of these methods also effectively treats any concomitant incubating (seronegative) syphilitic infection. Patients who are found to have negative screening tests for syphilis at the time they are treated for gonorrhea are usually considered to have received adequate treatment for both infections. Follow-up screening tests used to check on treatment for syphilis would not usually be carried out in such cases, although surveillance for repeated or inadequately treated syphilitic infections would be desirable, particularly where opportunities for reinfection are known to occur.

There is no evidence indicating transmission of *N. gonorrhoeae* in the dental office even where patients with laboratory-diagnosed oropharyngeal gonorrhea are concerned. As discussed in the following section on oral manifestations of gonorrhea, there is also little evidence to implicate oropharyngeal gonococcal infection as a source of transmission of gonorrhea in the community.

Genital Candidiasis

As described in more detail in Chapter 6 (Red and White Lesions of the Oral Mucosa), vulvovaginal infection with *Candida albicans* is a particularly prevalent infection. This fact is borne out by its appearance next after gonorrhea on the list of the most frequent sexually transmitted infections (see Table 28-1). *Candida* infection of the external genitalia in men, however, is less common. In women, it may manifest itself as a redness and itchiness of the perineal area with or without actual erosions and satellite pustules and vesicles. *Candida* vaginitis may be asymptomatic or the cause of itching, a discharge, and bad odor. Concomitant infection of other intertriginous and orificial areas is common. In men, especially those who are uncircumcised, candidiasis usually presents itself as a painful red balanitis, but the infection may also be difficult to distinguish clinically from a nonspecific urethritis. In both sexes, smears and cultures for *Candida* sp. or other yeasts (e.g. *Torulopsis*) are needed for accurate diagnosis.

While the source of the infection is not always clear and is probably frequently nonvenereal due to the widespread presence of these organisms as saphrophytes on skin, mucous membranes, and clothing, recurrences of infection following treatment have been traced to untreated genital infection in a sexual partner. Predisposing factors for genital candidiasis are similar to those described in Chapter 6 for candidiasis of the mouth and other skin surfaces. To this list should be added excessive humidity associated with tight underwear, especially those made of synthetic and relatively impermeable fabrics, elimination of natural vaginal flora by medications for trichomoniasis, and reduction in vaginal secretions after menopause.

Speculations have been made on the frequency with which genital candidiasis is acquired by sexual contact and the possible role of oral and vaginal strains of *Candida* in the etiology of oral and genital candidiasis. Currently, adequate markers do not seem to exist to allow any accurate answer to this question, and the main reason for listing candidiasis as a sexually transmitted disease is the frequency with which it occurs as an associated or primary problem in patients seeking treatment for genital infections.

Interrelationships between oral and genital candidiasis remain obscure, except for the fact that due to the frequency of candidal vulvovaginitis, female patients with oral candidiasis will often respond affirmatively to inquiries about a history of candidiasis, and the fact that symptoms of genital candidiasis will usually regress during treatment of oral candidiasis, when systemic antifungal therapy with one of the newer imidazole compounds is involved.

The principles of treatment of the various forms of candidiasis are outlined in Chapter 6.

Trichomoniasis and Other Protozoal Infections

Trichomoniasis is caused by the flagellated protozoan *Trichomonas vaginalis*. It is most commonly an infection of women characterized by an intense vaginitis with a frothy greenish offensive discharge and excoriation of the orificial tissues. Infection in males is almost always asymptomatic, but may be present as a balanitis or urethritis, and transmission between partners has been documented. It is almost always considered a sexually acquired infection. In women, the infection is most frequently diagnosed when there is an appearance of trichomonads in Papanicolaou smears, but the organism can also be identified in wet mounts with the light microscope and cultured in the laboratory to obtain increased yields for further studies. In men, diagnosis is difficult and culture is the only reliable method. Orally administered metronidazole* is commonly used to treat this infection, and sexual consorts as well as symptomatic patients should be treated concurrently.

The demonstration of *trichomonads in the oral cavity* has, from time to time, caused speculation as to their etiologic roles in oral lesions, gingivitis and periodontal disease in particular. There appears to be no evidence for such a role, even though at one time metronidazole was used for treatment of acute necrotizing ulcerative gingivitis. Suggestions

---

* Flagyl, Searle Consumer Products, Division of Searle Pharmaceuticals, Inc., Box 5110, Chicago, IL 60680.

Metryl, Lemmon Company, Sellersville, PA 18960

have also been made that *Trichomonas vaginalis* infections of the oral cavity may occur after orogenital contact. None of the cases reported to date, however, have provided adequate data to ensure identification of *T. vaginalis* in the presence of the usual saprophytic oral trichomonads *(Trichomonas tenax).* Ultrastructural studies are needed to make this distinction.

As discussed earlier, sexual transmission of other protozoal parasites has also been documented, and the relatively common intestinal parasites, *Giardia lamblia* and *Entamoeba histolytica* (causative agents of giardisis and amebic dysentery, respectively) have been added to the list of sexually transmitted infections. Some uncommon intestinal parasites of animals, *Cryptosporidium* and *Isospora,* which have been isolated from a number of male homosexual patients with the acquired immune deficiency syndrome, are also believed to be transmitted sexually.

Venereal Warts

The terms genital or venereal warts, or condyloma acuminatum, are used to describe pink fleshy papillomatous lesions developing on the external genitalia. Like warts elsewhere, they are of viral etiology and the virus-infected cells possess markers that are visible both under the light microscope and at ultrastructural levels. While it is recognized that human warts can be autoinoculated, venereal warts are almost always sexually acquired and are at least as prevalent as trichomoniasis. Their rate of growth is quite variable, although wart growth appears to be favored by the moist, warm environment of the perineal skin and mucosal surfaces. The urethral, vaginal, anorectal, and oral mucosae may also be affected by additional papillomatous lesions. Spectacular rates of growth and multiple florid lesions on the glans penis, vulva, perianal skin and oral mucosa are not uncommon, and cause patients who might otherwise consider warts as minor, if undesirable, skin blemishes, to seek prompt treatment. Recurrences are common due, possibly, to inadequate removal of infected tissue in some cases, but also to reinfection from a sexual partner with similar lesions.

A number of different types of warts viruses have been identified based on serologic characteristics, and are probably associated with the varied appearances of warts in different locations. Type 6 warts virus is said to be preferentially associated with genital warts. A number of cases of recurrent multiple warts of the lips and oral cavity, where the patient gave a history of orogenital sexual contact, have been identified as oral condyloma acuminatum (see the section on Oral Manifestations of Sexually Transmitted Disease, which follows).

Genital warts are treated by excision, electro- and cryosurgery, application of chemical agents such as podophyllin and cantharidin, and with 5-fluorouracil. Examination for, and treatment of, any genital warts in the sexual partner is an important step in the prevention of recurrences. A number of papers have documented the frequent association of genital warts with other sexually transmitted infections, such as nonspecific urethritis, candidiasis, syphilis, gonorrhea and pediculosis pubis, justifying the need to search for other sexually transmitted infections in any patient known to have genital warts.

Herpes Simplex Infections

Epidemiology

Epidemiologic studies carried out in the United States in the early 1970's confirmed the existence of two antigenically and biologically distinct types of herpes simplex virus (HSV-1 and HSV-2), and their association with oral and genital infections respectively. These initial studies, and similar studies carried out in Europe approximately 10 years later (see Table 28-3), reported that 90% to 95% of herpes simplex lesions above the waist were due to HSV-1 and about 85% of lesions below the waist were due to HSV-2. HSV-1 was therefore referred to as the "oral"strain of herpes simplex, and HSV-2 as the "genital" strain. A number of cases of HSV-2 infection "above the waist" were recognized, and an even larger number of "below the waist" lesions were known to be caused by HSV-1, but the "genital" strain was predominantly type-specific for genital infections, and HSV-2 infections were consid-

Table 28-3. Association of Herpes Simplex Virus Type 1 and Type 2 with Site of Clinical Involvement and Virus Isolation

Site of Clinical Involvement	Virus Isolation from	Nahmias et al 1970* # of Strains (n = 855)			Dundarov et al 1980† # of Strains (n = 700)		
		Type 1	Type 2	% Type 1	Type 1	Type 2	% Type 1
Herpes labialis	lip	84	0	100%	173	2	99%
Gingivostomatitis	mouth	142	3	98%	20	0	100%
Facial dermatitis	face	–	–	–	111‡	–	100%
Keratoconjunctivitis	cornea/conjunctiva	29	1	96%	14	0	100%
Genital tract	penis vulva/vagina	7	199	3%	0	223‡	0%
Dermatitis	buttocks extremities	18	91	18%	4‡	81	5%

* From Nahmias A et al: Antibodies to Herpesvirus homonis types 1 and 2 in humans. Am J Epidermiol 9:539, 1970. Johns Hopkins University Press, Baltimore

† From Dundarov S et al: Characterization of herpes simplex virus strains isolated from patients with various diseases. Archives of Virology 63:115, 1980; Springer-Verlag, Pub., New York

‡ 5 of the strains in these groups behaved antigenically intermediate.

ered to be sexually transmitted. Some recent studies, however, have reported an increasing number of genital infections with HSV-1, with ratios down to 1/1 for the incidence of both types of HSV in both locations. Appreciation of these differences is the result of more widespread use of virus cultures and type-specific serodiagnostic methods in the evaluation of both oral and genital herpes. Most importantly, they illustrate the fact that *both HSV-1 and HSV-2 can be transmitted sexually, and that the term, ''genital herpes'', should be used to designate an infection with HSV at a particular location, rather than one with a specific type of virus.*

Seroepidemiologic data derived from a variety of sources in the 1960's and 1970's (see Figure 28-5) indicated that the majority of infections with HSV occurred in early childhood, fairly soon after loss of any immunity passively transferred from the mother *in utero.* From about 9 to 12 months of age onward, children are non-immune and susceptible to infection with the virus, and the percentage of individuals developing antibodies to HSV rises at its steepest rate from age 1 through about 7 years. These infections in the preschool and kindergarten periods are associated with HSV-1 and are facilitated by the free exchange of salivary and nasal secretions characteristic of school and playtime contacts at this age, as well as close family contact between a susceptible child and a parent with recurrent oral herpes. These infections are non-venereal in nature.

Beyond this age, there is a gradual but smaller increase in the percentage of individuals in the population developing antibodies to HSV-1. The great majority of these infections probably also occur non-venereally, for example simply from kissing someone with infected oral secretions. Extended periods of kissing, as may occur with more intimate relationships, simply increase the opportunity for exchange of oral secretions and the risk of the susceptible partner acquiring herpes-simplex gingivostomatitis or pharyngitis. The antibody to HSV-2 begins to appear in a significant percentage of the population with the onset of adult-type sexual behavior, and accounts for the major increment of antibodies to HSV in the adult population. These HSV-2 infections are probably all acquired sexually, as are some of the infections acquired by adolescents and adults. By age 30, approximately 70% of most population samples exhibit antibodies to either HSV-1 or HSV-2.

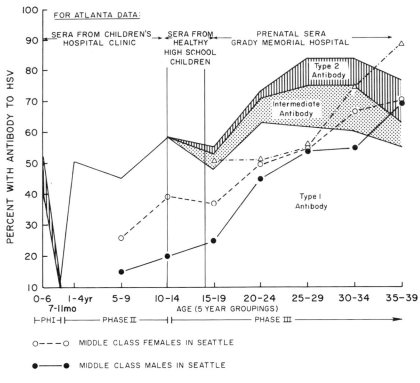

Fig. 28-5 Seroepidemiology of infections due to herpes simplex virus (HSV), types 1 and 2, shows the development of antibodies to HSV Type 1 in middle-class males and females in Seattle contrasted with the development of Type 1, Type 2, and intermediate antibodies in females of lower socioeconomic levels in Atlanta. (Data from Nahamais AJ et al: Antibodies to *Herpesvirus hominis* types 1 and 2 in humans. (I) Patients with genital herpetic infections. Am J Epidemiol 91:539, 1970; Wentworth BB and Alexander ER: Seroepidemiology of infections due to members of the herpes virus group. Am J Epidemiol 94:496, 1971) The intermediate antibody describes sera that react with both type 1 and type 2 herpes simplex virus. (Courtesy of The John Hopkins University Press, Baltimore)

Natural History

The method of acquisition and the natural history of herpes simplex infections are quite variable, although a number of characteristic patterns occur frequently enough to be of help in establishing a diagnosis of herpes simplex infection:

Non-venereal acute ulcerative herpetic gingivostomatitis in children. An acute febrile episode with sore mouth, refusal of food, and an ulcerative gingivostomatitis due to herpes simplex virus is a very common pediatric problem, which in most cases is a self-limiting infection, with the primary lesions and subsequent manifestations of recurrent viral infection restricted to the oral cavity and perioral tissues. A brief period of HSV viremia can be detected in most patients with primary herpes simplex gingivostomatitis, but dissemination of virus by the bloodstream with development of visceral or skin lesions at a distance from the mouth occurs very rarely, usually only in the neonatal period or in an immunologically compromised host. Herpes simplex infection thus differs from some other primary viral infections like chicken pox, in which disseminated skin lesions are the rule. Consequently, a child or adult with primary-herpes-simplex gingivostomatitis does not usually risk the development of genital lesions as a complication of the oral infection. Where this does occur, the spread of virus from oral to genital mucosa is usually due to direct contamination of the genital area with infected oral secretions transferred on the hands. This phenomenon does occur in young children and less rarely in adults, and accounts for the majority of non-venereal genital infections with HSV. Recurrences of herpes simplex are determined by latent virus infection of the sensory ganglion of the nerve that supplies each area involved in the original infection, and the potential for recurrences is always present following primary infection of the mouth, genital mucosa, or other skin or mucous membrane sites. However, recurrences at one site are not always matched with recurrences at all primary sites. While it is known that about 60% of individuals who have been infected with HSV will experience recurrent herpes labialis by their early twenties, no figures are available on the risk of recurrent genital herpes in the child or adult who acquires the infection non-venereally as just described.

Primary Herpes Simplex Gingivostomatitis and Pharyngitis Among High-School and College Students

These infections are also very common, and have been shown to account for as much as 40% of acute pharyngitis in the latter group. Kissing, petting, and developing adult sexual behavior account for the majority of these infections, and the term, "kissing disease," describes the herpes simplex infection in this age-group equally as well as it does infectious mononucleosis. The risk of developing genital infection along with the oral infection in this age-group as well as any older age group, is related to the extent of sexual contact that occurred, and specific inquiry about this topic is necessary if the adolescent's con-

cerns about possible genital infection are to be answered honestly. Figure 28-5 indicates that the development of an antibody to herpes simplex tends to occur later in children with a higher socioeconomic background, a phenomenon that has been noted in other epidemic orally transmitted infections such as poliomyelitis (prior to introduction of polio vaccine), and is believed to be related to a more stringent adherence to principles of hygiene and a smaller circle of close contacts in children of middle-class families. Coupled with the fact that the onset of adult-type sexual behavior also comes later in children of higher socioeconomic background, this difference probably accounts for a greater frequency of primary herpes infections (both oral and genital) in older high-school and college students.

Primary Herpetic Infections of the Oropharynx in Older Adults

Since the majority of primary herpes-simplex infections occur during childhood and adolescence, they are usually thought of as pediatric problems, and primary herpes simplex infections of the oropharynx in older adults are often misdiagnosed or considered to be very unusual, even when confirmed by virus isolation and development of specific antibody. Characteristically, such infections are seen in patients who did not acquire herpes simplex infection and immunity during childhood, and whose sexual contacts have previously been limited to one or a small number of like individuals. In such patients, primary herpes simplex infection is often acquired along with a new sexual partner and primary herpes simplex gingivostomatitis and pharyngitis, or genital infection, are seen by the clinician in the context of a divorce, a new partner, or the more traditional casual sexual encounter. As pointed out in Chapter 5, primary oropharyngeal infection of the adult with herpes simplex may present as an acute pharyngitis and tonsillitis with few or minimal oral lesions, and virus isolation and titration of acute and convalescent serums for antibody to the virus may be needed to establish the diagnosis when the circumstance suggests the possibility of primary herpes in the adult.

In the majority of cases, primary oropharyngeal herpes simplex in the adult is a result of contact with infected oral secretions or a freshly ruptured cold sore on the lips of a partner, and it is usually due to HSV-1. Less frequently, oropharyngeal lesions are the result of orogenital contact with a partner with recurrent genital herpes and then may be associated with either HSV-1 or HSV-2.

Genital Herpes (see Figures 28-6 and 28-7)

The primary lesions of genital herpes usually develop 3 to 6 days after exposure and develop as vesicular lesions that are often preceded by a burning, pricking sensation. Lesions may occur on the penis, vulva, perineal area, or anus. Lesions are more likely to be vesicular on well-keratinized surfaces, such as the shaft of the penis, but depending on the location, may pass more or less rapidly into superficial erosions that are very painful when touched or contaminated with urine. The urethra may be involved and an extremely painful dysuria may develop. The intense pain and functional distress that occur in some cases are even said to be deterrents to the patient's search for medical care during the acute phase for fear of the added discomfort during an examination. As in primary syphilis (q.v.) the regional lymph nodes are usually involved in a primary attack of genital herpes; constitutional symptoms, fever, malaise, and anorexia may also be present.

As with herpes simplex infection of the oropharynx, the majority of primary genital infections are either asymptomatic or go unrecognized as primary herpes. Patients often develop lesions bearing the features of a recurrent infection, yet with no history of a primary episode. This phenomenon is more common in the female, where it is often attributed to the primary, largely asymptomatic, episode having been on the cervix or vaginal mucosa. Like primary oropharyngeal infections, primary genital infections are associated with heavy virus secretion that is sometimes matched with a widespread acute vulvovaginitis or balanitis. Either HSV-1, HSV-2, or a combination of strains may be found in the infected secretions. Antibody to

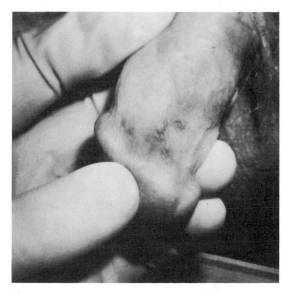

Fig. 28-6 Initial lesions of genital herpes simplex infection in the male. (Courtesy Burroughs Wellcome Co., Research Triangle Park, NC 27709).

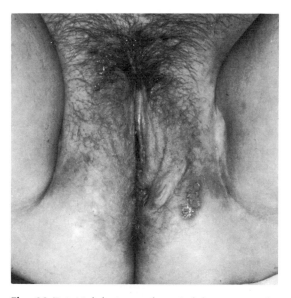

Fig. 28-7 Initial lesions of genital herpes simplex infection in the female. (Courtesy Burroughs Wellcome Co., Research Triangle Park, NC 27709).

the virus develops to a measurable titer 4 to 6 weeks after the primary infection, and may be detected by neutralization, complement fixation, immunofluorescence, or other suitable techniques. The presence of virus may be detected by an appropriate culture of scrapings, fluid from unbroken vesicles, or a sample of urogenital discharge. Tzanck smears prepared from scrapings of intact vesicles, and cervical and vaginal smears stained by Papanicolaou or other stains giving good nuclear differentiation, will reveal characteristic viral giant cells (see Chapter 3).

Recurrent genital herpes may be recognized either as recurring, localized areas of vesiculation and ulceration of the penis, vulva, anus and perineal tissues, or by the discovery of characteristic viral-infected cells in a routine Papanicolaou smear in the female. Recurrent infection is characterized by lack of associated systemic response, limited clinical lesions, smaller amounts of virus, and the presence of detectable specific antibody in both acute and convalescent serum specimens. A number of factors have been described as the stimuli for recurrences, *e.g.*, fever, trauma, other genito-urinary infections, intercourse, and menstruation. As with recurrent herpes labialis, however, there are few data available to confirm these anecdotal associations.

Complications

Complications of genital herpes are more apparent in the female and include transmission of the virus either *in utero* or at birth, and an increased risk of carcinoma of the cervix (and possibly carcinoma in situ of the vulva) in women with evidence of HSV-2 infection. Caesarian section is sometimes needed to reduce the risk of neonatal infection when active cervical or genital herpes is detected in late pregnancy. Annual cervical cytology is recommended for women with genital herpes in order to detect, as early as possible, any cellular atypia suggestive of malignancy. Concerns about sexual intercourse are an important complication of genital herpes, and probably account for the anxiety about this infection that can be observed in many patients with this problem. This issue has been described in numerous articles in the lay press (see Figure 28-8) in recent years. Concerns include anxiety that intercourse will promote recurrent lesions, or that

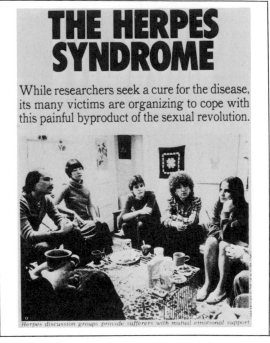

Fig. 28-8 The public press reveals concerns about herpes simplex infection as a sexually transmitted disease. A simulated group discussion about personal problems associated with genital herpes simplex infection (From the New York Times Magazine, Feb 21st, 1982, Courtesy of The New York Times, Co., New York. Artist: Sara Krulwich/NYT Pictures)

clinically latent virus will be transmitted to a sexual partner even during the period of remission of the infection. This latter concern is a real one, inasmuch as silent secretion of virus from cervical, vaginal, or urethral mucosa has been demonstrated in both males and females in the absence of external lesions. However, like the risk of acquiring herpes orally from silent oropharyngeal infections, this risk cannot be accurately measured, and the only certain protection is provided by abstention or use of barrier methods such as condom (with or without added spermicidal agents) and topical disinfectants. Silent secretion of virus in both oral and genital sites is usually minimal and discontinuous, so that even with daily vaginal swabbing and/ or Papanicolaou smears, evidence of the virus will usually be detected only on an isolated day. Recurrent lesions of genital herpes, however, have been documented as remaining positive for virus twice as long as those of recurrent herpes labialis.

Each of these patterns of natural history and virus secretion are characteristic of the patient with a normal immunologic response. In patients with chronic herpes simplex infection associated with an acquired immune deficiency, quite different patterns of lesions, and persistence of lesions and virus over long periods of time, can be expected.

Treatment

Until the licensing of the antiviral agent acyclovir,* in 1982, none of the treatments commonly used for genital herpes produced anything but a palliative effect, and the concern that herpes simplex infection was a major sexually transmitted disease rapidly rising to epidemic proportions was hard to separate from the concern that it was an untreatable and recurrent infection. Topical applications of ether, chloroform, idoxuridine or vidarabine (two previously available antiviral agents), photoinactivation with neutral red, and systemic administration of L-lysine were all used, based upon various demonstrated effects of these agents on herpes simplex virus *in vitro* or in tissue culture. While none of these has been shown to be effective against genital herpes infection *in vivo*, topical acyclovir has been shown to decrease the length of time that virus is detectable in the lesions of primary genital herpes, and to reduce the time it takes for crusting of the lesions. Controversy continues as to whether topical acyclovir had any effect on recurrent genital herpes, although this medication is commonly requested and prescribed for patients with recurrent herpes. The Food and Drug Administration has not approved it for this purpose. Intravenous acyclovir is also available for treatment of patients with disseminated herpes, herpes encephalitis, and extensive and persistent lesions of chronic herpes. Data are not available at this time on the effect of acyclovir in controlling transmis-

*Zovirax Ointment 5%, Burroughs Wellcome Co. 3030 Cornwallis Road, Research Triangle Park, NC 27709.

sion of this infection or on the epidemiologic pattern of genital herpes.

Sexually Transmitted Dermatologic Diseases—Pediculosis Pubis, Scabies, and Molluscum Contagiosum

These three dermatologic lesions occur as sexually transmitted infections with prevalences similar to that of genital herpes in the case of pediculosis pubis and scabies, and somewhat less frequently in the case of molluscum contagiosum. Pediculosis pubis (crabs) and scabies are caused by parasitic insects, *Phthirus pubis* (or crab louse), and *Acarus (Sarcoptes) scabei,* respectively; molluscum contagiosum is caused by a pox virus and is discussed with the two parasitic infections because of its dermatologic nature. Each of these infestations may also be transmitted by non-venereal routes, but in each case, close body contact, *e.g.,* sharing the same bed, or use of contaminated bed linen or clothing is essential.

Pediculosis Pubis

The crab louse is only one of several kinds of lice that can infest human body hair, but it is different from other lice, such as those associated with pediculosis capitis, by its characteristic microscopic morphology, its preferred location on the pubic hair (although it may infest all the body hair, including beard, moustache and eyebrows; but rarely, the scalp hair), its obligate parasitism, and its high rate of transmissibility. It is very easily passed from person to person during sexual contact. After an incubation period of about 30 days, the main symptom of infestation is itching, followed by urticarial macules, papules, vesicles, and secondary impetigo. Diagnosis is based on finding the adult lice (small brown motile flecks) or smaller nits (tiny non-motile flecks usually seen only with a hand lens) on the pubic hair. Microscopic observation of the characteristic morphology of the louse confirms the diagnosis. Some experience is needed in distinguishing nits from dandruff, particularly on other hairy areas, *e.g.* , the scalp, beard and eyebrows. Care should be used in making a diagnosis of *Phthirus pubis* infestation at extra-pubic locations simply because a history of pediculosis pubis has been noted and louse or nit-sized scales or particles on the head or facial hair have been observed. Epidemiologic studies indicate that patients showing up at venereal disease clinics for treatment of pediculosis pubis often have additional sexually transmitted infections, and should be at least examined and tested for syphilis and gonorrhea. Treatment of pediculosis pubis is usually effective in the absence of opportunities for reinfestation, and involves the use of pyrethrin substances (*e.g.*, RID Shampoo*) or lindane (Kwell Shampoo†) and usually does not necessitate shaving of the affected hair.

Scabies

Infestation with the mite, *Acarus (Sarcoptes) scabei*, produces small itchy erythematous areas on the skin, particularly between the fingers, and on the wrists, axillary folds, and buttocks. Examination with a hand lens may reveal small burrows (described as straight lines with a black dot at the end) in these locations. Lesions on the scrotum and penis are nodular but otherwise similar. Infestation of the female genitalia is rare. The face, neck and hand are rarely, if ever, involved. Diagnosis is usually made on clinical grounds (the appearance of lesions on the male external genitalia is usually considered pathognomonic), but may be confirmed by microscopic demonstration of the mite in scrapings from the surface of the skin lesions. Lindane (Kwell† lotion) with or without corticoste-

* Pfipharmecs Div., Pfizer Inc., 235 E. 42nd Street, New York, NY 10017

† Reed and Carnrick, 1 New England Ave, Piscataway, NJ 08854

Note: both of these preparations are also used for treatment of head lice infestations (pediculosis capitis). They contain highly toxic ingredients and contact with skin should be brief (10 minutes or less) whether the preparation is used as a hair shampoo or a scrub for contaminated upholstery on a dental chair. 10% household bleach and 75% alcohol are probably adequate for decontaminating plastic surfaces.

roids to control itching, is the usual method of treatment. A search is also made for evidence of other sexually transmitted infections when the infestation is suspected to be of venereal origin.

Molluscum Contagiosum

Clinically, this virus infection is characterized by multiple or isolated small waxy papules with a depressed center occurring on the skin of the inner thighs, lower abdomen, or external genitalia. It is seen as a dermatologic problem from time to time in pediatric clinics, usually with more than one member of the family who share sleeping accommodations being infected and having lesions. In venereal disease clinics, it is seen with a more specific perigenital location in patients who also have other sexually transmitted infections. In children, lesions have also been recorded on the face, eyelids, trunk, fingers, and arms; the linear distribution of lesions on some occasions suggest that autoinoculation of the virus occurs with scratching. Intraoral lesions have been described as rare findings (*q.v.*). Lesions on the skin are infrequently biopsied, but on occasions, histologic similarity to a variety of other dermatologic conditions, *e.g.*, histiocytoma, keratoacanthoma, sebaceous adenoma, Darier's disease, or nevus (see Chapters 6 and 8) may confuse the diagnosis, particularly if the core of the lesion with the characteristic molluscum bodies has been dislodged (see Figure 28–9).

Diagnosis is usually achieved solely on clinical grounds supplemented with Papanicolaou or gram-stained smears prepared from scrapings of the lesions or from contents of the lesion that have been crushed on a slide, thereby demonstrating the molluscum bodies. Scrapings or material curetted from the lesions will produce cytopathic changes in a variety of tissue cultures but propagation of the agent beyond the first passage has not been confirmed. Electron-micrographic examination of the lesions and the first passage tissue culture material reveals characteristic pox-virus type particles.

Most lesions of molluscum contagiosum resolve spontaneously in about 1–2 months and

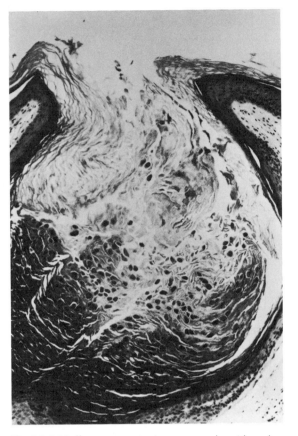

Fig. 28-9 Molluscum contagiosum papule with a plug of acanthotic and hyperkeratotic epidermis containing numerous intracytoplasmic inclusions and opening to the surface through an apical hole. (X75, hematoxylin and eosin stain) From Brown ST, Nalley JF, Kraus SJ: Molluscum contagiosum. Sex Trans Dis 8:227, 1981; Courtesy Am Vener Dis Assoc, 2350 Virginia Ave, Hagerstown, MD 21740)

the infection rarely persists longer than 3 years. Lesions are asymptomatic and are usually treated only when multiple, or when concerns about transmission to sexual partners are raised. Treatment includes curettage followed by some form of local cautery, cryotherapy, or topical application of caustics and irritants such as phenol, trichloracetic acid, podophyllin, cantharidin, and tretinoin. Systemic administration of griseofulvin, sulfonamides and tetracyclines is also used, but is not supported by controlled trials.

Syphilis and Other Treponemal Infections

Epidemiology

Syphilis is a chronic infectious systemic disease with a number of stages, caused by the spirochete, *Treponema pallidum*. In the developed countries of the world, infection with this organism occurs almost exclusively by venereal contact. In primitive overcrowed conditions (as existed in isolated communities in eastern Europe through the first half of this century, and which still exist in many developing third-world countries), infection by this organism and a number of closely related species *(Treponema pertenue* and *Treponema carateum)* also occurs by non-venereal routes. Under these circumstances the diseases that are produced, endemic syphilis (bejel), yaws, and pinta, are endemic diseases of children with destructive skin and bone lesions as tertiary manifestations in adults. Endemic syphilis, yaws and pinta are referred to as the *non-venereal treponematoses*, and eradication of these diseases, which on a worldwide basis are more prevalent than venereal syphilis, has been a particular concern of the World Health Organization and the United Nations Childrens Emergency Fund for some years.

T. pallidum continues to be susceptible to penicillin. The worldwide prevalence of venereal syphilis decreased considerably after the introduction of this antibiotic in the late 1940's (see Figure 28-1). Its prevalence has remained low and it has been surpassed as a major cause of sexually transmitted infections by each of the infections already considered in this chapter. However, a reservoir of cases persists among the sexually promiscuous, and minor epidemics continue to occur in urban areas where relative anonymity and a large transient population favors such behavior. Both heterosexual prostitution and male homosexual communities are prominent features of most large cities in Europe, North America, and elsewhere, and epidemic syphilis in these areas continues to be a concern of public health authorities. On occasions, individuals acquiring syphilis (and other sexually transmitted infections) in a urban area are also identified as the source of minor outbreaks in non-urban areas. While syphilis remains an important sexually transmitted disease (and a useful marker of exposure to other sexually transmitted diseases, because it can be screened for by relatively simple laboratory tests), the frequency with which the tertiary manifestations of the disease are seen continues to decrease as the result of using penicillin to treat the early infection. The tertiary manifestations of syphilis (see following) lead to considerable morbidity and mortality, and represented the major health care (hospitalization and domiciliary) costs associated with this infection in the past. The response of primary syphilis to penicillin and the disappearance of tertiary syphilis as a major health problem have probably contributed to syphilis dropping from sight as a major sexually transmitted infection in the last two decades. As discussed in the following section on Hazards of Non-Venereal Transmission of Sexually Transmissible Diseases in The Dental Office, accidental infection of clinical personnel (syphilis insontium or syphilis innocentum), through contact with lesions or secretions of patients with infectious syphilis, has also possibly been eradicated with the availability of penicillin for treatment of the infection and prophylaxis of contacts.

Despite the lack of prominence of syphilis in both clinical and epidemiologic settings at this time, continued surveillance is recommended for this infection, particularly at a time when antibiotics other than penicillin, which often are not equally effective as penicillin against *T. pallidum,* are being used for the treatment of gonorrhea, and screening tests for syphilis are no longer part of routine laboratory testing for all hospital admissions in many institutions.

Clinical Features of Acquired Syphilis*

The vast majority of syphilitic* infections are acquired by sexual contact in adult life. These infections are referred to as *acquired syphilis* to distinguish them from infections acquired

---

*The words lues and luetic infection are commonly used for syphilis and are used interchangeably with syphilis and syphilitic in this chapter.

in utero, which are referred to as *congenital syphilis,* because of the association of congenital abnormalities with infection by this route. (Congenital syphilis is described at the end of this section and in the section dealing with Oral, Pharyngeal, and Facial Manifestations of the Sexually Transmitted Diseases, which follows).

Acquired syphilis is classified according to the type of lesion and temporal course of the disease into primary, secondary, and tertiary syphilis.

Primary syphilis is the initial manifestation of the disease. The lesion is the chancre, a slightly raised, ulcerated, firm plaque, which is usually round and indurated with rolled raised edges. It begins as a papule before proceeding to ulceration, and may vary in size from 5 mm to several centimeters in diameter. It is usually painless unless superinfected. The chancre occurs at the site of entry of *T. pallidum,* which is most commonly on the genitalia but can be elsewhere (the mouth is the second most common site). Although a chancre may occur anytime from 10 to 90 days after exposure, the usual time is within 3 to 4 weeks. It spontaneously disappears without therapy after about 10 days, unfortunately giving the patient a false sense of security. The lesion is usually single, but multiple lesions do occur. At the same time, or shortly after, the appearance of the chancre, the regional lymph glands (usually the inguinal glands with genital chancres) become firm, enlarged, and non-tender. The combination of an indurated ulcer on an appropriate mucosal surface and enlarged non-tender regional lymph glands constitutes the classical sign of primary syphilis. Not all patients with primary syphilis develop a chancre however, and the chancre may also be concealed in the genital tract or anorectal area.

After entering the body at the primary focus, the organisms proliferate and spread by way of the bloodstream to produce lesions elsewhere. These lesions, *the secondary lesions,* usually appear within 3 to 6 weeks after the primary lesions. Their location is not related to the site of the primary lesion. When they appear on the skin, they are manifested as a fine macular or papular rash, sometimes accompanied by alopecia. The manifestations of secondary syphilis are varied and may mimic many types of skin diseases (although with the exception of those of congenital syphilis, syphilitic lesions are not vesicular or bullous). On the mucous membranes and moist skin areas, there are three possible types of lesions: the mucous patch, the split papule, and condyloma latum. Sometimes the disease may present only with fever and generalized lymphadenopathy. Laryngeal involvement may lead to hoarseness.

Mucous patches are small, smooth, erythematous areas or superficial grayish-white erosions found on the mucous membranes of the vulva, penis or oral cavity. On the palate and tonsil they have also been described as "snail-track ulcers." *Condyloma latum* are grayish, moist, flat-topped, extra-large papules, sometimes coalescing into plaques, which are usually found on moist mucocutaneous surfaces such as the vulva, anus, scrotum, thighs, axilla and other intertriginous areas. At intertriginous sites, such as skin folds and the angles of the mouth, the lesion may appear as a double papule and is then referred to as a *split papule*. The rashes of secondary syphilis are varied and pleomorphic, and may be misdiagnosed as an allergy, viral infection (roseola, infectious mononucleosis), or psoriasis. Characteristically, the syphilitic rash is described as pruritic. A number of patients have no, or only trivial, signs of the secondary stage, and this stage is then recognized only on the basis of the development of a positive serologic test (see Chapter 3).

Tertiary syphilis is usually asymptomatic. The lesion is the gumma, which may occur anywhere in the body including the oral cavity. Involvement of the cardiovascular or nervous systems produces the most serious damage. *Neurosyphilis* produces a wide variety of symptoms, depending on the location and the extent of the lesion, and is manifested as tabes dorsalis and/or general paresis. General paresis is syphilitic involvement of the cerebral tissue and tabes dorsalis is syphilitic involvement of the posterior root ganglia.

General paresis develops in approximately three percent of patients with syphilis, with a marked predominance in males. The symptoms of paresis are extremely varied, and they may mimic almost any disease. A single cerebral gumma may produce symptoms suggesting a brain tumor. Involvement of the cranial nerves results in pupils that react to accommodation but not to light—the Argyll Robertson pupil. Personality changes are often the first manifestations of paresis, with increased irritability, fatigue, mental sluggishness, and carelessness in personal habits. There is a loss of fine muscular coordination, as indicated by the inability to enunciate clearly or to perform delicate tasks with the hands. The patient may have ideas of grandeur, wealth, and ability far beyond his station in life. Occasionally, these euphoric symptoms have first suggested the diagnosis.

Involvement of the spinal cord (*i.e.*, tabes dorsalis) is a common late manifestation of untreated or inadequately treated syphilis, which occurs in 2% to 3% of all luetics. Symptoms develop usually in 10 to 20 years following the initial infection. A patient with tabes dorsalis soon loses the positional sense of his lower extremities and walks with a characteristic slapping step. This gait may be accompanied by burning or pricking sensations of the extremities, paresthesias, or, at times, actual anesthesia of the part. Such an individual is unable to stand erect unaided with his eyes closed, the positive Romberg's sign. Short, shooting, knifelike pains may be experienced in the abdominal region, the "tabetic crises." They result from involvement of the posterior root ganglia. These sporadic pains are at times mistaken for symptoms of organic disease in the structures supplied by these nerves. Occasionally, operations have been performed before the true nature of the symptoms was determined. Trophic changes consist of deep perforating ulcers and painless destruction of the larger joints (Charcot joint).

Involvement of the *cardiovascular system* in tertiary syphilis affects particularly the aorta or aortic valve. This involvement accounts for 80% of deaths due to syphilis. Obliteration of the vasa vasorum of the aorta and its larger branches as the result of syphilis leads to medial necrosis and destruction of elastic tissue in the walls of the large blood vessels. Aortitis, aortic regurgitation, aneurysm formation in the proximal aorta (ascending and arch segments), or narrowing of the ostia of the coronary arteries may result from these changes. About 10% of patients with un-treated tertiary syphilis experience such problems. Asymptomatic syphilitic aortitis may also be suspected on the basis of linear calcification of the ascending aorta demon-strated in chest radiographs. Aneurysms of the abdominal (descending) aorta are only rarely due to tertiary syphilis.

Early, Late, and Latent Syphilis

Syphilis is also classified into early and late stages on the basis of infectivity related to time. This classification is particularly useful for epidemiologic or public-health purposes.

Early syphilis is defined as syphilis 4 years or less after infection. This includes all cases of primary and secondary syphilis as well as the stage of early latent syphilis that follows. Early syphilis is infectious. It may be either symptomatic (with lesions present) or latent. Latent syphilis is an asymptomatic form and is diagnosed only by a positive blood test. The patient is susceptible to reinfection after treatment. *Late syphilis* is syphilis of more than 4 years' duration. It is not infectious, and the patient is probably immune to rein-fection. It may be symptomatic (cardiovas-cular or neurosyphilis or a gummatous le-sion) or asymptomatic (latent). The latter group comprise 60% to 70% of patients with late syphilis having no manifestations of the disease other than a positive serological test for syphilis.

After the primary and secondary stages, the surface lesions heal and the patient enters a long phase with no sign of the disease ex-cept a positive serologic test *(latent syphilis)*. Without adequate treatment, an unknown proportion of these relapse into contagious secondary syphilis, and approximately one-third ultimately undergo spontaneous cures with no further symptoms, and serologic tests revert to negative. Of the remaining two-thirds who remains seropositive, one-half develop the serious late effects of tertiary syphilis just described, and the others die of unrelated problems.

Latent syphilis is also sometimes divided into early and late stages (which differ some-what from the early and late stages of syphilis already described). *Early latent syphilis* (clini-cally symptomless syphilis with a positive se-rologic reaction and negative spinal fluid test) is arbitrarily defined as less than 2 years after infection. Such patients are potentially infec-tive and a danger to themselves as well as others. *Late latent syphilis* (more than 2 years after infection) is not usually infectious and any future adverse consequences affect the patient (and the community that supports the chronically ill patient) but *not* the patient's contacts.

Diagnosis of Syphilis

In primary syphilis, the blood test may not be positive. (See Chapter 3 for a review of the various types of blood tests, both reagin and treponemal, used in the diagnosis of sy-philis.) The Venereal Disease Research Lab-oratory test (VDRL) is positive in 76% of pri-mary cases and the fluorescent treponemal antibody absorption test (FTA-ABS) is posi-tive in 86%. The latter becomes positive to-ward the end of the primary stage. Because the blood test cannot always be relied upon to make a diagnosis in primary syphilis, it is sometimes necessary to do a darkfield ex-amination using exudate from the lesion and examining the exudate for the presence of living treponema under a darkfield micro-scope. This examination is useful in genital lesions, *but not* in oral lesions because of the presence of other treponema in the oral cav-ity that cannot be differentiated from *T. pal-lidum* by this method. The diagnosis of sec-ondary syphilis should be suspected on the basis of symptoms or signs and may be con-firmed by blood tests. Ninety-eight to one hundred percent of both reagin and trepo-nemal tests are positive during this stage. Since the reagin tests are known to be reac-tive sometimes in the absence of syphilis (biological false-positive), a treponemal test should be done if the validity of the positive reagin test is in doubt and not consistent with the patient's clinical symptoms.

Histopathology of Syphilitic Lesions

Histopathologic examination of primary le-sions shows perivascular plasma-cell and his-tiocytic infiltration, capillary endothelial proliferation, and obliteration of small blood vessels. *T. pallidum* may be demonstrated in sections of a chancre either by silver staining or by more precise immunofluorescent techniques. The organisms are usually found in spaces between epithelial cells, and in the process of phagocytosis by epithelial cells, fibroblasts, plasma cells, and endothelial cells, as well as by macrophages and polymorphs. Secondary cutaneous lesions are characterized by hyperkeratosis, capillary proliferation in the superficial corium and dermal papillae (with migration of polymorphs), and a perivascular infiltrate of plasma cells in the deeper dermis. Mucocutaneous lesions may resemble lichenoid reactions both clinically and histopathologically (see Chapter 6). Gummas (which are now widely stated to be quite rare and are considered to be highly penicillin-sensitive lesions) may be microscopic or grossly visible lesions, consisting of non-specific granulomatous inflammations with central necrosis, surrounded by mononuclear, epithelioid, fibroblastic and occasionally giant cells, with a surrounding zone of perivasculitis. *T. pallidum* organisms are only rarely demonstrated in gummas, but have been isolated from these lesions by inoculation of rabbits. Virtually any organ may be involved by gummatous changes. The skin, skeletal system, mouth, upper respiratory tract, larynx, liver, and stomach were identified as the most common sites in earlier studies. Delayed hypersensitivity to *T. pallidum* is an important component in the production of these lesions.

Congenital Syphilis

It has long been known that the lesions of congenital syphilis are related to transplacental infection occurring after the sixteenth week of gestation. Previously, it was believed that this was due to an increased permeability of the placenta to *T. pallidum* following degeneration of the Langerhans cell-layer of the placenta about this time. This has been shown not to be the case, however; transplacental transmission of *T. pallidum* may occur at any time after conception, and the time of development of the lesions of congenital syphilis is probably related to the development of immune competence rather than to any toxic effect of the organism. Despite the decreased prevalence of syphilis, the frequency of congenital syphilis in the United States has remained at about 5 cases for every 100 reported cases of primary and secondary syphilis. The persistence of this form of the infection is attributed to failure to seek prenatal care and to the acquisition of syphilis during pregnancy. The risk of congenital syphilis is less for the mother with evidence of late syphilis. Syphilis in pregnancy is often subclinical, though frequently leads to severe congenital manifestations or death of the fetus *in utero*. Routine serologic testing of pregnant women early in pregnancy and again at the time of delivery is an important means of controlling this problem.

Congenital syphilis may be manifested within the first 2 years of life (*neonatal congenital syphilis*), characteristically as a rhinitis and chronic nasal discharge (snuffles) with a maculopapular eruption, other mucocutaneous lesions, and loss of weight. These lesions include bullae, vesicles, and superficial desquamation with cracking and scaling of the reddened soles and palms, petechiae, and mucous patches and condyloma latum, as seen in secondary acquired syphilis in the adult. Osteitis, anemia, and a number of disorders involving the visceral organs may also occur. *Late manifestations of congenital syphilis* develop after 2 years of age and include interstitial keratitis and vascularization of the cornea, eighth nerve deafness, arthropathy, signs of congenital neurosyphilis, and gummatous destruction of the palate and nasal septum. The *stigmata* of congenital syphilis involve developing bone and tooth structure, and, for the most part, affect general skeletal, as well as individual, bone growth (*e.g.*, "saber shins," or anterior tibial bowing), with characteristic and classically described changes affecting the facial bones and dentition. These orofacial changes are described in the following section dealing with Oral, Pharyngeal and Facial Manifestations of the Sexually Transmitted Diseases. Unexplained nerve deafness, and retinal and corneal damage noted later in life, in a child born to a syphilitic mother, may also be attributed to congenital syphilis, and may be considered a stigmata of that infection.

Diagnosis of congenital syphilis is based on the knowledge that the child was born to a syphilitic mother together with the recognition of characteristic clinical lesions. All children born to mothers with positive tests for syphilis (either reagin or specific FTA-ABS) have positive tests at birth due to a passive transfer of antibody. Detection of IgM antitreponemal antibody in cord serum suggests the presence of active infection in the infant, since maternal IgM antibody does not cross the placenta. Screening tests for syphilis in congenitally infected children may remain positive throughout life, or convert to negative.

A number of other infections acquired *in utero* (*e.g.*, herpes simplex, rubella, cytomegalovirus, toxoplasmosis), and immunologic disease due to red blood cell incompatibilities between mother and fetus may also produce congenital abnormalities that are similar to those described as part of congenital syphilis.

Treatment of Syphilis

Current recommendations for the treatment of syphilis are as follow:*

Early Syphilis. The recommended regimen for treatment of early syphilis (primary, secondary, and latent syphilis of less than one year's duration) is: benzathine penicillin G, 2.4 million units intramuscularly at a single session. Penicillin-allergic patients should be treated with tetracycline hydrochloride 500 mg by mouth 4 times a day for 15 days. Penicillin-allergic patients who cannot tolerate tetracycline should be treated with erythromycin, 500 mg by mouth 4 times-a-day for 15 days.

Syphilis of More than One Year's Duration (excepting neurosyphilis) should be treated with: benzathine penicillin, 2.4 million units

intramuscularly once a week for three successive weeks. Penicillin-allergic patients should be treated with tetracycline Hydrochloride, 500 mg by mouth 4 times-a-day for 30 days. Penicillin-allergic patients who cannot tolerate tetracycline should be treated with erythromycin, 500 mg by mouth 4 times-a-day for 30 days.

Neurosyphilis. The antibiotic treatment of neurosyphilis is generally more intensive than that of early or late syphilis. Potentially effective regimens include: aqueous crystalline penicillin G, 12-24 million units intravenously for 10 days, followed by benzathine penicillin G, 2.4 million units intramuscularly, weekly for three doses, *or* aqueous procaine penicillin G, 2.4 million units intramuscularly daily, plus probenecid 500 mg by mouth 4 times-a-day for 10 days, followed by benzathine penicillin G, 2.4 million units intramuscularly, weekly for three doses, *or* benzathine penicillin G, 2.4 million units intramuscularly, weekly for three doses.

Follow-up to Therapy

Unless treated early in the disease, patients with syphilis may not revert to a negative serology subsequent to treatment. These patients are termed "sero-fast." Nonetheless, the antibody *titer* in the serologic test for syphilis in sero-fast patients should show a decrease in the number of dilutions subsequent to treatment, and this decrease in the number of dilutions can be used to monitor the effectiveness of treatment.

Clinical Features of the Non-venereal Treponematoses

Yaws, pinta and endemic syphilis are distinguished from venereal syphilis only on clinical and epidemiologic grounds. Pinta involves the skin alone; yaws affects skin and bone; and endemic syphilis affects skin, bone, and mucous membranes. Stages of these diseases are less well-defined than those of venereal syphilis. Congenital and late tertiary complications, such as the cardiovascular and central nervous system involvement described for venereal syphilis, do

---

*As published in MMWR 31:50S, 1982. Established by a group of consultative experts and staff at the United States Public Health Service Centers for Disease Control, and reviewed by a large group of physicians prior to publication.

not usually occur with the non-venereal tre-ponematoses. *Yaws* is a disease of children that occurs predominantly in the hot, humid environment of the tropics, with transmission favored by scanty clothing, poor hygiene and frequent skin trauma. In the western hemisphere, the focus of yaws persists in the West Indies, Central America, and the countries of northeastern South America. *Endemic syphilis* (bejel) is now restricted to arid subtropical climates in Africa, the Eastern Mediterranean, Central Asia, and the Arabian Peninsula. It is not known in the western hemisphere. Infection occurs by direct mouth-to-mouth contact or by infected communal drinking and eating utensils. *Pinta* is a less contagious dermatologic problem that affects older children and is confined to isolated Indian villages in Central America and northern South America. Individuals infected with any of these diseases have positive serologic tests for reagin and specific antigens of *T. pallidum* (FTA-ABS), which are indistinguishable from those in patients with venereal syphilis.

In addition to the cutaneous lesions characterizing these infections, destructive gummatous lesions, osteitis, and periostitis are late features of yaws and endemic syphilis. Orofacial involvement may be quite striking (see description of lesions in the following section dealing with Oral, Pharyngeal, and Facial Manifestations of the Sexually Transmitted Diseases).

Hepatitis B and Other Sexually Transmitted Viral Infections

Hepatitis B

The epidemiology, natural history and clinical features of hepatitis B infections are described in Chapter 20, and serologic procedures for diagnosis can be found in Chapter 3. Transmission of hepatitis B may be parenteral, transcutaneous or transmucosal, although non-parenteral modes of transmission usually require heavier doses and an open laceration or abrasion of the skin or mucosa. Transmission of hepatitis B has been documented following both heterosexual and homosexual intercourse, although simultaneous occurrence of intravenous drug abuse, and the long incubation period of the infection make it difficult to establish venereal transmission in individual cases. Exact figures for the prevalence of hepatitis B as a sexually transmitted infection are therefore not available. Infection with this agent has been found to be particularly prevalent among members of male homosexual communities, who as a group, cooperated with investigators and made important contributions to the better understanding of hepatitis B and to the development of an effective vaccine for this infection in recent years.

Other Viral Infections

A number of other viral infections have also been found to be prevalent among members of these communities, and are also considered to be sexually transmitted infections under these circumstances, even though non-venereal transmission of these agents also occurs. Included under this heading are *herpes simplex types 1 and 2, warts virus, and molluscum contagiosum virus* (see discussion earlier in this chapter), *cytomegalovirus* (CMV, virus of cytomegalic-inclusion body disease), Epstein-Barr virus (EB virus of infectious mononucleosis), and possibly *human T-cell leukemia* and other *retroviruses* (see following discussion of the acquired immune deficiency syndrome). Numerous other viral agents, including those associated with *common upper respiratory* and *gastrointestinal infections* are probably also transmitted under the circumstances of multiple casual sexual contact described for users of "gay bath houses" and "gay clubs" in large cities.

The Acquired Immune Deficiency Syndrome

Acquired Immune Deficiency and Opportunistic Infection

The name *acquired immune deficiency syndrome* (AIDS) is given to a severe and apparently irreversible acquired defect in cell-mediated immunity, which predisposes the affected individuals to multiple severe opportunistic infections and/or unusual neoplasms, such as Kaposi's sarcoma. This category excludes individuals who have similar defects in cell-mediated immunity as a result of another disease process, such as an inborn immune deficiency, any of those immune deficiencies secondary to lymphoma, leukemia or diabetes, or the result of treatment with cytotoxic, immunosuppressive, or lengthy broad spectrum antibiotic therapy. *The essence of the acquired immune deficiency syndrome, and the feature that distinguishes it from other types of acquired immune deficiency, is the development of one or more opportunistic infections, or the atypical presentation of an infection in an otherwise healthy person who should be resistant to infection with these particular organisms.*

The term "opportunistic infection" as defined elsewhere in this text, (see section on Candidiasis in Chapter 6), can refer to persistent and sometimes overwhelming infections with a great variety of microorganisms (viruses, bacteria, fungi, and protozoal parasites), which as a group, are non-pathogenic, saphrophytic members of the normal skin, gut and orificial flora of humans and animals (and common organisms in soil and water). The list of organisms of this type, which under unusual circumstances may be found as contaminants of skin and mucosal wounds, is quite extensive. However, certain of these organisms have been isolated from persistent skin, mucosal, and visceral infections in immune deficient patients frequently enough to be of primary concern in all acquired immune deficient states. As described in Chapter 6, these organisms include fungi such as *Candida, Aspergillus* and *Cryptococcus,* and protozoal parasites such as *Toxoplasma, Pneumocystis carinii, Cryptosporidium,* and *Isospora.* Another consequence of defective cell-mediated immunity is the failure of a host tissue to limit or contain a variety of infectious agents that usually produce only localized disease, but that may disseminate throughout the body of the immune deficient host and produce a variety of atypical clinical presentations. Included under this heading are infections with *herpes simplex virus, varicella-zoster virus, cytomegalovirus,* and infections with the so-called atypical mycobacteria (*Mycobacterium avium intracellulare* group of organisms).

Epidemiology and Proposed Etiologies

The acquired immune deficiency syndrome was first recognized as a result of surveillance by the United States Public Health Service Centers for Disease Control of patients for whom the restricted antibiotic, Pentamidine was requested for treatment of *Pneumocystis carinii* infections. *P. carinii* had been described as a cause of rare ("plasma cell") pneumonia for many years, but more recently it was noted as a prevalent infectious agent in the lungs, other visceral organs, and bone marrow of immune-suppressed patients. Investigators at the Centers for Disease Control noticed that a cluster of these infections was occurring in individuals without inborn immune deficiency or evidence of any disease likely to cause an acquired immune deficiency. All of these initial cases were in male homosexuals, many of whom reported multiple sexual contacts. Subsequently, numerous cases of atypical, and often overwhelming infections with one or more of the other opportunistic agents just listed, were reported in male homosexuals. *Kaposi's sarcoma* (an otherwise rare and indolent skin malignancy restricted to elderly individuals of Jewish or Mediterranean descent) was also noted frequently in young male homosexuals, where it manifested as a disseminated and rapidly fatal disease.

As of June 1983, 1450 cases of the acquired immune deficiency syndrome had been reported in the United States, with a case fatality rate of 39%. Among 78 cases, which were diagnosed at least two years earlier, the fatality rate was 82%. The disease has not been restricted to male homosexuals with multiple sexual contacts (71% of cases), but has also been seen in association with intravenous drug abuse (17%), repeated transfusions of blood or blood products in hemophiliacs (1%), and also in heterosexual contacts of men with the syndrome. An unusually large number of cases (5%) has also been recorded among allegedly heterosexual, recent Haitian immigrants to the United States, and unexplained cellular immune deficiency and opportunistic infections have been reported in infants born to mothers at high risk for the syndrome.

The distribution of cases of the acquired immune deficiency syndrome thus parallels that of hepatitis-B infection, and suggests that the syndrome may be due to an infectious agent, which like hepatitis B, is transmitted by blood or blood-contaminated bodily secretions, providing for both parenteral and sexual routes of transmission noted above. To date, no person-to-person transmission has been identified other than through intimate contact or parenteral routes, and no cases have been reported in clinical or laboratory workers exposed to patients with the acquired immune deficiency syndrome or their blood or tissues. No infectious agent specific for this syndrome has been identified, although recent evidence suggests that human T-cell leukemia virus (HTLV) or a related retrovirus (RNA viruses containing the enzyme reverse transcriptase, allowing production of a DNA copy of their RNA genome) may be involved. HTLV infection occurs in patients with the acquired immune deficiency syndrome, and HLTV can infect and terminally transform their T-helper lymphocytes, suggesting a basis for the defect in cell-mediated immunity. Further study is needed, however, to establish that HLTV and related retroviruses are not simply additional opportunistic infectious agents but etiologic agents of the acquired immune deficiency syndrome. Other hypotheses, also largely unsupported by critical data, have implicated cytomegalovirus infection, excessive doses of antigenically foreign semen, abuse of nitrites as mood enhancers, and chronic infection with hepatitis B or other unknown infectious agents.

Diagnosis and Clinical Features

There is currently no laboratory test to identify the patient with the acquired immune deficiency syndrome, and diagnosis is based on the finding of Kaposi's sarcoma in individuals under 50 years-of-age or finding life-threatening, opportunistic infections with no underlying cause for immune deficiency. The syndrome should be strongly suspected individuals from any of the high-risk categories (individuals with multiple homosexual or heterosexual contacts, those receiving multiple transfusions of blood or blood products, the offspring of individuals in high risk groups, intravenous drug abusers, and recent Haitian immigrants). Patients with atyp-

ical presentations of certain viral and bacterial infections (*e.g.*, chronic herpes simplex infection, disseminated herpes zoster, progressive pulmonary infection with *Mycobacterium avium*), should also be considered as possible cases of the syndrome, if no underlying cause for the atypical presentation can be found.

The exact nature of the cellular immune deficiency in patients with the syndrome has not been defined, but 95% of cases have been shown to have persistent and profound selective decrease in function as well as in number of T lymphocytes of the helper/inducer subset with relative or absolute increase of the suppressor/cytotoxic subset. Experimentally, this may be detected by determination of circulating T-lymphocyte subsets, by rosette formation, using specific antibody coated with sheep red blood cells, and by enumerating the so-called (OK) T4 and T8* subsets of lymphocytes in a fluorescence-activated cell sorter using monoclonal antibodies. While calculation of the T4/T8 ratio utilizing these techniques is becoming more widely available, and probably essential in any investigation of this syndrome, the cost of the procedure and uncertainty about interpretation of the results currently limits its usefulness (depression of T-lymphocyte subsets and reversal of the T4/T8 ratio also occur as transient phenomena with many minor upper-respiratory infections, and infectious mononucleosis, for example). There is also, usually, anergy to recall skin-test antigens (mumps, *Candida*, *Trichophyton* and streptokinase/streptodornase). The majority of cases of the acquired immune deficiency syndrome are diagnosed solely on clinical and epidemiologic grounds, with the assistance of conventional microbiologic isolation procedures. Humoral immunity remains intact, often with increase of serum immunoglobulin levels.

The clinical course of the syndrome varies considerably, depending on the nature of the opportunistic infectious agents and/or neoplasms involved. However, the disease usually begins wth malaise, weight loss, and unexplained lymphadenopathy, followed by

---

*Ortho Diagnostic Kit monoclonal antibody reagents. Ortho Diagnostics Inc., Division of Johnson & Johnson, Raritan, NJ, 08869

severe opportunistic infections, Kaposi's sarcoma or other unusual malignancies, such as EB virus associated lymphomas. Additional findings may include fever, leukopenia, and cutaneous anergy. An otherwise common infection such as oral or genital candidiasis may be the initial clinical presentation; conversely, pneumonia, persistent diarrhea, colitis, proctitis, or chronic herpes simplex may be the cause for additional evaluation of a patient for an underlying disease such as undiagnosed malignancy, diabetes, lymphoma, or unusual infectious agents. In many cases, the natural history of the syndrome involves multiple and recurring infections with gradual deterioration and development of complications secondary to the infections. Currently, there is no specific treatment for the syndrome other than the administration of appropriate antibiotic agents in the hope of controlling the multiple and repeated infections.

The lesions of Kaposi's sarcoma in this group of patients are described in the following section dealing with the Oral, Pharyngeal, and Facial Manifestations of the Sexually Transmitted Diseases. Lymph nodes removed from patients with the acquired immune deficiency syndrome show lymphoid and endothelial cellular proliferation, expanded germinal centers, large sheets of mature plasma cells and other evidences of B-cell activation.

Four stages of the syndrome have been defined. *Stage I* (asymptomatic) includes any defect in cellular immunity, with neutropenia detectable only by laboratory studies. *Stage II* (prodrome) involves fever of unknown origin, chronic diarrhea, unexplained weight loss, general malaise, oral candidiasis, and oral and perioral herpes simplex as characteristics of this stage. *Stage III* (generalized lymphadenopathy) involves cervical, axillary, and inguinal lymphadenopathy with reactive hyperplasia. *Stage IV* (final) includes Kaposi's sarcoma, opportunistic infections (usually pulmonary or gastrointestinal), and ocular lesions (viral retinitis and phlebitis). Cases where patient exhibits opportunistic infections are more likely to progress to fatal outcomes than are those where patients with Kaposi's sarcoma have no major opportunistic infections.

The "Minor Venereal Diseases"—Granuloma Inguinale, Lymphogranuloma Venereum, and Chancroid

The so-called "minor venereal diseases" (minor in comparison with the major diseases of syphilis and gonorrhea) are listed among the sexually transmitted diseases, even though their prevalence in western countries is very low and they are usually due to infection contracted while traveling in an area of the world where the infection remains endemic. Granuloma inguinale and lymphogranuloma venereum have, on occasion, been described in association with oral lesions (see following section); chancroid is a localized infection of the external genitalia and inguinal lymph nodes with no reported oral lesions.

Granuloma inguinale (donovanosis) is an infectious granuloma usually found in the inguinal and the anogenital regions. It is caused by a gram-negative bacterium, *Donovania granulomatis*, and is a chronic, slowly progressive, mildly contagious disease. The lesions begin as small papules that ulcerate, increase slowly in size, and eventually give rise to velvety, beefy, granulating, spreading ulcerative lesions of the inguinal and the anogenital regions. Constitutional symptoms like pain and suppuration are uncommon. The inguinale lymph nodes are not involved, although the lesions may spread to involve the inguinal creases. Diagnosis is made by demonstration of Donovan bodies in smears from deep scrapings or biopsy specimens of the lesions. In smears and sections, the organisms are recognized as large gram-negative oval bacteria with intense bipolar staining ("safety pin" appearance). They are usually surrounded by halos and are typically situated in mononuclear cells. These structures are referred to as Donovan bodies. One of the tetracycline drugs or streptomycin is usually used to treat the infection. Plastic surgery may be needed for correction of extensive scarring secondary to the large granulomatous lesions.

Lymphogranuloma venereum (also referred to as LGV, and *lymphopathia venereum*) is caused by an organism of the genus *Chlamydia* (LGV agent), which produces a regional lymphadenitis. In the male, the infection presents as a firm tender enlargement of the inguinal lymph glands: the overlying skin becomes reddened and dusky, and multiple purulent fistulas develop over the enlarged gland (the fully developed lesion being referred to as a bubo). Due to the different anatomic arrangement of lymphatic drainage in the female, the pararectal, rather than the inguinal, glands are usually involved. Constitutional disturbances may also occur. Marked scarring and local edema frequently develop secondary to the suppurative lymphadenitis, particularly in the female. Lymphogranuloma venereum is important in the differential diagnosis of inguinal adenopathy in both male and female, and of rectal stricture in the female. It is diagnosed by a complement fixation test on the patient's serum; the intradermal Frei test, which was previously used, is not specific for infection with the LGV agent. Both antibiotic therapy as well as surgical treatment of the buboes and secondary scarring may be needed.

Chancroid (or "soft sore") is caused by a small gram-negative bacillus, *Hemophilus ducreyi,* and is characterized by darkfield-negative (*i.e.* non-syphilitic) genital ulcers and inguinal buboes. Outbreaks of chancroid that occurred in California and Canada in recent years were traced to contacts with prostitutes, and demonstrated that the minor venereal infections have not disappeared in North America. Continued surveillance, follow-up and treatment of infected sexual contacts, and prophylactic treatment of members of high-risk groups, as traditionally practiced by the public health authorities, remain important keys to the control of all sexually transmitted diseases.

ORAL, PHARYNGEAL AND FACIAL MANIFESTATIONS OF THE SEXUALLY TRANSMITTED DISEASES

Pharyngeal Gonorrhea and Gonococcal Stomatitis

Gonococcal stomatitis was briefly mentioned in literature prior to the introduction of antibiotics. However, even Frazer, whose report of a case of gonococcal stomatitis in 1931 remained a classic description for over 35 years, admitted that it was a rare condition, and listed only 40 cases reported since Neisser discovered the gonococcus in 1879. A description of gonococcal stomatitis was included in early editions of this textbook, but from 1946 to 1977, all references to oropharyngeal infection with *N. gonorrhoeae* were deleted, and gonorrhea was dropped from the section dealing with venereal diseases of dental interest. Gonococcal pharyngitis and asymptomatic gonococcal pharyngeal infections were again described in the late 1960's, and in the following decade there were at least 20 papers dealing with the clinical spectrum of pharyngeal gonococcal infection, totaling well over 500 published cases. These represent only a fraction of the number of cases currently occurring yearly; and a clinical diagnostic laboratory in an urban medical center might handle as many gonococcus-positive throat cultures each year. Routine culturing of the throat (and anorectal mucosa), as well as the genitourinary secretions, is therefore now advised for all patients with suspected gonorrhea.

Pharyngeal Gonorrhea

This changed orientation to pharyngeal gonorrhea followed the introduction of a new antibiotic-containing selective medium for *N. gonorrhoeae* (Thayer Martin medium), which allowed more certain isolation of this fastidious species from the mixed population of saphrophytic *Neisseria* and other organisms constituting the normal oropharyngeal flora (see Table 28-4). A more liberal attitude to public discussion of sexual habits (homosexuality in particular) has also no doubt made the medical and dental profession more perceptive and aware of the likelihood of oropharyngeal sexually transmitted disease in particular situations. Prevalence rates for pharyngeal gonorrhea vary considerably depending on the group investigated, and rates of about 2% to 7% are found among unselected patients attending clinics for sexually transmitted diseases; higher rates are seen in pregnant women (2% to 15%) and in male homosexuals (20% to 25%). The highest prevalence rates are reported when case selection is based on a history of recent contact

Table 28-4. Selective Growth of *Neisseria* sp. and Other Microorganisms on Chocolate Agar and Thayer-Martin Medium*

Organisms	# of Strains	Growth on Chocolate Agar	Growth on Thayer-Martin Medium[†]
Staphylococcus aureus	6	6	0
Staphylococcus epidermidis	7	7	0
Sarcina lutea	2	2	0
Escherichia coli	1	1	0
Pseudomonas sp.	2	2	0
Bacillus sp.	3	3	0
Corynebacterium sp.	3	3	0
Listeria monocytogenes	2	2	0
Lactobacillus sp.	3	3	1
Acinebacter sp. (previously *Mima polymorpha*)	3	3	1
Neisseria sicca	5	5	0
Neisseria subflava (includes *N. flava, N. perflava*)	7	7	0
Neisseria flavescens	4	4	0
Branhamella catarrhalis (previously *Neisseria catarrhalis*)	6	6	1
Neisseria meningitidis (A, B & C)	4	4	4
Neisseria gonorrhoeae	50	50	50

* (Modified from Thayer JD and Martin JE Jr: Improved medium for selective cultivation of *N. gonorrheae* and *N. meningitidis*. Pub Health Reports 81:599, 1966; Courtesy of United States Public Health Service, Department of Health Education and Welfare)

[†] A medium for primary isolation of *N. gonorrheae* and *N. meningitidis* that is enriched with the antibiotics vancomycin, colistimethate, and nystatin to inhibit other saphrophytic urogenital and nasopharyngeal microbial flora, and encourage growth of the more fastidious pathogenic *Neisseria* sp. This medium with minor changes is now available commercially for clinical use as prepackaged agar plates that can be transported in Zip-loc bags with a carbon dioxide atmosphere. See Chapter 3 for further details.

with a sexual partner with gonorrhea (greater than 30%), or based on evidence of *N. gonorrhoeae* infection at other mucosal sites (*e.g.,* 39% to 96%, in different studies for pregnant women with gonorrhea). All studies have emphasized the necessity of orogenital contact in the acquisition of pharyngeal gonorrhea, but the possibility of other routes for colonization of the pharynx (*e.g.,* auto-inoculation, or ordinary kissing) have not been definitely excluded.

The term pharyngeal gonorrhea refers to all patients in whom *N. gonorrhoeae* is isolated from the nasopharynx, and includes those in whom the infection is asymptomatic (80%), as well as those in whom symptoms of sore throat or exudative pharyngitis are observed at the time of isolation and have been attributed to the sexually transmitted infection. Despite the availability of a selective me-

dium, the false-negative culture rate for pharyngeal *N. gonorrhoeae* is considered to be high, and accurate matching of particular symptoms with time of isolation has not been possible. Some investigators have questioned whether the presence of *N. gonorrhoeae* in the throat actually constitutes a disease, or rather a transient colonization of this specialized columnar epithelium by organisms better adapted to the urogenital mucosa. Even without treatment, asymptomatic pharyngeal carriers of this organism, who have no other evidence of gonorrhea, will lose the organism from the pharynx over a two-month period, and usually fail to transmit the infection through mouth-to-mouth contact (*c.f.* the old adage that gonorrhea is not acquired by kissing). Similarities have been seen between pharyngeal infection with *N. gonorrhoeae* and another closely related potential pathogen,

Neisseria meningitidis. Invasive disease caused by *N. meningitidis* is associated with lack of specific bactericidal antibody, and not simply with the presence of the organism in the nasopharynx.

Despite conflicting opinions concerning the local pathogenicity and transmissibility of pharyngeal gonococci, pharyngeal cultures positive for *N. gonorrhoeae* are considered to be evidence of gonorrhea, and the diagnostic laboratory is required to report such cases to local health authorities along with cases where genitourinary (and anorectal) cultures are positive. This practice is supported by a number of documented cases in which *N. gonorrhoeae* was isolated from the tonsillar/pharyngeal region only, and not from other mucosal sites. Disseminated gonococcal infection and gonococcal septicemia and arthritis have also been reported in association with positive pharyngeal cultures, and in patients whose pharynx was the only mucosal site positive for the organism.

Gonococcal Stomatitis

The clear evidence for the existence of nasopharyngeal gonorrhea, based upon isolation of the gonococcus on selective media has not been matched by equally critical evidence for the existence of gonococcal stomatitis following orogenital contact. In addition to the cases described in the 1930's, we are aware of some 12 papers that describe cases identified as "gonococcal stomatitis." In the great majority of these, the bacteriologic data provided either do not state if antibiotic-containing selective media were used, or clearly indicate the use of relatively nonselective media (*e.g.*, chocolate agar) and/or limited identification techniques. Both of these deficiencies could allow confusion between *N. gonorrhoeae* and saphrophytic oral gram-negative cocci (*e.g.*, *Neisseria catarrhalis*, now referred to as *Branhamella* sp.). There is thus considerable doubt as to whether most of the cases of gonococcal stomatitis described in the 1930's, and even many of the more recently described cases, are due to gonococcal infection. One of the cases described by Weisner and colleagues in which acute gingivitis developed around extraction sites in a patient who had practiced fellatio repeatedly four days after extensive dental extractions is a more convincing example of gonococcal stomatitis, since *N. gonorrhoeae* was isolated from the extraction site on Thayer Martin medium, and identified by exhaustive cultural, fermentation and serologic methods.

Very likely, the general availability of Thayer Martin medium, the continued epidemic of gonorrhea, and the increased awareness of pharyngeal gonorrhea will result in more confirmed cases of gonococcal stomatitis. At the moment, however, critical review of published data leaves some doubt as to the clinical spectrum of oral lesions that are associated with positive oral cultures for *N. gonorrhoeae*. The wide range of lesions described in the literature (isolated ulcers, gingivitis, and membranous gingivostomatitis, variously described as "fiery red," "yellowish," "greenish," and so forth) probably includes a number of cases of non-specific or traumatic lesions associated with orogenital sexual activity. This range suggests that caution should be used in making a diagnosis of gonococcal stomatitis (on the basis of a history of recent orogenital contact) without adequate confirmatory bacteriologic data. The resistance of stratified squamous epithelium versus columnar epithelium to penetration by *N. gonorrhoeae* also probably reduces the chance of gonococcal stomatitis developing, when gonococci are inoculated into the oral cavity. The more frequent association of symptomatic pharyngeal gonorrhea with a history of fellatio, as opposed to a history of cunnilingus, also suggests that at least some of the oral lesions described in patients following orogenital sexual contact are due to trauma to the oral mucosa rather than to any specific sexually transmitted agent.

Procedures for laboratory diagnosis of oropharyngeal infection with *N. gonorrhoeae* are described in Chapter 3. The relative resistance of pharyngeal gonorrhea to antibiotic therapies that are successful in the treatment of urogenital gonorrhea is well documented. Current regimens for treatment of pharyngeal gonorrhea specify that neither amoxicillin, ampicillin, or spectinomycin regimens be used, and that treatment with tetracycline hydrochloride (1.5 g initial dose followed by 500 mg by mouth 4 times a day for 7 days), or aqueous penicillin G (4.8 million units injected intramuscularly at two sites with 1 g of probenecid by mouth) be used.

Oral Candidiasis

The oral lesions of candidiasis are described in Chapter 6—Red and White Lesions of the Oral Mucosa.

Oral Condyloma Acuminatum

Condyloma acuminatum of the oral cavity has been described as involving the gingiva, cheeks, lips, hard palate, tongue (including the frenum), and the floor of the mouth (see Figure 28-10). The incidence of oral condyloma acuminatum, and of its simultaneous occurrence with genital condyloma acuminatum, is not known. It is probably more prevalent than a review of cases reported in literature might suggest. The occurrence of multiple oral warts, (their location on a mucosal surface likely to suggest orogenital sexual contact), a history of genital warts in sexual contact, recurrences following local excision, and a history of repeated orogenital contact can all be useful clues in the identification of oral warts as condyloma acuminatum. Surgical excision or cryotherapy are the preferred methods of treatment.

Herpes Simplex Infection of the Oropharyngeal Region

The oropharyngeal lesions caused by herpes simplex virus infection are described in Chapter 5. No consistent clinical differences have been noted between either primary or recurrent lesions due to type 1 versus type 2 herpes simplex virus. The literature contains case reports of primary oropharyngeal herpes infections due to either type 1 or type 2 virus acquired by orogenital contact with an infected sexual partner (as well as genital lesions resulting from contact with oral infection due to either type 1 or type 2). Clinically, primary infection of the oral region from this source may manifest as an acute gingivostomatitis, pharyngitis, or perioral vesicular rash, in each case usually with obvious constitutional symptoms of fever, malaise, and muscle pain. Alternatively, the primary oral infection may be asymptomatic and subclinical, and only manifest subsequently as re-

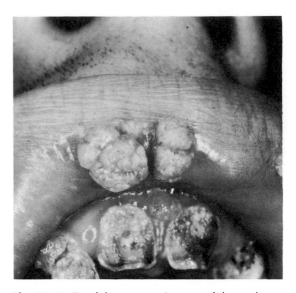

Fig. 28-10 Condyloma acuminatum of the oral cavity.

current herpes labialis. Concurrent oral and genital infection with identical strains of herpes virus confirmed by restriction–endonuclease analysis has been described.

Molluscum Contagiosum

Characteristic lesions of this superficial viral infection rarely occur on the face and usually occur only in children, as a result of nonvenereal but close contact associated with shared sleeping accommodations. Lesions located close to the eyes or on the conjunctiva may be associated with a marked foreign body reaction. Intraoral lesions of molluscum contagiosum are rare, but papillary eruptive lesions showing the histologic features of molluscum contagiosum have occasionally been noted on the lips, cheeks, and other regions in the oral cavity. An incidence for labial lesions of about 8% was recorded in studies of institutional epidemics of this infection at the turn of the century.

Oral and Facial Manifestations of Syphilis

Oral lesions may occur in all three stages of acquired syphilis as well as congenital syphilis. These lesions are of some dental importance, though the reason for their significance differs with the stage. The oral cavity is described as the most frequent site for an extragenital chancre in the primary stage (see Table 28-5), although the rarity of extragenital lesions of syphilis in recent years makes this more a matter of historical, rather than current, practical diagnostic interest. Oral mucosal lesions may be a prominent and important diagnostic clue for secondary syphilis and may occur with or without a more obvious skin rash and/or a history of a chancre. The palate was considered the common site for a gumma prior to the introduction of penicillin, and tertiary syphilis was an important consideration in the differential diagnosis of acquired palatal perforations. Many of the classic lesions of congenital syphilis also manifest in the craniofacial area and the dentition. The oral lesions that are seen in each of the three stages of acquired syphilis and in congenital syphilis are therefore described in some detail in this section, although at this time a clinician is most likely to encounter only the oral lesions of secondary syphilis, and perhaps occasionally the lesions of congenital syphilis. The oral lesions of primary and secondary syphilis are contagious; those of tertiary and congenital syphilis are not.

Oral Manifestations of Primary Syphilis

The oral lesion of primary syphilis is, as elsewhere, the chancre. Chancres have been described on the lips, oral mucosa, tongue, soft palate, tonsillar area, pharyngeal region, and gingiva (see Figure 28-11 A, B & C). The lip alone accounted for over one half of 68 extragenital chancres reported in one study in 1941. Since the introduction of penicillin, however, extragenital chancres in any location have become unusual events, and a number of authors have stated that they are rarely seeing them even in venereal disease clinics. In fact, the discovery of a chancre on the finger of a sailor in a Danish venereal disease clinic in recent years was considered so unusual that it warranted publication of the case. The reasons for the rarity of extragenital chancres are not clear, but they may relate to the widespread availability of antibiotics, which may abort the primary syphilitic lesion even with doses that are inadequate to cure the infection. Changes in the pathogenicity and contagiousness of *T. pallidum* may also possibly have occurred.

Extragenital chancres present interesting diagnostic problems, since the serologic test for syphilis is usually negative at the time. Chancres of the oral cavity may also not present as characteristic painless, brown-crusted indurated lesions found on the genitalia, because of the moisture, trauma, and microbial flora present in the mouth. Intraoral chancres are usually slightly painful (because of secondary infection) and are covered with a grayish white film. Extraoral portions of lip chancres may have the more typical brown-crusted appearance. Chancres of the lips may occur as multiple lesions; the literature contains conflicting information on the relative frequency with which the lower versus the upper lip is involved with a chancre. Induration of the underlying tissue is not as striking as it is on other body surfaces. A history

Table 28-5. Distribution of Extragenital Syphilitic Chancres by Site & Sex

SITE	MALES	FEMALES
Lip	8	5
Tonsil	—	2
Tongue	1	—
Mouth	—	1
Nose	—	1
Breast	—	1
Wrist	—	1
Finger	1	1
Abdomen	2	—
Groin	1	—
Totals	13	12

(Modified from Kampmeier R.H.: Essentials of Syphilology. Philadelphia, J.B. Lippincott 1943. In recent years, extragenital chancres have become rare lesions, except in the anorectal area.)

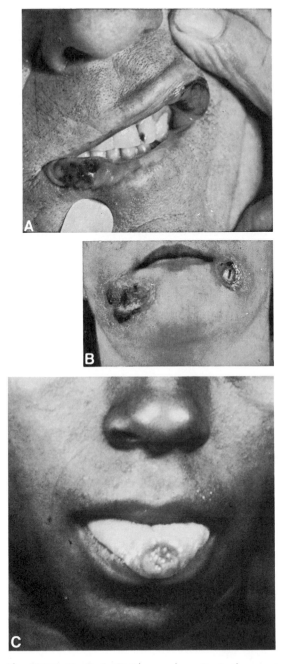

Fig. 28-11 (A, B & C) The oral cavity is the most common location for extragenital chancres, although these lesions have become rare since the introduction of penicillin therapy. (A) Multiple chancres appear in acute primary syphilis. (From Kampmeier RH: Essentials of Syphiology, Philadelphia, JB Lippincott, 1943) (B) Two chancres appear on the chin. (From Lever WF: Multiple extragenital giant chancres. New England Journal of Medicine 231:227, 1944) (C) A chancre appears on the tip of the tongue.

of exposure to infection is an important aid in making a tentative clinical diagnosis. The appearance of the lesion and the darkfield examination are not specifically diagnostic of intraoral chancres, since other spirochetes (*Treponema microdentium*) inhabit this region and make differentiation from *T. pallidum* difficult. The organism is also not adequately stained by aniline dyes, and it cannot be seen in smears or sections stained with Giemsa, Papanicolaou, or hematoxylin and eosin. Staining with fluorescein-labeled antitreponemal antibody, however, can provide positive identification of a chancre.

As with suspected genital chancres, herpes simplex infections must be considered in the differential diagnosis of chancres of the lip. The superficial crusting that occurs after the rupture of a large vesicle or a group of small vesicles of herpes may simulate a chancre. The history of onset of the herpetic lesion is usually characteristic. It is also usually more painful, of shorter duration, and frequently associated with an upper respiratory tract infection. Lymphadenopathy is uncommon. An "herpetic" lesion that requires more than 2 weeks for involution, especially if it is accompanied by unilateral adenopathy, should be suspected of being luetic in origin. An early malignancy may also have many of the characteristics of the syphilitic chancre.

Oral Manifestations of Secondary Syphilis

The oral lesions of secondary syphilis, as mentioned earlier are: mucous patches, split papules and, rarely, condylomata lata. The disease can be transmitted through contaminated salivary droplets from the patient with secondary syphilis.

Mucous Patches. Syphilitic mucous patches represent the mucous membrane analogue of the papular or macular skin eruption. They are found on the tongue, buccal mucosa, the tonsillar and the pharyngeal regions, and on the lips, yet are uncommon on the gingiva. They are considered the most highly infectious lesions of syphilis and appear as slightly raised, grayish-white lesions surrounded by an erythematous base (see Figure 28-12). When mucous patches are observed on the tongue, they have raised appearances in their early stages, with the partial loss of the lingual papillae over the lesions clearly demarcating them from the uninvolved tissue. They are often painless but may be mild-to-moderately painful when they develop on movable tissues, especially when they are exposed to the oral environment. This mild-to-moderate pain is disproportionate to the large area of oral mucosa involved; and if the mucous patches had been aphthous ulcers, the pain would have been considerably more

severe. Trauma to the surface of the lesions results in a raw, bleeding surface.

Oral mucous patches may be mistaken for healing herpetic, traumatic, fusospirochetal, or erythema multiforme lesions. The healing herpetic lesion has a yellow, opaque coating, as opposed to the grayish, translucent surface of the mucous patch. Fusospirochetal ulcerations are more acutely painful, and they are usually associated with typical gingival lesions. Erythema multiforme lesions are painful and usually involve the lips, with marked hemorrhage and eschar formation on the skin surface of the lip.

Recent studies have indicated that syphilitic mucous patches and other oral and skin lesions of secondary syphilis are rarely diagnosed correctly when first encountered. They are usually attributed to a variety of other infectious agents or allergic processes before the presence of a positive serologic test for syphilis suggests the diagnosis.

Papules. Split papules are raised papular lesions that develop at the commissures of the lips and develop a fissure separating the upper-lip portion of the papule from the lower-lip portion. They are often confused with cases of angular cheilitis. Papules have been described at other oral locations, *e.g.*, dorsum of the tongue. The clinical appearance of the lesion is usually non-specific, and the diagnosis is based on positive laboratory tests for syphilis and response of the lesion to penicillin.

Condylomata Lata. Condylomata lata, which may occur on the skin as well as on the mucosa, are flat, silver gray, wart-like papules sometimes having an ulcerating surface (see Figure 28-13). They are usually painless.

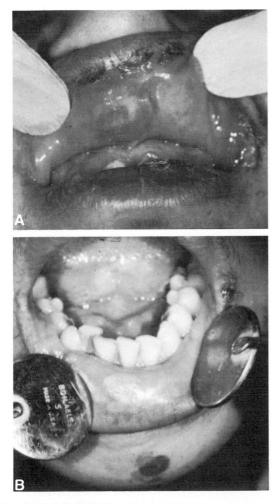

Fig. 28-12 (A & B) The mucous patch is a common intraoral lesion of secondary syphilis and may be accompanied by other skin and oral mucosal lesions. (A) Note the oval shape of the mucous patch of the upper lip and its translucent surface. (B) A split papule at the left oral commissure, a mucous patch on the lip, and a papular lesion on the chin are all present.

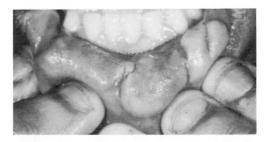

Fig. 28-13 Condylomatous types of secondary luetic lesions appear on inner surface of lower lip.

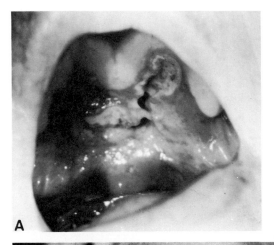

Fig. 28-14 (A & B) Intraoral gummas, the characteristic lesions of tertiary syphilis, are penicillin-sensitive and rarely seen since the introduction of penicillin therapy. These two illustrations from an earlier edition of this text show the characteristic features of this lesion. (A) Developing gumma of the palate. The marginal discoloration of the lesion is typical. Perforation of the palate was not complete at this time. (B) Another gumma of the palate.

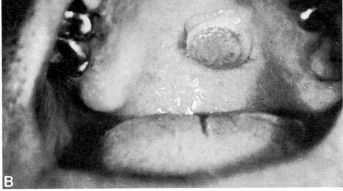

Oral Manifestations of Tertiary Syphilis

The oral lesions of tertiary syphilis occur most frequently on the palate and the tongue. Gummatous destruction of the palatal bones is a known cause of perforation of the palate, which is now rarely if ever seen (see Figure 28-14 A & B). Gummata have also been described as involving the salivary glands and the jaw bones.

Gummatous involvement of the tongue was at one time common in late untreated syphilis and a chronic ulcerated gumma often presented a difficult diagnostic problem. Malignant growths and tuberculous lesions had to be considered in the differential diagnosis. Numerous small healed gummata in the tongue resulted in a series of nodules or scars in the deeper areas of the organ, giving the tongue an "upholstered" or tufted appearance. A diffuse luetic involvement of this organ often resulted in complete atrophy of the papillary coating and a firm fibrous texture— a luetic bald tongue, also referred to as interstitial glossitis. Leukoplakia was frequently associated with luetic glossitis (see Figure 28-15 A & B), but the exact nature of the relationship has not been established (see discussion of leukoplakia of the tongue as a precancerous lesion in Chapters 6 and 10).

Delayed fracture healing (or nonunion) or a resistant osteomyelitis following oral surgery also suggested, at one time, the possibility of chronic syphilis (see Figure 28-16).

Severe neuralgic pains of the head and neck may occur in tabes dorsalis and must be differentiated from neuralgic pains secondary to dental or pharyngeal disease. Tertiary neurosyphilis must still be considered in the differential diagnosis for older patients with unexplained jaw and face pain who

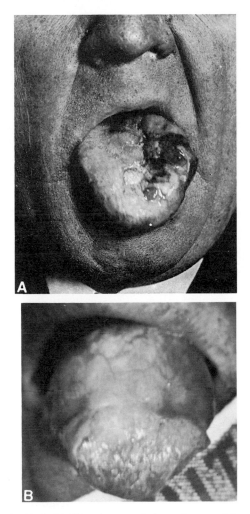

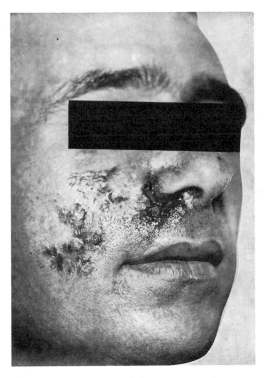

Fig. 28-16 Tertiary syphilitic osteomyelitis is associated with an impacted supernumerary tooth in the upper incisor region. Note the numerous fistulous openings.

Fig. 28-15 (A & B) The characteristic tertiary syphilitic lesions of the tongue are now rarely seen: (A) Syphilitic gumma of the tongue. Illustration is attributed to MacKee GM in Sutton RL, Sutton RL, Jr: Handbook of Diseases of the Skin. St. Louis MO, CV Mosby, 1949. (B) Syphilitic interstitial glossitis with associated leukoplakic changes and squamous cell carcinoma of the tip of the tongue is shown.

have a history of inadequately treated tertiary syphilis and a persistently positive serologic test for syphilis. It is not unusual for tabes dorsalis to involve a degeneration of the sensory portion of the fifth cranial nerve with complete integrity of the motor root. Loss of taste, and spontaneous necrosis of the alveolar process without any observable cause have also been recorded in tabetic patients. Paresthesia may occur in the lips, the tongue,

and the cheeks. Virtually painless ulcerations of the palate and the nasal septum are also reported. Spontaneous death of the dental pulp in the absence of recognizable precipitating factors and altered pulp-test responses have also been recorded in both tabetic and paretic patients.

The patient who has a damaged aortic valve secondary to luetic involvement is still occasionally seen, and should be given antibiotic prophylaxis before dental treatment in order to prevent bacterial endocarditis.

Oral and Facial Manifestations of Congenital Syphilis

The oral changes associated with syphilis acquired *in utero* represent visual evidence of this disease. Since these changes persist or are manifest years after the acute infection, the dentist may be the first to suspect congenital syphilis. The patient is seldom infectious during this stage of the disease. The oral features of congenital syphilis include postrhagadic scarring about the mouth, changes in the teeth, and other dentofacial abnormalities.

Postrhagadic Scarring and Syphilitic Rhagades

Postrhagadic scars are linear lesions found around the oral or anal orifices. They result from a diffuse luetic involvement of the skin in these parts from the third to the seventh week after birth. The lesions first appear as red or copper-colored linear areas covered with a soft crust. Rhagades are said to be seen more frequently on the lower lip because of the thinness of the epithelium covering this structure, and its greater mobility.

Healed syphilitic rhagades appear clinically as ordinary cicatrices, but histologic study reveals specific pathologic changes. The linear scars are radially arranged and perpendicular to the mucocutaneous junction (see Figure 28-17). They are most prominent on the lower lip near the angles of the mouth. Frequently, there is diminished coloring of the lip and lack of distinctness of the mucocutaneous border. Differentiation from perioral and nasolabial wrinkles and fissures associated with loss of teeth and occlusal vertical dimension is important; these latter signs usually increase with advancing age and follow the natural skin creases.

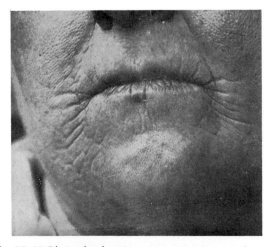

Fig. 28-17 Rhagades forming permanent scars radiate from the lips in congenital syphilis. (From Thoma, KH: Oral Pathology. St Louis, C V Mosby)

Changes in the Dentition

The deciduous dentition is rarely affected, since fetal luetic infection occurring during the formation of the crowns of these teeth usually results in abortion or stillbirth. Abnormalities in color, size, and shape of the deciduous teeth have been described, and Burket demonstrated histologic changes confined to the dentition in such teeth. Retarded root resorption of the deciduous dentition is noted frequently in congenital luetics.

In 1856, Sir Jonathan Hutchinson reported the typical defects, or "marring," of the permanent incisors associated with congenital syphilis, and in 1859 he described the diagnostic triad, which now bears his name. *Hutchinson's triad* includes the characteristic defects (hypoplasia) of the permanent incisors and first permanent molars, eighth nerve deafness and interstitial keratitis. The complete triad occurs in fewer than 1% of individuals with congenital syphilis.

The dental hypoplasia associated with congenital syphilis primarily affects the permanent incisors, the cuspids, and the first molars, since these teeth are being formed during the period of the acute luetic infection (see Figure 28-18 A, B & C). Bradlaw reported in the 1950's that 6% to 28% of the incisors and 3% to 37% of the molars were hypoplastic, with the morphology of the entire tooth being altered characteristically. There is a general constriction of the crown toward the incisal edge, which produces the "screwdriver" and "peg shaped" incisors frequently associated with this disease. There is also a rounding of the mesial and the distal incisal-line angles. The tip of the cuspid is frequently involved, and spacing between the incisors and this tooth is a common observation.

The molar lesions are characterized by a positioning of the cusps toward the central portion of the crown, giving the tooth a bud-shaped or a shrunken occlusal form (see Figure 28-19). The enamel covering the cusps may be intact, although marked defects are present in the grooves and the fissures of the tooth. A prominent accessory buccolingual cusp of the upper molars (Carabelli's cusp) was once erroneously believed to indicate prenatal lues.

There is speculation about whether these dental deformities are the direct result of *T.*

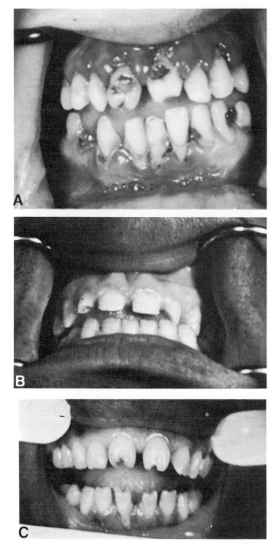

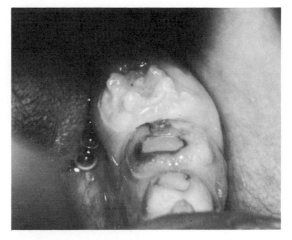

Fig. 28-19 A "mulberry molar," a hypoplastic tooth with a compressed fissured crown, appears in a 10-year-old child, who also exhibited a saddle nose deformity.

Fig. 28-18 (A, B & C) Hypoplastic defects of the permanent dentition are typical findings in congenital syphilis. (A) Notched incisors and peg-shaped teeth are present in a patient with congenital syphilis. (B) Screwdriver incisors, the spacing of the maxillary teeth, and the open-bite deformity are commonly found in individuals with congenital lues. (C) Notched incisors are found in another patient with congenital syphilis.

pallidum on the tooth bud, or whether they represent a more general interference resulting from endocrine or nutritional disturbances secondary to *T. pallidum* infection. Bauer demonstrated *T. pallidum* in the enamel organ of the developing teeth, but Hill and others were not as successful. Certainly,

luetic infections are sometimes associated with the hypoplasias described, but enamel hypoplasia produced by different agents have essentially the same histologic findings, and must be considered in the differential diagnosis of dental defects in the child with other evidence of congenital syphilis.

The dental changes associated with prenatal syphilis must be distinguished from those occurring as a result of rickets, tetracycline therapy, or the exanthematous fevers. The general morphology of the tooth is usually unaltered in the enamel hypoplasias associated with the latter conditions, and the defects are confined to linear or zonal areas on the labial or the cuspal surfaces. Although there may be marked local areas of hypoplasia of the enamel and the dentin, the typical constriction of the crowns of the teeth or the cusps is rarely seen except in prenatal syphilis.

The characteristic notching of the incisal edge of the permanent incisors has been demonstrated by means of a radiographic examination before the eruption of this tooth (see Figure 28-20 A). A less commonly described radiographic finding is the altered morphology of the mandibular first permanent molar (see Figure 28-20 B). The clinical crown and the root of this tooth are dwarfed. The mesiodistal diameter and the size of this tooth are usually smaller in prenatal luetics than the adjacent second molar—the reverse

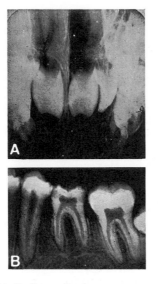

Fig. 28-20 (A & B) (A) Radiograph demonstrates Hutchinsonian incisors prior to their eruption. (From Stokes JH and Gardner BS: Demonstration of unerupted Hutchinson's teeth by roentgen ray. JAMA 80: 28, 1923) (B) Radiograph of mandibular molar area in a patient with congenital syphilis demonstrates the dwarfing of the crown and root of the first permanent molar.

of the usual condition. Although there may be marked hypoplasia of the crown of the first mandibular molar in rickets, the root of the tooth is usually of normal size and shape.

Dentofacial Changes (Syphilitic Stigmata)

Malocclusion is frequently observed in congenital luetics, and the "open bite," which may be found in these individuals, has been considered as having the same implication as the Hutchinsonian tooth. One author reported an "open bite" deformity in approximately one-third of the luetic children studied, the deformity resulting apparently from the lack of development of the premaxilla. Other authors, however, have denied that any characteristic malocclusion occurs with congenital syphilis.

An abnormal facies characterized by frontal bossing, saddle nose (see Figure 28-21), and the poorly developed premaxilla is also described as one of the *stigmata* of congenital syphilis. Similar bony abnormalities may oc-

cur in other congenital and inherited syndromes. *e.g.,* congenital ectodermal dysplasia, and are not specific for congenital syphilis.

Orofacial Manifestations of the Non-venereal Treponematoses

Oral and facial lesions occur in endemic syphilis and yaws, and may produce severe destruction and disfigurement of the oral and nasal structures. The skin of the face may contain lesions of pinta, but intraoral lesions have not been described. Since the primary infection with each of the non-venereal treponematoses occurs in childhood, and the phase of treponemal bacteremia has usually passed before adulthood, congenital lesions rarely occur with these three infections.

Endemic syphilis. The orofacial manifestations of endemic syphilis are similar to those of acquired venereal syphilis in the adult, except that primary lesions (extragenital chancres) in endemic syphilis are rarely seen. An intraoral mucous patch, split papule, or condyloma associated with a regional lymphadenopathy may be the earliest evidence of the infection. Treponemes are abundant in these lesions and in the regional nodes, and the infection may be spread to nursing mothers from infected children with oral lesions. Tertiary gummatous lesions subsequently develop and are similar to those seen in adult syphilis. Destructive gummatas, osteitis, and periostitis of the nasopharynx and adjacent tissues are said to be common.

Yaws. Oral lesions are described in all three stages of yaws. The primary lesion, which is analogous to the syphilitic chancre, and is referred to as the "mother yaw," usually occurs on the legs, which are more frequently exposed to trauma, but in less than 4% of cases, the mother yaw occurs on the head or face. Large papillomatous primary lesions of yaws are referred to as *frambesiform* (raspberry-like) *lesions.* The secondary stage of yaws is represented by a maculopapular rash or a recurrence of frambesiform lesions, which show a predilection for mucocutaneous junctions, and the lips and perioral area are often involved. Intraorally, papillom-

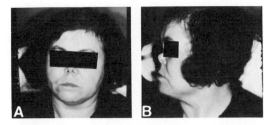

Fig. 28-21 (A & B) Front and profile views of the saddle nose facial deformity resulting from gummatous destruction of the nasal bones in a patient with congenital syphilis.

atous lesions of yaws have been described on the hard and soft palate and tonsils. However, intraoral lesions of secondary yaws are considered to be less frequent than intraoral lesions of secondary syphilis. Histologically these lesions show mononuclear cell infiltration, acanthosis, hyperkeratosis, and multiple treponemes. Tertiary lesions of yaws are similar to the gummatous lesions of syphilis, but have a tendency to be more destructive and to involve both soft and hard tissues. These lesions often begin as an ulcerating periostitis, which in the oro-nasal–pharyngeal area, may lead to a destructive mutilating nasopharyngitis, referred to as *gangosa* (or rhinopharyngitis mutilans). In this condition, soft tissues, cartilages, and bones of the nose and palate are destroyed from without. Hypertrophic osteitis and generalized maxillary periostitis have also been described in communities with endemic yaws, and are considered to be the cause of a characteristic facial appearance in the affected individual, referred to as *goundou*. Other authors have raised doubt as to whether goundou results from yaws, however. Differential diagnosis for rhinopharyngitis mutilans includes Wegener's granulomatosis, as well as leprosy and leishmaniasis, which are often endemic in the areas where yaws exists.

Pinta. Pinta is essentially a dermatologic problem that causes little disability other than a cosmetic disfigurement, which may be striking when the face is involved in depigmentation (the so-called porcelain white achromic lesions) that follow the secondary lesions (pintides). Primary and secondary lesions of pinta are often clinically and his-

tologically similar to lichen planus and must be considered a possible cause of lichenoid reactions (see Chapter 6) in individuals exposed to this infection.

Oral Manifestations of Hepatitis B and Other Sexually Transmitted Viral Infections

Hepatitis B

There are no specific oral manifestations of this infection, although *jaundice* may be detected with appropriate illumination in both oral and conjunctival mucous membranes as well as the skin during the icteric phase of the infection. However, laboratory studies of oral secretions of patients with acute hepatitis B infection, and chronically infected individuals, indicates that mixed saliva as well as serum is frequently positive for hepatitis B_s antigen. The antigen has not been detected in samples of saliva collected directly from the ducts of the parotid or submaxillary glands, and its presence in mixed saliva is believed to be due to transudation of serum in the gingival crevice or to inapparent minor intraoral hemorrhages. Saliva that is positive for hepatitis B_s antigen has also been shown to be infectious by appropriate animal inoculation. The saliva of patients whose serum is positive for hepatitis B_s antigen is assumed to be potentially infectious as long as the serum remains positive. As discussed in the following section, the degree of infectivity of saliva as regards transmission of hepatitis B infection is related to the extent of contamination of the oral cavity with blood.

Epstein-Barr (EB) Virus and Cytomegalovirus Infections

The viruses associated with these two infections may be detected in saliva either as an inapparent infection or in association with specific lesions. *EB virus* occurs in association with infectious mononucleosis (see Chapter 12) and the oral secretions are usually positive for the virus during the acute phase of the disease, irrespective of the presence of oral lesions. *Cytomegalovirus* may infect the major salivary glands as well as other visceral organs (pancreas, kidney, and liver, notably) and its presence in salivary gland tissue during autopsy was responsible for the designation "salivary gland virus" previously given to this agent. However, its presence in salivary gland tissue has never been associated with any clinical signs or symptoms, and there are still no oral lesions associated with infection with this agent. On occasion, the characteristic large intranuclear inclusions caused by this virus are detected in sections of tumors from the oropharynx, and as there is usually little associated tissue response, it is assumed to be simply an opportunistic infectious agent under these circumstances. Antigens of the EB virus (but only very rarely the characteristic inclusions) have also been detected in the lesions diagnosed as nasopharyngeal carcinomas and Burkitt's lymphoma, in which an oncogenic role for this virus seems more likely.

Oral Lesions Associated with the Acquired Immune Deficiency Syndrome

There are no oral lesions that are specifically associated with the acquired immune deficiency syndrome. However, a number of the opportunistic infections (*e.g.*, candidiasis and herpes simplex) associated with the syndrome may be manifested in oral lesions and can even be the presenting illness that results in recognition of the syndrome. In addition, atypical neoplasms associated with the syndrome, Kaposi's sarcoma most notably, may involve the oral cavity (see Figure 28–22).

Oral candidiasis in patients with the acquired immune deficiency syndrome may manifest simply as thrush or as chronic mucocutaneous candidiasis with or without systemic lesions. In one case recently described in the dental literature, oral candidiasis was the presenting complaint that preceded the recognition of other evidences of the syndrome (positive cytomegalovirus cultures, inverted T4/T8 lymphocyte ratios, perianal herpes simplex, a brain abscess, and a positive sputum culture for *P. carinii*). After a 10-weeks' illness, the patient died and the oral lesions were described as a severe candidal infection throughout the attached and unattached mucosa, with areas of ulceration on the hard palate. Smears were positive for

yeast and pseudohyphae. Herpes simplex infections associated with the acquired immune deficiency syndrome likewise may run a usual course or be characterized by chronic lesions with evidence of prolonged viral excretion.

Due to the lack of specificity about these oral lesions, and to their prevalence in otherwise healthy individuals without evidence of immune suppression, care must be taken in interpreting such oral infections as part of a syndrome such as AIDS without other evidence to support this diagnosis. At the time of writing, the acquired immune deficiency syndrome has been restricted to certain high-risk groups listed in the preceding section, and this syndrome should be considered in the differential diagnosis of one of these common oral infections only when a member of one of the high-risk groups is involved. As discussed in Chapter 6, there are numerous predisposing factors for oral candidiasis that must be excluded before a diagnosis of suspected acquired immune deficiency syndrome is considered on the basis of oral lesions alone.

Oral Lesions of Kaposi's Sarcoma

Kaposi's sarcoma was formerly considered a rare neoplasm (or multiple reactive lymphoreticular and endothelial cell proliferation, rather than a true neoplasm), which primarily affected the skin of the extremities and sometimes the gastrointestinal tract of certain genetically predisposed individuals of Jewish, Italian, or Bantu ancestry. The disease was almost never seen under age 60, and ran an indolent course, which was only occasionally complicated by visceral involvement, aggressive sarcomatous growth, or the development of leukemia or a lymphoma. Oral lesions of Kaposi's sarcoma were a great rarity. The disease was also occasionally seen in patients who had been treated with prolonged systemic corticosteroids or who had been intentionally immune suppressed.

Within the last 5 years, a more aggressive form of this neoplasm has occurred in epidemic form among members of male homosexual communities, and has been included as one of the features of the acquired immune deficiency syndrome. In these patients, the

Fig. 28-22 (A, B & C) Lesions of Kaposi's sarcoma appear on the (A) face and (B) palate of a 43-year-old male who exhibited many of the features of the acquired immune deficiency syndrome. The patient was described as an active homosexual with no history of sexual contacts in the preceding year and no history of intravenous drug abuse or transfusion. A seminoma was treated surgically with radiation to the chest and abdomen some years earlier with no evidence of recurrence. Symptoms included a recent history of weight loss, watery diarrhea with isolation of *Giardia sp*, and flat, nodular, pigmented lesions on chest wall, back, arms, trunk, and penis—diagnosed on biopsy as Kaposi's sarcoma. A three-week-old purplish mass, detected on the palate, had a similar histologic appearance on biopsy and increased rapidly in size, overlapping the partial upper denture. (C) illustrates florid oral candidiasis. No history or lymphoadenopathy was reported, but biopsy of lung lesion revealed granulomatous changes associated with disseminated infection with atypical mycobacteria. Chronic perianal ulcer responded to treatment with topical acyclovir, but was negative for herpes simplex virus on culture. Patient suffered anemia secondary to gastrointestinal blood loss, no neutropenia, and a T_4/T_8 ratio of 0.22 (normal range 1.8–2.0); (Courtesy Drs. M. S. Greenberg and S. Gary Cohen, Philadelphia PA).

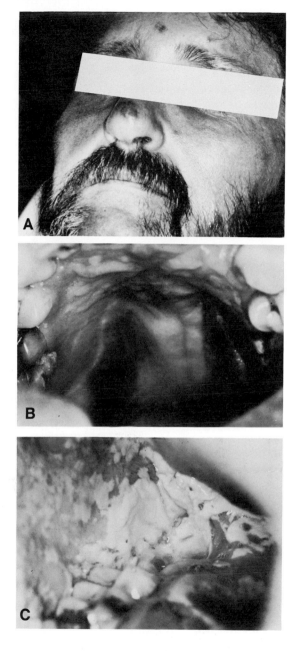

Kaposi's lesions are frequently disseminated over wide areas of the body and also involve the lymph nodes, gastrointestinal tract, and, occasionally, the lungs. The gastrointestinal tract is usually involved with multiple lesions, and in a number of these patients, oral submucosal lesions have been recorded. These oral lesions of disseminated Kaposi's sarcoma have occurred on the gingiva, hard and soft palates, base of the tongue, and posterior pharynx, and have usually been described as flat or slightly raised deep purple papular or diffuse lesions. Deposits of hemosiderin around older lesions may give them a pink to brown appearance. Differential diagnosis from hematomas of the palatal tissue is important, but the clinical appearance of the Kaposi's lesions is generally stated to be distinctive. Histologically, these lesions show an extensive network of irregular blood vessels with areas of spindle-cell and endothelial-cell proliferation and a patchy mononuclear infiltrate.

Oral Manifestations of Granuloma Inguinale and Lymphogranuloma Venereum

Oral Manifestations of Granuloma Inguinale

Donovan first described the oral lesions in 1905 on the basis of their typical granulomatous appearance and his demonstration of the intranuclear Donovan bodies in scrapings. Lesions of the lip were characterized by extensive superficial ulceration with a well-defined elevated granulomatous margin (see Figure 28–23 A, B, C & D). Hunter reported a case of granuloma inguinale with severe oral and laryngeal lesions, dysphagia, and "bilateral ankylosis of the jaws."

Lesions of granuloma inguinale confined to the gingiva of the lower jaw were observed by Burket in a 25-year-old man who came to the clinic because of "bleeding and a feeling of fullness of the lower gums" (see Figure 28–24). A small granular area had been noted on the mandibular gingiva about 5 months

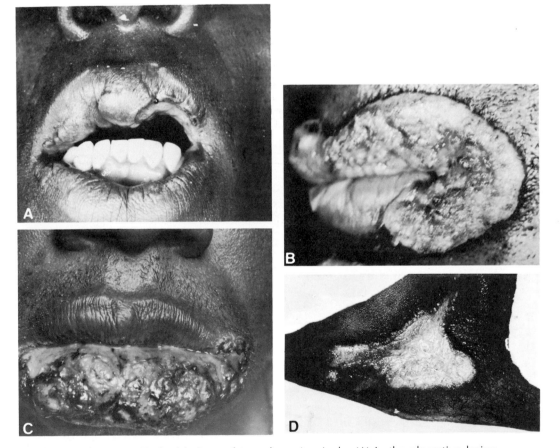

Fig. 28-23 (A, B, C & D) Oral lesions of granuloma inguinale. (A) In the ulcerative lesion, the buccal mucosa, pharynx and vocal cords were involved. (B) The same lesions are viewed from the side to demonstrate involvement of oral commissure. (C) In the exuberant type of lesion, the patient's oral lesions were further complicated by using copper sulphate as a mouthrinse. (D) Lesions of granuloma inguinale are found in the inguinal region. (From Ferro ER and Richter JW: Oral lesions of granuloma inguinale: Report of three cases. J Oral Surg 4:121, 1946)

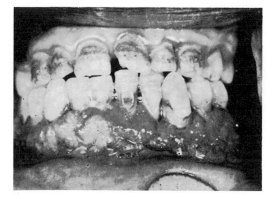

Fig. 28-24 Granulomatous lesions of granuloma inguinale may affect the mandibular gingiva. The oral lesions are a result of self-inoculation of the gums from the anal lesions.

previously. During the intervening time, the previously normal gingival tissues increased markedly in size, bled easily and turned bluish-red. The labiobuccal and the lingual mandibular alveolar gingivae were composed of a mass of bluish purple tissue, which bled on the slightest trauma. The tissues could be separated readily from the teeth and the alveolar process. There were no visible areas of necrosis or ulceration. The mandibular teeth were loose. Radiologic examination of the teeth and the jaws revealed a moderate degree of alveolar resorption, which was more extensive in the lower jaw. Bacterial smears, using appropriate staining methods, demonstrated no etiologic agent. The serologic tests for syphilis and the Frei test were repeatedly negative. Donovan bodies were observed in a biopsy of the affected gingival tissues. Physical examination revealed a shallow ulceration extending from the anal region, with a granulomatous margin extending on the right buttock. Biopsy of this lesion presented a histopathologic picture similar to that of the gingival biopsy. The mandibular gingival lesion was assumed to have been autoinoculated.

Oral Manifestations of Lymphogranuloma Venereum

The oral lesions may result from orogenital contact or autoinoculation. A symptomatic triad consisting of iritis, aphthoid lesions of the mouth and the penis, and a positive Frei test, has been described.

The tongue is reported to be a common site of oral involvement. The lesions in this location consist of small, slightly painful, superficial ulcerations with non-indurated borders, which appear on the tip of this organ. In cases of long-standing infection, there are zones of cicatricial retraction, dark-red areas, with loss of the superficial epithelium or opaque lichenoid grayish papules. Dysphagia, red soft palate, and small red granulomatous lesions accompanied by regional lymphadenopathy are commonly associated symptoms. Cervical adenopathy is a prominent symptom when the infection enters through the mouth. The skin covering the swollen nodes is violaceous and indurated, and usually presents one or more sinuses. Lymphogranuloma venereum infections of the cervical region must be differentiated from actinomycosis, tuberculous adenitis, blastomycosis, and cat-scratch fever. The tongue lesions must be differentiated from syphilitic gumma and from those of actinomycosis and tuberculosis. The diagnosis of oral lesions can be suspected on the basis of a suggestive history, particularly when anogenital lesions are present.

HAZARDS OF NON-VENEREAL TRANSMISSION OF THE SEXUALLY TRANSMISSIBLE DISEASES DURING DENTAL TREATMENT

While the diagnostic features of oropharyngeal, sexually transmitted diseases are of interest to the dentist when he is called upon to identify unusual changes in the oral mucosa, greater concern is often expressed about the risk of the dentist and his staff becoming infected with a sexually transmissible infection through contact with the oral secretions of dental patients. To some extent, this concern no doubt reflects the fact that a dentist is only rarely called upon to treat the oral lesions of a sexually transmitted disease. However, attitudes about syphilis and gonorrhea, which were developed by the dental profession before antibiotics became available, still persist, and also underlie much of our current professional anxiety about oropharyngeal, sexually transmitted infections. The final section of this chapter examines the background behind these concerns and evaluates them in the light of what has been described in the preceding pages about the epidemiology of individual sexually transmitted diseases and their oropharyngeal manifestations.

At this time, hepatitis B and herpes simplex infections have been demonstrated to be occupational hazards of dental practice. Historically, syphilis was considered an occupational hazard, though currently it should only be a minor concern. The oral secretions of patients with oropharyngeal gonorrhea, infectious mononucleosis, cytomegalovirus infections, and the acquired immune deficiency syndrome pose a theoretical hazard for dental personnel treating patients with these infections, but to date, no specific evidence of infection of dental or medical personnel by non-venereal routes has been documented. Except in immune compromised individuals or those with chronic dermatitis, candidiasis is rarely an infection of the hands or skin surfaces, and almost never a source of airborne pulmonary infection, and is not a hazard in the dental office. For the remaining sexually transmitted infections (non-specific urethritis, pediculosis pubis, scabies, granuloma inguinale, lymphogranuloma venereum, chancroid) infection of the oropharynx or head and neck area is either non-existent or sufficiently infrequent to justify speculation on any particular hazard to dental personnel.

Any consideration of the hazards of non-venereal transmission of these infections in the dental office must also include the hazards of transmission between patients in the dental setting. For the most part, the microbial agents associated with the sexually transmitted diseases have only brief existences outside the host. Standard measures for controlling cross infection in dental offices, *e.g.,* hand washing, sterilization of instruments, and disinfection of contaminated work surfaces and objects such as pens and telephone receivers, is adequate enough to control any potential cross infection with these agents. Hepatitis B, however, resists heat and drying

fairly well, and special attention is needed to prevent cross infection with this agent.

The hazards of non-venereal transmission of *gonorrhea, herpes simplex, hepatitis B, syphilis,* and the *acquired immune deficiency syndrome* are described in the following paragraphs:

Gonorrhea

N. gonorrhoeae has been isolated from the pharynx, and on occasions, from the oral cavities, of individuals with both symptomatic and asymptomatic pharyngeal gonorrhea, as well as those considered to have gonococcal stomatitis (see preceding section). The skin lesions of disseminated gonococcemia are positive for *N. gonorrhoeae,* and any oral lesions occurring simultaneously would likewise be expected to contain this organism transiently. Blood cultures from patients with acute gonococcemia are usually positive for *N. gonorrhoeae* prior to antibiotic treatment. Despite these various sources of contamination of oral secretions, and the known prevalence of gonorrhea, we know of no reports of non-venereal transmission of this infection to either dental or medical personnel. There is no explanation for this lack of confirmation of the theoretical hazard, although the relative resistance of stratified squamous epithelium to this organism may be involved. Age-stratified serologic data that might document previous contact with this microorganism are not readily available for either dental or other medical personnel (*c.f. Figure 28–26, which illustrates data of this type for hepatitis B*). Non-venereal transmission of gonorrhea would be expected to be a greater hazard for those conducting rectal, urologic, and gynecologic examinations than for dentists; the incidence of gonorrhea infection of the hands among the former is also negligible.

A history of treatment for gonorrhea elicited from a dental patient provides evidence of exposure to sexually transmitted infection, as well as evidence that the possibility of other similar infections exists. In the absence of clear proof of such infections however, and with the knowledge that the gonococcal infection has been treated, no specific hazard is associated with providing dental treatment for the patient. In the patient whose exposure

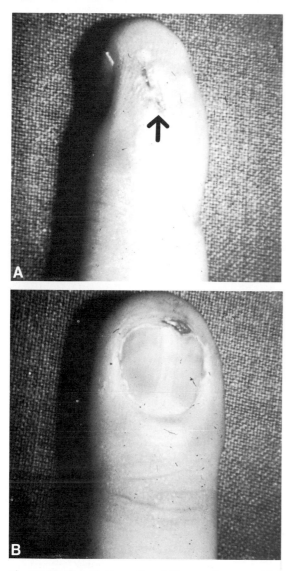

Fig. 28-25 (A & B) Herpetic whitlow and paronychial infection developed on the index finger of a dental intern six days after he lacerated it while extracting a molar tooth. Note the small vesicles on the palmar surface of the finger (arrow). Clear fluid and a cheesy yellowish material obtained from these vesicles were positive for herpes simplex virus, and "viral" giant cells were demonstrated in a Tzanck smear (see Fig. 3-25). The patient began to develop serum-neutralizing antibodies to the virus by day 17. (From Brightman VJ and Guggenheimer JG: Herpetic paronychia: Primary herpes simplex infection of the finger. J Amer Dent Assoc 80:112, 1970. Courtesy American Dental Association, Chicago IL 60611)

to gonorrhea has been recent, and under circumstances where oropharyngeal contamination with this organism is a good possibility, dental treatment might well be delayed until the patient has received adequate diagnosis and/or antibiotic treatment if appropriate.

Herpes Simplex

Traumatic infection of the dentist's fingers (herpetic paronychia, herpetic whitlow) is the main documented hazard associated with transmission of this infection in dental practice (see Figure 28–25). The great majority, if not all, of the lesions of this type that have been documented by viral isolation and typing of isolates, are associated with herpes simplex virus type 1. This association reflects the predominance of this virus type in oral infections. Some primary oropharyngeal infections with herpes simplex virus in dental personnel are also very probably acquired through contact with infected secretions from a dental patient.

The lesions of primary herpes simplex gingivostomatitis contain very large numbers of virus particles, and mixed saliva from patients with this acute infection may contain 10^6 or more particles of virus per cc for up to 5–7 days after onset of symptoms. By contrast, the vesicle fluid of recurrent herpes labialis, and the saliva of the patient with recurrent intraoral herpes simplex infection, as well as the silent oropharyngeal secretor of this virus, contain very little infectious virus (usually fewer than 10 viral particles per cc of saliva or vesicle fluid), and the virus can usually be detected for only 1 or 2 days at a time. It is postulated that primary herpes simplex gingivostomatitis is acquired on occasion from kissing an individual with recurrent herpes, and the likelihood of acquiring an infection of the fingers while providing dental treatment on the same individual might be expected to be less. However, it is rare for a case of herpetic paronychia to develop following known contact with a patient with primary herpes gingivostomatitis or acute pharyngitis. Most cases seem to follow inapparent infection acquired from silent carriers or other recurrent infections. Extent of

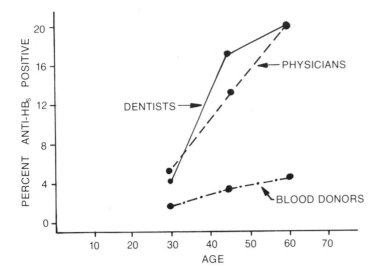

Fig. 28-26 A higher prevalence of antibodies to hepatitis B surface antigen (anti-HB$_s$) was found in dentists and physicians than in socioeconomically comparable first-time volunteer blood donors. (From Smith JL et al: Comparative risk of hepatitis B among physicians and dentists. J Infec Dis 133:705, 1976. Courtesy Univ of Chicago Press, Chicago IL 60637)

contact with the patient and trauma to the dentist's hands while he provides dental treatment may help to explain this paradox.

As with other acute viral infections, the presence of circulating antibody to the virus may be interpreted as a measure of immunity to subsequent challenges by the organism. Herpetic paronychia has been documented as a relatively common problem among a variety of medical and dental personnel. In most cases (*e.g.*, medical, dental and nursing students) the percentage of individuals entering medical, dental, and nursing school who have detectable anti-herpes antibody is well below 50%. Given the increased opportunity for contacting herpes simplex virus that clinical activities provide, the prevalence of herpetic paronychia among these professional groups is understandable.

Brightman and Ship found that the frequency of antibody to herpes simplex type 1 among freshman dental students at the University of Pennsylvania in 1964 was 28%; and among freshman nursing students at The Philadelphia General Hospital in 1971, it was 44%. Sophomore medical students at the University of Pennsylvania School of Medicine in 1980 had frequencies of 50% for antibody to type 1 and some also had antibody to type 2. By the senior year of dental school, an incidence of 5% for new infections with herpes simplex (herpetic paronychia, acute herpetic gingivostomatitis and pharyngitis, and subclinical infections) had been recorded for the dental students who lacked antibody to herpes simplex type 1 as freshman. Even higher figures for the annual rate of seroconversion to a positive antibody titer for herpes simplex have been quoted for other groups studied: 10% for college students and 16.5% for nurses and students working in a neurosurgical ward. Because of the age group involved however, it is difficult to determine how many of these infections among professional school students are nosocomial and how many are due to social contacts (see earlier discussion on herpes simplex infection as a sexually transmitted infection in adolescents and young adults).

In general, measurement of circulating antiherpes antibody in clinical personnel identifies those who are non-immune and at special risk and need to take added precautions. Due to the sharing of some antigens by both herpes type 1 and herpes type 2 strains, infection with one type of virus may give some, though not complete, protection against infection with the other type. Since infections with herpes type 2 are far less common than those with type 1, special care should perhaps be taken in treating patients with active type 2 infections of the oral cavity.

A vesicular perioral eruption and an acute herpetic gingivostomatitis have been documented in an intern who provided mouth-to-mouth resuscitation for a patient who was subsequently shown to have a herpes simplex virus pneumonia due to type 2 virus.

The lesions of herpetic paronychia are described in Chapter 5, Ulcerative, Vesicular, and Bullous Lesions. These lesions are frequently mistaken for staphylococcal infections, and may also have been incorrectly diagnosed as extragenital chancres in the past, when syphilitic infection of the dentist's fingers was reportedly more frequent.

Hepatitis B

Hepatitis B is probably the major occupational infectious hazard associated with dental practice at this time. This belief is based on numerous cases of clinically apparent infection with this virus among dentists and dental personnel, as well as the increased frequency with which antibody to hepatitis B virus is detected among dentists with increase in age (see Figure 28–26). The occupational risk for infection with the virus is similar for physicians, clinical laboratory workers, and dental hygienists. The risk of acquiring infection from this virus is related to the degree of exposure to blood or blood-contaminated bodily secretions, and is greatest for those dental specialties with most day-to-day exposure to blood (*e.g.,* oral surgery, periodontal surgery). Approximately 20% of dentists and physicians acquire markers for hepatitis-B infection over the normal span of practice. The relative annual percentage rates for development of serologic markers for hepatitis B infection are dentists (0.5%), physicians (0.46%), hygienists (0.40%), and blood donors in the general population (0.087%).

The majority of infections with hepatitis B among dentists are subclinical and most of these infections, whether they are subclinical or accompanied by jaundice, malaise, and other evidence of hepatitis (see Chapter 20), are self-limited infections from which the patient recovers in 1–2 months with no detectable sequelae. A small percentage, however, fail to eliminate the virus and chronic infection may result. Chronic infection carries with it the risk of transmission of the infection to close contacts and a low-but-definite risk for development of hepatocellular carcinoma as a result of the chronic infection. Currently, there are no easily achievable means for eliminating chronic infection with this virus once it is established.

The Risk of Transmission of Hepatitis B from Dentist to Patient

The risk of transmission of this infection from a chronically infected dentist to his patient has been shown to be quite high at times. When detected, chronic infection with this virus almost always requires some modification of the way in which a dentist practices, and on occasions, may lead to restriction of practice. Considerable attention has been given in the medical literature to a relatively small number of episodes in which a localized outbreak of hepatitis B infection has been traced to chronically infected dental personnel. Such episodes, however, appear to be the exception rather than the rule, and the risk of transmission of hepatitis B from dentist to patient appears to be considerably less than the risk of transmission from infected patient to dental personnel. Retrospective analysis of antecedent events for infections with hepatitis B versus hepatitis A (see Table 28-6) fail to demonstrate any significant role for dental treatment in the etiology of either of these infections, and prospective study of the patients of chronically infected dentists usually fails to demonstrate any evidence for transmission of the infection.

The risk of transmission of hepatitis B virus from dentist to patient is correlated with the amount of trauma involved in the dental procedure (*e.g.,* a traumatic extraction or impaction carries a greater risk than a routine restorative procedure) and the presence of abrasions or chronic dermatitis on the dentist's hands. A total of seven such episodes were studied by The United States Public Health Service Centers for Disease Control through mid-1982. All the dentists identified in these episodes were chronic carriers and had positive serum titers for both hepatitis B_s antigen and hepatitis B_e antigen; 60% were oral surgeons. Gloves were not used routinely by any of the dentists involved in the

Table 28-6. Antecedent Events in Acute Hepatitis B & Hepatitis A Infections*

	% HEPATITIS B (n = 8194)	% HEPATITIS A (n = 13,159)	RELATIVE TRANSMISSION RATE[†]
Dental procedures prior to clinical hepatitis	14.1	14.2	1.0[‡]
Oral surgery prior to clinical hepatitis	3.3	2.2	1.5[†]
History of drug abuse	8.8	2.5	3.5
Hemodialysis associated	2.0	0.3	6.6

* (Data courtesy of Dr. J. Ahtone, United States Public Health Service, Centers for Disease Control, Atlanta GA).

[†] Relative transmission rate = $\dfrac{\text{\% acute hepatitis B with antecedent event}}{\text{\% acute hepatitis A with antecedent event}}$

[‡] Not significant

episodes of transmission, and following institution of routine gloving for all procedures, no additional episodes of transmission were recorded.

Knowledge that a dentist is a chronic carrier of hepatitis B is not considered a barrier to practice, although it is essential that gloves be worn at all times when treating patients, and special care be taken to control opportunities for contamination of items that might subsequently be used in treating a patient. In most cases, evidence that a dentist or other health care worker, has been the source of infection to patients places the dentist under surveillance by local health authorities. In some cases where a number of a dentist's patients have been infected, opportunities for the dentist to practice have been restricted, either by adverse local feeling or recommendations of the health authorities. It is interesting to note that in the eight episodes studied by the United States Public Health Service Centers for Disease Control the only restrictions placed on the chronic carrier dentist were the wearing of gloves while treating patients and the requirement that patients be notified of a possibility that they might acquire hepatitis infection as a consequence of treatment by the dentist. In most cases where this was done, the warning to patients appeared to have little influence on the volume of patients seen in the practice.

Historically, dentists have been identified as playing an important role in the transmission of hepatitis B, because of the frequency with which local anesthetic injections are used in dental treatment. Outbreaks of hepatitis B ("serum jaundice") have been traced to the use of multiple dose syringes, multiple dose containers of vaccines and drugs, and to contaminated blood products, but the opportunity for this to happen in dental practice has become almost non-existent, since the use of disposable needles and local anesthetic carpules became routine dental practice some 20 years ago. Prior to this, multiple-dose anesthetic vials were used and inadequate sterilization of reusable needles undoubtedly occurred. However, as a result of the recognition that hepatitis B virus was unusually heat resistant, and because the occurrence of a number of major outbreaks of infection were traced to the use of multiple dose containers of medication in medical practice, there has been almost universal acceptance of the obligation to use disposable needles and single-dose cartridges of anesthetic. It is still commonplace to question a patient who develops jaundice and hepatitis about his dental visits. This procedure is still carried out, even though the reason for involving the dental office as a hazard for transmission of this virus no longer exists, and even though dental visits are demonstrably of little relevance to the acquisition of hepatitis B in the vast majority of cases.

Risk or no risk, the routine use of disposable syringes and needles and sterilization of all instruments by either dry heat or autoclaving after use, removes any opportunity for transmission of this infection in dental practice.

The Risk of Transmission of Hepatitis B from Patient to Dentist

A variety of approaches are used for the control of this hazard in dental practice; screening of patients with a history of hepatitis and those in high-risk groups for acquiring hepatitis B infection; increased use of barrier techniques for control of cross-infection in dental practice; and use of active and passive immunization techniques for dental personnel.

Screening of Patients for Evidence of Chronic Infection with Hepatitis B

This screening is achieved by testing for the presence of hepatitis B_s antigen in the patient's serum. The presence of hepatitis B_s antigen in serum is interpreted as a risk that infectious virus is also present and will appear in the mixed saliva when it is contaminated with serum. A negative test for hepatitis B_s antigen in the serum is evidence that neither acute nor chronic infection with hepatitis B is present. When such screening is limited to patients with a history of hepatitis or jaundice, individuals who developed into chronic carriers following subclinical infection will be missed. One study based on a small population sample estimated that approximately one half of the cases of chronic hepatitis B among patients registering for treatment at a dental school would be missed by this approach. However, the chance of detecting carriers is greatly increased if screening for hepatitis B_s antigen is broadened to include *individuals in high-risk groups for this infection.* These include: hemodialysis patients and patients who have received a renal transplant, individuals who have been institutionalized for mental treatment or penal service for over 6 months, individuals on methadone or similar replacement therapy for narcotic addiction, individuals showing evidence of parenteral drug abuse such as multiple forearm scars, military personnel or others who have lived "off-base" for longer than 6 months in Mediterranean, tropical, S.E. Asian, and other countries where the prevalence of hepatitis B is known to be high (see Figure 28–27), migrants from these countries (*e.g.,* refugee "boat people" from S.E. Asia), and individuals reporting multiple sexual contacts, whether of a heterosexual or homosexual nature.

Screening of prospective dental patients as described above is intended to identify the hepatitis-B carrier, so that special attention can be given to controlling the hazards of infectious transmission associated with dental care. The main disadvantage of this approach, however, is that it identifies a group of individuals who are often stigmatized on this account, and who subsequently find it very difficult if not impossible to obtain dental care unless they hide the fact that they are hepatitis-B carriers.

Use of Barrier Techniques for Control of Cross Infection with Hepatitis B in Dental Practice

Dental care can be provided safely and efficiently for chronic hepatitis-B carriers provided that attention is given to the control of infectious hazards by doing any of the following: using barrier techniques (double gloving, mask and gown, draping of large pieces of equipment likely to be contaminated by saliva or blood); limiting the use of water, the use of air sprays, and the opportunity for rotating instruments to produce aerosols of saliva and blood; utilizing dental instruments and supplies that can either be sterilized by hot air, steam in an autoclave, or ethylene oxide, or disposed of and incinerated; and by avoiding opportunities for puncture of gloves and laceration of the operator's fingers by needles, blades, burrs, sharp cavity margins, bone spicules, and so forth. Other commonly used precautions include: scheduling hepatitis B carrier patients at the end of the day's clinic session; wiping down all exposed surfaces; mopping floor and walls of the operatory with a 10% household bleach solution at the conclusion of treatment; and excluding

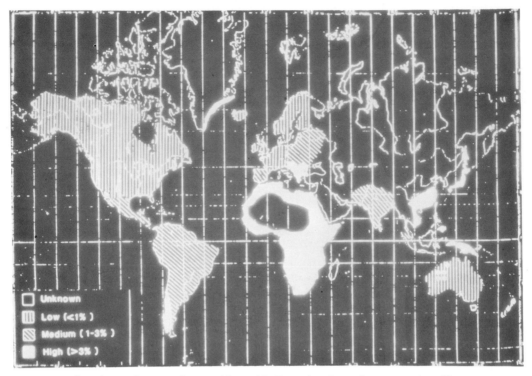

Fig. 28-27 This shows the prevalence of hepatitis B carriers in various countries. (Courtesy Dr. Blumberg BS, Institute for Cancer Research, Philadelphia PA 19111)

other personnel from the operatory while treatment is in progress. All potentially contaminated articles from the operatory should either be sterilized or wiped down with bleach or disposed of in double thickness bags plainly marked "Contents - Infection Hazard" with specific instruction to janitorial personnel on their handling and disposal. Disposable needles should be discarded unsheathed into autoclavable containers and sterilized before disposal; dental impressions should be poured in the operatory and the casts sterilized by ethylene oxide or overnight exposure to formalin vapor before they are released to the laboratory. Sterilizable dental hand pieces and prophylaxis heads should always be used.

Active and Passive Immunization Techniques

By far the greatest advance in controlling the transmission of hepatitis-B virus to dental personnel has been the availability of a highly purified, sub-particulate, inactivated hepatitis-B vaccine.*

This vaccine produces antiviral antibody in over 95% of recipients (see Table 28-7) and has been shown to be an effective protection against infection with hepatitis B in several groups at high risk for this infection, such as male homosexuals and clinical personnel in hemodialysis units. Its use has been approved and strongly recommended by the United States Public Health Service Food and Drug Administration, Centers for Disease Control, and the American Dental Association Council on Dental Therapeutics for administration to all individuals at high risk for hepatitis-B infection. Dental clinic personnel and dental laboratory technicians have been specified as being of major concern in this regard. Since this vaccine, which consists of purified hepatitis B_s antigen, is obtained by fractionation of human serum from chronic carriers of hepatitis B (see Figure 28–28),

* Heptavax B. Merck, Sharp and Dohme. Division of Merck & Co. Inc. West Point, PA 19486

there have been speculations that the vaccine might transmit other virus infections and the acquired immune deficiency syndrome. The multiple purification and inactivation steps involved in the production of Heptavax B exclude any likelihood of its containing other active virus particles. Table 28-8 illustrates the key steps in preparing the vaccine.

Follow-up studies, some four years after the prelicensing-controlled clinical trials of the vaccine in male homosexuals, have demonstrated that these speculations are unfounded. No cases of the acquired immune deficiency syndrome have occurred in vaccine recipients other than members of male homosexual communities who are at particular risk for this disease. Moreover, among the 10,000 male homosexuals in New York City and Los Angeles who participated in the Heptavax B trials, the incidence of the acquired immune deficiency syndrome has been significantly higher in those who received only saline injections ("control vaccine") than in those who received Heptavax B. The very low incidence of other complications in vaccine recipients also has established that this vaccine, by virtue of its unique multistep purification procedure, is probably the least hazardous of all vaccines currently available. The occurrence of a small number of cases of a demyelinating disease of the central nervous system, the Guillain-Barré syndrome, following administration of Heptavax B, is considered to be unrelated to the vaccine.

Administration of this vaccine to all dental clinical and laboratory personnel, and to all dental and oral hygiene students before they commence clinical training, is strongly recommended, and is likely to be a major factor in the control of transmission of hepatitis B to dental personnel in future years. Development of widespread immunity to hepatitis B among the dental profession by this means should also remove many of the problems currently associated with provision of dental care for the chronic hepatitis-B carrier.

No untoward effects result from administration of the vaccine to those who already have a naturally acquired immunity to hepatitis B. Among groups of individuals who are likely to have naturally acquired immunity, screening for hepatitis B_s antibody prior to vaccination will save some cost and will prevent waste of a vaccine that is still in short supply; for those groups with low frequency of naturally acquired immunity, such as dental students, screening is usually omitted. There are also no untoward effects when the vaccine is administered to hepatitis-B carriers or to those incubating the infection. Since carriers already have circulating levels of hepatitis B_s antigen, which have failed to elicit antibody formation, the additional antigen provided by the vaccine also fails to elicit a response. Heptavax B, therefore, does not eliminate the carrier state. On the other hand, there is some evidence to suggest that administration of the vaccine during the incubation period for this infection may abort or modify the severity of any subsequent infection.

Table 28-7. Development of Antibody to Hepatitis B_s Antigen in 111 Faculty, Staff and Students at the University of Pennsylvania School of Dental Medicine Following Three Doses of Heptavax B§

Time After First Dose of Heptavax B†	Males Seroconversion Rate # with HB_s antibody / # vaccinated	GMT‡	Females Seroconversion Rate # with HB_s antibody / # vaccinated	GMT‡
3 mos	71/79 (89.9%)	294	29/32 (90.6%)	276
6 mos	72/78 (92.3%)	427	30/32 (93.8%)	551
7 mos	73/77 (94.8%)	8,427	31/32 (96.9%)	10,285

* (Data from Brightman VJ et al: Immunization of Dental Personnel with Inactivated Hepatitis B Vaccine. Proc Am Acad Oral Pathol Ann Mtg, Reno NV, May 1982)
† Vaccine administered at times zero, one month and six months.
‡ Geometric mean titer of serum antibody to hepatitis B_s antigen (responders only).
§ Merck, Sharp & Dohme, Div. of Merck & Co. Inc., West Point PA 19486.

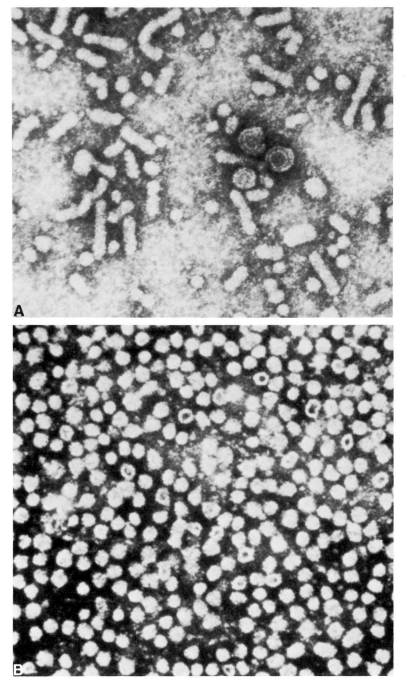

Fig. 28-28 (A & B) (A) Electron micrograph shows a serum sample containing hepatitis B virus. Three different morphologic forms can be seen. One is a double-shelled structure with an outer surface and an inner core; this is the virus itself and is referred to as the Dane particle. It exists in relatively small numbers compared with the vast supply of additional protein material known as the outer coat, or surface antigen, of incomplete virus particles. This hepatitis B_s antigen occurs both as small spheres and long tubules. (B) Electron micrograph shows a purified hepatitis B vaccine (Heptavax B) composed only of hepatitis B_s antigen particles. It contains no intact infectious virus, no e antigen and none of the viral enzyme DNA polymerase. When mixed with an alum adjuvant, it is non-infectious, very immunogenic, and highly effective in preventing infection with hepatitis B; see text of this chapter and Chapter 3 for further details. (From Dienstag JL: A Visual Exploration of Hepatitis B and Immunization. Courtesy Merck, Sharp & Dohme Inc, Div of Merck & Co., West Point PA 19486)

Table 28-8. Key Steps in Preparing Human Hepatitis B Vaccine

Plasma from Hepatitis B Carriers
↓
Defibrination (with Added Calcium)
↓
Ammonium Sulfate Precipitation (Concentration)
↓
Isopycnic Banding (Sodium Bromide)
↓
Rate Zonal Sedimentation (Sucrose Gradient)
↓
*Pepsin Digestion, pH2 (10-fold Purification)
↓
*Urea, 8 Molar (Denature-Renature)
↓
Gel Filtration (Molecular Sieve)
↓
*Formalin 1:4000 (72 hrs., 36°C.)
↓
Vaccine. 20 μg Surface Antigen/Dose With 0.5 mg Al^{+++} (Alum)
in 1.0 ml and Thimerosal

*Critical Inactivation Steps

(Courtesy Merck, Sharp and Dohme, Div. Merck and Co. Inc., West Point PA 19486)

Passive immunization against hepatitis B with both immune-serum globulin* and hepatitis-B hyperimmune globulin[†] is described in Chapter 20 and remains available as post-exposure prophylaxis for individuals who have been in contact with patients with hepatitis B, and who may have acquired the infection in the clinical setting by inadvertent needle sticks, finger lacerations, or contamination of mucosal surfaces with infected secretions from a carrier or acutely infected patient. Administration of a vaccine, either with or without prior passive immunization, is also used for postexposure prophylaxis.

Syphilis

There is a fairly extensive and sobering literature that describes extragenital syphilitic lesions of the hands and face acquired by dentists, physicians, midwives, and other health professionals while treating patients. The paper by Salzman and Appleton published in 1932 (see Figure 28–29) is an example of this classical literature that describes numerous syphilitic infections that were acquired in this fashion, and also sometimes

* Immune serum globulin (human) U.S.P.
[†] Hep-B-Gammagee. Merck, Sharp and Dohme. Division of Merck & Co. Inc. West Point, PA 19486

PROCEEDINGS
OF THE
FIRST DISTRICT
DENTAL SOCIETY

Syphilis Insontium: Acquired by the Operator During Dental Treatment *†

By J. A. Salzmann, D.D.S., and J. L. T. Appleton, Jr., B.S., D.D.S.

From the School of Dentistry, University of Pennsylvania, Philadelphia, Pa.

"No one who deals with syphilis day in and day out can fail to realize the tragic incidence and the deplorable outcomes of the disease among those whose professions bring them in contact with it. Several facts have high significance here. Syphilis is the Dangerous Unexpected. It is not the syphilologist who acquires it, even from a lifetime of potentially dangerous contacts. It is the practicing doctor, secure in ignorance, of a low index of suspicion, of a mistaken casualness and bravado, and irresponsible in treatment, who meets ruin in this way."[1]—STOKES, 1931.

This study has been aided by a grant from the Research Fund of the Academy of Stomatology, Philadelphia, Pa.
†Read before the Section on Pathodontia of the First District Dental Society of New York as part of a Symposium on Syphilis, February 16, 1932.

Fig. 28-29 (A & B & C) (A) Title page of an article published in 1932 describes the risks of syphilis insontium (innocentum) during dental treatment. (B) Figure from the same article illustrates the relative frequency of location of points of entry of syphilitic infection, as seen in a palmar view. Most of these sites are also involved in herpetic whitlow or paronychia, and it is possible that some of the lesions attributed to syphilis at this time may have been due to herpes simplex virus infection. (C) Extragenital chancre is seen on the finger of a health professional. (From Salzman JA and Appleton JT Jr: Syphilis insontium acquired by the operator during dental treatment. NY J Dent 2:269, 1932, A & B; C—Courtesy Willcox RR, London, England)

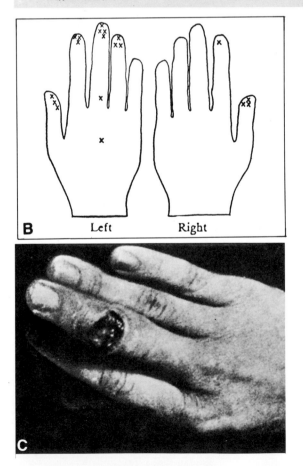

subsequently transmitted to the practitioner's family. However, this literature ends in the early 1940's (the last reference to syphilis insontium in a dentist that we are aware of was described in the paper by Liefer in 1942; subsequent papers on this topic are simply reviews of the problem as it existed before that time*). At about the same time, the literature on venereally acquired extragenital lesions of syphilis also tapered off. (Wile's and Holman's review of 68 cases collected over the preceding 25 years apparently was the last large series of cases reported.) More recent authors comment on the infrequency with which extragenital syphilitic chancres are seen apart from those in the anorectal region. Much of this change is no doubt related to the introduction of penicillin as an antisyphilitic therapy in the 1940's, although it is also possible that the control of syphilis that has been achieved as a result of antibiotic

* Some literature references to syphilis insontium after this date are also concerned with the non-venereally acquired skin lesions of endemic syphilis (see section on the Non-venereal Treponematoses).

therapy in the last 30 years accounted for some of the decrease in its contagiousness.

Thorough examination of the oral mucosa, and a high index of suspicion and appropriate consultation concerning otherwise unexplained mucosal lesions, are still important bits of advice for the dentist. A recent increase of cases of syphilis in urban areas suggests that this infection should always be considered in the differential diagnosis of solitary ulcers, nodules of the lips, tongue, and fauces, intraoral enanthems, lichenoid lesions and unexplained areas of mucositis. Evaluation of such lesions should always be done with a gloved finger, and routine use of gloves by personnel in dental screening (oral diagnosis) clinics is justified by the fact that lesions of this type (and other infections) may be asymptomatic and not listed as a dental complaint by a patient prior to examination. Inquiries regarding sexual contacts are also fully justified as part of the evaluation of such lesions and may be quite important in establishing a correct diagnosis. Despite this need for caution in the diagnosis of oral lesions, *the likelihood that a dentist or his assistants could acquire syphilis innocently, even following direct contact with the saliva of a patient in the primary or secondary stages of the disease, now seems quite low.* Patients with latent or tertiary syphilis are, by definition, non-infectious. Prompt treatment of infected wounds of the hands and fingers with systemic antibiotics (as is customary) further lowers the likelihood that any primary syphilitic infection of the hands will become established as a systemic infection.

While *routine* testing of hospital patients for serologic evidence of syphilis has been discontinued in many institutions, dental schools have required for many years that patients with a history of syphilis or other venereal disease undergo a serologic test for syphilis prior to acceptance for dental treatment, if there is no evidence of any negative test results subsequent to the original infection. Patients who are found to have persistently positive Rapid Plasma Reagin, Kline, Kahn, or Wasserman tests, for example, are then either tested with more specific reagents (*e.g.,* FTA-ABS), referred elsewhere for medical evaluation, or evaluated in conjunction with the local public health authority to de-

termine if additional antisyphilitic treatment is needed. Because of the relatively low prevalence of syphilis at this time, this practice is now largely a public health gesture aimed at ensuring adequate treatment for a disease known to be associated with the insidious onset of late stages of the infection, which can bring disastrous consequences *to the patient.* For the reasons given above, the serologic test for syphilis is not justified as a screening procedure solely for the purpose of protecting staff and students against an occupational infectious hazard (*c.f.,* screening of dental patients for hepatitis B infection).

Acquired Immune Deficiency Syndrome

At the time this book was written no cases of the acquired immune deficiency syndrome (with few exceptions) have been identified outside of the high-risk groups for this infection listed earlier in this chapter, and no clear evidence of transmission of the syndrome to health-care workers by non-venereal routes has been reported.

Due to the unknown etiology of the syndrome and the high fatality rate associated with it, guidelines for clinical management of patients suspected of having this syndrome have been published by the United States Public Health Service Centers for Disease Control. In general, the guidelines are similar to those used for management of carriers of hepatitis-B virus and include gowning and wearing gloves for contact with body fluids, blood, secretions, and excreta of these patients, thorough hand-washing after contact, and sterilization, or disposal by incineration, of all supplies and instruments used. Surfaces contaminated by blood, saliva, and other body fluids, should be washed with 10% household bleach. Hospitalized patients are housed in a single room with specific hazard precautions posted. Likewise, dental patients should not be treated in an open clinic, and adjacent equipment should be draped as described for treatment of hepatitis-B carriers. Special care must be taken when handling and disposing of sharp-edged and pointed instruments in order to avoid needle sticks and lacerations.

BIBLIOGRAPHY

General References and Epidemiology of Sexually Transmitted Diseases

Adler MW: Sexually transmitted disease statistics. J R Soc Med 75:4, 1982

Allen AL and Organ RJ: Occult blood accumulation under the fingernails: a mechanism for the spread of blood-borne infection. JADA 105:455, 1982

Appleton JLT: Bacterial Infection, 2nd ed, Lea & Febiger, Philadelphia 1938, pp. 309–310

Arndt KA: Battling sexually transmitted diseases. Patient Care Apr 15 1981

Arthes F: Some Aspects of the Epidemiology of Venereal Diseases, in Castelazo-Ayala L and MacGregor C (eds). Gynecology & Obstetrics, Proc VIII World Congress of Gynec. & Obs., Mexico City, Oct. 17–22, 1976. Excerpta Med, Amsterdam, 1977

Backman LA: Infection control in the hospital dental clinic. Inf Control and Urological Care 7:22, 1982

Castelazo-Ayala L and MacGregor C (eds): Gynecology and Obstetrics, Proc VIII World Congress of Gynecology and Obstetrics, Mexico City, Oct 17–22, 1976; Excerpta Med, Amsterdam 1977

Catterall RD and Nicol CS: Sexually Transmitted Diseases, Proc of a Conf Sponsored by Roy Soc Med and Roy Soc Fdn, June 23–25, 1975, Academic Press. New York 1976

Centers for Disease Control: Sexually transmitted diseases guidelines. MMWR 31:25, 1982

Chapel TA et al: Simultaneous infection with *Treponema pallidum* and herpes simplex virus. Cutis 24:191, 1979

Danielsson D et al (eds): Genital Infections and Their Complications, Proc Wellcome Fdn Sympos. Stockholm Oct 9–11, 1974; Almqvist and Wiksell, Stockholm Sweden.

Felman YM: Relative incidence of sexually transmitted diseases in New York City Social Hygiene Clinics 1977–79. Bull NY Acad Med 56:715, 1980

Fichtner RR, Aral SO, et al: Syphilis in the United States: 1967–1979. Sex Transm Dis 10:77, 1983

Fiumara NJ: Venereal disease of the oral cavity. J Oral Med 31:36, 55, 1976

Johnstone T: WHO Workshop on Sexually Transmitted Diseases, Suva, Fiji Apr 2–12, 1979. N Z Med J 90(640):78, 1979

Judson FN: Screening for syphilis and gonorrhea in the gay baths of Denver Colorado. Am J Pub Health 67:740, 1977

Judson FN (ed) Symposium: Venereal disease and gay men. Sex Trans Dis 4:49, 76, 1977

Judson FN: The importance of coexisting syphilis, chlamydial, mycoplasma and trichomonal infection in treatment of gonorrhea. Sex Trans Dis 6:112, 1979

Noble RC et al: Recidivism among patients with gonococcal infection presenting to a venereal disease clinic. Sex Trans Dis 4:39, 1977

Sparling PF: Current problems in sexually transmitted diseases. Adv Int Med 24:203, 1979

Willcox RR: The management of sexually transmitted diseases: a guide for the general practitioner. EURO Reports and Studies WHO, Copenhagen 1979

Zaidi AA, Aral SO et al: Gonorrhea in the United States: 1967–1979, Sex Transm Dis 10:72, 1983

Non-Specific Urethritis

Arya OP et al: Post-gonococcal cervicitis and post-gonococcal urethritis. A study of their epidemiological correlation and the role of *Chlamydia trachomatis* in their etiology. Br J Ven Dis 57:395, 1981

Bouis PJ Jr et al: Nongonococcal urethritis: A clinical problem of the 80's. J Fla Med Assoc 68:965, 1981

Cassell GH et al: Microbiologic study of infertile women at the time of diagnostic laparoscopy. Association of Ureaplasma urealyticum with a defined subpopulation. N Engl J Med 308:502, 1983

Eschenbach DA: Epidemiology and diagnosis of acute pelvic inflammatory diseases. Obstet Gynecol 55:142S, 1980

Holmes KK: The Chlamydia epidemic. JAMA 245:1718, 1981

Kousa M: Clinical observations on Reiter's disease with special reference to the venereal and non-venereal etiology. Acta Dermatovenerol 58:Suppl 81, 1978

Munday PE et al: Clinical and microbiological study of non-gonococcal urethritis with particular reference to non-chlamydial disease. Br J Ven Dis 57:327, 1981

Newhall WJ et al: Analysis of the human serological response to proteins of chlamydia trachomatis. Infect Immun 38:1181, 1982

Oriel JD et al: Epidemiology of chlamydial infections of the human genital tract: evidence for the existence of latent infection. Eur J Clin Microbiol 1:69, 1982

Pindborg JJ, Gorlin RJ and Asboe-Hansen G: Reiter's syndrome. Review of the literature and report of a case. Oral Surg 16:551, 1963

Quinn TC et al: *Chlamydia trachomatis* proctitis. N Engl J Med 305:195, 1981

Schachter J: Chlamydial infections. N Engl J Med 298:428, 490, 540, 1978

Thelin I: Diagnosis and treatment of chlamydial venereal disease. Infection 10:553, 1982

Wølner-Hanssen P et al: Laparoscopy in women with chlamydial infection and pelvic pain: a comparison of patients with and without salpingitis. Obstet Gynecol 61:299, 1983

Gonorrhea

Austin TW et al: Oropharyngeal gonorrhea. Disseminated gonococcal disease. Can Med Assoc J 117:438, 1977

Bro-Jørgensen A and Jensen T: Gonococcal pharyngeal infection: report of 110 cases. Br J Ven Dis 49:491, 1973

Caldwell et al: Sensitivity and reproducibility of Thayer-Martin culture medium in diagnosing gonorrhea in women. Am J Obstet Gynecol 109:463, 1971

Catterall RD: The Situation of Gonococcal and Infections in the United Kingdom, in Castelazo-Ayala L and MacGregor C (eds). Gynecology & Obstetrics. Proc VIII World Congress of Gynec. & Obs., Mexico City, Oct. 17–22, 1976. Excepta Med, Amsterdam, 1977

Centers for Disease Control: Gonorrhea - United States. MMWR 28:533, 1979

Chue PWY: Gonorrhea: its natural history, oral manifestations, diagnosis, treatment and prevention. JADA 90:1297, 1975

Cooke DB et al: Gonococcal endocarditis in the antibiotic era. Arch Intern Med 139:1247, 1979

Corman LC: The high frequency of pharyngeal gonococcal infection in a prenatal clinic population. JAMA 230:568, 1974

Cowan L: Gonococcal ulceration of the tongue in the gonococcal dermatitis syndrome. Br J Ven Dis 45:228, 1969

Felman YM and Nikitas JA: Nongonococcal urethritis. A clinical review. JAMA 254:381, 1981

Fiumara NJ et al: Gonorrheal pharyngitis. N Engl J Med 276:1248, 1967

Frazer AD and Menton J: Gonococcal stomatitis. Br Med J 1:1020, 1931

Jamsky RJ: Gonococcal tonsillitis—report of a case. J Oral Surg 44:197, 1977

Jewitt JF: Non-sexual acquisition of genital gonococcal infection. N Engl J Med 301:1347, 1979

Kohn SR et al: Primary gonococcal stomatitis. JAMA 219:86, 1972

Kraus SJ: Incidence and therapy of gonococcal pharyngitis. Sex Transm Dis 6 (Suppl):143, 1979

Merchant HW et al: Oral gonococcal infection. JADA 95:807, 1977

Osborne NG and Grubin L: Colonization of the pharynx with Neisseria gonorrhoeae: experience in a clinic for sexually transmitted diseases. Sex Trans Dis 6:253, 1979

Owen RL and Hill JL: Rectal and pharyngeal gonorrhea in homosexual men. JAMA 220:1315, 1972

Schmidt H, Hjørting-Hansen E and Philipsen HP: Gonococcal stomatitis. Acta Dermatovenerol 41:324, 1961

St John RK et al: Treatment of gonococcal infections, revisited. Sex Transm Dis 6:87, 1979

Wiesner PJ et al: Clinical spectrum of pharyngeal gonococcal infection. N Engl J Med 288:181, 1973

Wiesner PJ and Thompson SE: Gonococcal Diseases. Disease-A-Month, Year Book Medical Publishers, Chicago IL 1980

Candidiasis (see also Chapter 6)

Gottlieb MS et al: Pneumocystis carinii pneumonia and mucosal candidiasis in previously healthy homosexual men: evidence of a new acquired cellular immunodeficiency. N Engl J Med 305:1425, 1981

Trichomoniasis and Other Protozoal Sexually Transmitted Infections

Blumencrantz H et al: The role of endoscopy in suspected amebiasis. Am J Gastroenterol 78: 15, 1983

Butler T et al: Isospora belli infection in Australia. Pathol 13:593, 1981

Centers for Disease Control: Human crytosporidiosis–Alabama. MMWR 31:252, 1982

Editorial: Sexual transmission of enteric pathogens. Lancet 12:1329, 1981

Hager WD et al: Metronidazole for vaginal trichomoniasis. Seven day vs. single-dose regimens. JAMA 244:1219, 1980

Harries J: Amoebiasis: a review. J R Soc Med 75:190, 1982

Patterson M et al: The presentation of amoebiasis. Med Clin North Am 66:689, 1982

Phillips SC et al: Sexual transmission of enteric protozoa and helminths in a venereal disease clinic population. N Engl J Med 305:603, 1981

Rein MF: Current therapy of vulvovaginitis. Sex Trans Dis 8:316, 1981

Spence MR et al: The clinical and laboratory diagnosis of Trichomonas vaginalis infection. Sex Trans Dis 7:168, 1980

Verm RA: Gastrointestinal parasites I. Protozoal infections. Am Fam Phys 25:170, 1982

Venereal Warts (Condyloma Acuminatum)

Bruegil PJ et al: 5-fluorouracil cream 5% in the treatment of intraurethral condylomata acuminata. Br J Urol 54:295, 1982

Jenson AB et al: Frequency and distribution of

papilloma–virus structural antigens in verrucae, multiple papillomas and condylomata of the oral cavity. Am J Pathol 107:212, 1982

Judson FN: Condyloma acuminatum of the oral cavity: a case report. Sex Trans Dis 8:218, 1981

Powell LC: Condyloma acuminatum: recent advances in development, carcinogenesis and treatment. Clin Obstet Gynecol 21:1061, 1978

Shafer EL Jr et al: Oral condyloma acuminatum. A case report with light microscopic and ultrastructural features. J Oral Pathol 9:163, 1980

von Krogh G: Podophyllotoxin for condylomata acuminata eradication. Clinical and experimental comparative studies on *Podophyllin* lignans, colchicine and 5-fluorouracil. Acta Derm Venereol 98 (Suppl):1, 1981

Herpes Simplex Virus Infections (see also Chapter 5)

Bleckman H and Pascher F: Primary herpes simplex virus infection in an adult. J Oral Surg 12:185, 1959

Brightman V, Green LH and Ship II: Immunity to herpes simplex among freshmen dental students. Proc. IADR 44th Ann Mtg. Miami FL, 1966, Abs. #414

Brightman VJ and Guggenheimer JG: Herpetic paronychia: primary herpes simplex infection of the finger. JADA 80:112–5, 1970

Brooks SC et al: Prevalence of herpes simplex virus disease in a professional population. J Am Dent Assoc 102:31, 1981

Bryson YJ et al: Treatment of first episodes of genital herpes simplex virus infection with oral acyclovir: a randomized double-blind controlled trial in normal subjects. N Engl J Med 306:916, 1983

Buchman TG et al: Restriction endonuclease fingerprinting of herpes simplex virus DNA: a novel epidemiological tool applied to a nosocomial outbreak. J Infect Dis 138:488, 1978

Burkhart CG: Persistent cutaneous herpes simplex infection. Int J Dermatol 20:552, 1981

Chang TW: Herpetic angina following orogenital exposure. J Am Ven Dis Assoc 1:163, 1975

Corey L et al: A trial of topical acyclovir in genital herpes simplex virus infection. N Engl J Med 306:1313, 1982

Dundarov S, Andonov P and Bakalov B: Characterization of herpes simplex virus strains isolated from patients with various diseases. Arch Virol 63:115, 1980

Eberle R and Courtney RJ: Assay of type-specific and type-common antibodies to herpes simplex virus types 1 and 2 in human sera. Infec Immun 31:1062, 1981

Embil JA et al: Concurrent oral and genital infection with an identical strain of herpes simplex virus type 1: restriction endonuclease analysis. Sex Trans Dis 8:70, 1981

Evans AS and Dick EC: Acute pharyngitis and tonsillitis in University of Wisconsin students. JAMA 190:699, 1964

Evrard JR: Orogenital transmission of herpes simplex type 1. Obstet Gynecol 44:593, 1974

Field HJ et al: Isolation and characterization of acyclovir resistant mutant's of herpes simplex virus. J Gen Virol 49:115, 1980

Glezen WP et al: Acute respiratory disease of university students with special reference to the etiologic role of herpes virus hominis. Am J Epidemiol 101:111, 1975

Guinan ME et al: The course of untreated recurrent genital herpes simplex infection in 27 women. N Engl J Med 304:759, 1981

Hambrick GW Jr et al: Primary herpes simplex infection of finger of medical personnel. Arch Dermatol 85:583, 1972

Hendricks AA: Primary herpes simplex virus infection following mouth-to-mouth resuscitation. JAMA 243:257, 1980

Louis DS: Herpetic whitlow. J Hand Surg 4:90, 1979

Luby J: Therapy in genital herpes. N Engl J Med 306:1356, 1982

McDonald AD et al: Neutralizing antibodies to herpes virus types 1 and 2 in carcinoma of the cervix, carcinoma in situ and cervical dysplasia. Am J Epidemiol 100:130, 1974

Merchant VA, Molinari JA, Sabes WR: Herpetic Whitlow: Report of a case with multiple recurrences. Oral Surg 55:568, 1983

Mogabgab WJ: Acute respiratory illness in university (1962–1966), military and industrial (1962–1963) populations. Am Rev Respr Dis 98:359, 1968

Nahmias AJ and Norrild B: Oncogenic potential of herpes simplex viruses and their associations with cervical neoplasia, in Rapp F (ed) Oncogenic Herpes Viruses VII 1980, CRC Press, Boca Raton FL

Nahmias AJ et al: Antibodies to herpes virus hominis types 1 and 2 in humans. I. Patients with genital herpetic infections. Am J Epidemiol 91:539, 1970

Rapp F: Herpes simplex virus type 2 and cervical cancer. Curr Probl Cancer 6:1, 1981

Reeves WC et al: Risk of recurrence after first episode of genital herpes: relation to HSV type and antibody response. N Engl J Med 305:315, 1981

Scott TF et al: Some comments on herpetic infection in children with special emphasis on unusual clinical manifestations. J Pediatr 41:835, 1952

Shoham MA: Herpetic infection of the finger. A risk to the endoscopist. Gastro Endosc 25:26, 1979

Sogbetun AO: Herpes virus hominis antibodies among children and young adults in Ibadan. Br J Ven Dis 55:44, 1979

Stern H et al: Herpetic whitlow, a form of cross-infection in hospitals. Lancet 2:871, 1959

Symposium: Oral herpes simplex virus infection. J R Soc Med 72:126, 1979

Thygeson P et al: Observations on herpetic keratitis and keratoconjunctivitis. Arch Ophthal 56:375, 1956

Wentworth BB and Alexander ER: Seroepidemiology of infections due to members of the herpes virus group. Am J Epidemiol 94:496, 1971

Whitney RJ et al: The natural history of herpes simplex virus infection of mother and newborn. Pediatrics 66:489, 1980

Young EJ et al: Acute pharyngo-tonsillitis caused by herpes virus type 2. JAMA 239:1885, 1978

Pediculosis Pubis, Scabies and Molluscum Contagiosum

Berson RB: Head lice infestation and pedodontic practice. J Dent Child 48:201, 1981

Brown ST et al: Molluscum contagiosum. Sex Trans Dis 8:227, 1981

Couch JM et al: Diagnosing and treating Phthirus pubis palpebrarum. Surv Ophthal 26:219, 1982

Kincaid MC: Phthirus pubis infestatioon of the lashes. JAMA 249:590, 1983

Knowles FC: Molluscum contagiosum: report of an institutional epidemic of 59 cases. JAMA 53:671, 1909

Lynfield YL et al: Molluscum contagiosum: an unusual presentation. Cutis 30:321, 1982

Nelson JF: Molluscum contagiosum of the lower lip: report of a case. J Oral Med 35:62, 1980

Schiff BL: Molluscum contagiosum of the buccal mucosa. Arch Dermatol 78:90, 1958

Shacter B: Treatment of scabies and pediculosis with lindane preparations: an evaluation. J Am Acad Dermatol 5:517, 1981

Syphilis

Bara J: Les manifestations bucco-maxillo-faciales de la syphilis tertiaire. Actual Odontostomatol 13:7, 1951

Beecher SB, et al.: Dental hypoplasias in relation to congenital syphilis. J Ven Dis Inform 32:70, 1951

Bradlaw RV: The dental stigmata of prenatal syphilis. Oral Surg 6:147, 1953

De Koning GAJ, Blog FB and Stolz E: A patient with primary syphilis of the hand. Brit J Ven Dis 53:386, 1977

Fiumara NJ: Oral lesions of gonorrhea and syphilis. Cutis 17:689, 1972

Fiumara NJ: Treatment of primary and secondary syphilis: serologic response. JAMA 243:2500, 1980

Fiumara NJ and Berg M: Primary syphilis in the oral cavity. Br J Ven Dis 50:463, 1974

Fiumara NJ and Lesele S: Manifestations of late congenital syphilis. An analysis of 271 patients. Arch Dermatol 102:78, 1970

Fiumara NJ and Walker EA: Primary syphilis of the tonsil. Arch Otolaryngol 108:43, 1982

Fiumara NJ, Grande DJ and Giunta JL.: Papular secondary syphilis of the tongue. Oral Surg 45:540, 1978

Glatt MM: Neurosyphilis again. Br Med J 19:796, 1981

Holmes KK: Spirochetal Diseases, Ch 177 in Petersdorf RG et al (eds): Harrison's Principles of Internal Medicine, 10th ed., NY 1983, p. 1034

Huebsch RF: Gumma of the hard palate. Oral Surg 8:690, 1955

Kingon RJ and Weisner PJ: Premarital syphilis screening: weighing the benefits. Am J Pub Health 71:160, 1981

Meyer I and Abbey LM: The relationship of syphilis to primary carcinoma of the tongue. Oral Surg 30:678, 1970

Meyer I and Shklar G: The oral manifestations of acquired syphilis. Oral Surg 23:45, 1967

Moore MG, Jr: The epidemiology of syphilis. JAMA 186:71, 1963

Nathan AS and Lawson W: Syphilitic osteomyelitis of the mandible. Oral Surg 17:284, 1964

National Communicable Disease Center. Venereal Disease Program. Syphilis: a Synopsis. USPHS Publicn #1660, US Govt Printing Office 1968

Putkonin T: Dental changes in congenital syphilis. Acta Derm Venereol 42:44, 1962

Rathbun KC: Congenital syphilis. Sex Trans Dis 10:93, 102, 1983

Walter P et al: The placental lesions in congenital syphilis. A study of six cases. Virchows Arch 397:313, 1982

Wynder EL, Bross IJ and Feldman RM: A study of the etiological factors in cancer of the mouth. Cancer 10:1300, 1957

Ysuf H et al: Syphilitic osteomyelitis of the mandible. Br J Oral Surg 20:122, 1982

Syphilis Before the Introduction of Penicillin

Anderson BG: Dental defects in congenital syphilis. Am J Dis Child 57:52, 1939

Barnett CW, and Kulchar GV: The infectivity of

saliva in early syphilis. J Invest Dermatol 2:327, 1939

Bauer WH: Tooth buds and jaws in patients with congenital syphilis. Am J Pathol 20:297, 1944

Campbell DK: Dental deformities in children of parents with Hutchinson's teeth. D Cosmos 75:348, 1933

Carr MW: Condylomata lata of the tongue in congenital syphilis. J Oral Surg 6:179, 1948

Combes FC, and Bluefarb SM: Annular papular syphilis of the tongue. Arch Dermatol Syph 43:383, 1941

DeWilde H: Stigmata of congenital syphilis in the deciduous dentition. Am J Orthod 29:368, 1943

Downing JG: Incidence of extragenital chancres. Arch Dermatol Syph 39:50, 1939

Epstein CM and Zeisler EP: Chancre of the gingiva. JADA 20:2228, 1933

Greenbaum SS: Syphilis insontium. Dent Cosmos 72:937, 1930

Hill TJ: An investigation on spirochetosis of the anlage in congenital syphilis. Am J Pathol 7:515, 1931

Hutchinson J:On the influence of hereditary syphilis on the teeth. Lancet 9:449, 10:187, 1856

Hutchinson J: Report on the effects of infantile syphilis in marring the development of the teeth. Trans Pathol Soc London 9:449, 1858

Hutchinson J: Hutchinson's triad. Trans Pathol Soc London 10:287, 1859

Hutchinson J: Heredito-syphilitic struma and the teeth as a means of diagnosis. Br Med J 1:515, 1861

Hutchinson J: Syphilis-diagnosis in the late periods of the teeth. Trans Pathol Soc London 38:85, 1887

Johnston WD et al.: Effects of congenital syphilis on the teeth and associated structures in children. Am J Orthod and Oral Surg 27:667, 1941

Karnosh LJ: Histo-pathology of syphilitic hypoplasia of the teeth. Arch Dermatol Syph 13:25, 1926

Leifer W: Accidental syphilitic infection of dentists, report of two cases. JADA 29:435, 1942

Lever WF: Multiple extragenital giant chancres. N Eng J Med 231:227, 1944

Pentz WR: Vital reactions of the pulp of teeth in syphilis produced by induced currents. Arch Dermatol Syph 28:163, 1933

Pentz WR and Borman MC: Dental sensation in syphilis of the central nervous system. Arch Neurol Psychiat 16:629, 1926

Salzmann JA and Appleton LT Jr: Syphilis insontium: acquired by the operator during dental treatment. New York State Dent J 2:269, 1932

Sarnat BG et al: Roentgenologic diagnosis of congenital syphilis. JAMA 116:2745, 1941

Stathers FR: Congenital syphilis and malocclusion of the teeth. Am J Orthod 28:138, 1942

Stokes JH and Gardner BS: The demonstration of unerupted Hutchinson's teeth by roentgen ray. JAMA 80:28, 1923

Straith FE: Chancre of the gingivae. JADA 24:926, 1937

Strakosch EA: Postrhagadic scars. Arch Dermatol Syph 43:664, 1941

Strauss I: Masseter and temporal muscle tenderness in syphilitic trigeminal neuritis. J Mt Sinai Hosp 8:1060, 1942

Sutton IC: The need for caution in the diagnosis of Hutchinson teeth. Am J Syph 9:94, 1925

Tucker HA and Mulherin JL: Extragenital chancres: survey of 219 cases. Am J Syph 32:345, 1948

Vonderlehr RA and Usilton LJ: Syphilis among men of draft age in the United States. JAMA 120:1369, 1942

Wile UJ and Holman HH: A survey of 68 cases of extragenital chancres. Am J Syph 25:58, 1941

Non-Venereal Treponematoses

Editorial: Yaws again. Br Med J 281:1090, 1980

Ginestat G et al: Gangosa. Ann Clin Plast Surg 5:275, 1960

Hollander DH: Treponematosis from pinta to venereal syphilis revisited-hypothesis for temperature determination of disease patterns. Sex Transm Dis 8:34, 1981

Holmes KK and Perine PL: Nonvenereal treponematoses: yaws, pinta and endemic syphilis. Chap 178 in Petersdorf RG et al (eds): Harrison's Principles of Internal Medicine, 10th edit, New York 1983, p 1045

Hopkins DR: Yaws in the Americas, 1950-1975. J Infect Dis 136:548, 1977

Hudson EH: Non-Venereal Syphilis: A Sociological and Medical Study of Bejel. Edinburgh, E & S Livingstone, 1958

Manson-Bahr PH: Manson's Tropical Diseases, ed 14. Cassel & Co. London 1954

Marquez F, Rein CR and Arias O: Mal del pinto in Mexico. Bull WHO 13:299, 1955

Mazunder JK: Survey of oral manifestations of tropical diseases. Int Dent J 4:209, 1953

Hepatitis B & Other Viral Sexually Transmitted Diseases

Dienstag JL and Ryan DM: Occupational exposure to hepatitis B virus in hospital personnel: infection or immunization. Am J Epidemiol 115:26, 1982

Drew WL et al: Prevalence of cytomegalovirus infection in homosexual men. J Infect Dis 143:188, 1981

Fleischer GR et al: Intrafamilial transmission of Epstein-Barr virus infections. J Pediatr 98:16, 1981

Fleischer GR et al: Vaccination of pediatric nurses with live attenuated cytomegalovirus. Am J Dis Child 136:294, 1982

Gerety RJ: Hepatitis B transmission between dental or medical workers and patients. Ann Int Med 95:229, 1981

Griffiths PD et al: A prospective study of primary cytomegalo-virus infection in pregnant women. Br J Obstet Gynaecol 87:308, 1980

Guadagnino V et al: Risk of hepatitis B virus infection in patients with eczema or psoriasis of the hand. Br Med J 284:84, 1982

Hadler SC et al: An outbreak of hepatitis B in a dental practice. Ann Int Med 95:133, 1981

Hentzer B et al: Viral hepatitis in a venereal clinic population. Relation to certain risk factors. Scand J Inf Dis 12:245, 1980

James SP and Sampliner RE: Hepatitis B in the dental setting: dental hygienists. J Md State Den Assoc 21:26, 1978

Judson FN: Epidemiology of sexually transmitted hepatitis B infections in heterosexuals: a review. Sex Transm Dis 8 (Suppl):336, 1981

Mosley JW and White E: Viral hepatitis as an occupational hazard of dentists. JADA 90:992, 1975

Perrillo RP and Aach RD: The clinical course and chronic sequelae of hepatitis B virus infection. Semin Liver Dis 1:15, 1981

Saemundsen AK et al: Documentation of Epstein-Barr virus infection in immunodeficient patients with life-threatening lymphoproliferative diseases by Epstein-Barr virus complementary RNA/DNA and viral DNA/DNA hybridization. Cancer Res 41:4237, 1981

Stause M: Cytomegalovirus and the otolaryngologist. Laryngoscope 91:1995, 1981

Syndman DR et al: Infectious mononucleosis in an adult progressing to fatal immunoblastic lymphoma. Ann Int Med 96:737, 1982

Szmuness W et al: A controlled clinical trial of the efficacy of the hepatitis B vaccine (Hepatavax B): a final report. Hepatology 1:377, 1981

Thestrup-Pederson K et al: Epstein-Barr virus-induced lymphoproliferative disorder converting to fatal Burkitt-like lymphoma in a boy with interferon-inducible chromosomal defect. Lancet 2:997, 1980

Tzukert A and Gandler SG: Dental care and spread of hepatitis B virus infection. J Clin Microbiol 8:302, 1978

Urmacher C et al: Outbreak of Kaposi's sarcoma

with cytomegalovirus infection in young homosexual men. Am J Med 72:569, 1982

Williams SV et al: Dental infection with hepatitis B. JAMA 232:1231, 1975

The Acquired Immune Deficiency Syndrome

Centers for Disease Control. Acquired immune deficiency syndrome (AIDS): precautions for clinical and laboratory staffs. Morb Mort Wkly Reps 31:577, 1982

Centers for Disease Control: Acquired immunodeficiency syndrome (AIDS) update: United States. MMWR 32:309, 1983

Centers for Disease Control: An evaluation of the acquired immunodeficiency syndrome (AIDS) reported in health-care personnel: United States. MMWR 32:358, 1983

Centers for Disease Control: Human T-cell leukemia virus infection in patients with acquired immune deficiency syndrome: preliminary observations. MMWR 32:233, 1983

Centers for Disease Control: Immunodeficiency among female sexual partners of males with acquired immune deficiency syndrome (AIDS)—New York. MMWR 31:697, 1983

Centers for Disease Control: Prevention of acquired immune deficiency syndrome (AIDS): report of interagency recommendations. MMWR 32:101, 1983

Centers for Disease Control: Task Force on Kaposi's Sarcoma and Opportunistic Infections: epidemiologic aspects of the current outbreak of Kaposi's sarcoma and opportunistic infections N Eng J Med 306:248, 1982

Fauci AS: The acquired immune deficiency syndrome: the ever-broadening clinical spectrum. JAMA 249:2375, 1983

Fiale M et al: The role of lymphocytes in infections due to Epstein-Barr virus and cytomegalovirus. J Infect Dis 146:300, 1982

Friedman-Kien AE et al: Disseminated Kaposi's sarcoma in homosexual men. Ann Int Med 96:693, 1982

Gallo RC et al: Isolation of human T cell leukemia virus in acquired immune deficiency syndrome (AIDS). Science 220:865, 1983

Gotlieb GJ and Ackerman AB: Kaposi's sarcoma: an extensively disseminated form in young homosexual men. Hum Pathol 13:883, 1982

Gottlieb MS et al: *Pneumocystis carinii* pneumonia and mucosal candidiasis in previously healthy homosexual men: evidence of a new acquired cellular immunodeficiency. N Engl J Med 305:1425, 1981

Heidelman JF, Armstrong W and Graham L: Acquired-cell immune deficiency syndrome. Oral Surg 55:452, 1983

Henrickson RV et al: Epidemic of acquired immunodeficiency in rhesus monkeys. Lancet 1:388, 1983

Kornfeld H et al: T lymphocyte subpopulations in homosexual men. N Engl J Med 307:729, 1982

Mildvan D et al: Opportunistic infections and immune deficiency in homosexual men. Ann Int Med 96:700, 1982

Rubenstein A et al: Acquired immunodeficiency with reversed T4/T8 ratios in infants born to promiscuous and drug-addicted mothers. JAMA 249:2350, 1983

Seigal FP et al: Severe acquired immunodeficiency in male homosexuals, manifested by chronic perianal ulcerative herpes simplex lesions. N Engl J Med 305:1439, 1981

The Minor Venereal Diseases (Granuloma Inguinale, Lymphogranuloma Venereum and Chancroid)

Hall TB: Granuloma inguinale: report of cases of involvement of upper lip and depigmentation and edema of vulva. Arch Dermatol Syph 38:245, 1938

Hammond GW et al: Epidemiologic, clinical, laboratory and therapeutic features of an urban outbreak of chancroid in North America. Rev Infect Dis 2:867, 1980

Margolies RJ et al: Chancroid: diagnosis and treatment. J Am Acad Dermatol 6:493, 1982

Mauff AC et al: Problems in the diagnosis of lymphogranuloma venereum. A review of six cases. S Afr Med J 63:55, 1983

Rao et al: Oral lesions of granuloma inguinale. Oral Surg 34:1112, 1976

Index